ORAL AND MAXILLOFACIAL SURGERY

VOLUME ONE

The biomedical and clinical basis for surgical practice

DANIEL M. LASKIN
D.D.S., M.S.

Professor and Head, Department of Oral and Maxillofacial Surgery, College of
Dentistry, and Clinical Professor, Department of Surgery, College of
Medicine, University of Illinois at the Medical Center; Director,
University of Illinois Temporomandibular Joint and Facial Pain
Research Center; Head, Department of Dentistry, and Chief, Division
of Oral and Maxillofacial Surgery, University of Illinois Hospital;
Deputy Chairman, Department of Oral and Maxillofacial Surgery, Cook
County Hospital; Head, Department of Oral Surgery, Edgewater
Hospital, Chicago, Illinois; Diplomate, American Board of
Oral and Maxillofacial Surgery

with **714** illustrations, including **23** in color

The C. V. Mosby Company

ST. LOUIS · TORONTO · LONDON   1980

VOLUME ONE

Copyright © 1980 by The C. V. Mosby Company

All rights reserved. No part of this book may be reproduced in any manner without written permission of the publisher.

Printed in the United States of America

The C. V. Mosby Company
11830 Westline Industrial Drive, St. Louis, Missouri 63141

Library of Congress Cataloging in Publication Data

Main entry under title:

The biomedical and clinical basis for surgical practice.

    (Oral and maxillofacial surgery; v. 1)
    Bibliography: p.
    Includes index.
    1. Mouth—Surgery. 2. Maxilla—Surgery. 3. Face—Surgery. I. Laskin, Daniel M. II. Series.
RK529.066 vol. 1   617'.522'008s [617'.522]   79-18723
ISBN 0-8016-2822-9

C/CB/B 9 8 7 6 5 4 3 2   01/A/058

Contributors

John F. Cleall, B.D.S., D.D.S., M.D.S., F.R.C.D.

Professor and Head, Department of Orthodontics, University of Illinois College of Dentistry, Chicago, Illinois

R. Bruce Donoff, D.M.D., M.D.

Associate Professor of Oral and Maxillofacial Surgery, Harvard School of Dental Medicine; Associate Visiting Oral Surgeon, Massachusetts General Hospital, Boston, Massachusetts

Fred G. Emmings, D.D.S., Ph.D.

Associate Professor of Clinical Dentistry, and Chairman, Dental Research, University of Rochester School of Medicine and Dentistry; Dentist-in-Chief, Strong Memorial Hospital, Rochester, New York

David S. Evaskus, D.D.S., M.S.

Associate Professor, Department of Oral and Maxillofacial Surgery, University of Illinois College of Dentistry, Chicago, Illinois

Gary F. Gates, M.D.

Director of Nuclear Medicine, Good Samaritan Hospital and Medical Center; Clinical Associate Professor of Radiology, University of Oregon School of Medicine, Portland, Oregon

William Greenfield, D.D.S.

Professor of Oral and Maxillofacial Surgery and Head, Division of Medical and Surgical Sciences, Associate Dean for Hospital and Extramural Affairs, New York University College of Dentistry, New York, New York

John M. Gregg, D.D.S., Ph.D.

Professor of Oral and Maxillofacial Surgery, The University of North Carolina School of Dentistry, Chapel Hill, North Carolina

Arthur V. Kroeger, Ph.D.

Professor, Department of Microbiology and Immunology, University of Illinois at the Medical Center, Chicago, Illinois

Judith C. Kusek, Ph.D., D.D.S.

Assistant Professor, Department of Pharmacology, University of Illinois at the Medical Center, Chicago, Illinois

Daniel M. Laskin, D.D.S., M.S.

Professor and Head, Department of Oral and Maxillofacial Surgery, College of Dentistry, and Clinical Professor, Department of Surgery, College of Medicine, University of Illinois at the Medical Center, Chicago, Illinois

Jeffrey L. Laskin, D.D.S., M.S.

Assistant Professor, Department of Oral and Maxillofacial Surgery, University of Florida College of Dentistry, Gainesville, Florida

Victor J. Matukas, D.D.S., M.D., Ph.D.

Professor of Dentistry, School of Dentistry; Associate Professor of Surgery, University of Alabama School of Medicine, Birmingham, Alabama

Louis G. Mercuri, D.D.S., M.S.

Assistant Professor, Department of Oral and Maxillofacial Surgery, Medical College of Virginia/Virginia Commonwealth University School of Dentistry and Medical College of Virginia Hospital, Richmond, Virginia

Alan M. Miller, D.D.S.

Associate Professor, Department of Radiology, University of Illinois College of Dentistry, Chicago, Illinois

Jerry E. Patterson, D.D.S., M.D.

Private Practice and Part-Time Clinical Instructor, Department of Oral Diagnosis, The University of North Carolina School of Dentistry, Chapel Hill, North Carolina

Frederick J. Schoen, M.D., Ph.D. (Materials Science)

Formerly, Assistant Professor, Department of Dental Biomaterials, College of Dentistry; Presently, Fellow, Department of Pathology, College of Medicine, University of Florida, J. Hillis Miller Health Center, Gainesville, Florida

Norman Trieger, D.M.D., M.D.

Chairman, Department of Dentistry and Oral Surgery, Montefiore Hospital Medical Center; Professor of Surgery, Albert Einstein College of Medicine, Bronx, New York

Edward E. Vicher, Ph.D.

Professor Emeritus, Department of Microbiology and Immunology, University of Illinois at the Medical Center, Chicago, Illinois

Matisyohu Weisenberg, Ph.D.

Ben-Gurion University of the Negev, Faculty of Health Sciences, Beersheva, Israel

Richard D. Zallen, D.D.S., M.D.

Director of Dentistry and Oral Maxillofacial Surgery, Denver General Hospital; Associate Professor of Oral Surgery, University of Colorado School of Dentistry, Denver, Colorado

To my friend
LEONARD J. ROBINSON who taught me how to be a student

To my mentor
BERNARD G. SARNAT who gave me the opportunity to become a surgeon

To my wife
EVIE whose encouragement and sacrifice helped
to make it all possible

Preface

It was over 30 years ago that Kurt H. Thoma authored the first edition of his book *Oral Surgery*. In the subsequent years this text underwent four revisions, the last in 1969. During that time there were many changes in the scope of oral surgery, but Dr. Thoma's book expanded along with the specialty to maintain its position as the most comprehensive treatise on the subject. The death of Kurt Thoma in 1972 not only left a great professional void but also brought to an end his continuation of this classic textbook.

Initially, when asked by the publisher to accept the responsibility for revival of the book, I intended to assume the entire task of revision. To my chagrin, it soon became apparent that what one man had been able to accomplish originally was no longer possible to do in a reasonable period. In fact, in retrospect it is difficult to conceive how one person was able to accomplish this task in the first place. So what began as an individual endeavor in 1948 became an endeavor involving about 50 people in 1979. This fact alone is a testimonial to the talent and genius of Kurt H. Thoma.

The field of oral surgery has changed considerably over the last 30 years, but perhaps more so in the past decade. Major progress has occurred, particularly in the areas of orthognathic surgery, reconstructive bone grafting, and preprosthetic surgical preparation of the jaws. Coupled with these advances have been great improvements in the techniques of anesthesia and other methods of pain control, the use of chemotherapeutic agents, and the general management of the surgical patient. Diagnostic techniques have also become more sophisticated, and our understanding of disease mechanisms has increased. Along with these advances have been changes in the educational process so that the oral and maxillofacial surgeon has attained new levels of academic and technical achievement. In fact, the complexity of the field has reached the stage where we are beginning to see individuals developing special areas of interest and expertise. It was this explosion in knowledge and technology that led to the decision to make this essentially a new, multiauthored book rather than a revision of its predecessor.

There are many textbooks dealing with varying aspects of oral and maxillofacial surgery. Each serves a specific purpose and deals with the subject in its own particular way. The purpose of this book is to permit authorities in various areas to present a comprehensive review of available information. The authors were given no limitations on length of chapters, use of illustrations, or number of references. They were also advised to describe all reasonable approaches to a problem rather than their own preference. In this way, the book becomes a reference text rather than merely a documentation of individual capability and accomplishment. The contributors are to be commended for their compliance with these requests.

The results of using a comprehensive approach to the subject of oral and maxillofacial surgery has led to an accumulation of material that makes publication in a single volume impossible. The information has therefore been divided into three parts. Volume One deals with the biomedical and clinical basis for surgical practice; Volume Two covers those procedures that generally fall within the scope of oral surgery; and Volume Three is concerned with maxillofacial procedures. Such a division not only provides a logical separation of the subject but also permits individuals besides oral and maxillofacial surgeons to have easy access to specific material. Thus the book should be useful to dental students; general practitioners; other dental specialists such as the periodontist, pedodontist,

and endodontist; as well as to otolaryngologists and plastic surgeons.

An undertaking of this magnitude obviously involves the cooperation of many individuals. My sincere thanks to all of the contributors who gave so unselfishly of their time and knowledge. Finally, and most importantly, my deep appreciation to my wife, Evie, for her personal sacrifice in permitting me to undertake and accomplish this almost impossible dream.

Daniel M. Laskin

Contents

Introduction to volume one

Surgery is a science as well as an art. The complete surgeon must not only be able to perform the technical aspects of his profession, but he must also have a broad knowledge of the biological and biomedical sciences that form the foundation on which these procedures are based. He must know the principles and techniques of diagnosis and their application, because knowing when to operate is equally as important as knowing how. He must understand the pathogenesis of disease so that he is able to institute the necessary corrective measures at the proper time and provide appropriate preoperative and postoperative care. He must be thoroughly familiar with the means of controlling pain and anxiety so as to eliminate suffering and assure patient comfort. Last, but not least, he must understand the psychological aspects of behavior so that he is able to relate to his patients and their problems. This volume of *Oral and Maxillofacial Surgery*, as its subtitle implies, is devoted to these basic biomedical and clinical aspects of surgical practice.

The material is divided into four parts. Part One deals with the biomedical sciences; Part Two discusses basic principles of oral and maxillofacial surgery; Part Three covers examination and diagnosis; and Part Four relates to control of pain and anxiety. Many of the subjects covered under these headings are not found in most textbooks on oral and maxillofacial surgery or are only provided in an abbreviated manner. For example, there are detailed chapters on such topics as embryology, craniofacial growth and development, immunobiology, biomaterials, radionuclide diagnosis, and psychological aspects of pain and anxiety control. This approach is in keeping with the expressed philosophy that such information forms the essential basis for the technical aspects of practice. Although basic material on these subjects can be found in other books, the emphasis in these chapters is on specific application to oral and maxillofacial surgery — information generally not found in such books. Moreover, combining this material in one place provides easy access and permits ready reference to the basic background information when reading the subsequent clinical sections.

There have been great technical advances in oral and maxillofacial surgery in recent years. In general, these advances have been based on an increased knowledge and understanding of the basic biomedical sciences. Thus improved technology and science go hand-in-hand. To say one aspect is practical and the other theoretical is untrue. Practical means useful, and both technology and science fit this definition. The pragmatic reader should need no further impetus to recognize that he should spend as much time, or even more, on this volume as on the following volumes that deal with the more procedurally oriented aspects of oral and maxillofacial surgery.

PART ONE

APPLIED BIOMEDICAL SCIENCES

CHAPTER 1

Surgical anatomy

John M. Gregg

In-depth knowledge of structure is the necessary starting place for the surgeon and a prerequisite for understanding physiology and pathology. It is also the basis for planning and carrying out safe surgical operations. In the case of the oral and maxillofacial region, certain anatomic features that have much influence on surgery in this area set it apart from other body regions. First, the organization is complex when compared to the ordered segmentation of other parts of the body. The head and upper neck contain 29 bones, 24 muscles, 2 bilateral arterial systems, 2 parallel systems for venous drainage, 12 bilateral mixed cranial nerves in addition to cervical and autonomic extracranial additions, 4 bilateral subdivided paranasal sinuses, and over 50 named foramina or canals. The complexity reflects the multiple embryologic origins of the tissue masses that have migrated long distances as concentric and overlapping compartments. The complexity also reflects the high functional demands of a region that participates simultaneously in most of the body's vital functions, including alimentation (mastication, digestion), respiration, communication, sensation, sexual activity, and protection of the brain. Two interdependent joints serve this region, and they have the unique combination of an articular disc, one fibrocartilaginous and one bony articular surface, and a condyle developed from intramembranous bone with an endochondral-like adaptive structure. The oral and maxillofacial region is much more vascular than most other body areas and collateralization to the facial muscles, skeleton, and mucosa permits tissue grafting and osseous surgery that cannot be carried out in other body regions (Bell and Kennedy, 1976; Bosma, 1970). The vascularity also increases the hazards for uncontrolled hemorrhage and spread of blood-borne pathology. The sensory innervation density of the perioral region is the highest in the body, and neuromuscular motor units of the masticatory system are among the smallest and most sensitive (Bosma, 1970). All these structures must adapt to an extremely high lifelong rate of attrition from inevitable infection of dental, periodontal, and paranasal tissues, direct trauma to the prominent parts, and extensive aging atrophy.

REGIONAL TOPOGRAPHY

It is useful to divide the head and neck surface into natural zones defined by prominent landmarks (Sicher and DuBrul, 1975; Woodburne, 1975). In the neck a series of natural triangles occur as a result of major muscle and bone placement (Fig. 1-1). The *anterior triangle* is defined posteriorly and inferiorly by the sternocleidomastoid muscle, medially by the midline, and superiorly by the inferior border of the mandible. This triangle subdivides above the hyoid bone into the *submandibular* and *submental triangles*, adjacent regions separated from one another by the deeply placed anterior belly of the digastric muscle. Orientation to these regions is important for surgical manipulations of

3

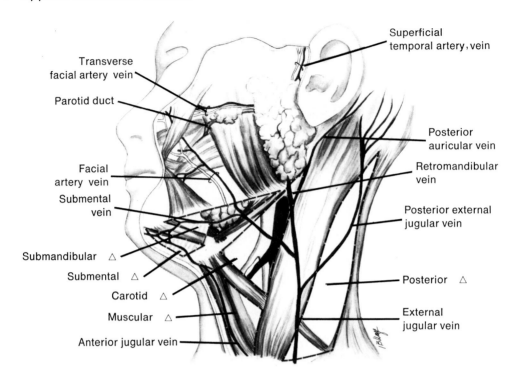

Fig. 1-1. Surgical boundaries and superficial vessels.

Transverse facial artery vein

Parotid duct

Facial artery vein

Submental vein

Submandibular △

Submental △

Carotid △

Muscular △

Anterior jugular vein

Superficial temporal artery, vein

Posterior auricular vein

Retromandibular vein

Posterior external jugular vein

Posterior △

External jugular vein

the submandibular gland, access to the inferior border and angle of the mandible for orthognathic and trauma surgery, and approach to deeper muscular compartments in the control of spreading odontogenic infection. The inferior border of the submandibular triangle is formed by the posterior digastric and stylohyoid muscular sling, which also forms the superior border of the important *carotid triangle*. This triangle is bounded anteriorly by the omohyoid muscle and is the surgical access region to the carotid arterial system. It also contains the internal jugular vein and the vagus, hypoglossal, and cervical sympathetic nerves. The inferior part of the anterior triangle, defined by the body of the hyoid bone above and the sternal notch below, is designated the *infrahyoid* or *muscular triangle*. It contains the infrahyoid muscles, thyroid gland, trachea, and esophagus.

The *posterior triangle* of the neck is bounded anteriorly by the sternocleidomastoid muscle, posteriorly by the margin of the trapezius muscle, and inferiorly by the middle one third of the clavicle

(Fig. 1-1). Superficially this region contains the external jugular venous system and in the inferior region provides access to suprathoracic structures such as the subclavicular artery and brachial nerve plexus.

In contrast to the neck, where muscles predominate as surface landmarks, areas in the head are defined by the prominent bones (Figs. 1-2 and 1-5). The maxillary zone is bounded above by the *nasomaxillary* complex and more posteriorly by the *zygomaticotemporal* region. *Auricular, occipital, parietal, frontal, orbital,* and *mandibular* regions make up the remainder of the surface landmarks and form a palpable outer framework for a series of deeper lying compartments.

The skin of the head and neck is firmly attached only at the ear cartilages and the alae of the nose. Elsewhere it is freely movable and forms natural folds beneath bony prominences and in smaller *Langer's lines* that radiate concentrically toward the midline from the auricular and occipital regions. Whenever possible, surgical incisions in the skin of the head and neck should be made in the

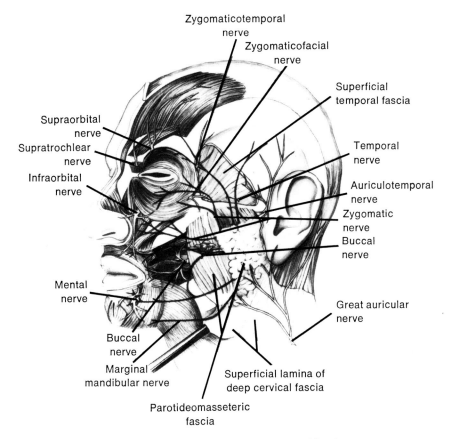

Zygomaticotemporal
nerve

Zygomaticofacial
nerve

Superficial
temporal fascia

Supraorbital
nerve

Supratrochlear
nerve

Infraorbital
nerve

Temporal
nerve

Auriculotemporal
nerve

Zygomatic
nerve

Buccal
nerve

Mental
nerve

Great auricular
nerve

Buccal
nerve

Marginal
mandibular nerve

Superficial lamina of
deep cervical fascia

Parotideomasseteric
fascia

Fig. 1-2. Superficial nerves, muscles, and fascia.

natural skin folds and creases and be designed to accommodate the movability of the facial skin.

The skin of this entire region is unique in containing the voluntary skeletal muscles of facial expression, which arise from underlying bones and insert in the subcutaneous tissue. In the neck this function is assumed by the platysma muscle, a thin continuous sheet that arises from the clavicle and sternal notch and inserts in the skin overlying the lateral mandible as far anterior as the angle of the mouth. In the face individual specialization of the facial muscles is seen; the majority of these muscles insert in the perioral and periorbital regions. All of the muscles of facial expression are innervated by the seventh cranial or *facial nerve*, which fans across the face to approach the muscles from their deep aspect.

In the neck the platysma muscle layer is superficial to the major veins and nerves. In the scalp the subcutaneous

epicranial muscles underlie the neurovascular bundles, whereas in the face the vessels course both superficial and deep to the separate muscles.

FASCIAL LAYERS

A series of connective tissue sheaths are found in the head and neck that contain and protect nerves, vessels, and glands; permit free movement of individual muscle and bone groups; and define the boundaries of natural tissue compartments for the surgeon (Sicher and Du-Brul, 1975; Woodburne, 1975). The fascial layers are also important because they form natural planes of dissection for the surgeon and direct the spread of hemotomas and infections (Granite, 1976).

The fasciae are logically divided into layers most easily observed in the neck (Fig. 1-3). The *superficial fascia* is a delicate and poorly defined layer that lies just beneath the skin. It contains the platysma in the neck and the muscles of expression in the face and can rarely be identified as a distinct surgical plane.

The deep cervical fascia consists of six separate but interdependent sheets: the superficial lamina or investing fascia and the prevertebral, middle cervical, cervical visceral, alar, and carotid sheath fasciae (Fig. 1-3).

The first and best defined layer of the deep cervical fascia is the *superficial lamina,* or *investing fascia.* In the neck this lamina lies just beneath the platysma as a firm, semitransparent cylinder that arises inferiorly from the medial clavicle and posteriorly from the spines of the cervical vertebrae. It is continuous across the midline where it attaches inferiorly on both the deep and superficial surfaces of the *manubrium sternae* and as a result forms the small *suprasternal space* (of Burns). Laterally the superficial lamina splits to enclose the entire sternocleidomastoid and trapezius muscle masses (Fig. 1-3). In the submandibular region it contributes to the loose *submandibular gland capsule,* then continues superiorly to attach along the entire inferior border

of the mandible. Anteriorly it divides to encircle the body and symphysis of the mandible as a periosteal sheath. Posteriorly the upward extension is designated as the *parotideomasseteric* fascia because it forms an adherent sheath laterally over the *masseter muscle* and provides the *parotid gland* with its capsule (Figs. 1-2 and 1-4). It then fuses posteriorly along the mastoid process and is attached in the midline to the external occipital process. Anteriorly it attaches to the zygomatic arch and zygoma. Above this level it extends as the outer layer of *temporalis muscle fascia* and it terminates at the temporal crest. Beneath the mandible the superficial lamina covers the medial aspect of the ramus and the medial and lateral pterygoid muscles. It is continuous in the retromandibular region with the *sphenomandibular ligament,* the *styloglossus, stylohyoid,* and *posterior digastric muscles,* and the parotid capsule. These combined fascial and muscular structures form a thick, hammocklike retromandibular barrier, the *stylomandibular diaphragm* (Fig. 1-4).

The superficial lamina of the deep

Fig. 1-3. Cervical fasciae.

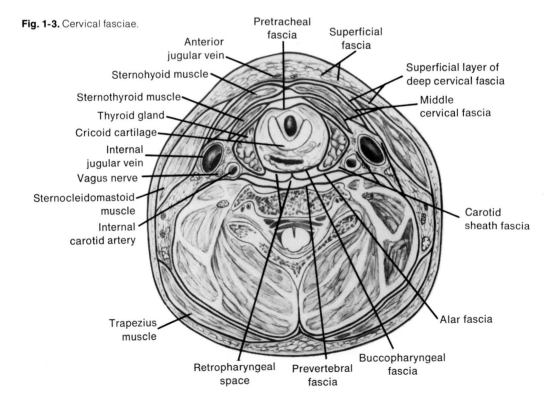

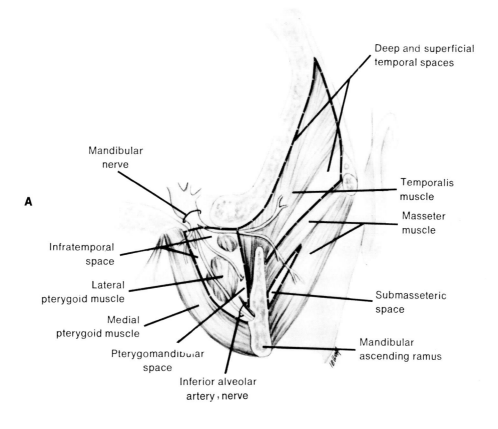

A

Deep and superficial temporal spaces

Mandibular nerve

Temporalis muscle

Masseter muscle

Infratemporal space

Lateral pterygoid muscle

Medial pterygoid muscle

Submasseteric space

Pterygomandibular space

Mandibular ascending ramus

Inferior alveolar artery, nerve

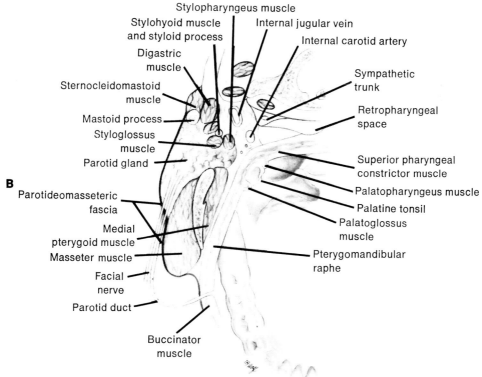

B

Stylopharyngeus muscle

Stylohyoid muscle and styloid process

Internal jugular vein

Digastric muscle

Internal carotid artery

Sympathetic trunk

Sternocleidomastoid muscle

Mastoid process

Retropharyngeal space

Styloglossus muscle

Parotid gland

Superior pharyngeal constrictor muscle

Palatopharyngeus muscle

Parotideomasseteric fascia

Palatine tonsil

Medial pterygoid muscle

Palatoglossus muscle

Masseter muscle

Pterygomandibular raphe

Facial nerve

Parotid duct

Buccinator muscle

Fig. 1-4. Surgical spaces. **A,** Frontal; **B,** horizontal.

cervical fascia is especially important in surgical approaches to the inferior border of the mandible because the parotid and submandibular glands, the seventh cranial and cervical cutaneous nerves, the facial and retromandibular veins, and the facial arteries are all located either within or just beneath this fascial layer. There may be unnecessary damage to these structures if the lamina is cut at any place other than its fusion line with the mandible. The fascia also serves as a plane for direct spread of infection from perioral structures into the neck and determines the course of postoperative hematomas. It also provides a plane of spread for subcutaneous emphysema introduced by high-speed air devices during oral surgery.

The deep layer of the cervical fascia, also named the *prevertebral fascia,* is a complete cylinder within the larger one formed by the superficial lamina (Fig. 1-3). It surrounds the deep neck muscles, the cervical spinal cord, and the vertebral bodies and attaches superiorly to the basilar part of the occipital bone.

The *middle cervical fascia* sheathes the infrahyoid muscles, with one layer for the more superficial sternohyoid and omohyoid muscles and a second for the deeper sternothyroid and thyrohyoid muscles (Fig. 1-3). In the midline this fascia blends with the superficial fascia and laterally it blends with the carotid sheath. Inferiorly this fascia is prolonged behind the sternum and eventually onto the pericardium.

In the central part of the neck the pharynx, esophagus, larynx, trachea, and parathyroid and thyroid glands are surrounded by a cylindric covering named the *cervical visceral fascia* (Fig. 1-3). This consists of the pretracheal fascia anteriorly and the buccopharyngeal fascia posteriorly. The smooth pretracheal portion covers the larynx and trachea and splits to enclose the thyroid gland. It attaches superiorly to the hyoid bone and blends inferiorly with the middle cervical fascia behind the sternum. Laterally, the pretracheal fascia blends with the buccopharyngeal fascia along the line of attachment of the pharyngeal constrictor muscles to

the hyoid bone and thyroid cartilages. The *buccopharyngeal fascia* is an external covering for the upper alimentary tract beginning superiorly from an attachment on the pharyngeal tubercle of the occipital bone. From this midpoint a thin layer called the *pharyngobasilar fascia* extends laterally to the medial pterygoid plate and then covers the *superior pharyngeal constrictor muscle.* It continues to an insertion on the *pterygomandibular raphe* and finally extends forward as the external covering of the *buccinator muscle* (Fig. 1-4). Inferiorly it covers the surface of the *middle* and *inferior pharyngeal constrictor muscles.*

The *alar fascia* is a delicate wall interposed in the space between the prevertebral fascia and the buccopharyngeal fascia to which it is attached at the midline (Fig. 1-3). This fascia blends laterally with the carotid sheath.

The *carotid sheath* is a loosely defined but functionally important complex of connective tissue that surrounds and cushions the internal and common carotid arteries, the internal jugular vein, and the vagus and sympathetic nerve trunks (Figs. 1-3 and 1-4). Its fibers are continuous with most of the other deep cervical fasciae, and it thereby becomes an important potential avenue for the spread of pathologic processes from the base of the skull to the chest.

SURGICAL FASCIAL SPACES

In the preantibiotic era the surgeon often viewed the maxillofacial region as a series of autonomous fascia-lined spaces that tended to limit the spread of infection. Now, those infections that limit themselves to smaller spaces are readily managed by chemical antibiosis and selective surgical drainage. The "modern infections" characterized by virulent, resistant strains of organisms now seem to have little respect for thin fascial barriers. This, as well as the great displacement of masticatory structures in current orthognathic procedures, has produced a different view of the surgical fascial spaces (Granite, 1976).

The fascial spaces can be understood as divisions of two major complexes: (1)

the *masticatory complex,* with masticatory, buccal, submasseteric, parotid, infratemporal, temporal, and pterygopalatine extensions, and (2) the *peripharyngeal complex,* which encompasses submandibular, paralingual, lateral pharyngeal, and retropharyngeal extensions. The dividing line between these two complexes is the medial upward extension of the superficial lamina of the deep cervical fascia, the parotideomasseteric fascia, which splits at the inferior mandibular border and extends posterosuperiorly to attach on the lateral base of the skull.

The *masticator space* proper is the central nidus for the masticatory complex. It contains the ascending ramus of the mandible, temporomandibular joint, zygomatic arch, and medial and lateral pterygoid, masseter, and temporalis muscles (Fig. 1-4). It is bounded laterally by the parotideomasseteric fascia and medially by the pterygoid fascia. It terminates superiorly at the temporalis attachment to the temporal bone; anteriorly at the margin of the masseter, temporal tendon insertion, and medial pterygoid muscle; and posterolaterally it is bounded by the deep component of the parotid fascia. Posteromedially, the space communicates with the lateral pharyngeal space. The buccal fat pad is a multilobular structure that occupies much of the looser regions of the masticator space.

The *submasseteric space* is a small recess of the masticator complex that lies just lateral to the mandibular ramus. It is bounded by the superficial belly of the masseter laterally and inferiorly and laterally and above by the deep belly attachments (Fig. 1-4). The anterior boundary is the mucosa of the retromolar trigone area of the mandible, a common source for spread of infection to the submasseteric space owing to third molar pathoses. Posteriorly it is bounded by the parotideomasseteric fascia as it splits to envelop the parotid gland.

The *buccal space* is another anterior and superior outpouching of the masticator complex that contains portions of the buccal fat pad (Fig. 1-4). It is bounded laterally by the attachments of the buccinator muscle to the maxilla and mandible and medially by the masseter muscle. Odontogenic infections or postoperative hematomas from the dentoalveolus that have dissected the sparse buccinator attachments will fill this expansile space and bulge the cheek externally.

The masticator space is continuous anteriorly with the *space of the body of the mandible,* which is also enveloped by the split superficial lamina fascia. This space contains the mandibular body; the inferior alveolar nerve, artery, and vein; and the dentoperiodontal apparatus.

Two superior pouches of the masticator complex are the superficial and deep temporal spaces (Fig. 1-4). The *superficial temporal space* is bounded laterally by the firm fascial covering on the lateral aspect of the temporalis muscle, which arises high on the temporal bone and terminates at the zygomatic arch. The temporalis muscle surface is the medial boundary of this space, which contains the superficial temporal vessels and auriculotemporal nerve. The *deep temporal space* is bounded laterally by temporalis muscle and medially by the fascia that covers its medial face and contains the deep temporal arteries and veins that supply the muscle mass. Infections contained in this deep space, rather than presenting externally, may compress deeper peripharyngeal structures and even erode portions of the adjacent temporal bone.

The posterior extension of the masticator complex is the *parotid space,* which is also bounded by the split parotideomasseteric fascia laterally and medially where it is reinforced by the sphenomandibular and stylomandibular ligaments (Fig. 1-4). The parotid gland occupies this space and extends both medially and laterally around the posterior border of the mandibular ramus. This space is traversed by the facial and auriculotemporal nerves; the external carotid, superficial temporal, and maxillary arteries; and the retromandibular vien.

The *infratemporal space* is an important upward and posterior side-compartment of the masticator complex that contains a number of important structures: the pterygoid plexus of veins, maxillary artery and branches, pterygoid muscles, and mandibular nerve and branches. This space is bounded medially by the lateral pterygoid plate, the inferior portion of lateral pterygoid muscle, and the lateral pharyngeal wall. Superiorly, it is bounded by the infratemporal surface of the greater wing of the sphenoid bone, and laterally it is bounded by the temporal tendon and coronoid process. The posterolateral boundary is the mandibular condyle, temporalis and lateral pterygoid muscles, and medial aspect of the parotid capsule. Its most inferior part is the *pterygomandibular space*, a wedge-shaped region between the medial aspect of the ramus of the mandible and the lateral aspect of the medial pterygoid muscle. Infections introduced into the infratemporal space mainly from the maxillary dentition spread to the postzygomatic portion, where localization and surgical access is difficult. This space is important because the lingual and mandibular neurovascular elements are concentrated together here and can be easily approached for anesthetic blockade. It is also an area where an osteotomy for orthognathic surgery can be made through an intraoral incision along the temporal crest of the ramus.

The *pterygopalatine space* communicates with the infratemporal and the masticator spaces as an upward extension behind the maxillary tuberosity. It is bounded above by the bony orbit and anteriorly by the posterior sinus wall. Its medial terminus is the pterygomaxillary fissure, which is continuous above with the inferior orbital fissure. This space contains the maxillary nerve and sphenopalatine ganglion, posterior superior alveolar nerves and vessels, and terminal portions of the maxillary artery.

The *peripharyngeal complex* lies deep to the masticator complex and consists of four interdependent spaces that form a ring around the pharynx (Fig. 1-4). The *submandibular space* lies medial to the entire length of the body of the mandible and extends to the midline raphe of the mylohyoid muscle attachments. The posterior part of the mylohyoid muscle, hyoglossus, and superior pharyngeal con-

strictor muscles form the roof of this space and separate it from the sublingual space above. Posteriorly, it is bounded loosely by the stylohyoid and posterior belly of the digastric muscles. Anteriorly, the bilateral anterior bellies of the digastric muscles further separate the submandibular spaces from the *submental space*. The submandibular space contains the submandibular gland and numerous lymph nodes and is traversed by the facial artery and vein.

The *sublingual space* contains the loose connective tissue between the muscles of the tongue, submandibular (Wharton's) duct, sublingual gland, lingual and hypoglossal nerves, and lingual vessels (Figs. 1-4 and 1-7). The space lies completely above the mylohyoid muscle, is bounded posteriorly by the hyoglossal muscle attachments and laterally and anteriorly by the mandibular body, and is loosely subdivided in the midline by the median raphe of the mylohyoid and intrinsic tongue muscles. Infections in the sublingual space readily spread across the midline and deep to the submental and submandibular spaces because of the sparse barrier provided by the mylohyoid muscle fibers. Bilateral infections involving all of these spaces are termed "Ludwig's angina" and are life-threatening because of their potential to occlude the airway and spread further to the lateral and retropharyngeal spaces.

The *lateral pharyngeal space* is an irregular space bounded entirely by soft tissues except at its superior terminus at the base of the skull near the petrous portion of the temporal bone and its inferior extent at the level of hyoid bone (Fig. 1-4). The lateral wall of the pharynx, formed by the *superior pharyngeal constrictor muscle*, makes up the medial boundary that extends anteriorly to the point of juncture of the constrictor muscle with the buccinator muscle, the *pterygomandibular raphe*. The lateral boundary is the internal fascia of the medial pterygoid muscle and the deep capsule of the parotid gland. The space terminates posteriorly with the contents of the carotid sheath and the stylohyoid, styloglossus, and stylopharyngeus muscles.

The important contents of this space are found posteriorly behind the plane of the styloid muscles and consist of the internal carotid artery, internal jugular vein and associated deep jugular lymphatic chain, and the glossopharyngeal, vagus, spinal accessory, hypoglossal, and sympathetic chain nerves. There is potential for direct communication with the submandibular space and also deeper into the neck along the carotid sheath to the retropharyngeal space. Surgical access to this space is possible through an intraoral incision at pterygomandibular raphe and dissection along the lateral aspect of the superior pharyngeal constrictor muscle, or by penetrating anterior to the sternocleidomastoid muscle through the superficial lamina of the deep cervical fascia.

The *retropharyngeal space* is located between the prevertebral fascia and the posterior wall of the pharynx. It extends from the base of the skull above, behind the esophagus, and into the superior mediastinum. The space contains no major structures but represents a potentially dangerous avenue for the spread of infection or lymphogenous spread of neoplasia from lesions in the base of the tongue, nasopharynx, and tonsillar fossae as well as direct spread of pathoses from the lateral pharyngeal spaces (Granite, 1976; Kruger, 1974).

MAXILLOFACIAL SKELETON

The maxillofacial skeleton is structurally and functionally divided into three regions: (1) the lower face, consisting of mandible, temporomandibular joint, and hyoid bone, (2) the midface, made up of nasal, ethmoidal, palatal, sphenoidal, zygomatic, and maxillary bones with associated paranasal sinuses, and (3) the upper face, consisting of the temporal and orbital complexes and the skull and its basilar complex of bones. The differences among these regions are especially evident in their response to trauma. The mandible, for example, resembles a long bone. It is most vulnerable to shearing fractures at the weak neck of the condyloid process (18% to 36%), at the angle (20% to 31%), and at points of weakness in the body (21% to 36%) caused by pa-

thoses such as impacted teeth and cysts (Dingman and Natvig, 1964; Kruger, 1974). Fractures of the mandible tend to be displaced by the attached muscles, especially the opposing actions of the inferomedial displacers (lateral pterygoid, mylohyoid, anterior digastric, suprahyoid muscles) versus the pull of the superolateral (masseter and temporalis muscles) or superomedial (medial pterygoid) displacers. The midfacial complex, by contrast, is not a single exposed unit, nor is it significantly displaced by attached muscles after trauma. Because it is highly compartmented with rows of thin bones set against the solid base of the skull, trauma to the midfacial region causes comminution and posterior collapse in accordion-like fashion, most commonly along lines weakened by foramina, sutures, or pneumatization. A further contrast is the upper face and skull. The orbital bones are usually protected from direct blows but respond in explosive fashion to rapid compressions of the eyeball. The skull, on the other hand, is a spherical complex of basically flat bones that absorb and spread trauma over the entire vault, developing denting kinds of responses to blunt trauma. Because of the relative strength of the cranial vault, compared to the thin superstructure of the midface, a shearing separation between midface and upper basilar complexes may occur (Rowe and Killey, 1968).

Mandible

The mandible is a single bone with four anatomically distinct regions: a body, alveolar process, ramus, and condyloid process (Figs. 1-5 to 1-7). The horizontal, U-shaped *body* has a dense basilar portion that contains the neurovascular bundle and provides for muscle attachments and an *alveolar* portion that is hollowed out by the teeth and is largely dependent on them for its development and maintenance. The vertical *ramus* is a thin, dense structure with little marrow that is entirely sheathed by masticatory muscles. Its anterosuperior projection, the *coronoid process*, provides attachment for the temporalis mus-

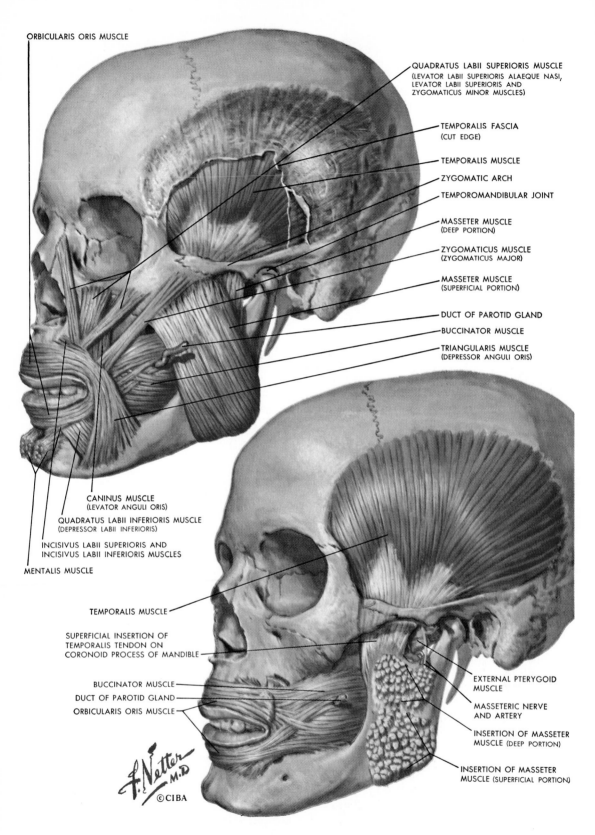

Fig. 1-5. Muscles of mastication. (© Copyright 1959, CIBA-GEIGY Corporation. Reproduced with permission. All rights reserved.)

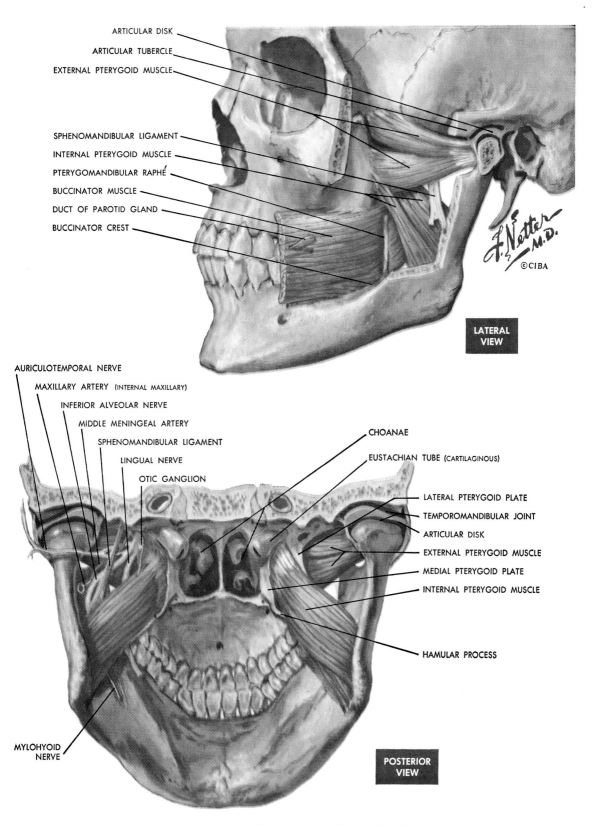

ARTICULAR DISK

ARTICULAR TUBERCLE

EXTERNAL PTERYGOID MUSCLE

SPHENOMANDIBULAR LIGAMENT

INTERNAL PTERYGOID MUSCLE

PTERYGOMANDIBULAR RAPHÉ

BUCCINATOR MUSCLE

DUCT OF PAROTID GLAND

BUCCINATOR CREST

LATERAL VIEW

AURICULOTEMPORAL NERVE

MAXILLARY ARTERY (INTERNAL MAXILLARY)

INFERIOR ALVEOLAR NERVE

MIDDLE MENINGEAL ARTERY

SPHENOMANDIBULAR LIGAMENT

LINGUAL NERVE

OTIC GANGLION

CHOANAE

EUSTACHIAN TUBE (CARTILAGINOUS)

LATERAL PTERYGOID PLATE

TEMPOROMANDIBULAR JOINT

ARTICULAR DISK

EXTERNAL PTERYGOID MUSCLE

MEDIAL PTERYGOID PLATE

INTERNAL PTERYGOID MUSCLE

HAMULAR PROCESS

MYLOHYOID NERVE

POSTERIOR VIEW

Fig. 1-6. Muscles of mastication. (© Copyright 1959, CIBA-GEIGY Corporation. Reproduced with permission. All rights reserved.)

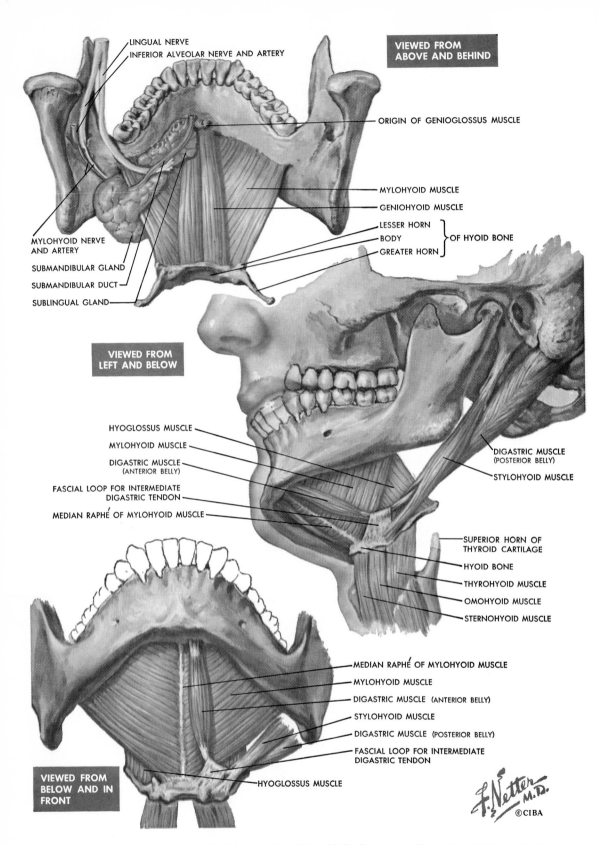

Fig. 1-7. Floor of mouth. (© Copyright 1959, CIBA-GEIGY Corporation. Reproduced with permission. All rights reserved.)

cle. The mandibular *condyle* rests on the ramus on a thin neck and articulates with a portion of the temporal bone, the *glenoid fossa*. It has its own fibrous capsule and an avascular articular surface of fibrocartilage. The mandible grows most rapidly during puberty, especially in males, where the greatest change is seen as a lengthening of the body, parasymphysis region, and condylar neck. Trauma to the adult mandible, therefore, tends to produce more damage in the body and subcondylar regions as compared to the infant or child, where forces are transmitted to the soft condyle and more often produce mushrooming intracapsular injuries (Irby, 1977; Rowe and Killey, 1968).

Two bilateral foramina, the mandibular and mental, penetrate the mandible. The *mandibular foramen* is located on the medial side of the ramus and is the site of entry of the inferior alveolar nerve, artery, and vein. A small fossa is found at the opening, and it is opposed by a pyramidal bony projection from the fossa rim, the *lingula*, which lies anteromedial to the neurovascular bundle and provides attachment for the thin, tough *sphenomandibular ligament*. The mandibular foramen is usually located at a point two-thirds the distance from the anterior border of the ramus at the junction of the middle and upper thirds. Its location is variable, however, and may be as high as just below the mandibular notch or well below the continuation of the occlusal plane of the teeth. It is important that the surgeon recognize this variability because the lingula is a key landmark for performing anesthetic blockade of the inferior alveolar nerve and for completing the intraoral cuts in certain mandibular osteotomies.

The mental foramen opens laterally from the basilar bone of the body at a point typically just below the apex of the second premolar tooth. The mental nerve, artery, and vein exit at this point and fan into the vestibular mucosa, gingiva, lower lip, and chin. With severe atrophy of the alveolar bone, the mental foramen and its neurovascular contents may come to lie close to the crest of the mandibular ridge, a condition that may com-

plicate routine dentoalveolar surgery and require surgical correction before a denture prosthesis can be worn comfortably.

A series of ridges, bony projections, and fossae are palpable on the inner aspect of the mandibular body. The *mylohyoid ridge* is an oblique overhang that provides attachment for the mylohyoid muscle and posteriorly for an attachment of the *pterygomandibular raphe*. In the midline two bilateral *genial tubercles* provide attachment superiorly for the genioglossus muscles and inferiorly for the geniohyoid muscles. Each of these tubercles may be quite prominent and require reduction in floor of the mouth vestibuloplasty procedures. A long, oval *sublingual fossa* is palpable just lateral to the genial tubercles and contains the sublingual gland. Below the posterior mylohyoid ridge, a larger depression contains the lateral bulging of the *submandibular gland*. Together these fossae cause a thinning of the mandible that results in radiolucencies that must be differentiated from cystic, developmental, or neoplastic conditions that may also occur in these locations.

The external aspect of the mandible is supplied by three main arteries. Inferiorly, the *facial artery* provides *sublingual* and *submental branches;* the *lingual artery* provides medial branches, and the ramus region is supplied by the *masseteric* and *mylohyoid* branches of the *maxillary artery*. The internal aspect of the mandible is supplied mostly by the *inferior alveolar* branch of the maxillary artery with additional supply from perforating branches of the *sublingual artery*. The mandibular cortex is more dense and less perfused when compared to the maxilla, especially in the posterior body region. This may account for the greater tendency for localized osteitis, osteomyelitis, and avascular necrosis of grafted materials to occur in the mandible.

Hyoid bone

The hyoid bone is located at the base of the submandibular triangles as a small, U-shaped body with posterolateral extensions, the *greater* and *lesser horns* (Fig. 1-7). The body provides attachment superiorly for the geniohyoid muscles and, at its junction with the lesser horn, for the tendinous sling of the digastric muscle and for the stylohyoid muscle. The middle pharyngeal constrictor and hyoglossus muscles arise from the hyoid bone beneath this plane. Functionally, the hyoid bone provides stability to the upper neck for the actions of mandibular opening, tongue protrusion, and pharyngeal constriction.

Temporomandibular joint

The articulation of the mandible with the cranium consists of a fossa, a condyle, a separating articular disc, a joint capsule, and a series of extracapsular check ligaments (Fig. 1-6) (Choukas and Sicher, 1960; Kreutziger and Mahan, 1975; Sicher and DuBrul, 1975). In cross section, the *mandibular or glenoid fossa* and the articular eminence of the temporal bone form a "lazy S" posteroanteriorly. Lateral to the eminence is a bony knob on the zygomatic arch, the *articular tubercle,* which provides attachment for the reinforced *lateral capsular ligament.* The fossa as well as the condyle is lined by a dense, avascular fibrocartilage that is thickest in the posterior fossa. The bone is thin enough in the depth of the fossa that, in rare instances of high impact to the mandible, the temporal bone may be fractured into the middle ear chamber or the fractured condyle may be displaced into the middle cranial fossa (Kallal, Gans, and Lagrotteria, 1977).

The mandibular condyle is a cylindroid structure, narrowest front to back, and approximately 2 cm across in its broadest mediolateral dimension. Its long axis is directed medially and somewhat posteriorly, and it rests on the thin neck of the condyloid process. The condyle is roughened on its medial and lateral poles where the *articular disc* and combined fibers of the *capsule* are attached. It was formerly believed that the fibrocartilage covering the condyle functioned like an epiphyseal plate and was a primary determinant of overall mandibular growth. However, it has since been shown that condylar growth is mainly an adaptive response to changes in the "functional matrix" of surrounding masticatory muscles and other soft tissues (Moss and Rankow, 1968; Sorensen and Laskin, 1975). In cases where there is a restricted stimulus from the soft tissues as a result of early trauma, destructive infections, or congenital neuromuscular anomalies, the condylar growth response will also be restricted and a progressive retrognathia will occur. A similar situation will also occur from direct injury to the condylar cartilage.

An *articular disc* separates the joint cavity into lower and upper chambers. The disc consists of interwoven connective tissue bundles with scattered basophilic cells. The avascular central part of the disc is thinner than the periphery and may become perforated with advancing age and chronic trauma. Posteriorly, the disc continues into a thick layer of vascularized connective tissue, the *retrodiscal pad,* that fuses with the posterior wall of the articular capsule. The pad region is most significant because sensory branches of the *auriculotemporal* nerve are abundant here, and the highly responsive *Golgi tendon organs* and *encapsulated mechanoreceptors* function as the primary proprioceptors for maintaining physiologic joint position (Schmid, 1969). Disturbance of the retrodiscal pad region during joint surgery will interfere with proper mandibular positional senses and require a retraining of mandibular movements (Kreutziger and Mahan, 1975).

The *fibrous capsule* consists of thin, separable fibers that attach above on the entire circumference of the mandibular fossa, including the articular tubercle, and insert below the condyle around the neck of the condyloid process. It is reinforced by the *temporomandibular ligament,* which extends down and back from the articular tubercle and inserts on the mandibular neck.

The *stylomandibular ligament* is located posterior to the joint and is a thickening of the deep parotid fascia. The *sphenomandibular ligament* is a thin, flat but strong span that arises on the sphenoid spine as well as the adjacent petrotympanic fissure and inserts on the lingula on the medial aspect of the mandible. Neither of these ligaments limits the joint. However, the sphenomandibular ligament is an important surgical landmark because the maxillary artery and auriculotemporal nerve pass between it and the mandibular neck.

The blood supply to the lateral joint comes from the superficial temporal artery, although the majority of vessels are concentrated deep and posteriorly in the retrodiscal capsular part as terminal deep auricular, posterior auricular, and masseteric branches of the maxillary artery. The condyle itself is penetrated by nutrient foramina vessels that enter the joint with the lateral pterygoid muscle attachments. The lateral pterygoid vascular pedicle appears to be adequate by itself to maintain the viability of the condyle detached during mandibular osteotomy (Path et al., 1977).

Two basic movements occur in the human temporomandibular joint: (1) a rotatory *hinge axis* movement that results from a pivoting of the condyle relative to the articular disc in the lower joint chamber and (2) a gliding *translational* action in the upper joint chamber in which the articular disc slides along the surface of the mandibular fossa and eminence. Hinge opening is accomplished mainly by action of the geniohyoid and anterior digastric muscles. Translatory protrusion is due to action of the lateral pterygoid, and retrusion is carried out by the deep head of masseter and posterior fibers of temporalis muscles. This is made possible through the action of paravertebral muscles that maintain the position of the cranial base and the stylohyoid, geniohyoid, and infrahyoid muscles that fix the position of the hyoid bone. Closure is achieved by action of the masseter, medial pterygoid, and temporalis muscles.

Ordinary hinge opening in the adult is in the range of 20 to 25 mm of interdental width, which, combined with translation action, brings the normal opening range to 35 to 45 mm. Pathologic hypermobility of the joint may result from congenital or acquired defects in the capsular ligaments or from spastic dyskinesias (Irby, 1977). In such cases the problem may be simply a *subluxation* in which the condyle is displaced out of the mandibular fossa but can be replaced spontaneously. This is in contrast to true *dislocation* in which the condyle is displaced from the fossa, most often anterior to the articular eminence, and cannot be replaced without the use of external force.

Midface

The skeleton of the central face consists of an outer *zygomaticomaxillary* buttress and a deeper midline *palatonasal* complex of bones (Figs. 1-5, 1-6, and 1-8). The paired maxillae are broad three-sided pyramids with a central body and four processes that abut at suture lines with the zygomatic, palatine, nasal, sphenoid, and smaller orbital bones. The maxillae function as a base for containing the teeth, support for the nasal cartilages, attachment of the facial muscles, as the shell for the maxillary sinus, and as the major plates of the bony palate and floor of the orbit. Its anterior limit is the prominent *anterior nasal spine* and its lateral continuation is the sharp margined *piriform rim*. The firm, vascular epithelium of the nasal floor is loosely attached along this rim and can easily be elevated to expose the roof of the palatine process of the maxilla as is often necessary in maxillary orthognathic surgery (Bell et al., 1975). A concavity of the midanterior maxillary surface, the *canine fossa*, is a common zone for localization of odontogenic infections. Such infections have the potential for hematogenous spread, since the *angular vein* traverses the fossa and anastomoses with the inferior ophthalmic plexus superiorly. The *infraorbital nerve, artery, and vein* enter into the upper aspect of the canine fossa from the *infraorbital foramen*.

The lateral maxilla expands upward to meet the zygomatic bone, forming the *malar eminence*. Posteriorly, the *maxillary tuberosity* abuts against the *pterygoid process* of the sphenoid bone at the sharply defined *pterygopalatine fissure*. This fissure is an important site in the mobilization of the maxilla during midface orthognathic advancement surgery (Nelson et al., 1977). Above, the fissure

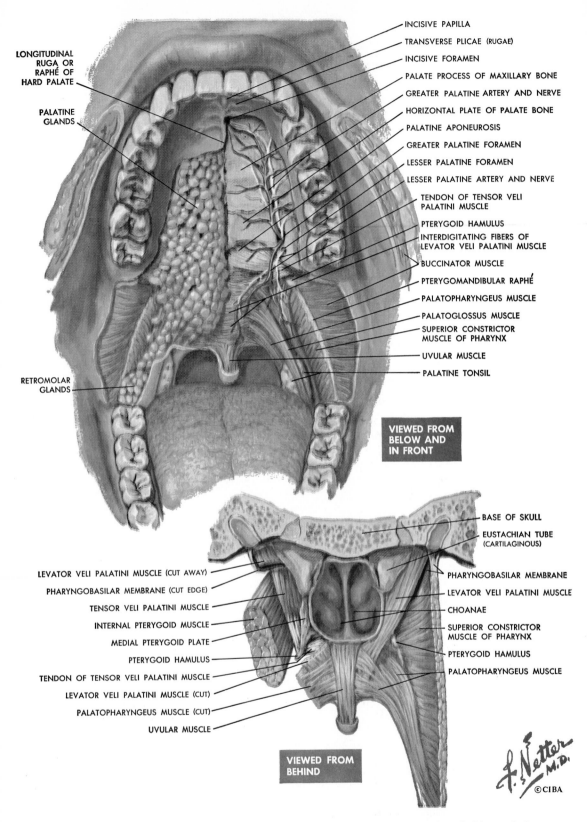

INCISIVE PAPILLA

TRANSVERSE PLICAE (RUGAE)

INCISIVE FORAMEN

PALATE PROCESS OF MAXILLARY BONE

GREATER PALATINE ARTERY AND NERVE

HORIZONTAL PLATE OF PALATE BONE

PALATINE APONEUROSIS

GREATER PALATINE FORAMEN

LESSER PALATINE FORAMEN

LESSER PALATINE ARTERY AND NERVE

TENDON OF TENSOR VELI PALATINI MUSCLE

PTERYGOID HAMULUS

INTERDIGITATING FIBERS OF LEVATOR VELI PALATINI MUSCLE

BUCCINATOR MUSCLE

PTERYGOMANDIBULAR RAPHÉ

PALATOPHARYNGEUS MUSCLE

PALATOGLOSSUS MUSCLE

SUPERIOR CONSTRICTOR MUSCLE OF PHARYNX

UVULAR MUSCLE

PALATINE TONSIL

LONGITUDINAL RUGA OR RAPHÉ OF HARD PALATE

PALATINE GLANDS

RETROMOLAR GLANDS

VIEWED FROM BELOW AND IN FRONT

BASE OF SKULL

EUSTACHIAN TUBE (CARTILAGINOUS)

PHARYNGOBASILAR MEMBRANE

LEVATOR VELI PALATINI MUSCLE

CHOANAE

SUPERIOR CONSTRICTOR MUSCLE OF PHARYNX

PTERYGOID HAMULUS

PALATOPHARYNGEUS MUSCLE

LEVATOR VELI PALATINI MUSCLE (CUT AWAY)

PHARYNGOBASILAR MEMBRANE (CUT EDGE)

TENSOR VELI PALATINI MUSCLE

INTERNAL PTERYGOID MUSCLE

MEDIAL PTERYGOID PLATE

PTERYGOID HAMULUS

TENDON OF TENSOR VELI PALATINI MUSCLE

LEVATOR VELI PALATINI MUSCLE (CUT)

PALATOPHARYNGEUS MUSCLE (CUT)

UVULAR MUSCLE

VIEWED FROM BEHIND

f. Netter M.D.

©CIBA

Fig. 1-8. Roof of mouth. (© Copyright 1959, CIBA-GEIGY Corporation. Reproduced with permission. All rights reserved.)

opens into the *pterygopalatine fossa,* which connects with the orbit superiorly through the *inferior orbital fissure.* The pterygopalatine fossa is important as the passageway for the major nerves and vessels of the maxilla, nasal fossa, and palate. The neural contents of the pterygopalatine fossa are accessible for local anesthetic blocks from four different directions: directly laterally by using the pterygoid plate as a landmark or by passing the needle obliquely behind the maxillary tuberosity, and indirectly by applying topical cocaine in the posterior nasal fossa behind the middle concha at the point where the sphenopalatine foramen opens or by passing an injection needle up the descending palatine canal.

The *zygomatic bone* gives prominence to the lateral face, provides attachment for the masseter muscle, and forms the floor and that part of the lateral wall of the orbit where the *lateral suspensory ligament* that gives support for the eyeball and the *lateral rectus muscle* attaches. The zygoma is attached at the broad *zygomaticomaxillary* suture and the thin *zygomaticofrontal* and *zygomaticotemporal* sutures. Separation occurs along these three sutures in the typical "trimalar" zygomatic fracture and results in facial flattening and diplopia. The zygomatic arch is also vulnerable to lateral trauma that may collapse the arch medially into the temporal space where it can restrict the translatory opening movements of the mandible by impinging on the coronoid process (Rowe and Killey, 1968).

The *palatonasal complex* is made up of small interdigitating and compartmentalized bones: the palatal and nasal portions of the *maxilla, palatine, vomer, ethmoid,* and *inferior concha* bones and *pterygoid plates of the sphenoid bone.* The hard palate is made up of the arched *palatine processes* of the maxillary bones, which in the adult are joined by a calcified midline suture and are continuous posteriorly across the transverse *palatomaxillary* suture with the horizontal plates of the *palatine bones.* In the anterior midline of the palate the *incisive*

canal opens as one or more *incisive foramina* that transmit the terminal branches of the *nasopalatine nerves* and *sphenopalatine arteries.* The posterior hard palate is grooved laterally by the greater palatine nerves and arteries, which course forward toward the incisive region from their point of emergence from the *greater palatine foramina* in the palatine bones (Fig. 1-8). The *lesser palatine foramina* are smaller, variable in number, and transmit lesser palatine arteries and sensory nerves that distribute to the soft palate and paratonsillar region. The palatine bones that make up the posterior hard palate are very thin except laterally where a thickened *pyramidal process* forms a junction with the *pterygoid process of the sphenoid bone.* The pterygoid process is an important fulcrum for a number of deep oropharyngeal muscles. It is split posteriorly into a wide, short lateral plate whose outer surface gives origin to the *lateral pterygoid muscle,* and a shorter medial plate that ends below in a thin hooklike projection, the *pterygoid hamulus,* which is palpable in the lateral soft palate. The inferior end of the hamulus serves as the upper attachment for the *pterygomandibular raphe,* a fascial fold into which the *superior pharyngeal constrictor muscle* terminates and from which the *buccinator muscle* arises. Between the medial and lateral pterygoid plates a deep depression, the *pterygoid fossa,* gives origin to the *medial pterygoid muscle.* At the root of the medial plate a shallower depression, the *scaphoid fossa,* gives origin to the *tensor veli palatini muscle.* The tensor muscle passes inferiorly and becomes tendinous as it makes a 90 degree medial turn around the hamulus, then fans out and becomes interspersed in the *palatal aponeurosis,* the fibrous "skeleton" of the soft palate.

Clefts of the soft palate disturb speech and swallowing functions by breaking the continuity of the palatal aponeurosis and aborting the actions that the tensor and levator muscles exert on these tissues. The horizontally directed fibers of the tensor cannot form the firm transverse barrier of soft tissue, nor can the levator elevate this barrier to make contact with the pharyngeal constrictors of the posterior pharynx to create the *velopharyngeal sphincter.* Surgical correction of cleft deformities in this region has the dual purpose of establishing a transverse tensor veli palatini action and also assuring anteroposterior velopharyngeal contact. Some cleft palate surgeries gain midline muscular closure by fracturing the pterygoid hamuli medially and relaxing the tensor veli palatini muscles as they turn into the aponeurosis. Other procedures gain length by mobilizing the palatine bones and aponeurosis posteriorly and then filling the void at the end of the hard palate with an "island flap" of hard palate tissue based on a *greater palatine arterial pedicle* (Hayward, 1974).

The external *nasal skeleton* is suspended from the frontal bone by the paired, thin nasal bones. Below, the midline *septal cartilages* and the *lateral* and *alar cartilages* are joined by fibrous attachments. The septal cartilage is continuous posteriorly with the *perpendicular plate of the ethmoid bone* and joins the *vomer* and the *anterior nasal spine of the maxilla* below to make up the *nasal septum.* The nasal septum, therefore, is a continuous unit that terminates posterosuperiorly in a thin rectangular section of the ethmoid bone, the *cribriform plate,* that is fused between the greater wings of the sphenoid bones in the floor of the anterior cranial fossa. This plate is relatively weak and may fracture as a result of trauma to the nasal septum spilling cerebrospinal fluid into the nasal chambers. Because many fibers of the *first cranial (olfactory) nerve* also perforate through the cribriform plate, injury to this region may also result in anosmia (Rowe and Killey, 1968).

The *lateral wings* of the *alar cartilages* are concave and are based inferiorly on the *piriform rim* of the maxilla. In combined cleft lip and palate this nasomaxillary junction is directly in the line of the cleft, causing formation of oronasal fistulae and collapse of the external nares, both of which must be repaired surgically.

The lateral nasal wall is made up of the vertical plates of the maxillary and palatine bones and is usually subdivided by three irregular overhanging projections, the *conchae.* The inferior concha is a separate bone of the skull whereas the middle and superior conchae are part of the *ethmoid bone.* The conchae subdivide the nasal cavity into horizontal groovelike passages, *meatuses.* The *inferior meatus,* which is most accessible to examination contains the slitlike opening of the *nasolacrimal duct* about 1 cm posterior to the front edge of the inferior concha. The recess anterior to the inferior concha is the site at which antrostomy openings are made to establish effective nasal drainage for an obstructed maxillary sinus. Posterior to the inferior concha and in direct line with the inferior meatus may be found the orifice of the *cartilaginous auditory tube.* In the *middle meatus* a bulging mass called the *ethmoidal bulla* has a series of perforating canals that lead to various of the *ethmoid air cells.* Below the bulla a deep partially open groove, the *semilunar hiatus,* provides the opening for the *frontonasal duct* from the *frontal sinus* anteriorly and in its midportion the large *ostium of the maxillary sinus.* The mucoperiosteum in the entire nasal cavity and especially over the conchae is thick, highly vascular, and lined with a mucus-secreting, pseudociliated epithelium. Hemorrhage control in these membranes is difficult because the feeding vessels converge from diverse sources: the ophthalmic, maxillary, pharyngeal, and palatal arteries.

Paranasal sinuses

A bilateral series of four pneumatic areas, the *sphenoid, ethmoid, frontal,* and *maxillary sinuses,* span the central portions of the face (Sicher and Dubrul, 1975). All are lined by a thin membrane that is a fusion of periosteum and a stiff pseudostratified columnar epithelum. The primary functions of the sinuses are to reduce the bulk of the facial skeleton, to warm incoming air, and to assist in cleaning the air by secreting an adherent mucin that is moved by ciliary action into the nasal chambers for discharge. The sinuses develop as outpouchings of the nasal fossa that are less than one-tenth their adult size at birth. With aging, the cavitations expand into adjacent areas such as edentulous parts of the maxilla and the palatine and frontal bones. This makes the mid- and upper facial skeleton more prone to comminution from trauma, and in the case of the maxillary sinus it makes it more likely that disease processes in the alveolus will extend into it than at an earlier age.

The *sphenoid sinus* is the smallest, most posterior, and inaccessible sinus. It is located immediately below the *hypophyseal fossa*. It is cube-shaped, irregular, and divided in the midline by a thin septum. A short canal connects the sphenoid sinus with the *sphenoethmoidal recess* in the superior meatus.

The *ethmoid sinuses* are highly variable in size, number from 3 to 18, and communicate with the nasal fossa by several openings in the middle and superior meatuses. With aging, they extend into adjacent areas of the ethmoid, sphenoid, lacrimal, and palatine bones on either side of the superior bony septum. This makes surgical reconstruction of the damaged or deficient interorbital skeleton very difficult.

The *frontal sinus* is flat, highly variable in its upward extension, and divided by an irregular midseptum. It communicates with the anterior aspect of the middle meatus through the thin *frontonasal canal*. Although the outer table of the frontal bone is very thick, it may be fractured into the sinus and usually separates at the *frontonasal suture* line. The inner table is much thinner and vulnerable to puncture or even erosion by chronic sinus infection. Therefore this is a possible avenue of microbial spread into the adjacent anterior cranial fossa.

The *maxillary sinus*, or *antrum*, is the largest of the paranasal sinuses, occupying the entire body of each maxilla in the adult. It is pyramidal with a floor at or below the level of the nasal floor and a roof that slopes anterolaterally and is flat except for a distinct ridge formed by the *infraorbital canal*. The floor may be partitioned by bony septae, especially in the

posterior one-third, which may hinder the retrieval of foreign bodies such as tooth roots that may have been displaced into the sinus. The *maxillary ostium* opens into the semilunar hiatus in the middle meatus at a level that is close to the roof of the sinus cavity, an arrangement that does not favor drainage in the erect position. Thus it is sometimes necessary to provide dependent drainage for a hematoma or purulence by penetrating the sinus wall either medially in the inferior meatus or intraorally in the canine fossa, the so-called Caldwell-Luc procedure.

Upper face

The upper facial skeleton is made up of the orbitofrontal and the basilar skull bones. The bony *orbit* is pyramidal and formed by parts of seven bones: maxillary, zygomatic, frontal, lacrimal, ethmoid, palatine, and sphenoid. Its outer rim is dense and perforated inferiorly by the medially directed *infraorbital foramen*, which transmits the infraorbital branch of the maxillary artery and the infraorbital nerve of the maxillary division of the trigeminal nerve (V_2). The superior rim is notched by the *supraorbital foramen* and the *supratrochlear notch*, which transmit similarly named arterial branches of the *ophthalmic artery* and branches of the ophthalmic division of the trigeminal nerve (Fig. 1-2). The *nasolacrimal duct* begins in a groove just inside the medial rim. Behind this depression the lacrimal and ethmoid bones are paper thin and perforated by *anterior* and *posterior ethmoid* branches of the *superior ophthalmic artery*. The *suspensory ligaments* and *medial palpebral ligaments* take origin from small tubercles on the medial anterior wall. Therefore, comminution of the thin bones of this region may result in significantly impaired ocular function. The lateral orbit is also weakened by the *zygomaticofrontal suture*, a point of separation in midfacial LeForte II and III type fractures. A foramen is also found in the lateral wall of the orbit through which the *zygomatico-orbital* nerve branch of V_2 enters the zygomatic bone, divides, and exits the bone again as the *zygomaticotemporal and zygo-*

maticofacial sensory nerves. The floor of the orbit is very thin because of the underlying *maxillary sinus* and the infraorbital canal that traverse it. Direct trauma to the eyeball may on rare occasions produce a "blowout" fracture of the midorbital floor, allowing the soft tissues of the orbit to herniate into the maxillary sinus, resulting in double vision. More often, trauma that disrupts the walls of the orbit will interfere with extraocular muscle function because of entrapment of these muscles, especially the *inferior oblique, inferior rectus,* and *lateral rectus muscles.*

In the floor of the posterior orbit, the *infraorbital fissure* gives access to the orbit for the *infraorbital* and *zygomatico-orbital* nerves, the infraorbital terminations of the maxillary artery, and a connecting vein from the pterygoid plexus to the *inferior ophthalmic* vein. The borders of this fissure also provide attachment for Muller's muscle, a largely vestigial smooth muscle that helps maintain the eyeball in its proper anteroposterior position.

In the upper lateral apex of the orbit the *superior orbital fissure* provides access for cranial nerves III, IV, V, and VI, the sympathetic postganglionic fibers from the cavernous sinus plexus, and the ophthalmic veins. Bleeding or pressure from pathosis in the orbit may compress these structures as they pass through the narrow bony opening and produce the *superior orbital fissure syndrome* of ophthalmoplegia, pupillary constriction, enophthalmos, and ptosis of the eyelid (Kronsclenabel, 1974).

The *optic foramen,* found in the most superior recess of the orbit, conducts the *optic nerve* (II) and the *ophthalmic artery* and is better protected from trauma.

Basilar skull

The zygomaticomaxillary, palatonasal, and orbitofrontal bony complexes of the face rest on a common foundation, the *sphenoid bone.* The sphenoid consists of a body and three processes, the *greater wings,* the *lesser wings,* and the *pterygoid processes.* The sphenoid body is dense, box-shaped, hollowed out by the *sphenoid sinus,* and continuous posteriorly and laterally with the saucer-shaped *occipital* and *temporal* basilar bones. Its superior surface is a saddle-shaped *hypophyseal fossa* that contains the pituitary gland. The fossa is grooved anteriorly by the *optic canals,* which meet in the midline where the *optic chiasm* of the cranial nerve II rests. On the lateral walls of the body of the sphenoid a reticular semirigid structure, the *cavernous sinus,* is formed between the meningeal and the periosteal layers of the dura. The sinus is the passageway for cranial nerves III, IV, VI, and parts of the ophthalmic and maxillary divisions of the cranial nerve V on their way to the orbit and face. The *internal carotid artery* enters the sinus posteriorly and arches out again just behind the chiasm. In the anterolateral junction of the sphenoid body with the greater and lesser wings the slitlike *superior orbital fissure* provides communication between the orbit and the cavernous sinus and the middle cranial fossa for transmittal of *cranial nerves III, IV,* and *VI,* the *ophthalmic branch* of V, *sympathetic fibers* of the cavernous plexus and the *ophthalmic vein.*

Immediately behind the superior orbital fissure, the *greater wing of the sphenoid* bone forms the floor of the middle cranial fossa. The *foramen rotundum* is found most anteriorly, transmitting the maxillary division of cranial nerve V, and the larger *foramen ovale* through which the mandibular division of cranial nerve V passes lies posterior and laterally. In the same line posteriorly, the *foramen spinosum* transmits the *middle meningeal* branch of the *maxillary artery.* On the most medial slope of the greater wing a large bony depression contains the trigeminal ganglion, and just posterior to the fossa the *foramen lacerum* provides entry to the cavernous sinus for the internal carotid artery. A groove and *hiatus of the facial canal* is situated between the foramen spinosum and foramen lacerum and contains the *greater superficial petrosal nerve.* A series of *emissary veins* connect the face with the dural venous sinuses in the region of the hypophyseal fossa and the middle cranial fossa. Veins from the pterygoid plexus perforate near the hiatus of the facial canal, through the foramen ovale and foramen lacerum, and occasionally through the foramen spinosum. Direct venous communication is also found between the superior and inferior ophthalmic veins and the cavernous sinus through the superior orbital fissure.

The sphenoidal basal structures may figure prominently in surgical pathology of the maxillofacial region. The emissary vein system, devoid of internal valves, is a potential avenue for spread of blood-borne bacterial emboli from the face and jaws to the cavernous sinus region. Infratemporal space infections may involve the pterygoid plexus. More commonly, infections in the lateral nasal, palatal, and canine fossa may gain access to the intracranium by progressing from the *angular facial vein* to the *inferior* or *superior ophthalmic veins,* and through the superior orbital fissure to the cavernous sinus (Evans, 1965; Kronsclenabel, 1974).

Severe mid- and upper face trauma may result in separation of the palatomaxillary, nasoethmoidal, and orbitofrontal complexes from the sphenoidal basilar skull, producing the classical LeForte III fracture. The sphenoid bone, weakened by the line of foramina from the superior orbital fissure posteriorly to foramen spinosum, may fracture along this plane, rupture emisssary veins or even the middle meningeal artery, produce progressive deficits in cranial nerves that pass through these fissures and foramina, and potentially influence hypothalmic and pituitary functions in the hypophyseal fossa (Rowe and Killey, 1968).

NEUROMUSCULAR APPARATUS

Orofacial tissues perform a number of simultaneous crucial motor functions. Mastication of food involves sucking, grasping, chewing, and swallowing that is accomplished by a series of visceral sphincters that assist the powerful muscles that move the mandible. Communication is aided through expressive facial movements, articulation of sounds, and the velopharyngeal control of air flow within nasal, oral, and pharyngeal chambers. The neuromuscular apparatus also serves in respiration by maintaining patency of the upper airway and assists in sensation by positioning and protecting the sensory organs for vision, smell, taste, and tactile exploration. In managing surgical disorders of this region each of these major functions must be preserved or enhanced.

Masticatory muscles

The muscles that bring about the chewing actions of the mandible are the masseter, medial pterygoid, temporalis, and lateral pterygoid muscles and the suprahyoid group of geniohyoid, mylohyoid, and anterior digastric muscles (Table 1-1) (Figs. 1-5 to 1-9).

The *masseter* muscle attaches by a superficial and a deep head to the lower one fourth of the mandibular ramus. It functions synergistically with the *medial pterygoid muscle* in forming a sling that pulls the mandible upward and forward. The deep belly origins of the masseter muscle intermingle with the superficial fibers of the temporalis muscle along the *external oblique ridge* of the mandible. Irritation of these muscle fibers attributable to pericoronal inflammation in the mandibular molars commonly causes myospasm and trismus. Root fragments from the mandibular third molar may be displaced during surgery and pass subperiosteally deep to the attachment of the medial pterygoid muscle. Both the medial pterygoid and the masseter muscles are often detached from the angle of the mandible when mandibular fractures are repaired or when osteotomy of the mandibular ramus is done. This can be accomplished safely because the neurovascular supply to both muscles enters their deep aspects near their superior bony insertions. The *masseteric nerve,* a branch of motor V_3, and the *masseteric artery,* a branch of the maxillary artery, reach the muscle belly by coursing through the *mandibular* or *sigmoid notch* of the mandible behind the temporalis muscle. Both the masseter and medial pterygoid appear to have influence on the shape of the mandibular bone, since changes brought about to the angle region by osteotomy will return to their preoperative state in a

Table 1-1. Neuromuscular units of the maxillofacial region

Cranial nerve	Muscles	Actions
III	Medial rectus, superior rectus, inferior rectus, inferior oblique	Eyeball rotation (medial, up, down and in)
	Levator palpebrae superioris	Lid elevation
IV	Superior oblique	Eyeball rotation down and out
VI	Lateral rectus	Eyeball rotation lateral
V	Masseter	Mandibular elevation
	Medial pterygoid	Mandibular elevation
	Temporalis	Mandibular elevation, retraction
	Lateral pterygoid	Mandibular anterior translation
	Mylohyoid	Mandibular depression
	Anterior digastric	Mandibular depression
	Tensor veli palatini	Palatal aponeurosis stabilization
VII	Frontalis, auricular, orbicularis oculi, orbicularis oris, buccinator, zygomaticus, platysma, posterior digastric, stylohyoid	Facial expression, ocular and oral sphincter, mandibular depression
IX	Stylopharyngeus	Pharyngeal widening
X	Superior, middle, inferior pharyngeal constrictor	Pharyngeal narrowing
	Palatoglossus	Pharyngeal narrowing
	Palatopharyngeus	Pharyngeal narrowing
	Levator veli palatini	Palatal elevation
	Musculus uvulus	Uvular contraction
XI	Sternocleidomastoid	Head rotation
	Trapezius	Shoulder elevation
XII, $C_{1, 2}$	Intrinsic tongue	Tongue movement
	Styloglossus	Tongue retraction
	Hyoglossus	Tongue depression
	Genioglossus	Tongue protraction
	Geniohyoid	Mandibular retraction

matter of months following muscular reattachment.

The *temporalis muscle* is fan-shaped and arises above from the temporal fossa. Its anterior fibers are directed almost vertically downward to insert on the mandible and therefore have an elevating action. Its posterior fibers, however, run almost horizontally and then bend in front of the articular eminence to exert a retracting action on the mandible. The temporalis fibers become organized into two thick tendons as they approach the mandible. The superficial tendon inserts along the *external oblique ridge* and the anterior crest of the *coronoid process,* whereas the larger deep tendon inserts along the medial temporal crest and *internal oblique ridge* as far inferiorly as the *retromolar trigone* region. In certain osteotomy procedures the coronoid process is sectioned from the mandible,

which then permits the temporalis muscle to retract the free segment superiorly. In cases of oblique "unfavorable" mandibular fractures of the body and anterior angle, the combined powerful elevator action of masseter, medial pterygoid, and temporalis muscles will displace the proximal segments superiorly and act in opposition to the suprahyoid group of mandibular depressor muscles (Kruger, 1974).

One head of the *lateral pterygoid muscle* arises from the lateral pterygoid plate and the other from the scaphoid fossa region of the sphenoid body. Because of its insertion on the neck of the condyloid process and into the meniscus and joint capsule, it exerts both an opening and translating action on the mandible and also causes lateral shifting with the aid of the medial pterygoid muscle. Fractures low on the neck of the condyloid

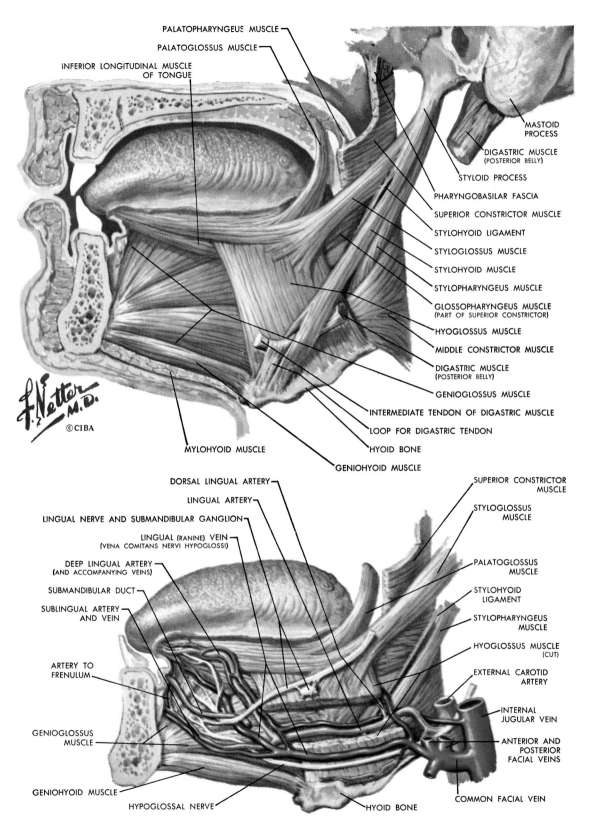

PALATOPHARYNGEUS MUSCLE

PALATOGLOSSUS MUSCLE

INFERIOR LONGITUDINAL MUSCLE
OF TONGUE

MASTOID
PROCESS

DIGASTRIC MUSCLE
(POSTERIOR BELLY)

STYLOID PROCESS

PHARYNGOBASILAR FASCIA

SUPERIOR CONSTRICTOR MUSCLE

STYLOHYOID LIGAMENT

STYLOGLOSSUS MUSCLE

STYLOHYOID MUSCLE

STYLOPHARYNGEUS MUSCLE

GLOSSOPHARYNGEUS MUSCLE
(PART OF SUPERIOR CONSTRICTOR)

HYOGLOSSUS MUSCLE

MIDDLE CONSTRICTOR MUSCLE

DIGASTRIC MUSCLE
(POSTERIOR BELLY)

GENIOGLOSSUS MUSCLE

INTERMEDIATE TENDON OF DIGASTRIC MUSCLE

LOOP FOR DIGASTRIC TENDON

MYLOHYOID MUSCLE

HYOID BONE

GENIOHYOID MUSCLE

DORSAL LINGUAL ARTERY

LINGUAL ARTERY

LINGUAL NERVE AND SUBMANDIBULAR GANGLION

LINGUAL (RANINE) VEIN
(VENA COMITANS NERVI HYPOGLOSSI)

DEEP LINGUAL ARTERY
(AND ACCOMPANYING VEINS)

SUBMANDIBULAR DUCT

SUBLINGUAL ARTERY
AND VEIN

ARTERY TO
FRENULUM

GENIOGLOSSUS
MUSCLE

GENIOHYOID MUSCLE

HYPOGLOSSAL NERVE

HYOID BONE

SUPERIOR CONSTRICTOR
MUSCLE

STYLOGLOSSUS
MUSCLE

PALATOGLOSSUS
MUSCLE

STYLOHYOID
LIGAMENT

STYLOPHARYNGEUS
MUSCLE

HYOGLOSSUS MUSCLE
(CUT)

EXTERNAL CAROTID
ARTERY

INTERNAL
JUGULAR VEIN

ANTERIOR AND
POSTERIOR
FACIAL VEINS

COMMON FACIAL VEIN

F. Netter
M.D.
©CIBA

Fig. 1-9. Muscles controlling tongue. (© Copyright 1959, CIBA-GEIGY Corporation. Reproduced with permission. All rights reserved.)

process will permit the lateral pterygoid muscle to tip the condyle medially and anteriorly completely out of the mandibular fossa and into the infratemporal space.

The suprahyoid group of *geniohyoid, mylohyoid,* and *anterior digastric muscles* have the common features of mandibular depressor action, origin on the hyoid bone, and insertion on the anterior mandible. They are assisted in their action by the stylohyoid muscle, which tends to fix the hyoid bone in position so that the other suprahyoid muscles may open the mouth forcefully. In certain of the facial deformities, such as mandibular retrognathia and open bite, the actions of suprahyoid muscles may be detrimental to the stability of the surgical repairs, and therefore they may have to be partially released along their inferior mandibular insertions (Steinhauser, 1973).

The *mylohyoid muscle* forms the *floor of the mouth* and inserts posteriorly along the mylohyoid ridge as far as the second or third molar region. In cases of mandibular alveolar atrophy, where preprosthetic reconstruction requires floor of the mouth vestibuloplasty, the mylohyoid fibers can be completely detached without change in speech. This also reduces mylohyoid displacement of the denture.

Visceral muscles

Two functional sphincters are formed by an intertwining of facial and parapharyngeal muscles (Figs. 1-8 and 1-9). An anterior sphincter is formed from the buccinator, orbicularis oris, and lingual muscles and functions in grasping, sucking, and positioning food for mastication and also in speech articulation. A posterior sphincter is formed by the palatoglossus, palatopharyngeus, levator and tensor veli palatini, and superior and middle pharyngeal constrictor muscles and functions mainly in swallowing and vocalization.

The *buccinator muscle* arises from a horseshoe-shaped line that begins on the posterior alveolar bases of the maxilla and mandible and is continuous over the pterygoid hamulus and into a tendinous fold, the *pterygomandibular raphe,* which also provides the anterior attachment for the *superior pharyngeal constrictor muscle.* Anteriorly the upper and lower buccinator fibers converge and some cross just before inserting in the mucosa at the corner of the mouth where they intermingle with crossing fibers of the orbicularis oris muscle. This common zone of muscle termination is semitendinous and important to the oral sealing functions of the anterior sphincter. Lacerations or burns that interrupt this zone are very debilitating, and surgical repairs must strive to minimize scarring and recreate the crossing-fiber pattern.

The *orbicularis oris muscle* makes up the entire lips and has no skeletal attachments. Its deepest fibers are circular and continuous across the midline. The superficial fibers of the upper lip insert in a vertical subcutaneous fold on each side of the midline, forming the *philtrum.* Both the buccinator and orbicularis oris muscles are innervated by branches of the *facial nerve (VII)* and must function in coordination with the tongue, which is innervated entirely by the *hypoglossal nerve (XII).* Dysfunctions of the facial nerve, as in Bell's palsy or from lateral facial trauma, will disturb anterior sphincter coordination.

The *tongue* is a muscular organ with both *intrinsic muscles* that are longitudinal, transverse, and vertical in orientation, and deeper *extrinsic muscles,* the styloglossus, hyoglossus, and genioglossus muscles, which arise from skeletal points and fan into the tongue (Figs. 1-9 and 1-10). The *styloglossus muscle* arises from the styloid process and enters the lateral mass of the tongue at the base of the palatoglossal arch. Its fibers are horizontal and reach nearly to the tip of the tongue to act as retractors. The *hyoglossus muscle* arises mainly from the greater horn of the hyoid bone, forms a thin vertical sheet that intermingles with the styloglossus muscle, and acts as a depressor of the tongue. The *genioglossus muscle* is a relatively strong protractor and depressor of the tongue tip that arises from the genial tubercle on the mid-inner aspect of the mandible. Large portions of the mid-

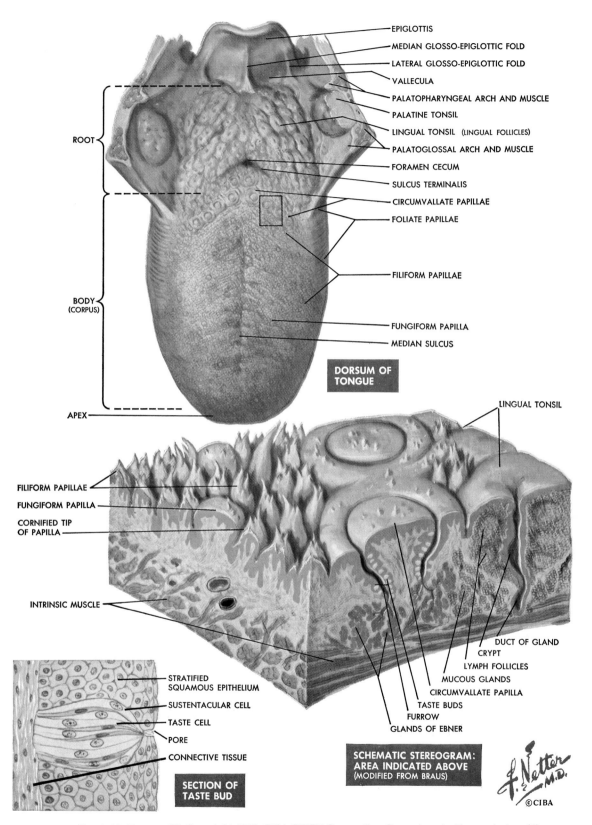

Fig. 1-10. Tongue. (© Copyright 1959, CIBA-GEIGY Corporation. Reproduced with permission. All rights reserved.)

and upper portions of the tongue may be resected, if necessary over one third of the total mass, without major impairment of tongue function (Wickwire, White, and Proffit, 1972). Excision of tongue tissue laterally and inferiorly, however, is not well tolerated because of the specific extrinsic muscle bellies found there.

The muscles of the *palate* are the small, unpaired *musculus uvulus,* which arises from the posterior nasal spine and palatal aponeurosis, and the paired *tensor veli palatini* and *levator veli palatini muscles* (Fig. 1-8). The tensor takes origin from the greater wing of the sphenoid bone, the adjacent scaphoid fossa of the pterygoid process, and the *cartilaginous auditory tube.* It descends vertically from its origin, turns 90 degrees medially around the pterygoid hamulus, and inserts into the posterior palatine bony shelf and the *palatal aponeurosis.* The tensor has two important functions: by changing the tension on the auditory tube, it adjusts air pressure in the middle ear; and because of its pulleylike insertion on the palate, it makes the anterior part of the soft palate rigid and actually depresses it slightly. The *levator* takes origin just posteromedial to the tensor, but descends diagonally to insert above and behind the palatal aponeurosis. It lifts the posterior soft palate into contact with a corresponding bulge on the posterior pharyngeal wall. On lateral view the combined action of tensor and levator, therefore, forms a lazy "S" configuration. Some cleft palate surgeries attempt to enhance the "S" configuration and assist the levator in its action by attaching "pharyngeal flaps" pedicled from the superior pharyngeal constrictor to the top of the posterior soft palate.

The palatal sphincter is coordinated with the muscles of the pharynx proper, which consist of the pharyngeal constrictors and three vertical muscle groups: the small stylopharyngeus, the palatoglossus, and the palatopharyngeus.

The *superior pharyngeal constrictor* is the uppermost of the cylindric muscles that are continuous across the midline posteriorly where a connective tissue raphe anchors them to the vertebral column. It arises anteriorly from the pterygoid hamulus, the pterygomandibular raphe, and the mylohyoid ridge terminus on the mandible. Anesthetic injections, and even dissections for preprosthetic surgery, may inadvertently penetrate the anterior portions of the superior pharyngeal constrictor and may result in complications, since both the ascending pharyngeal and ascending palatine arteries are located on the deep aspect at this level. The *stylopharyngeus muscle* is the only pharyngeal muscle innervated solely by nerve IX and it interdigitates with superior pharyngeal constrictor fibers posteriorly.

The remaining vertical muscles of the pharynx act as part of the lateral palatal sphincter. The *palatoglossus muscle* makes up the *anterior palatine arch* or faucial pillar on the anterior face of the superior constrictor, and the *palatopharyngeus muscle* forms the *posterior palatine arch.* Between the two arches, the *tonsillar fossa* contains the palatine tonsil.

With the exception of the *tensor veli palatini,* which is innervated by a motor branch of the trigeminal nerve, and the stylopharyngeus muscle, which is innervated by nerve IX, all the remaining palatal and pharyngeal muscles are innervated by the pharyngeal plexus branches of the vagus nerve (X). Because of the diffuseness of this motor supply and its origins deep and superiorly, major dysfunctions of the palatopharyngeal sphincter are not usually caused by peripheral surgical lesions but rather by intracranial lesions.

MOTOR NERVES OF MAXILLOFACIAL REGION

The skeletal muscles of the craniofacial region are activated by clusters of large neurons called *cranial motor nuclei,* which are found in a longitudinal column throughout the midventral brain stem (Table 1-1) (Crosby, Humphrey, and Lauer, 1962). The motor nuclear column spans from anteriorly in the midbrain, where the motor nuclei of III and IV arise, through the level of the pons, where the *trigeminal* (V) and facial (VII) nuclei arise, to the lower *medulla* and upper *spinal cord* segments for the spinal accessory (XI) and hypoglossal (XII) motor nuclei. All the motor nuclei send out their uncrossed thick roots ventrolaterally from the brain stem, except for the trochlear (IV) nerve, which emerges dorsally and crosses to the undersurface. The motor roots course individually through foramina in the base of the skull to innervate the motor end-plates of the cranial muscles. Because these lower motor neurons and their nerve roots are the final common pathway to the muscles, surgical or pathologic lesions to them will produce paresis or paralysis in all muscles innervated by the lesioned nerve. Thus trauma to the facial nerve in its peripheral course in the *facial canal* or at its point of emergence from the *stylomastoid foramen* will produce a "lower motor lesion" and disturb function in all facial muscles of that side. So-called upper motor lesions of cranial nerves may be seen in which only certain segments of the total muscle group innervated by a given cranial nerve are disturbed. This is because the central nervous system tracts that converge on the motor nuclei as upper motor neurons are often incomplete bilateral systems, and central lesions such as trauma, strokes, or tumors will therefore produce only partial involvement.

The major input to the masticatory motor nuclei arises first from stretch receptors in the masticatory, facial, and lingual muscles as well as proprioceptors in the mucosa, the periodontal membrane, and especially from the temporomandibular joint capsule. Impulses from these receptors travel primarily as part of the mandibular branch of the trigeminal nerve through the *foramen ovale* and terminate in the *mesencephalic nucleus of V* in the midbrain where the cell bodies are located. Because the motor nerve fibers to all the masticatory muscles are also part of the mandibular branch of V, direct surgical damage to this deeply placed trunk is unlikely. Most deficits seen in masticatory proprioceptive-motor function, therefore, are due to

middle cranial fossa or more central lesions.

The cranial nerves supplying the *extra-ocular muscles* are the *oculomotor* (III), the *trochlear* (IV), and the *abducens* (VI), which traverse the cavernous sinus in close association with the trigeminal ganglion and enter the orbit through the *superior orbital fissure* (Table 1-1). The *oculomotor nerve* branches into superior and inferior divisions before passing through the fissure and is well protected from direct orbital trauma. The *abducens nerve,* because it courses in the lateral orbit and terminates in the *lateral rectus muscle,* can potentially be damaged in a severe lateral orbital comminution. However, direct trauma to these nerves is relatively uncommon. More often, traumatic ophthalmoplegia caused by III, IV, and VI nerve dysfunction is seen transiently as a result of pressure ischemia in the region of the superior orbital fissure that has resulted from intraorbital edema or hematoma.

The motor root of the trigeminal (V) emergences from the pons, passes as a distinct trunk ventral to the trigeminal ganglion in the middle cranial fossa, and exits through foramen ovale as part of the *mandibular division of V.* The nerve immediately divides into five named branches to eight different muscles (Fig. 1-11). The *medial pterygoid nerve* branches first, penetrating the dorsomedial attachment of the muscle and also sending branches to the adjacent *tensor veli palatini muscle* and through the cartilaginous auditory tube to reach the *tensor tympani muscle.* The *masseteric nerve* passes laterally above the lateral pterygoid muscle, penetrates the fascia of the *mandibular notch* with the *masseteric artery,* and innervates the deep surface of masseter near its attachments to the zygomatic arch. The *deep temporal nerves,* usually two in number, course on the infratemporal surface of the cranium upward over the infratemporal crest and finally reach the deep bellies of the temporalis muscle. The *nerve to the lateral pterygoid muscle* is a small terminal branch that may be combined with the sensory *buccal nerve* before entering the

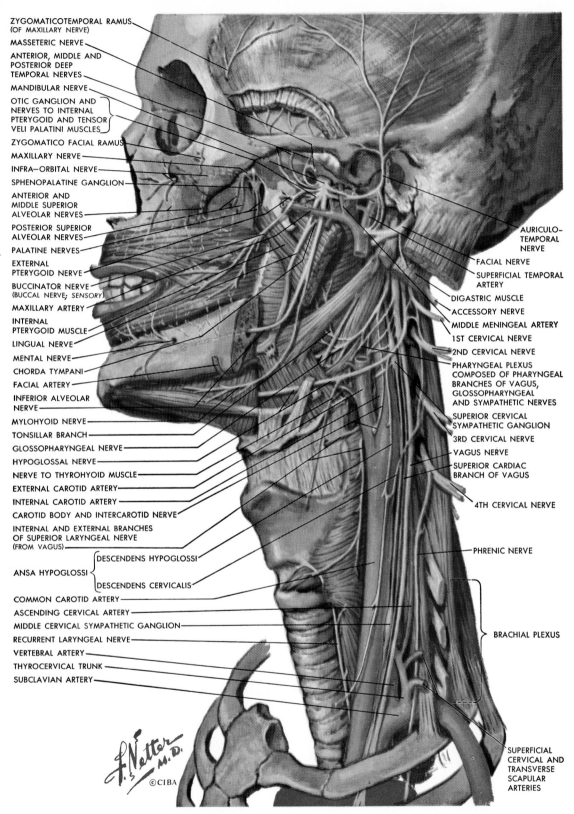

ZYGOMATICOTEMPORAL RAMUS
(OF MAXILLARY NERVE)

MASSETERIC NERVE

ANTERIOR, MIDDLE AND
POSTERIOR DEEP
TEMPORAL NERVES

MANDIBULAR NERVE

OTIC GANGLION AND
NERVES TO INTERNAL
PTERYGOID AND TENSOR
VELI PALATINI MUSCLES

ZYGOMATICO FACIAL RAMUS

MAXILLARY NERVE

INFRA-ORBITAL NERVE

SPHENOPALATINE GANGLION

ANTERIOR AND
MIDDLE SUPERIOR
ALVEOLAR NERVES

POSTERIOR SUPERIOR
ALVEOLAR NERVES

PALATINE NERVES

EXTERNAL
PTERYGOID NERVE

BUCCINATOR NERVE
(BUCCAL NERVE; SENSORY)

MAXILLARY ARTERY

INTERNAL
PTERYGOID MUSCLE

LINGUAL NERVE

MENTAL NERVE

CHORDA TYMPANI

FACIAL ARTERY

INFERIOR ALVEOLAR
NERVE

MYLOHYOID NERVE

TONSILLAR BRANCH

GLOSSOPHARYNGEAL NERVE

HYPOGLOSSAL NERVE

NERVE TO THYROHYOID MUSCLE

EXTERNAL CAROTID ARTERY

INTERNAL CAROTID ARTERY

CAROTID BODY AND INTERCAROTID NERVE

INTERNAL AND EXTERNAL BRANCHES
OF SUPERIOR LARYNGEAL NERVE
(FROM VAGUS)

ANSA HYPOGLOSSI {
DESCENDENS HYPOGLOSSI
DESCENDENS CERVICALIS

COMMON CAROTID ARTERY

ASCENDING CERVICAL ARTERY

MIDDLE CERVICAL SYMPATHETIC GANGLION

RECURRENT LARYNGEAL NERVE

VERTEBRAL ARTERY

THYROCERVICAL TRUNK

SUBCLAVIAN ARTERY

AURICULO-
TEMPORAL
NERVE

FACIAL NERVE

SUPERFICIAL TEMPORAL
ARTERY

DIGASTRIC MUSCLE

ACCESSORY NERVE

MIDDLE MENINGEAL ARTERY

1ST CERVICAL NERVE

2ND CERVICAL NERVE

PHARYNGEAL PLEXUS
COMPOSED OF PHARYNGEAL
BRANCHES OF VAGUS,
GLOSSOPHARYNGEAL
AND SYMPATHETIC NERVES

SUPERIOR CERVICAL
SYMPATHETIC GANGLION

3RD CERVICAL NERVE

VAGUS NERVE

SUPERIOR CARDIAC
BRANCH OF VAGUS

4TH CERVICAL NERVE

PHRENIC NERVE

BRACHIAL PLEXUS

SUPERFICIAL
CERVICAL AND
TRANSVERSE
SCAPULAR
ARTERIES

Fig. 1-11. Nerve supply of mouth and pharynx. (© Copyright 1959, CIBA-GEIGY Corporation. Reproduced with permission. All rights reserved.)

deep aspect of the muscle. The *mylohyoid nerve* is the final motor trigeminal branch that diverges from its association with the inferior alveolar nerve above the level of the mandibular foramen, descends in its own groove on the medial aspect of the mandible, and innervates the deep side of the *mylohyoid muscle* beneath the *submandibular gland*. It also branches at this point to supply the anterior belly of the *digastric muscle*. Although damage to these nerves may occur, especially to the *masseteric nerve* during condylar surgery and the *mylohyoid-digastric* branches during floor of the mouth surgery, they tend to be well protected by entering the muscle masses on their deep sides, and permanent surgery-induced paresis or paralysis of the masticatory muscles is rare.

The motor root of the *facial nerve* (VII) emerges from the pons, enters the *internal acoustic meatus*, then runs a looping course through the *facial canal* to exit from the *stylomastoid foramen* behind the earlobe. Within the facial canal the nerve is especially vulnerable to compression from edema or bleeding, which will produce a hemifacial palsy of the muscles of facial expression. Just after exiting from the stylomastoid foramen the facial nerve gives off the *posterior auricular* branch and branches to the *stylohyoid* and *posterior digastric muscles*. Behind the angle of the mandible the facial nerve trunk immediately enters the substance of the *parotid gland* where it typically divides just below the tragus of the ear into equal parts: the *temporofacial* and *cervicofacial divisions*. These two divisions diverge and run nearly vertically at the posterior border of the mandible, then turn more horizontally to surround the *isthmus* between the deep and superficial lobes of the parotid gland. Surgery on the parotid gland or the posterior mandible requires careful retraction of the facial nerve, but because of the intertwining of nerve and gland, it is best to identify the nerve either proximal or distal to the parotid capsule. Within the gland the two major divisions intercommunicate and then emerge from the gland as five named branches: *temporal, zygomatic, buccal, mandibular,* and cer-

vical (Fig. 1-2). The *temporal branches* course with the *superficial temporal artery* and supply the *auricular, frontalis,* and eyebrow *corrugator* muscles and, along with the *zygomatic branches*, the *orbicularis oculi* muscle. If these fibers are cut, regeneration is usually satisfactory, but there is an interim risk of damage to the cornea because of the inability to forcefully close the eyelids. The *buccal branches* course parallel to the *parotid duct* and supply the *buccinator, orbicularis oris,* and smaller perioral muscles. The *mandibular branches* run parallel with the lower border of the mandible and one sub-branch, the *marginal mandibular nerve*, loops below the inferior border 20% of the time and then recrosses the mandible in direct association with the *facial artery and vein*. Dissections in the region of the inferior mandibular border for trauma repair or orthognathic surgery must be done by layers in order to identify these neurovascular structures that lie beneath the platysma muscle and embedded within the *superficial lamina of the deep cervical fascia*.

The *glossopharyngeal nerve* (IX) gives motor supply to the *stylopharyngeus* muscle and contributes a few fibers to the *vagus nerve* (X) somatic efferent component to make up the *pharyngeal plexus*, which supplies the *tensor veli palatini, palatopharyngeus,* and all the *pharyngeal constrictor muscles* from their deep aspect (Fig. 1-14).

The *hypoglossal nerve* (XII) runs a deep looping course after exiting the *hypoglossal canal* in the base of the skull and finally enters the oral cavity slightly above the *posterior digastric* tendon at the posterior border of the mylohyoid muscle. The nerve courses with the *sublingual vein* on the superomedial surface of mylohyoid, then fans out to innervate all of the muscles of the tongue. The nerve is a potential hazard in posterior floor of the mouth, salivary gland, and duct dissections and should be protected by retracting the tongue mass medially.

SENSORY NERVES OF THE MAXILLOFACIAL REGION

Sensory functions of the head and neck consist of general somatic senses that include tactile discrimination and heat-pain sense (nociception), position sense (proprioception), and the special senses of vision, hearing, smell, and taste (Crosby, Humphrey, and Lauer, 1962). The general somatic functions are served mainly by the trigeminal nerve complex with minor contributions in the lateral face from sensory branches of VII, IX, X, and the upper cervical spinal segments. The primary cell bodies are located in *sensory ganglia*, the *trigeminal* or *semilunar* (V), *geniculate* (VII), *petrosal* (IX), and the *jugular* (X), which lie in bony crypts adjacent to the brain stem. There are no synapses in these ganglia and their cells send off two processes: a peripheral process, which exits through a bony foramen and terminates in the sensory receptor, and a central sensory root fiber, which penetrates the brain stem and collects into the *spinal tract of* V before ending in synapses in the *chief sensory nucleus of* V for touch senses and in the *spinal tract nucleus* of V for the more crude tactile and pain senses. All of the general somatic afferent fibers from the head and neck converge on the distal portions of the spinal tract of V before synapsing, which may explain some of the patterns of referred pain that characterize many facial disorders.

The *trigeminal ganglion* is ensheathed in a sleeve of dura and rests in *Meckel's cave*, a depression in the floor of the middle cranial fossa. The small *trigeminal motor root* passes through the ventral part of the ganglion where it mingles with fibers of the mandibular division of V. Although the ganglion is well-protected from facial trauma in this position, it is surrounded by vascular structures that may have great pathologic influence. A variable number of *emissary veins* that originate in the *pterygoid venous plexus* in the infratemporal fossa pass through various foramina to surround the ganglion and terminate in the dural venous sinuses, primarily the *cavernous sinus*. Infections in the infratemporal fossa may spread along these venous routes intracranially to produce a trigeminal neuritis. Similar spread of local anesthetics can induce major sensory changes by acting on the periganglionic emissary plexus. The ganglion may be even more directly affected by arteries that lie near it. The *internal carotid artery* arches through the floor of the middle cranial fossa just below and medial to the ganglion. Branches of the *superior cerebellar artery* loop against the superior aspect of the ganglion and sensory root. Pathologic aging changes in these vessels that cause degeneration of the trigeminal neural tissues may be a causative factor in paroxysmal facial pain syndromes.

Three peripheral nerve divisions branch from the trigeminal ganglion: the ophthalmic (V_1), maxillary (V_2), and mandibular (V_3). The peripheral sensory trigeminal nerves arise in receptor plexuses that are among the densest of any body region. The peripheral fibers span from very small C and A delta fibers, which range in size from 1 to 4 microns in diameter and serve crude touch, heat, and pain senses, to large, heavily myelinated fibers of 8 to 18 microns in diameter, which mediate fine tactile and proprioceptive senses (Bosma, 1970). Local anesthetics applied to these fibers will often produce a complete block of the smaller fibers while the larger fiber functions are maintained.

The *mandibular division of the trigeminal* (V_3) exits from the sphenoid bone through the *foramen ovale* at approximately a 45 degree downward and forward direction. Once free of the foramen ovale, it gives off the small *meningeal nerve* branch that reenters the cranium through the *foramen spinosum* to innervate the dura. The *auriculotemporal nerve* arises next from the mandibular nerve as two roots that encircle the middle meningeal artery, then reunite to pass posteriorly between the *sphenomandibular ligament* and the *capsule* of the *temporomandibular joint* (Figs. 1-11 and 1-12). Sensory fibers are given off to the capsule and the main nerve continues laterally through the upper *parotid gland* and over the zygomatic arch to terminate in the skin in the region of the external ear and the temporal scalp. Preauricular surgical approaches to the mandibular condyle or neck will routinely expose the terminal

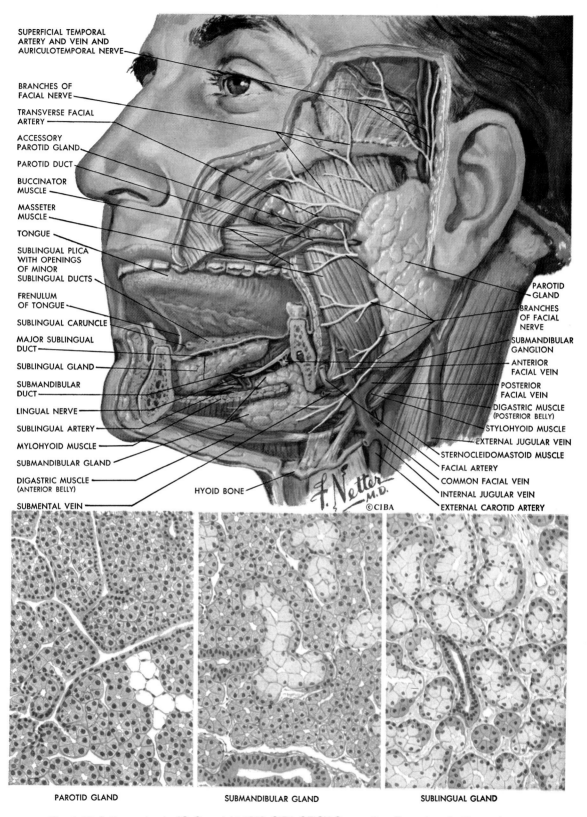

SUPERFICIAL TEMPORAL ARTERY AND VEIN AND AURICULOTEMPORAL NERVE

BRANCHES OF FACIAL NERVE

TRANSVERSE FACIAL ARTERY

ACCESSORY PAROTID GLAND

PAROTID DUCT

BUCCINATOR MUSCLE

MASSETER MUSCLE

TONGUE

SUBLINGUAL PLICA WITH OPENINGS OF MINOR SUBLINGUAL DUCTS

FRENULUM OF TONGUE

SUBLINGUAL CARUNCLE

MAJOR SUBLINGUAL DUCT

SUBLINGUAL GLAND

SUBMANDIBULAR DUCT

LINGUAL NERVE

SUBLINGUAL ARTERY

MYLOHYOID MUSCLE

SUBMANDIBULAR GLAND

DIGASTRIC MUSCLE (ANTERIOR BELLY)

SUBMENTAL VEIN

HYOID BONE

PAROTID GLAND

BRANCHES OF FACIAL NERVE

SUBMANDIBULAR GANGLION

ANTERIOR FACIAL VEIN

POSTERIOR FACIAL VEIN

DIGASTRIC MUSCLE (POSTERIOR BELLY)

STYLOHYOID MUSCLE

EXTERNAL JUGULAR VEIN

STERNOCLEIDOMASTOID MUSCLE

FACIAL ARTERY

COMMON FACIAL VEIN

INTERNAL JUGULAR VEIN

EXTERNAL CAROTID ARTERY

F. Netter M.D.
©CIBA

PAROTID GLAND

SUBMANDIBULAR GLAND

SUBLINGUAL GLAND

Fig. 1-12. Salivary glands. (© Copyright 1959, CIBA-GEIGY Corporation. Reproduced with permission. All rights reserved.)

auriculotemporal nerve trunk as it courses in a common sheath with the *superficial temporal artery.*

The *buccal nerve* branches near the auriculotemporal nerve but diverges anteriorly to follow the tendon of the temporalis muscle and cross lateral to the external oblique line of the mandible to reach the skin overlying the buccinator muscle. Some of the buccal branches innervate the skin while others penetrate the muscle to supply the mucosa of the mandibular vestibule and lateral gingiva. Although the buccal nerve branches intermingle with the motor VII nerve fibers to the buccinator muscle, the buccal nerve is strictly sensory, and local anes-

thetic blocks to it will not impair muscle function.

Another major mandibular branch, the *lingual nerve,* arises medial to the lateral pterygoid muscle and descends medially in the pterygomandibular space. It penetrates the fibers of the *superior pharyngeal constrictor muscle* just below the terminus of the *mylohyoid ridge* where it enters the *paralingual space.* In the floor of the mouth the lingual nerve courses from lateral to medial, crossing below the *submandibular duct* as it ascends from the submandibular space. The nerve usually crosses the duct at approximately the first molar level and is a helpful point of orientation during floor of the

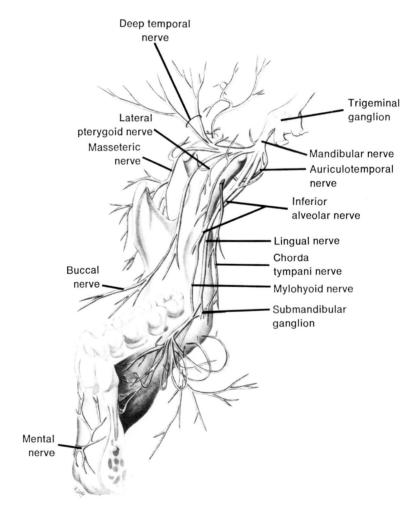

Fig. 1-13. Mandibular division of trigeminal nerve.

mouth surgery such as gland extirpation, vestibuloplasty, and sialolithotomy (Fig. 1-9).

The main branch of the mandibular division is the *inferior alveolar nerve,* which courses directly downward in the lateral pterygomandibular space and enters the ramus of the mandible through the *mandibular foramen* just lateral to the *lingula* and the attachment of the *sphenomandibular ligament.* The point of nerve entry into the mandibular foramen is important as the site of inferior alveolar block anesthesia and for orientation during orthognathic surgery. Within the mandible, the inferior alveolar nerve courses in its own canal from medial to lateral in the third molar area. As it enters the body of the mandible, it remains lateral beneath the apices of the teeth. Most of its fibers exit from the *mental foramen* in the apical region of the second premolar as the *mental nerve,* which terminates in the lateral vestibule, gingiva, and the entire thickness of the lower lip and chin.

The mandibular division is overlapped by several other cranial sensory nerves. The external auditory meatus is innervated by the auriculotemporal nerve as well as branches of the facial and glossopharyngeal nerves. At the angle of the mandible there is overlapping between V_3 and the *great auricular* nerve (C_2, C_3); this may be significant in attaining anesthesia for surgery in the third molar region (Fig. 1-13) (Woodburne, 1975).

The *maxillary division of* V exits through the *foramen rotundum* directly forward and almost immediately enters the *pterygopalatine fossa* where its three main branches, the *zygomatic, pterygopalatine trunk,* and *infraorbital nerves,* are given off (Fig. 1-14). The thin *zygomatico-orbital nerve* passes directly through the *inferior orbital fissure,* then usually divides into two branches, the *zygomaticotemporal* and the *zygomaticofacial* nerves, both of which run anteriorly on the lateral and inferior wall of the orbit. They reenter the zygomatic

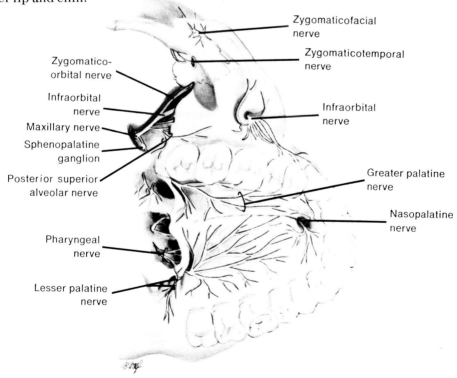

Fig. 1-14. Maxillary division of trigeminal nerve.

bone through variable zygomatico-orbital and -facial foramina, then finally re-emerge on the lateral face, the zygomatico-temporal fibers terminating in the skin of the anterior temporal region, and the zygomaticofacial fibers supplying the skin over the prominence of the cheek (Fig. 1-2). Trauma to the zygomatic bone and orbit may damage these sensory nerves and also induce changes in tearing, since communicating autonomic nerves to the *lacrimal gland* travel via the zygomatic nerves.

The second branches of the maxillary division are the two pterygopalatine trunks, which descend in the pterygopalatine fossa, become attached to the *sphenopalatine ganglion,* and then give off a series of palatine and nasal nerves. The *greater palatine nerve* descends in the *greater palatine canal* with the *descending palatine artery* and emerges onto the posterior hard palate through the anteromedially directed *greater palatine foramen.* The nerve runs anteriorly in the lateral palate, supplying the mucosa and gingiva as far as the incisive papilla region where some of its terminal fibers communicate with the *nasopalatine nerve. Lesser palatine nerve* branches descend with the greater palatine nerve but diverge posteriorly as they near the palate and emerge through the *lesser palatine foramina* to distribute to the *soft palate* and *palatine tonsil.* An anesthetic may be injected through a needle passed up the descending palatine canal to produce a nearly total block of the maxillary division.

The *posterior superior lateral nasal* branches pass medially through the *sphenopalatine foramen* and distribute in part to the posterior ethmoidal and middle concha mucosa. The main trunk continues to arc over the roof of the nasal fossa to reach the nasal septum as the *nasopalatine nerve.* The nasopalatine nerve courses obliquely downward on the vomerine septum to terminate through the *incisive foramen* in the anterior palate, gingiva, and occasionally the pulps of the incisor teeth.

The direct continuation of the maxillary division is the *infraorbital nerve,* which passes through the inferior orbital fissure and then enters the *infraorbital canal* along with the *infraorbital artery.* Just before entering the orbit, the *posterior superior alveolar nerve* is given off inferiorly. It swings laterally out of the pterygopalatine fossa and inferiorly around the maxillary tuberosity, which is penetrated by most of the nerve's fibers, and finally distributes to the posterior molar teeth and vestibular mucosa. The *middle superior alveolar nerve* is variable in size, number of branches, and course. It is usually given off within the posterior infraorbital canal, courses through thin canals in the lateral wall of the maxillary sinus, and sends terminal fibers to the sinus membrane, premolar teeth, and adjacent gingiva. The larger *anterior superior alveolar nerve* diverges from the infraorbital nerve just before it emerges from the infraorbital canal and then descends in the anterior wall of the maxillary sinus before innervating the canine and incisor teeth and adjacent gingiva. The terminal branches of the infraorbital nerve distribute as *lateral nasal fibers* and *superior labial fibers* to the entire substance of the lip. Anesthetic injections into the infraorbital canal can be expected to block the *anterior superior alveolar* and *infraorbital nerves.*

Overlap of the maxillary division by the *ophthalmic division* of V is minimal. The ophthalmic division is also entirely sensory, enters the orbit through the *superior orbital fissure,* and quickly gives off the *lacrimal nerve,* which supplies the upper lateral eyelid, skin, and conjunctiva; the *frontal nerve,* which branches as the *supraorbital* and *supratrochlear nerves* through fissures to supply the skin above the orbit; and the *nasociliary nerve* branches, which supply sensory fibers to the eyeball, conjunctiva, and much of the ethmoidal mucosa. These nerves are rarely damaged directly by surgery or trauma because of their deep origin, but they may undergo transient degenerative response to ischemia caused by hematoma and edema pressures exerted at the superior orbital fissure (Kronsclenabel, 1974).

The special visceral sense of smell is

mediated by the filamentous *olfactory nerve* (I) receptors, which penetrate the *cribriform plate* in the *sphenoethmoidal recess*. The olfactory cells are relatively sparse in man, numbering fewer than 20,000, and since the bipolar receptor neurons are located on the roof of the cribriform plate, in direct connection with the *olfactory bulb*, smell functions are especially vulnerable to permanent disruption when this plate is badly comminuted in facial trauma (Rowe and Killey, 1968).

Taste functions are primarily mediated by the *chorda tympani branch of VII* for the anterior two thirds of the tongue, the *glossopharyngeal nerve* (IX) for the posterior one third of the tongue, and the *superior laryngeal* branch of the *vagus* nerve (X) for the epiglottic and glottic taste receptors. The *chorda tympani nerve*, carrying visceral efferent fibers to the salivary glands as well as its taste afferent fibers, takes origin in the petrous portion of temporal bone, passes through the *petrotympanic fissure*, courses medial to the trigeminal nerve and ganglion, and exits the skull into the infratemporal fossa where it joins the *lingual nerve*. The chorda tympani maintains a loose association with the lingual nerve throughout its terminal course, and surgical injuries to the lingual nerve will usually also involve the chorda tympani. Regeneration of such injuries may be faulty as cross-innervations between general somatic lingual fibers become mixed with special visceral chorda tympani fibers (Crosby, Humphrey, and Lauer, 1962).

AUTONOMIC NERVE SUPPLY TO THE MAXILLOFACIAL REGION

The main autonomic functions of the maxillofacial region are salivation, lacrimation, ocular accommodation, and peripheral vascular and sweat control. The autonomic nervous system, like the general somatic motor system, has a higher central nervous system control and a peripheral effector system. Central regulatory nuclei are located mainly in the hypothalamus and send fiber tracts to cranial nerve nuclei and spinal cord nuclei,

which make up the origins of the peripheral autonomic system (Crosby, Humphrey and Lauer, 1962). The peripheral autonomic neurons are organized as two parallel divisions, the *sympathetic* and *parasympathetic*, both of which are two-neuron circuits with a first neuron (preganglionic) arising in the central nervous system and the second arising in a peripheral ganglion (Table 1-2).

Preganglionic sympathetic neurons arise in the *intermediolateral gray* columns of spinal cord segments T_1 to T_3, emerge with the ventral roots to take short courses to synapse in the *middle and superior cervical chain ganglia*, which are lodged in the medial fascia of the *carotid sheath*. Postganglionic fibers emerge from these ganglia and become enmeshed in the adventitia of the carotid arteries, which they follow as the *internal and external carotid sympathetic plexuses*. Most of the sympathetic nerves to maxillofacial tissues are terminal branches of the external carotid subplexuses, although two notable contributions are made from the internal carotid plexus: the *deep petrosal* and *ciliary nerves*. The *deep petrosal nerve* arises from the internal carotid plexus and passes through the middle cranial fossa and into the pterygoid canal to become, with parasympathetic fibers, part of the *nerve of the pterygoid canal*. Sympathetic fibers then pass into the *pterygopalatine fossa* where they join the maxillary (V_2) nerve branches to supply the nasal mucosa, soft palate, palatine glands, and pulps of the upper teeth. The ciliary nerve arises in part from the cavernous sinus sympathetic plexus and passes into the orbit and completely through the ciliary ganglion to terminate mainly in the dilator pupillae muscle of the eye. Trauma or surgical lesions to either the cervical sympathetic trunk or to branches from the internal carotid plexus that enter the orbit will result in *Horner's syndrome*, the predominant features of which are miosis (pupillary constriction), partial ptosis, and ipsilateral vasodilation and anhidrosis.

The *preganglionic parasympathetic neurons* for the maxillofacial region arise

Table 1-2. Autonomic nervous system units of the maxillofacial region

Preganglionic cells	Preganglionic nerves	Peripheral ganglia	Postganglionic nerves	Organ functions
Intermediolateral gray column, T_1 to T_3	T_1 to T_3, sympathetic chain	Superior cervical ganglion	External carotid plexus, internal carotid plexus (deep petrosal nerve to nerve of pterygoid canal)	Vascular smooth muscles, sweat glands, mucous salivary glands, dilator pupillae muscle
Edinger-Westfall nucleus (midbrain)	Oculomotor nerve (III)	Ciliary, episcleral ganglia	Short ciliary nerves	Ciliary and sphincter pupillae
Superior salivatory nucleus (pons-medulla)	Nervous intermedius (VII) branches (greater petrosal; nerve of pterygoid canal)	Sphenopalatine ganglion	With maxillary nerve distribution	Nasal, palatine, and lacrimal glands
Superior salivatory nucleus (pons-medulla)	Nervous intermedius (VII) branches (chorda tympani with lingual nerve)	Submandibular, diffuse submandibular ganglia	With lingual nerve distribution	Submandibular and sublingual salivary glands
Inferior salivatory nucleus (medulla)	Glossopharyngeal nerve (IX) branches (tympani, lesser petrosal)	Otic ganglion	With auriculotemporal nerve distribution	Parotid salivary gland

in a column of separate nuclei in the brain stem and send out roots that become components of cranial nerves III, VII, and IX (Table 1-2). The postganglionic neurons for these nerves are located in the *ciliary* (III), *episcleral* (III), *submandibular* (VII), *sphenopalatine* (VII), and *otic* (IX) ganglia. Oculomotor preganglionic neurons arise in the midbrain, course directly from the midbrain as part of the *ciliary nerve*, and synapse in part in the *ciliary ganglion*, which is located on top of the eyeball between the optic nerve and lateral rectus muscle. Other of the fibers pass through to synapse in the *episcleral ganglion* on the surface of the sclera. Postganglionic fibers from these ganglia distribute to the *ciliary muscles* for altering the lens diameter and to the dilator pupillae muscles of the iris. All of the autonomic nerves that enter the orbit through the superior orbital fissure are important in normal light reflexes and ocular accommodation.

Parasympathetic fibers of nerve VII arise in the pons and branch as two nerves: the *greater superficial petrosal* and the *chorda tympani*. The *greater superficial petrosal* nerve branches in the internal acoustic meatus, passes beneath the trigeminal ganglion, and enters the pterygoid canal along with deep petrosal sympathetic fibers. The parasympathetic fibers continue to the *sphenopalatine ganglion* within the *pterygopalatine fossa* where they synapse. The postganglionic fibers distribute with the maxillary nerve sensory fibers to the nasal and palatal mucosa, palatine glands, and lacrimal gland. The *chorda tympani nerve* arises from nerve VII within the facial canal and loops back through the middle ear and out of the cranium through the *petrotympanic fissure* behind the mandibular condyle where it joins the *lingual nerve sheath*. At the posterior border of the mylohyoid muscle some of the fibers of the chorda tympani synapse in the *submandibular ganglion*, whose postganglionic fibers then rejoin the lingual nerve to distribute to the *sublingual gland*. Other chorda tympani fibers enter the substance of the submandibular gland where they synapse within the *diffuse plexus* (of

Langley) and innervate the gland. Surgical lesions of the chorda tympani nerve are commonly associated with lingual nerve damage and produce the clinical pattern of diminished serous salivary flow and absent taste senses on the anterior two thirds of the tongue on that side.

The *lesser superficial petrosal nerve* arises as part of the *glossopharyngeal nerve* (IX) in the medulla, is joined by branches of nerve VII while in the petrous portion of the temporal bone, and eventually leaves the cranial cavity through a variable sphenoid foramen to terminate in the *otic ganglion*. The latter lies medial to the mandibular nerve trunk, and its postganglionic fibers quickly join and distribute with the *auriculotemporal nerve* to the *parotid gland*, vascular smooth muscles, and sweat glands over the lateral face. Because of the intermingling of sensory, sweat, and salivatory fibers, auriculotemporal nerves regenerating from surgical transection may undergo functional transposition and result in *gustatory sweating*, a condition in which fibers originally destined for the parotid gland terminals have relocated in sweat gland effectors.

SALIVARY GLANDS

Three major salivary glands, the *parotid, submandibular,* and *sublingual,* function mainly as exocrine organs, with the parotid fluids being mainly serous, the sublingual fluids being mainly mucous, and the submandibular fluids being mixed (Sicher and Dubrul, 1975). The rate and type of secretion are controlled by the dual *sympathetic* and *parasympathetic* innervation. A series of *minor salivary glands* populate the submucosa of the lips, hard and soft palate, buccal pouch, retromolar trigone, tonsillar pillar, and the ventral apex of the tongue. The minor glands secrete a thick mucin and are of little surgical significance except when their short ductal systems become traumatized and salivary retention cysts form. By contrast, the parotid and submandibular glands have long, superficial ducts that predispose the glands to chronic adenitis and ductal obstructions.

The *parotid gland* is the largest; it is triangular and wedges into the retromandibular fossa (Fig. 1-2). It has a deep and superficial lobe connected by an isthmus that marks the level of the temporofacial and cervicofacial divisions of the facial nerve as they enter the gland. An inferior (cervical) lobe extends into the concavity between the angle of the mandible and the sternocleidomastoid muscle and may be a surgical hazard during dissections to the mandible using the submandibular (Risdon) approach. The gland extends anteriorly onto the masseter muscle, and accessory lobes may be found along the course of the *parotid (Stensen's) duct*. The parotid duct typically runs about 1 cm below and parallel to the zygomatic arch, turns medially around the anterior margin of the masseter, and penetrates the buccinator muscle and oral mucosa adjacent to the maxillary second molar tooth. The duct may be severed during trauma, and it is important that the cut ends be identified and sutured or that a new ductal exit be made intraorally to avoid a retention cyst or a salivary fistula. The *parotid capsule* is the upward extension of the superficial lamina of the deep cervical fascia and is very firmly attached by numerous intraglandular septae, which make clean extirpation of parts of the salivary gland a tedious process. The *external carotid artery, retromandibular vein,* and *facial nerve* are embedded at certain loci within the parotid gland or capsule and present obvious hazards to the surgeon.

The *submandibular gland* is a round, bilobed gland with a main body that lies posterior in the submandibular triangle on the outer surface of the hyoglossus muscle and a lesser lobe that is folded around the free border of the mylohyoid muscle. The *submandibular (Wharton's) duct* runs a folded course around the mylohyoid, and mucous retention plugs and sialoliths are especially likely to occur at this location. The duct continues forward in the floor of the mouth to be joined by smaller sublingual ducts and terminates near the anterior midline in the *sublingual caruncle*. The lingual nerve is a hazard during glandular or ductal surgery because it loops from above laterally, then medially around the submandibular duct. The glandular capsule is distinct and loosely attached, making extirpation of the gland relatively easy. The *facial artery* enters a groove on the inferomedial surface of the gland, gives off *sublingual* branches within the gland capsule, and exits again at the inferior border of the mandible. In cases of hemorrhage it is advisable to ligate the facial artery either before it enters the gland or after it emerges at the mandibular border.

The *sublingual gland* is actually a series of thinly encapsulated glands. Its main body is long and flattened and lies within the sublingual fossa of the mandible. In addition, there are five to fifteen lesser glands that are scattered anteriorly lying on the mylohyoid fibers. The major *sublingual (Bartholin's) duct* arises posteriorly and usually joins the submandibular duct anteriorly. Other lesser ducts (Rivini) also join the main duct or individually perforate the mucosa in the crest of the *sublingual fold*. This complex duct arrangement and the superficial location of the glands make them vulnerable to damage, which may result in the formation of mucous extravasation cysts that occasionally greatly distend the thin overlying mucosa to form ranulas.

VASCULATURE OF
THE MAXILLOFACIAL REGION
Arteries

The arterial supply to the head and neck is remarkable in its richness when compared to other body regions (Castelli and Huelke, 1965). The major branches overlap, collateralize, and even cross the midline, especially in the nasal and pharyngeal regions. Vestigial channels from the internal carotid system also have the potential to open into the external carotid distribution. This rich vascularity affords increased opportunity for grafting or creation of soft tissue pedicles and also accounts for the great powers of repair and resistance to infection seen in these tissues. However, the risk of hemorrhage is also greater and arteriovenous anomalies appear unpredictably throughout the region and may create life-threatening situations (Rappaport and Yim, 1973).

The primary arterial supply to the maxillofacial structures comes from the *external carotid artery,* which arises from the common carotid trunk under cover of the anterior border of the sternocleidomastoid muscle at the general level of the superior border of the *thyroid cartilage* (Fig. 1-15). The external carotid artery may be ligated at this point to control hemorrhage by retracting the sternocleidomastoid muscle posteriorly, separating the artery from the internal jugular vein in the carotid sheath, and tying it off above the first branch, the *superior thyroid artery.* An alternative external carotid ligation can be accomplished higher behind the angle of the mandible deep to the reflected parotid tail. However, neither type of external carotid ligation will assure a dry field in the ipsilateral maxillofacial tissues because of the rapid takeover of collateral channels from the contralateral external carotid and vestigial internal carotid arteries.

Eight major branches are given off from the external carotid: the anteriorly branching *superior thyroid, lingual,* and *facial arteries;* the posteriorly coursing *occipital* and *posterior auricular* arteries; the medial branching *ascending pharyngeal* and terminal arteries; and the *superficial temporal* and *maxillary* arteries (Figs. 1-15 and 1-16).

The *lingual artery* branches at the level of the greater horn of the *hyoid bone,* sometimes in common with the *facial artery (linguofacial trunk).* It courses forward horizontally into the submandibular triangle deep to the hyoid attachments of the posterior digastric belly and the hyoglossus muscle and parallels the hypoglossal nerve and its accompanying vein that lie on the outside of the hypoglossus. This is the target area for ligation of the lingual artery because distal to this point it turns deeper and superiorly over the free border of the *mylohyoid muscle* to enter the floor of the mouth. In the posterior mylohyoid region a *dorsal lingual* branch supplies the base of the tongue and anterior tonsillar pillar, and the large *sublingual artery* is given off from the main artery and terminates medially in the deep muscular plexus of the tongue.

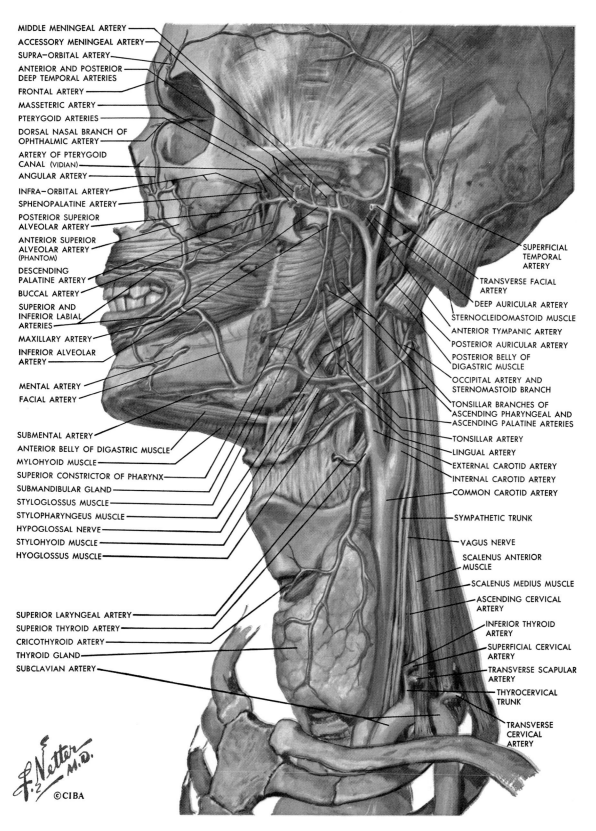

MIDDLE MENINGEAL ARTERY

ACCESSORY MENINGEAL ARTERY

SUPRA-ORBITAL ARTERY

ANTERIOR AND POSTERIOR DEEP TEMPORAL ARTERIES

FRONTAL ARTERY

MASSETERIC ARTERY

PTERYGOID ARTERIES

DORSAL NASAL BRANCH OF OPHTHALMIC ARTERY

ARTERY OF PTERYGOID CANAL (VIDIAN)

ANGULAR ARTERY

INFRA-ORBITAL ARTERY

SPHENOPALATINE ARTERY

POSTERIOR SUPERIOR ALVEOLAR ARTERY

ANTERIOR SUPERIOR ALVEOLAR ARTERY (PHANTOM)

DESCENDING PALATINE ARTERY

BUCCAL ARTERY

SUPERIOR AND INFERIOR LABIAL ARTERIES

MAXILLARY ARTERY

INFERIOR ALVEOLAR ARTERY

MENTAL ARTERY

FACIAL ARTERY

SUBMENTAL ARTERY

ANTERIOR BELLY OF DIGASTRIC MUSCLE

MYLOHYOID MUSCLE

SUPERIOR CONSTRICTOR OF PHARYNX

SUBMANDIBULAR GLAND

STYLOGLOSSUS MUSCLE

STYLOPHARYNGEUS MUSCLE

HYPOGLOSSAL NERVE

STYLOHYOID MUSCLE

HYOGLOSSUS MUSCLE

SUPERIOR LARYNGEAL ARTERY

SUPERIOR THYROID ARTERY

CRICOTHYROID ARTERY

THYROID GLAND

SUBCLAVIAN ARTERY

SUPERFICIAL TEMPORAL ARTERY

TRANSVERSE FACIAL ARTERY

DEEP AURICULAR ARTERY

STERNOCLEIDOMASTOID MUSCLE

ANTERIOR TYMPANIC ARTERY

POSTERIOR AURICULAR ARTERY

POSTERIOR BELLY OF DIGASTRIC MUSCLE

OCCIPITAL ARTERY AND STERNOMASTOID BRANCH

TONSILLAR BRANCHES OF ASCENDING PHARYNGEAL AND ASCENDING PALATINE ARTERIES

TONSILLAR ARTERY

LINGUAL ARTERY

EXTERNAL CAROTID ARTERY

INTERNAL CAROTID ARTERY

COMMON CAROTID ARTERY

SYMPATHETIC TRUNK

VAGUS NERVE

SCALENUS ANTERIOR MUSCLE

SCALENUS MEDIUS MUSCLE

ASCENDING CERVICAL ARTERY

INFERIOR THYROID ARTERY

SUPERFICIAL CERVICAL ARTERY

TRANSVERSE SCAPULAR ARTERY

THYROCERVICAL TRUNK

TRANSVERSE CERVICAL ARTERY

Fig. 1-15. Arterial supply of mouth and pharynx. (© Copyright 1959, CIBA-GEIGY Corporation. Reproduced with permission. All rights reserved.)

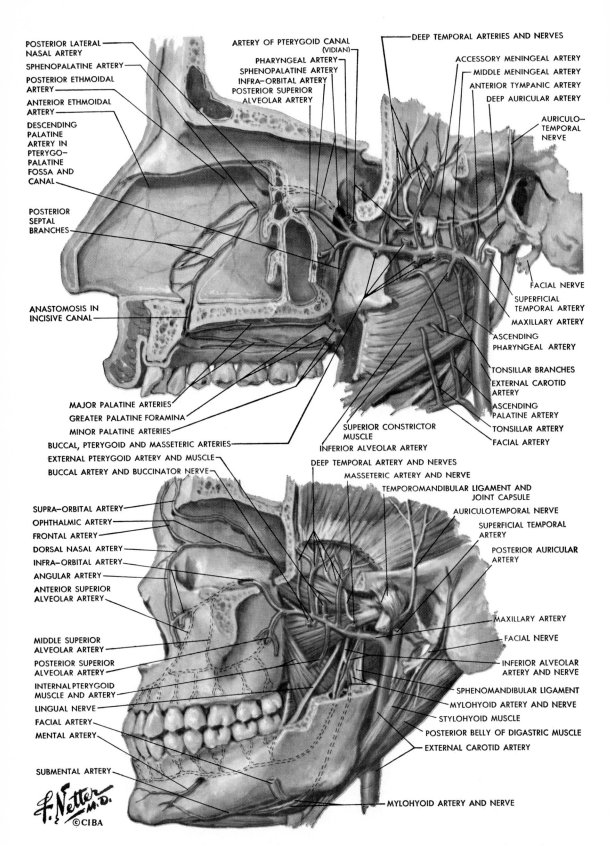

Fig. 1-16. Arterial supply of mouth and pharnyx. (© Copyright 1959, CIBA-GEIGY Corporation. Reproduced with permission. All rights reserved.)

The *sublingual artery* courses forward next to the hypoglossal nerve (XII), then parallels the medial aspect of the sublingual gland and submandibular duct that it supplies. The *submental artery*, a terminal branch of the *facial artery*, runs a parallel course with the *sublingual artery* but on the deep side of the mylohyoid muscle. These two vessels penetrate the muscle and anastomose at a number of points. Therefore it is often necessary to check the flow from both sublingual and submental vessels to control hemorrhage in the floor of the mouth.

The *facial artery* arises just beneath the posterior belly of the digastric muscle, gives off *ascending palatine branches*, and then crosses diagonally into the submandibular triangle superficial to the styloglossus and hyoglossus muscles under cover of the *submandibular gland*. Proximal ligation of the facial artery must be accomplished along this course because the artery next penetrates a notch in the deep aspect of the *submandibular gland* and gives off *glandular* and *submental arteries*. The main trunk swings superficially from the upper border of the gland to cross onto the lateral mandible just in front of the masseter muscle insertion. At this point it is paralleled in a common sheath by the *facial vein*. Both vessels follow a diagonal course within the facial muscles. The first branches on the face are the *inferior* and *superior labial arteries*, which lie close to the free mucocutaneous junction of the lips within the orbicularis oris muscle and anastomose across the midline. The main artery gives off the *lateral nasal artery*, some of whose branches anastomose within the *infraorbital canal* and finally terminate in the *angular artery* in anastomosis with branches of the *ophthalmic artery*.

All of the facial artery branches are loose and tortuous because of their relationship to the highly mobile facial muscles. Interruption of the facial artery flow by injury or during surgery is usually not significant since its zone of supply is rapidly taken over by *transverse facial artery* branches and also the *buccal, infraorbital*, and *sphenopalatine* branches of the *maxillary* artery.

After giving off its cervical branches,

the main external carotid trunk runs a straight vertical course behind the mandible where it lies next to the *retromandibular vein* on the outer surface of the *stylomandibular diaphragm* and in the deep capsule of the *parotid gland*. The *transverse facial artery* is a small and variable branch that emerges from behind the *mandibular neck* to cross on the surface of the masseter muscle parallel to the *parotid duct*. Beneath this point the external carotid artery divides into its terminal branches, the *maxillary* and the *superficial temporal arteries*.

The *maxillary artery* is the largest external carotid branch and is classically described in reference to three anatomic regions, the *mandibular, pterygoid*, and *pterygopalatine portions* (Fig. 1-12). The first, (mandibular) portion courses horizontally between the neck of the condyloid process and the *sphenomandibular ligament* adjacent to the *auriculotemporal* nerve. While still within the parotid fascia it gives off the *deep auricular* and *anterior tympanic arteries*. The *middle meningeal* artery passes upward from the maxillary trunk superficial to the sphenomandibular ligament and enters the middle cranial fossa through the *foramen spinosum*. The *inferior alveolar artery* also arises from the mandibular portion of the maxillary artery and descends in the pterygomandibular space, giving off a *lingual branch* near its origin and a *mylohyoid branch* just before it enters the *mandibular foramen* accompanied by the *inferior alveolar nerve* and *vein*. In the mandibular canal the artery distributes in the same manner as the nerve and also terminates as the *mental artery* in anastomosis with the inferior labial artery. The mandibular division of the maxillary artery and its branches are vulnerable during surgical procedures such as condylectomy or transoral osteotomies of the ascending ramus. In addition to the potential for significant hemorrhage, there may also be interference with trigeminal sensory and visceral motor functions in the parotid and lateral facial region because of the close relationships of maxillary artery branches with the *auriculotemporal nerve* and the *otic ganglion*.

The second (pterygoid) portion of the

maxillary artery passes upward and forward through the infratemporal fossa and gives off the muscular branches: masseteric, anterior and posterior deep temporal, pterygoid, and buccal arteries. Each of these distribute parallel to the named motor branches of the trigeminal nerve and generally enters the muscles on their deep aspect. The *masseteric artery* passes through the *mandibular notch* and may be damaged by joint injections or during coronoidectomy. The *buccal artery,* although small, is often cut by intraoral incisions along the anterior coronoid crest because the artery swings anteriorly around the crest to penetrate and supply the buccinator muscle.

The terminal *(pterygopalatine)* portion of the maxillary artery provides branches to the maxilla, maxillary teeth, nasal cavity, and palate. Its six branches, the posterior superior alveolar, infraorbital, descending palatine, artery of the pterygoid canal, pharyngeal, and sphenopalatine arteries, all distribute in company with the previously described branches of the *maxillary nerve.* The *posterior superior alveolar* artery enters the *pterygopalatine fossa* and descends laterally on the back of the maxillary tuberosity where needles used to inject local anesthetics may puncture it causing a rapid swelling of the cheek and buccal vestibule. The *infraorbital artery* is the direct continuation of the maxillary artery trunk and passes into the orbit through the inferior orbital fissure. Within the *infraorbital groove and canal* it gives off *anterior* and *middle superior alveolar* branches to supply the maxillary sinus, alveolus, and teeth and then terminates on the face in communication with the facial artery branches. The *descending palatine artery* passes vertically down in the descending palatine canal, divides into *greater* and *lesser* branches, and supplies the mucosa of the hard and soft palate as well as the palatine tonsil. The greater palatine artery courses anteriorly on the palate to anastomose in the incisive canal with the *sphenopalatine artery.* The sphenopalatine artery courses into the nasal cavity in company with the *nasopalatine nerves* and supplies the lateral

nasal wall and adjacent sinuses and then passes diagonally forward in a groove in the vomer to supply the nasal septum and much of the premaxillary palate. In cases of bilateral cleft lip and palate, the sphenopalatine supply often assumes extra responsiblity for perfusing the incisor teeth, bone of the premaxilla, upper lip, and external nasal tip. Corrective surgery must be planned accordingly (Hayward, 1974). The entire pterygopalatine portion of the maxillary artery becomes important during maxillary orthognathic surgery such as the Le Forte I osteotomy procedure. The success of this procedure relies on the preservation of some of these branches, particularly the sphenopalatine and descending palatine, yet there is potential for their damage as the maxilla is disarticulated from the pterygoid plates and the nasal septum is horizontally sectioned during the procedure (Nelson et al., 1977).

The *superficial temporal artery* is the terminal direct continuation of the external carotid artery beyond the retromandibular fossa. It gives off *articular* branches to the temporomandibular joint capsule, then emerges from the capsule of the *parotid gland* to cross the root of the zygomatic arch and divide into *parietal* and *frontal branches.* The parietal and frontal branches are superficial and tortuous and terminate over the scalp and above the eye in anastomoses with the *supraorbital, posterior auricular,* and *occipital* arteries. During the preauricular approach to condylar surgery, the superficial temporal trunk is identified along with the accompanying *auriculotemporal nerve* and retracted or tied.

Veins

The veins of the maxillofacial region serve certain unique functions in addition to return of deoxygenated blood to the heart via the *superior vena cava.* They are designed to cushion the associated arteries from the compressing movements of the jaws and pharynx and therefore are organized as *periarterial plexuses* throughout much of the region. They also protect against excessive intracranial pressure by permitting bidirectional flow between deep *maxillary veins* and *intracranial venous sinuses.* To accomplish this, the cranial veins have few if any valves, a design that unfortunately allows pathoses such as blood-borne bacterial emboli or cancer cells to spread more easily. It may also account for the uncontrollable bleeding that may come from arteriovenous anomalies in the jaws (Rappaport and Yim, 1973).

The *internal jugular vein* is the largest channel of the head and neck, beginning at the *jugular foramen* as a continuation of the *sigmoid dural sinus.* It runs a straight course in the carotid sheath and terminates behind the clavicular attachments of the sternocleidomastoid muscle in the *brachiocephalic vein.* Its main tributaries from superior to inferior are the inferior petrosal sinus and the lingual, vena comitans hypoglossus, pharyngeal, facial, and superior and middle thyroid veins.

The *facial venous* terminal is quite variable, however, and its flow may be more superficial, to the *external jugular vein* (Fig. 1-17). It originates in the *angular vein* on the side of the nose where important anastomoses with the *infraorbital* and *superior ophthalmic veins* occur. Blood-borne infections in the nose or maxillary teeth have been known to spread from the *angular* vein to the *superior ophthalmic* vein, backward through the medial orbit and *superior orbital fissure* to the *inferior ophthalmic vein,* and finally into the cavernous sinus. Bacterial emboli in the cavernous sinus may cause life-threatening thromboses and meningitis (Evans, 1965; Limongelli, Clark, and Williams, 1977).

The *facial vein* also has anastomoses to the deep face via the *infraorbital vein* and the *deep facial vein,* which course from the facial trunk at the corner of the mouth between the *buccinator* and *masseter muscles* to reach the *pterygoid plexus* of veins in the infratemporal fossa. This vein is a very common source of bleeding following oral surgery that involves the posterior vestibule lateral to the mandible.

The terminus of the facial vein is variable. After crossing the inferior border of

the mandible in company with the *facial artery* and the *marginal mandibular branch* of the *facial (VII) nerve,* it winds superficially through the *submandibular gland* capsule, then terminates in either the *internal jugular* or a *communicating vein* to the external jugular in the posterior submandibular triangle.

The remainder of the maxillofacial tissues are drained by two other plexuses, the *external jugular* and *anterior jugular* systems. Both of these are superficial and visible in the neck just below the fibers of the *platysma muscle.* The *external jugular* is usually formed at the level of the mandibular angle by the junction of the *retromandibular* and *posterior auricular veins.* The trunk runs diagonally over the *sternocleidomastoid muscle* and is eventually joined in the *supraclavicular fossa* by a variable communicating branch of the *anterior jugular vein* before terminating in the *subclavian vein.* The *retromandibular vein* parallels the posterior border of the mandible and receives the *superficial temporal* and *maxillary veins.* The *maxillary vein* empties behind the neck of the condyloid process in a common sheath with the *maxillary artery.* But unlike the precisely named branches of the artery, the maxillary vein is formed from the large and very dense *pterygoid plexus,* which envelops the artery throughout its course in the infratemporal fossa on the lateral surface of the *medial pterygoid muscle* and completely surrounds the *lateral pterygoid muscle.* The *pterygoid plexus* drains all of the masticatory muscles as well as the pterygopalatine, middle meningeal, and articular regions. A number of important *emissary veins* course between the pterygoid plexus and the cranial *dural sinuses,* usually passing through foramina with the cranial nerves. Hematomas or intravascular injections occur on occasion in the pterygoid plexus region, and maxillary infections that spread into the infratemporal fossa may use the emissary veins to spread further centrally.

The *anterior jugular veins* usually arise in the submental region, have some anastomoses with the external or internal jugular systems in the submandibular trian

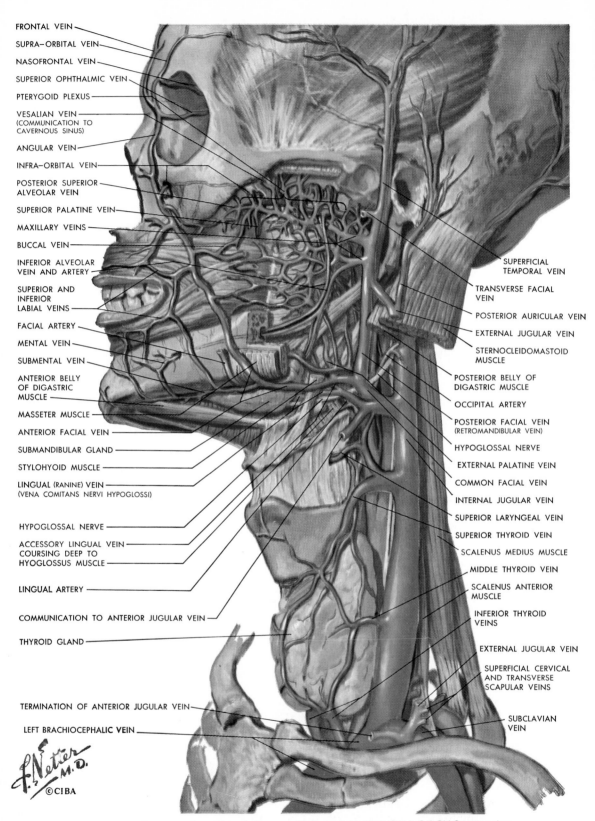

FRONTAL VEIN

SUPRA-ORBITAL VEIN

NASOFRONTAL VEIN

SUPERIOR OPHTHALMIC VEIN

PTERYGOID PLEXUS

VESALIAN VEIN
(COMMUNICATION TO
CAVERNOUS SINUS)

ANGULAR VEIN

INFRA-ORBITAL VEIN

POSTERIOR SUPERIOR
ALVEOLAR VEIN

SUPERIOR PALATINE VEIN

MAXILLARY VEINS

BUCCAL VEIN

INFERIOR ALVEOLAR
VEIN AND ARTERY

SUPERIOR AND
INFERIOR
LABIAL VEINS

FACIAL ARTERY

MENTAL VEIN

SUBMENTAL VEIN

ANTERIOR BELLY
OF DIGASTRIC
MUSCLE

MASSETER MUSCLE

ANTERIOR FACIAL VEIN

SUBMANDIBULAR GLAND

STYLOHYOID MUSCLE

LINGUAL (RANINE) VEIN
(VENA COMITANS NERVI HYPOGLOSSI)

HYPOGLOSSAL NERVE

ACCESSORY LINGUAL VEIN
COURSING DEEP TO
HYOGLOSSUS MUSCLE

LINGUAL ARTERY

COMMUNICATION TO ANTERIOR JUGULAR VEIN

THYROID GLAND

TERMINATION OF ANTERIOR JUGULAR VEIN

LEFT BRACHIOCEPHALIC VEIN

SUPERFICIAL
TEMPORAL VEIN

TRANSVERSE FACIAL
VEIN

POSTERIOR AURICULAR VEIN

EXTERNAL JUGULAR VEIN

STERNOCLEIDOMASTOID
MUSCLE

POSTERIOR BELLY OF
DIGASTRIC MUSCLE

OCCIPITAL ARTERY

POSTERIOR FACIAL VEIN
(RETROMANDIBULAR VEIN)

HYPOGLOSSAL NERVE

EXTERNAL PALATINE VEIN

COMMON FACIAL VEIN

INTERNAL JUGULAR VEIN

SUPERIOR LARYNGEAL VEIN

SUPERIOR THYROID VEIN

SCALENUS MEDIUS MUSCLE

MIDDLE THYROID VEIN

SCALENUS ANTERIOR
MUSCLE

INFERIOR THYROID
VEINS

EXTERNAL JUGULAR VEIN

SUPERFICIAL CERVICAL
AND TRANSVERSE
SCAPULAR VEINS

SUBCLAVIAN
VEIN

Fig. 1-17. Venous drainage of mouth and pharynx. (© Copyright 1959, CIBA-GEIGY Corporation.
Reproduced with permission. All rights reserved.)

gle region, and then course down toward the suprasternal notch. These veins are highly variable and frequently cross the midline where they may pose a minor problem during emergency airway surgery at the level of the *cricothyroid membrane.*

Lymphatics

The *lymphatic vessels* of the maxillofacial region, as elsewhere in the body, accompany blood vessels and as such are divided into deep and superficial node and channel systems. As a general rule, lymph vessels that take origin close to the midline often cross to the opposite side, particularly in areas such as the lips, tongue, and palate. Overlap between deep and superficial drainage systems is also seen at midoral depths. Therefore the posterior hard palate, buccal mucosa, premolar region of both jaws, and posterior part of the anterior tongue are marginal zones that drain both anteriorly to superficial plexuses and posteriorly to deep node groups. These lymphatic drainage patterns are of considerable surgical importance because spreading infections and malignant tumors tend to be propagated along the lymphatics. Knowledge of normal anatomy is necessary for proper diagnosis and therapy.

A series of *lymphatic organs* occupy the pharynx and are known collectively as the *lymphatic ring of Waldeyer.* They consist of the *pharyngeal, tubal, palatine, and lingual tonsils.* The *pharyngeal tonsils* (adenoids) occupy the entire breadth of the posterior pharyngeal wall between the *cartilaginous auditory tube* openings. They are continuous with the *tubal tonsils* at the openings of the tubes and tend to atrophy with age. The palatine tonsils are ovoid, clefted, and encapsulated masses that lie bilaterally between the arches of the *palatoglossal* and *palatopharyngeal folds.* They are continuous medially onto the base of the tongue with the *lingual tonsils,* which are occasionally mistaken for malignant tumors, especially in the region directly behind the foramen cecum.

The *deep cervical plexus* of lymphatic channels is the final common pathway for all head and neck drainage, terminating in the *thoracic duct* on the left and the junction of *internal jugular* and *subclavian veins* on the right. Its superior portion occupies the carotid triangle and generally lies lateral and posterior to the internal jugular vein. Four prominent node groups, the retropharyngeal, deep parotid, jugulodigastric and jugulo-omohyoid nodes, are part of the deep cervical chain. The *retropharyngeal nodes* are scattered at the superior end of the *carotid sheath* and in the *retropharyngeal space.* They drain the posterior nasal fossae, paranasal sinuses, and hard and soft palate and therefore are diagnostically inaccessible channels of "silent" metastasis for malignant lesions in these posterior tissues. The *deep parotid* nodes lie in the deep capsule of the *parotid gland* and in the adjacent *lateral pharyngeal space* and drain the external acoustic meatus, tympanic membrane, and lateral soft palate. A large node grouping, the *jugulodigastric,* is located anterior to the internal jugular vein just below the angle of the mandible where the posterior belly of the digastric muscle crosses. This important group drains the base of the tongue and palatine tonsillar fossa. It also receives some drainage from the superficial submandibular nodes before it continues deep along the internal jugular chain. All of the deep jugular drainage passes to the *jugulo-omohyoid nodes* along with some separate anastomoses from the superficial nodes in the submental and tongue tip regions. The *jugulo-omohyoid nodes* finally empty into the *supraclavicular* nodes, which together are important as the so-called sentinel cervical nodes for detecting metastatic lesions that have arisen above (Sicher and DuBrul, 1975).

The superficial nodes of the head are the occipital, retroauricular, anterior auricular, superficial parotid, and facial nodes. The *anterior auricular nodes* lie just anterior to the tragus and drain into the more numerous *superficial parotid* nodes within the superficial parotid capsule. These nodes drain the external ear, external acoustic meatus, temporofrontal skin and temporomandibular joint, eyelids, cheek, and nose and then pass deep toward the jugulodigastric complex. The *facial nodes* lie along the course of the facial arteries and veins and tend to cluster as infraorbital, corner of mouth (buccal), and lateral mandibular groups. Most of this drainage goes to *submandibular nodes*, but lateral and deep drainage to the *superficial parotid* plexus allows alternate escape of fluid and cells. Pressure dressings placed following maxillofacial surgery should avoid closing off both avenues of lymphatic drainage from the face.

In the neck, superficial lymphatic drainage proceeds through the submental, submandibular, external jugular, and anterior jugular node groups. The *submental* nodes lie superficial to the mylohyoid muscle between the anterior digastric muscle bellies and receive drainage from the anterior skin, lower lip, cheek, anterior gingiva, anterior teeth, and tip of the tongue. These nodes drain either to the *submandibular nodes* or directly down the *anterior jugular* channels. The submandibular nodes lie within the superficial capsule of the submandibular gland and distribute to both deep and superficial channels. The *external jugular* nodal chain lies on the sternocleidomastoid muscle and accumulates drainage from the submandibular and parotid plexuses. Finally, the *anterior jugular* chain is highly asymmetric and drains the submental complex above. It is usually palpable on either side of the *thyroid* and *cricoid cartilages* and as far inferiorly as the *suprasternal notch* where the channels turn laterally and deep to terminate in the inferior deep internal jugular lymphatic trunk. Metastatic lesions from the tip of the tongue and anterior floor of the mouth usually propagate along the anterior or external jugular plexuses, but because of the variability in drainage in the carotid triangle, these metastases may spread deep into the internal jugular system.

REFERENCES

Bell, W. H., et al. 1975. Bone healing and revascularization after total maxillary osteotomy, J. Oral Surg. 33:253.

Bell, W. H., and Kennedy, J. W. 1976. Biological basis for vertical ramus osteotomies—a study of bone healing and revascularization in adult rhesus monkeys, J. Oral Surg. 34:215.

Bosma, J. A., ed. 1970. Oral sensation and perception; second symposium, Springfield, Ill., Charles C Thomas, Publisher.

Castelli, W. A., and Huelke, D. F. 1965. The arterial system of the head and neck of the rhesus monkey with emphasis on the external carotid system, Am. J. Anat. 116: 149.

Choukas, N. C., and Sicher, H. 1960. The structure of the temporomandibular joint, J. Oral Surg. 13: 1203.

Crosby, E. C., Humphrey, T., and Lauer, E. W. 1962. Correlative anatomy of the nervous system, New York, MacMillan Inc.

Dingman, R. O., and Natvig, P. 1964. Surgery of facial fractures, Philadelphia, W. B. Saunders Co.

Evans, H. W. 1965. Cavernous sinus thrombosis, Lancet 85: 109,

Freedus, M. S., Ziter, W. D., and Doyle, P. K. 1975. Principles of treatment for temporomandibular joint ankylosis, J. Oral Surg. 33:757.

Granite, E. L. 1976. Anatomic considerations in infections of the face and neck: review of the literature, J. Oral Surg. 34: 34.

Hayward, J. R. 1974. In Kruger, G. D. Textbook of oral surgery, St. Louis, The C. V. Mosby Co.

Irby, W. B. 1977. Current advances in oral surgery, St. Louis, The C. V. Mosby Co.

Kallal, R. H., Gans, B. J., and Lagrotteria, L. B. 1977. Cranial dislocation of mandibular condyle, Oral Surg. 43: 2.

Kelsey, C. C. 1968. Radiographic cephalometric study of surgical corrected mandibular prognathism, 1975. J. Oral Surg. 26:239.

Kreutziger, K. L., and Mahan, P. E. 1975. Temporomandibular degenerative joint disease: anatomy, pathophysiology, and clinical description, J. Oral Surg. 40:165.

Kronsclenabel, E. F. 1974. Orbital apex syndrome due to sinus infection, Laryngoscope 84:353.

Kruger, G. D. 1974. Textbook of oral surgery, ed. 5, St. Louis, The C. V. Mosby Co.

Limongelli, W. A., Clark, M. S., and Williams, A. C. 1977. Panfacial cellulitis with contralateral orbital cellulitis and blindness after tooth extraction, J. Oral Surg. 35:38.

Moss, M. L., and Rankow, R. 1968. The role of the functional matrix in mandibular growth, Angle Orthod. 39:95.

Nelson, R. L., et al. 1977. Quantitation of blood flow after LeFort I osteotomy, J. Oral Surg. 35:10.

Path, M. G., et al. 1977. Blood flow changes after sagittal split of the mandibular ramus, J. Oral Surg. 35:98.

Rappaport, I., and Yim, D. 1973. Congenital arteriovenous fistulas of the head and neck, Arch. Otolaryngol. 97:350.

Rowe, N. L., and Killey, H. C. 1968. Fractures of the facial skeleton, ed. 2., Baltimore, The Williams & Wilkins Co.

Schmid, F. 1969. On the nerve distribution of the temporomandibular joint capsule, J. Oral Surg. 28:63.

Sicher, H., and DuBrul, E.L. 1975. Oral anatomy, ed. 6, St. Louis, The C. V. Mosby Co.

Siegel, M. I. 1974. The role of the cartilaginous nasal septum in mid-facial growth, Am. J. Phys. Anthropol. **41:**503.

Sorensen, D. C., and Laskin, D. M. 1975. Facial growth after condylectomy or ostectomy in the mandibular ramus, J. Oral Surg. **33:**746.

Steinhauser, E. W. 1973. Advancement of the mandible by sagittal ramus split and suprahyoid myotomy, J. Oral Surg. **31:**516.

Wickwire, N. A., White, R. P., Jr., and Proffit, W. R. The effect of mandibular osteotomy on tongue position, J. Oral Surg. **30:**184.

Woodburne, T. T. 1975. Essentials of human anatomy, ed. 5, New York, Oxford University Press, Inc.

CHAPTER 2

Surgical embryology

John M. Gregg

The human face and jaws do not result, as was thought, from a simple enlargement of a miniature preformed man ("homunculus") contained within the sperm cell. Nor do they appear in a single gradual precipitation like a photographic print. As a product of millions of years of evolution, the human maxillofacial region develops through a dynamic series of tissue divisions, expansions, migrations, fusions, and involutions. Adult human anatomy, variations from normal, and gross congenital malformations are better understood and dealt with surgically when the dynamics of this embryology are known. For example, the manner in which the facial nerve fans across the lower lateral face to innervate the facial muscles becomes more clear when it is known that facial muscles have migrated into the face embryologically from the lateral neck, carrying their innervation with them. The surgeon is also better able to predict patterns of collateral blood supply to a given region and deal more effectively with vascular malformations when it is known that at a critical stage of development the maxillofacial tissues are served by both extracranial and intracranial vessels. Benign congenital anomalies such as median rhomboid glossitis are more easily recognized and distinguished from pathoses when it is known that the midbase of the tongue in the embryo, known as the tuberculum impar, is a normal structure that usually invaginates deep to the lateral branchial arch tongue masses in the seventh week of embryogenesis. The management of facial clefts is also im-

proved when the surgeon understands how midfacial development depends on a crucially timed fusion of processes with different origins and growth vectors.

GENERAL EMBRYOLOGY

The prenatal development of the head and neck organizes naturally into three successive periods: *predifferentiation,* *embryonic,* and *fetal* (Langman, 1975). The predifferentiation period begins with ovulation, fertilization, and implantation, followed by rapid cell division and the formation by the end of the first week of a fluid-filled sphere of cells called the *blastula.* Next, through continued cell cleavage and a migration of cells from the outer surface inward, a bilayered and finally trilayered organism forms by the middle of the third week. These three *germ layers,* named ectoderm, mesoderm, and entoderm, form the origins of all adult tissues. From them, the primitive body plan takes shape, and the stage is set for the critical 4 to 8 weeks ahead, when major organ systems will emerge.

In terms of relevance to craniofacial malformations, the predifferentiation period is of little significance. Despite the fact that a very high natural rate of abnormality, estimated at greater than 33%, is suspected during the predifferentiation phase (Hertig, 1967), abnormal blastulas usually fail to implant. There is no recognizable face or neck yet, and either teratogens that act during this time damage so many cells that death occurs, or embryonic cells are capable of adapt-

50

ing completely and no permanent malformation will be seen at birth.

It is the crucial embryonic period of 4 to 8 weeks development when the primitive three-layered body plan is remolded, the human facial masses take shape, and the adult organ systems are produced. It is also at this time that the embryo is most vulnerable to teratogenic factors and when most of the known malformations seen at birth have their origin. During this period great migrations of tissues are seen flowing ventrally into the facial region from vital areas such as the dorsal neural crest, and the major organ systems are seen to emerge sequentially (Johnston, Bhakdinaronk, and Reid, 1974). Although most teratogens acting during embryogenesis have the potential to affect many organ systems simultaneously to produce the common multisystem anomaly syndromes, in most cases a single predominant organ system is affected. Each organ system seems to progress through its own most crucial period of development independent of other systems and therefore has a specific time when it is most vulnerable to teratogens. The general progression of system susceptibility is central nervous, heart, skeletal, urinary, peripheral, and vascular (Langman, 1975). At the same time that the internal systems are undergoing their crucial changes, the external masses are likewise passing through progressive phases. In general, external facial form progresses dorsal to ventral, cephalo-caudal, and superficial to deep.

The fetal period of development, 3 to 9 months gestation, is characterized by maturation and growth of all systems and relatively little differentiation. Only late and slow-developing organ systems such as the cerebral cortex, cerebellum, and urogenital system are still differentiating during this period. Therefore malformations that arise during the fetal period of development usually do not threaten life or produce major agenesis syndromes. Rather, the malformations tend to be distortions of basically established systems. An example of a deformity produced in the fetal period is the mandibular micrognathia component of the Pierre Robin

syndrome, which appears to be a result of intrauterine space restrictions (Poswillo, 1966).

EXTERNAL FORM

The human embryo of 4 weeks has no discernible face or neck, and the cranium is clearly divisible into two parts: a *neurocranium* containing the brain and eventually the associated sense organs and a *viscerocranium* containing upper alimentary and respiratory structures and eventually the face and jaws. Throughout the embryonic and early fetal period the neurocranium is vastly larger than the viscerocranium, and even at birth there is a ratio of 8 to 1 as compared with the eventual 2.5 to 1 relationship of the adult (Enlow, 1975). At birth the cranial vault volume is 65% complete and the orbital diameters are 75% complete.

The general plan of the face arises in the fourth week from two widely separated origins: a midline downward expansion from the *frontal process* and a medial ingrowth of a series of barlike ridges that appear on the ventrolateral surface of the head, called the *pharyngeal* or *branchial arches* (Fig. 2-1). The mouth and associated internal structures also form from combinations of both frontal and branchiomeric tissues as well as outgrowths from the primitive gut. In the earliest embryogenesis the future orofacial structures are paired saclike swellings in the ventral midline that are generally separated from one another by epithelial linings (Fig. 2-2). In the intermediate stages of 5 to 9 weeks of embryogenesis these linings break down as the facial processes merge to form the definitive orofacial structures. In the later fetal stages of development the main growth additions are made laterally and in the anteroposterior dimensions of the viscerocranium.

Branchial arch (branchiomeric) derivatives

Early in the fourth week a series of five barlike ridges appear laterally on the head. At the same levels the entodermal lining of the pharynx bulges out to unite with the surface ectoderm, thereby form-

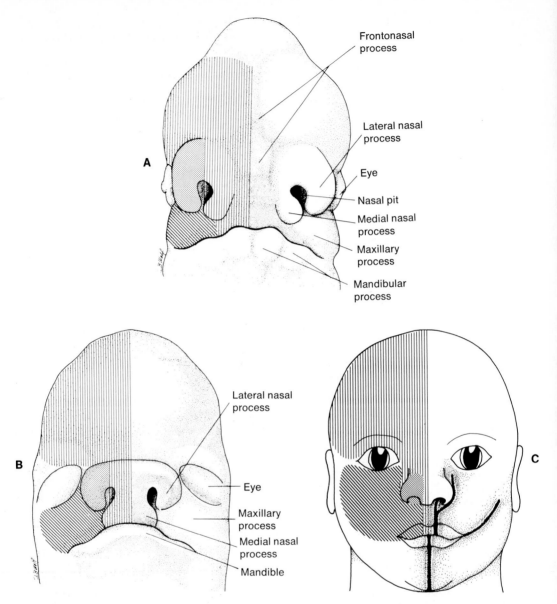

Fig. 2-1. External facial form development at **A,** 5½ weeks; **B,** 7½ weeks; and **C,** birth, showing possible lines of clefting. Major facial processes are seen as frontonasal (vertical lines), lateral nasal (dots), maxillary process (diagonal lines).

ing a series of epithelial plates or grooves that separate the branchial arches. The branchial arches correspond to the gill arches of fishes and some amphibians but are never destined to function as such. Instead the arches expand or bifurcate, then fuse, and in the process obliterate the epithelial linings of the branchial grooves. Cell migrations occur rapidly within the matrix of the branchial arches. In particular, *neural crest cells*, which originate lateral to the dorsal neural tube, flow ventromedially and on reaching the midline, interact with local available mesenchyme to initiate the development of tissue and organ systems within each

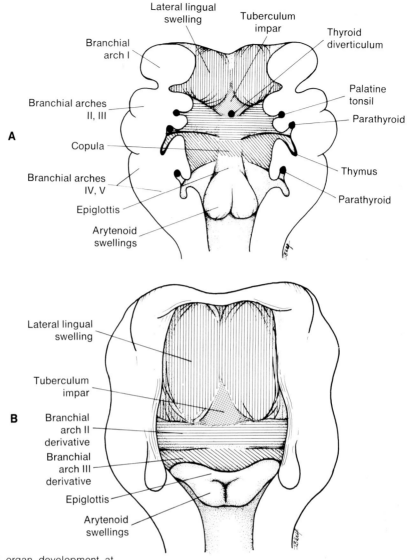

Lateral lingual swelling

Branchial arch I

Branchial arches II, III

Copula

Branchial arches IV, V

Epiglottis

Arytenoid swellings

Tuberculum impar

Thyroid diverticulum

Palatine tonsil

Parathyroid

Thymus

Parathyroid

A

Lateral lingual swelling

Tuberculum impar

Branchial arch II derivative

Branchial arch III derivative

Epiglottis

Arytenoid swellings

B

Fig. 2-2. Oropharyngeal organ development at **A,** 6 weeks; **B,** 8 weeks; and **C,** birth, showing tongue landmarks. Major derivatives are seen as lateral lingual swellings (vertical lines), tuberculum impar (dots), branchial arch II (horizontal lines), and branchial arch III (diagonal lines).

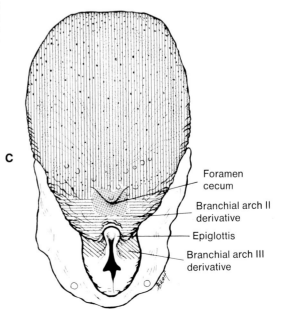

C

Foramen cecum

Branchial arch II derivative

Epiglottis

Branchial arch III derivative

arch (Poswillo, 1975; Pratt, Larsen, and Johnston, 1975).

Each branchial arch contains sets of arteries called aortic arches, nerves, muscles, either cartilage or bone, and glands that are specific to that arch and will persist in part as postnatal structures (Table 2-1). The first branchial arch, the *mandibular arch*, expands medially and fuses with its opposite arch in the fifth week. The mandibular member continues to differentiate forming a transient cartilaginous bar, *Meckel's cartilage*, and the primordia of the *mandible*, the masticatory muscles and their primitive neurovascular network, and the primordia of the body of the tongue, thyroid gland, external ear, and first two ossicles. At about this time budlike swellings are seen on the most lateral aspects of the mandibular arches, which are known as the *maxillary processes* (Fig. 2-1). The lateral *maxillozygomatic* process, *secondary palate*, and *maxillary sinus* will be derived from this process. The sinuses do not appear as outgrowths of nasal epithelium until about the fourth month and they remain as pea-sized chambers even at birth. The second branchial arch, or *hyoid arch*, and the third, fourth, and fifth branchial arches similarly expand lateral to medial to fuse in the midline and carry their specific vital structures with them.

Derivatives of the branchial arches and clefts (pouches) are:

First arch: maxilla, mandible, masticatory muscles, malleus and incus, trigeminal nerve, Rathke's pouch, thyroid diverticulum, anterior tongue and tuberculum impar, Meckel's cartilage, auricle of external ear, middle ear chamber, sphenomandibular ligament

First cleft: tympanic cavity, auditory tube

Second arch: hyoid bone, hyoid cartilages (lesser), stapes, hyoid muscles, muscles of facial expression, facial nerve, styloid process, Reichert's cartilage, tongue base

Second cleft: palatine tonsil

Third to fifth arches: tongue base, laryngeal cartilages, laryngeal muscles, hyoid cartilages (greater)

Third to fifth clefts: parathyroid glands I to IV, thymus, ultimobranchial bodies

Superiorly, in the prominent *frontal* region of the 4-week embryo, tissue masses are flowing ventrally and laterally to merge with the borders of the first branchial arch. An important series of bilateral thickenings called *placodes* are seen on the surface ectoderm at this stage. They include the *lens placode*, which marks the future site of the eyes; the *auditory placodes*, around which the ears will develop; and the *nasal placodes*, which will serve as a nidus for nasal development (Fig. 2-1). The lens placode responds to the internal stimulus of the evaginating forebrain optic fields by beginning differentiation of the lens and cornea. The eyes at this stage are set laterally on the head at an axis of 180 degrees to one another. Between 3 months and birth the head broadens mainly by additions to the lateral face, and little change is brought about in the interorbital distance. Consequently, the eyes and orbits undergo a relative convergence that positions the orbits anteriorly and permits human binocular vision. The eyes and orbits, similar to the brain, grow very precociously in the embryo and are three-fourths their final adult diameters at birth.

The auditory placode rapidly invaginates from its position just above and behind the first branchial cleft and forms the *auditory vesicle*, the forerunner of the inner ear. The tract left by the invagination process serves as a nidus around which the *external ear*, *middle ear*, and *tympanic membrane* develop from mandibular arch mesenchyme.

The *nasal placodes* at 5 weeks of age appear ventrolaterally in the frontal process surrounded by rapidly expanding horseshoe-shaped ridges called *nasal swellings* (Fig. 2-1). As the nasal swellings grow, the previous placode tissues sink into the future nose. The nasal pits and eventually the placodal membranes break down as the external nasal passages enlarge. The posterior floor of the nasal pit at this stage is a transient oronasal membrane that soon disintegrates to bring about a continuous oronasal cavity behind the forming external nares. Externally the nasal swellings are expanding rapidly with a *medial nasal limb* that merges with its contralateral medial limb at approximately 6 weeks. The fused medial nasal limbs will result in the formation of the nose midline, the philtrum of the lip, and the premaxillary portion of the anterior palate, including the maxillary incisor teeth. Meanwhile the *lateral nasal limbs* are forming the primordial nasal alae and undergoing fusion with the expanding maxillary processes along an oblique line that will form the eventual roof of the nasolacrimal ducts. Inferiorly the lateral nasal limb, maxillary process, and medial nasal limb fuse to complete the upper lip in the sixth week (Fig. 2-1). As was the case with the eyes and orbits, the nasolabial complex appears to move from lateral to medial in the facial mass during the later fetal stages of development owing to the greater growth additions to the lateral face.

The *embryonic mouth* appears in the fourth week in the junction area of the first branchial arch and the frontal process. It is seen as a blind ectoderm-lined sac, the *stomodeum*, which soon ruptures at the approximate level of the future *palatoglossal pharyngeal membrane* (anterior fauces) to establish continuity with the entodermally-lined foregut. Thus the future nasal passages, palate, front parts of the tongue, and oral vestibule are lined by surface ectoderm, and the palatine tonsil, root of the tongue, and cartilaginous auditory tube are lined by foregut entoderm.

The anterior two thirds of the tongue develops at 6 weeks from the right and left first (mandibular) arches where they join in the floor of the pharynx by the fusion of paired lateral *lingual swellings* and a midline swelling, the *tuberculum impar* (Fig. 2-2). The posterior two thirds of the tongue is derived from the lateral swellings of the second through the fourth branchial arches and midline masses, the *copula,* which also contribute to future formation of the *epiglottis.* As development proceeds, the thyroid gland, which arises in the groove be-

tween the copula and the tuberculum impar invaginates into the neck carrying the tuberculum impar with it and leaving a permanent midline depression at the point of the adult *foramen cecum.* In this region the embryonic boundary between first and second branchial arch structures can be seen clearly in the V-shaped adult *sulcus terminalis.* The *posterior palatal shelves* form from the medial aspect of each maxillary process and are situated vertically and pointing inferiorly on either side of the tongue, which at the sixth week occupies the entire oral cavity and nasal fossae (Fig. 2-3). Anteriorly and separated from the palatal shelves, the premaxillary segment of the medial nasal limb is seen attached at its base to the *nasal septum.* Between $6\frac{1}{2}$ and $7\frac{1}{2}$ weeks, dramatic changes in oral cavity size take place, the embryonic head and neck begin to move reflexly in extension-flexion, and a rapid growth and flowing movement is seen in the medial aspects of the palatal shelves. In a matter of a few hours the shelves flow laterally around the tongue to take up a horizontal position where they fuse in the midline and also anteriorly with the premaxillary (primary) palatal mass to form the adult pattern of separate oral and nasal chambers (Fig. 2-3).

Postnatal implications

The fact that the face, neck, and internal oral tissues do not develop from a single process but as a result of the crucially timed convergence of masses from greatly different origins sets the stage for postnatal anomalies along the lines of normal fusion. Orofacial clefting is a well-known abnormality; the most common form is the *secondary palatal cleft,* followed by *lip clefts* and *primary cleft palate* (Gorlin, Pindborg, and Cohen, 1976). The embryologic basis for these separations, of course, lies in the origin of the palatolabial structures from three separate tissue masses, the palatal shelves of the maxillary process, and the medial and lateral nasal limbs of the frontal process (Figs. 2-1 and 2-3). *Oblique facial clefts* may also appear along the embryonic fusion line of the lateral nasal limb and the

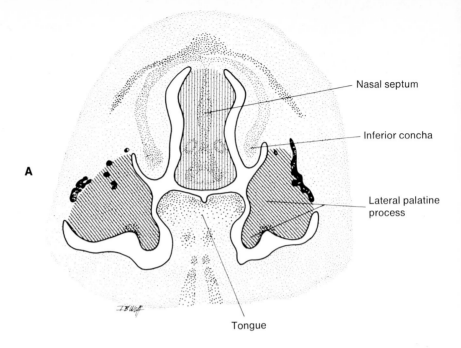

Nasal septum

Inferior concha

Lateral palatine process

A

Tongue

Fig. 2-3. Nasopalatal development at, **A,** 6½ weeks; **B,** 10 weeks; and, **C,** birth, showing lines of possible clefting.

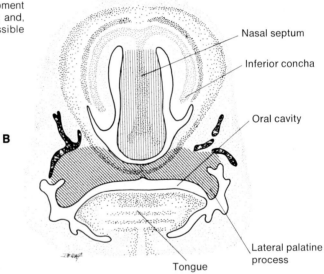

Nasal septum

Inferior concha

Oral cavity

B

Lateral palatine process

Tongue

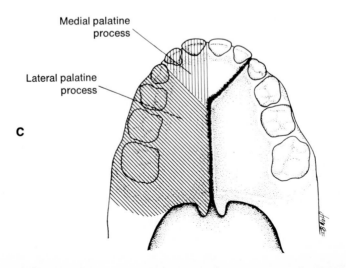

Medial palatine process

Lateral palatine process

C

superior maxillary process. *Midline clefts* of the nose, philtrum, and mandible are known to occur and reflect the very earliest stages of external facial development, but they are extremely rare. Congenital *macrostomia* may occur if the maxillary and mandibular processes fail to rejoin completely or the maxillary process becomes displaced from its mandibular arch origins. If there is excessive fusion of these processes, *microstomia* will result.

The teratologic mechanisms of facial clefting are not completely known. However, they appear to involve combinations of factors such as genetic deficiencies in available mesenchyme (Johnston, Bhakdinarouk, and Reid, 1974; Pratt, Larsen, and Johnston, 1975), abnormal fusion or breakdown of adjacent epithelial membranes, and local interferences with the movement or development of growing tissue masses (Poswillo, 1966). One recently proposed source of interference may be intraembryonic hematomas, the probable result of hypoxia (Ingalls, Curley, and Prindle, 1952; Poswillo, 1975). Other interferences may be mechanical, such as the impacted position of the tongue within the nasal fossa and between the vertical palatal shelves. Failures in embryonic flexion-contraction movements may maintain tongue impaction at the crucial time that the palatal shelves should be free to elevate (Humphrey, 1968). Recent demonstrations of the oral cleft teratogenicity of certain CNS neuromuscular depressants in humans lends even more support to this possible mechanism (Safra and Oakley, 1975; Seip, 1973).

Other common but more benign abnormalities may result from problems in the fusion process. *Developmental cysts* and *fistulas* may occur along any of the fusion lines, the most significant of which is the *branchial cleft cyst* or *fistula*, which forms along the junction line of the first and second arches (Gorlin, Pindborg, and Cohen, 1976). Other common cysts are found at the junction of embryonic medial and lateral nasal limbs and develop as *nasolabial* and *nasoglobular cysts* later in life. The most benign

remnant of facial fusion appears to be the *epithelial pearl*, which represents entrapped collections of former surface ectoderm.

The segmental origins of the head and neck tissues may also result in rather specific patterns of agenesis in which the only structures missing will be those derived from a single embryonic process. For example, the so-called *first arch syndrome* produces unilateral and often isolated deficits only in the mandibular bone, attached masticatory muscles, fifth nerve motor supply, mandibular vessels, external ear structures, and stapes (McKenzie, 1968; Smith, 1970). Other isolated anomalies may center on zygomaticomaxillary and lateral orbital structures, as in the *Treacher Collins* syndrome, and spare the independently developing adjacent nasal and mandibular structures (Gorlin, Pindborg, and Cohen, 1976).

MUSCULOSKELETAL SYSTEM

The craniofacial skeleton begins forming in the fifth and sixth weeks when a mass of dense mesenchyme envelops the cranium of the embryo. During the next 4 weeks a soft osteoid cranial vault, middle face, and rudimentary mandible will form. This is accomplished by three different growth processes: (1) *endochondral formation*, in which the future skeleton is first laid down in cartilage and then undergoes internal resorption and bone deposition much like an epiphyseal plate of a long bone; (2) *intramembranous formation*, in which bone forms directly within highly vascular ossification centers without any intermediate cartilaginous stage; and (3) *branchiomeric (mixed) formation*, in which intramembranous bone forms adjacent to and around temporary cartilaginous bars that also contribute endochondral centers (Table 2-1).

The earliest cranial skeleton to be established is endochondral in type and appears first with the differentiation of cartilaginous plates in the future occipital and sphenoidal regions. Shortly a cartilaginous capsule surrounds the internal ear and a straight appendage develops as the nasal septum. By the third month a saucerlike *chondrocranium* with attached otic and nasal capsules has formed. Gradually these cartilages are replaced by a dense internal trabeculation of bone, a process that continues well into the fetal period with the formation of the petrous portion of the temporal bone. As in the case of the ethmoid bone, the septal cartilage remains largely uncalcified until well into adult life. Some of the endochondral bones are secondarily invaded by invaginations of the surface epithelium, which stimulate the resorption of bone and form the paranasal sinuses and mastoid air cells.

Intramembranous bones of the head consist of the bilateral parietal bones, squamosal and tympanic portions of the temporal bones, and the vomer, nasal, and lacrimal bones (Table 2-1). They take origin in the ninth week as clusters of mesenchymal cells that organize the surrounding jellylike ground substance into collagen matrices. Calcium salts are then precipitated into fanlike spicules that coalesce with other spicules to form a meshwork of trabeculae. The trabecular network is rapidly invested by an osteoblast-lined *periosteal membrane,* which then becomes the primary formation organ for appositional growth of these bones. All of the intramembranous bones gradually join with one another. The intramembranous maxillary, zygomatic, and palatal bones fuse in the tenth and eleventh weeks to form continuous growing units. However, in some regions such as the frontal and parietal skull the centers of ossification remain separated until after birth and the intervening spaces exist as membrane-covered areas called *fontanelles.*

Bones derived from branchial arch tissues are preceded by bilateral bars of cartilage: the mandibular arch *(Meckel's cartilage),* the second arch *(Reichert's cartilage),* and similar structures contained within the third, fourth, and fifth arches. Meckel's cartilage is the most prominent and extends around the entire arch length and into the tympanic cavity. By the eighth week the future mandible has begun to be laid down through intramembranous bone deposition just lateral to and surrounding Meckel's cartilage. The most distal portions of the cartilage are incorporated into the forming mandibular symphysis and body, and the proximal ends emerge from the bony mandible at the future site of the *mandibular foramen* along with the inferior alveolar nerves. The proximal portions of Meckel's cartilage subsequently atrophy but remain attached to the mandible as the *sphenomandibular* ligament, and the portion contained within the tympanic cavity is converted to the first two auditory ossicles, the *incus and malleus.*

The *mandibular condyle* develops rather differently from the rest of the mandible. It appears entirely separate from Meckel's cartilage as an intramembranous outgrowth of the ramus. Soon, however, in apparent response to the compressive forces of opposition with the temporal bone, a secondary endochondral type of bone deposition appears within the expanding fibrous articular surface region. Therefore the condylar process forms both from an intramembranous process and through a slow secondary endochondral replacement.

The second branchial arch cartilage, Reichert's cartilage, is replaced by en-

Table 2-1. Origins of bones of the head and neck

Endochondral	Membrane
Occipital	Nasal
Sphenoid	Lacrimal
Ethmoid	Vomer
Temporal	Frontal
(petrous)	Parietal
Ear ossicles*	Temporal
Hyoid*	(squamosal)
Mandible*	Maxilla*
(condyle)	Palatine*
Temporal*	Zygomatic*
(styloid)	Mandible*
	(body)
	Temporal*
	(tympanic)

*Branchiomeric relation.

dochondral bones that make up the *stapes, styloid process,* and *lesser horn of the hyoid bone,* and remnants of cartilage make up the *stylohyoid ligament* (Table 2-1). The third arch cartilaginous bar is replaced by endochondral bone and remains as the greater horn of the *hyoid bone.*

Muscles of the head and neck appear in the sixth to eighth week and are of biphasic origin (Table 2-2). Most of the muscles are derived from mesenchyme of the branchial arches. The mandibular (first branchial) arch supplies the deeper *muscles of mastication,* which solidify in direct relation to the masticatory bones and are innervated by the fifth cranial nerve. The *facial muscles,* innervated by the seventh cranial nerve, are derived from the second branchial arch, which remains superficial as a subcutaneous specialization that is drawn out over the entire developing face, epicranium, and neck and then separated into sheetlike muscles only later in the fetal period. A few of the muscles of the head and neck appear to be derived from ventral portions of the segmented *somite* masses that are the source of musculature for the remainder of the body trunk (Enlow, 1975; Langman, 1975). The future muscles of the tongue supplied by the twelfth nerve, the infrahyoid muscles, and the extraocular muscles originate in the ventral aspects of the occipital somites, migrate deep to the branchial masses of the first three arches, and then take up their final positions.

VASCULAR SYSTEM

In the early predifferentiation period the primordia of future blood vessels exist as random pools of undifferentiated red blood cells and angioblasts called "blood islands." By the second week, a delicate capillary network connects the blood islands throughout the embryo. In the next few days this network differentiates into functional arteries and circulatory veins on the basis of both genetic predisposition and from the stimulus of hemodynamic flow.

In the ventral thorax primitive cells begin contracting individually even before they coalesce to form a tubular one-chamber heart late in the second week. Vessels extending cephalad from the heart enlarge and split early into paired "dorsal aortae" that loop through the primitive cranium, then turn caudally to enter the extraembryonic circulation before returning to the heart as the pericardial veins (Fig. 2-4). Early in the third week a series of six "aortic arches" begin to extend from the base of the heart anteriorly and dorsally to reach the dorsal aortae. The aortic arches are important intermediate structures in embryonic development because certain ones are destined to persist as adult cranial arteries. In particular, the paired third aortic arches gradually enlarge to become the internal carotid arteries by 3½ weeks of age (Fig. 2-4). At this stage of development the maxillofacial mass is still very rudimentary and lies directly opposite the thorax. The entire cranial region is sup-

Table 2-2. Embryologic origins of muscles and cartilages of the head and neck

First branchial arch	Second branchial arch	Third branchial arch	Fourth to fifth branchial arches
Temporalis	Facial muscles	Stylopharyngeus	Cricothyroid
Medial pterygoid	Hyoglossus	Pharyngeal constrictors	Pharyngeal constrictors
Lateral pterygoid	Stylohyoid	Posterior tongue*	Posterior tongue*
Masseter	Posterior tongue*		Palatine
Anterior tongue	Posterior digastric		Levator veli palatini
Anterior digastric	Stapedius		Tensor veli palatini
Tensor tympani	Reichert's cartilage		Thyroid cartilage
Meckel's cartilage	(degenerate)		
(degenerate)			

*Believed to be derived also from occipital somite masses.

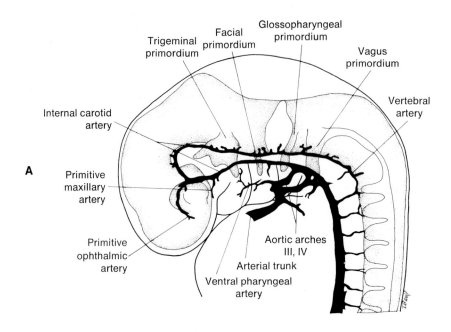

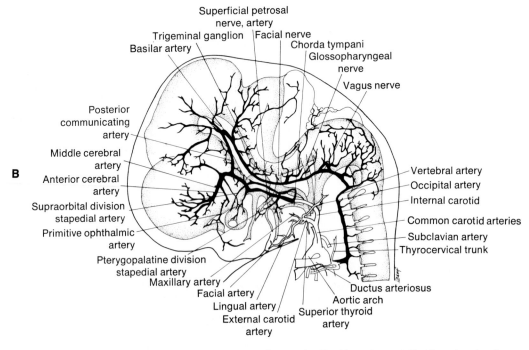

Fig. 2-4. Craniofacial arterial development at, **A,** 4 weeks; **B,** 5½ weeks; and, **C,** 10 weeks, showing common and external carotid derivatives (clear vessels), internal carotid-vertebral derivatives (solid vessels), and transitional stapedial derivatives (lined vessels).

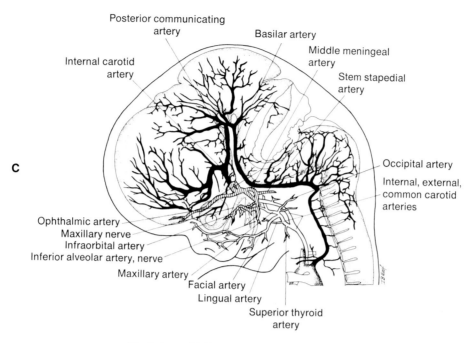

Posterior communicating artery

Basilar artery

Middle meningeal artery

Internal carotid artery

Stem stapedial artery

C

Occipital artery

Internal, external, common carotid arteries

Ophthalmic artery
Maxillary nerve
Infraorbital artery
Inferior alveolar artery, nerve
Maxillary artery
Facial artery
Lingual artery
Superior thyroid artery

Fig. 2-4, cont'd. For legend see opposite page.

plied by branches of the third arch-internal carotid artery as well as contributions from the ingrowing vertebral arteries, which eventually link with terminal portions of the internal carotid artery to form the basilar artery and circle of Willis (Padget, 1948).

A large vessel called the pterygopalatine or stapedial artery arises dorsally from the internal carotid artery, courses deep to the tympanic bulla through the primordial stapes, and then passes medial to the trigeminal ganglion, finally passing through the foramen lacerum region to distribute to the developing pterygoid, mandibular, and especially palatal, ethmoidal, and ophthalmic tissue masses (Fig. 2-4). During the fourth week when the ventral face and mandible take shape, the paired external carotid arteries bud off from the common carotid stems and are carried into the face with the medially migrating branchial and somitic muscle masses. As the external carotid branches enter the region, they overlap with the terminal branches of the pterygopalatine artery, which almost immediately begin to atrophy or are simply annexed by the ingrowing external carotid branches. In the final adult form, therefore, certain of the terminal portions of the maxillary artery such as the middle meningeal artery and the orbital-infraorbital and descending palatine arteries were formerly branches of the internal carotid system that were "taken over" by the late-arriving external carotid system (Padget, 1948). Other remnants of atrophic extracranial internal carotid branches exist in the form of the adult pharyngeal artery and particularly the artery of the pterygoid canal (vidian artery).

Craniofacial venous system development generally parallels the transformation in arterial patterns. In the early differentiation period little difference is seen between venous and arterial microstructure, and bidirectional flow is common. Venous drainage in the 4-week embryo is mainly along intracranial and dorsal spinal routes. These intracranial systems eventually become the dural sinus-internal jugular system, and it is only in the fifth and sixth weeks that venous flow from the jaws and face toward the sinus system diminishes and the adult form of external jugular flow takes over. Remnants of these embryonic maxillofacial-to-intracranial vein connections are quite numerous in the adult and are represented by the "emissary" veins that communicate primarily from pterygoid, mastoid, and ethmoid venous plexuses.

Postnatal implications

The great variety and peculiar characteristics of many head and neck vascular anomalies become more understandable when viewed in terms of vascular embryology. Arteriovenous fistulas and central hemangiomas of the face and jaw are often poorly differentiated as to vessel type and display bidirectional flows that resemble the early differentiation phase of development (Stark et al., 1965). The extreme richness of the collateral blood supply of the head and neck may in part be a by-product of the alternate patterns of vascular development and overlapping blood supplies that characterize the embryonic state. Certain of the major vascular anomalies appear to reflect the original contributions of the intracranial vessels to maxillofacial arteries and veins. An extreme example is the Sturge-Weber or encephalofacial angiomatosis syndrome, which is characterized by hemifacial direct communications between poorly differentiated extracranial and intracranial vessels (Gorlin, Pindborg, and Cohen, 1976). Cases are known in which the pterygopalatine (stapedial) artery persists in the adult as a major artery and reverse-direction middle meningeal arteries supplying maxillary tissues are suspected (Steffan, 1968). In other cases vertebral arterial branches supplying mandibular region tissues have been seen (Smith, 1970).

The role of vascular maldevelopment as a mechanism in major deformities is still unclear, but recent experimental models have stressed that the orderly transition from an internal to an external carotid-based system may be important in first branchial arch syndromes including congenital microsomia, mandibular hypoplasia, and cleft palate (Gregg and Avery, 1971; Poswillo, 1975; Stark et al., 1965).

NERVOUS SYSTEM

The brain and cranial sensorimotor innervations have their origins in the pre-differentiation period from three ectodermal sources: *dorsal neural tube, neural crest,* and surface *epithelial placodes.* The neural tube flexes and segments itself first into a three-vesicle stage, and then by 7 weeks into five vesicles, the *telencephalon, diencephalon, mesencephalon, metencephalon,* and *myelencephalon.* The ventral half of the metencephalon and myelencephalon are destined to be the future pons and medulla and, along with the upper spinal cord, will be the source of all outgrowing motor nerves (V, VII, IX, X, XI, and XII) of the head and neck.

The specialized sensory functions including vision, hearing, and smell are associated with dorsal aspects of the brain stem and especially the more anteriorly placed diencephalon and mesencephalon. The general sensory ganglia, primarily trigeminal (V) and also geniculate (VII) and ganglia IX and X, appear as bipolar cells of both neural crest and surface placode origin in the fourth and fifth weeks. Their central cell processes grow rapidly, penetrate the metencephalon, then grow caudally in the brain stem to make up the *spinal tract of* V and terminate in the caudal myelencephalon and upper spinal cord (Humphrey, 1968). Simultaneous with this central ingrowth, the peripheral process of the ganglion cells grows outward to make anatomic and functional contact with primitive subepithelial networks that have developed as specializations of the surface placodes.

By the fifth and sixth weeks a full complement of twelve paired *cranial nerves* has been established, but unlike the spinal nerves, which are all fundamentally alike, the cranial nerves have intermingled sensory, motor, and autonomic components and undergo complex peripheral migrations that reflect the nonsegmental origins of the head and neck structures. The general motor components of cranial nerves V, VII, IX, and X, for example, do not appear segmentally from superior to inferior. Rather, they appear in succes-

Table 2-3. Development of fetal reflex activity

Gestational age (in weeks)	Activity	Morphologic basis	Motor connections
6	*Myogenic*—muscle contraction in response to direct stimulation	Orofacial muscle differentiation	
6½	*Neurogenic*—sharply localized response to electrical stimulation of motor neuron	Primitive neuromuscular connections established	
7½	*Reflexogenic*—stimulation of oral region elicits overt response	Differentiation of subnucleus caudalis in upper cervical cord	
Total pattern responses	Contralateral neck flexion and head turning Contralateral arm and shoulder extension Contralateral trunk rotations	Downgrowth (caudal) of afferent V tracts into medulla and cervical cord; connection with already differentiated secondary and motor arms	Spinal XI to sternocleidomastoid and trapezius
9½	*Spontaneous activity*		
9½ 10-10½ 12½ Partial pattern responses	Lowering of mandible Swallowing Lip closure, momentary	Caudal to rostral differentiation of subnuclei caudalis, interpolaris, and rostralis; connections with caudorostral developing motor divisions of cranial nerves	Cervical plexus to infrahyoid muscles; XI, X, IX to palatal, laryngeal, pharyngeal area; XII to tongue
13 13	Lip closure, maintained Mouth closure, chewing movements		Motor division of V
15½	Perioral muscle movement; lip protrusion and pursing		VII nerve to facial muscles
29	Audible sucking		Coordinated cranial motor connections

sive layers and run courses that reflect their origins laterally within the branchial arches. The seventh nerves are seen most superficially, fanning lateral to medial across the face and neck from their postauricular point of exit from the skull. At the next layer motor V branches course from lateral to medial and surround the final pharyngeal and palatal muscular masses innervated by nerves IX and X. In contrast, the general sensory and specialized sensory branches of these same nerves run grossly different courses from their motor branches. The sensory V nerve divides into three main trunks just distal to the ganglion, which reflects the separate origin of these different embryonic processes: the mandibular, maxillary, and fronto-ophthalmic. Special fibers for taste to the anterior part of the tongue, although originating centrally as nerve VII fibers, are drawn far medially to join the peripheral trunk of the lingual branch of V.

The functional development of the head and neck nervous system reflects the early predominance of oral sensation and feeding abilities in the fetus (Table 2-3). The first body area to demonstrate reflex sensitivity is, in fact, the small zone immediately around the lip, tip of the tongue, and nares (Humphrey, 1968). From the initial responsiveness in the seventh week, the zone of reflex sensitivity enlarges concentrically over the face, and central synaptic connections become functional in the caudal myelencephalon between sensory nerve V and all motor cranial nuclei, thereby producing a recognizable feeding reflex by the twelfth week in utero. The feeding reflex is the first organized human activity, far advanced over later arriving digital or even respiratory reflexes. Swallowing movements have been observed in fetuses younger than 4 months and may be important not only in preparation for postnatal survival but also as a stimulus to continued fetal development of perioral tissues, tongue, and palate.

Myelination, which appears first in the trigeminal nerves at 12 weeks, continues especially in the motor nerves of mastication, speech, and facial expression until the third and fourth years of life (Langman, 1975).

Postnatal implications

Isolated abnormalities of the peripheral portions of the cranial nerves are extremely rare, more often being associated with agenesis or faulty migration of branchiomeric or somitic muscle masses. Because of the extreme precociousness of the orofacial sensory apparatus and its anatomic association with early developing and vital brain stem structures, any major deficiency in this system would not be consistent with life. For these same reasons grossly deformed infants such as congenital anencephalics are often seen with well-developed feeding abilities. It is the more refined oro-facial neuromuscular activities such as precise dental mastication, speech articulation, and vocalization that require long-term nerve myelination and cerebral control, and on which teratogens have their greatest effect.

PARAORAL STRUCTURES

A series of important structures develop as surface specializations of the primitive oropharyngeal epithelium, forming the oral vestibules and teeth; the salivary, pituitary, thyroid, and parathyroid glands; the tonsils; thymus; and ultimobranchial bodies.

A thickening of epithelial layers is seen first in the anterior mouth but eventually spreads laterally to separate the lips and the expanding mound of gum tissue. This partition, the *labial lamina*, then gradually breaks down to form the oral *vestibule*, separating lips from jaws by the tenth week. Remnants of the labial lamina are seen in the newborn as weblike *frenulae*.

Teeth

The primordia of the teeth arise from an epithelial plate, the *dental lamina*, adjacent to the labial lamina at the junction of the vestibule and the gum margin. The dental lamina consists of cells of neural crest and surface ectoderm origin, which are gradually engulfed by the expanding mound of gum tissues. Early in the third month knoblike thickenings of the dental lamina and the *enamel organs* invaginate in the jaws to form cuplike structures that contain dense accumulations of mesenchymal cells. This mesenchyme, the *dental papilla*, will eventually form *dentin, cementum,* and *dental pulp,* whereas the enamel organ will form the *enamel* of the teeth. Ten of these primordia of the *deciduous* teeth will have formed in each dental arch by the tenth week and will begin calcifying by the sixteenth week. The dental lamina that remains connected to the individual enamel organs by a stalk of epithelium persists in some areas to provide enamel organs for the future permanent teeth. Most of the cells of the lamina and its stalks, however, normally have broken down and disappeared by birth.

Salivary glands

All of the paired salivary glands have common planes of origin. The primordia arise as buds of epithelium from the oral vestibule and floor of the mouth and then grow by local branching to produce bushlike structures near the sites of oral invagination. Parts of the epithelial buds become canalized to form ducts. The ducts are then greatly lengthened and in some cases are stretched over developing masticatory muscles. In the case of the parotid, the gland itself remains in its original developmental position at the lateral base of the first branchial arch and *Stensen's* (parotid) *duct* is drawn out over the masseter muscle. The *submandibular gland* becomes subdivided by the horizontal mylohyoid muscle into portions that occupy both the mandibular and paralingual spaces. The basic plan of the major salivary glands is established at 3 months.

Pituitary gland

The pituitary gland (hypophysis) is an endocrine gland with a dual origin; one part, the future *anterior lobe,* is the result of an outpouching of oral stomodeal ectoderm, and the other part, the *posterior* or *neurohypophyseal lobe,* is a specialized outgrowth of the brain wall. Early in the fourth week a midline outpouching called *Rathke's pouch,* is seen in the dorsal aspect of the stomodeal cavity just in front of the still intact pharyngeal membrane. Rathke's pouch elongates and flattens into contact with the floor of the forebrain. The stalk of epithelium called the *craniopharyngeal duct* normally atrophies by the eighth week, and the original point of invagination of Rathke's pouch is ultimately located in the roof of the adult nasopharynx at the caudal border of the nasal septum.

Thyroid gland

The thyroid gland is the earliest of the glands to develop, beginning as the *thyroid diverticulum* or *sac* in the third week. The sac is a midline bilobed outpouching of the ventral pharyngeal floor between the swellings of the first branchial pouches (Fig. 2-2). The gland is quickly separated from the surface but maintains communication by a narrowing neck, the thyroglossal duct, which opens within the mass of the tuberculum impar of the tongue. The duct becomes a solid stalk and fragments in the sixth week, but its point of origin in the tongue remains in the adult as a distinct pit, the *foramen cecum.* Meanwhile, the thyroid sac further differentiates and descends into contact with the primitive aortic stem. As a result of forward growth of the pharynx and larynx during the seventh week, the gland settles posterolaterally in the neck with a narrowed *thyroid isthmus* joining the two lobes across the midline. The gland is joined at about this time by the *parathyroid glands* and *ultimobranchial bodies.* By the eighth week cavitations appear within the beaded outgrowths of the gland and *thyroid follicles* form that will contain colloid by the third month.

Tonsils

In the fifth and sixth weeks a series of glandular structures arise as outgrowths or sacculations of the lateral recesses of pharyngeal pouches two, three, four, and five (Fig. 2-2). At the level of the second pouch a ring of lymphoid tissue begins to accumulate early in the third month. First to be seen are the *palatine* tonsils, solid outgrowths of the lateral second pouch surface. The *lingual* tonsils elevate from the midline arches II and III just behind the foramen cecum, and the *pharyngeal* tonsils complete the circle of tonsils in the fourth month.

Thymus

The thymus actually begins its development in advance of the tonsils. Near the end of the sixth week, ventral sacculations are seen in each third pharyngeal pouch. The two primordia sink rapidly in the neck, join with one another at their lower ends in the eighth week, and attain their permanent position attached to the pericardium in the thorax. The superior origins of the thymus gradually atrophy during this time and the characteristic small cell lymphocytes and thymocytes begin appearing toward the end of the third month. The thymus will not begin to retrogress until puberty.

Parathyroid glands

The dorsal aspects of the third and fourth pouches thicken into solid cellular masses in the fourth week as the beginnings of the parathyroid glands. The pair from the fourth pouch become detached and are drawn down by the migrating thymus, finally taking up permanent position in the thyroid capsule as the *inferior* parathyroids. The *superior* parathyroids are actually derivatives of the fourth pharyngeal pouch, which do not change their basic position but simply become embedded in the thyroid capsule.

Ultimobranchial bodies

In the fifth week multiple saclike structures, the ultimobranchial bodies, expand from the fifth pouches. In the seventh week these bodies are joined by the detached parathyroid glands and both sets of glands are brought into contact with the downgrowing thyroid gland. The ultimobranchial bodies become lost in the thyroid mass and are believed to supply active *parafollicular*, calcitonin-secreting *cells* to the thyroid gland long before birth.

Postnatal implications

Nearly all of the paraoral structures arise from the surface epithelium, prolif-

erate and invaginate, and then the original stalks of epithelium that connected them to the oral cavity atrophy. Because of this process, a number of accessory and potentially abnormal tissues may be seen along the course of embryonic invagination. In the case of the invaginating dental lamina, ectopic epithelial remnants may appear in the newborn as *epithelial pearls* or *supernumerary teeth*. *Accessory salivary glands* may occur at any point along the major parotid or submandibular ducts. Unobliterated remnants of Rathke's pouch and the craniopharyngeal duct may be the source of neoplastic cells of the *pituitary ameloblastoma*, which tends to make its appearance before puberty. Persistence of portions of the thyroglossal duct may give rise to *accessory thyroid glands, thyroglossal duct cysts,* and *fistulas,* which may occur at any point on the midline course of gland migration from the base of the tongue to just below the hyoid bone.

TERATOLOGY

Congenital malformations are of obvious significance to the surgeon. It is estimated that 2% to 3% of all live born infants show one or more significant malformations, and this figure doubles by the end of one year because of the discovery of defects indiscernible at birth (Hertig, 1967). Cleft lip and palate alone occur once in every 850 to 1,000 live births, second only to clubfoot among major malformations (Gorlin, Pindborg, and Cohen, 1976; Langman, 1975). Six general classes of congenital malformations are recognized:

1. *Agenesis,* in which there is complete developmental failure, for example, limb agenesis, congenital absence of teeth
2. *Incomplete development,* in which some portion or quantity of tissue is lacking, for example, dwarfism, cleft palate, micrognathia
3. *Excessive development,* in which there is congenital overgrowth, for example, hypertelorism, premaxillary clefting, maxillary hyperplasia
4. *Embryonic survival,* in which there is failure of involution of an em-

bryonic structure, for example, thyroglossal duct cyst, retained stapedial artery

5. *Hamartoma*, in which there is a misplacement of normal tissue, for example, lingual thyroid
6. *Blastoma*, in which there is atypical differentiation of embryonic tissue, for example, trigeminal teratoma

It was formerly thought that congenital malformations were the result only of genetic defects. Since the 1940's, however, when rubella virus was first implicated in the production of congenital malformation (Gregg, 1941), a growing list of potential environmental teratogens has been recognized. It is now estimated that approximately 10% of all malformations are the result purely of environmental factors, 10% are caused solely by the expression of abnormal genetic chromosomal factors, and 80% are attributable to a complex interplay of environmental factors and genetic predispositions (Wilson, 1973). A wide range of environmental teratogens have been identified. Infectious agents, particularly the rubella, (Gregg, 1941), cytomegalovirus, (Weller and Handshaw, 1962), herpes simplex, (Fuecillo and Sever, 1973), and other viruses are best known, (Hakosolo and Saxen, 1971), although congenital syphilis and toxoplasmosis are also known teratogens (Wilson, 1973). Radiation was first shown to be a strong factor through investigation of the offspring of Hiroshima atomic bomb victims, and since that time it has been verified many times with experimental animals (Carter, Lyon, and Phillips, 1958; Wood, Johnson, and Omori, 1967). In more recent years chemicals and drugs have been increasingly correlated with malformations. The best known example is the sedative thalidomide, (Somers, 1962), but there is a growing list of rather commonly used agents including the anorexigenic drugs (dextroamphetamines), tetracyclines, ethyl alcohol, tobacco, antihistamines, and the tricyclic antidepressants (Barnes, 1968; Bongiovanni and McPadden, 1960). Antiepileptic drugs have been implicated among populations in which facial clefts were seen 29 times more frequently

(Seip, 1973), and cleft lip and palate deformities have been found to be four times more frequent among offspring of mothers taking benzodiazepine tranquilizers (Safra and Oakley, 1975). Exogenous hormone preparations have also been implicated as possible teratogens (Bongiovanni and McPadden, 1960). Synthetic progestins and severe insulin metabolic disruptions among diabetic mothers have been linked with pelvic and extremity anomalies, (Passarge and Lenz, 1966), and the corticosteroids have been implicated in the pathogenesis of cleft lip and palate since the early demonstration that 100% clefting could be induced among experimental rodent embryos following maternal cortisone injections (Fraser et al., 1954; Kalter and Warkany, 1959). Nutritional deficiencies and hypoxia are classic teratogens in experimental animals, although the limits of human tolerance have not been defined as yet (Barnes, 1968; Ingalls, Curley, and Prindle, 1952). There is much controversy about the possible role of pesticides and defoliants as teratogens, but to date the best documented relationship is that of organic mercurials and multiple neurologic malformations (Snyder, 1971; Wilson, 1973).

A wide range of hereditable generalized defects are known to be associated with anomalies in the dentition. These include dentinogenesis imperfecta and retarded eruption with cleidocranial dysostosis. Genetically related defects of other oral tissues include ankyloglossia, oral and facial clefts, mucosal-hemorrhagic telangiectasia, facial angiomatosis with Sturge-Weber disease, gargoylism, mandibulofacial dysostosis, Crouzon's disease, multilocular cystic fibrous dysplasia, and circumoral pigmentation with gastrointestinal polyposis (Peutz-Jeghers syndrome) (Gorlin, Pindborg, and Cohen, 1976; Smith, 1970).

The current view of craniofacial dysmorphogenesis therefore is that a multitude of environmental agents may act with certain genetic predispositions to cause malformations (Barnes, 1968; Wilson, 1973). The actual mechanisms through which teratogens act, however, are probably few in number. In most cases of tissue deficiency, particularly facial clefts, a local shortage in mesenchymal tissue mass is believed to exist. These deficiencies, in turn, are likely caused by failure in the flow of cells dorsally from the neural crest into the ventrally positioned facial tissue masses (Johnston, Bhakdinaronk, and Reid, 1974). Recent research has documented the important contributions of the neural crest in forming facial structures as well as peripheral nerves, endocrine glands, and dental tissues. It has been shown that genetically determined mesenchymal substrates consisting primarily of hyaluronic acid guide the flow of the critical neural crest cells (Pratt, Larsen, and Johnston, 1975). A specific example of the genetically based mesenchymal deficiency may be the mandibulofacial dysostosis syndrome. A functional but deficient periosteal matrix exists in this condition, but it provides an asymmetric hypoplastic skeleton (Smith, 1970).

Intrauterine postural factors have also been implicated in the mechanism of mesenchymal deficiency. For example, inadequate amniotic sac space may result in excessive contact between flexed embryonic structures such as the face and thorax, thereby preventing migration of mesenchyme into the facial processes. Experimental models based on this concept have been developed that produced restriction of natural embryonic movements by withdrawing amniotic fluid, resulting in "molding" anomalies of clubfoot, congenital dislocation of the hip, syndactyly, cleft palate, and mandibular micrognathia and high arched palates reminiscent of the human Pierre Robin syndrome (Poswillo, 1966). Other postural mechanisms have been proposed in which maldevelopment of cranial base endochondral bone and the cervical vertebrae, as seen in the Klippel-Feil syndrome, produce immobilization of the head against the chest and inhibit the normal migration of facial-cervical tissues (Gorlin, Pindborg, and Cohen, 1976; Smith, 1970). A related hypothesis of secondary palate closure suggests that intraembryonic mandibular reflex openings are necessary to mobilize the tongue from within the nasal fossa, thereby permitting elevation of the palatal shelves and subsequent development of the nasomaxillary complex (Humphrey, 1968).

Vascular mechanisms may also be important factors in craniofacial teratology. During the crucial 4 to 8 weeks of organogenesis, the craniofacial arterial network undergoes a transformation in source from a dorsal aortic arch – internal carotid base to a predominantly external carotid-based origin. Interference with this vascular transformation, most probably on the basis of hypoxia-induced hematomas, has been hypothesized as a mechanism in the production of craniofacial anomalies, especially second branchial arch syndromes (Gregg and Avery, 1971; Ingalls, Curley and Prindle, 1952; Stark et al., 1965).

REFERENCES

Barnes, A. C. 1968. The fetal environment: drugs and chemicals. In Barnes, A. C., ed.: Intrauterine development, Philadelphia, Lea & Febiger, p. 362.

Bongiovanni, A. M., and McPadden, A. J. 1960. Steroids during pregnancy and possible fetal consequences, Fertil. Steril. **11**:181.

Carter, T. C., Lyon, M. F., and Phillips, R. J. 1958. Genetic hazard of ionizing radiations, Nature (Lond.) **182**:409.

Enlow, D. H. 1975. Handbook of facial growth, Philadelphia, W. B. Saunders Co.

Fraser, F. C., et al. 1954. Experimental production of cleft palate with cortisone and other hormones, J. Cell. Comp. Physiol. **43** (Suppl. 1):237.

Fuccillo, D. A., and Sever, L. J. 1973. Viral teratology, Bacteriol. Rev. **37**:19.

Gorlin, R. J., Pindborg, J. J., and Cohen, M. 1976. Syndromes of the head and neck, ed. 2, New York, McGraw-Hill Book Co.

Gregg, G. H. 1941. Congenital cataract following German measles in mothers, Trans. Ophthalmol. Soc. Aust. **3**:35.

Gregg, J. M. and Avery, J. K. 1971. Experimental studies of vascular development in normal and cleft palate mouse embryos, Cleft Palate J. **8**:101.

Hakosalo, T., and Saxen, L. 1971. Influenza epidermic and congenital defects, Lancet **2**:1346.

Hertig, A. T. 1967. The overall problem in man. In Benirschke, K., ed.: Comparative aspects of reproductive failure, New York, Springer-Verlag, p. 11.

Humphrey, T. 1968. The development of mouth opening and related reflexes involving the oral area of human fetuses, Ala. J. Med. Sci. **5**:126.

Ingalls, T. H., Curley, F. J., and Prindle, R. A. 1952. Experimental production of congenital abnormalities, timing and degree of anoxia as factors causing fetal deaths and congenital abnormalities in mouse, N. Engl. J. Med. **247**:758.

Johnston, M. C., Bhakdinaronk, A., and Reid, Y. C. 1974. An expanded role of the neural crest in oral and pharyngeal development. In Bosma, J. F., ed.: Fourth symposium on oral sensation and perception, Washington, D.C., U.S. Government Printing Office.

Kalter, H., and Warkany, J. 1959. Experimental production of congenital malformations in mammals by metabolic procedure, Physiol. Rev. **39**:69.

Langman, J. 1975. Medical embryology, ed. 3, Baltimore, The Williams & Wilkins Co.

McKenzie, J. 1968. The first arch syndrome, Arch. Dis. Child. **33**:477.

Padget, D. H. 1948. The development of the cranial arteries in the human embryo, Contrib. Embryol. **32**:205.

Passarge, E., and Lenz, W. 1966. Syndromes of caudal regression in infants of diabetic mothers, Pediatrics **37**:672.

Poswillo, D. 1966. Observations of fetal posture and causal mechanisms of congenital deformity of palate, mandible, and limbs, J. Dent. Res. **45**:584.

Poswillo, D. 1975. Causal mechanisms of craniofacial deformity, Br. Med. Bull. **31**:101.

Pratt, R., Larsen, M. A., and Johnston, M. C. 1975. Migration of cranial neural crest cells in a cell-free hyaluronate-rich matrix, Dev. Biol. **44**:298.

Safra, M. J., and Oakley, G. P. 1975. Association between cleft lip with or without cleft palate and prenatal exposure to diazepam, Lancet **2**:7933:478.

Seip, M. 1973. The effects of antiepileptic drugs in pregnancy on the fetus and newborn infant, Ann. Clin. Res. **5**:205.

Smith, D. W. 1970. Recognizable patterns of human malformation, Philadelphia, W. B. Saunders Co.

Snyder, R. D. 1971. Congenital mercury poisoning, N. Engl. J. Med. **284**:1014, 1971.

Somers, G. S. 1962. Thalidomide and congenital abnormalities, Lancet **1**:912.

Stark, R. B., et al. 1965. The role of vascular deficiency in the production of congenital malformation, Plast. Reconstr. Surg. **35**:478.

Steffan, T. N. 1968. Vascular anomalies of the middle ear, Laryngoscope **78**:171.

Warkany, J., and Kalter, H. 1961. Congenital malformations, N. Engl. J. Med. **265**:993.

Weller, T. H., and Hanshaw, J. B. 1962. Virologic and clinical observations on cytomegalic inclusion disease, N. Engl. J. Med. **266**:1233.

Wilson, J. G. 1973. Environment and birth defects, New York, Academic Press, Inc.

Wood, J. W., Johnson, K. G., and Omori, Y. 1967. In utero exposure to the Hiroshima atomic bomb: an evaluation of head size and mental retardation twenty years later, Pediatrics **39**:385.

CHAPTER 3

Postnatal craniofacial growth and development

John F. Cleall

That the adult craniofacial complex is not simply a uniform enlargement of the infant's head must have been well recognized early in man's history. However, documentation of the dimensional changes involved is a fairly recent occurrence and seems to have stemmed from the work of the earlier anthropologists' efforts to measure the craniofacial region in different human racial groups and from comparative craniofacial anatomy.

Scammon (1927) published an extensive paper in which he reviewed the literature up until that time relating to physical growth and development. Between the years 1500 and 1700 he found only 41 references. After that time, however, the literature became extensive.

Morphologists have been concerned largely with growth changes in size and shape. However, in the late nineteenth century it was recognized that changes in body composition could also be expected with growth (Von Bezold, 1857). Other, earlier workers in the field of chemical maturation included Moulton (1923). A review by Shohl (1939) evaluated the work recorded up to that time. More recent works include the text edited by Cheek (1968).

CRANIOMETRY AND CEPHALOMETRY

The availability of large numbers of dried human skulls and those of other animals provided excellent material for comparative qualitative and quantitative studies. Physical anthropology achieved recognition as a scientific discipline during the eighteenth century, and as a result the craniofacial relationships of a large number of ethnic groups were documented. The "head spanner" and other measuring instruments were used extensively and resulted in a vast amount of numerical data. The accumulation of these data during the second half of the nineteenth century resulted in little change in basic concepts, which, in part, led to the present lack of interest in this type of study.

The use of dead material necessarily resulted in cross-sectional investigations, which, while useful in characterizing the morphology of the craniofacial structures, gave no information on the process of growth. Lack of accurate age determination and the concern that a "dead" child may not have been undergoing normal growth were further limitations.

Camper (1792) made one of the first attempts at classifying the facial profile. The methods of assessing facial prognathism were reviewed by Topinard (1890). He noted that some 15 reference planes had been suggested by various workers during the nineteenth century. This plethora of possible planes of orientation was the forerunner to the past and ongoing difficulties facing the radiographic cephalometrician. Van Hering and Merkel, as referred to by Brown (1965), defined a reference plane passing through the center of the external acoustic meatus and the lower point of the intraorbital margin. The subsequent adoption of this plane, with some modification, at a conference in 1884 brought some degree of standardization into the literature. This plane became known as the "Frankfort horizontal" plane and is still used in cephalometric radiography. Once standardized landmarks and measurements were developed, much useful information resulted from craniometry.

Despite the cross-sectional nature of the studies, several workers made major contributions to the early understanding of the morphologic age changes of the human head. The study by Keith and Campion (1922), while using only a very small sample, attempted to define the sites of growth in the human skull. Hellman (1927a, b) used dental age to group a sample of skulls. The facial region was subdivided into parts for descriptive and measurement purposes and resulted in excellent comparative data. The work of Todd (1930) and his co-workers is also noteworthy for that time.

The limitations of these cross-sectional "growth" studies were noted and led to considerable interest in cephalometry — the study of head dimensions in the living. Much of the instrumentation was similar to that used in craniometry, but despite the possibility of following individual subjects longitudinally throughout their postnatal growth period, the presence of variable amounts of covering soft tissues proved a severe drawback. Smyth and Young's study (1932) showed high correlations between the pattern of facial growth and age, height, and body weight in groups of children. Also, sex differences were observed and documented. Subsequent studies by Goldstein (1936), Davenport (1941), and the more recent and excellent publication by Krogman (1970) have provided much of our information on the overall morphologic changes occurring during postnatal craniofacial growth and development. The literature on human growth studies, up until the development of the radiographic cephalometer, is well reviewed by Brader (1956).

CEPHALOMETRIC RADIOGRAPHY

Soon after clinical radiography became an acceptable medical technique it was suggested that profile radiographs would be most useful in the field of physical anthropology. Pacini (1922) reported that radiographs taken in *norma lateralis* gave rise to many recognizable midsagittal landmarks. Standardization is the most important aspect of cephalometric radiography, and it was not until the independent works of Broadbent (1931) and Hofrath (1931) were published that the system became a useful tool for craniofacial growth research. The progression from craniometry to cephalometry to radiographic cephalometry was a logical sequence. This allowed the orderly transfer of anatomic landmarks and reference planes to be passed on to our current system of clinical craniofacial growth analysis. Modifications of the original technique by such researchers as Higley (1936), Margolis (1940), Weingart (1948), Downs (1948), Koski (1951), Coben (1955), and Krogman and Sassouni (1957) have made the technique useful for both research and clinical patient assessment. Salzman (1960a) and Krogman and Sassouni (1957) have published excellent reviews of most of the currently used cephalometric analyses.

The equipment consists basically of a cephalostat or head-holding device that is engineered to have a constant relationship to an x-ray generator (Fig. 3-1). A subject's head is positioned by means of adjustable ear rods, and most machines are capable of making exposures in both the lateral and posteroanterior views. Magnification errors are reduced by using a long anode-patient distance and short patient-film distance. The resulting radiographs are traced using a fine, hard pencil on thin, matte acetate. Measurements can then be made of this tracing. Alternatively, some investigators prefer to measure directly on the film, and, more recently, computerized systems have been devised to record and process the data numerically (Chebib, Cleall, and Carpenter, 1976; Cleall and Chebib, 1971; Walker and Kowalski, 1971). The errors of cephalometric radiography have

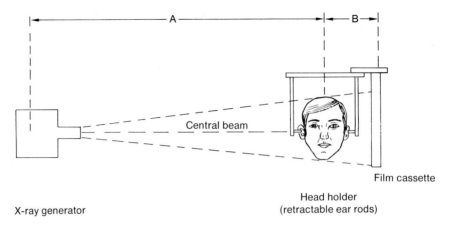

Fig. 3-1. Diagram showing arrangement of components of typical radiographic cephalometer. **A,** Anode to midsagittal plane (approximately 5 feet). **B,** Midsagittal plane to film cassette (may be variable or fixed at a standard distance).

been studied and documented by several investigators. Adams (1940) noted the importance of maintaining an exact and standardized technique. Thurow (1951) suggested refinements to assist in determining the magnification errors.

As a clinical research tool, cephalometric radiography has proved to be the greatest single influence on the direction and volume of craniofacial growth research. As a diagnostic aid for assessing craniofacial morphology and treatment changes, it has also proved its worth. The reader is directed to standard texts for a review of the various analyses in use today (Anderson, 1955; Graber, 1966; Krogman and Sassouni, 1957; Salzman, 1960a; and Thurow, 1970).

It should be remembered that the cephalometric radiography technique gives little information regarding the specific sites of growth. It simply gives the changing relationships of a series of indentifiable osteologic or soft tissue landmarks as a function of time. The technique was greatly improved for use in craniofacial growth research with the advent of metallic implants (Björk, 1955), wherein small, inert, metal pins were driven into the mandible and maxilla using an intraoral approach by means of a specially designed implanting device. Apart from the limitations imposed by the possible loss or movement of some of the implants, it is possible by using this technique to follow the remodeling changes in the facial bones by superimposing successive radiographs on the implants. This technique has also been found to be most useful in experimental animals (Gans and Sarnat, 1951; Henry, 1974).

These later studies have the obvious advantage in that the overall patterns of growth can be followed cephalometrically and the information can then be verified by subsequent sacrifice of the animal followed by histologic examination. This dual approach is not practical in normal human subjects, but histologic studies of biopsy specimens of selected growth sites have been most useful in helping substantiate clinical or cephalometric information (Melsen, 1975).

BONE GROWTH STUDIES

Early bone growth research was helped greatly by the observation of Belchier (1736) that madder-fed pigs developed red-stained bones. Hunter (1771) used this method to study the growth of the mandible in pigs. In his classic study he described the mandible as increasing in length by apposition at the posterior border of the ramus with concomitant resorption of the anterior border together with condylar and coronoid process growth. He noted that exfoliation of teeth is always accompanied by resorption of the alveolar bone, while tooth eruption is

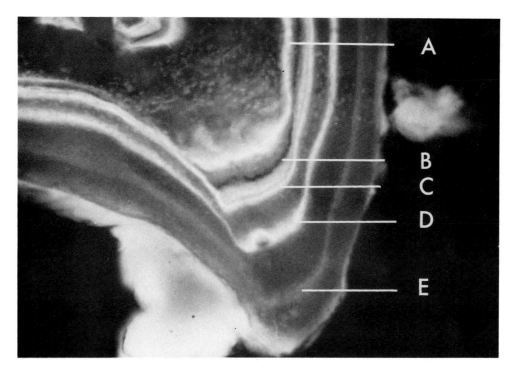

Fig. 3-2. Ultraviolet light photomicrograph of coronal section of hard palate of rat in region of incisive foramen. Bone-marking agents appear as different colors through microscope. *A,* Terramycin; *B,* alizarin red S; *C,* Terramycin and alizarin red S; *D,* Terramycin and trypan blue, *E,* alizarin red S. Detailed data on magnitude and direction of bone growth assessed in this manner is not available from cephalometric radiographic studies.

accompanied by alveolar bone growth. These observations are still largely accepted today.

Brash (1924) extended Hunter's vital-staining work to the upper face and cranial vault. His observations on bone-surface reactions led him to conclude that the cranial vault grows by apposition on the external surface and by resorption internally. The use of alizarin red S (an active staining compound in madder) by workers such as Moore (1949), Massler and Schour (1941), Baer (1954), and Craven (1956) has added much to our current knowledge. The use of multiple bone-marking agents (Cleall, 1964) has expanded the technique for longitudinal bone growth studies (Fig. 3-2).

Histologic studies have provided much of our basic descriptive craniofacial growth information and a major contributor in recent years has been Enlow (1968). His examination (macroscopically and microscopically) of skull material in both

monkeys and humans has demonstrated a pattern of appositional and resorptive changes that shows not only the detailed complexity of skeletal changes with growth but also the individual variation, thus supporting the radiographic studies by Björk (1963).

FACTORS INFLUENCING POSTNATAL GROWTH AND DEVELOPMENT

The process of growth is a cellular phenomenon and depends on the complex interactions of genes, nutrition, and environment as functions of time. Growth is fastest early in prenatal life and continues at an ever-diminishing rate. Once maturity is reached, the replication of DNA to produce new cells becomes relatively low in most tissues. Negative growth then occurs as cells die or their functions become reduced, leading to old age and, eventually, death.

The genetic material in each cell determines its range of functions and its general morphology. However, as with all populations, a fair degree of variability exists and this gives groups of cells the necessary flexibility to react to external factors. Growth and function, therefore, consist of an intricate and often subtle balance between genetic and environmental factors.

Reproducibility of morphologic traits from one generation to another underlines the importance and relative constancy of the genetic influence. However, in the past, a concentration of effort on the study of genetically simple situations has to a degree hindered progress. While this approach has helped order our thinking, it has resulted in an oversimplistic view of gene action. Certainly, in the craniofacial region, the morphologic characters making up the human head are polygenic in nature. For example, limiting discussion to only the skeletal structures, it is possible that for much of the skeleton the possible "fields" of gene action may be quite large. However, in the craniofacial complex these "fields" could well be very small. Considerable latitude, therefore, may exist in this region for the various functional influences to modify the shape of the structures.

The morphologic and functional complexity of the craniofacial region in large measure is related to the phylogenetic history of the region. The aggregation of the brain and special sense organs and the openings of the respiratory and digestive systems at the cephalic end of the organism have made the region complex in its phylogenetic and ontogenetic development. Form and functional modifications relating to binocular vision, bipedal locomotion, and the attainment of an upright posture also have led to far-reaching implications in man.

On this phylogenetic history and genetic blueprint plays the ever-present and important factor of environment. Postnatally, the environment of the developing craniofacial structures may vary greatly during each child's growth and from child to child. Because of the enormous diminution of the relative rate of cell division postnatally, the effects of environmental factors postnatally may be far less than the effects prenatally. Postnatal en-

vironmental influences are usually recognizable only in gross conditions. The growth processes have a built-in mechanism to return aberrant growth to a normal, orderly pattern, and this ability will vary from child to child, again leading to great individually different responses.

General factors, such as geographic and climatic conditions, seem to have little measurable effect on general postnatal growth and development. While statements to the contrary (Mills, 1944) have suggested a retardation of growth in children living in tropical climates, it should be noted that often these children also are from relatively poor socioeconomic groups whose general nutrition is substandard. There does, however, seem to be a seasonable variation in growth rates; for example, growth in height seems to be greatest in the spring. This seasonable difference has not been noted in the craniofacial region, probably because of the small magnitude of change and inaccuracy in our measurement systems.

Socioeconomic factors are important in influencing overall height and weight (Greulich, 1958) but are probably recognizable to a lesser degree in the craniofacial region. These same factors are operating in the demonstrable secular trend in the Western world and are evidenced by the increase in height and weight of individuals in sequential generations (Meredith, 1950). Nutrition, therefore, seems to play an important role in optimal postnatal growth. Both the quantity and types of nutrients needed, including protein, fats, carbohydrates, minerals, and vitamins, must be considered. While in the Western world gross malnutrition is only occasionally observed, the long-term, subclinical effects of inadequate dietary intake must be taken into consideration.

The effects of a disturbance on the internal environment caused by a hormonal imbalance should be noted. The pituitary, thyroid, parathyroid, and adrenal glands, gonads, and perhaps also the pancreas, thymus, and pineal gland and their interactions, may all be expected to have some influence on the growth process. While general body growth disturbances may occur in many instances, specific effects on the jaws and teeth may also be observed.

Normal cell metabolism is necessary throughout the period of growth if a child is to achieve his or her full potential. The general health of the individual is thus an important factor in growth. The acute, mild, illness experienced by most children probably has little effect on growth of the craniofacial region. Skeletal development and functional maturation is, however, almost certain to be affected by chronic conditions. This is especially true if the illness occurs in the early years of life. While some diseases, notably the endocrine disorders, may result in an abnormal acceleration of growth, most often the result is a retardation.

The capacity for growth, especially in early life, is great. This, coupled with the functional adaptability of the tissues and structures, provides a homeostatic mechanism that resists any permanent and adverse structural and functional change. This ability to respond to adverse conditions permits some degree of "catchup" growth to occur following illness or other growth-retarding conditions (Prader, Tanner, and Von Harnack, 1963).

As form and function are inextricably interwoven, the function of the craniofacial structures must play an important part in their overall growth and development. The precise mechanism controlling the interaction of form and function is controversial. Extensive changes in the functional aspects of the craniofacial region are readily observed, but the more minor alterations in function acting for a long period are the ever-present, if hard to detect, factors of importance to the clinician. The dynamic functions of respiration, deglutition, head posture, and mastication are obvious sources of influence, while the presence and function of the soft tissues of the developing brain and respiratory tissues are more subtle but have far-reaching consequences relating to the finer details of craniofacial skeletal development.

MECHANISMS OF CRANIOFACIAL GROWTH AND DEVELOPMENT

The concepts of craniofacial growth in the past have dealt largely with the

modes of bone growth rather than the underlying mechanisms. Controversy existed largely regarding the relative importance of growth in cartilage, sutures, and appositional changes. Hunter (1771) and Brash (1924), using madder feeding, felt that most of the craniofacial skeletal growth resulted from a combination of appositional and resorptive changes on the surfaces of the growing bones. Staining at the sutures of the cranium was stated by Brash (1924) to result from secondary reformation to maintain the relative position of the suture during increase in size. However, it should be noted that in the pig (the animal studied by Brash) sutural growth is completed very early. Brash considered the growth of the cranial base as being analogous to that of the long bones.

Sutural changes were first emphasized when Keith and Campion (1922) described the morphologic differences among three skulls of differing ages. Regarding facial growth, they implied that active growth changes in the circummaxillary system of sutures was primarily responsible for the downward and forward displacement of the midfacial region. Weinmann and Sicher (1955) carried this concept further by noting the relatively parallel orientation of the frontomaxillary, zygomaticomaxillary, pterygopalatine, and zygomaticotemporal sutures. They suggested that growth in these sutures would then carry the maxillary region downward and forward. They failed to observe that in the deeper aspects of some of these sutures, the approximating surfaces of the bones are far from parallel. Support for this sutural concept is found in the vital-staining experiments on rats and monkeys by Massler (1944).

Cartilage was held to be under genetic control and, therefore, a self-determining and most predictable tissue in terms of craniofacial growth. The cranial base with its synchondroses has, therefore, traditionally been used as a stable area from which to assess growth in adjacent structures. Weinmann and Sicher (1955) emphasized the importance of cartilage in growth of the cranial base. Broadbent (1937), Brodie (1941), and many subse-

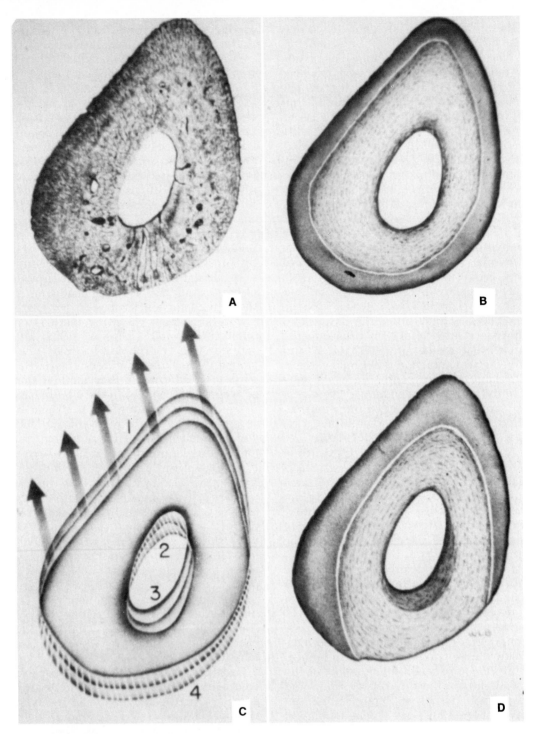

Fig. 3-3. Cortical drift. Sequence of remodeling changes that produced arrangement seen in photomicrograph **A** are schematized in succession. Beginning with original stage seen in **B,** consisting of outer zone of periosteal bone enclosing inner layer of endosteal bone, entire cortex "drifts" in direction of arrows, shown in **C.** Periosteal bone is added at surface *1.* Inner margin of cortex is undergoing resorption at surface *2.* Endosteal bone is added at surface *3,* and periosteal resorption occurs at surtace *4.* Resulting arrangement of structure is seen in **D,** which is comparable with photomicrograph **A.** (From Enlow, D. H. 1963. Principles of bone remodeling, Springfield, Ill., Courtesy of Charles C Thomas, Publisher.)

quent workers have used the cranial base as a so-called stable reference area. Scott (1953) evolved a "septum theory" around the growth of the cartilaginous nasal capsule and nasal septum and considered cartilage to be the prime mover of midfacial growth. Growth of the mandible has also been ascribed largely to growth of the condylar cartilage with concomitant appositional changes at the alveolus, posterior border, coronoid process, and lower border.

The concept of strict genetic control and unalterable expression of cartilage growth has recently been placed in some doubt(Charlier, Petrovic, and Herrmann-Stulzmann, 1969; Enlow, 1975, McNamara, 1972; Petrovic, 1972). Certainly, cartilage is programmed to undergo rapid and well-ordered cell division (Felts, 1959; Koski, 1971; Lacroix, 1952) and is most resistant to pressure, but the rate and direction of this growth would seem to be actively alterable by external modifying phenomena. The site of the growing cartilage and its embryologic origin, for example, whether it is a primary or secondary cartilage, would seem important. In the craniofacial complex these points can be exemplified by considering the difference in modes of growth of the cartilage plates in the cranial base on the one hand and the appositional type of growth occurring in the condylar cartilage on the other hand (Duterloo, 1967; Duterloo and Walters, 1972; Koski and Rönning, 1965, 1970; Meikle, 1973; Melchor, 1971; Vilmann, 1971). Condylar cartilage (a secondary cartilage) studied by Charlier, Petrovic, and Herrmann-Stulzmann (1969), McNamara (1972), and Durkin, Heeley, and Irving (1973) does not parallel the modes of growth of the synchondroses, a fact that leaves its role in the growth of the mandible uncertain.

The changes occurring in terms of appositional bone growth and resorptive changes (bone remodeling) would seem to be an intricate and well-controlled system sensitive to both intrinsic and extrinsic factors (Cleall, Wilson, and Garnett, 1968; Enlow, 1963). The nature of some of these factors has been extensively studied and includes such influences as the piezoelectric effect as demonstrated by Bassett and co-workers (1961, 1962, 1968). These studies have shown that deformation of bone produces measurable piezoelectric potentials that increase with tension and decrease with pressure. Apposition of bone seems to be promoted in electronegative areas.

Sutures, while in the past held to be primary sites of growth, have now been relegated to an important but adaptive role (Baer, 1954; Cleall, et al., 1965; Cleall, Wilson, and Garnett, 1968; Watanabe, Laskin, and Brodie, 1957). The importance of appositional and resorptive changes as a mode of bone growth has been well-known and was emphasized by some of the early workers. However, a well-defined description of the process involved had been lacking until Enlow (1962, 1966, 1968) published a series of papers on the subject. His data were primarily derived from the histologic study of skull bones. Each bony component of the skull undergoes an individual process of remodeling growth. This is carried out by a complex balance of periosteal and endosteal deposition and resorption and involves most of the inside and outside surfaces of the bone. Thus a bone may "drift" by progressive deposition on one side and resorption on the other; it may rotate by a disproportionate change, and, as the whole process is three-dimensional, areas of a bone may be relocated in virtually any direction (Fig. 3-3). However, these changes are well controlled and are capable of accurate description and even prediction for a given bone.

As the bones of the craniofacial region continue to grow, they are also simultaneously displaced away from each other. Displacement or translation may be primary (that is, a local displacing movement) or secondary (that is, moved by the growth of structures often far-removed from the bone in question) (Fig. 3-4).

While Enlow has tended to separate and characterize these various remote and local modes of growth, it must be remembered that not only the overall size, shape, and growth pattern of the craniofacial region but also the ultimate

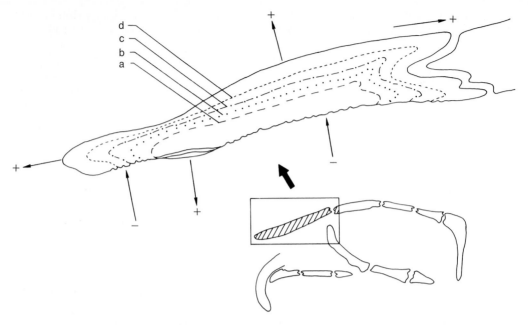

Fig. 3-4. Displacement. Parasagittal section of rat skull showing growth changes demonstrated by sequential bone-marking agents. Appositional growth on superior surface of nasal bones with concomitant intranasal resorption results in local displacement of bone in space. Bone is also displaced anteriorly by growth on nasal side of frontonasal suture. Adjacent bone (frontal bone) also contributes to this displacement. *a,* Terramycin, *b,* alizarin red S; *c,* Terramycin and alizarin red S; *d,* Terramycin and trypan blue.

size, shape, and growth progress of the individual bones are a combination of these well-integrated processes. Also, these changes themselves are the result of the interactions of the form and functions of the region being studied. Enlow's approach is most useful but is qualitative in nature. Quantitative data, such as are required for clinical work, still must come from other sources, for example, the prevalent, but often misunderstood literature based on cephalometric radiography.

The present concepts of craniofacial growth have shifted from the consideration of where and how the craniofacial bones grow to the more general and biologically sound approach of "why" these changes occur and in what relationship to the functional activities of the region. Much of our current thinking has been prompted by the papers of Moss (1962, 1969) and is embodied in his "functional matrix theory," which was, to a degree, based on the earlier concepts of Van Der Klaauw (1946, 1948). Although supported

by often inconclusive evidence, Moss' concepts have provided considerable stimulus to other workers in the field. His work and suggestions by Dullemeijer (1968) and Van Limborgh (1972) have provided us with a more holistic and viable approach to the riddle of craniofacial growth. The study of "abnormal" growth in subjects with craniofacial anomalies (nature's experiments) (Pruzansky, 1961) has also added greatly to our knowledge.

MORPHOLOGIC CRANIOFACIAL AGE CHANGES
General aspects

Growth proceeds at an ever-diminishing rate from conception to maturity. In terms of successive cell divisions, for example, it has been estimated roughly that prenatally some 44 successive cell divisions take place compared to only 4 during postnatal life. It, therefore, becomes apparent that in terms of the shape and function of structures most of the important growth changes occur prior to birth. Postnatally, the overall growth rate

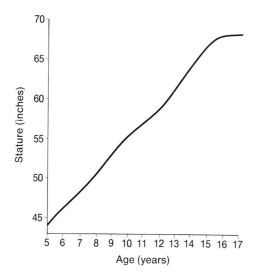

Fig. 3-5. Usual distance curve for increase in height as function of age.

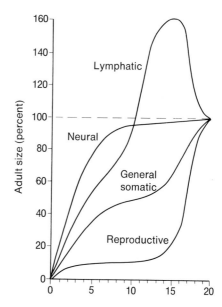

Fig. 3-6. General growth curves are shown for several body systems. Note early development of brain and nervous system and relative late maturation of genital system.

gradually decreases, but with recognizable periods of relative acceleration such as the pubertal "growth spurt" (Fig. 3-5).

Sexual dimorphism exists for some growth parameters, and individual tissues or systems decelerate at differing rates. The classic example of this latter point was presented by Scammon (1930). The distance curve of general body growth shows the relative pubertal growth acceleration, and this should be contrasted with the relative changes in the brain, head, and reproductive system. These differential growth rates are also reflected in changes in overall body proportions during growth (Fig. 3-6). At birth, the head has already grown to approximately 65% of its adult size. However, the individual's height at birth is only about 30% of that which is finally attained at maturity. The head, therefore, is relatively well-developed at birth. This cephalocaudal growth gradient appears to hold true for many species, including man, as well-demonstrated by Scammon and Calkins (1929). However, Ford (1955) has shown that this growth gradient in man is reversed anterior to the limit of the notochord (embedded in the future cranial base) and, as such, would account for several of the later, relatively

extensive changes in the facial region with growth.

While major species differences do exist, there seems to be ample evidence that postnatal craniofacial growth in the human follows, in general terms, a pattern similar to other mammals. The brain and neurocranium demonstrate an early rapid period of growth, while the facial region grows more slowly for an extended period and tends to follow the general somatic growth curve. Gradients of growth also exist in terms of postnatal facial proportions. Again, in general terms, an increase in craniofacial depth tends to exceed an increase in height, which in itself often appears to be greater (at least in the face) than the width increase. Krogman's (1951) data substantiate these differential growth changes, demonstrating that postnatally the viscerocranium in the human undergoes 65% to 70% of its total growth in depth, 55% to 60% in height, and 40% to 45% in width.

Within the craniofacial structures, the postnatal differential growth gradients account for the changes that are the major concerns for those clinicians responsible for following or altering the morphology or function of the craniofacial region.

Maturity indicators

The changes in the size and shape of the craniofacial structures from birth to maturity are measured as a function of time. However, our standard references of time in days, months, and years have little to do with the biologic passage of time in the growing tissues of an individual. Therefore efforts have been made to consider biologic indicators of time. These maturity indicators include height and weight age, bone age, and dental age.

Most height and weight tables simply use mean data derived from normal, healthy, growing children and relate the numerical data to chronologic age. The problem with the use of these tables is that they do not take into consideration the fact that children do not all reach the same size and therefore during development could also be expected to vary in size. The Wetzel grid (1943) for evaluating physical fitness is a more sophisticated system of assessing the overall growth of a child. Growth progress is assessed using this system by comparing the individual's growth curve with a subgroup of children having a similar physique. While this maturity indicator gives some indication of the overall growth progress and the effects of such relative accelerations as the pubertal "growth spurt," overall growth may not be well-correlated with facial growth. However, when used in conjunction with the other indicators, it has proved useful to clinicians for many years.

Bone age has been used for some time as an indication of the degree of skeletal maturation. Radiographic standards have been developed to determine the order, rate, time of appearance, and progress of ossification of the bones in several areas of the body (Greulich and Pyle, 1959; Hoerr and Pyle, 1955; Pyle and Hoerr, 1955; Todd, 1937). Using these systems, the clinician obtains a standardized radiograph of the skeletal structures being assessed and compares this with the standard films reproduced in the at-

las. An indication is thereby gained as to the degree of retardation, or otherwise, of the subject's bony skeleton. It is assumed that bone maturation in one region of the skeleton reflects the overall bone age (Tanner, Whitehouse, and Healy, 1962a). More recently, Acheson (1954) and Tanner (1962a,b) developed a series of standard stages through which each bone passes. Identifiable bones in the hand and wrist radiographs are matched with these standards, giving a maturation score.

A simplified modification of the Oxford method (Acheson, 1954) has proved useful in orthodontics for assessing the adolescent "growth spurt" and thereby assisting the clinician in timing his treatment to use the period of maximal growth. In this system, various stages of skeletal maturation are assessed from the hand-wrist film and related to body height. While helpful around the pubertal growth period, it must be pointed out that although correlation of wrist maturation to body height is fairly reliable, the nature of any relationship to facial growth is, as yet, unclear. These maturation indicators cannot be relied on to predict accurately the onset of such clinically important parameters as the pubertal growth spurt, the magnitude of growth increments, or the duration of growth.

Many oral procedures require that an assessment of dental age be made. The eruption of the dentition provides a useful measure of dental maturation and tables were published as early as 1837 (Saunders). Longitudinal studies have been reported by several authors, including Stones and co-workers (1951), Fulton and Price (1954), and Carr (1962). The radiographic assessment of tooth development would seem to be more reliable than tooth eruption, and the works of Bengston (1935), Pinney (1939), Gleiser and Hunt (1955), Garn and co-workers (1958), Nolla (1960), and Fanning (1961) have resulted in fairly consistent and reliable data.

Because none of the maturation indices so far developed has a very high statistical correlation with the timing of growth in all facial structures, the clinician would be wise to use some or all of those mentioned, if an effort is to be made to assess the growth period that an individual patient has reached. Certainly, a reliance on only chronologic age to assess the postnatal stage of development would seem to be inadequate.

Overall craniofacial growth changes

Postnatal growth of the craniofacial region has been studied and described in terms of both the overall changes and by considering the growth of related parts. As has been discussed, growth mechanisms operate both generally and locally, with a multitude of regulatory and interacting feedback systems. Therefore, growth of one part, in a strict morphologic sense, cannot be considered without also concurrently considering the growth interactions with other parts. Functional "fields" may cross bony or soft tissue structural boundaries, and individual bones or organs may involve more than one functional activity. The following description of postnatal craniofacial growth will adhere to the traditional regional approach for no other reason than ease of presentation.

The craniofacial structures at birth appear to be small with little facial depth, the face being tucked-in under the cranium, and the overall features showing a more rounded appearance than in the adult. The decelerating rate of postnatal enlargement of the cranial base and calvaria becomes dominated by the relatively more rapid enlargement of the facial structures. The brain, with its capsule, probably triples in volume in the first 2 years of life, and then growth slows down. After the seventh year, growth is minimal and may well have ceased by puberty. The facial skeleton, however, not only grows faster than the brain case postnatally, but it also continues to grow for a much longer period (perhaps, in some regions, into the third decade of life) (Colby, 1972).

A stable reference point must be selected in order to follow the overall changes in the spatial relationships of the craniofacial structures during the postnatal growth period. Ideally, this site will not be growing or changing. No such re-

gion exists in absolute terms, and, therefore, one must settle for the area showing the least postnatal growth change. An area related to the earlier developing brain, and perhaps to the more primitive (phylogenetically) regions of the brain, would seem to be logical. The bony elements lend themselves to the measurement techniques available (for example, radiography and histology). Therefore it is not surprising that a position somewhere in, or near, the cranial base has been a traditional orientation site. In the coronal plane, midline cranial base structures seem to offer the most promising starting points for width and height assessments; the sagittal plane aspect involves the sella turcica, ethmoid complex, basisphenoid, and frontonasal region.

When related to the middle of the cranial base, in general terms, the upper face and nasal structures move forward with growth, thus reducing the apparent bulging of the infant's forehead. The upper face increases in the vertical direction, with a considerable increase in the size of the nasal cavity. The large eyes of the child become relatively less apparent as the surrounding hard and soft tissue facial structures develop. The base of the skull in the region of foramen magnum moves downward and backward, and at a faster rate than the petrous temporal region. Hence, in effect, the ears are higher in the adult. A major and obvious change occurs in the lower facial region, where the chin moves downward and forward. The dentition drops back in the face. Collectively, these differential growth rates are reflected in the facial profile as a progressive flattening, and from the frontal view as a lengthening of the face with a well-developed dental area and wider mandible.

Growth of the craniofacial region is a three-dimensional process. The literature is replete with descriptive and statistical data (mainly from cephalometric radiography) on the growth changes, as assessed from the lateral aspect (Fig. 3-7). On the other hand, information on changes in the frontal plane are relatively few in number. Fortunately, as most post-

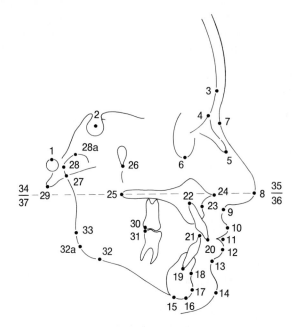

Fig. 3-7. Several commonly used cephalometric landmarks are shown. Interrelationship of these landmarks is used to assess both growth changes, as diagnostic aid to assess facial abnormalities, and to evaluate orthodontic or surgical treatment changes. *Key: 1*, porion; *2*, sella turcica; *3*, frontale; *4*, nasion; *5*, tip of nasal bone; *6*, orbitale; *7*, soft tissue nasion; *8*, pronasale; *9*, soft tissue "A" point; *10*, upper lip; *11*, lip contact; *12*, lower lip; *13*, soft tissue "B" point; *14*, soft tissue pogonion; *15*, menton; *16*, gnathion; *17*, pogonion; *18*, "B" point; *19*, apex of lower central incisor; *20*, incisal edge of upper incisor; *21*, incisal edge of lower incisor; *22*, apex of upper central incisor; *23*, "A" point; *24*, anterior nasal spine; *25*, posterior nasal spine; *26*, pterygomaxillary fissure; *27*, articulare; *28*, posterior surface of condyle; *28a*, condylion; *29*, basion; *30*, distobuccal cusp of maxillary first permanent molar; *31*, disto-buccal cusp of mandibular first permanent molar; *32*, posterior inferior border of mandible; *32a*, gonion; *33*, posterior border of ramus; *34, 35, 36,* and *37*, maxillary and mandibular transfer axes (for computer analysis).

natal growth is greatest and growth abnormalities more frequent in the anteroposterior or vertical directions, the relative lack of width data is less a handicap to the clinician than it might appear at first sight.

A few years after the advent of cephalometric radiography, Broadbent (1937) published a composite pattern of facial growth, which showed that the face moved downward and forward from under the cranial base in an orderly and consistent manner. Tracings of successive films were superimposed on the cranial base. The growth vectors were such that there appeared to be a straight-line pattern of landmark migration during growth. Broadbent contended that growth of the face was not as complex or erratic as it had seemed to be from earlier

craniostatic studies. More recently, a complete analysis of his data has been published (1975). Computer-derived polygon plots, using this published mean data for boys and girls combined, are presented in Fig. 3-8.

Brodie (1941), using some of Broadbent's material in a longitudinal study of children from the age of 3 months to 8 years, and again, in 1953, using a sample from 8 years to 17 years, concluded that the change in position of the cephalometric landmarks in the face, with time, were integrated such that the anatomic points fell on a series of straight lines. The data were interpreted to show that the morphologic pattern of the head was established early in postnatal life and, therefore, remained constant. Unfortunately, both Broadbent and Brodie based

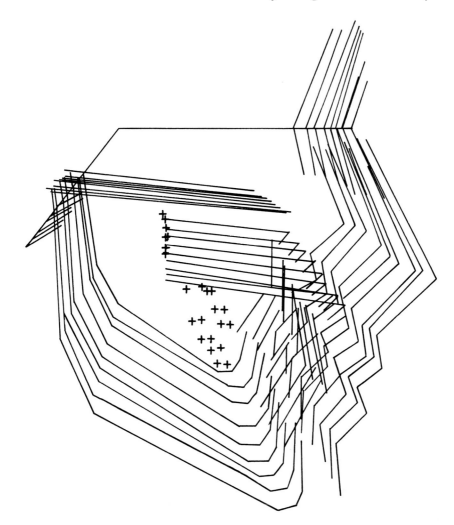

Fig. 3-8. Selected, computer-derived, polygon plots of mean data for boys and girls combined. Age sequence is 1, 2, 3, 5, 7, 9, 12, 14, and 17 years. (From Broadbent, B. H. 1975. Bolton standards of dentofacial developmental growth, St. Louis, The C. V. Mosby Co.)

their conclusions on mean data, which precluded the demonstration of any individual variation. Brodie, unlike Broadbent, however, did recognize that individual variations occurred.

Baum (1951) felt that the face of a child did not have the same proportions as the face of a young adult; the child tends to have a more convex face, with a more protrusive dentition. His description seems to contradict the idea of constancy of facial growth and supports the work of Hellman (1935). This "constancy" concept was finally discounted by Björk

(1955) who, with the aid of cephalometric radiography supplemented with metallic implants, verified the existence of individual facial variation within the craniofacial structures during growth.

Cranial base

The cranial base consists of the basioccipital, sphenoid, and ethmoid bones. It partitions the brain from the deep structures of the face. Despite its phylogenetic background, the frontal bone is included as a part of the anterior cranial base by several authors. To a degree, this inclusion relates to the use of nasion as a cephalometric landmark in growth studies (Fig. 3-7).

During the late prenatal period of development, the cranial base consists of a number of separate bony elements, with possibly a fair degree of individual freedom of movement. There appears to be some variability in shape at this time, although a general tendency is for the cranial base to flatten with growth.

At the time of birth, the nonbony elements of the midline cranial base region, which ossify in cartilage, have been reduced to the synchondroses between the sphenoid and occipital bones and between the presphenoid and ethmoidal complex. While the role of these cartilages is still unclear, it would seem that differential growth at these sites may be responsible for some of the changes in the cranial base seen during postnatal growth (DuBrul and Laskin, 1961; Vilmann, 1971). However, remodeling changes in the bones themselves have also been amply demonstrated by Enlow (1968) in the human and are noted in other species by Cleall and co-workers (1968).

On the average, the cranial base seems, postnatally, to undergo a gradual flexure, and this is coincident with the late stages of brain growth. At approximately 10 years of age, the brain has reached almost its full size and the cranial base appears to be reaching its final shape. However, while the morphologic pattern of the cranial base remains relatively stable with age, Björk (1969) has demonstrated from cephalometric radiographic studies that this region does change even through adolescence and the late teens and that the changes are individual in nature. He points out that any rotation of the cranial base can influence the anteroposterior position of the mandible.

Fusion of the several ossification centers in the various components of the developing cranial base occurs at or shortly before birth. Development proceeds thereafter in two stages according to Scott (1958) and Ford (1958). The two sphenoid centers are united at birth, and ossification of the cribriform plate and ethmoid bone occurs between the first and third years. The sphenoethmoidal synchondrosis closes early in life, and this area of the anterior cranial base seems to become relatively stable in terms of growth thereafter. However, the area between the foramen cecum and nasion may not show this stability (according to some authors) and, consequently, measurements from nasion could be affected by subsequent growth changes. Several authors have observed the continued thickening of the frontal bone during postnatal growth (Ford, 1958; Scott, 1958; and Stramrud, 1959), again perhaps making this region suspect in terms of its use as a stable landmark for measurements.

The posterior cranial base (often measured from basion to sella) is often referred to as having a skeletal rather than a neural growth pattern (Brodie, Jr., 1955; Ford, 1958; and Stramrud, 1959) in that it exhibits continued growth to adulthood. The spheno-occipital synchondrosis is an important contributor to this growth and appears to be active into late adolescence. Most authors feel that bony fusion occurs somewhere between 17 to 25 years of age, although this wide range may be on the high side according to Powell and Brodie (1963). The slightly different growth behavior of the anterior and posterior cranial base regions may account for some of the lack of uniformity reported from radiographic growth studies that use different parts of the cranial base as reference points to assess facial changes.

Remodeling growth changes in the cranial base are subtle but important (Fig. 3-9). The intracranial surface is largely resorptive, with bone apposition occurring on the extracranial surface (mainly on the inferior surfaces of the sphenoid). This area, therefore, is drifting inferiorly and anteriorly. The pterygoid plates are good examples of the mode of appositional growth in this region in that the pterygomaxillary fissure is situated at the posterior surface of the maxillary complex.

Cranial vault

The cranial vault functions to protect and support the brain. As such, it follows

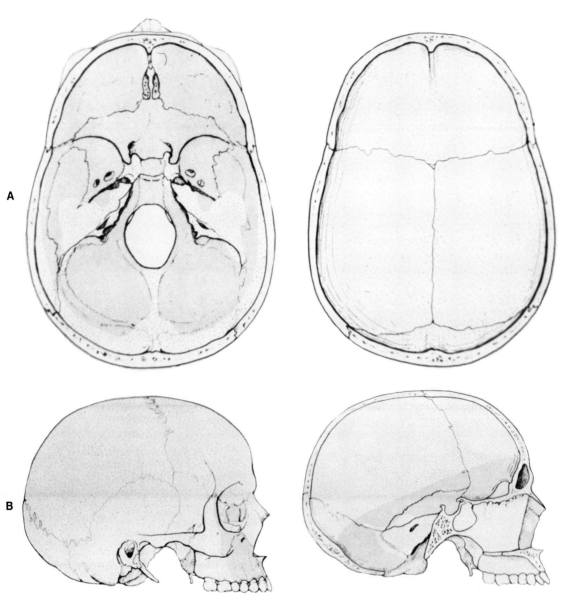

Fig. 3-9. Distribution of resorptive (dark stippled area) and depository (light stippled area) periosteal surfaces of cranium. **A,** Dorsal view of cranial floor (left) and inner side of cranial vault (right). **B,** These views are of lateral external surface (left) and lateral internal surface (right). (From Enlow, D. H., 1968. The human face, New York, Hoeber Medical Division, Harper & Row, Publishers, Inc.)

the neural pattern of growth to a considerable degree. The cranial vault is made up of bones that have ossified in membrane and consists of the frontal, the parietal, the squamous part of the occipital, the temporal, and a portion of the greater wings of the sphenoid bone.

This region enlarges by sutural changes and by appositional growth and includes extensive remodeling concomitant with brain enlargement as the bones drift apart. Differential growth at different parts of the sutures plus remodeling changes on the flat surfaces of the bones

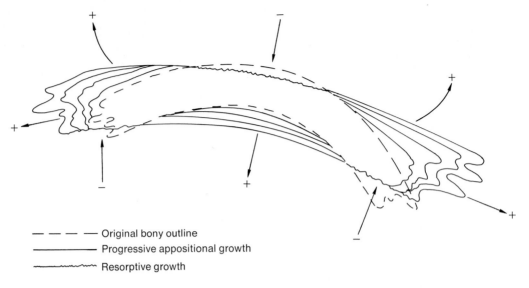

— — — — Original bony outline

———————— Progressive appositional growth

∼∼∼∼∼∼∼ Resorptive growth

Fig. 3-10. Diagrammatic representation of parasagittal section of rat calvarium in which sequential bone-marking agents were deposited. Remodeling changes over 66-day period beginning with 90 gm rats show progressive flattening of parietal bone. Note disproportionate appositional changes near the center and extremities of bone. Adjustments also occur in sutures between adjacent bones.

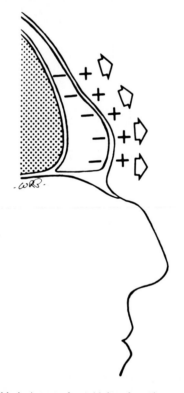

Fig. 3-11. As long as frontal lobe of cerebrum continues to grow, inner table of forehead also continues to drift in anterior direction. By sixth or seventh year, frontal lobe enlargement slows and ceases; and growth of inner table also terminates. Outer table continues its forward drift, thus permitting frontal sinus to enlarge. (From Enlow, D. H., 1975. Handbook of facial growth, Philadelphia, W. B. Saunders Co.)

allow the skull to flatten during growth (Fig. 3-10). A reversal line encircles the intracranial surface of the cranium (Fig. 3-9, *A*). Above this line, apposition of bone occurs, while below the line the surface is resorptive (Enlow, 1968). The skull bones thicken with age and the extra-cranial surfaces vary from resorptive (where flattening is to occur) to passive, through to appositional (for example, at the site of some muscle attachments). No diploë exists in the thin skull bones at birth, but with subsequent growth and remodeling of the inner and outer tables, space is developed for an extensive diploë. As the brain enlarges, extensive changes occur at the sutures. These act as adjustment sites and seem to adapt in amount and type of reaction to the demands established by growth.

The infant's forehead appears to be prominent and rounded, with the most anterior bulge being higher than in the adult. During childhood, the outer plate of the frontal bone increases in thickness and drifts anteriorly, producing the frontal eminences and allowing the frontal sinus to develop (Fig. 3-11).

The zygomatic arch serves as an important site of muscle attachment and also as a flying buttress to transmit functional forces from the facial skeleton backward to the cranium. Bizygomatic width increases during postnatal life almost until adulthood. Apart from cranial base and cranial sutural growth in width, which possibly carries the zygomatic arch laterally, there are important growth changes in the structure itself. The zygomaticotemporal suture continues to grow for a longer time than any other facial suture (Scott, 1956) and would seem, therefore, to represent an important adjustment site between lateral cranial growth and facial growth.

Upper and midfacial skeleton

The upper and midfacial skeleton region consists of several bones having different origins. Most are membranous bones, including the maxillary, lacrimal, palatine, and zygomatic bones. Others, including the ethmoid and inferior turbinates, ossify in cartilage. Growth research relating to the midfacial skeleton has centered around the controversy mentioned earlier as to the importance of the sutures and the cartilaginous nasal septum.

The nasomaxillary complex of bones is carried forward by growth of the anterior cranial base, which satisfies several functional requirements including an increase in depth of the upper airway. Growth of the cartilaginous nasal capsule prenatally and continued growth of the nasal septum postnatally also would seem to be of importance especially in early childhood (Schundy, 1964; Scott, 1953). Scott observed the upper part of the nasal cavity to be well developed at birth, while noting that the lower part continues to grow until adulthood. He also states that the width dimensions of the upper nasal cavity are approximately 75% of the adult size by 1 year of age and are fully developed by about 10 years of age. The lower part, on the other hand, continues to develop in both width and height beyond the first decade of life.

The importance of the septal cartilage is also emphasized by Sassouni and Forrest (1971), who report that the septal cartilage is rarely deviated before 7 years of age. They consider the deviations seen later to be caused by continued growth of the nasal septum with a lack of concomitant adjustment at the surrounding sutures.

Much experimental work has been done to establish the role played by the nasal septal cartilage in growth of the midface (Babula, 1970; Moss et al., 1968; Wexler and Sarnat, 1965). According to Moss, the growth of the nasal septum is secondary and compensatory to the primary growth of the nasal cavity. Thus he contends that the septal cartilage is basically passive and grows in response to the related orofacial functional matrices. Sarnat and Wexler (1966), on the other hand, believe that their septal resection experiments support the concept that the septum is a primary growth site. The conflicting results from some of these studies and also including additional research by Jarabak and Thompson (1949), Gianelly and Moorrees (1965), Hall-Craggs and Lawrence (1969), and Sarnat (1971) have left the role of cartilage in growth somewhat undecided.

The role played by the sutures in the postnatal development of the region cannot be denied. However, most evidence seems to point to the conclusion that these sites serve as major remodeling areas and are capable of considerable variability in terms of the amount and direction of their adjustment. Both clinical (Haas, 1970; Issacson and Ingram, 1964; Wertz, 1970) and animal (Henry, 1973; Starnback, et al., 1966) studies suggest that through the use of heavy orthodontic force systems, the facial sutures are capable of considerable modification during growth (Figs. 3-12, and 3-13). The sutures appear to be major sites of bone apposition in the midfacial region and would, therefore, seem to present ideal target sites for therapeutically induced facial growth modification or for compensatory modification when functional or other growth processes are abnormal.

Local surface appositional and resorptive changes play a large part in the postnatal shaping and increase in size of the midfacial region. The predominant direction of maxillary growth, for example, is posteriorly and superiorly with corre-

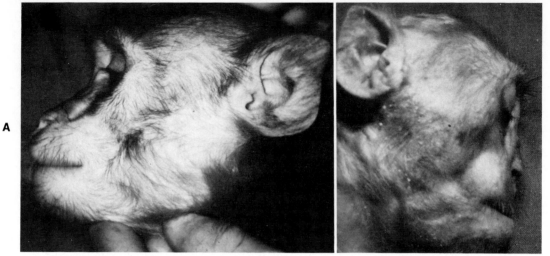

Fig. 3-12. A, Facial profile of rhesus monkey prior to application of "orthopedic" headgear. **B,** Animal after application of heavy forces to maxillary complex using tooth and soft tissue-borne appliance for several months.

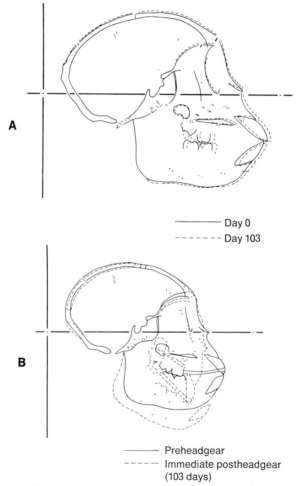

——— Day 0
- - - - - Day 103

——— Preheadgear
- - - - - Immediate postheadgear
(103 days)

Fig. 3-13. Tracings of radiographs of monkey subjected to "orthopedic" headgear therapy. **A,** Superimposed tracings (registered on cranial base metallic implants) of normally growing, untreated animal. **B,** Superimposed tracings of experimental animal to which approximately 800 gm per side of force were applied to maxillary complex for stated time interval. Note great distortion in pattern of facial growth. (From Henry, H. L. 1973. Craniofacial changes induced by "orthopedic forces" in the Macaca mulatta rhesus monkey. Thesis. University of Manitoba.)

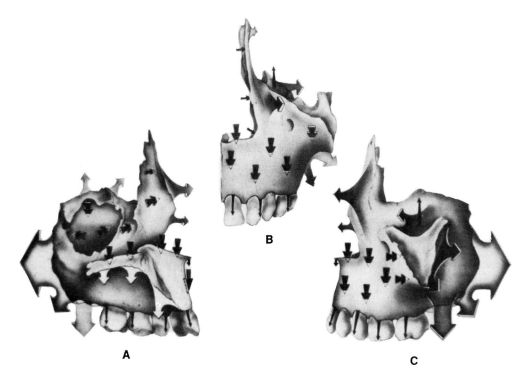

Fig. 3-14. Diagram showing details of maxillary growth as ascertained by Enlow. **A,** Medial surface; **B,** frontal view; **C,** lateral aspect. (From Enlow, D. H. 1968. The human face, New York, Hoeber Medical Division, Harper & Row, Publishers, Inc.)

sponding anterior and inferior displacement. However, very specific and detailed remodeling is continually occurring on most surfaces of all the facial bones (Fig. 3-14). An example of the interactions of sutural and remodeling changes during palatal and maxillary incisor eruption is shown in Fig. 3-15. This diagram is made from parasagittal sections of a series of growing rats that had received sequential injections of bone-marking agents. There are differing amounts of growth occurring at each side of both the premaxillary-maxillary suture and the maxillary-palatine suture. The bone apposition on the oral surface of the hard palate is complemented by resorption on the nasal surface such that the palate drifts toward the oral cavity. Similar changes in the human, although hard to quantify, are well-documented by Enlow and Bang (1965) and are shown in an overall manner in Fig. 3-16.

The nasomaxillary region is complex in its phylogenetic origin, having changed from a triangular shape to that of a more boxlike structure. Also, the complexity of the functional activities associated with the region would suggest that no single driving force, for example, growth of the nasal septum, could be responsible for growth in this area. Moss' "functional matrix theory" (1962) has done much to help us understand the possible interactions of soft tissue growth, growth of the hard tissue structures, and the functional activities of the area.

As the nasomaxillary region becomes displaced forward and downward, extensive bone apposition occurs on the posterior surface, especially in the area of the tuberosity. This allows the dental arch to be increased in length and thus permits the accommodation of successive posterior teeth. Differing modes of bone growth can be observed in the bones themselves as the whole complex is carried downward and forward away from the cranial base. The surfaces of the bones forming the nasal cavity, associated mainly with

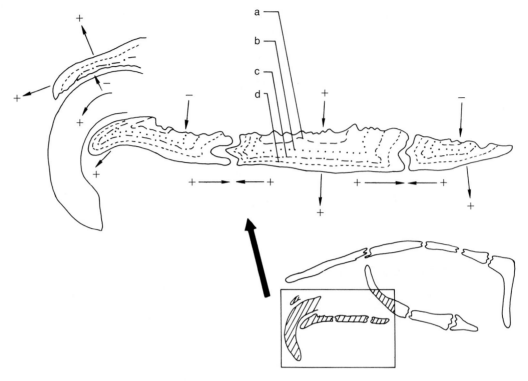

Fig. 3-15. Pattern of bone growth as shown by sequential bone-marking agents in hard palate region in rat. Positive signs indicate bone apposition and negative signs show areas of bone resorption. *a,* Terramycin; *b,* alizarin red S; *c,* Terramycin and alizarin red S; *d,* Terramycin and trypan blue; *e,* alizarin red S.

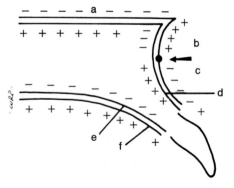

Fig. 3-16. Surface *a* is resorptive; *b* is depository. Reversal occurs precisely at "A" point (indicated by arrow; this is common cephalometric landmark). Periosteal surface *c* is resorptive; *d* is depository; surface *e* is resorptive; and periosteal surface *f* is depository. (From Enlow, D. H., 1975. Handbook of facial growth, Philadelphia, W. B. Saunders Co.)

respiratory function, largely show resorption (the vertical plate of the ethmoid being an exception). The oral surfaces, on the other hand, basically show apposition.

The bony orbits undergo complex postnatal changes. It has been shown by Ford (1958) that the interorbital growth in width of skulls exceeds 10 mm from age 2 years to adulthood. Much of the bone growth in the orbit is appositional. The lateral surface and inferior walls show this, while considerable remodeling changes occur in the lacrimal bones and

several of the surrounding facial sutures to permit the downward and outward displacement of the whole complex and the increasing dimensions of the openings. Extensive appositional changes occur on the rims of the orbits, thus permitting the orbital cavities to become deeper. The neural content of the orbits, however, is well developed early in childhood and with orbital growth the

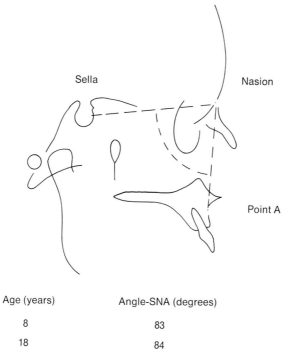

Age (years)	Angle-SNA (degrees)
8	83
18	84

Fig. 3-17. Minimal change in angular relationship of point "A" to anterior cranial base measured cephalometrically. This is an average figure for a group of subjects and may increase or decrease slightly depending on individual variation in summation of all related growth sites.

eyes tend to become less prominent. This region, therefore, seems to develop not only in relationship to the eyes themselves but also to the nasal cavity, oral area, and developing brain.

The combination of forward and downward displacement, posterior appositional growth, and addition of bone at facial sutural margins suggests that the midface should become increasingly protrusive relative to the cranial base. However, cephalometric measurements, for example, the angle between the anterior cranial base (sella nasion) to nasion point A on the maxilla, show a relative constancy with growth (Fig. 3-17). In part, this can be accounted for by some forward appositional growth in the upper face at nasion, but it is also attributable to the fact that in man much of the change in the facial surface of the maxilla and premaxilla is resorptive (other mammals, especially long-snouted animals, show apposition). The net effect, then, of all these changes

is that the midfacial region grows in a largely downward direction. Cephalometric studies have demonstrated this point. Coben (1955) reported that the midfacial region increased more in height than it did in depth. In a longitudinal study of 52 males, Savara and Singh (1968) also showed this. They described the dimensions of height as having the most rapid rate of growth in the maxillary complex, followed by length and width, respectively. Ricketts' (1961) data also support this assumption of midfacial growth. He reported that forward growth of the maxilla was similar to forward growth at nasion, as measured along the nasion-sella line, and amounted to approximately 1 mm per year, while the vertical growth of the maxilla was approximately one third of the total increase in facial height. The contribution in height made by the midface to the total facial height has been examined by Cannon (1970) and, while the picture is far from clear, it appears likely that at least during childhood the nasal area increases vertically at a greater rate than does the total face.

This downward vector of growth is further emphasized by the vertical component of growth in the maxillary alveolus. As major appositional growth occurs at the crest of the ridge, some additions are made at the lateral and posterior surfaces. However, in the anterior part of the arch, resorption is considered to take place (Enlow and Bang, 1965). To some degree these changes are reflected in the changes seen in the dentition, in which some buccal expansion occurs with growth, while the anterior part of the dental arch flattens and the incisors become less proclined anteriorly. The vomer, like the maxilla, shows growth in an upward and backward direction and is thereby displaced downward and forward, being specially adapted to slide on the anteroinferior surface of the sphenoid (Takagi, 1964).

Growth of the palatine processes of the maxilla and, in general, also the palatine bone is well-integrated into these downward growth vectors. The hard palate grows backward by addition to the posterior surface and resorption on the nasal surface. The combined effects of lowering the hard palate and downward movement of the maxilla account largely for the great increase in the vertical dimension of the nasal cavity with growth. The lateral growth in the region is related to growth in the midpalatal suture and to remodeling changes.

The growth changes just mentioned, if occurring alone, would result in a relatively massive structure, whereas even a superficial examination of the midface impresses the observer with the delicate nature of many of the bones. The development of the sinuses in the maxilla and ethmoid are important in this respect, and the overall architectural arrangement in the midface is an excellent example of economy of calcified tissue, but with well-developed stress pathways that permit the maintenance of structural integrity to support the functional requirements of the region.

The zygomatic bone is described by Weinmann and Sicher (1955) as having three processes (frontal, temporal, and maxillary), and thereby it has growth and functional associations with the cranial vault, cranial base, and the midfacial structures. As a site for major muscle attachment and a stress pathway, it would be expected to increase in size considerably and undergo precise remodeling changes. The anterior malar portion of the bone drifts backward along with the posterior shift of the zygomatic process of the maxilla and seems to keep pace with the elongation of the tuberosity. The anterior surface undergoes resorption, and this serves to move the lateral orbital rim posteriorly. Despite this resorption, adjustments in the sutures allow the region to be displaced anteriorly and inferiorly along with the whole maxillary complex. The lateral surface of the bone shows appositional growth and, with concomitant medial resorption, the result contributes to an increase in bizygomatic width.

Lower face

The mandible is the skeletal component of the lower face. Studies using cephalometric radiography have often inferred that the mandible grows downward and forward. However, over 200 years ago Hunter (1771) recognized that this bone actually grows in a predominantly upward and backward direction toward the base of the skull.

The mandible, at birth, may be present as two halves connected by fibrous tissue. Union of the two halves occurs during the first year and, whereas in many animals this area may provide a growth and often a functional adjustment site, in the human all subsequent change must involve remodeling in other parts of this single unit. During postnatal life, growth changes involve almost all surfaces of the bone.

The mandible, on the average, is carried downward and forward. Much of the bone growth relating to this change occurs at the condyle. However, Brodie (1941) showed that the glenoid fossa was carried inferiorly and posteriorly with growth, a change that in itself would contribute to a vertical displacement of the mandible. Björk (1955) in his implant studies showed that a rotation of the cranial base would also affect the temporal bones and, hence, the mandible. According to Björk, depending on the direction of this rotation, the glenoid fossa would move downward and forward or upward and backward. Mandibular and maxillary position would be similarly affected.

Most authors agree that anteroposterior and vertical growth changes in the mandible occur predominantly at the condyles (Björk, 1955; Brodie, 1941; and Sassouni, 1958). As the condylar cartilage grows upward and backward, or upward and forward, it is replaced by bone and the whole mandible translates in a downward and forward direction. In opposition to those who visualize the condyle as a primary site of mandibular growth, Moss (1962) and Moss and Salentijn (1969) contend convincingly that the mandible is composed of several functional components, including an alveolar portion, the coronoid process, the gonial region, the condylar area, and a basilar portion, and that all of these respond to the needs of the teeth, nerves, muscles, and blood vessels. Moss considers the condylar cartilages simply to be centers where secondary compensatory growth changes can occur in response to forward translation of the mandible. A similar conclusion was reached by Sorenson and Laskin (1975) based on studies involving condylectomy and subcondylar ostectomy.

While constancy of the gonial angle with growth has been claimed by some authors (Björk, 1947; Brodie, 1941; and Weinmann and Sicher, 1955) and rejected by others (Jensen and Palling, 1954), Björk (1963) (with the aid of implants) and Maj and Luzi (1964) have shown cephalometrically that this response is variable and may depend on growth vectors elsewhere (for example, at the condyle), or that a change may be masked by compensatory changes in the ramus or body of the mandible.

That an ongoing series of remodeling changes occurs has been well-documented histologically by Enlow (1968) in human skulls and by Cleall and Chelib (1971) in rats (Figs. 3-18 and 3-19). In the human these necessary remodeling changes were demonstrated in the condyle by Enlow who showed that as the condyle grows upward and backward, apposition of bone occurs on both the anterior and posterior surfaces of the neck of the condyloid process, thus increasing the depth of this area as the neck blends into the ramus. But the condyle is broad laterally so that with upward and backward growth, as the bone progressively becomes relocated into the neck, the medial and lateral sides of the neck undergo resorption. These latter changes are compensated for by bone apposition on the endosteal surfaces of the neck.

The lateral surface of the coronoid process shows resorption that, with apposition on the medial side, allows this structure to maintain its relationship to the adjacent cranial and midfacial structures as a muscle attachment while the condyle grows posteriorly. The anterior border of the ramus is also predominantly a resorptive area, although rotational changes in the mandible may make this variable. The posterior and lateral surfaces of the ramus (below the condylar neck and coronoid process) are basically appositional. As the apposition on the posterior surface exceeds the resorption on the anterior border, the ramus generally becomes wider. The medial surface of the ramus behind the coronoid process, however, is largely resorptive, which along with the lateral apposition tends to flare the posterior margin and gonial angle laterally.

Traditionally, for descriptive purposes, the mandible has been divided into two parts: the ramus and the body. This division, while anatomically acceptable, is, however, an arbitrary one and different partitions may be more appropriate when considered on a functional and/or phylogenetic basis. In terms of its postnatal morphogenesis, the division into ramus and body also loses its impact when it is realized that a sizable proportion of the body is developed by the progressive remodeling of the ramus.

As the ramus grows posteriorly, apposi-

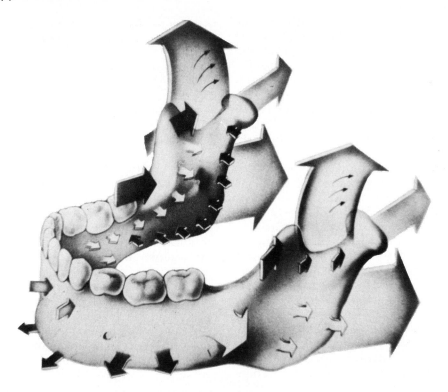

Fig. 3-18. Regional growth and remodeling changes in human mandible. Arrows represent direction and approximate magnitude of changes. (From Enlow, D. H., and Harris, A. 1964. Am. J. Orthodont. **50:**25, 1964).

tional growth occurs on the medial side of the body near the alveolar border, this area serving to support the posterior end of the dental arch as the rami grow apart. Below this region the lingual surface in the human shows resorption (Enlow, 1968). The lateral surface of the body undergoes largely appositional remodeling and, although variable, this is often quite prominent in the chin region.

The height of the body of the mandible increases during postnatal growth and this is accomplished by extensive apposition at the alveolar border and probably some apposition on the lower border. Björk (1969), however, has suggested that the lower border changes are variable, and perhaps in some subjects it undergoes considerable resorption, especially in the posterior region near the angle. The antegonial notch moves posteriorly with posterior ramal growth. The mental foramen tends to be variable in its direction of movement with growth. Lateral apposi-

tion in this region will tend to move the foramen in the direction in which the neurovascular bundle exits the bone, and this region is, as a consequence, a dubious landmark for assessing dental changes.

Temporomandibular joint

The temporomandibular joint is unique in the body and differs from other synovial joints in several respects. During prenatal life the morphology of this structure lags behind other synovial joints both in terms of the timing of its appearance and also its progress such that at birth the joint is still largely underdeveloped.

The articular surfaces of both the condyle and temporal bones are covered with fibrous connective tissue at the time of birth. Later this is slowly converted to fibrocartilage as the fossa deepens and the condyle develops under functional influences. Extensive remodeling changes

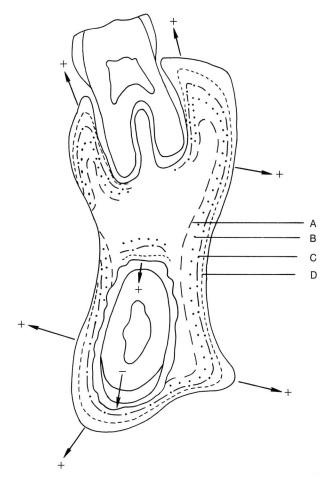

Fig. 3-19. Diagramatic representation of cross section at third molar region of rat. Appositional growth changes are shown by sequential bone-marking lines. Note growth of alveolus and lower border. Passive area on lingual surface just below alveolus is also of interest. *A*, Terramycin; *B*, alizarin red S; *C*, Terramycin and alizarin red S; *D*, Terramycin and trypan blue; and *E*, alizarin red S.

occur during postnatal life. Changes involving an increase in the posterior slope of the articular tubercle and an increase in the depth of the mandibular fossa are reported up to the fourth decade of life (Moffett, 1966).

The complex phylogenetic background of the temporomandibular joint, the fusion of the two sides of the mandible in man, and the lack of cuspal wear (in "civilized" man) all pose intriguing physiologic and pathologic problems for the clinician.

Postnatal remodeling changes occur in bone adjacent to the joint in harmony with mandibular growth and growth of the cranial base and temporal bone. Neuromuscular and occlusal changes are also reflected in discrete bony and functional changes in the joint region.

Dentition

Growth of the jaws in many species seems to be closely related to the development of the teeth and the maintenance of their occlusion. This is most obvious in animals with continuously growing incisors, such as the rat, where the jaws appear to be composed largely of the teeth, with a minimal amount of surrounding bone. Human craniofacial morphologists rarely place this importance on the teeth

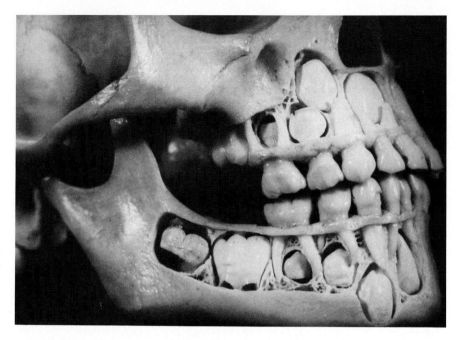

Fig. 3-20. Photograph of dissected skull of child in late primary dentition period. Note large number of erupted and developing teeth present in both maxilla and mandible.

and yet even a superficial examination of the child's skull will in fact reveal the relative enormity of the amount of dental units, relative to bone, in the region. The jaws are literally "stacked" with erupted or unerupted teeth during childhood, and one must be amazed at the manner in which these dental units manage to move into orderly, functional positions during growth (Fig. 3-20).

The position of the developing teeth is initially determined prenatally by the dental lamina, but as this structure becomes enclosed by the bone of the developing jaws a host of position-influencing factors become operable. Prenatal and postnatal variability of the development of the primary and permanent teeth and occlusions becomes manifest and is characterized by such things as bilateral asymmetry in shape, size, and position of teeth, sexual dimorphism, and differences in eruption timing.

The primary teeth begin to erupt at about 6 months of age and the primary dentition is usually complete approximately 2 years later (Table 3-1). Eruption

Table 3-1. Eruption of primary teeth*

Age (months)	Number of teeth
6	One third of children have 1 or more teeth
9	Mean: 3 teeth; 80% have between 1 and 6 teeth
12	Mean: 6 teeth; 50% have between 4 and 8 teeth
18	Mean: 12 teeth; 85% have between 9 and 16 teeth
24	Mean: 16 teeth; 60% have between 15 and 18 teeth
30	Mean: 19 teeth; 70% have all primary teeth

*Adapted from Meredith, H. V. 1946. J. Dent. Res. **25**:43.

of the individual teeth does not begin until root formation has started and this process of primary tooth – root formation is usually complete by about 3 years of age. The primary tooth eruption sequence, while somewhat variable, usually conforms to the following pattern: lower central incisor, upper central incisor, upper lateral incisor, lower lateral incisor, lower and upper first molars, lower and upper canines, lower second molar, and upper second molar.

Dental development and the timing of eruption are variable between individuals and can be used, as mentioned earlier, as an indication of dental maturity. The development of a good occlusion or of possible malocclusion would seem to be related more to the sequence of tooth eruption in an individual than the time of eruption per se.

Once the primary teeth come into occlusion the child develops an "occlusal sense" and masticatory movements become orderly. The shape of the dental arches and the relationship of the individual teeth seem to be less variable in the primary dentition than in the permanent dentition, and this point is substantiated by the lower incidence of malocclusion observed for the primary dentition.

The arch form during the primary dentition period (2½ years to 6 years) tends to be ovoid, and owing to differential upper and lower second molar sizes, there usually is a flush terminal plane distal to the molars. Spacing between the anterior teeth often exists, and although this may increase toward the end of this developmental period (perhaps because of marked attrition of the tapering incisor crowns), the total arch circumference in fact is progressively reduced (Arnold, 1954). During the later part of this period, considerable occlusal wear may occur and the overbite and overjet may be reduced to a minimum.

With the eruption of the first permanent molars at approximately 6 years of age, the mixed dentition period begins. This transitional period is most important to the clinician in that changes of major importance relating to the final achievement of an acceptable permanent occlusion or signs of future malocclusion take place during this period. The mean ages of permanent tooth eruption for boys and girls, as ascertained by Hurme (1949), are shown in Fig. 3-21. A permanent tooth may begin to erupt once its crown is fully formed and it usually reaches the level of the alveolar crest when two thirds of the root is formed and erupts into the mouth when three-fourths has developed (Shumaker and El Hadary, 1960). Use of defined stages of tooth development (Nolla, 1960) and the timing of these events (Fanning, 1961) has led to useful eruption prediction indices.

The sequence of permanent tooth eruption is more variable than for the primary dentition. Knott (1966) has established that about 50% of children develop the sequences of 3, 8, 7, 5, 4, 6, 2 and 14, 9, 10, 12, 11, 13, 15 in the maxillary arch. In the mandible, sequences of 30 and 25, 26, 27, 28, 29, 31 and 19 and 24, 23, 21, 22, 20, 18 include over 40% of children. Generally, eruption of the mandibular tooth precedes eruption of the similar maxillary tooth. The usual sequence for boys is as follows: lower first molar, upper first molar, lower central incisor, upper central incisor, lower lateral incisor, upper lateral incisor, upper first premolar, lower canine, lower first premolar, upper second premolar, lower second premolar, upper canine, lower second molar, and upper second molar. The sequence in girls is similar, except that the lower canine often precedes the eruption of the upper first premolar. The eruption schedule for girls usually is ahead of that for boys by several months.

Owing to the presence of the second primary molars, the first permanent molars tend to be limited in their positional adjustments soon after eruption. They may have a cusp-to-cusp relationship if a flush terminal plane of the primary second molars exists. This arrangement usually alters during the mixed dentition period, relating possibly to subsequent mandibular growth, closing of the "primate" spaces, or loss of the "leeway" space (Baume, 1950; Moorrees, 1954; Nance, 1933; Sillman, 1953).

Most studies on the development of occlusion have used plaster models, often with no coincident examination of cephalometric radiographs; consequently they have emphasized the anteroposterior changes that occur with growth. However, it must be remembered that changes in the vertical dimension in the oral region far outweigh these anteropos-

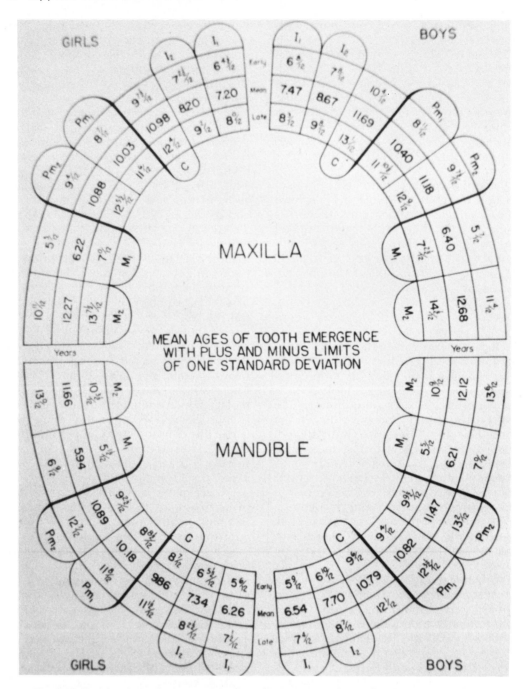

Fig. 3-21. Eruption times of permanent dentition. (From Hume, V. O., and The Forsyth Dental Center. 1949. J. Dent. Child. **16**:11.)

terior adjustments. The occlusal table may be likened to a joint with sutures on each side (the periodontal supporting structures) and confluent with two rapidly growing bony structures (the maxilla and mandible). The complex nature of occlusal adjustments and their degree of integration with the other growth parameters in the region provide fertile ground for therapeutic experimentation but difficulty in accurate prediction.

Changes in the dimensions of the dental arches are usually described in the anteroposterior direction as arch length changes (usually measured at the midline from the mesial aspect of the central incisors to a line tangent to the distal aspect of the second primary molars or mesial to the first permanent molars). Arch width is a measure of the lateral dimension and may be expressed from comparable teeth on each side of the arch or from the midline (median raphe in the maxilla or its projection vertically for the mandibular arch). Arch width is often measured in the canine and molar regions. Another important arch dimension for the clinician is arch circumference, which is usually expressed as the length of the line (in a smooth curve) from the distal aspect of the primary second molar or mesial aspect of the permanent first molar on one side around the arch through the contact points and incisal edges to a comparable point on the other side. The development of asymmetries in the form of the arches may become of concern, and the vertical relationship of the teeth, measured as incisor overbite or "open bite," and the curve of Spee, may pose important dimensional growth and diagnostic problems for the clinician.

During the mixed dentition period the mandibular arch circumference undergoes several interesting changes. The permanent lower incisors often erupt lingually to the relatively "upright" lower primary incisors and then tip labially as they continue to erupt (Milne and Cleall, 1970), thus producing a slight increase in the anterior circumference of the arch. However, in the late mixed and early permanent dentitions, these teeth upright along with continued forward mandibular growth and continued vertical growth of the alveolus. These changes coupled with the loss of the larger mandibular primary molars, which are replaced with the smaller premolars, result in a reduction in lower arch circumference (Knott, 1961; Speck, 1950). This generally is true for both sexes.

The maxillary arch behaves somewhat differently. While there is a slight reduction in arch length in the buccal segments in the late mixed dentition period owing to the differential in primary and permanent tooth size (as in the mandible), this is often offset by an increase in the circumference from canine to canine owing to the relative proclination of the permanent upper incisors and their vertical change at this angulation. Later, during adolescence, these teeth do upright, but the net effect is either a slight overall increase in maxillary arch circumference or, at most, a small decrease.

Dental arch width increases during the mixed dentition and early permanent dentition stages. This change is more pronounced in the maxilla. While lateral dentoalveolar changes (DeKock, 1972; Woods, 1950) and growth of the midpalatal suture are important, the great vertical component of alveolar growth combined with the divergence of the buccal segments must play a large part in the increase in width of the maxillary arch (Cleall, 1974).

The edge-to-edge or minimal overbite incisor relationship often noted at the end of the primary dentition stage of development usually is followed by a great increase in overbite, which is often followed during adolescence with a slight reduction in this parameter. Associated changes in the curve of Spee are also noted. These dimensional changes are the usual or average changes. However, the variability on an individual basis is great and it behooves the clinician to recognize and evaluate this individual variation before any therapeutic procedure, for example, orthodontic treatment or serial extraction, is instituted.

Dental arch dimensional changes with growth are three-dimensional, as are all craniofacial growth changes. Changes in one dimension will be associated with, or elicit compensatory changes in, another dimension. This important consideration must be remembered by the clinician. For example, the oral and maxillofacial surgeon who wishes to change the anteroposterior relationship in a mandibular prognathism must remember that unless an existing deep overbite or an arch width or length discrepancy is not corrected (often orthodontically), his efforts may prove to be partially acceptable in terms of facial esthetics but disastrous in terms of the dentition.

The changing relationship of the mandible to the maxilla with growth and the continuous remodeling of facial bones with extensive sutural adjustments are related to a whole host of associated dental changes. While few comprehensive studies combining dental changes as assessed from dental casts and skeletal changes determined cephalometrically are available, much interesting data from separate studies are in the literature and a knowledge of the possible interactions is mandatory for any clinician concerned with predicting and treating dentofacial growth problems.

Integumental profile

The integumental profile is made up of the soft tissues covering the facial skeleton. Growth of these tissues has a variable relationship to the growth of the underlying bones, depending on the area under consideration. This, in part, is responsible for some of the problems in interpreting direct clinical measurements made on growing children.

The skeletal profile tends to become less convex with age. The denture becomes less protrusive and the incisors upright. These changes are, however, only partially mirrored in the soft tissue profile. This point was demonstrated by Subtelny (1959) in a cephalometric radiographic study in which he showed that while the skeletal profile becomes less convex with age, the total soft tissue profile, if the nose is included, becomes more convex. If, on the other hand, the nose is excluded, the soft tissue profile remains relatively stable in its degree of convexity. Hambleton (1964) largely concurs with these findings, noting that as the mandible is translated forward, the soft tissue follows it. He also observed a thickening and lengthening in the lips and, like Subtelny, emphasized the importance of the growth of the nose.

The nose grows downward and forward. In childhood the tip of the nose is somewhat retruded, but this is followed by its swinging out from under the cranium. The dorsum tends to elevate with continued growth of the nasal bones during adolescence (Chaconas, 1969; Kiser, 1960; Subtelny, 1959).

Growth of the soft tissue covering bony nasion and the bony chin seems to follow the underlying skeletal structures more closely with growth. The lips and anterior teeth also bear a fairly consistent relationship with growth. It would seem, therefore, that a clinician seeking a mandibular or maxillary change as a result of treatment might expect a fairly harmonious concomitant soft tissue change with continued growth; however, he must be aware of the relatively independent type of change to be expected in the nose (especially during adolescence).

FUNCTIONAL MATURATION

While the morphologic changes occurring with postnatal growth are fairly well documented in the literature, the detailed changes in the functional activities in the region are poorly recorded. The importance of function is well recognized, but our ability to describe and measure maturational changes and the interactions of these with the growing facial skeleton is limited. The vital functions of airway maintenance and deglutition and the lesser functional significance of mastication and the overlayed function of speech seem to undergo degrees of maturational change closely related to the alterations in the size and shape of the craniofacial structures.

The maintenance of an adequate airway during growth to sustain the need for oxygen would seem to be of prime consideration. The development of protective reflexes are life-sustaining, and some of the morphologic/physiologic interactions in childhood have been examined in detail (Bosma, 1973). The early development and extensive degree of neuromuscular control of the pharyngeal region is well demonstrated in the cinefluorographic records of the patient shown in Fig. 3-22. This baby with Pierre Robin syndrome had a tracheotomy tube in place that bypassed the upper airway. Selected frames from the cinefluorographic film show the great ability to open the collapsed airway when the tube

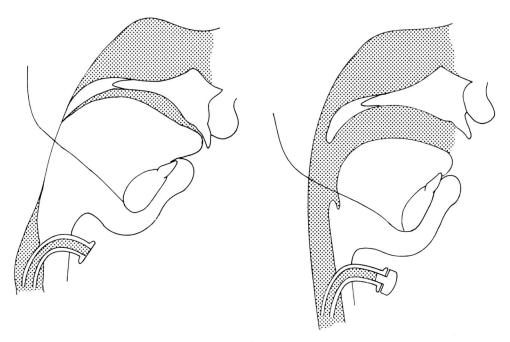

Fig. 3-22. Changes in airway following temporary blockage of tracheotomy tube used to bypass upper airway. Tracings are shown from selected cinefluorographic film frames.

is temporarily blocked. These extensive alterations in function may well be reflected in structural changes over the long term.

An infant has the ability to suckle and swallow and still breathe at the same time. With neck and cranial base growth, the proximity of the soft palate and epiglottis in the infant is lost and these coincidental functional abilities no longer exist. This is an interesting example of a form/function interrelationship that changes during maturation.

The relationship of mouth breathing and the presence of enlarged and inflamed tonsils and adenoids has long posed a difficult diagnostic question for the clinician. At the present time (as a generalization) the consensus is that no firm cause and effect relationship can be ascribed to these conditions and the development of dentofacial abnormalities and malocclusion. However, animal studies involving nasal airway restriction do suggest subtle but measurable changes (Chalk, 1974) and one is left with the feeling that our clinical measurement

systems are largely too inaccurate to record the changes taking place.

Cross-sectional studies considering airway, tongue size and position, head posture, and morphologic interactions are available (Cleall, Alexander, and McIntyre, 1966; Yip and Cleall, 1971). However, there are few longitudinal studies in humans. The tongue does seem to drop back slightly and come to occupy relatively less of the oral cavity with growth. This and similar changes in position and perhaps function are presumably closely related to structural changes with growth.

Coordinated swallowing movements occur before birth. The presence of amniotic fluid in the stomach of the neonate confirms this statement. Protective reflexes in the pharynx and well-controlled functional movement patterns during swallowing (a function that has protective aspects to it as well as ingestive) are noted at birth. Apart from loss of the ability to breathe and swallow at the same time, mentioned earlier, functional changes in the region with growth are well ordered and are coincident with local morphologic changes. The neuromuscular control of the anterior aspect of the oral cavity may be less well developed in early childhood than the pharyngeal region. Lip and tongue control during suckling is such that considerable loss of fluids from the mouth is normal. The infant's tendency to drool saliva is also evidence of this.

During childhood the lips, tongue, and mandible come to act in well-coordinated movement patterns. Before the eruption of the teeth, the tongue and lips make contact during swallowing. Following eruption, the tongue tends to remain behind the teeth and swallowing becomes a characteristic fluid motion (Fig. 3-23).

While the muscles of mastication do serve to stabilize the mandible during suckling, the jaw movements during this function do not seem to be closely related to those later associated with mastication. An "occlusal sense" develops rapidly as the teeth erupt. Rhythmic jaw movements during mastication develop, the details of which would seem to be closely related to the positions of the teeth and the morphology of the jaws and muscle masses. The range of postural positions of the mandible or the movements during mastication are very flexible during childhood. Rapid and often transitory changes occur as the local occlusal relationships change. Long-term changes are also manifest and relate to the differential rates of jaw growth and to the development of the temporomandibular joint.

Speech, as an overlayed function of the oropharyngeal region, uses the structures primarily designed for the more vital functions (Bosma, 1975). Successful speech development relies on adequate structural form and neuromuscular con-

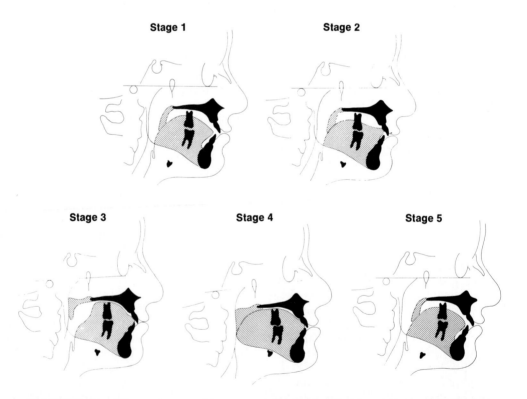

Fig. 3-23. Series of diagrams prepared from mean data for series of subjects with normal swallowing patterns. Standardized lateral cinefluorographic records were made of saliva clearance swallows. *1,* Rest prior to swallowing; *2,* tongue tip elevation; *3,* dorsum of tongue rolls back to junction of hard and soft palate; *4,* hyoid bone in most superoanterior position; *5,* structures return to rest position after swallowing sequence.

trol in the region, including good velopharyngeal valving and the development of finely controlled lip, tongue, and mandibular movements.

GROWTH PREDICTION

Knowing, in general terms, the sites and directions of craniofacial growth and being able to quantitate many of the changes using cephalometric radiography, it would seem logical to apply this knowledge and predict growth prospects for our clinical patients. This ability would enable the dentist to plan accurately any therapeutic procedures should a developing deformity be recognized.

Unfortunately, while useful as a guide to future growth, the predictive systems in use today (Schulhof and Bagha, 1975) are not accurate enough to permit the clinician to rely heavily on them (Harris, 1976; Horwitz and Hixon, 1966). These systems essentially use the average increment of growth for each measurable parameter using "norms" just as the diagnostician may use standards to assess the characteristics of a craniofacial deformity. However, the individual growth variability is of such magnitude that no good clinician will blindly follow the dictates set by mean data. Correlations of craniofacial structures with each other during growth are not high and, therefore, the use of prediction tables based on these correlations is also of only limited value. Most forecasting systems in use assume that the individual will grow the average amount and that the pattern of growth will remain stable. Many individual patients do not conform to these assumptions thus rendering any growth prediction suspect. As more is learned regarding the variations of growth, so the predictive ability of the clinician will increase.

REFERENCES

Acheson, R. M. 1954. The Oxford method of assessing skeletal maturity, Clin. Orthop. **10**:19.

Adams, J. W. 1940. Correction of error in cephalometric roentgenograms, Angle Orthod. **10**:3.

Anderson, G. 1955. Practical orthodontics, ed. 8., St. Louis, The C. V. Mosby Co.

Arnold, E. 1954. A study of the significance of the interdental spacing in the primary dentition.

Thesis. Horace H. Rackham School of Graduate Studies, University of Michigan, Ann Arbor.

Babula, W. J. 1970. Role of the cartilaginous nasal septum in midfacial growth, Am. J. Orthod. **58**: 250.

Baer, M. J. 1954. Patterns of growth of the skull as revealed by vital staining, Hum. Biol. **26**:80.

Bassett, C. A. L. 1968. Biological significance of piezoelectricity, Calcif. Tissue Res. **1**:272.

Bassett, C. A. L., and Becker, R. O. 1962. Generation of electric potentials by bone in response to mechanical stress, Science **137**:1063.

Bassett, C. A. L., and Hermann, I. 1961. Influence of oxygen concentration and mechanical factors on differentiation of connective tissue in vitro, Nature **190**:460.

Baum, A. T. 1951. Cephalometric evaluation of the normal skeletal and dental patterns of children with excellent occlusion, Angle Orthod. **21**:96.

Baume, L. J. 1950. Physiological tooth migration and its significance for the development of occlusion, J. Dent. Res. **29**:123.

Belchier, J. 1736. An account of the bones of animals being changed to a red color by ailment only, Philosoph. Tr. **39**:286.

Bengston, R. G. 1935. A study of the time of eruption and root development of the permanent teeth between six and thirteen years, Northwestern Univ. Bull. **36**:3.

Björk, A. 1947. The face in profile, Sven, Tandlak. Tidskr. **40**:56.

Björk, A. 1955. Facial growth in man, studied with the aid of metallic implants. Acta Odontol. Scand. **13**:9.

Björk, A. 1963. Variations in the growth pattern of the human mandible: longitudinal radiographic studies by the implant method, J. Dent. Res. **42**: 400.

Björk, A. 1969. Prediction of mandibular growth rotation, Am. J. Orthod. **55**:535.

Bosma, J. F., ed. 1973. Oral sensation and perception, U.S. Department of Health, Education, and Welfare, Bethesda, Md.

Bosma, J. F. 1975. Anatomic and physiologic development of the speech apparatus. The nervous system, vol 3. Human communication and its disorders, New York, Raven Press.

Brader, A. C. 1956. Historical review of research findings of growth and development prior to the introduction of roentgenographic-cephalometry, Angle Orthod. **26**:1.

Brash, J. C. 1924. The growth of the jaws, normal and abnormal, in health and disease, London, Dental Board of the United Kingdom.

Broadbent, B. H. 1931. A new x-ray technique and its application to orthodontia, Angle Orthod. **1**:45.

Broadbent, B. H. 1937. The face of the normal child, Angle Orthod. **7**:183.

Broadbent, B. H. 1975. Bolton standards of dentofacial developmental growth, St. Louis, The C. V. Mosby Co.

Brodie, A. G. 1941. On the growth pattern of the human head from the third month to the eighth year of life, Am. J. Anat. **68**:209.

Brodie, A. G. 1953. Late growth changes in the human face, Angle Orthod. **23**:146.

Brodie, A. G., Jr. 1955. Behavior of the cranial base and its components as revealed by serial cephalometric roentgenograms, Angle Orthod. **25:**148.

Brown, T. 1965. Craniofacial variations in a central Australian tribe. Master's thesis. University of Adelaide, South Australia.

Camper, P. 1792. Dissertation sur les varietes naturelles qui caracterisent la physionomie des hommes des divers climats et des differents ages, suivie de reflexions sur la beaute, particulierement sur celle de la tete; avec une maniere nouvelle de dessiner toute sorte de tetes avec la plus grande exactitude. Traduct du hollandais par H. J. Jansen; on y a joint une dissertation du meme auteur sur la meilleune forme des souliers, Paris, Francart.

Cannon, J. 1970. Craniofacial height and depth increments in normal children, Angle Orthod. **40:**202.

Carr, L. M. 1962. Eruption ages of permanent teeth, Aust. Dent. J. **7:**367.

Chaconas, S. J. 1969. A statistical evaluation of nasal growth, Am. J. Orthod. **56:**403.

Chalk, W. N. 1974. The effect of unilateral nasal blockage on the growth of the rat craniofacial complex—a quantified gross and histological microscopic assessment. Thesis. University of Manitoba, Winnipeg, Man.

Charlier, J. P., Petrovic, A., and Herrmann-Stulzmann, J. 1969. Effects of mandibular hyperpropulsion on the prechondroblastic zone of young rat condyle, Am. J. Orthod. **55:**71.

Chebib, F. S., Cleall, J. F., and Carpenter, K. S. 1976. On-line computer system for the analysis of cephalometric radiographs, Angle Orthod. **46:**305.

Cheek, D. B. 1968. Human growth, Philadelphia, Lea & Febiger.

Cleall, J. F. 1964. Bone marking agents for the longitudinal study of growth in animals, Arch. Oral Biol. **9:**627.

Cleall, J. F. 1972. Circumstances limiting the development and verification of a comprehensive theory of craniofacial morphogenesis, Acta Morphol. Neerl. Scand. **10:**115.

Cleall, J. F. 1974. Growth of the palate and maxillary dental arch, J. Dent. Res. **53:**1226.

Cleall, J. F., and Chebib, F. S. 1971. Coordinate analysis applied to orthodontic studies, Angle Orthod. **41:**214.

Cleall, J. F., Alexander, W. J., and McIntyre, H. M. 1966. Head posture and its relationship to deglutition, Angle Orthod. **36:**335.

Cleall, J. F., Wilson, G. W., and Garnett, D. S. 1968. Normal craniofacial skeletal growth of the rat, Am. J. Phys. Anthropol. **29:**225.

Cleall, J. F., et al. 1965. Expansion of the midpalatal suture in the monkey, Angle Orthod. **35:**23.

Coben, S. E. 1955. The integration of facial skeletal variants, Am. J. Orthod. **41:**407.

Colby, W. B. 1972. Cephalometric analysis of the Northern Foxe Basin Eskimo: a cross-sectional study. Thesis. University of Manitoba, Winnipeg, Man.

Craven, A. H. 1956. Growth in width of the head of the Macaca Rhesus monkey as revealed by vital staining, Am. J. Orthod. **42:**341.

Davenport, C. B. 1940. Postnatal development of the head, Proc. Am. Phil. Soc. **83:**1.

DeKock, W. H. 1972. Dental arch depth and width studied longitudinally from 12 years of age to adulthood, Am. J. Orthod. **62:**56.

Downs, W. B. 1948. Variations in facial relationships: their significance in treatment and prognosis, Am. J. Orthod. **34:**812.

DuBrul, E. L., and Laskin, D. M. 1961. Preadaptive potentialities of the mammalian skull: an experiment in growth and form, Am. J. Anat. **109:**117.

Dullemeijer, P. 1968. Some methodology problems in an holistic approach to functional morphology, Acta Biotheor. **18:**203.

Durkin, J. F., Heeley, J. D., and Irving, J. T. 1973. The cartilage of the mandibular condyle, Oral Sci. Rev. **2:**29.

Duterloo, H. S. 1967. In vivo implantation of the mandibular condyle of the rat. Doctoral dissertation. University of Nymegen, Nymegen, Netherlands.

Duterloo, H. S., and Walters, J. M. 1971. Experiments of the significance of articular function as a stimulating chondrogenic factor for the growth of secondary cartilages of the rat mandible, Eur. Orthod. Soc. Trans. **1971:**103, 1972.

Enlow, D. H. 1962. A study of postnatal growth and remodeling of bone, Am. J. Anat. **110:**79.

Enlow, D. H. 1963. Principles of bone remodeling, Springfield, Ill., Charles C Thomas, Publisher.

Enlow, D. H. 1968. The human face: an account of the postnatal growth and development of the craniofacial skeleton, New York, Hoeber Medical Division, Harper & Row, Publishers.

Enlow, D. H. 1975. Handbook of facial growth, Philadelphia, W. B. Saunders Co.

Enlow, D. H., and Bang, S. 1965. Growth and remodeling of the human maxilla, Am. J. Orthod. **51:**446.

Enlow, D. H., and Hunter, W. S. 1966. A differential analysis of sutural and remodeling growth in the human face, Am. J. Orthod. **52:**823.

Fanning, E. A. 1961. A longitudinal study of tooth foundation and root resorption, N.Z. Dent. J. **57:**202.

Felts, W. J. L. 1959. Transplantation studies in skeletal organogenesis. 1. The subcutaneously implanted immature long-bone of the rat and mouse, Am. J. Phys. Anthropol. **17:**201.

Ford, E. H. R. 1955. The growth of the foetal skull. M.D. thesis. University of Cambridge.

Ford, E. H. R. 1958. Growth of the human cranial base, Am. J. Orthod. **44:**498.

Fulton, J. T., and Price, B. 1954. Longitudinal data on eruption and attack of the permanent teeth, J. Dent. Res. **33:**65.

Gans, B. J., and Sarnat, B. G. 1951. Sutural facial growth of the Macaca rhesus: a gross and serial roentgenographic study by means of metallic implants, Am. J. Orthod. **37:**829.

Garn, S. M., et al. 1958. The sex difference and tooth calcification, J. Dent. Res. **37:**561.

Gianelly, A. A., and Moorrees, C. F. A. 1965. Condylectomy in the rat, Arch. Oral Biol. **10:**101.

Gleiser, I., and Hunt, E. E. 1955. The permanent

mandibular first molar: its calcification, eruption, and decay, Am. J. Phys. Anthropol. **13**:253.

Goldstein, M. S. 1936. Changes in dimension and form of the face and head with age, Am. J. Phys. Anthropol. **22**:37.

Graber, T. M. 1966. Orthodontics: principles and practice, Philadelphia, W. B. Saunders Co.

Greulich, W. W. 1958. Growth of children of the same race under different environmental conditions, Science **127**:515.

Greulich, W. W., and Pyle, S. I. 1959. Radiographic atlas of skeletal development of the hand and wrist, ed. 2, Stanford, Stanford University Press.

Haas, A. J. 1970. Palatal expansion: just the beginning of dentofacial orthopedics, Am. J. Orthod. **57**:219.

Hall-Craggs, E. C. B., and Lawrence, C. A. 1969. The effect of epiphyseal stapling on growth in length of the rabbit's tibia and femur, J. Bone Joint Surg. **51B**:359.

Hambleton, R. S. 1964. Soft tissue covering the skeletal face as related to orthodontic problems, Am. J. Orthod. **50**:405.

Harris, J. E. 1976. All in the family: use of familial information in orthodontic diagnosis, case assessment and treatment planning, Am. J. Orthod. **69**:493.

Hellman, M. 1927a. A preliminary study in development as it affects the human face, Dent. Cosmos **71**:250.

Hellman, M. 1927b. Changes in the human face brought about by development, Int. J. Orthod. Oral Surg. **13**:475.

Hellman, M. 1935. The face in its developmental career, Dent. Cosmos **77**:1.

Henry, L. H. 1973. Craniofacial changes induced by orthopedic forces in the Macaca mulatta rhesus monkey. Thesis. University of Manitoba, Winnipeg, Man.

Henry, L. H., and Cleall, J. F. 1974. Radiographic cephalometric method of assessment of craniofacial growth in monkeys, J. Dent. Res. **53**:369.

Higley, L. B. 1936. A new and scientific method of producing temporomandibular articulation radiograms, Int. J. Orthod. Oral Surg. **22**:983.

Hoerr, N. L., and Pyle, S. I. 1955. Radiographic atlas of the skeletal development of the foot, Springfield, Ill., Charles C Thomas, Publisher.

Hofrath, H. 1931. Bedeutung der roentgenfern-und abstandsoufnahme fur die diagnostik der kieferanomolien, Fortschr. der Ordhod. **1**:232.

Horowitz, S. L., and Hixon, E. H. 1966. The nature of orthodontic diagnosis, St. Louis, The C.V. Mosby Co.

Hunter, J. 1771. Natural history of the human teeth, London, John Johnson.

Hurme, V. O. 1949. Ranges of normalcy in the eruption of permanent teeth, J. Dent. Res. **28**:11.

Issacson, R. J., and Ingram, A. H. 1964. Forces produced by rapid maxillary expansion, Angle Orthod. **34**:261.

Jarabak, J. R., and Thompson, J. R. 1949. Cephalometric appraisal of the cranium and mandible of the rat following condylar resection, J. Dent. Res. **28**:655.

Jensen, E., and Palling, M. 1954. The gonial angle, Am. J. Orthod. **40**:120.

Keith, A., and Campion, G. G. 1922. A contribution to the mechanism of growth of the human face, Int. J. Orthod. Oral Surg. **8**:607.

Kiser, J. V. L. 1960. A serial radiographic cephalometric study on the growth of the soft and hard tissue of the nose in the midsagittal plane. Thesis. Chicago, Ill., Northwestern University.

Knott, V. B. 1961. Size and form of the dental arches in children with good occlusion studied longitudinally from age 9 years to late adolescence, Am. J. Phys. Anthropol. **19**:263.

Knott, V. B. 1966. Statistics on eruption of the permanent dentition from serial data for North American white children, Angle Orthod. **36**:68.

Koski, K. 1951. Roentgenographic cephalometric methods used in diagnosis of developmental disturbances of the dentofacial complex. A critical review, Odontol. Tidskr. **59**:11.

Koski, K. 1971. Some characteristics of craniofacial growth cartilages. In Moyers, R. E., and Krogman, W. M., ed.: Cranio-facial growth in man, Oxford, Pergamon Press.

Koski, K., and Rönning, O. 1965. Growth potential of transplanted components of the mandibular ramus of the rat III, Suom. Hammaslaak. Toim. **61**:292.

Koski, K. and Rönning, O. 1970. Growth potential of intracerebrally transplanted cranial base synchondroses in the rat, Arch. Oral Biol. **15**:1107.

Krogman, W. M. 1951. The problem of "timing" in facial growth, with special reference to the period of the changing dentition, Am. J. Orthod. **37**:253.

Krogman, W. M. 1970. Growth of head, face, trunk and limbs in Philadelphia White and Negro children of elementary and high school age, Monogr. Soc. Res. Child Dev., Serial No. 136, **35**:1.

Krogman, W. M., and Sassouni, V. 1957. Syllabus in roentgenographic cephalometry, Philadelphia, Philadelphia Center for Research in Child Growth.

Lacroix, P. 1952. The organization of bones, London, J. & A. Churchill, Ltd.

Maj, G., and Luzi, C. 1964. Longitudinal study of mandibular growth between nine and thirteen years as a basis for an attempt of its prediction, Angle Orthod. **3**:220.

Margolis, H. I. 1940. Standardized x-ray cephalographics, Am. J. Orthod. **27**:725.

Massler, M. 1944. Postnatal growth pattern of the facial skeleton as measured by vital injection of alizarin red S, J. Dent. Res. **23**:193.

Massler, M., and Schour, I. 1941. The growth of the cranial vault in the albino rat as measured by vital staining with alizarin red S, Anta. Rec. **110**:83.

McNamara, J. A., Jr. 1972. Neuromuscular and skeletal adaptations to altered orofacial function. Monograph No. 1. Craniofacial growth series, Center for Human Growth and Development, Ann Arbor, University of Michigan.

Meikle, M. C. 1973. In vivo transplantation of the mandibular joint of the rat—an autoradiographic investigation into cellular changes at the condyle, Arch. Oral Biol. **18**:1011.

Melcher, A. M. 1971. Behavior of cells of condylar

cartilage of foetal mouse mandible maintained in vitro, Arch. Oral Biol. **16:**1379.

Melson, B. 1975. Palatal growth studied on human autopsy material, Am. J. Orthod. **68:**42.

Meredith, H. V. 1946. Order and age of eruption for the deciduous dentition, J. Dent. Res. **25:**43.

Meredith, H. V. 1950. Measurements of Oregon school boys, Hum. Biol. **23:**24.

Mills, C. A. 1944. Climatic factors in health and disease. In Glasser, O., ed. Medical physics, Chicago, Year Book Publishers, Inc. p. 232.

Milne, I. M., and Cleall, J. F. 1970. Cinefluorographic study of functional adaptation of the oropharyngeal structures, Angle Orthod. **40:**267.

Moffett, B. 1966. The morphogenesis of the temporomandibular joint, Am. J. Orthod. **52:**401.

Moore, A. W. 1949. Head growth of the Macaque monkey as revealed by vital staining, embedding, and undecalcified sectioning, Am. J. Orthod. **35:**654.

Moorrees, C. F. A. 1954. Biometrics of crowding and spacing of the teeth in the mandible, Am. J. Phys. Anthropol. **12:**77.

Moss, M. L. 1962. The functional matrix. In Kraus, B. S., and Riedel, R. A., eds.: Vistas in orthodontics, Philadelphia, Lea & Febiger.

Moss, M. L., and Salentijn, L. 1969. The primary role of functional matrices in facial growth, Am. J. Orthod. **55:**566.

Moss, M. L., et al. 1968. The passive role of nasal septal cartilage in mid-facial growth, Plast. Reconstr. Surg. **41:**536.

Moulton, C. R. 1923. Age and chemical development in mammals, J. Biol. Chem. **57:**79.

Nance, H. N. 1933. Limitations of orthodontic treatment, Am. J. Orthod. Oral Surg. **4:**177.

Nolla, C. M. 1960. The development of the permanent teeth, J. Dent. Child. **27:**254.

Pacini, A. J. 1922. Roentgen ray anthropometry of the skull, J. Radiogr. **42:**230;322;418.

Petrovic, A. 1972. Mechanisms and regulation of condylar growth, Acta Morphol. Neerl. Scand. **10:**25.

Powell, T. W., and Brodie, A. G. 1963. Laminographic study of the sphenooccipital synchondrosis, Anat. Rec. **147:**15.

Prader, A., Tanner, J. M., and Von Harnack, G. A. 1963. Catch-up growth following illness or starvation, Pediatrics **62:**646.

Pruzansky, S. 1961. Congenital anomalies of the face and associated structures, Springfield, Ill., Charles C Thomas, Publisher.

Pyle, S. I., and Hoerr, N. L. 1955. Radiographic atlas of skeletal development of the knee, Springfield, Ill., Charles C Thomas, Publisher.

Ricketts, R. M. 1961. Cephalometric analysis synthesis, Angle Orthod. **31:**141.

Salzmann, J. A. 1960a. The research workshop on cephalometrics, Am. J. Orthod. **46:**834.

Salzmann, J. A. 1960b. Roentgenographic cephalometrics. Proceedings of the second research workshop, Philadelphia, J. B. Lippincott Co.

Sarnat, B. G. 1971 Surgical experimentation and gross postnatal growth of the face and jaws, J. Dent. Res. **50:**1462.

Sarnat, B. G., and Wexler, M. R. 1966. Growth of the face and jaws after resection of the septal cartilage in the rabbit, Acta. Anat. **118:**755.

Sassouni, V. 1958. Diagnosis and treatment planning via roentgenographic cephalometry, Am. J. Orthod. **44:**433.

Sassouni, V., and Forrest, E. J. 1971. Orthodontics in dental practice, St. Louis, The C. V. Mosby Co.

Saunders, E. 1837. The teeth as a test of age, considered with reference to the factory children; addressed to the members of both houses of parliament, London, H. Renshaw.

Savara, B. S., and Singh, I. J. 1968. Norms of size and annual increments of seven anatomical measures of maxillae in boys from three to sixteen years of age, Angle Orthod. **38:**106.

Scammon, R. E. 1927. The literature on the growth and physical development of the fetus, infant and child: a quantitative summary, Anat. Rec. **35:**241.

Scammon, R. E. 1930. The measurement of the body in childhood. In Harris, J. A., et al.: The measurement of man, Minneapolis, University of Minnesota Press.

Scammon, R. E., and Calkins, L. A. 1929. The development and growth of the external dimensions of the human body in the foetal period, Minneapolis, University of Minnesota Press.

Schulhof, A. B., and Bagha, L. 1975. A statistical evaluation of the Ricketts and Johnston growth-forecasting methods, Am. J. Orthod. **67:**258.

Schundy, F. F. 1964. Vertical growth versus anteroposterior growth as related to function and treatment, Am. J. Orthod. **34:**75.

Scott, J. H. 1953. The cartilage of the nasal septum. A contribution to the study of facial growth, Br. Dent. J. **95:**37.

Scott, J. H. 1956. Growth at facial sutures, Am. J. Orthod. **42:**381.

Scott, J. H. 1958. The cranial base, Am. J. Phys. Anthropol. **16:**319.

Shohl, A. T. 1939. Mineral metabolism, New York, Reinhold.

Shumaker, O. B., and El Hadary, M. S. 1960. Roentgenographic study of eruption, J.A.D.A. **61:**535.

Sillman, J. H. 1953. An analysis and discussion of oral changes related to dental occlusion, Am. J. Orthod. **39:**246.

Smith, H. G. 1974. Experimental alteration of the coronal sutural area: A histological and quantitative microscopic assessment. Thesis. Winnipeg, Man., University of Manitoba.

Smyth, C., and Young, M. 1932. Facial growth in children with special reference to dentition. Medical Research Council, Special Report Series No. 171. London, HMSO.

Sorenson, D. C., and Laskin, D. M. 1975. Facial growth after condylectomy or ostectomy in the mandibular ramus, J. Oral Surg. **33:**746.

Speck, N. I. 1950. A longitudinal study of developmental changes in human lower dental arches, Angle Orthod. **20:**215.

Starnbach, H., et al. 1966. Facioskeletal and dental changes resulting from rapid maxillary expansion, Angle Orthod. **36:**152.

Stones, H. H., et al. 1951. Time of eruption of permanent teeth and time of shedding of deciduous teeth, Br. Dent. J. **90:**1.

Stramrud, L. 1959. External and internal cranial base. A cross-sectional study of growth and association in form, Acta Odontol. Scand. **17:**239.

Subtelny, J. D. 1959. A longitudinal study of soft tissue facial structures and their profile characteristics, defined in relation to underlying skeletal structures, Am. J. Orthod. **45:**481.

Takagi, Y. 1964. Human postnatal growth of vomer in relation to base of cranium, Ann. Otol. Rhinol. Laryngol. **73:**238.

Tanner, J. M. 1962. Growth at adolescence, ed. 2, Oxford, Blackwell, Scientific Publications Ltd.

Tanner, J. M., Whitehouse, R. H., and Healy, M. J. R. 1962. A new system for estimating skeletal maturity from the hand and wrist, with standards derived from a study of 2,600 healthy British children. Part II. The scoring system, Paris, International Children's Centre.

Thurow, R. C. 1951. Cephalometric methods in research and private practice, Angle Orthod. **21:** 104.

Thurow, R. C. 1970. Atlas of orthodontic principles, St. Louis, The C. V. Mosby Co.

Todd, T. W. 1930. Facial growth and mandibular adjustment, Int. J. Orthod. Oral Surg. Radiol. **16:** 1243.

Todd, T. W. 1937. Atlas of skeletal maturation, St. Louis, The C. V. Mosby Co.

Topinard, P. 1890. Anthropology, London, Chapman & Hall, Ltd.

van der Klaauw, C. J. 1946. Cerebral skull and facial skull. A contribution to the knowledge of skull structure, Arch. Neerl. Zool. **7:**16.

van der Klaauw, C. J. 1948. Size and position of the functional components of the skull. A contribution to the knowledge of the architecture of the skull, based on data in the literature, Arch. Neerl. Zool. **9:**1.

Van Limborgh, J. 1972. The role of genetic and local environmental factors in the control of postnatal craniofacial morphogenesis, Acta Morphol. Neerl. Scand. **10:**37.

Vilmann, H. 1971. The growth of the cranial base in the Wistar Albino rat studied by vital staining with alizarin red S, Acta Odontol. Scand. (Suppl) **29:**59.

Von Bezold, A. 1857. Uhlersuchungen über die verlheilung von wasser, organischer materie und anorganische verbindungen im thierreiche, Z. Wiss. Zool. **8:**486.

Walker, C. H., and Kowalski, C. J. 1971. A two-dimensional coordinate model for the quantification, description analysis. Prediction and simulation of craniofacial growth, Growth **35:**191.

Watanabe, M., Laskin, D. M., and Brodie, A. G. 1957. The effect of autotransplantation on growth of the zygomatico-maxillary suture, Am. J. Anat. **100:**319.

Weingart, A. M. 1948. A simplified cephalometric head positioner, Am. J. Orthod. **34:**362.

Weinmann, J. P., and Sicher, H. 1955. Bone and bones, ed. 2, St. Louis, The C. V. Mosby Co.

Wertz, R. A. 1970. Skeletal and dental changes accompanying rapid midpalatal suture opening, Am. J. Orthod. **56:**41.

Wetzel, N. C. 1943. Assessing physical condition of children: I, case demonstration of failing growth and the determination of "par" by the grid method, J. Pediatr. **22:**82.

Wexler, M. R., and Sarnat, B. G. 1965. Rabbit snout growth after dislocation of nasal septum, Arch. Otolaryngol. **81:**68.

Woods, G. A. 1950. Changes in width dimensions between certain teeth and facial points during human growth, Am. J. Orthod. **36:**676.

Yip, A. S. G., and Cleall, J. F. 1971. Cinefluorographic study of velopharyngeal function before and after removal of tonsils and adenoids, Angle Orthod. **41:**251.

CHAPTER 4

Microbiology

Arthur V. Kroeger and Edward E. Vicher

It has been pointed out by Bartels (1968) that infections of the oral cavity are most often caused by microorganisms that are indigenous members of the normal flora. Thus the oral microbiota can act as opportunistic pathogens that incite disease when the normal state of the oral tissues is altered or the ecologic balance of the flora is upset. In addition, exogenous microorganisms may cause oral lesions when they enter the mouth by direct contact with infected people or animals or by the ingestion of contaminated food or polluted water. The lesions that result may be primary, or they may represent secondary manifestations of systemic infections.

The capacity of the normal flora to act as opportunistic pathogens is aptly exemplified by the study of Sabiston and his colleagues (1976). The results of their investigation of the flora isolated from 58 dental abscesses is presented in Table 4-1. From inspection of the data, it is evident that a wide variety of bacterial species may be involved in pyogenic oral infections. It appears that the facultative streptococci were found with a greater frequency than any other group of microorganisms. Both anaerobic gram-positive and gram-negative bacilli were isolated in a significant number of the specimens of pus. Facultative gram-negative bacilli were rarely encountered in this study. The authors pointed out that most of the specimens of pus contained a mixture of bacterial species. This observation could signify that most of the species may be incapable of producing infections

by themselves. There is no doubt that the data from this investigation emphasize that anaerobic techniques are essential in culturing the flora involved in oral pyogenic infections.

Because oral lesions may be elicited by both endogenous and exogenous microorganisms, it is important to be familiar with the normal flora and to understand those systemic diseases that present oral manifestations. It is also important to know the proper method of collection and handling of specimens that may be submitted to the laboratory for diagnosis and to have a basic understanding of the procedures that are used to identify the various types of etiologic agents.

ECOLOGIC NICHES OF THE NORMAL ORAL FLORA

The human oral cavity is normally colonized by a wide variety of microorganisms (Hardie and Bowden, 1974). The density of microorganisms in the adult mouth is quite high. For example, saliva has been reported to contain between 43 $\times$ 10^6 and 55 $\times$ 10^8 bacteria per ml (Burnett and Scherp, 1968), while dental plaque and debris from the gingival crevice contain 2.5 $\times$ 10^{11} and 1.7 $\times$ 10^{11} bacteria per gram wet weight, respectively (Gibbons et al., 1963; Socransky et al., 1963).

At birth the oral cavity is frequently bacteriologically sterile, but after several hours the number of microorganisms increases rapidly. McCarthy, Snyder, and Parker (1965) found that species of *Streptococcus, Staphylococcus, Veillonella,*

Table 4-1. Bacteria isolated from dental abscesses of periodontal or pulpal origin*

Species, genus, or group	Number of specimens from which isolated	Percentage of positive cultures from which isolated
Anaerobic gram-positive rods unidentified	1	1.7
Eubacterium lentum	1	1.7
Eubacterium alactolyticum	2	3.4
Eubacterium species	2	3.4
Lactobacillus species	8	13.8
Actinomyces species	10	17.2
Bifidobacterium species	6	10.3
Anaerobic gram-negative rods unidentified	15	25.9
Bacteroides oralis	3	5.2
B. ruminicola s.s. brevis	8	13.8
B. melaninogenicus s.s. intermedius	8	13.8
B. melaninogenicus s.s. melaninogenicus	2	3.4
Bacteroides species	3	5.2
Fusobacterium nucleatum	14	24.1
Fusobacterium species	1	1.7
Anaerobic gram-positive cocci unidentified	8	13.8
Peptococcus magnus	2	3.4
Streptococcus morbillorum	5	8.6
Peptostreptococcus anaerobius	9	15.5
Peptostreptococcus micros	13	22.4
Streptococcus constellatus	2	3.4
Streptocuccus intermedius	5	8.6
Anaerobic gram-negative cocci		
Veillonella parvula	6	10.3
Veillonella alcalescens	4	6.9
Facultative gram-positive rods unidentified	4	6.9
Lactobacillus species	6	10.3
Actinomyces species	3	5.2
Facultative gram-negative rods unidentified	3	5.2
Facultative gram-positive cocci		
Streptococci — catalase-negative, unspeciated	41	70.7
Streptococcus pyogenes	1	1.7
Staphylococcus epidermidis	8	13.8
Staphylococcus aureus	2	3.4
Facultative gram-negative cocci unidentified	5	8.6
Other unidentified bacterium	1	1.7
Yeast (not Candida albicans)	1	1.7
Spirochetes (phase-contrast microscopy)	7	12.1

*From Sabiston, C. B., Jr., et al. 1976. Oral Surg. **41**:430.

and *Neisseria* could be isolated from all infants studied by 1 year of age. Species of *Actinomyces, Fusobacterium, Nocardia (Rothia)*, and *Lactobacillus* could be cultured from more than half of the subjects studied, while species of *Bacteroides, Candida, Corynebacterium*, and *Leptotrichia* and coliforms were isolated from less than half of the infants by 1 year of age. *Streptococcus salivarius* is most frequently detected in the mouth of the newborn, since it has a predilection for the dorsum of the tongue (Carlsson et al., 1970; McCarthy, Snyder, and Parker, 1965).

Socransky and Manganiello (1971) have tabulated the major cultivable bacteria that are found in the oral cavity of the human adult. These data, presented in Table 4-2, were derived from the work of several different investigators (Gibbons et al., 1963; Gibbons et al., 1964; Gordon and Gibbons, 1966; Gordon and Jong, 1968; Richardson and

Table 4-2. Mean percentages of cultivable organisms in the adult oral cavity*

	Gingival crevice area	Dental plaque	Tongue	Saliva
Gram-positive facultative cocci	28.8	28.2	44.8	46.2
Streptococci	27.1	27.9	38.3	41.0
Streptococcus salivarius	N.D.	N.D.	8.2	4.6
Enterococci	7.2	–	N.D.	1.3
Staphylococci	1.7	0.3	6.5	4.0
Gram-positive anaerobic cocci	7.4	12.6	4.2	13.0
Gram-negative facultative cocci	0.4	0.4	3.4	1.2
Gram-negative anaerobic cocci	10.7	6.4	16.0	15.9
Gram-positive facultative rods	15.3	23.8	13.0	11.8
Gram-positive anaerobic rods	20.2	18.4	8.2	4.8
Gram-negative facultative rods	1.2	N.D.	3.2	2.3
Gram-negative anaerobic rods	16.1	10.4	8.2	4.8
Fusobacterium	1.9	4.1	0.7	0.3
Bacteriodes melaninogenicus	4.7	N.D.	0.2	N.D.
Vibrio sputorum	3.8	1.3	2.2	2.1
Other *Bacteroides*	5.6	4.8	5.1	2.4
Spirochetes	1.0	N.D.	N.D.	N.D.

N.D. = not detected.
*From Socransky, S. S., and Manganiello, S. D. 1971. J. Periodontol. **42**:485.

Jones, 1958; Socransky et al., 1963). It is apparent that the bacterial flora are both complex and variable. The gram-positive facultative cocci appear to be the most common group of bacteria found in all areas of the mouth, although there is considerable variation in the numbers of different species depending on the site that is sampled. Strict anaerobic organisms also comprise a significant proportion of the normal flora, and these bacteria commonly reside in the gingival crevice and in dental plaque. Hardie and Bowden (1974) have pointed out that the quantitative counts of the mixed flora of the mouth reported in the literature should not be regarded as absolute values but merely as an indication of the relative proportions of microorganisms in any given sample. In the first place it is extremely difficult to obtain adequate dispersion in an oral specimen. Secondly, investigators have employed a wide variety of selective and nonselective media in their studies, and the identification procedures used often have been rudimentary.

Table 4-3 emphasizes the differences in the distribution of several well-recognized species of bacteria in various sites in the human mouth. These differences are thought to reflect the capacity of a

Table 4-3. Distribution ranges of various oral bacteria in plaque and on the tongue*

Organism	Dental plaque	Saliva	Dorsum of tongue
Streptococcus mutans†	0–50	<1	<1
Streptococcus sanguis†	30–40	10–20	5–15
Streptococcus mitis†	30–40	30–40	10–20
Streptococcus salivarius†	<1	40–60	40–60
Lactobacilli‡	0–0.04	0–1	0–2
Veillonella‡	1–3	5–10	10–15

*From Gibbons, R. J., and van Houte, J. 1973. J. Periodontol. **44**:347.
†Data expressed as a percent of the facultative streptococcal flora.
‡Data expressed as a percent of the total flora cultivable on anaerobically incubated blood agar plates.

given organism to adhere to or be retained at a given site (Socransky and Manganiello, 1971), and this has generated the concept that certain species have a specific "primary ecologic niche" in the mouth. *Streptococcus salivarius* is more prominent on the dorsum of the tongue, and the high numbers in saliva are thought to result from mechanical dislodgment. *Streptococcus sanguis* is prominent in plaque and saliva. On the other hand *Streptococcus mutans* is found in a greater percentage in plaque than in the other ecologic niches. The lactobacilli are numerically scant in noncarious plaque (van Houte, Gibbons, and Pulkkinen, 1972) and saliva. Thus retention or adherence to the oral tissues is an important factor that governs the distribution of microorganisms in the oral environment. Organisms that are unable to adhere are swept away by the flow of saliva and swallowed or ingested with food and fluids (Gibbons, van Houte, and Liljemark, 1972).

Gibbons and Nygaard (1970) have pointed out that at least two types of adherence exist, adherence of organisms to the teeth or epithelial surfaces and adherence of microorganisms to one another. The adherence of cariogenic strains of *Streptococcus mutans* to the teeth in vivo and to smooth surfaces in vitro as a result of the synthesis of extracellular polysaccharides in the presence of sucrose has been most intensively studied (Germaine and Schachtele, 1976; Gibbons and Banghart, 1967; Gibbons and Nygaard, 1968; Guggenheim and Newbrun, 1969; McCabe and Smith, 1975). In addition, adherence has been demonstrated to occur between organisms of the same species or different species (Bourgeau and McBride, 1976; Gibbons and Nygaard, 1970; Newman and McKay, 1973). These bacterial interactions appear to be of great importance in the ecology of the oral flora and have been reviewed in detail by Gibbons and van Houte (1973, 1975).

PRINCIPAL GROUPS OF ORAL MICROORGANISMS
Gram-positive cocci
Staphylococcus

The organisms of the genus *Staphylococcus* are spherical, gram-positive cocci about 0.8 μm in diameter that are nonmotile and nonsporulating and produce the enzyme catalase. They are facultative anaerobes that produce acid from glucose under both aerobic and anaerobic conditions. This characteristic differentiates the genus from the *Micrococcus*, which only oxidizes glucose. The genus *Staphy-*

lococcus is tolerant to high salt concentrations and will grow in or on media containing 7.5% to 15% sodium chloride. Such media are often used for the selective isolation of staphylococci from clinical material. They are one of the most resistant of the vegetative bacteria and are often used to test the potency of germicides. Several species of the genus *Staphylococcus* have been isolated from the human mouth: *Staphylococcus candidus, Staphylococcus citreus, Staphylococcus epidermidis, Staphylococcus salivarius,* and *Staphylococcus aureus* (Gordon, 1967; Ikeda, Isoda, and Iidako, 1964; Taplin and Goldsworthy, 1958). The last species is the one most frequently involved in human infections. *Staphylococcus epidermidis,* a normal resident of the skin, is usually differentiated from the more highly pathogenic *Staphylococcus aureus* by the fact that the latter usually ferments the carbohydrate mannitol, coagulates citrated mammalian plasma, produces a heat-stable DNase and the enzyme lysozyme, and elaborates staphylococcal protein A. Bacteriophage typing (Wentworth, 1963) has proved useful in epidemiologic studies, particularly in tracing carriers of *Staphylococcus aureus.* The increasing frequency of isolation of antibiotic-resistant, coagulase-negative staphylococci from human infections has brought about an increased interest in the potential pathogenicity of *Staphylococcus epidermidis* (Andriole and Lyons, 1970; Marsik and Parisi, 1973).

Humans are the most important reservoir for the dissemination of *Staphylococcus aureus* (Elek, 1959). The organism may be found on the mucous membranes of the anterior nares, oral cavity, nasopharynx, and gastrointestinal tract in the absence of disease. The nose is considered to be the principal site of multiplication, and roughly 50% of the human population are carriers. Knighton (1962) obtained 864 nasal and 864 oral cultures from 74 students over a period of 14 months and found that 48.5% of the nasal cultures showed coagulase-positive staphylococci and 46.5% of the oral cultures showed coagulase-positive staphylococci. Both oral and nasal cultures were constantly negative from 12.2% of the individuals studied. Of those individuals from whom positive cultures were obtained, 77.9% contained 10 to 1000 colony-forming units per milliliter of saliva, and only 4.5% contained over 10,000 colony-forming units per milliliter of saliva. Handelman and Mills (1965) have also reported relatively low numbers of staphylococci in human saliva. Thus it appears that while staphylococci are frequently present in the human oral cavity, they represent only a small proportion of the total oral flora.

The pathogenicity and virulence of *Staphylococcus aureus* appear to be attributable to a variety of extracellular toxins and enzymes, including coagulase, enterotoxin, exfoliative toxin, several hemolysins, hyaluronidase, leukocidin, and staphylokinase or fibrinolysin. However, no single enzyme or toxin alone can account for the virulence of the organism, with the possible exception of enterotoxin in the case of staphylococcal food poisoning (Casman, 1971) and the exfoliative toxin produced by strains of *Staphylococcus aureus* causing the scalded skin syndrome (Melish and Glasgow, 1970; Melish, Glasgow, and Turner, 1972).

Staphylococcus aureus can invade any organ or tissue of the body; the localized lesions are characterized by inflammation, necrosis, and abscess formation. The skin is the most common site of infection; furuncles and carbuncles develop most frequently on the face, nose, axillae, neck, and buttocks. Osteomyelitis is one of the most serious infections caused by *Staphylococcus aureus* and accounts for at least 50% to 60% of all cases (Waldvogel, Medoff, and Swartz, 1970 a, b, and c). This infection may follow dental procedures such as extractions; injection of local anesthetics; fractures; or spread of infection from a facial, periapical, or periodontal abscess. The mandible is more frequently involved than the maxilla (Nolte, 1973). *Staphylococcus aureus* is not uncommonly isolated from infected root canals (Winkler and van Amerongen, 1959). Genitourinary tract infections, pneumonia, endocarditis, sep-

ticemia, and enterocolitis may also be caused by *Staphylococcus aureus*.

One of the most serious problems associated with staphylococcal infections has been the emergence and dissemination of antibiotic-resistant strains of the organism. It has been recognized for many years that 85% to 95% of the strains of *Staphylococcus aureus* associated with hospital-acquired infections are resistant to penicillin G (Oven, Kirsten, and Bulow, 1969). On the other hand the incidence of resistant strains in the community at large has been considerably lower; however, a definite increase has been reported for several years (Barrett et al., 1970; Ross et al., 1974). Most, if not all, penicillin G– , penicillin V– , or ampicillin-resistant strains of staphylococci produce the enzyme penicillinase, which hydrolyzes the beta-lactam ring of the molecule, thereby destroying the antimicrobial activity. It is now recognized that the capacity to elaborate penicillinase depends on the presence of a plasmid that can be transmitted from resistant to susceptible strains by means of transducing bacteriophages. Because of the frequency of antibiotic-resistant mutants in most staphylococcal strains, all pathogenic staphylococci isolated from human infections should be tested for antibiotic susceptibility, since they may be resistant to other antibiotics as well as the penicillins (Myrvik, Pearsall, and Weiser, 1974).

Peptococcus

The organisms of the genus *Peptococcus* (Rogosa, 1974b) are spherical, gram-positive bacteria about 0.5 to 1 μm in diameter. In stained smears they are arranged singly, in pairs, in packets of four, in irregular masses, and rarely as short chains. They are nonmotile and do not produce spores. All species are anaerobes that utilize peptones and amino acids as an energy source. Their capacity to ferment carbohydrates is usually quite limited. The catalase reaction is usually negative or weak, and they do not produce the enzyme coagulase. Although some species are occasionally beta hemolytic, most are not hemotytic on blood agar plates. The genus is separated into species on the basis of various biochemical reactions and by the analysis of organic acids by means of gas chromatography following cultivation of pure cultures in a peptone-yeast-glucose broth (Martin, 1974).

These organisms have been isolated from the human mouth (Kantz and Henry, 1974), respiratory and intestinal tracts, and female urogenital tract (Rogosa, 1974). The pathogenicity of the genus is not well established, since they are frequently recovered from sites where other opportunistic pathogens are present.

Streptococcus

The genus *Streptococcus* is composed of a large and biologically diverse group of gram-positive bacteria. The cells are spherical or ovoid and occur in pairs or chains; the length of the chains is variable and depends on the environmental conditions of growth. Long chains of cocci are observed when the organisms are grown in liquid or semifluid media. Species of the genus *Streptococcus* are facultative anaerobes that are catalase-negative.

The earliest system of classification was based on three different types of hemolytic reactions observed when the organisms were grown on the surface of blood agar streak plates or in blood agar pour plates. These were termed "alpha," "beta," and "gamma." Colonies of alpha-hemolytic streptococci are surrounded by a zone of partial lysis of the red blood cells in the medium that often has a green discoloration; they have been referred to as the "viridans" or greening streptococci. The green appearance is dependent on the species of animal blood that is used in the preparation of the medium; sheep blood agar plates usually show more greening and less lysis than do human blood agar plates. Colonies of the beta-hemolytic streptococci are surrounded by a clear zone of complete hemolysis of the erythrocytes in the blood agar medium. Colonies of the so-called gamma streptococci characteristically give no hemolytic reaction on blood agar plates. Such organisms are more appropriately referred to as indifferent or simply nonhemolytic streptococci.

The next major advance in the classification of the genus *Streptococcus*, developed by Lancefield (1933), was based on the presence of specific carbohydrate antigens present in the cell wall of beta-hemolytic streptococci. Soluble antigens were extracted from cultures of a variety of different sources using hot 0.2 N HCl. Following neutralization and clarification, the extracts would give a positive precipitin ring test with homologous antiserum prepared by injecting rabbits with whole, killed streptococci. Using this technique, several distinct groups of beta-hemolytic streptococci could be differentiated with respect to their origin or source. These groups were designated by capital letters: A, B, C, D, E, F, G, H, and so forth. However, later investigation revealed that some of the cell wall antigens were also present in some but not all isolates of alpha-hemolytic and nonhemolytic streptococci.

Sherman (1937) proposed that the streptococci be separated into four divisions on the basis of various cultural reactions. These divisions were referred to as the pyogenic, viridans, enterococcus, and lactic streptococci. The organisms of the enterococcus division could be placed into Lancefield's group D, and the lactic division could be placed into Lancefield's group N. Some of the organisms of the viridans group could not be placed into any of the known Lancefield groups. The majority of the organisms of the pyogenic or lactic divisions could be placed into Lancefield's groups A, B, C and E, F, G, H and K through V. Groups A, B, C, and D are the most frequent cause of acute human streptococcal infection.

The eighth edition of *Bergey's Manual of Determinative Bacteriology* (Buchanan and Gibbons, 1974) has omitted these physiologic divisions from the key, since newly recognized species cut across the broad lines of Sherman's divisions. Therefore we have elected to use the species officially recognized in *Bergey's Manual* in discussing the genus *Streptococcus*. One exception to this rule has been the inclusion of the species *Streptococcus*

Table 4-4. Species of the genus *Streptococcus* commonly found in the oral cavity

Species	Blood agar reaction	Serologic group	Usual habitat	Human disease association
Streptococcus faecalis	γ	Lancefield D	Human mouth; animal and human feces	Infected root canal, subacute bacterial endocarditis, urinary tract infections
Streptococcus mitis	α	None	Human mouth, throat, feces	Infected root canal, subacute bacterial endocarditis
Streptococcus mutans	α or γ	Bratthall a, b,c,d,e,f,g	Human mouth	Caries, infected root canal, subacute bacterial endocarditis
Streptococcus salivarius	γ	Lancefield K	Human mouth and throat	Infected root canal, subacute bacterial endocarditis
Streptococcus sanguis	α	Lancefield H	Human mouth	Infected root canal, subacute bacterial endocarditis

mutans. Table 4-4 lists the hemolytic reaction, serologic group, usual habitat, and human diseases associated with some of the currently recognized species of the genus *Streptococcus* that are found in the mouth.

The streptococci represent from 30% to 60% of the total bacterial populations residing in the various ecologic niches of the human mouth. (Carlsson, 1967; Gibbons et al., 1964; Gordon and Gibbons, 1966; van Houte, Gibbons and Banghart, 1970) (Fig. 4-1). Most of the oral species are alpha hemolytic or nonhemolytic. The four most commonly encountered species are *Streptococcus salivarius*, *Streptococcus sanguis*, *Streptococcus mutans*, and *Streptococcus mitis*.

Streptococcus salivarius produces an extracellular levan or polyfructan from the utilization of sucrose, and large mucoid or "gumdrop" colonies result when this organism is grown on sucrose containing media such as mitis-salivarius agar. Identification of this species may be difficult in the case of strains that do not produce the typical colonial morphology, because physiologic tests are frequently negative or variable (Hardie and Bowden, 1974). Some strains possess the Lancefield group K antigen (Williams, 1956). The levans produced are soluble and may be degraded and utilized by other oral bacteria as an energy source (Leach et al., 1972). *Streptococcus salivarius* makes up a high percentage of the facultative streptococci that can be cultured from the dorsum of the tongue, but it comprises less than 1% of the streptococci in dental plaque (Carlsson, 1967; van Houte, Gibbons, and Pulkkinen, 1971). This organism is a frequent cause of subacute bacterial endocarditis.

Streptococcus sanguis produces extracellular glucans from the utilization of sucrose. While this species may be isolated from the various ecologic niches of the mouth, it is a prominent inhabitant of dental plaque and is sometimes the cause of subacute bacterial endocarditis (White and Niven, 1946). The antigenic structure of *Streptococcus sanguis* appears to be complex (Rosan, 1973), and some isolates possess the Lancefield group H antigen (Farmer, 1954).

Isolates of the species *Streptococcus mitis* (*Streptococcus mitior*) are alpha hemolytic on blood agar, and they do not usually produce extracellular polysaccharides from the utilization of sucrose. There appears to be a lack of uniformity with respect to their biochemical activity and carbohydrate fermentation reactions (Guggenheim, 1968), and this species has been identified essentially by a process of elimination. Colman and Williams (1972) have shown that the cell walls of *Streptococcus mitis* are characterized by the absence of rhamnose and the presence of ribitol teichoic acid; this appears to be distinctive for this species. Like the other oral streptococci, *Streptococcus mitis* may be involved in the etiology of subacute bacterial endocarditis.

Clarke (1924) observed the presence of a streptococcus on 72% of all culture

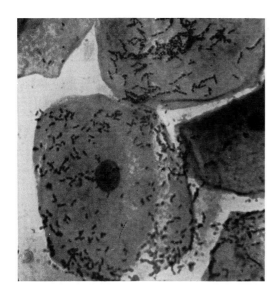

Fig. 4-1. Desquamated epithelial cells from gingiva with chains of streptococci.

plates inoculated with material from human carious lesions and considered this organism to be important in the etiology of dental caries. He described some of the morphologic and cultural reactions of the organism and named it *Streptococcus mutans,* because bacillary-like as well as coccal forms were observed in pure cultures.

While *Streptococcus mutans* has been strongly associated with dental caries in experimental animals as well as humans (Gibbons et al., 1974; Ikeda and Sandham, 1971, Littleton, Kahehashi, and Fitzgerald, 1970; Loesche et al., 1975; Shklair, Keene, and Simonson, 1972; Shklair, Keene, and Cullen, 1974; Street, Goldner, and LeRiche, 1976), other species have also been implicated as a cause of caries. According to Gibbons (1972), several investigators have demonstrated that *Streptococcus sanguis, Streptococcus salivarius, Streptococcus mitis,* and certain isolates of the enterococci can induce carious lesions in experimental animals. However, these species were not so highly cariogenic as *Streptococcus mutans.*

In view of the importance of *Streptococcus mutans* as a major etiologic agent of dental caries, there has been considerable interest in the development of a vac-

cine against this organism. However, considering the apparently contradictory results obtained by different investigators, further studies would appear to be necessary before immunization of humans against *Streptococcus mutans* becomes practical.

Two less common streptococci encountered in the oral cavity are *Streptococcus pyogenes* and *Streptococcus faecalis. Streptococcus pyogenes,* the prototype species of Lancefield's group A streptococci, is rare in the oral cavity of normal individuals; however, it has been isolated from the saliva of people suffering from streptococcal sore throat as well as from asymptomatic carriers (Ross, 1971). *Streptococcus faecalis* and several other similar species comprise a relatively small proportion of the streptococcal flora in the human. The isolation of enterococci from various sites in the human mouth has been reported by several investigators (Bahn et al., 1960; Williams et al., 1950; Winkler and van Amerongen, 1959). More recently, Gold, Jordan, and van Houte (1975) have observed that enterococci could be detected in 60% to 75% of the subjects whom they studied. The species most frequently isolated was *Streptococcus faecalis.*

Peptostreptococcus

The genus *Peptostreptococcus* can be viewed as the anaerobic counterpart of the genus *Streptococcus.* The organisms of the genus *Peptostreptococcus* (Rogosa, 1974) are gram-positive, spherical to ovoid cells about 0.7 to 1 μm in diameter. In stained smears they are arranged in pairs or short or long chains. They are nonmotile and do not form spores. The catalase reaction is negative. Most species ferment carbohydrates with the production of various organic acids and gas. While lactic acid is produced by some species (Martin, 1974), acetic, formic, isovaleric, succinic, and other organic acids are the most common fermentation end products. The hemolytic reaction on blood agar is variable; some species produce an alpha hemolysis while others produce a beta hemolysis. The genus is divided into species on the basis of fermentation reactions and by the analysis of organic acids by means of gas chromatography.

The peptostreptococci are prominent in the human mouth (Gibbons et al., 1964; Youmans, Paterson, and Sommers, 1975) and may be isolated also from the normal female genital tract. They may be involved in the etiology of puerperal sepsis and pyogenic and wound infections. Indeed, Finegold et al. (1972) have described the peptostreptococci as frequent etiologic agents of a great variety of human infections.

Gram-negative cocci
Neisseria and Branhamella

Gram-negative, nonmotile, nonspore-forming, coffee bean–shaped diplococci that are aerobic and possess the enzyme cytochrome oxidase are common bacterial parasites of the mucous membranes of the human oral cavity and upper respiratory tract. The genus *Neisseria* is divided into the pathogenic species, *Neisseria gonorrhoeae* and *Neisseria meningitidis*, and several commensal species, *Neisseria sicca*, *Neisseria subflava*, *Neisseria flavescens*, and *Neisseria mucosa*, principally on the basis of carbohydrate fermentation reactions. The species formerly called *Neisseria catarrhalis* has recently been placed into a newly created genus called *Branhamella*. *Branhamella catarrhalis* differs from the *Neisseria* species in that the former does not produce acid from the carbohydrates glucose, maltose, sucrose, and fructose. Also, the DNA base ratios of guanine plus cytosine are 40 to 45 moles %, while the DNA base ratios of guanine plus cytosine for the latter range from 47 to 52 moles % (Buchanan and Gibbons, 1974). The commensal species of the genus *Neisseria* are considered nonpathogenic or weakly virulent for the human, although instances of subacute bacterial endocarditis (Hudson, 1957) and purulent meningitis (Losli and Lindsey, 1963) have been reported.

Morris (1954a) and Pike et al. (1962) have described the properties of isolates from the human mouth and observed that most of the oral isolates can be classified as *N. pharyngis* or *N. catarrhalis* (*Branhamella catarrhalis*). Ritz (1967) has studied their occurrence in dental plaque and has been able to localize the distribution of one species in frozen, sectioned dental plaque by means of the fluorescent antibody staining technique (Ritz, 1969).

The two pathogenic species of the genus *Neisseria*, *Neisseria gonorrhoeae* and *Neisseria meningitidis*, are not normal residents of the human oral cavity. However, *Neisseria gonorrhoeae* may cause a primary stomatitis, parotitis, or pharyngitis as a result of oral-genital contact (Metzger, 1970; Schmidt, Hjørting-Hansen, and Philipsen, 1961; Wiesner et al., 1973) or autoinoculation from a primary genital infection via the fingers.

Veillonella

The genus *Veillonella* is divided into two species: *Veillonella alcalescens* and *Veillonella parvula* (Holdeman, Cato, and Moore, 1977). These organisms are about 0.5 μm in diameter, nonmotile, gram-negative, oxidase-negative, anaerobic diplococci. They do not ferment carbohydrates but utilize lactic, succinic, and some other organic acids as an energy source for growth (Rogosa, 1964). A selective medium devised by Rogosa (1956) has facilitated the primary isolation of the organisms from clinical specimens. The *Veillonella* are part of the normal flora of the human oral cavity as well as the intestinal and urogenital tracts. They are present in the human mouth in large numbers and may be found in variable proportions in the major ecologic niches (Hardie and Bowden, 1974).

The *Veillonella* are not considered to be frank pathogens, but they may be isolated as a part of a mixed bacterial flora from patients with appendicitis, periodontitis, pulmonary gangrene, and tonsillitis (Nolte, 1973). The role played by the *Veillonella* in the pathogenesis of these mixed infections is not clear; however, lipopolysaccharide possessing endotoxic activity is a part of the cell wall of these organisms (Hofstad and Kristoffersen, 1970; Mergenhagen and Varah, 1963;

Mergenhagen, Zipkin, and Varah, 1962), and the extracted endotoxin has been demonstrated to prepare and provoke a local Shwartzman reaction in the skin (Mergenhagen, 1960; Mergenhagen, Hampp, and Scherp, 1961) and palatal mucosa (Rizzo and Mergenhagen, 1964) of rabbits. Since the *Veillonella* occur in dental plaque and are present in the human gingival crevice, the endotoxin associated with these organisms may play a role in the pathogenesis of chronic marginal gingivitis and chronic marginal periodontitis via the activation of the complement cascade (Snyderman, 1973).

Gram-positive rods and filaments
Actinomyces, Arachnia, Bifidobacterium, Bacterionema, and *Rothia*

The genera *Actinomyces, Arachnia, Bifidobacterium, Bacterionema,* and *Rothia* are currently classified in the family Actinomycetaceae. With the exception of the genus *Bifidobacterium,* the biology and pathogenicity of the above genera have been discussed in great detail in the monograph by Slack and Gerencser (1975). The Actinomycetaceae are gram-positive bacteria that are mainly diphtheroid or club-shaped rods that tend to form branched filaments in infected tissue or under some in vitro cultural conditions (Fig. 4-2). Diphtheroid or coccoid forms may be produced when the filaments fragment. The organisms are nonmotile, do not form endospores, and are not acid-fast. The majority of the species are facultative anaerobes, although some are strict anaerobes and at least one species grows best under aerobic conditions. The enzyme catalase may or may not be produced.

Table 4-5 lists the oxygen requirements, the capacity to produce catalase, the presence of diaminopimelic acid (DAP) in the cell walls, the production of propionic acid from glucose, and the human diseases associated with the species found in the human mouth. The species *Actinomyces bovis* has been omitted, since it has not been isolated from

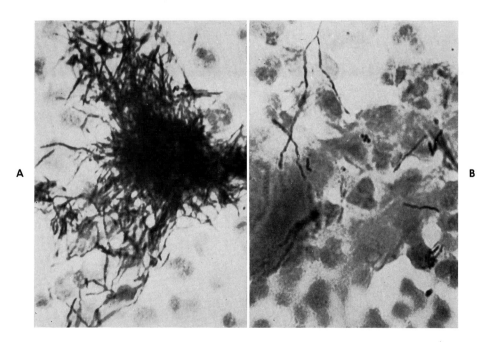

Fig. 4-2. A, Smear from skin fistula from patient with actinomycosis showing a mass of stained filaments. **B,** Smear from skin fistula in atypical actinomycosis showing a few filaments with other microorganisms.

Table 4-5. Oral bacteria of the family Actinomycetaceae*

Organism	Oxygen requirements	Catalase production	Presence of DAP in cell walls	Propionic acid from glucose	Human disease association
Actinomyces israelii	Anaerobe	−	−	−	Actinomycosis
Actinomyces naeslundii	Facultative anaerobe	−	−	−	Actinomycosis; root caries
Actinomyces odontolyticus	Facultative anaerobe	−	−	−	Actinomycosis
Actinomyces viscosus	Facultative anaerobe	+	−	−	Actinomycosis; root caries
Arachnia propionica	Facultative anaerobe	−	+	+	Actinomycosis; lacrimal canaliculitis
Bifidobacterium adolescentis var. B	Anaerobic	−	−	−	Not firmly established; has been isolated from carious lesions
"Bifidobacterium dentium group"	Anaerobic	−	−	−	Not firmly established; has been isolated from carious lesions
Bifidobacterium ericksonii	Anaerobic	−	−	−	Actinomycosis
Bacterionema matruchotii	Facultative anaerobe	+	+	+	None reported
Rothia dentocariosa	Aerobe to facultative anaerobe	+	−	−	Not firmly established; root caries?

*Data derived from Buchanan and Gibbons (1974), Georg (1974), Holdeman, Cato, and Moore (1977), Scordovi et al. (1971), and Slack and Gerencser (1975).

humans and appears to be an animal parasite (Slack and Gerencser, 1975). The characteristics listed allow only a preliminary categorization of these genera, and separation into species requires the study of colonial and microscopic morphology, use of fermentation and other biochemical tests, analysis of fermentation end products by means of gas chromatography, and various serologic techniques. Practical procedures for the isolation and identification of *Actinomyces, Arachnia,* and *Rothia* have been summarized by Slack and Gerencser (1975).

The most common etiologic agent of actinomycosis in the human is *Actinomyces israelii* (Georg, 1970; Holm, 1950; Slack, 1942); however, other species of the genus *Actinomyces* and *Arachnia propionica* have been implicated (Brock et al., 1973; Georg and Coleman, 1970). The organisms are introduced into the tissues by the extraction of teeth and other surgical procedures, jaw fractures, exposure of the tooth pulp as a result of caries, aspiration into the lungs, hematogenous extension, or trauma. Clinically, several types of infections are recognized: cervicofacial (Everts, 1970; Hartley and Schatten, 1973; Hertz, 1960; Hunter and Westrick, 1957; Kapsimalis and Garrington, 1968), thoracic (Coodley, 1969; Foley, Dines, and Dolan, 1971; Prather et al., 1970; Slade, Slesser, and Southgate, 1973), and abdominal (Adar et al., 1972; Pheils, Reid, and Ross, 1964; Putman, Dockerty, and Waugh, 1950). The cervicofacial type of infection occurs most frequently. Infection of the central nervous system (Fetter, Klintworth, and Hendry, 1967), bone (Cope, 1951), and skin and wounds (Cullen and Sharp, 1951) have been reported. Classically, actinomycosis is characterized by the insidious development of chronic granulomatous abscesses; sinus tracts develop that discharge pus and necrotic material to the outside. In the pus or tissue the organisms appear either as tangled masses of branched and unbranched wavy filaments (Fig. 4-2) or as "sulfur" granules (Fig. 4-3). The latter have a yellow appearance when present in the discharge. The presence of clubbed gran-

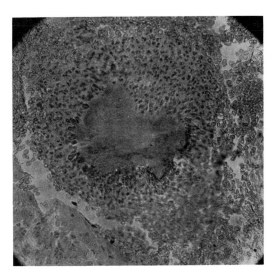

Fig. 4-3. Sulfur granule of actinomyces showing club-like peripheral extension surrounded by lymphocytes.

ules is not exclusively associated with infection by *Actinomyces* species, however, and may be observed in infections caused by other bacteria such as *Nocardia brasiliensis* (Macotela-Ruiz and Gonzalez-Angulo, 1966), *Staphylococcus aureus* (Spier, Mitchener, and Galloway, 1971), and *Streptomyces madurae* (Emmons, Binford, and Utz, 1970); therefore laboratory identification of the causative agent is important for proper treatment. Although actinomycosis is not a reportable disease, reported deaths have averaged 25 annually for the years 1949 to 1969 (Slack and Gerenscer, 1975).

In addition to actinomycosis, several species of the genus *Actinomyces* have been shown to produce periodontal pathosis in experimental animals or have been implicated in human root surface or deep dentinal caries. Socransky, Hubersak, and Propas (1970) were able to induce periodontal destruction in germfree rats with an isolate of *Actinomyces naeslundii* of human origin. However, the relationship of this organism to human periodontal disease has not been shown.

The species now called *Actinomyces viscosus* (formerly *Odontomyces viscosus*) was first isolated by Howell (1963) from gingival plaque of hamsters with periodontal disease. Subsequently, Jordon and Keyes (1964) and Jordan, Keyes, and Bellack (1972) demonstrated that this organism could induce periodontal disease in hamsters and gnotobiotic rats. Syed and co-workers (1975) found that *Actinomyces viscosus* was the dominant bacterial species isolated from human plaque samples obtained from tooth surfaces that exhibited typical lesions of root surface caries. This organism produces significant quantities of extracellular polysaccharides (Rosan and Hammond, 1974) in the absence of sucrose, which may account for its capacity to form dental plaque (Jordon, Keyes, and Lim 1969).

Actinomyces odontolyticus was initially isolated and described by Batty (1958). Since many of the 200 isolates studied were derived from human carious lesions, the organism appeared to be associated with dental caries. However, a firm etiologic relationship has yet to be established.

Arachnia propionica, formerly *Actinomyces propionicus*, is a common inhabitant of the human mouth (Slack, Landfried, and Gerencser, 1971). It was initially isolated from a case of lacrimal canaliculitis by Pine and Hardin (1959) who identified it as *Actinomyces israelii*. Subsequently, *Arachnia propionica* has been shown to be an important etiologic agent of both localized and systemic human infections (Brock et al., 1973; Georg, 1974).

The bacteria of the genus *Bifidobacterium* (Rogosa, 1974) are gram-positive, nonmotile, nonsporeforming rods that are extremely variable in their morphology. Freshly isolated strain may be uniform or branched; bifurcated Y, V, and club forms may be observed. The morphology appears to be influenced by nutritional conditions, and staining is often irregular. The organisms ferment a variety of carbohydrates, and gas is not produced; acetic and lactic acid are the main end products from glucose fermentations. They are anaerobic, although some may tolerate oxygen in the presence of CO_2. These organisms are usually found as normal inhabitants of the intestinal tract and vagina of humans and animals, al-

though the species listed in Table 4-5 have been isolated from the human mouth (Holdeman, Cato, and Moore, 1977; Scardovi et al., 1971).

The genera *Bacterionema* (Gilmour, 1961; Gilmour and Beck, 1961; Gilmour, Howell, and Beck, 1961; Howell and Pine, 1961) and *Rothia* (Georg and Brown, 1967) each consist of a single species: *Bacterionema matruchotii* and *Rothia dentocariosa*. *Bacterionema matruchotii* can be regularly isolated from mature dental plaque and calculus, but it has not been established as an etiologic agent of human disease. Since this filamentous organism has the capacity to convert intracellular calcium to hydroxyapatite (Ennever, 1963; Ennever, Vogel, and Takazoe, 1968; Takazoe, Vogel, and Ennever, 1970), it appears to be important in the formation of dental calculus. *Rothia dentocariosa* was first isolated from carious dentine by Onisi (1949). It has also been isolated from human abscesses, blood, and spinal fluid (Brown, Georg, and Waters, 1969); however, its role as an agent of human disease has not been firmly established.

Eubacterium and Propionibacterium

The organisms currently classified in the genus *Eubacterium* (Holdeman and Moore, 1974) are gram-positive, nonsporeforming, uniform or pleomorphic rods that may or may not be motile. All species are strict anaerobes. They usually produce mixtures of organic acids such as butyric, acetic, or formic acid from the utilization of carbohydrates or peptone. Some species of the genus occur in the cavities of man and other animals. Kantz and Henry (1974) have isolated *Eubacterium alactolyticum* from intact pulp chambers of nonvital human teeth. This species has also been encountered in various types of infections such as purulent pleurisy, jugal cellulitis, postoperative wounds, and abscesses of the brain, intestinal tract, lung, and oral cavity (Holdeman and Moore, 1974).

The bacteria comprising the genus *Propionibacterium* (Moore and Holdeman, 1974) are gram-positive, nonmotile, nonsporeforming rods. They are diphtheroid or club-shaped, and pleomorphism is usual. Coccoid, elongated, bifid, or branched cells may be observed in some cultures, and the cells may be arranged singly, in pairs, in V and Y configurations, or in clumps resembling "Chinese characters." Propionic acid is a characteristic fermentation end product as are acetic, formic, isovaleric, succinic, or lactic acids. Most species of this genus are strict anaerobes, but some are aerotolerant. *Propionibacterium avidum* has been isolated from brain, blood, infected wounds, and tissue abscesses including submandibular abscesses (Moore and Holdeman, 1974). *Propionibacterium acnes,* which is a normal inhabitant of the human skin and intestine, has been found in blood, wounds, and soft tissue abscesses (Moore and Holdeman, 1974) and the pulp of nonvital teeth (Kantz and Henry, 1974).

Lactobacillus

The organisms of the genus *Lactobacillus* are gram-positive, nonsporulating rods; most are nonmotile. The majority of the species are facultative anaerobes, although some are strict anaerobes. They may be divided into two groups on the basis of the end products produced from the fermentation of glucose. The homofermentative species produce lactic acid as the main end product, while the heterofermentative species produce acetic acid, carbon dioxide, ethanol, and lactic acid. A number of different species are parasitic for man as well as other animals; in the human they occur in the oral cavity, gastrointestinal tract, and vagina as a part of the normal flora. Under normal circumstances the lactobacilli are present in the normal mouth in low numbers apparently because they do not adhere well to the oral tissues (van Houte, Gibbons, and Pulkkinen, 1972).

Their association with dental caries (Enright, Friesell, and Trescher, 1932) in the human has been recognized for many years, although a direct etiologic relationship has not been proved (Loesche, 1974). It appears that one of the reasons for implicating these organisms in the causation of dental caries is related to the fact that they can grow and survive at pH 5. Under in vitro conditions enamel is not demineralized at pH values much above this value. Also, elevated counts of salivary lactobacilli generally correlate with the state of caries activity (Snyder et al., 1962; Snyder et al., 1963), and restoration of all carious lesions usually results in a noticeable decline in the lactobacillus count (Kesel et al., 1958; Shklair et al., 1956). However, the insertion of complete dentures (Shklair and Mazarella, 1961) and orthodontic appliances (Bloom and Brown, 1964; Owen, 1949; Sakamaki and Bahn, 1968) also results in an increase in the numbers of oral lactobacilli. Currently, the consensus appears to be that the lactobacilli are not the specific cause of human dental caries (Sims, 1970b) and that increased numbers of lactobacilli reflect conditions that favor an acidic environment and provide mechanical retention sites (van Houte, Gibbons, and Pulkkinen, 1972). Even though this view may be correct, the lactobacilli may contribute to the progression of the carious lesion, since they are not uncommonly isolated from root canal cultures (Winkler and van Amerongen, 1959).

Gram-negative rods and filaments

Gram-negative rods and filaments exhibit great variation in morphology, staining patterns, motility, biochemical activity, and antigenic structure. None of these produces endospores. The majority of the organisms are aerobes and facultative anaerobes, although those genera that are present regularly in the oral cavity in greatest numbers are obligate anaerobes. Although the aerobes and facultative anaerobes give rise to infections in the mouth, the role of anaerobic gramnegative bacilli in oral pathologic processes has been fully appreciated only recently.

Aerobes and facultative anaerobes

Coliforms. The coliform organisms of the family Enterobacteriaceae are not regular or predominant inhabitants of the human mouth of individuals residing in the western world. Although the coliforms have been isolated with some frequency from normal mouths, they are generally regarded as transient inhabitants. However, they may give rise to infection of the oral tissues. Often this occurs as a result of the use of antibiotics that suppress the gram-positive flora. In some instances these organisms are present in mixed infections. Mashberg, Carroll, and Morrissey (1970) reported an osteomyelitis of the mandible caused by a mixed flora in which *Enterobacter aerogenes* was the predominant organism along with *Escherichia coli* and alpha-hemolytic streptococci.

Klebsiella. The *Klebsiella* genus of the family Enterobacteriaceae comprises organisms that characteristically produce large polysaccharide capsules. The type species *Klebsiella pneumoniae* is divided into more than 80 serotypes on the basis of the antigenic determinants of the polysaccharide moiety.

Klebsiella pneumoniae is responsible for about 1% of the bacterial pneumonias. This organism was reported by Agranat (1969) as the cause of chronic osteomyelitis of the mandible. Faucett and Miller (1948) reported stomatitis in infants caused by this organism. A similar stomatitis associated with diarrheal disease in infants was also reported by Sternberg, Hoffman, and Zweitler (1951). A suppurative infection of the carotid space was reported by Mashberg, Carroll, and Morrissey (1970) to be caused by an unidentified species of the genus *Klebsiella*. *Klebsiella* species have also been isolated from a small proportion of root canal cultures (Fox and Isenberg, 1967). Heitman and Brasher (1971) reported the case of a patient who developed swelling and erythema of the right side of the palate 4 days following periodontal osseous surgery. A purulent exudate was readily expressed from the mesiopalatal aspect of the maxillary right first molar. Culture revealed that the predominant organism was *Klebsiella pneumoniae,* which was resistant to erythromycin in in vitro tests. Since the patient had been treated prophylactically with erythromycin prior to and following the surgery, it is possible that the antibiotic administration may have been a predisposing factor in the

development of this infection by disrupting the ecologic balance of the normal flora.

Klebsiella rhinoscleromatis has been recovered from rhinoscleroma, a chronic and destructive granuloma of the nose and pharynx that may involve the upper lip, cheeks, soft and hard palate, and the superior alveolar process. However, the etiologic role of this organism in the pathogenesis of this syndrome is uncertain. The syndrome cannot be evoked in laboratory animals, and the organism can be isolated from healthy individuals.

Proteus. Members of this genus of the family Enterobacteriaceae are responsible for disease in various parts of the body, and the infections present special problems in therapy because of the marked resistance of the etiologic isolates to most antibiotics. *Proteus vulgaris,* one of the most frequently isolated species from infectious processes, has been reported in a few cases of submandibular abscesses (Kirner et al., 1969). It has been reported as a rarely occurring organism in infected root canals (Slack, 1953), and it has been occasionally isolated from cases of bacterial parotitis (Rose, 1954).

Pseudomonas. The organisms of the genus *Pseudomonas* are nonfermentative and are rather unique in that they grow and multiply with minimal nutritional sources. They have been found as contaminants in parenteral saline solutions and even in aqueous solutions of benzalkonium chloride. Most species are motile by means of a single or tufted monopolar flagella. *Pseudomonas aeruginosa* produces the water-soluble pigment, pyocyanin, and the fluorescing pigment, fluorescein, while *Pseudomonas fluorescens* produces only the latter.

The pseudomonads are primarily water and soil parasites. *Pseudomonas aeruginosa,* the type species, was for many years the only member of the genus that was accurately delineated and considered to be a potential pathogen in man. In the past 15 years, many other species such as *Pseudomonas cepacia* and *Pseudomonas stutzeri* have been accurately characterized and isolated from all types of infectious processes in man. These have been principally involved in noso-comial infections or infections in the compromised host.

Pseudomonas aeruginosa is apparently the species most commonly reported in the literature to colonize the mouth and to be involved in oral infection. Shklair, Losse, and Bahn (1963) indicated that it occurs in a small proportion of the American population as an established member of the oral microbiota. The study by Clement (1953) showed a relatively high incidence of the organism in the oral cavity of African natives living under primitive conditions. In a study of 350 individuals Sutter, Hurst, and Landucci (1966) observed that *Pseudomonas* species, especially *Pseudomonas aeruginosa*, were present in the saliva of about 8% of the subjects.

Fox and Isenberg (1967) isolated *Pseudomonas aeruginosa* from a small percentage of infected root canals. On occasion it was found to be present in nonvital teeth. Neonatal suppurative parotitis caused by *Pseudomonas aeruginosa* is rare but has been observed by Leake and Leake (1970). Such infections apparently result from the invasion of the tissues following a septicemia. Acute suppurative parotitis caused by a mixed infection involving staphylococci and pseudomonads has been reported in the adult (Hecht and Work, 1970).

Pseudomonas bacteremia (Goldberg, 1968) and oral infections owing to *Pseudomonas aeruginosa* following oral surgical procedures have been reported (Goldberg, 1966). The latter publication also describes the occurrence of a mandibular infection following extraction of impacted molars and infection in the mandibular molar region of a patient undergoing endodontic and periodontic treatment at the same site. Chronic osteomyelitis with sequestrum formation of the maxilla in an adult has been reported to be caused by a *Pseudomonas* species (Reade and Radden, 1963).

Klyhn and Gorrill (1967) reported on the steadily increasing rate of pseudomonad infection in hospitals. These occur most frequently in debilitated patients or in individuals whose immune systems have been depressed. The urinary tract and burned skin are especially prone to infection in the compromised host. It appears that *Pseudomonas aeruginosa* colonizes the gastrointestinal tract and that autoinfection may occur from the feces by way of the patient's hands. Such infected individuals are thus in part responsible for contamination of hospital equipment used by them. Equipment too large or intricate to be readily sterilized after use may become a source of new infections (McNamara et al., 1967). The use of humidifying equipment for newborn infants with respiratory problems has resulted in *Pseudomonas* infections that have been serious and frequently fatal. Hoffman and Finberg (1955) reported an infection of the lips of an infant that progressed to a noma involving the cheeks and nose; death resulted in spite of antibiotic therapy. Autopsy revealed scattered abscesses of the pleura of the lung.

Campylobacter. The genus *Campylobacter* comprises slender, curved, motile, gram-negative bacteria that are microaerophilic. They do not grow aerobically as surface colonies nor do they grow under strictly anaerobic conditions. They do not ferment carbohydrates. At present four species are delineated. Most of them are essentially animal pathogens, but some have been recovered from human infectious processes. The species now recognized are *Campylobacter fetus fetus*, *Campylobacter fetus venerealis*, *Campylobacter coli*, and *Campylobacter sputorum sputorum*. The latter species, along with *Fusobacterium nucleatum*, has been found to be present in the inflamed gingival crevice in a significantly higher proportion than in the normal gingival crevice (van Palenstein Helderman, 1975). The author has suggested that an increase in the number of gram-negative bacteria might act as an accelerative factor in the local inflammatory response of this area.

Hemophilus. Members of the *Hemophilus* genus of small gram-negative bacilli are no longer considered to be species of the family Brucellaceae. They are classified in the eighth edition of *Ber-*

gey's Manual (Buchanan and Gibbons, 1974) as a genus of uncertain affiliation.

Hemophilus influenzae is carried in the human nasopharynx and oropharynx and can be also isolated from saliva. Morris (1954b) reported occasional isolates of *Hemophilus* species from the mouth. Sims (1970a) showed that hemophili are frequently present in saliva, on mucosal surfaces, and in dental plaque. Based on a study of 100 specimens, this investigator reported a mean salivary level of 31.8×10^2 hemophili per ml; 92.8% of the isolates were V factor (nicotinamide adenine dinucleotide) dependent, while the remaining strains required both V factor and X factor (hemin).

A fulminating meningitis in infants and young children 6 months to 2 years of age is the most serious disease manifestation caused by *Hemophilus influenzae*. Occasionally in this situation oral manifestations may result in a cellulitis localized in the face, especially the cheek. The buccal mucosa may be pale and slightly edematous on the affected side; there may be teething associated with the onset of the cellulitis, and the tonsils may be enlarged and injected (Feingold and Gellis, 1965; Green and Fousek, 1957). *Hemophilus influenzae,* along with *Streptococcus pneumoniae* and anaerobic bacteria, were frequently recovered in sinusitis from the maxillary antrum in a study of 25 adults (Evans et al., 1975).

Miscellaneous bacteria. Some members of the group of gram-negative bacteria have been designated according to genus and species while others have not. Their morphology varies considerably among genera and groups. Some produce acid from carbohydrates either by fermentation or oxidation. About 35 organisms may be placed into this miscellaneous category, which includes the genera *Acinetobacter, Achromobacter, Alcaligenes, Eikenella, Flavobacterium,* and *Moraxella.* Others have been designated as "Group IIk," "Group Va," "Group Ve," "Group M-l," and so forth. These are described in the *Manual of Clinical Microbiology* (Lennette, Spaulding, and Truant, 1974). A variety of media, cultural conditions, and techniques are employed to recover these bacteria from

various sites in the human body, and an appropriate selection of these will allow for their isolation and identification. Many of these organisms have been isolated from both the normal and infected oral cavity and lesions of the face and neck. Some of these have been responsible for severe nosocomial infection, particularly in the compromised host.

Three cases involving mixed infections with *Eikenella corrodens* and other oral bacteria were reported by Glassman and Simpson (1975). A brain abscess developed in one patient who had several congenital cardiac anomalies about 1 month following a dental restoration and prophylaxis. Another patient with a known glucose-6-phosphate dehydrogenase deficiency developed a submandibular and sublingual abscess following extraction of a mandibular right third molar. In the third case an abscess developed on the anterior aspect of the neck several months after radiotherapy had been administered for treatment of a laryngeal carcinoma. The authors pointed out that dental practitioners should be alert to the role of *Eikenella corrodens* in mixed infections, because they present difficult problems with respect to treatment.

Anaerobes

The isolation and properties of the anaerobic gram-negative rods and filaments found in the human mouth have been reviewed by Bowden and Hardie (1971). The classification of the *Bacterioides* has been in a confused state for a number of years. Several taxonomic studies and identification schemes have been published (Loesche, Socransky, and Gibbons, 1964; Sawyer, Macdonald, and Gibbons, 1962; Barnes and Goldberg, 1968; Spiers, 1971; Werner, Pulverer, and Reichertz, 1971). However, the most recent information on the techniques for cultivation and biochemical characterization has been presented in detail by Holdeman, Cato, and Moore (1977).

Bacteroides. Twenty-two species and a number of subspecies or serotypes of the genus *Bacteroides* are delineated in *Bergey's Manual* (Buchanan and Gibbons,

1974). These microorganisms may be motile or nonmotile. Cells with terminal and central swelling and vacuoles may be observed; filamentous forms are common. However, individual cultures usually show a minimal variation in morphology.

A number of species have been isolated from the oral cavity, particularly from the gingival crevice area. Only a few members of this genus are true pathogens, but some are important as opportunistic pathogens. *Bacteroides oralis* has been isolated from infections of the mouth and respiratory and genital tracts. *Bacteroides melaninogenicus,* which produces a black pigment when grown on blood agar, is present in the oral cavity. Since this species elaborates the enzyme collagenase, its involvment in the pathogenesis of chronic periodontitis has been postulated. In a few instances it may appear in the oral cavity before the teeth erupt (Hurst and Fenderson, 1969), but it is universally present only upon the development of the gingival sulci following tooth eruption. Kelstrup (1966) concluded that there was no correlation between its presence and inflammation of the sulci. Other reports indicate that when the oral sites colonized by *Bacteroides* species are damaged or injured, the organisms gain entrance into the lymphatics and blood circulation, giving rise to involvement of the lungs, liver, bone, and joints (Brown, Williams, and Herrell, 1941). A number of *Bacteroides* species have been isolated from pyogenic infections of dental origin by Sabiston, Grigsby, and Sagerstrom (1976).

Fusobacterium. Sixteen species of the genus *Fusobacterium* are delineated in *Bergey's Manual* (Buchanan and Gibbons, 1974). These organisms may be motile or nonmotile. They are very pleomorphic and size varies from 1 to 20 μm long; classic morphologic forms may be spindle-shaped, club-shaped, straight, or curved. Some may be centrally or terminally swollen; others may be vacuolated.

Fusobacterium species are members of the normal oral microbiota and ordinarily exhibit low pathogenicity. However,

Hadi and Russell (1968) showed that the viable count of fusiforms in saliva from subjects with acute ulcerative gingivitis was significantly higher than in the saliva of normal subjects.

Leptotrichia. The genus *Leptotrichia* currently consists of only a single species, *Leptotrichia buccalis.* These organisms are straight or slightly curved rods, 1 to 1.5 μm wide by 5 to 15 μm long. One or both ends may be rounded or pointed. No club or branching forms are seen. Some cells show gram-positive granules. *Leptotrichia buccalis* is an anaerobe, and the presence of 5% carbon dioxide is considered essential for isolation and optimal growth.

Leptotrichia buccalis is not currently recognized to be specifically associated with oral disease. In comparison to the total number of fusiform organisms, Hadi and Russell (1969) found that *Leptorichia buccalis* was present in very low concentration in all cases of acute ulcerative gingivitis and advanced chronic periodontal disease that they studied.

Selenomonas. Originally, these organisms were considered to be members of protozoan families. They are gram-negative pleomorphic forms, exhibiting curved to helical rods whose ends are usually tapered and round to make then appear as crescent-shaped short cells. (This morphology is thus akin to certain protozoan forms—*Toxoplasma* species, *Leishmania* species, and so on.) Long cells and chains of cells may exhibit this helical form. Strains exhibit marked differences in size.

The cells are motile with an active tumbling motion (again akin to certain protozoans). Up to 16 flagella may be present as a tuft near the center of the concave side of the crescent form. Long cells may exhibit several such tufts similarly located. Their optimal growth temperature is within the normal bacterial range (35 to 40°C); however, they grow optimally at a lower pH range, pH 4.5 to 5.

Two species and three subspecies are delineated in *Bergey's Manual* (Buchanan and Gibbons, 1974). *Selenomonas sputigena* is found in the human oral cavity. Wantland, Wantland, and

Winquist (1963) reported finding *Seleno-monas* species during microscopic examination of oral specimens.

Spirochetes, mycoplasma, yeasts, and protozoa

Treponema

Spirochetes belonging to the genus *Treponema* are common inhabitants of the human oral cavity, particularly in the gingival crevice. Smibert (1974) describes the bacteria of this genus as unicellular, helical rods characterized by tight regular or irregular spirals. These motile cells possess axial fibrils that are inserted at each end of the protoplasmic cylinder. Most species stain well with silver impregnation methods, although dark-field microscopy is most frequently employed for microscopic examination. The oral species, *Treponema denticola*, *Treponema macrodentium*, *Treponema orale*, *Treponema scoliodontum*, and *Treponema vincentii* may be isolated under strict anaerobic conditions by the membrane-filter technique described by Holdeman, Cato, and Moore (1977). Separation into species is accomplished by fermentation and other biochemical tests as well as analysis of fermentation end products by means of gas chromatography.

With the exception of the symbiotic invasion of the gingivae by *Treponema vincentii* (formerly classified as *Borrelia vincentii*) and fusiform bacilli in acute necrotizing ulcerative gingivitis and in noma, none of the above species has been definitely established as an etiologic agent of human disease. However, Löe, Theilade, and Jensen (1965) have observed that a reversible gingivitis develops in human subjects within 10 to 21 days following withdrawal of all measures of oral hygiene. Using an impression smear technique and only microscopic observation, these investigators showed that vibrios and spirochetes appeared in plaque that accumulated at the gingival margin after about 2 weeks of no oral hygiene. While coccal and filamentous forms were also present in the plaque, it is tempting to speculate that the spirochetes contributed to the development of the gingivitis, since endotoxin has

been extracted from oral treponemes (Mergenhagen, Hampp, and Scherp, 1961). In addition Gibbons et al., (1963) indicated that spirochetes were present in the gingival crevice debris from subjects with periodontal disease in concentrations three times greater than that observed in normal subjects.

Mycoplasma

The bacteria of the genus *Mycoplasma* are the smallest prokaryotic organisms that can be cultivated on sterile artificial media. In contrast to other bacteria, they lack a cell wall, and as a result, they are extremely pleomorphic. Electron micrographs (Boatman and Kenny, 1971) of *Mycoplasma pneumoniae* show coccal, bacillary, and beaded filamentous forms; the smallest reproductive forms measure about 125 to 250 nm in diameter. However, their precise size is somewhat difficult to ascertain because of their pleomorphism.

The *Mycoplasma* were originally isolated from infectious pleuropneumonia in cattle, and they were initially referred to as pleuropneumonia organisms. Since these organisms were not trapped by bacterial filters, they were believed to be viruses. When similar organisms that caused disease in other animals as well as humans were isolated, they were referred to as pleuropneumonia-like organisms or PPLO. In 1967 it was proposed that a new class, Mollicutes, and genus, *Mycoplasma*, be created to accomodate these organsims.

The medium required for growth of the *Mycoplasma* is complex and contains peptones, yeast extract, and serum. The colonies that are formed are very small, ranging from 10 to 100 μm in diameter, and they often display the so-called fried egg appearance. This results from the growth of the organisms in the center of the colony into the agar. The techniques for isolation and staining are different from those employed for other bacteria and have been presented in some detail by Kenny (1974). These organisms are divided into groups on the basis of biochemical reactions and oxygen requirements and into species on the basis of inhibition of growth by specific antiserum. Since they lack a cell wall, none is susceptible to the action of the penicillins.

Apparently, Morton and co-workers (1951) were the first investigators to report the isolation of mycoplasmas from the human oral cavity. Subsequently, other investigators (Engel and Kenny, 1970; Fox, Purcell, and Chanock, 1969; Razin, Michmann, and Shimshoni, 1964; Shklair et al., 1962; Taylor-Robinson et al., 1964) described the presence of various species of mycoplasma in the mouth. The oral species of the genus Mycoplasma, *Mycoplasma orale, Mycoplasma pharyngis,* and *Mycoplasma salivarium* are microaerophilic to anaerobic and are considered to be normal flora without pathogenic effects.

The only species definitely proved to cause disease in humans is *Mycoplasma pneumoniae,* which is the major etiologic agent of primary atypical pneumonia (Grayston, Foy, and Kenny, 1959). The tiny or "T" strains of mycoplasma are often isolated from cases of nongonococcal urethritis (Lee et al., 1973; McCormack et al., 1973), but their significance in the pathogenesis of this syndrome is uncertain.

Candida and other yeasts

Microscopic fungi that exist as single, independent cells are referred to as yeasts. Morphologically, they are usually ovoid or round and are generally larger than bacteria. They differ from bacteria in that they are eukaryotic, that is possess a true nucleus separated from the cytoplasm by a nuclear membrane. The yeasts of dental importance reproduce primarily by an asexual process called budding or blastospore formation (Fig. 4-4). However some species, such as *Candida albicans,* may form chlamydospores and produce pseudomycelia as well as true mycelia (Fig. 4-5). They may be cultivated on a variety of media including Sabouraud agar. The latter is composed of peptone, glucose, water, and agar. Since the pH of 5.6 is inhibitory to many bacteria, it is a standard isolation medium in the mycology laboratory. Several other media are also employed for isolation or identification. Separation of the yeasts

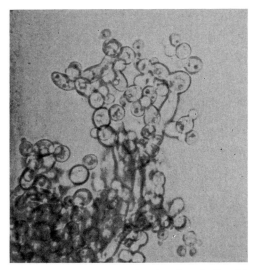

Fig. 4-4. Photomicrograph of cultured *Candida albicans* showing budding cells. Unstained. (×640.)

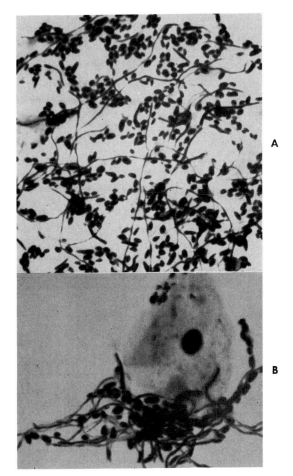

A

B

Fig. 4-5. A, *Candida albicans* with threadlike structures that are filaments of mycelium. **B,** Epithelial cell surrounded by organisms.

into species is accomplished mainly by carbohydrate fermentation and assimilation tests, nitrogen utilization, and the production of extracellular substances and enzymes (Rippon, 1974).

Yeasts comprise a small proportion of the normal flora of the mucous membranes of the mouth, gastrointestinal tract, and vagina of humans and some animals. Bartels and Blechman (1962) surveyed 320 saliva specimens from 160 individuals ranging in age from 20 to 30 years for the presence of yeasts. Yeasts were found in 40% of the specimens; 75.8% were identified as species of the genus *Candida. Candida albicans* was the species most frequently isolated (60%), although other species such as *Candida krusei, Candida tropicalis, Candida paropsilosis*, and *Candida guilliermondi* were present less frequently. In addition species of the genus *Cryptococcus* and *Saccharomyces* were found in some specimens. About 97% of the positive specimens contained between 10 and 500 yeast colony–forming units per milliliter of saliva, and only 2.4% of the specimens contained counts greater than 1000 colony-forming units per milliliter. Schmitt (1971) cultured the mouths of 103 volunteers using a gargle-rinse technique and observed that *Candida albicans* could be isolated from about 34% of the subjects. Therefore it appears that *Candida* species are present in the mouths of some, but not all, individuals.

Entamoeba and Trichomonas

Although several investigators including Barrett (1914), Kofoid (1929), and Beatman (1933) reported the occurrence of protozoa in the human mouth, the most extensive studies have been conducted by Wantland and co-workers (1958, 1960, 1963). These investigators have shown that both *Entamoeba gingivalis* and *Trichomonas tenax* may colonize relatively "clean and healthy" mouths and that the incidence increases with the age of the subjects studied. In patients with advanced periodontitis, *Entamoeba gingivalis* was observed in 100% of the subjects and *Trichomonas tenax* in 80% of the subjects; both were found in 80% of

the subjects. Wantland and Lauer (1970) found that the incidence of oral colonization was correlated with the amount of calculus present, the degree of coating on the dorsum of the tongue, and the progression of periodontal disease. These two oral protozoa are usually considered to be nonpathogenic and their presence appears to reflect the degree of oral hygiene and the increased presence of bacteria associated with chronic periodontitis. Their role in the pathogenesis of periodontal disease is questionable. Gottlieb and Miller (1971) did not observe *Entamoeba gingivalis* within histologic sections of viable gingival tissue in patients with advanced periodontal disease; they appeared to be confined to the surface of the crevicular epithelium or within dental plaque adjacent to the epithelial and connective tissue in the gingival crevice.

BACTERIAL, MYCOTIC, PROTOZOAN, AND VIRAL INFECTIONS
Systemic bacterial infections presenting oral manifestations
Scarlet fever

Scarlet fever is caused by strains of Lancefield's group A beta-hemolytic streptococci *(Streptococcus pyogenes)* that elaborate an erythrogenic toxin. The oral manifestation is termed "stomatitis scarlatina." The oral mucosa, especially that of the palate, becomes congested and appears fiery red. The tonsils exhibit a white coating as do the faucial pillars; they are swollen and a grayish exudate is seen. The changes in the tongue are pathognomonically important. The tongue develops a white coating; edematous and hyperemic fungiform papillae are observed. This is clinically described as a "strawberry tongue." This coating is lost first from the tip and lateral margins of the tongue, and then the tongue looks deep red, glistening, and smooth. However, hyperemic papillae are still apparent. Clinically, this is termed "raspberry tongue." If the case of scarlet fever is extremely severe, ulceration of the buccal mucosa and palate develops; this reaction is most likely caused by secondary infection. Complications may arise as a result of local, lymphatic, or circulatory dissemination of the cocci. Hypersensitivity reactions may be a further complication attributed to bacterial toxins.

Rheumatic fever is one of the most serious sequelae that may follow untreated infections caused by Lancefield's group A serotypes of *Streptococcus pyogenes.* Streptococcal infections include not only scarlet fever but also cellulitis, erysipelias, otitis media, puerperal sepsis, septic sore throat, sinusitis, and tonsillitis. Rheumatic fever is thought to result from immunologic injury in that antibodies formed against antigens of the group A streptococci cross react with antigens of a similar or identical antigenic nature in the tissues of the human heart. This immune attack causes cardiac inflammation and damage. A serious characteristic of this disease is its tendency to recur following later infections with other "M" types of the group A beta-hemolytic streptococci. It is important that the oral and maxillofacial surgeon be aware of a history of rheumatic fever in patients he or she treats, because such patients are more prone to develop subacute bacterial endocarditis as a result of entrance of oral bacteria into the bloodstream following surgical procedures. The incidence of bacteremia of oral origin is highest in patients who have multiple extractions of the teeth, although it may also result from a variety of dental procedures including prophylaxis and endodontic treatment.

Diphtheria

Toxigenic strains of *Corynebacterium diphtheriae* are involved in the etiology of diphtheria. The first sign may often be the development of a "diphtheritic membrane" on the tonsils. This membrane enlarges and becomes confluent. In reality it is termed a "pseudomembrane" and appears grayish, thick, and fibrinous. A gelatinous-appearing exudate accompanies this manifestation. The membrane and exudate consist of dead cells, leukocytes, and bacteria overlying necrotic, ulcerated areas of the mucosa and covering the tonsils, pharynx, and larynx. It is extremely adherent, and if an attempt is made to strip it off, a bleeding surface results.

The membrane may form on the uvula, soft palate, and gingiva. Infrequently, it may occur at the site of erupting teeth and on the buccal mucosa. Paralysis of the soft palate may develop. If there is extensive spreading of the membrane, for example, to produce a laryngeal pseudomembrane, a mechanical respiratory obstruction results. If this is not cleared away, the patient is in danger of death caused by suffocation.

Tuberculosis

Mycobacterium tuberculosis is the etiologic agent of tuberculosis. Lesions of the oral cavity are said to occur uncommonly. Farber, Friedland, and Jacobs (1940) reported less than 0.1% incidence in the patients they studied. On the other hand, Katz (1941) reported that 20% of 141 patients examined at autopsy had unrecognized oral lesions, primarily at the base of the tongue.

There appears to be general agreement that the oral lesions are secondary to pulmonary disease. It also has been stated that tubercle bacilli may reach these sites by hematogenous spread. Another strong possibility is that the organisms may enter the oral tissues through minor breaks in the surface of the mucous membranes.

Although the tongue is the site most frequently involved, lesions may occur elsewhere, including the palate, lips, buccal mucosa, gingiva, and frenula. The lesion appears as an irregular, superficial, painful ulcer and increases in size. Occasionally it begins in an area of trauma. Tuberculosis of the bone is an unusual manifestation, but it may occur. The bone of the maxilla or mandible may become involved. One possible mode of entry is said to be into an area of periapical inflammation by way of the bloodstream. It has also been said that organisms may enter the periapical area by direct immigration through the pulp chamber and root canal. Such entry could give rise to a tuberculous periapical granuloma or a tuberculoma. Oral lesions of tubercular origin are usually noted late in the disease and are normally consistent with an unfavorable prognosis.

The possibility of infection of the surgeon is of great clinical significance. Viable acid-fast bacilli in washings or swabs of the oral mucosa may certainly be recovered. Abbott, Briney, and Denaro (1955) reported their recovery from 45% of 300 samples of water used to wash patients' teeth; there was also good recovery from 111 gingival swabs.

Leprosy

The etiologic agent of leprosy is *Mycobacterium leprae*. The lesions reported in the oral cavity are generally tumorlike masses (lepromas) that may be observed on the tongue, lips, and palate. These lesions tend to break down and ulcerate. Gingival hyperplasia with a loosening of the teeth may occur. Epker and Via (1969) and Reichart (1976) have most recently discussed the oral manifestations of leprosy.

Tularemia

The etiologic agent of tularemia, *Francisella tularensis,* is one of the smallest nonsporeforming gram-negative bacilli. This disease has its reservoir in the wild rodent population and rabbits. It occurs in man by accidental transmission of the organism from the animal host. Very often this involves handling an infected animal or its skin. Necrotic ulcers of the oral mucosa or pharynx may be observed, and these are usually painful. On occasion a generalized stomatitis may be seen rather than a localized lesion. Such a manifestation may develop into multiple abscesses. Commonly a regional submandibular and cervical lymphadenitis is part of the clinical picture.

Melioidosis

Pseudomonas pseudomallei is the etiologic agent of melioidosis. This disease is endemic in certain areas of the Far East such as Burma, Ceylon, India, Indochina, Malaysia, Thailand, and Indonesia. Its significance was increased when the United States conducted military operations in these areas; however, it has now become a worldwide problem (Dodin, 1976).

There are two forms of melioidosis—the acute and chronic. In the acute form, no oral lesions are manifest. The chronic disease develops in individuals who survive the acute form of the infection. Involvement of the cervicofacial area may be observed, and these lesions resemble those of fungal infection or tuberculosis. For the most part, cases seen in the United States have been in American servicemen who had returned from duty in Southeast Asia.

Syphilis

Syphilis is caused by the spirochete *Treponema pallidum.* From 1958 to 1969, a greater than 200% increase in reported cases of primary and secondary syphilis was noted in the United States. In essence the disease is currently being seen in increasing numbers. Much of the astonishing upsurge is among teenage individuals. Syphilis is most frequently contracted as a venereal disease. Occasionally dentists working with infected patients may contract the disease.

If untreated, three distinctive stages of syphilis are recognized: the primary, secondary, and tertiary stages. In the *primary stage* the lesion is the chancre that commonly occurs on the penis in the male and the vulva or cervix in the female. However, lesions of the lips, tongue, palate, gingiva, and tonsils are of particular interest to the oral and maxillofacial surgeon. Chancres have been reported as developing at the site of a fresh extraction wound. The usual lesion is an elevated, ulcerated nodule, exhibiting local induration and producing a regional lymphadenitis. Such a lesion on the lip may have a brownish, crusted appearance. The chancre usually heals spontaneously in 3 weeks to 2 months.

An intraoral chancre normally appears as an ulcerated lesion covered by a grayish-white membrane. Usually a syphilitic chancre is not painful unless it is secondarily infected. The chancre abounds with spirochetes and is highly infectious. *Treponema pallidum* may be seen on dark-field examination. *Treponema denticola* is one of the nonpathogenic treponemes that inhabit the oral cavity, and it is impossible to distinguish this organism from *Treponema pallidum* on the basis of morphology. It has become dictum that dark-field examination should not be done on exudate from lesions contaminated with saliva. Instead, dark-field examination should be made on fluid aspirated from a regional lymph node. Enlarged nodes are almost always found along the lymphatics draining the area of a chancre. It is important to note that not every patient presenting a primary syphilitic lesion will exhibit a positive serologic test for syphilis despite the existence of a spirochetemia.

The *secondary* or *metastatic stage* of syphilis begins approximately 6 weeks after the primary lesion. This stage is characterized by diffuse eruptions of the skin and mucous membranes. On the skin one most often observes macules or papules. The oral lesions, called "mucous patches," are usually multiple, painless, grayish white plaques overlying an ulcerated surface. They occur most frequently on the tongue, gingiva, or buccal mucosa. They appear ovoid or irregular and are surrounded by an erythematous zone. Mucous patches are highly infectious; they contain large numbers of spirochetes. In the secondary stage serologic tests for syphilis are positive. Usually spontaneous remission occurs within a few weeks, but exacerbations may continue to occur for months or several years.

In the *tertiary stage* lesions usually do not appear for several years and the cardiovascular and central nervous systems as well as certain other tissues and organs are chiefly involved. The "gumma" is the principal localized lesion, and it occurs most frequently in the skin, mucous membranes, liver, testes, and brain. It appears as a focal granulomatous inflammatory process with central necrosis. Such a lesion may vary in size from several millimeters to several centimeters in diameter.

Intraoral gumma most frequently involves the tongue and palate. It is a nodular mass in the tissue that may subsequently ulcerate. In lesions of the palate, perforation may result owing to sloughing of necrotic tissue masses. Occasionally this may be the manifestation of a Jarisch-Herxheimer reaction following the initiation of antibiotic therapy.

Meyer and Shklar (1967) reported oral manifestations in 81 cases of acquired syphilis. They stressed the fact that lesions of the tertiary stage are more common than primary or secondary stage lesions in the oral cavity. They also emphasized that atrophic or interstitial glossitis is one of the most important characteristic manifestations of syphilis.

Congenital or *prenatal syphilis* should be mentioned in spite of the fact that it is a rare disease today. However, Fiumara and Lessell (1970) reported a 168% increase in the number of reported cases of congenital syphilis in children under 10 years of age in the United States between 1960 and 1969.

Persons with congenital syphilis manifest a variety of lesions. The investigators cited above reported that 87% of a series of 271 patients manifested frontal bosses; 76% showed short maxilla; 76% had a high palatal arch; 73% were "saddle-nosed"; 70% had "mulberry molars"; 26% exhibited relative protrusion of the mandible; 39% had irregular thickening of the sternoclavicular portion of the clavicle; and 4% had "saber shins." Considered pathognomonic of congenital syphilis is "Hutchinson's triad": hypoplasia of the incisors and molars, eighth nerve deafness, and interstitial keratitis. In the study by Fiumara and Lessell (1970), 75% of the individuals had one or more components of this triad, but it was unusual for all three components to be observed in one individual.

Gonorrhea

The etiologic agent of gonorrhea is *Neisseria gonorrhoeae*. Gonorrhea is a venereal disease primarily infecting the male and female genital tracts. However, an increasing number of extragenital infections, including gonococcal stomatitis, are being reported in the literature. Schmidt, Hjørting-Hansen, and Philipsen (1961) have pointed out that the oral lesions caused by *Neisseria gonorrhoeae* may appear clinically similar to those of erythema multiforme, erosive or bullous lichen planus, and herpetic stomatitis.

Diagnosis cannot be made by examination of Gram-strained smears of the oral lesions, since nonpathogenic *Neisseria* species are a part of the normal oral flora. A complete and select bacteriologic culture workup must be made, and history of proclivity of the patient must be a part of the diagnostic picture.

Granuloma venereum

Granuloma venereum is a chronic, infectious, granulomatous disease caused by bacilli designated under the species name *Donovania granulomatis*. It is a venereal disease, considered only mildly contagious. (It should not be confused with another venereal disease, lymphogranuloma venereum, which is of chlamydial etiology.) It is most prevalent in tropical zones but is also found in the southern portions of the United States. Primary lesions appear on the external genitalia and in the inguinal region. The oral lesion is the most common extragenital form of granuloma venereum; lesions may occur on the oral mucous membranes. These lesions are said to be the result of autoinoculation rather than primary infection. Lesions have been observed on the pharynx, esophagus, and larynx; extragenital lesions are observed in approximately 6% of the cases. Metastatic spread to bone and soft subcutaneous tissue from oral lesions has been reported.

Lesions may occur in any location: lips, buccal mucosa, or palate with diffuse involvement of mucosal surfaces. The clinical appearance varies and three types are recognized: ulcerative, exuberant, and cicatricial. The ulcerative and exuberant lesions may be painful and bleeding; otherwise proliferative granulomatous masses with intact epithelial covering are manifest.

Pathognomonic for the disease is the presence of large mononuclear phagocytes, each containing tiny intracytoplasmic cysts within which are found "Donovan's bodies." These are tiny, elongated basophilic and argyrophilic rods and are present intracellularly in profuse numbers.

Rhinoscleroma (scleroma)

Rhinoscleroma is an unusual chronic infectious disease, presumably caused by *Klebsiella rhinoscleromatis*. The lesions appear chiefly in the upper respiratory tract, but involvement of the lacrimal glands, orbit, skin, colon, paranasal sinuses, and brain has been described. The oral lesions appear as proliferative granulomas.

Gangrenous stomatitis (noma, cancrum oris)

Gangrenous stomatitis is a rapidly spreading gangrene of the oral and facial tissues. It is a disease of the compromised host, occurring in debilitated or nutritionally deficient patients, chiefly children. Predisposing factors play a role in its development. Children debilitated by such infections as diphtheria, measles, and scarlet fever and patients who have had pneumonia, tuberculosis, or syphilis are subject to this syndrome. It seems appropriate to consider "noma" as a secondary complication of systemic disease.

Most likely noma originates as an infection by the same organisms involved in acute necrotizing ulcerative gingivitis, namely *Treponema vincentii* and fusobacteria. The acute necrotizing gingivostomatitis is followed by rapid secondary invasion by many other organisms including streptococci, staphylococci, and diphtheria or diphtheria-like bacilli.

The syndrome begins as a small gingival mucosal ulcer that rapidly spreads to involve surrounding tissues of the jaws, lips, and cheeks by gangrenous necrosis. The initial site may be an area of stagnation around a fixed bridge or crown; the overlying skin becomes inflamed and edematous, and finally, large necrotic masses of tissue may slough, leaving the jaw exposed. The commencement of a gangrene is noted by blackening of the skin. An extremely foul odor results from the gangrenous tissue. Occasionally the tongue and palate are involved. Patients are seriously febrile during the disease course and suffer secondary infections with death from pneumonia or anoxemia. The mortality rate in the absence of antibiotic therapy is about 75%. Prognosis becomes better with selected therapeutic measures and, whenever possible, correction of the factors that compromised the host.

Systemic mycotic infections presenting oral manifestations

North American blastomycosis

The etiologic agent of North American blastomycosis is the dimorphic fungus *Blastomyces dermatitidis.* The disease may occur as a primary pulmonary infection, in a chronic cutaneous form as a generalized systemic disease, or as a self-limiting primary infection termed "inoculation blastomycosis." The last may result from a laboratory accident or from accidental implantation during the autopsy or embalming of a patient who had succumbed to the infection.

Lesions of the oral cavity may be manifested as tiny ulcers; on occasion abscess formation may occur. The oral lesions may be primary or secondary to lesions occurring elsewhere in the body. Ranier (1951) reported initial lesions that occurred in the larynx. Witorsch and Utz (1968) reported that 25% of a group of 40 patients had oral or nasal mucosal lesions. Bell, Gambler, and Garrington (1969) also reported that oral lesions could be observed as the first manifestation of blastomycosis and that this manifestation occurred more frequently than has been observed or reported.

Microabscesses are frequently found in organs. Organisms in the tissue phase (yeast cells) may be 5 to 15 μm in diameter and may be seen often as budding cells. An identifying feature is the double refractile capsule. These may be observed in the giant cells that are a part of the classic histologic appearance of these lesions.

South American blastomycosis

Blastomyces brasiliensis is the etiologic agent of South American blastomycosis. The types of infection are similar to those of North American blastomycosis.

Bogliolo (1950) reported that organisms may enter the body through the periodontal tissues, subsequently reach regional lymph nodes, and produce a severe, generalized lymphadenopathy. He was able to demonstrate organisms in the periodontal membrane and in a periapical granuloma and culture them from these sites. The fungus has been shown to penetrate the tissues and establish infection after extraction of teeth; in this instance papillary lesions of the oral mucosa are observed. Widespread oral ulceration may be a common finding.

Blastomyces brasiliensis in the yeast phase in infected tissues may vary in size from 10 to 60 μm in diameter (Fig. 4-6).

Histoplasmosis

Histoplasmosis, caused by *Histoplasma capsulatum,* is a very common granulomatous disease of worldwide distribution. Approximately 75% of cases are subclinical or benign. The remaining cases often develop a chronic progressive lung disease, which usually leads to scattered, calcified nodules. A small number of patients develop systemic disease or an acute, fulminating, rapidly fatal infection often presenting cutaneous manifestations.

In the United States, the disease is endemic in the Mississippi valley and the Northeast. Up to 75% of the population in these endemic areas has had a primary but subclinical infection. It is contracted by inhalation of dust contaminated with spores of the fungus (source to soil is bird excreta).

Oral lesions are present in a high percentage of cases. Weed and Parkhill (1948) reported that 33% of 73 cases had oral lesions as presenting complaints. Patients had been reported as having a small lesion of the tongue. Levy (1945) and more recently Stiff (1963) reviewed the oral manifestations of the disease. In addition to lesions of the tongue, patients exhibit lesions of the buccal mucosa, gingiva, palate, or lips. The ulcerated areas are indurated and usually covered with a nonspecific gray membrane.

The yeast or tissue phase of this dimorphic fungus may be demonstrated in histologic sections in many but not all cases (Fig. 4-7). It is wise therefore, as in the instances of tissue biopsy in any deep

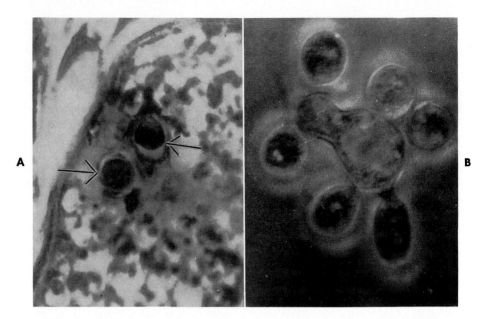

Fig. 4-6. South American blastomycosis. **A,** Photomicrograph of a lesion showing giant cell with round-bodied *Blastomyces*. **B,** Cultured *Blastomyces* producing buds. (From Salman, L., and Sheppard, S. M. 1962. Oral Surg. **15:**671.

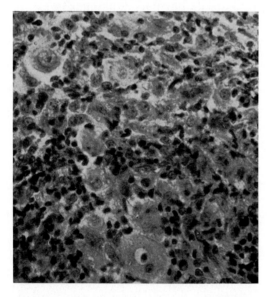

Fig. 4-7. Histologic section showing *Histoplasma capsulatum* in cytoplasm of phagocytic cells. (From Nutman, N. N. 1949. Oral Surg. **2:**1562.)

mycosis, to preserve a piece of tissue without formalin for culture purposes. Appropriate culture techniques will grow out viable yeasts at 37° C, or in the mycelial phase at room temperature, on Sabouraud agar.

Coccidioidomycosis

The etiologic agent of coccidioidomycosis is *Coccidioides immitis*. Coccidioidomycosis is now recognized as a common fungal disease endemic in the United States chiefly in the Southwest—Arizona, California, Nevada, New Mexico, Texas, and Utah. It is also seen in Mexico and Central and South America and occasionally in Europe. Similar to the situation existing with histoplasmosis, large numbers of the population in the endemic areas have developed subclinical infections. The disease is contracted by man and animals by inhalation of dust contaminated with the arthrospores of *Coccidioides immitis*.

Two forms of the disease are recognized: a primary nondisseminated form and a progressive disseminated coccidioidomycosis. In the primary form the patients develop a syndrome suggestive of a respiratory disease—cough, pleural pain, headache, and anorexia. This syndrome is self-limiting, running its course within 10 to 14 days. About 20% of these cases develop skin lesions (erythema nodosum or erythema multiforme). In a small percentage of cases pulmonary cavitation, calcified nodules, or pulmonary fibrosis may remain.

The disseminated form runs a rapid course, and dissemination extends from the lungs to the viscera, bones, joints, skin, and central nervous sytem; in the last instance meningitis is a frequent cause of death. Dissemination occurs in only about 1% of cases of the disease, and mortality rate of this form is about 50%.

Lesions of the head and neck including the oral cavity occur with some frequency as reported by Frauenfelder and Schwartz (1967). The lesions of the oral mucosa are proliferative, granulomatous and ulcerative lesions, nonspecific in clinical appearance. Marked chronicity is often a feature. They usually heal by hyalinization and scarring.

The organisms are found within the cytoplasm of the giant cells that are scattered throughout the lesion in histologic section. They may also be seen free in the tissue. Histologic section examination reveals a great variation in size and generally no budding is observed. The endospores and large endospherules can be readily recognized. Again, the organism can be cultured in the laboratory, although great caution must be used since the mycelial phase of the organism is highly infectious. Spherules, the tissue phase, may be observed in histologic sections or when grown on highly specialized media.

Cryptococcosis

The etiologic agent of cryptococcosis is *Cryptococcus neoformans*. Cryptococcosis is a chronic disease, and widespread lesions may be observed in the skin, oral mucosa, subcutaneous tissues, lungs, joints, and particularly the meninges. Since the organisms can often be found on the skin of healthy persons, it is not always clear whether an infection is of exogenous or endogeneous origin.

The first evidence of infection with *Cryptococcus neoformans* is lesions of the skin; dissemination via the blood frequently occurs. However, some investigators feel that visceral lesions are the primary manifestations of infection and skin lesions are secondary. Lung lesions produce symptoms of nonspecific pneumonitis, while meningeal involvement produces a variety of neurologic signs.

Occasional cases of oral cryptococcosis have been reported in patients with visceral or cutaneous lesions. The oral lesions may appear as a nonspecific solitary lesion, although multiple ulcers may be observed in some cases. Newman and Rosenbaum (1962) reported that oral lesions were the first evidence of infection in a patient suffering from lymphatic leukemia. Such a manifestation may be mistaken for the widespread ulceration often seen in leukemia. The immunologic systems of leukemic patients are depressed, and infections develop readily.

The tissue reaction is essentially a granulomatous response. Budding yeast-like cells with a thick gelatinous capsule, measuring 5 to 20 μm in diameter, are seen in histologic sections of the lesions. The capsule stains intensely with the periodic acid-Schiff's reagent. Organisms may be cultured on Sabouraud agar.

Candidosis (candidiasis, moniliasis, thrush)

The etiologic agent of candidosis is most frequently *Candida albicans* although other species of the genus may be involved. The yeastlike fungus, *Candida*, is a relatively common inhabitant of the normal oral cavity and gastrointestinal tract. However, the mere presence of the organism is not productive of disease; it must actually penetrate the tissues. Usually the tissue invasion is superficial. Although oral candidosis or thrush most often remains a localized infectious process, it may occasionally extend to the larynx or even the lungs. In addition to thrush, infection of the skin, vagina, lungs, and gastrointestinal and urinary tracts occurs.

Candidosis is most frequently observed in infants or in patients whose host defense mechanisms are compromised, for instance, debilitated individuals and patients with uncontrolled diabetes. Nutritional deficiencies such as avitaminoses may also predispose to the development of *Candida* infection. Infection with *Candida albicans* has become more common since the advent of antibiotics. Since this organism is not susceptible to antibiotics used in the treatment of bacterial infections, a super-infection may result from the elimination of the microbiota that are normally antagonistic to it.

The oral lesions of candidosis are characterized as soft, white, elevated plaques that most frequently occur on the buccal mucosa and tongue. The lesions may also be observed on the palate and the floor of the mouth. The plaques have been described as grossly resembling milk curds, and they consist chiefly of tangled masses of fungal pseudohyphae. In severe cases the entire oral cavity may be involved, although *Candida* cheilitis (Jansen, Dillaha, and Honeycutt, 1963) usually involves the lips without producing intraoral lesions.

The observation that stripping off the plaque leaves a raw bleeding surface is often considered pathognomonic, because other plaquelike lesions such as those of leukoplakia cannot be peeled off. Roed-Petersen, Renstrup, and Pindborg (1970) reported a high incidence of *Candida* organisms in a survey of 225 patients with leukoplakia.

Geotrichosis

Various species of the genus *Geotrichum* are involved as the etiologic agents of geotrichosis. The most common lesions are those of the lung and oral mucosa, but on occasion the skin and intestinal tract may be involved. The disease is similar to candidosis in that infections occur primarily in the compromised host as a result of a superinfection. The oral lesions are essentially identical to those of thrush; they may be isolated or diffuse in distribution. Differential diagnosis depends on microscopic examination of scrapings from the oral mucosa and preferably culture of the etiologic agent.

Aspergillosis

Aspergillosis broadly defined is a group of diseases in which members of the genus Aspergillus are involved. Some ten species have been associated with the infectious process in man; *Aspergillus fumigatus* is considered the most virulent and invasive. Clinical diseases documented include pulmonary aspergillosis, disseminated aspergillosis, central nervous system aspergillosis, naso-orbital aspergillosis, and iatrogenic aspergillosis.

Aspergillus infection in patients with debilitating diseases such as tuberculosis, diabetes, malignancies, and immunodeficiency (for example, leukemias, lymphomas) has been recognized for some 50 years. More recently aspergillosis has been reported in patients under therapy with antibiotics, cytotoxins, corticosteroids, and immunosuppressive agents; in patients undergoing irradiation; and following a variety of surgical transplantation procedures (Rippon, 1974).

A striking, yet not atypical, case of fungal infection in the compromised host has been reported by Erlichman and Trieger (1978) (Figs. 4-8 and 4-9). A 40-year-old female was first seen in the dental clinic with the chief complaint of "a lump under the chin." The lesion was a nontender submental swelling. Repeated culture of specimens of a purulent aspirate was negative for acid-fast organisms and aerobic and anaerobic bacteria. *Aspergillus fumigatus* was observed in KOH mounts and grown in culture. This patient had lupus erythematosus and had been hospitalized previously for glomerulonephritis and pleural effusion. She had been under steroid therapy and had developed diabetes. A short time later she died of *Cryptococcus neoformans* infection in spite of concerted antifungal therapy.

Phycomycosis (mucormycosis)

Numerous saprophytic fungi of the class Phycomycetes, especially species of the genera *Rhizopus, Mucor,* and *Absidia,* are involved as the etiologic agents of phycomycosis. This acute, frequently fatal infection is almost always seen in individuals with lowered resistance. Diabetes mellitus, malnutrition, kwashiorkor, blood dyscrasias, renal insufficiency, cirrhosis, malignancies, and administration of corticosteroids, cytotoxic drugs

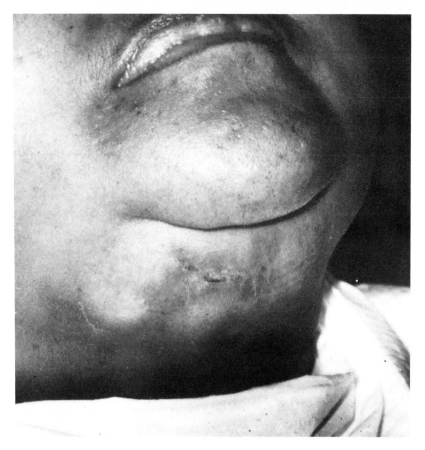

Fig. 4-8. Patient with aspergillosis. There is diffuse, doughy, nontender swelling in submental area. Patient is edentulous with no intraoral source of infection evident. (From Erlichman, M. C., and Trieger, N. 1978. J. Oral. Surg. **36:**978.)

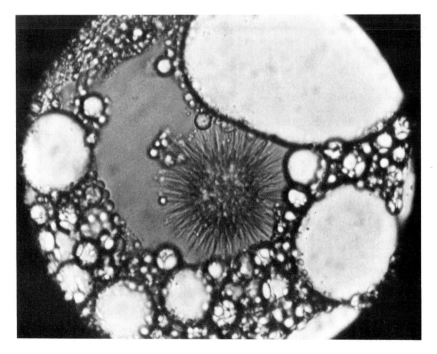

Fig. 4-9. Aspergillus fumigatus in KOH preparation of pus aspirated from submental swelling. (×200.) (From Erlichman, M. C., and Trieger, N. 1978. J. Oral. Surg. **36:**978.)

and antibiotics for extended periods are considered predisposing factors. However, diabetes mellitus is the most frequent antecedent. A thorough review of the literature was published by Hutter (1959), and the craniofacial form has been discussed and reviewed by Green, Goldberg, and Wohl (1967), Landau and Newcomer (1963), and Taylor and co-workers (1969). A rare case of mucocutaneous mucormycosis that followed dental extractions in a patient with uncontrolled diabetes has been described by Limongelli and co-workers (1975). In this instance the infection was successfully resolved by controlling the diabetes, administration of antibiotics, and surgical excision of the necrotic tissue.

Two forms of mucormycosis are commonly seen: (1) superficial, involving the external ear, fingernails, and skin, and (2) visceral, involving the pulmonary or gastrointestinal tracts or cervicofacial structures. Mucormycosis of the central nervous system is characterized by the clinical triad of uncontrolled diabetes, unilateral periorbital infection, and meningoencephalitis. The organisms enter the tissues through the nasal mucosa and extend to the paranasal sinuses, pharynx, palate, orbit, and brain.

Phycomycosis of the maxillary sinus may be seen clinically as a mass in the maxilla. Typical cases have been described by Faillo, Sube, and Anderson (1959) and Green, Goldberg, and Wohl (1967). Surgical exploration reveals masses of necrotic tissue and the causative organisms can be observed in histologic sections.

Rhizopus infections of the skin following the use of nonsterile Elastoplast bandage have been reported by several investigators, including Gartenberg and co-workers (1978). The cutaneous lesions have varied from vesiculopustular eruptions to ulceration with eschar formation; in certain cases necrosis of the skin with subcutaneous involvement has occurred. These infections have been attributed to contamination of the bandage material with species of the genus *Rhizopus* and have occurred most frequently in individuals whose immune systems were compromised. It is important to note that an Elastoplast bandage should not be used to cover open wounds nor should it be placed in contact with a sterile field when aseptic conditions are to be maintained.

Sporotrichosis

Sporothrix schenkii is the etiologic agent of sporotrichosis. The most common infections seen involve the skin, subcutaneous tissues, and oral, nasal, and pharyngeal mucosa. Occasional visceral involvement has been reported. Lesions of the skin have been termed "sporotrichal 'chancres'."

Oral manifestations are seen as nonspecific, ulcerative lesions of the oral, nasal, and pharyngeal mucous membranes. Regional lymphadenophathy usually accompanies the lesions. When healing occurs, soft pliable scars remain. The tissue reaction is a granulomatous one.

It should be emphasized that the organism is seldom recognized in histologic section. It becomes necessary therefore to include the culture of the specimen or biopsy to establish a diagnosis of sporotrichosis.

Rhinosporidiosis

Rhinosporidiosis, caused by *Rhinosporidium seeberi*, is a rare infection, affecting the oropharynx and nasopharynx. On occasion the larynx, skin, eye, and genital mucosa may be infected.

Oronasopharyngeal lesions appear as soft, red growths of a tumorlike nature, which spread to the pharynx and larynx. The lesions are accompanied by a mucoid discharge, are vascular, and bleed easily. An unusual case involving the parotid duct was reported by Topazian (1966).

The organism appears as a sporangium containing large numbers of endospores 5 to 7 μm in diameter; these may be seen on a smear preparation or in histologic sections.

Angular cheilitis (perlèche, angular cheilosis)

Numerous studies have reported that *Candida albicans*, staphylococci, and streptococci are usually isolated from patients with angular cheilitis, but not all of these were found at the same time in individual cases. *Candida* species have been assumed to be the most frequent and significant etiologic agent of angular cheilitis. However, a recent study (MacFarlane and Helnarska, 1976) of 100 patients revealed that the syndrome was of infective etiology in only 68 of the cases. *Candida* species were isolated from 44% of these individuals while beta-hemolytic streptococci were recovered from 15% of the cases. *Staphylococcus aureus* was isolated from 79% of the lesions. Thirty-two patients yielded negative cultures.

Dentures that result in improper vertical dimension and overclosure of the jaws in edentulous patients have been considered to be a predisposing factor. As a result of this condition, saliva collects in a fold that is produced at the corners of the mouth, and the skin becomes macerated, fissured, and secondarily infected. It has been reported that correction of these errors, for example, increasing the vertical bite, has resulted in resolution of this syndrome.

A deficiency of the vitamin riboflavin has also been associated with angular cheilitis. This avitaminosis with a superimposed candidal or bacterial infection has been suggested as being involved in the etiology of the syndrome. Such a theory appears to be supported by the observation that administration of B complex vitamins often leads to a resolution of the infection. Cawson (1963) reported on a series of patients with perlèche associated with "denture sore mouth." *Candida* species or related organisms were isolated. He suggested that these cases were associated with intraoral infection with *Candida*.

Angular cheilitis may occur in children or adults. A burning sensation and feeling of dryness at the corners of the mouth are presenting symptoms. The epithelium at the commissures is wrinkled in appearance and exhibits maceration. The wrinkling develops into one or more deep fissures that appear ulcerated. The tendency to bleed is minimal, although a superficial exudative crust may form.

There is no involvement of the mucosal surface of the commissure inside the mouth; the lesion stops at the mucocutaneous junction. Even in the absence of treatment there is a tendency to spontaneous regression. However, the lesions rarely disappear completely and exacerbation may occur.

Protozoan infections presenting oral manifestations

There are a few protozoan diseases that on occasion manifest oral involvement. These manifestations are most significant to the oral and maxillofacial surgeon whose practice exists in the areas of endemic occurrence of these infections. They may also be of great importance to the oral surgeon in the United States, however, because certain of these diseases, once restricted to areas outside the United States, are becoming cosmopolitan because of jet-age travel and military involvement of our forces in the countries where protozoan diseases are important infectious disease problems. This does not necessarily mean that such diseases will become endemic in the United States, because the necessary vectors or reservoirs do not exist in this country. It does mean, however, that individuals infected with these organisms may be seen and in certain instances may even present an infectious hazard. The major diseases of protozoan origin that will be discussed here are leishmaniasis and American trypanosomiasis.

Mucocutaneous leishmaniasis (American leishmaniasis)

Leishmania brasiliensis, which is the etiologic agent of mucocutaneous leishmaniasis seen in the Western hemisphere, produces a variety of skin and mucous membrane lesions. In warm, moist areas of the Americas, ulcerating lesions of both the skin and mucous membranes are observed in this infection. These are usually accompanied with simultaneous erosion of the nasal septal and palatine tissues. This syndrome is referred to as "mucocutaneous leishmaniasis" or "espundia." On occasion the mucocutaneous manifestations may appear decades after healing of the primary skin lesion.

Certain sandflies of the genus *Phlebotomus* are the chief vectors of the disease; forest rodents are infected and are reservoirs in endemic areas. Other biting flies may mechanically transmit the organism, which they pick up when they alight on weeping lesions of an infected individual.

Hyperplasia, inflammation, and edema characterize the lesions. The "young" lesions are painful, and ulcers have a granulating base. Involvement of the mucous membranes results in mutilating deformity and paves the way for secondary bacterial invasion. In other manifestations of disease caused by *Leishmania brasiliensis* such as "Chiclero ulcer" and "uta," nasopharyngeal metastasis has not been reported to occur.

Diagnosis is confirmed by demonstration of the protozoan in direct smears or culture of material from the lesion or the aspirate of lymph nodes draining the area of infection.

Visceral leishmaniasis (kala-azar)

The etiologic agent of this disease is *Leishmania donovani*. Visceral leishmaniasis is endemic in semitropical and tropical areas, and the organism is transmitted by the bite of certain *Phlebotomus* flies. Infected individuals and possibly certain domestic animals may be reservoirs of the infection.

This disease particularly involves the reticuloendothelial system. Hyperplasia of tissues and organs is manifest. Edema of the skin and bleeding of the gingivae and other mucous membranes are observed.

Confirmation of infection depends on demonstration of protozoans in direct smears or culture of material obtained from organs by aspiration or biopsy. Serologic tests are a confirmatory aid.

Trypanosomiasis

African trypanosomiasis, caused by *Trypanosoma gambiense* or *Trypanosoma rhodesiense*, is not known to produce oral manifestations of significance. However, American trypanosomiasis may involve the head, neck, and parts of the esophagus.

American trypanosomiasis or Chagas' disease is caused by *Trypanosoma cruzi*. Damage to nerves and ganglia in the muscular walls of the viscera results in dilation and atony of any part of the gastrointestinal tract; one of these manifestations that may come to the attention of the oral and maxillofacial surgeon is megaesophagus. The acute form of American trypanosomiasis is characterized by an initial red-hot, tender, plaquelike lesion, the chagoma, which is seen at the site of the infective bite. This lesion is characteristically but not exclusively located on the face. On the upper eyelid the lesion is pathognomonic and is known as "Romaña's sign." To our knowledge, specific oral involvement has not been reported in the literature.

Diagnosis in early disease may be confirmed by the observation of leishmanial forms in scrapings obtained from a chagoma. Clinical signs and serologic tests are perhaps most useful in making a confirmatory diagnosis.

Viral infections causing oral ulceration

Viral infections exhibiting oral manifestations are comparatively common (Shklar, 1971). While some viral diseases may appear to be confined to the oral mucosa, others may produce lesions of the skin or other tissues of the body. The herpesvirus group, including the herpes simplex and the varicella-zoster agents, and the coxsackieviruses are the viruses most frequently associated with ulcerative lesions in the human oral cavity (Lennette and Magoffin, 1973). Table 4-6 summarizes the clinical syndromes and the types of lesions that can result from infection with these agents.

Herpesvirus infections

The herpes simplex virion measures about 150 to 200 nm in diameter and possesses a capsid displaying icosahedral symmetry that is surrounded by a lipoprotein envelope. The nucleic acid of the virion is DNA, and the virus replicates in the nucleus of the infected cells (Fenner and White, 1976). Two antigenic types of

Table 4-6. Viral infections associated with intraoral ulcerative lesions*

Causative virus(es)	Primary or recurrent infection	Clinical syndrome	Systemic signs of acute infection	Intraoral lesions		Skin lesions	
				Discrete lesions	Diffuse inflammation	Localized	Disseminated
Herpes simplex (type I) (Herpesvirus hominis)	Primary	Gingivostomatitis	Yes	Yes	Yes	No	Rarely†
Herpes simplex (type I) (Herpesvirus hominis)	Recurrent	Herpes labialis	No	Concurrent in some instances	No	Yes	Rarely†
Herpes simplex (type I) (Herpesvirus hominis)	Recurrent	Intraoral herpes	No	Yes	No	Concurrent herpes labialis in some instances	No
Varicella-zoster (Herpesvirus varicellae)	Primary	Chickenpox	Yes	Yes	No	No	Yes
Varicella-zoster (Herpesvirus varicellae)	Recurrent	Herpes zoster	No	May occur	No	Yes	Rarely
Coxsackieviruses, group A Types 2-10; 16; 22	Primary	Herpangina	Yes	Yes	No	No	No
Type 16; less often 5, 10	Primary	Hand-foot-mouth syndrome	Yes	Yes	No	No	Yes
Type 10	Primary	Lymphonodular pharyngitis	Yes	Yes (nodular, nonulcerative)	No	No	No

*From Lennette, E. H., and Magoffin, R. L. 1973. J. Am. Dent. Assoc. **87**:1055. Copyright by the American Dental Association. Reprinted by permission.
†Erythema multiforme (Stevens-Johnson syndrome) or clinically indistinguishable disseminated mucocutaneous disease has been reported both in association with primary herpetic gingivostomatitis and after recurrent herpes labialis.

herpes simplex virus are currently recognized: herpes simplex virus, type 1, and herpes simplex virus, type 2 (Nahmias and Roizman, 1973). The latter is most frequently associated with genital infection, and the former is most frequently associated with oral infection. However, both types may produce a wide variety of clinical syndromes.

At about 6 months of age, following the decline in neutralizing antibodies acquired from the mother, the infant becomes susceptible to infection with herpes simplex virus. The initial or primary infection is frequently, but not always, acquired in childhood by close contact with individuals who are shedding the virus. The primary infection may or may not result in clinically recognizable disease; in fact it has been estimated that only 1% to 10% of these primary infections elicit clinical disease (Lennette and Magoffin, 1973). Acute gingivostomatitis is the most common manifestation of primary clinical disease. The gingivae are swollen and red, and bleeding occurs readily. Multiple lesions can occur anywhere in the oral cavity; these begin as vesicles that collapse and develop into ulcers surrounded by an erythematous zone. Local pain is usually present. Fever and other systemic signs of disease generally accompany the oral lesions. The process of vesiculation and ulceration may continue for several days, but the lesions usually heal without scar formation within 1 or 2 weeks. However, in some primary infections the virus may produce a dermatitis, eczema herpeticum, keratoconjunctivitis, and vulvovaginitis. Occasionally the virus spreads throughout the body, giving rise to visceral involvement, encephalitis, or meningoencephalitis, which may carry a high mortality rate. These serious complications occur most frequently in premature infants or neonates whose mothers lacked neutralizing antibody or in adults whose immune systems are compromised. It should be emphasized that specific viral neutralizing antibodies appear in the blood following either a clinical or subclinical infection. The study of Smith, Peutherer, and MacCallum (1967) confirmed the observation of several other investigators that the incidence of complement-fixing and neutralizing serum antibodies to herpes simplex virus, type 1, is widespread. In children under 6 months of age the incidence of neutralizing antibody was about 75% to 100%. This declined to 19% at 6 to 11 months. Thereafter it rose slowly to 65% to 69% at 15 to 25 years of age. At the age of 60 the incidence was 97%. However, the incidence of neutralizing antibody in the sera from 131 fourth-year medical students (average age, 22 years) and 75 student nurses (average age, 19 years) was only 40% to 48%, respectively.

Shklar (1971) has pointed out that three conditions should be considered in the differential diagnosis of herpetic gingivostomatitis: herpangina, aphthous stomatitis, and erythema multiforme. In herpangina the lesions appear in the oropharynx and posterior areas of the mouth; the gingivae are not involved. In aphthous stomatitis the gingivae are not involved, and the ulcers are recurrent and have no preceding vesicular phase. Erythema mutliforme, an acute vesicular disease, presents systemic manifestations. Vesicles are prominent on the lips, although they may occur in the mouth and oropharynx. Acute gingivitis is absent, but disseminated lesions of the skin are usually observed at least in adults.

Localized herpetic infection of the skin of the fingers following trauma is recognized as an occupational hazard of medical (Hambrick, Cox, and Senior, 1962; Rustigian et al., 1966) and dental personnel (Snyder, Church, and Rickles, 1969). These infections are usually manifested as a herpetic whitlow or paronychia. Rosato, Rosato, and Plotkin (1970) recommend that the operator wear rubber gloves when administering oral or pharyngeal care to patients exhibiting herpetic lesions.

Following a primary herpetic infection, the virus may persist in the body in a latent form in the epithelial cells of the oral cavity and in certain sensory nerve ganglia (Baringer, 1974; Baringer and Swoveland, 1973; Bastion et al., 1972; Merigan, 1974). Also, some individuals shed herpesvirus from the respiratory tract or oral cavity in spite of the fact that their blood serum contains viral specific antibody and they display no apparent clinical signs of infection (Douglas and Couch, 1970. Lindgren, Douglas, and Couch, 1968). Under stressful situations, including section of the posterior root of the trigeminal nerve (Ellison, Carton, and Rose, 1959), the latent virus may become activated, travel along the neural routes, and produce vesicular lesions followed by ulceration on the operated side of the skin of the face, lips, nose, oral mucosa, or cornea. The last is by far the most serious manifestation of secondary or recurrent herpesvirus infection, and it is characterized by dendritic or geographic ulcers of the cornea (Locatcher-Khorazo and Seegal, 1972). It is interesting to note that secondary or recurrent infection occurs in individuals who have high levels of neutralizing antibodies in their blood serum. Since immunoglobulin molecules cannot penetrate living body cells, the virus is thought to spread from cell to cell without coming into contact with specific serum immunoglobulins. Colds, fever, exposure to sunlight, menstruation, mechanical trauma, emotional disturbances, and topical corticosteroids are believed to act as precipitating factors (Blank and Rake, 1955) in secondary or recurrent herpesvirus attacks. Topical application of ethyl ether (Nugent and Chow, 1973; Pasricha, Nayyar, and Pasricha, 1973; Sabin, 1975) has been reported to be useful in the treatment of recurrent herpesvirus skin lesions. Pain is reduced, and healing occurs rapidly when compared to other methods of treatment.

The oral manifestations of herpes simplex virus infection and recurrent aphthous ulcers have been succinctly delineated by Lennette and Magoffin (1973), and these data are presented in Table 4-7. Recurrent aphthous ulcers, commonly called "canker sores," were thought for many years to be an intraoral manifestation of herpes simplex virus infection. However, the studies of Dodd and Ruchman (1950) demonstrated that herpesvirus could not be consistently isolated from recurrent aphthae. Other causative agents have been suggested as being involved in the pathogenesis of aphthous stomatitis, but none has been proved conclusively. The literature on this subject is quite voluminous and has been reviewed by Francis (1970) and Lehner (1977).

Attention has been focused on the immunologic aspects of aphthous ulcers in the last decade. The work of Graykowski and co-workers (1966) and Oppenheim and Francis (1970) has suggested that the lesions may represent a delayed type of hypersensitivity or cellular immune reaction to a bacterial species that is a part of the normal oral flora, namely *Streptococcus sanguis*. On the other hand the data of Lehner (1969, 1972) suggest that an autoimmune reaction may account for the pathogenesis of these lesions. Dolby (1969) has demonstrated that peripheral blood lymphocytes from patients with recurrent aphthous stomatitis were more lethal to oral epithelial cells under in vitro conditions than those from normal subjects. Taken together, these observations appear to lend support to the hypothesis that immunologic phenomena are involved in the pathogenesis of these lesions. Levamisole, an antihelmintic drug that increases both cellular and humoral immune responses, was reported by Olson and his colleagues (1976) to be of value in the treatment of recurrent aphthous stomatitis in 62% of the 50 patients they studied.

Varicella-zoster virus infections

Another agent of the herpesvirus group that may elicit lesions in the oral cavity is the varicella-zoster virus. This virus is similar in size and structure to the herpes simplex virion, and it is difficult to distinguish between these two viruses under the electron microscope. They are antigenically different, and antiserum prepared against one of these will not neutralize the other; however, these two agents possess common antigenic components (Schmidt, Lennette, and Magoffin, 1969).

This virus is recognized as the etiologic agent of at least three different clinical

Table 4-7. Oral manifestations of herpes simplex virus infection and recurrent aphthous ulcers, origin undetermined*

Clinical syndrome	Primary herpetic gingivostomatitis	Recurrent labial herpes	Recurrent intraoral herpes	Recurrent aphthous ulcers
Predisposing factors	None	Febrile illness Emotional stress Trauma Sunlight	Same as recurrent labial herpes	Emotional stress Trauma History allergy Familial history
General symptoms	Fever, anorexia	None	None	Usually none
Local symptoms	Sore mouth Fetid breath Salivation Regional lymphadenopathy	Local paresthesia Irritation or pain	Local irritation or pain; usually not severe	Oral pain, usually intense
Lesions	Multiple vesicles, yellow plaques, become shallow ulcers, 1-3 mm Diffuse erythema Diffuse oral edema Swollen red gingiva	Papules, vesicles, yellow crusts with erythematous base Labial swelling	Few to multiple small vesicles 1-3 mm, often in clusters; form shallow punctate ulcers; may coalesce to form large shallow ulcer	One or two to 20 lesions, 3-10 mm initial papule; erodes to form ulcer Gray or white center Erythematous halo
Location	Labial mucosa Buccal mucosa Tongue Gingiva	Lips, mucocutaneous junction, and adjacent skin	Hard palate Alveolar ridges Attached gingiva Less often buccal or labial mucosa	Buccal mucosa Labial mucosa Buccal sulci Tongue Soft palate
Histopathology	Swelling of epithelial cells; "ballooning degeneration," intranuclear inclusions; multinuclear giant cells; polymorphonuclear inflammatory cell infiltrate	Same as primary herpetic lesions	Ballooning degeneration Giant cells	Erosion of mucosal epithelium and corium Thin necrotic membrane Lymphocytes predominate in early inflammatory infiltrate

*From Lennette, E. H., and Magoffin, R. L. 1973. J. Am. Dent. Assoc. **87**:1055. Copyright by the American Dental Association. Reprinted by permission.

syndromes: varicella, or chickenpox; herpes zoster, or shingles; and herpes zoster ophthalmicus (Krugman and Ward, 1973). The primary infection with the varicella-zoster virus is manifested as chickenpox; however, in some instances the infection may be subclinical. Chickenpox most frequently occurs in children, but some individuals escape infection until they have reached adulthood. After an incubation period of about 2 weeks, fever develops that is followed shortly by the appearance of a rash, first on the trunk and then on the extremities and face (Krugman and Ward, 1973). The cutaneous lesions progress through several stages: pink maculopapules, vesicles, collapsed vesicles, and finally crusts (Lennette and Magoffin, 1973). Intraoral lesions usually accompany the skin lesions and occur most frequently over the palate. They begin as vesicles that rupture to form small ulcers about 2 to 4 mm in diameter surrounded by a red zone. Healing occurs within 10 to 14 days (Shklar, 1971).

Herpes zoster is thought to be caused by the activation of latent varicella-zoster virus in individuals who have previously experienced a clinical or subclinical attack of chickenpox. The evidence to indicate that varicella and zoster are different manifestations of the same virus has been summarized by Krugman and Ward (1973). It has been estimated that zoster occurs annually in about 0.3% and 0.5% of the human population (Fenner and White, 1976). The incidence of the disease increases with age, and about half the cases occur in individuals over 50 years old. However, zoster has been reported to occur in infants and children (Brunell, 1967; Winklemann and Perry, 1959).

The clinical manifestations of zoster are quite varied and appear to depend on the location of the neural ganglia in which the virus is presumably latent. Following activation of the latent virus, the virions may travel to the cutaneous or mucosal surface by a neural route. While the exact pathway has not yet been established, it does appear to involve passage along the axons (Merigan, 1974). Zoster is characterized by the abrupt development of painful lesions of the skin or mucous membranes that follow the pathway of the sensory nerve distribution of dorsal root ganglia or the ganglia of cranial nerves. The lesions resemble those of varicella but are unilateral and terminate abruptly at the midline; the skin of the face and trunk are the anatomic sites most frequently affected. Lesions appearing on the trunk indicate the involvement of dorsal root ganglia, while those appearing on the shoulders, arms, and neck indicate the involvement of the second to fifth cervical ganglia.

When the virus has remained latent in the fifth cranial (trigeminal) nerve, activation, axonal passage, and viral replication may result in intraoral or ocular lesions. If the maxillary division of the trigeminal nerve is involved, the lesions occur on the soft palate, uvula, and tonsillar area. Involvement of the mandibular division results in lesions that appear on the buccal mucosa, floor of the mouth, and anterior portion of the tongue (Krugman and Ward, 1973). In contrast to herpes labialis or intraoral herpes, attacks of herpes zoster are rarely recurrent. From a clinical standpoint the prominence of pain and the unilateral distribution of the intraoral lesions are an aid in differentiating between herpes zoster and herpes simplex (Nally and Ross, 1971).

When the ophthalmic division of the trigeminal nerve is involved, the lesions appear on the skin of the forehead, and in about half the cases of herpes zoster ophthalmicus the lesions also appear on the palpebrae and the cornea. Clinically, hyperesthesia and sharp cutting or tearing pain precede the development of the skin rash by several days. Involvement of the seventh cranial (facial) nerve or geniculate ganglion results in unilateral pain; a vesicular eruption on the external ear, in the external auditory canal, or sometimes on the tongue; and facial paralysis on the affected side. The last usually resolves with time but may occasionally be permanent (Krugman and Ward, 1973; Lennette and Magoffin, 1973).

Herpes zoster is a common complication in patients whose host defense mechanisms have been compromised by immunosuppressive drugs or reticuloendothelial malignancies (Schimpff et al., 1972). In such instances the infection may be acutely debilitating or life-threatening if the viscera are involved as a result of dissemination of the virus (Goffinet, Glatstein, and Merigan, 1972; Merselis, Kaye, and Hook, 1964). Intravenous therapy with adenine arabinoside has been reported useful in immunosuppressed patients with herpes zoster (Whitley et al., 1976).

Coxsackievirus infections

The coxsackieviruses, echoviruses, and polioviruses are currently classified as subgroups of the enterovirus group (Jawetz, Melnick, and Adelberg, 1976) because of their similarity in size, structure, and biochemical characteristics. The coxsackieviruses are among the smallest animal viruses; they measure about 28 nm in diameter under the electron microscope. The virions contain a core of ribonucleic acid that is surrounded by a protein capsid possessing cubic symmetry. In contrast to the herpesviruses they have no outer lipoprotein envelope and are resistant to inactivation by ether and other organic lipid solvents; they multiply in the cytoplasm of the infected cells. They are divided into groups A and B on the basis of the types of lesions produced following injection into suckling mice. Among the group A coxsackieviruses about 24 different antigenic types are recognized, whereas the group B coxsackieviruses consist of only 6 antigenic types. The majority of the group A serotypes cannot be isolated from clinical specimens by the inoculation of in vitro cell cultures, and the laboratory must employ newborn mice for this purpose.

The coxsackieviruses are responsible for a variety of human illnesses, including aseptic meningitis, pleurodynia, myocarditis and pericarditis, and the common cold (Acton et al., 1974). In addition three clinical syndromes (herpangina; hand, foot, and mouth disease; and acute lymphonodular pharyngitis) present vesiculoulcerative lesions of the oral cavity and pharynx. These infections are seen most often in children under 10 years old, and they occur usually, but not always, during the summer and fall of the year. The oral lesions are acccompanied by fever and other systemic manifestations of acute infectious diseases.

The serotypes of the coxsackieviruses that are most frequently implicated in infection in which oral manifestations are observed are listed in Table 4-6. Among the serotypes of group A coxsackieviruses, type 4 has been most frequently involved in the etiology of herpangina, although types 2, 5, 6, 7, 8, 10, 16, and 22 may also give rise to this syndrome (Lennette and Magoffin, 1973). Several types of group B coxsackieviruses and echoviruses (Debre and Celers, 1970) are occasionally associated with herpangina. Coxsackievirus A16 is usually involved in the etiology of hand, foot, and mouth disease; types A4, A5, and A10 are less frequently involved (Magoffin, Jackson, and Lennette, 1961; Mink and Winter, 1970; Robinson and Rhodes, 1961). Acute lymphonodular pharyngitis has been reported to involve only type A10 (Lennette and Magoffin, 1973).

Some of the characteristics of herpangina; hand, foot, and mouth disease; and acute lymphonodular pharyngitis are summarized in Table 4-8. The oral lesions of herpangina and hand, foot, and mouth disease are similar, but the latter syndrome may be distinguished clinically by the presence of lesions on the buccal mucosa and gingivae and the presence of a skin rash on the abdomen, buttocks, palms and fingers of the hands, and soles and toes of the feet. In acute lymphonodular pharyngitis (Steigman, Lipton, and Braspennickx, 1962), discrete, raised nodules are observed on the anterior pillars, posterior pharynx, and uvula. These lesions do not form vesicles nor do they ulcerate; they usually resolve within 6 to 10 days after onset of the clinical signs.

Viral hepatitis

While a number of bacterial, chemical, and viral agents may give rise to an inflammation of the liver, two different viruses currently referred to as hepatitis A

Table 4-8. Oral and systemic manifestations of some coxsackievirus infections*

Clinical syndrome	Herpangina	Hand, foot, and mouth disease	Acute lymphonodular pharyngitis
Systemic signs and symptoms	Anorexia, fever	Anorexia, fever, skin rash	Anorexia, fever
Local signs and symptoms	Dysphagia, sore throat	Dysphagia, sore throat	Sore throat
Lesions			
Oral	Two to 15 or more gray-white papular vesicles, 1-2 mm in diameter, vesicles rupture to form punctate ulcers with bright red margin.	Similar to herpangina	Discrete, raised, solid nodules, white to yellow, surrounded by zone of redness 3-6 mm in diameter.
Cutaneous	None	Maculopapular rash with some vesiculation	None
Location			
Oral	Generally on anterior pillars of the fauces; less frequent on soft and posterior hard palate, tonsils, tongue, or uvula. Buccal mucosa and gingivae spared.	Similar to herpangina but vesicles more frequently present on tongue, buccal mucosa, and gingivae.	Anterior pillars, posterior pharynx, and uvula
Cutaneous	None	Papulovesicular rash on abdomen, buttocks, and extremities, notably the palms and fingers of hands and soles and toes of feet.	None
Histopathology	Cells scraped from lesions show non-specific hyper-chromatic large nuclei.	Vesicles seen first within the epidermis, later beneath the epidermis. Ballooning degeneration of epithelial cells, subepidermal eosinophil infiltration; no inclusion bodies.	Nodules tightly packed with lymphocytes

*Derived from Lennette and Magoffin, 1973; Mihm, 1971; Shklar, 1971; and Steigman, Lipton, and Braspennickx, 1962.

virus (HAV) and hepatitis B virus (HBV) appear to be frequently involved in the etiology of viral hepatitis. The diseases caused by these agents were formerly referred to as infectious hepatitis and serum hepatitis, respectively. Now the terms "viral hepatitis, type A" and "viral hepatitis, type B" are used (Krugman and Ward, 1973).

Reliable and repeated cultivation of HAV in cell cultures in vitro has been documented recently by Provost and Hilleman (1979). Two previous investigations (Moritsugu et al., 1976; Provost et al., 1975b) reported purifying and characterizing HAV from infected marmoset sera and from feces of infected humans. It has been concluded that HAV

is a small virion 27 nm in diameter that seems to be closely related to the enterovirus group. The viral genome appears to be ribonucleic acid. It is now possible to qualitatively and quantitatively assay for hepatitis A antigen (HA Ag) and antibody to HA Ag (anti-HA) by immune electron microscopy, complement fixation, immune adherence hemagglutination, and microtiter solid-phase radioimmunoassay (Dienstag, Alling, and Purcell, 1976; Feinstone, Kapikian, and Purcell, 1973; Krugman, Friedman, and Lattimer, 1975; Miller et al., 1975; Provost et al., 1975a; Purcell et al., 1976). A few of these procedures are now available in some viral diagnostic laboratories.

Since the discovery of the Australia

antigen (Au Ag) by Blumberg and his colleagues (1965) and the subsequent association of this antigen with hepatitis type B infection (Blumberg, Alter, and Visnich, 1965; Gocke and Kavey, 1969; Prince, 1968), the antigenic structure of HBV has been demonstrated to be quite complex. The current knowledge on the structure of HBV has been summarized by McAuliffe, Purcell, and LeBouvier (1976) as follows: The complete virion is thought to be the 43 nm "Dane" particle (Dane, Cameron, and Briggs, 1970), which is composed of a 27 nm core called the hepatitis B core antigen or HB$_c$Ag. Within the core a DNA-dependent DNA polymerase and a double-stranded circular DNA molecule serving presumably as the viral genome are present. The core is surrounded by a 7 to 8 nm coat that is antigenically distinct and is referred to as the hepatitis B surface antigen or HB$_s$Ag (formerly Au Ag). HB$_s$Ag is also associated with the 22 nm–diameter spherical and tubular particles, which are more numerous in the serum of chronic carriers and patients with active hepatitis B virus infection. These particles are thought to represent excess virus coat protein that is released from HBV-infected hepatocytes. While the HB$_s$Ag detected in the sera of different individuals possesses a common antigenic determinant, subspecific determinants are recognized (Le Bouvier and McCollum, 1970; Nielsen, Le Bouvier, and The Copenhagen Hepatitis Acute Program, 1973).

Another antigen system that may be found in the serum of certain HB$_s$Ag-positive patients was initially demonstrated by Magnius and Espmark (1972) and was termed the "e" antigen. This antigen differs from the HB$_s$Ag in that it is smaller, has a molecular weight of about 300,000 daltons, and seems to be a soluble protein (Magnius, 1975). It appears in the serum during the acute phase of HBV infections (Magnius et al., 1975) and persists in some individuals in whom chronic persistent or chronic active hepatitis develops (Nielsen, Dietrichson, and Juhl, 1974) or in some asymptomatic carriers (Okada et al., 1976).

HB$_s$Ag or anti-HB$_s$ can be detected in the blood serum of individuals with acute or chronic active hepatitis or in individuals who are chronic carriers by a variety of immunologic procedures. They include agar gel diffusion, counter electrophoresis, complement fixation, hemagglutination, and radioimmunoassay. Many of these tests are now routine in viral diagnostic laboratories; the details of these techniques may be found in the publication by Ashcavai and Peters (1973). More recent diagnostic tests involve the detection of DNA polymerase activity (Kaplan et al., 1973) and antibody to HB$_c$Ag (Hoofnagle, Gerety, and Barker, 1973) in human serum. The latter test appears to be of considerable importance because the presence of anti-HB$_c$ is said to reflect an ongoing virus replication (Hoofnagle et al., 1974; Krugman et al., 1974).

Table 4-9 presents some of the major differences between these two infections. Type A hepatitis is more common in children than in adults and is usually transmitted by the oral-fecal route by the ingestion of contaminated food and water. Type B hepatitis is more common in adults and is predominantly transmitted via the parenteral route by the transfusion of blood or plasma and by penetration of human tissues by instruments contaminated with the virus. However, it has been recognized for some time that both types can be transmitted by parenteral as well as nonparenteral routes (Krugman, Giles, and Hammond, 1967). Nonparenteral transmission of HBV may occur between members of families who are carriers of HB$_s$Ag (Szmuness et al., 1973); saliva appears to be the vehicle of infection in such situations (Villarejos et al., 1974). In addition, vertical transmission of hepatitis B virus from asymptomatic carrier mothers to their infants has been documented by Fawaz and co-workers (1975), Stevens and co-workers (1975), and Okada and co-workers (1976). In the United States it has been estimated that about 150,000 cases of type B hepatitis occur annually and that there are hundreds of thousands of chronic carriers of the HB$_s$Ag (Gerin, 1976).

The risk of contracting type B hepatitis

Table 4-9. Viral hepatitis types A and B—comparison of clinical, epidemiologic, and immunologic features*

Features	Type A	Type B
Incubation period	15 to 40 days	50 to 180 days
Type of onset	Usually acute	Usually insidious
Fever	Common; precedes jaundice	Less common
Age group affected	Usually children and young adults	All age groups
Jaundice	Rare in children; more common in adults	Rare in children; more common in adults
Abnormal SGOT	Transient—1 to 3 weeks	More prolonged—1 to 8+ months
Thymol turbidity	Usually increased	Usually normal
IgM levels	Usually increased	Usually normal
HB$_s$ Ag (Australia antigen) in blood	Not present	Present in incubation period and acute phase; occasionally may persist
Virus in feces	Present during late incubation period and acute phase	Probably present but no direct proof
Virus in blood	Present during late incubation period and early acute phase	Present during late incubation period and acute phase; occasionally persists for months and years
Immunity		
Homologous	Present	Present
Heterologous	None	None

*From Krugman, S., and Ward, R. 1977. Infectious diseases of children and adults, ed. 6, St. Louis, The C. V. Mosby Co.

is apparently greater among health-care workers than it is among the population at large (Byrne, 1966; Feldman and Schiff, 1975; Mosley and White, 1975; Trumbull and Greiner, 1951). The survey conducted by Mosley and his associates (1975) demonstrated that 0.9% of 1245 dental practitioners were positive for HB$_s$Ag and 12.7% were positive for anti-HB$_s$. Among individuals who had had clinical hepatitis while in dental school or subsequently in practice, 53% were positive for anti-HB$_s$. The data also indicated that the frequency of evidence of prior hepatitis B virus infection increased with the years of dental practice.

Hepatitis B surface antigen has been demonstrated to be present in saliva by Ward and co-workers (1972). Villarejos and his associates (1974) reported that HB$_s$Ag occurred in the saliva of 76% of patients with acute hepatitis during the first 3 weeks after clinical onset and intermittently in 86% of chronic carriers. It appears that the dental practitioner may contract type B hepatitis as a result of

puncture of the skin of the fingers or possibly by the aerosolization that occurs during drilling. The use of rubber gloves when treating patients may reduce the risk to the operator of contracting type B hepatitis.

The question of the risk of transmission of HBV by HB$_s$Ag-positive health-care workers to patients has been the subject of several retrospective investigations (Garibaldi et al., 1972; Levin et al., 1974). The rather limited study by Alter and his associates (1975) failed to demonstrate transmission in this fashion, although the authors cautioned that additional data must be accumulated before the question can be firmly resolved.

The prevention or prophylaxis of type B hepatitis in individuals exposed to the virus by the administration of hepatitis B immunoglobulin (HBIG) and standard immune serum globulin (ISG) has been the subject of numerous reports. The results of three carefully conducted clinical trials (Grady and Lee, 1975; Prince et al., 1975; Redeker et al., 1975) comparing the effectiveness of HBIG and ISG have suggested that HBIG was effective in reducing the incidence of the disease in some high-risk situations, but none of the studies demonstrated total protection.

LABORATORY DIAGNOSIS

It should be apparent from the preceding sections of this chapter that the oral and maxillofacial surgeon may be confronted with disease processes that are caused by a variety of microorganisms—aerobic, facultative anaerobic, and anaerobic bacteria; yeasts and molds; viruses; and protozoa. Usually, but not always, the technology involved in the isolation and identification of bacterial species is the most conducive to reasonably rapid microbiologic diagnosis. The etiologic agents of mycotic infections, although often recognizable from wet mount or stained smear preparations or histologic section of the lesion site, may take longer to identify because of the slower growth of most of these organisms on culture media. Isolation of mycoplasmal, rickettsial, and viral agents requires more specialized and sophisticated technology, and longer periods of time may be required for final identification of the etiologic agent or confirmation of the disease entity. Protozoans are usually recognized in wet mount or smear preparations. Some may be grown on culture media, and often culture is an integral part of the confirmation of the etiologic agent of the disease.

Specimens for culture may be collected either from sites normally free of normal flora or from sites that teem with a mixture of organisms colonizing certain sites. The latter is certainly true of the oral cavity. Selective culture media and specialized isolation procedures may not only be necessary but mandatory. For the recovery of certain fastidious organisms, it may be necessary to collect specimens in a manner that utilizes specialized approaches, as in the recovery and isolation of obligate anaerobic bacteria.

Different types of bacteria and fungi may require specific culture media and unique incubation conditions for growth and confirmation of species identity. If such conditions are not met, the etiologic agents may not be recovered or identified in spite of the presence of the organisms in reasonably large numbers at the infected site. In every situation the need for prompt processing of the collected specimen cannot be overemphasized. The more rapidly the specimen is inoculated onto or into appropriate culture media, the greater is the likelihood that the etiologic agent or agents will be recovered.

Bacterial infections
Collection of specimens

There is a large variety of methods for collecting specimens for culture. In lesions in the oral cavity we are most often dependent on gathering exudative material either by aspiration with a needle and syringe or by use of a swab. In certain infections we may have to carefully scrape the surface area of a specific portion of the infected site, for example the periphery of the lesion. In any instance where the possibility of infection exists, a specimen directly from the infected site must be obtained, and contamination from parametric areas must be avoided.

If swabs are to be used, several factors should be borne in mind. Although cotton swabs are inexpensive and readily available, cotton may contain small amounts of lipoproteins that may be toxic to fastidious bacteria. One may avoid this situation by using swabs made of polyester or calcium alginate fibers. In the latter instance calcium alginate swabs may be dissolved in a sodium hexametaphosphate solution, thus liberating essentially all organisms picked up from the lesion. This technique is not routinely employed by most diagnostic laboratories; higher cost and the extra effort required to dissolve the fiber are probably the main reasons.

There is available at this time a "swab unit" known as the "Culturette"*(Fig. 4-10). It is a complete sterile unit ready to use. It consists of one rayon-tipped swab and an ampule containing modified

---

*Available from Scientific Products, Division of American Hospital Supply Corporation, 1430 Waukegan Road, McGaw Park, Ill. 60085.

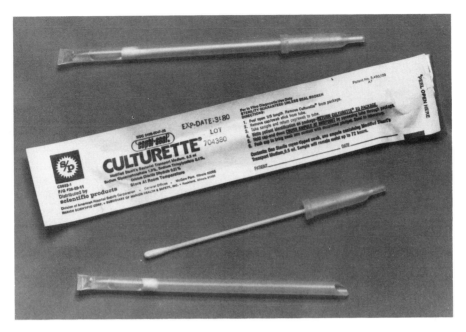

Fig. 4-10. "Culturette." (Photographed and reproduced with permission of Marion Scientific Corporation, Kansas City, Mo. 64114)

Stuart transport medium. The package is peeled open and a cardboard cap is squeezed to grasp the stick end of the swab, which may be withdrawn ready for use. The specimen is taken, and the swab is returned to the tube. The ampule containing the transport medium is crushed by a squeeze of the tube. The swab is then pushed into the medium to bring it into contact with a moistened cotton pledget, which is placed just above the ampule. This results in a swab specimen protected from drying and whose organisms maintain viability for a reasonable period of time. This unit is not recommended for use in the recovery and isolation of obligate anaerobes.

In certain instances a transport medium should be used when the specimen cannot be immediately inoculated onto primary culture media. Such a medium does not contain carbohydrate or nitrogen sources, and the overgrowth of a fastidious etiologic agent by contaminating flora is temporarily subdued. Transport media are buffered. Occasionally they are semisolid in consistency; this may be accomplished by the addition of low concentrations of agar. They may also contain a variety of compounds designed to favor the survival of specific microbial species. The primary function of a transport medium is to prevent organisms in the collected specimen from dying rapidly due to a drying out process and to inhibit overgrowth by contaminants. The transport of specimens to be cultured for obligate anaerobes poses a very special problem (see p. 157).

Microscopic examination of the specimen

Preparation of smears. Prior to staining, wherein the bacterial cells themselves are "colored" with one or another of the basic dyes or by a combined staining, decolorizing, and counterstaining procedure, a smear of the specimen is made as follows: A clean glass slide is used, one from which all traces of fatty substance are "burned off" by passing the slide through the flame of a Bunsen burner. If the specimen is an exudate, a sterile wire loopful of the liquid is spread evenly over the center one third of the slide. The resulting smear should be reasonably thin in nature, yet should represent a good sampling of the specimen. Next the smear should be air-dried. To prevent the smear from being washed off the slide during the staining process, it is "fixed" by passing the slide over the Bunsen burner flame three times. The slide should not be allowed to become too hot. This technique results in a binding of the specimen and bacterial protein to the glass.

If the specimen is taken with a swab, the primary plating media and broth media of choice should be inoculated first; "rolling" the swab over a clean non-sterile slide will contaminate the specimen with organisms from the environment. If deemed appropriate and possible, with certain exceptions, the swab may be immersed in a small amount of sterile isotonic saline solution or preferably a transport medium—type menstruum, and the specimen material from the swab may be suspended or emulsified in the liquid. The swab may be rolled with moderate pressure over the clean glass slide to make the smear, and is then discarded. The workup of the specimen is continued using the liquid remaining in the tube. The steps of the procedure may be reversed—the swab appropriately moistened with specimen suspension (not dripping) may be used to inoculate the culture media, and the suspension remaining in the tube may be employed to make the smear.

The Gram stain. There are a number of modifications of both the Gram stain reagents* and the Gram staining procedure. These can be found in several microbiology textbooks and in diagnostic laboratory manuals such as the *Manual of Clinical Microbiology* (Lennette, Spaulding, and Truant, 1974). The Gram stain procedure may be carried out as follows:
1. Flood the smear with crystal violet solution. Let stand for 1 minute.
2. Wash the smear briefly with tap water. Drain off excess water.
3. Flood the smear with the iodine solution. Let stand for 1 minute. Wash with tap water and drain off excess water.
4. Decolorize with acetone-alcohol

---

*Prepared reagents are available from Difco Laboratories, P. O. Box 1058A, Detroit, Mich. 48232.

just until the solvent flows colorlessly from the smear. This is a most crucial step; do not overdecolorize.
5. Wash briefly with tap water. Drain off excess water.
6. Counterstain with safranin for 10 seconds. Wash with water and carefully blot dry.

The stain is now ready for microscopic examination using the oil immersion objective. Gram-positive organisms appear blue or purple; gram-negative organisms appear red. It should be noted that certain anaerobic gram-negative species counterstain weakly when stained with safranin; carbolfuchsin makes an excellent counterstain in these instances.

In the preparation and interpretation of Gram stains several important points should be borne in mind. Lack of familiarity with the procedure or with the evaluation and interpretation may lead to errors. Simultaneous staining of a specimen of saliva may serve as a control to evaluate the staining technique. Since saliva contains both gram-positive and gram-negative microorganisms, both types should be observed in the stained smear if the procedure has been correctly performed. One must remember that gram-positive organisms become gram-negative as the cells age or die. The age of the culture at which this change occurs varies with the species, growth medium, and so on. One must also be aware of the variation in size of cells of different bacterial species. Such knowledge and its pertinent use may serve to aid in making a presumptive morphologic identification.

Other important information may be gained from the observation of a Gram stained smear. The presence and type of inflammatory cells should be noted. Neutrophils in large numbers denote an infection primarily controlled by phagocytosis and intracellular killing, for example, pneumococci and *Hemophilus influenzae*. Smears of clinical specimens devoid of inflammatory cells should be interpreted with caution. Often epithelial cells may be observed. Such an observation usually indicates lack of an infectious or invasive process.

Gram stains may be helpful in the

rapid, presumptive identification of a number of acute infections. Staphylococcal and streptococcal infections as well as a nocardial abscess may be cited as examples of this interpretation of a Gram stained smear. When organisms are seen on Gram stained smears that are not recovered on culture, it may signify that inadequate cultural procedures have been employed. This point has been emphasized in the study by Sabiston, Grigsby, and Sagerstrom (1976).

Other stains. Certainly the Gram stain is the most important in relation to the presumptive diagnosis of many oral infections. However, if one is confronted with oral lesions attributable to *Mycobacterium tuberculosis* or with nocardial abscesses, the acid-fast stain must be employed. The term "acid-fast" refers to the fact that the cells of certain microorganisms are lipid-rich and resist decolorization with alcohol, acetone-alcohol, or acid alcohol. Such organisms have a strong affinity for certain dyes such as phenolized carbolfuchsin and resist decolorization with a 4% hydrochloric acid alcohol for a specific period of time. The staining technique most commonly employed is the Ziehl-Neelsen method. However, the acid-fast staining method of Kinyoun may be substituted.

Other specialized staining techniques are used on occasion for a variety of purposes, usually to aid in the classification or identification of a microbial species, for example, spore stain, flagella stain, or capsule stain. Certain organisms such as *Mycobacterium tuberculosis* may be stained by the fluorochrome auramine-rhodamine. Examination by fluorescent microscopy by an experienced individual may offer a method that is more rapid and in some instances more specific for detection of these organisms in a smear preparation. The details of these techniques may be found in the *Manual of Clinical Microbiology* (Lennette, Spaulding, and Truant, 1974).

Other techniques of microscopic examination

Dark-field microscopy. There are a few situations in which the examination of a "wet mount" by dark-field microscopy is pertinent and of specific diagnostic val-ue. The examination of the exudate from a syphilitic chancre is the outstanding example. The technology and its application in diagnosis are discussed in the *Manual of Clinical Microbiology* (Lennette, Spaulding, and Truant, 1974).

Immunofluorescence. In many instances, fluorescence microscopy is a valuable tool in the diagnosis of infections. The technique involves the use of immunologic reagents that have been labeled with fluorescent moieties. Immunofluorescence combines the advantages of microscopic sensitivity and immunologic specificity. Certain bacterial species can be identified, or different strains serotyped by treating a specially prepared smear with specific antibody preparations conjugated with a fluorescing dye, such as rhodamine-lissamine, and examined by the technique of immunofluorescence microscopy. These are termed the "fluorescent antibody" (FA) methods. Streptococci may be grouped, strains of *Escherichia coli* may be serotyped, and other microorganisms may be identified by this technique. Fluorescent antibody staining procedures are useful not only for rapid diagnosis but in epidemiologic surveys as well. Currently there appears to be some possibility that certain obligate anaerobic species may be identified by these methods. Identification in these instances makes use of the "direct" method. Modifications allow the examination of a patient's serum or body fluids for specific antibodies, thus serving to confirm the existence of an infectious process. This is termed the "indirect" method. The best example of this important modification is the confirmatory serologic test for syphilis—the FTA-ABS test (Fig. 4-11). A complete discussion of this technology appears in the *Manual of Clinical Microbiology* (Lennette, Spaulding, and Truant, 1974).

Culture of specimens

Preparation of specimens for primary culture. Generally the oral and maxillofacial surgeon need not concern himself with special preparation of a collected specimen. However, when a piece of tissue is submitted for microbiologic

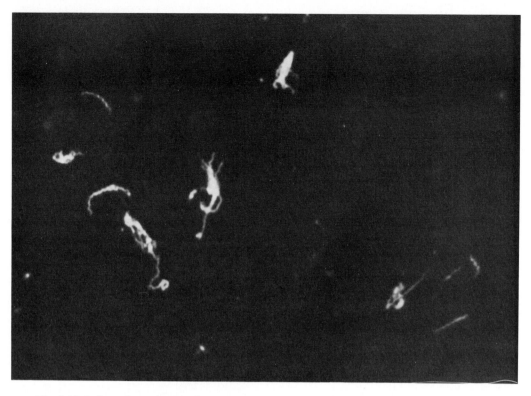

Fig. 4-11. Indirect fluorescent antibody staining of *Treponema pallidum.* (Courtesy L. J. LeBeau, Ph.D.)

analysis, it should be cut into small pieces or, if available, a tissue grinder or homogenizer may be employed for maceration. This must be done using aseptic techniques. In certain instances where tissues may also be sent to the pathologist for histologic examination, consideration of a microbiologic culture workup must preclude the formalinization of the biopsy specimen. If the material submitted is extremely viscous, an equal volume of *N*-acetyl cysteine or amyl acetate may be added. Such treatment frees the organisms within the specimen and does not inhibit the growth of the bacteria.

Media for primary culture. Certain media are routinely employed for the isolation of organisms from infectious processes in the oral cavity. The first of these is a blood agar plate. The usual concentration of blood is 5%; commercially available sheep blood is preferable, although outdated human bank blood is commonly used. Some laboratories employ resuspended human erythrocytes in specific concentration to prepare blood agar plates.

In certain instances chocolate agar may be required for primary isolation. The concentration of blood is again 5%. The blood may be added to a variety of agar bases, which may be prepared in the laboratory or are commercially available. After the blood is added aseptically to the previously sterilized base, the mixture is carefully heated to 80° C for 15 minutes or until the color of the media is chocolate brown.

There may be occasions where it is desirable to suppress the growth of aerobic and facultatively anaerobic gram-negative bacilli. In this instance sodium azide or sodium tellurite may be employed in specific concentrations as additives to a basal medium. On occasion one may also desire to suppress the growth of gram-positive organisms to select gram-negative bacilli. Media containing bile, bile complexes, or bile salts will suppress the growth of most gram-positive bacteria. The newest group of agents used in selective media are the antimicrobial agents such as cycloheximide, sulfonamides, trimethoprim, and nalidixic acid as well as the antibiotics neomycin, colistin, and vancomycin.

Certain reducing agents may be incorporated to promote anaerobiosis and thus enhance the growth of obligate anaerobes and microaerophilic bacteria. The most commonly employed are sodium thioglycollate and cysteine. Specific concentrations are used and added to basic enriched formulations. On occasion 0.5 to 1 gm of agar per liter is added to a broth formulation; convection currents are limited by the "semisolid" medium, and thus for some organisms suitable growth conditions are provided.

The large variety of media that fulfill these requirements are fully discussed in authoritative microbiology texts such as Lennette, Spaulding, and Truant (1974) and Finegold, Martin, and Scott (1978) as well as in the literature available from media manufacturers.

Inoculation of media. The bacteriologic inoculating loop is the best tool for inoculation of media when a homogeneous inoculum or specimen is available. It is also useful when a small volume of specimen, for instance an aspirate, is obtained. A small drop or two from the syringe may be placed on the surface of the medium somewhere near the periphery and then appropriately dispersed with a sterile inoculating loop.

If the specimen is material collected on a swab, the swab is gently but firmly "rolled" over one small segment of the plated medium. The plate is then streaked with a sterile inoculating loop. To obtain isolated colonies, the inoculum is streaked back and forth over the surface of approximately one quarter of the plate with the loop held loosely between the thumb and index finger. After the first quadrant has been inoculated, the loop is flamed and the plate is turned 90 degrees. Streaking is resumed at right angles to and across the first quadrant for several excursions to pick up some inoculum; then the streaking is continued over the second quadrant avoiding the previously inoculated area. The loop is then flamed again and the procedure is repeated until all four quadrants of the plate have been streaked.

Incubation of inoculated media. Following the inoculation of appropriate media, the culture must be placed in an incubator at the optimal temperature and humidity as rapidly as possible. For pyogenic infections of the oral cavity, isolation of organisms is optimal at 37° C. Some bacterial pathogens such as the gonococcus are known to grow optimally at 35° C and primary isolation is best accomplished at that temperature. Other pathogens require a carbon dioxide atmosphere for primary isolation, for example the gonococcus, meningococcus, *Brucella abortus*, and so on. Certain organisms of importance in dental pyogenic infections, the obligate anaerobic bacteria, require the complete absence of atmospheric oxygen. The techniques necessary for their recovery and isolation are discussed on p. 157.

In most instances organisms will grow out adequately for follow-up bacteriologic procedures in 18 to 24 hours. The usual laboratory procedure allows an overnight incubation period, after which the plates are examined and the colonial growth evaluated. In dealing with certain obligate anaerobic species, however, it is wise to allow 48 hours for the first incubation period of primary cultures.

Examination of cultures for presumptive recognition and identification of isolates. Following incubation at the optimal temperature and humidity for the optimal time period, the organisms are recognized presumptively by colonial characteristics (Fig. 4-12). Recognition of a significant bacterial species in an infectious process that is a member of the normal flora is of considerable importance; yet species that colonize the various tissues of the oral cavity may be the causative agents of pyogenic infections, particularly in a compromised host.

The absence of growth on a primary plating medium or in a broth may be a presumptive finding. However, culture results that differ from a presumptive

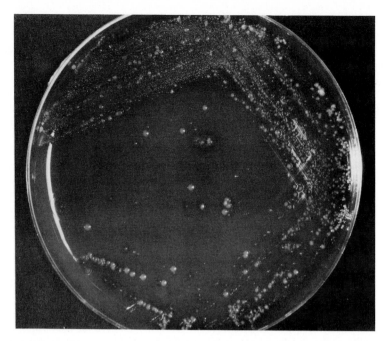

Fig. 4-12. Streak plate showing well-isolated colonies. (Courtesy L. J. LeBeau, Ph.D.)

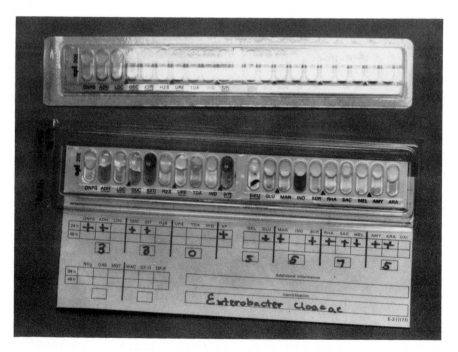

Fig. 4-13. Differentiation of *Enterobacteriaceae* by biochemical tests using API 20E System. The API 20E strip consists of small plastic tubes containing sterile dehydrated media. Tubes are inoculated with suspension of pure bacterial culture and incubated. Results are read, generally after 18 to 24 hours, when indicator systems are affected by bacterial metabolic products or added reagents. (Reproduced with permission. API 20E is a registered trademark of Analytab Products, Division of Ayerst Laboratories, Inc., Plainview, N. Y.)

diagnosis, especially when based on interpretation of a Gram stained smear, may indicate inadequate culture conditions. For example, an obligate anaerobic species may be noted in the smear, particularly if staining characteristics and morphology are unique, but the organism will not grow under aerobic or microaerophilic conditions. Such discrepancies must be noted in the final diagnosis.

Once the etiologic agents are isolated, various identification procedures are then required. These differ with the various groups (family and genus) to which the bacterium belongs. The procedures include the use of specific substrate media to establish the biochemical pattern of the isolate (for instance, the final pH of a culture, recognition of an intermediate or an end product metabolite, recognition of a single enzyme's activity — catalase, oxidase, urease, and so on). Rapid methods and/or micromethods are frequently used to facilitate identification. One of these is shown in Fig. 4-13. Often it may be necessary to confirm speciation or subspeciation by antigenic analysis — determination of a streptococcal group, a pneumococcal type, or a *Salmonella* species serotype. This depends on specific results of serologic reactions such as precipitation, agglutination, and so forth.

The techniques involved may be found in detail in authoritative microbiology texts (Lennette, Spaulding, and Truant, 1974; Rose and Friedman, 1976; Finegold, Martin, and Scott, 1978).

Isolation and identification of anaerobic bacteria

Both gram-positive and gram-negative obligate anaerobic bacteria are of importance as potential pathogens in pyogenic oral infections. Within the past 15 years, the methods of isolation of obligate anaerobic bacterial species have dramatically improved. Methods of characterization according to genus and species involve biochemical characterization using special media and gas-liquid chromatography for analysis of volatile and nonvolatile acid metabolites such as acetic acid, propionic acid, lactic acid, succinic acid, and so forth. By interpretation of a chromatogram, organisms are delineated as to genus and species. Detailed information is available in the *Manual of Clinical Microbiology* (Lennette, Spaulding and Truant, 1974), the *Anaerobe Laboratory Manual* (Holdeman, Cato, and Moore, 1977) and the *Wadsworth Anaerobic Bacteriology Manual* (Sutter, Vargo, and Finegold, 1975).

Collection of specimens. The procedures involved in collection and processing of clinical specimens suspected of containing anaerobic organisms are presented in Fig. 4-14. The majority of specimens related to anaerobes involved in pyogenic oral infections are subject to contamination with normal oral microbiota, because the oral mucosa teems with microorganisms. Therefore a needle introduced into the lesion (for example, an abscess) and withdrawal of pus into the syringe afford the most efficient approach. Minimal contact of the anaerobic bacteria with atmospheric oxygen is mandatory. The technique employed must preclude, for example, allowing a bubble of air to be mixed with the specimen in the syringe.

The gathering of material from a lesion by a swab is still an acceptable procedure when aspiration is not possible. Anaerobic bacteria in a pus specimen may remain viable for 4 to 24 hours, depending on the species involved. Pus itself provides a reduced, protective environment that allows for reasonable persistence of viability.

Specimen transport. As previously mentioned, some anaerobes are moderately resistant to oxygen contact and may survive for an extended period of time if only kept moist. On the other hand others may not tolerate even brief exposure to air. Consequently, special transport methods have been devised to increase survival of all anaerobes in clinical material. Obligate aerobes and facultative anaerobes remain viable in an anaerobic environment; therefore the universal carrier for the specimens under discussion, where anaerobic bacteria are sought, should be an anaerobic container.

The material collected in a syringe should be injected into a tube or bottle

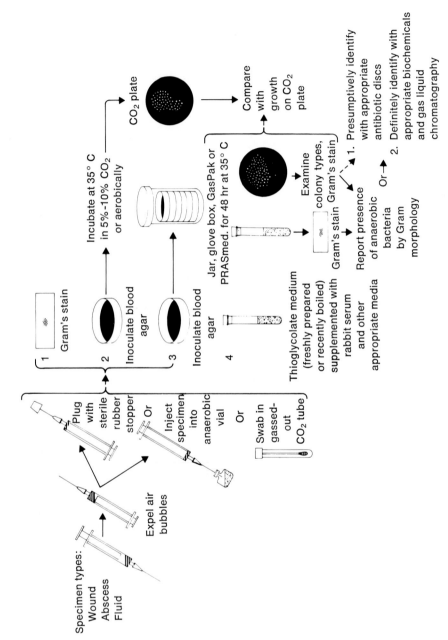

Fig. 4-14. Flowchart for processing specimens suspected of containing anaerobic organisms. (Redrawn and reproduced with permission from Anaerobic specimens: from patient to laboratory, 1975, The Upjohn Company, Kalamazoo, Michigan; and from BBL Manual of Products and Laboratory Procedures, ed. 5, p. 60, 1968, BBL Microbiology Systems, Division of Becton, Dickinson and Company, Cockeysville, Md. 21030.)

containing oxygen-free gas. These should be empty containers, since dilution of specimens with liquids reduces proportionately the chance of recovery of obligate anaerobes present and promotes the overgrowth of facultative species. It is desirable that these containers have a small amount of oxidation-reduction indicator within them (for example, aqueous reazurin, final concentration 0.0003%); they should be stored in the dark to preserve the indicator.

A syringe and needle may be taken directly to the laboratory if the needle is inserted into a sterile rubber stopper or if it is bent at a 90-degree angle to shut off access of air into the syringe. Prompt delivery and processing of such a specimen is necessary, because the plastic syringe gradually admits air. A container may be made anaerobic for tissue scrapings and biopsy specimens by using a portable "gassing-out" device.

The swab method is least desirable for collection of specimens for anaerobic bacteriologic workup, and its use should be limited to those situations where aspiration is impossible or extremely difficult. A recommended technique involves the use of two tubes of oxygen-free carbon dioxide. One tube contains a swab and should be rubber- or neoprene-stoppered. The other tube contains semisolid Cary-Blair transport medium. After the specimen is collected using the swab in the first tube, that swab is then immediately inserted into the transport medium. The insertion is made holding the tube in an upright position. Since carbon dioxide is heavier than air, the atmosphere within the tube remains oxygen-free.

All specimens should be cultured promptly. Refrigeration may be used to slow down the growth of facultative species if the culture cannot be set up within 2 hours.

Direct examination. Direct examination of clinical material suspected of containing obligate anaerobes is invaluable. The unique morphology of many of these organisms (fusiform bacilli, branching forms, granular cells, and so on) serves to alert the clinician to the possibility of infection with these bacteria. In turn this evaluation serves as a guide for the microbiologist in selection of the special media and technology. A rough quantitation of various types of organisms may also be made. The direct examination also serves as a check on the adequacy of the anaerobic techniques in use; there should be reasonable correlation between what is seen microscopically and what is cultured from a specimen.

Gram stained smears will provide, in the main, most of the necessary direct examination information required. Gram staining reaction, shape, size, morphology including branching and the presence of spores and their shape and position in the cell are features that may be delineated by the careful examination of the Gram stained smear. Some gram-negative obligate anaerobic species stain very lightly; safranin counterstaining reveals a light red or pink bacterial cell. The use of carbolfuchsin as a counterstain stains the gram-negative cells more deeply. Decolorizing procedures may dictate the use of 95% alcohol instead of acetone-alcohol.

Identification of anaerobic species. The identification procedures involve the characterization of four groups of anaerobic bacteria: the members of the genus *Clostridium,* the anaerobic cocci, the gram-negative nonsporeforming bacilli, and the gram-positive nonsporeforming bacilli. The species belonging to each group are delineated by employing a variety of techniques—Gram staining reaction, morphology, biochemical characterization, immunofluorescent techniques, and gas-liquid chromatography. The reader is referred to the *Manual of Clinical Microbiology* (Lennette, Spaulding, and Truant, 1974), the *Anaerobe Laboratory Manual* (Holdeman, Cato, and Moore, 1977), and the *Wadsworth Anaerobic Bacteriology Manual* (Sutter, Vargo, and Finegold, 1975) for the details of these procedures.

Blood culture

Since both transient, inconsequential and serious bacteremias result in a sufficient number of instances following pyogenic oral infections or traumatic manipulations in the oral cavity (for instance, tooth extraction and other surgical procedures), a discussion of blood culture as a laboratory diagnostic method is necessary.

A septicemia is suspect when the patient manifests certain signs and symptoms. The onset of chills, prostration, hypertension, and increase in the patient's temperature and pulse rate may be the first indications for the necessity of blood culture. A prolonged mild and intermittent fever in association with a heart murmur may be the indication of an endocarditis or arteritis. A bacteremia may be continuous as in an uncontrolled infection or endocarditis, or it may be intermittent. In the latter instance the time of the collection of the blood culture can be important. And yet the timing of the collection of a blood specimen may be a problem. The bacteremia usually precedes the onset of fever and chills. If a rhythm exists, correct timing may be possible; if it does not exist, proper timing is difficult.

If bacterial endocarditis is suspected, three separate cultures have been shown to be sufficient to isolate the etiologic agent in the majority of instances. Collection at no less than hourly intervals within a 24-hour period is preferential. In intermittent bacteremias three cultures collected over a 24- to 48-hour period usually result in isolation of the organism. Intervals between cultures may usually be determined by the clinical circumstances. Patients who have received antimicrobial agents prior to blood collection may present a problem; increased numbers of blood cultures may be necessary to isolate the causative organism.

Since resident skin microflora may result in false-positive blood cultures, an antiseptic should be applied to the skin prior to venipuncture. A 2% iodine tincture followed by removal with 70% ethyl alcohol or an iodophor, such as povidone iodine (Betadine), are considered to be the most effective skin antiseptics. Alcohol should *not* be used alone for this purpose! The agent of choice should be left in contact with the skin for at least 1 minute; "instant" antisepsis never occurs. The venipuncture site must not be touched unless the fingers used for palpation are similarly treated with an iodine compound.

Ten to 20 ml of blood should be collected for cultures; a lesser volume may result in lower recovery rates, since most bacteremias are of low magnitude. In infants and children the collection of 1 to 5 ml may be satisfactory.

In the majority of instances the blood is inoculated directly into culture media at the moment the specimen is drawn. Inoculation of blood into culture media should be on a 10% vol/vol basis; this allows sufficient dilution of the blood to counteract normal antibacterial activities of both chemical and cellular mediators of immunity. The addition of 0.05 to 0.025% sodium polyanethanol sulfonate (SPS) normally serves to neutralize residual antibacterial activity and acts as an anticoagulant and an anticomplementary and antiphagocytic agent.

A number of nutritionally adequate broth media may be used for blood culture; these include tryptic digest broth, trypticase soy broth, or brain-heart infusion broth. Columbia broth has been shown to support the growth of aerobes as well as anaerobic organisms (Blazevic, Stemper, and Matsen, 1975). Commercially available media are generally bottled under vacuum with carbon dioxide and contain 0.025% SPS. Bottles containing 50 to 100 ml of medium are most frequently employed.

If only one blood culture bottle is used, it should not be vented. However, it is preferable to use two bottles, one of which should be vented. Venting is accomplished by aseptic insertion of a sterile, cotton-plugged needle through the bottle's rubber stopper. The needle is withdrawn when the vacuum in the bottle has been replaced by air. Blood culture bottles* are available from several commercial sources including Difco Laboratories.

Cultures are incubated at 35° C and examined daily for at least 7 days for evidence of growth. Turbidity, hemoly-

---

*Bacto Blood Culture Bottles, Difco Laboratories, P. O. Box 1058A, Detroit, Mich. 48232.

sis, gaseousness, or presence of discrete colonies may be growth indicators. Ninety-five percent of clinically significant organisms are recovered within this time period. For certain infections (for example, brucellosis), blood cultures are held for 21 to 30 days, because a slow-growing organism may take extended periods of time to grow out. Also, when the patient has been under antibiotic therapy with little or no clinical response, longer periods of incubation may be necessary for growth of the etiologic organism.

Once evidence of growth is noted, a Gram stained smear of a suspect positive culture is made. Microscopic examination and interpretation of the smear then determines necessary subculture procedures for identification of the organism. The first subculture should always be both aerobic and anaerobic; anaerobes and microaerophilic bacteria may grow out in the depths of the blood culture bottle. Antibiotic susceptibility tests may then be performed if such are deemed necessary. For detailed information the reader is referred to the *Manual of Clinical Microbiology* (Lennette, Spaulding, and Truant, 1974).

There are special instances where variations of methodology may be necessary. These include the use of pour plates in addition to blood culture in broth, addition of penicillinase to broths for penicillin inactivation when the patient is under penicillin therapy, and change in incubation temperature (for example, 30° C for leptospiroses).

Another special technique is blood culture for anaerobic organisms. Anaerobic bacteria account for 12% to 27% of positive blood cultures and for 20% to 25% of patients clinically manifesting signs of bacteremia. As previously emphasized, collection, transport, media used, and examination of cultures are unique to this group of organisms.

New rapid techniques are also available for the detection of bacteremia. The use of ^{14}C-glucose radiometrically to detect early bacterial growth in blood is one method. This technique can detect growth of bacteria in blood culture as early as 4 to 6 hours after inoculation. Reports indicate that the method is very sensitive, and a unit that performs this new technique on a number of blood cultures at the same time is commercially available. For a detailed discussion, Prier, Bartola, and Friedman (1976) may be consulted.

Antimicrobial susceptibility testing of aerobes and facultative anaerobes

Antibiotic or chemotherapeutic agent susceptibility tests should be performed with all microorganisms contributing to an infectious process for which antimicrobial therapy is warranted, unless the microorganism's susceptibility is predicted by its identity. If the causative agent's capability to exhibit resistance to a commonly used antibiotic or chemotherapeutic agent has been established, for example, *Staphylococcus aureus* and *Pseudomonas* species, susceptibility or its lack should be determined. Susceptibility tests are rarely necessary for organisms such as the group A beta-hemolytic streptococcus or *Streptococcus pneumoniae*, which are almost always susceptible to penicillin or other highly effective antibiotics.

A number of susceptibility test methods are available and in use today. The diffusion procedure in standard use now has been accepted by the Food and Drug Administration and proposed as a tentative standard by the Antibiotic Susceptibility Testing Subcommittee of the National Committee on Clinical Laboratory Methods. Standardized dilution techniques have been recommended by an international collaborative study group (Ericsson and Sherris, 1971) on antibiotic susceptibility testing. When performed as recommended, these methods give intralaboratory and interlaboratory reproducibility.

Diffusion test procedures. Standardized representative concentrations of the antimicrobial agents are available on filter paper discs, which are placed on agar plate medium that has been freshly seeded over its entire surface with a diluted culture or a standardized suspension of the bacterial species whose susceptibility is being sought. A concentric zone of inhibition results; the size of the zone is subject to many factors that influence diffusibility in the medium—the molecular size of the agent, the concentration of the agent, the nature of the medium, and so forth. Standardization of the procedure and correlation of the in vitro test results with clinical therapeutic response have resulted in a procedure that is currently recommended (Bauer et al., 1966).

The test consists of inoculating a Mueller-Hinton agar medium with a turbidimetrically standardized 2- to 5-hour broth culture or a saline suspension of the bacterial species. A sterile cotton swab is used, and a standardized inoculating procedure is recommended. After the inoculated plate is allowed to dry, antimicrobial discs of standardized and recommended concentration for each agent are applied to the surface of the inoculated plate by hand with sterile forceps or by a commercially available dispenser.

After a 16- to 18-hour incubation period at 35° C, the plates (Fig. 4-15) are examined and the diameter of the zones of complete inhibition is measured to the nearest whole millimeter by use of a sliding caliper, ruler, or a template prepared for this purpose. The end point in all reading systems is complete inhibition of growth as determined by visual observation. Faint growth or tiny colonies that can be detected by close scrutiny are ignored. On the other hand, large colonies growing within the zone of inhibition may represent resistant variants or a mixed inoculum. Retesting or reidentification of the bacterial species is required in these instances.

The zone diameters for individual antimicrobial agents are converted into "susceptible," "intermediate," or "resistant" categories by reference to an interpretative table. The interpretations are those recommended by the FDA for antibiotics and by other sources for the chemotherapeutic agents.

Dilution test procedures. Dilution test procedures are employed to determine the minimal inhibitory concentration of an antimicrobial agent required to kill or inhibit the growth of a microorganism.

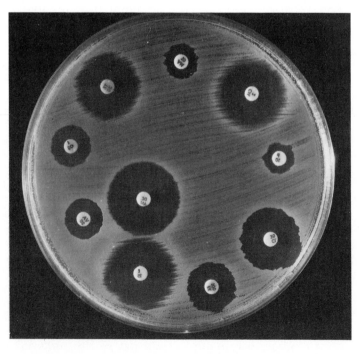

Fig. 4-15. Disc diffusion method for antibiotic susceptibility testing. (Courtesy L. J. LeBeau, Ph.D.)

The minimal inhibitory concentration (MIC) is the lowest concentration that prevents apparent growth. It is a "tube" or "broth" dilution test or an "agar plate" dilution test dependent on whether the test is performed in liquid or solid media.

The major goal to be attained using a dilution test is one of quantitation. These tests are most often performed to assure proper management of antimicrobial therapy. Qualitative data obtained from the disc diffusion test are adequate for guiding the therapy of most infections. Quantitative data may be needed when a drug dosage schedule must be maintained; in this instance disc tests are inapplicable, equivocal, or unreliable. Dilution tests are also useful for slow-growing organisms and confirmation of specific susceptibility, particularly with certain antibiotics such as polymyxin B or E. They should be performed when tests on strains fall into the intermediate susceptibility category, if treatment with potentially toxic agents is under consideration. There are instances when the disc tests appear to show that an organism is resistant to a relatively nontoxic drug. Broth dilution tests could determine the MIC of such a drug quantitatively, and then massive, yet safe, doses of such an agent can be employed to treat the infection.

Dilution tests were the first used for antibiotic susceptibility testing. As demands for tests increased and the laboratory load became large, setting up broth dilution tests was tedious and time-consuming. The disc diffusion test was then the alternate method of choice. At this time dilution tests may again become practical and economical for routine purposes because microtests and semiautomated broth dilution technology and agar dilution techniques utilizing inoculum replicators have been devised.

Agar dilution method. This procedure is convenient for testing a number of strains of bacteria simultaneously. It possesses the inherent ability to detect microbial heterogeneity or contamination. It has shown slightly better reproducibility than the broth dilution procedures.

Serial dilutions of the antimicrobial agent are prepared in each of a series of agar plates, for example, 128 μg/IU/ml, 64 μg/IU/ml to 0.25 μg/IU/ml. The base medium recommended is Mueller-Hinton agar, and it may be supplemented with 5% blood, preferably sheep blood. Usually supplementation is unnecessary; exceptions may include *Hemophilus* species, *Neisseria gonorrhoeae*, and so on. These plates are inoculated with a loop calibrated to deliver 0.001 to 0.002 ml per spot; one may note that many organisms may be tested on one plate of an antimicrobial agent medium at specific concentration at the same time. A Steers replicator may be used to facilitate performance of the tests. After inoculation of the plate, the spots are allowed to dry at room temperature, and the plates are incubated at 35° C for 16 to 20 hours.

The MIC of the agent in question against the organisms in question is the lowest concentration at which complete inhibition of growth occurs. A very fine, barely visible haze or single colony is disregarded.

Of course a variety of quality control procedures must be performed routinely to show stability of the agents in the plate media, possible variability in medium from batch to batch, and so forth. Controls are always run with each test series. An excellent coverage of the technique is afforded in the *Manual of Clinical Microbiology* (Lennette, Spaulding, and Truant, 1974).

Broth dilution method. This procedure is useful for testing rapidly growing aerobic and facultatively anaerobic bacteria. Mueller-Hinton broth is useful in most instances; a few fastidious species may require more enrichment, for example, as provided by a casein soy peptone medium.

Serial dilutions of an antimicrobial agent are prepared directly in the test tubes and a specific volume of standard inoculum of the microorganism is added to each tube. The tubes are incubated at 35° C for 16 to 20 hours.

The lowest concentration of the antimicrobial agent resulting in complete inhibition of growth represents the MIC. A faint turbidity or a small clump of growth is generally disregarded; a large cluster of growth or a definite turbidity means no inhibition. The minimum lethal concentration (MLC) is the lowest concentration of antimicrobic required to kill the microorganism. An inoculum control is included in each test.

Antimicrobial susceptibility testing of obligate anaerobes

The improved methods of isolation and identification of obligate anaerobic bacterial species and the antimicrobial therapy of infections caused by them have brought about a greater demand for information related to the in vitro testing procedures. In most instances initial therapy is determined empirically, since cultivation of clinically significant anaerobic species usually requires 3 to 4 days. There is a high-level predictability of antimicrobial susceptibility of these anaerobes, which forms the basis of appropriate initial therapy. However, it must be kept in mind that changing patterns of susceptibility to certain agents have been recognized for a number of years.

At present the conditions for testing of anaerobes have not been standardized; much work on these procedures is now in progress. Several problems associated with susceptibility testing of anaerobes are unique to this group. Anaerobiosis appears to decrease the activity of aminoglycoside antibiotics. The presence of carbon dioxide in the atmosphere will lower the pH of the medium and affect the activity of many antibiotics.

Within the past several years, agencies such as the FDA that are involved in the improvement and standardization of susceptibility test methods for aerobes and facultative anaerobes have recommended use of a dilution method for anaerobic species. No general agreement among workers as to dilution series, choice of medium, age and density of inoculum, or conditions or length of incubation has come about. A few studies directed toward standardization of a single disc technique have been made. These studies are referred to in the *Manual of Clinical Microbiology* (Lennette, Spaulding, and Truant, 1974).

Broth dilution tests. A broth dilution technique for rapidly growing strains (for example, *Bacteroides fragilis*, most *Clostridium* species) and one for slower growing strains (anaerobic cocci, *Eubacterium* species and many fusobacteria) are described in the *Manual of Clinical Microbiology* (Lennette, Spaulding, and Truant, 1974). A thioglycollate medium without indicator is enriched with hemin, sodium bicarbonate, and vitamin K (THCM); this medium is used for growth of the organisms. Each culture is then diluted with *Brucella* broth to a specific density with minimal aeration; slow-growing organisms require longer periods of growth for initial culture. On the day of the test, several two-fold dilutions of an antimicrobial agent are prepared in *Brucella* broth and equal volumes of inoculum are added. Tubes are incubated at 35° C in a GasPak jar for 48 hours. The MIC is the lowest concentration of the drug with no visible growth.

Agar dilution tests. The inoculum is prepared as for the broth dilution test. On the day of the test, dilutions of antibiotic solutions are incorporated into 5% laked blood or whole defibrinated sheep blood agar plates (*Brucella* agar base or BHI agar base with vitamin K supplement).

Plates are spot inoculated with a 0.001 ml calibrated loop or Steers replicator, allowed to dry, and incubated at 35° C in a GasPak jar for approximately 48 hours. The MIC is the lowest concentration yielding no growth, one or two colonies, or a fine, barely visible haze.

Mycotic infections

Fungi grow more slowly than the bacterial species. Considerable weight can be put on the morphologic characteristics of these microorganisms to establish not only a presumptive but often a final identification. In most instances these identifying characteristics can be recognized with a microscope, using a high power (×450) magnification.

Collection and handling of specimens

Collection of specimens for identification of fungi is similar to that for bacteria.

However, it is important to remember that if a biopsy specimen is to be cultured for yeasts or fungi, it should not be placed in formalin. As with specimens for bacteriologic diagnosis, prompt handling of freshly collected specimens is of the greatest importance. The selection of primary plating media is critical; it is important to plate each specimen on a battery of media, including simple nutrient media, enriched media, and selective media. The inoculation of these plates is in essence identical to the inoculation of primary plating media in the isolation of bacterial species. It is usual practice to incubate cultures both at 37° C and at 25° to 30° C (room temperature).

The incubation of primary cultures involves holding the cultures at incubation temperatures for at least 2 weeks and preferably 4 weeks or longer. Even though organisms, such as *Candida albicans*, may appear on the culture medium after several days of incubation, the plates should not be discarded because slower growing pathogens may require an extended time period before colonies can be observed. This extended incubation period means that dehydration must be prevented. The modern incubators of today handle the problem of relative humidity; otherwise, keeping a pan filled with water in the bottom of the unit will suffice. Dehydration of the media is also prevented by a partial seal of each Petri dish; the appropriate use of masking tape will accomplish this purpose. The seal must not be a complete one, because an aerobic environment is mandatory for most human pathogenic fungi. The use of screw-cap tubes is considered routine in mycologic diagnostic procedures; however, again, caps must be kept partially loosened to provide proper growth conditions.

Identification of fungi

Identification of fungi is accomplished by noting the development of their colonies and their gross and microscopic morphology. The surface texture, color, and growth rate of fungal colonies, and the pigmentation of the reverse side of the colony are important identifying characteristics.

Speciation involves inducing a fungus to display its characteristic spores, such as ascospores, blastospores, chlamydospores, macroconidia, and microconidia, or other distinguishing morphologic features. This usually requires the use of special media that serve to bring out these characterizing phases of growth. Biochemical tests have become routine and useful for the identification of species, especially the yeasts.

Fungi are easily differentiated into two types on the basis of macroscopic appearance of their colonies. Those that produce cottony, woolly, fluffy, or powdery aerial growth are termed "molds"; those that produce opaque, creamy, or pasty colonies are called "yeasts." There is a third group called the "dimorphic fungi," which develop as yeasts when cultured at 37° C and as molds when cultured at 25° to 30° C. The main systemic human pathogens are dimorphic. It is essential that conversion from one phase to another be accomplished for exact identification of these species.

Microscopically, the molds are observed to be multicellular organisms whose cells are joined together to make up long tubelike filaments called "hyphae." In certain instances hyphae that elongate form crosswalls, or "septa," behind the hyphal tip. Other hyphae do not form septa; these are termed "coenocytic." As hyphae multiply, they intertwine to form a "mycelium" or mold colony. The mycelial portion that penetrates the substrate or medium is called the "submerged" mycelium. The portion that grows above the substrate is called the "aerial" mycelium.

The true fungi reproduce sexually and asexually. Sexual reproduction involves the fusion of specialized cells called gametes. The fusion results in the development of a fruiting body in which "spores" are produced. The growth state induced by sexual combination is referred to as the "perfect state"; it provides the basis for the classification of fungi as *Phycomycetes*, *Ascomycetes*, or *Basidiomycetes*. A fourth class, the *Deu-*

teromycetes, or "Fungi Imperfecti," was established to comprise those species for which the perfect state is not recognized.

Asexual reproduction occurs by the formation of vegetative spores; types of these spores vary. Size, shape, color, and arrangement as seen microscopically are the most important laboratory identification criteria. Source and method of spore formation classify the type of spore—thallospore, blastospore, chlamydaspore, and so on. Vegetative spores, formed on specialized hyphal branches called "conidiophores", are termed "conidia." There are many kinds of conidia; if they are small and unicellular, they are "microconidia," if large and multicellular, "macroconidia."

Conidia and other spores may be demonstrated by removing a small piece of spore-bearing mycelium from a mold colony with a hooked needle and gently teasing it apart in a drop of lactophenol cotton blue, a dye mounting solution that stains the fungal cells. Size, shape, and color can be readily observed microscopically.

The technique just described may result in disruption of the true morphologic depiction because of difficulty in maintaining the intact structures. The "slide culture" technique ideally solves this problem. A small block of appropriate agar medium is placed on a sterile microscope slide supported on a bent glass rod in a sterile Petri dish. The agar block is inoculated on all four sides with the fungus under study, and a sterile coverslip is placed on the agar block. Water is added to the sterile filter paper on the bottom of the dish to prevent dehydration. The culture is incubated at 25° to 30° C.

The slide may be removed from the dish at any time to view the growth microscopically; one can study progressive growth in situ. When the fungus is fully developed, a permanent mount can be prepared by removing the coverslip from the agar and placing it face down in a drop of lactophenol cotton blue. The edges of the coverslip are then sealed with a nail polish or other mounting medium.

Microscopic observation

In dealing with the yeasts or yeast-phases of the dimorphic fungi, either a wet mount or a stained preparation is examined microscopically. In the latter instance differential staining is not an overall necessity. The concern is with the size and shape of the cell, whether or not budding occurs, and the shape and size of the daughter cells. Ascospores may be observed in stained smears; the true yeasts *(Ascomycetes)* produce ascospores under proper conditions of nutrition, temperature, and sexual mating. In some species elongation to form pseudomycelia occurs under certain environmental conditions (for example, *Candida albicans* on cornmeal agar); these may be observed in stained smears but most often are not sought by these staining techniques. Capsules may be the distinguishing morphologic characteristic for the identification of some important pathogenic species (for example, *Cryptococcus neoformans*). A capsule may be observed by the examination of a stained smear; most commonly a wet India ink mount or another type of wet mount preparation is utilized. The periodic acid–Schiff (PAS) stain, which takes advantage of the fact that the polysaccharide moieties attach to Schiff's base resulting in purple-red stained structure, may also be used to demonstrate capsules and cell walls of yeast cells. The cell walls of chitinous fungi also contain polysaccharide moieties and they too will be stained. The PAS stains are used mainly for the observation of the cells in tissue.

Observation of an inoculum from a yeast colony in a wet mount, using lactophenol cotton blue as the mounting and staining menstruum, is the method of choice. The characterization of species is based on the same features discussed in the preceding paragraph.

As indicated previously, the intent of this section was to present a pertinent, informative summary of laboratory diagnostic techniques of mycotic infections. The information provided may be supplemented by detailed authorative information in the *Manual of Clinical Microbiology* (Lennette, Spaulding, and Truant,

1974) and *Medical Mycology* (Rippon, 1974).

Immunologic techniques

Immunologic techniques are of importance in the diagnosis of mycotic infections. They serve as diagnostic aids and in certain instances as the diagnostic method. Two major difficulties are inherent in the application of these techniques: (1) sensitive and specific antigens for all fungus diseases are not commercially available and (2) there is a broad-based cross-reactivity of antigens. The latter makes the interpretation of test results difficult. Problems of mycoserologic or mycoimmunologic diagnoses result not from the type of test employed but from the crudeness and complexity of the antigens used in the tests.

Immunologic technology for diagnosis of fungal disease involves (1) skin testing to detect and evaluate hypersensitivity, (2) detection of circulating antibodies and antigens in the patient's serum by complement fixation, immunodiffusion tests, and so forth, and (3) in vitro and in vivo identification of fungi by immunofluorescent technology (Lennette, Spaulding, and Truant, 1974; Rippon, 1974).

Protozoan infections

To achieve correct diagnosis of protozoan infections, two basic necessities must be considered: (1) preparation of suitable smears (stained smears and wet mounts) of the blood, stool, or other appropriate specimens and (2) making an adequate systematic search of each or both to find the diagnostic stage of the organism. Some of the species will grow on artificial media or in tissue cell cultures, and certain of these techniques are employed by some laboratories. Immunologic procedures play a major role or contribute significantly to the diagnosis of amebiasis, toxoplasmosis, malaria, and a few other infections.

The microbiologist is concerned with morphology and identification of phases of the protozoan. The greatest diagnostic problems comprise *missed diagnoses* and *misdiagnosis*. Laboratory errors involve failure to detect the organisms, confusion of artifacts (especially in stool specimens), or confusion of a commensal protozoan with the pathogen.

Failure to detect the organisms most often results when proper illumination is not used. Amoebae may be missed if the microscopic field is too brightly illuminated; insufficient light fails to clarify important identifying features (morphologic details). There is an established routine for microscopic examination of diagnostic protozoan smears or wet mounts. The wet mount is carefully observed at ×450 magnification, followed by examination of a portion of the preparation using oil immersion at ×950 magnification. The stained smears are examined under the same conditions and in the same thorough manner. It should be emphasized that a careful, methodical search is required to complete a satisfactory stool examination. The same approach should be employed for the examination of blood smears or various aspirated specimens. Because artifacts may be minimally present, the recognition of diagnostic forms is not difficult.

For more detailed information on the collection and processing of specimens the reader is referred to the *Manual of Clinical Microbiology* (Lennette, Spaulding, and Truant, 1974) or other authoritative texts on parasitic diseases and tropical medicine.

Viral infections

Three general laboratory procedures can be employed to aid the clinician in the diagnosis of oral lesions in which a viral etiology is suspected. The first of these involves the cytologic examination of smears of cells scraped from the lesion(s). The second procedure involves the isolation and identification of the virus from clinical material. The third procedure involves the demonstration of at least a four-fold rise in the antibody titer to a given virus in serum specimens obtained from the patient during the acute and convalescent phases of the illness.

Preparation of smears

Smears of cells from the base of vesicular lesions may be prepared as follows

(Lennette, Spaulding, and Truant, 1974): The lesions should be swabbed lightly with sterile isotonic saline solution and allowed to dry. A fresh vesicle that is free of purulent material is incised at the periphery with a scalpel, and the top of the lesion is deflected. After the excess fluid has been removed by gentle blotting, the base of the lesion is scraped with a scalpel and the cellular material is smeared evenly over two 0.5 to 1 cm areas on clean microscope slides, allowed to air dry, and sent to the laboratory. If the smears are to be examined by the fluorescent antibody staining technique, at least three separate smears should be prepared to allow for necessary controls to be carried out.

The laboratory may be requested to stain the smear with Giemsa stain or by Papanicolaou's method. The stained smears are examined under the microscope for pathologic changes and the presence of cytoplasmic or intranuclear inclusions. These procedures do not constitute a specific virologic diagnosis, but they may aid in differentiating between recurrent aphthae and oral lesions caused by the herpesvirus group, that is, herpes simplex or varicella-zoster viruses. Medak and his associates (1971) reported that smears stained by Papanicolaou's technique were an aid in distinguishing between the oral lesions of bullous pemphigoid, Darier's disease, erythema multiforme, herpes simplex virus, lichen planus, and pemphigus vulgaris.

The fluorescent antibody staining technique is a specific diagnostic tool that has a wide variety of applications. It may be used to differentiate the oral or skin lesions caused by the herpes simplex virus from those caused by the varicella-zoster virus (Griffin, 1963; Schmidt et al., 1965). Fluorescent antibody staining is not practical in the diagnosis of herpangina or hand, foot, and mouth disease because of the multiplicity of antigenic types of the coxsackieviruses that may be involved in these syndromes.

Collection of specimens for virus isolation

Preferably specimens for virus isolation should be obtained aseptically within 3 days after the onset of the illness. Specimens obtained later than 7 days after onset of the illness are less likely to yield infectious virus. Sterile cotton swabs may be used to obtain specimens from the oral cavity or throat. The tonsils and posterior pharynx are rubbed with a dry swab or one that has been moistened with sterile transport broth. To obtain specimens from the oral cavity, the swabs should be rubbed over the mucosa of both cheeks opposite the upper molars and over the floor of the mouth anterior to the tongue. In both instances the swabs should be broken off just above the cotton tip and immediately placed into a screw-capped or tightly stoppered tube containing about 5 ml of sterile tryptose phosphate broth to which 1% gelatin or bovine serum albumin has been added. The latter aids in stabilizing the virus. Tissue culture medium containing 2% fetal bovine serum or 1% gelatin may also be used as a transport medium. Washings from the throat can be obtained by allowing the patient to gargle with about 10 ml of tryptose phosphate or nutrient broth. The patient then expectorates the fluid into a clean or sterile cup, and the washing is poured into a sterile stoppered or screw-capped vial. The tubes containing the specimens should be labeled with the patient's name, the source of the specimen, the date, and some indication of the kind of infection that is suspected. In all instances the specimens should be refrigerated at once and transported to the laboratory within 2 or 3 hours. If this is inconvenient, they may be frozen at −70° C.

In some instances it may be desirable to aspirate fluid from one or more fresh cutaneous or mucosal vesicles. This procedure can be carried out as follows: First, the vesicles are rinsed gently with sterile isotonic saline solution and the fluid aspirated by means of a 26- or 27-gauge needle attached to a tuberculin syringe. The collected fluids are then dispensed into 1 or 2 ml of tissue culture medium to prevent clot formation. In addition cellular material may be gently scraped from the base of opened vesicles and added to the tube containing the vesicular fluid. The specimens should be refrigerated and transported to the laboratory within several hours after collection or stored at −70° C until they can be processed. It is important to reiterate that material from vesicular lesions will rarely yield infectious virus unless the specimens are taken during the first 3 days of the eruption.

Titration of acute and convalescent sera

A retrospective diagnosis of many viral infections may be made by demonstrating a rise in the antibody titer of the patient's serum against a given virus during the course of an illness. The acute phase blood specimen should be collected from 1 to 7 days after onset of the illness, and the convalescent phase blood specimen should be collected between 14 and 28 days after onset. Approximately 10 ml of blood should be drawn aseptically; "Vacutainer" tubes* are convenient for this purpose. Anticoagulants or preservatives should not be used, and the whole blood should not be frozen, since this will result in red cell lysis. Each blood specimen should be appropriately labeled with the patient's name, date of collection, and an indication of the suspected disease and promptly sent to the laboratory. The laboratory will then separate the serum from the clot and store it at 4° or −20° C until the serologic tests can be carried out simultaneously on both the acute and convalescent serum samples. The results are considered to be of diagnostic significance only if the antibody titer of the convalescent phase serum shows a four-fold or greater rise in the titer over that of the acute phase serum. It should be noted that a rise in antibody titer is generally seen in primary herpetic, varicella-zoster, and coxsackievirus infections. However, this is not usually observed in secondary or recurrent herpes simplex virus infections.

Additional information on specimen collection and handling and the procedures employed by the diagnostic laboratory is available from several publications (Lennette and Schmidt, 1969; Lennette, Spaulding, and Truant, 1974; Pumper and Yamashiroya, 1975).

REFERENCES

Abbott, J. N., Briney, A. T., and Denaro, S. A. 1955. Recovery of tubercle bacilli from mouth washings of tuberculous dental patients, J. Am. Dent. Assoc. **50:**49.

Acton, J. D., et al. 1974. Fundamentals of medical virology for students of medicine and related sciences, Philadelphia, Lea & Febiger.

Adar, R. E., et al. 1972. Abdominal actinomycosis, Isr. J. Med. Sci. **8:**148.

Agranat, B. J. 1969. Friedlander's osteomyelitis of the mandible: report of a case, J. Oral. Surg. **27:**293.

Alter, H. J., et al. 1975. Health-care workers positive for hepatitis B surface antigen: are their contacts at risk? N. Engl. J. Med. **292:**454.

Andriole, V. T., and Lyons, R. W. 1970. Coagulase-negative staphylococcus, Ann. N.Y. Acad. Sci. **174:**533.

Ashcavai, M., and Peters, R. L. 1973. Manual for hepatitis B testing, Philadelphia, W. B. Saunders Co.

Bahn, A. N., et al. 1960. Incidence of oral group D streptococci, J. Dent. Res. **39:**686.

Baringer, J. R. 1974. Recovery of herpes simplex virus from human sacral ganglions, N. Engl. J. Med. **291:**828.

Baringer, J. R., and Swoveland, P. 1973. Recovery of herpes-simplex virus from human trigeminal ganglions, N. Engl. J. Med. **288:**648.

Barnes, E. M., and Goldberg, H. S. 1968. The relationships of bacteria within the family Bacteroidaceae as shown by numerical taxonomy, J. Gen. Microbiol. **51:**313.

Barrett, F. F., et al. 1970. Bacteriophage types and antibiotic susceptibility of *Staphylococcus aureus:* Boston City Hospital, 1967, Arch. Intern. Med. **125:**867.

Barrett, M. T. 1914. The protozoa of the mouth in relation to pyorrhea alveolaris, Dent. Cosmos. **56:**948.

Bartels, H. A. 1968. Introduction and bacterial incitants. In Nolte, W. A., ed.: Oral microbiology, ed. 1, St. Louis, The C. V. Mosby Co., p. 59.

Bartels, H. A., and Blechman, H. 1962. Survey of the yeast population in saliva and on evaluation of some procedures for identification of *Candida albicans,* J. Dent. Res. **41:**1386.

Bastion, F. O., et al. 1972. Herpesvirus hominis: isolation from human trigeminal ganglion, Science **178:**306.

Batty, I. 1958. *Actinomyces odontolyticus,* a new species of actinomycete regularly isolated from deep carious dentine, J. Pathol. Bacteriol. **75:**455.

Bauer, A. W., et al. 1966. Antibiotic susceptibility testing by a standardized single disk method, Am. J. Clin. Pathol. **45:**493.

Beatman, L. H. 1933. Studies on *Trichomonas buccalis,* J. Dent. Res. **13:**339.

Bell, W. A., Gamble, J., and Garrington, G. E. 1969. North American blastomycosis with oral lesions, Oral Surg. **28:**914.

---

*Available from Scientific Products, Division of American Hospital Supply Corporation, 1430 Waukegan Road, McGaw Park, Ill. 60085.

Blank, H., and Rake, G. 1955. Viral and rickettsial diseases of the skin, eye, and mucous membranes of man, Boston, Little, Brown & Co.

Blazevic, D. J., Stemper, J. E., and Matsen, J. M. 1975. Effect of aerobic and anaerobic atmospheres on isolation of organisms from blood cultures, J. Clin. Microbiol. **1:**154.

Bloom, R. H., and Brown, L. R. 1964. A study of the effects of orthodontic appliances on the oral microbial flora, Oral Surg. **17:**658.

Blumberg, B. S., Alter, H. J., and Visnich, S. 1965. A "new" antigen in leukemia sera, J.A.M.A. **191:**541.

Boatman, E. S., and Kenny, G. E. 1971. Morphology and ultrastructure of *Mycoplasma pneumoniae* spherules, J. Bacteriol. **106:**1005.

Bogliolo, L. 1950. South American blastomycosis (Lutz's disease), Arch. Dermatol. Syph. **61:**470.

Bourgeau, G., and McBride, B. C. 1976. Dextran-mediated interbacterial aggregation between dextran-synthesizing streptococci and *Actinomyces viscosus*, Infect. Immun. **13:**1228.

Bowden, G. H., and Hardie, J. M. 1971. Anaerobic organisms from the human mouth. In Shapton, D. A., and Boald, R. G., eds.: Isolation of anaerobes, London, Academic Press, Inc.

Brock, D. W., et al. 1973. Actinomycosis caused by *Arachnia propionica:* report of 11 cases, Am. J. Clin. Pathol. **59:**66.

Brown, A. E., Williams, H. L., and Herrell, W. E. 1941. Bacteroides septicemia: report of a case with recovery, J.A.M.A. **116:**402.

Brown, J. M., Georg, L. K., and Waters, L. C. 1969. Laboratory identification of *Rothia dentocariosa* and its occurrence in human clinical material, Appl. Microbiol. **17:**150.

Brunell, P. A. 1967. Varicella-zoster infections in pregnancy, J.A.M.A. **199:**315.

Buchanan, R. E., and Gibbons, N. E. 1974. Bergey's manual of determinative bacteriology, ed. 8, Baltimore, The Williams & Wilkins Co.

Burnett, G. W., and Scherp, H. W. 1968. Oral microbiology and infectious disease, ed. 3, Baltimore, The Williams & Wilkins Co., p. 273.

Byrne, E. B. 1966. Viral hepatitis: an occupational hazard of medical personnel, J.A.M.A. **195:**362.

Carlsson, J. 1967. Presence of various types of non-haemolytic streptococci in dental plaque and other sites of the oral cavity in man, Odontol. Revy **18:**55.

Carlsson, J., et al. 1970. Early establishment of *Streptococcus salivarius* in the mouths of infants, J. Dent. Res. **49:**415.

Casman, E. P. 1971. Staphylococcal enterotoxin, Ann. N.Y. Acad. Sci. **128:**124.

Cawson, R. A. 1963. Denture sore mouth and angular cheilitis, Br. Dent. J. **115:**441.

Clarke, J. K. 1924. On the bacterial factor in the aetiology of dental caries, Br. J. Exp. Pathol. **5:**141.

Clement, A. J. 1953. Field studies in the Southern Kalahari: August, 1951, J. Dent. Res. **32:**697.

Colman, G., and Williams, R. E. O. 1972. Taxonomy of some human viridans streptococci. In Wannamaker, L. W., and Matsen, J. M., eds.: Streptococci and streptococcal diseases, New York, Academic Press, Inc., p. 281.

Coodley, E. L. 1969 Actinomycosis: clinical diagnosis and management, Postgrad. Med. **46:**73.

Cope, V. Z. 1951. Actinomycosis of bone with special reference to infection of vertebral column, J. Bone Joint Surg. **33-B:**205.

Cullen, C. H., and Sharp, M. E. 1951. Infection of wounds with *Actinomyces*, J. Bone Joint Surg. **33-B:**221.

Dane, D. S., Cameron, C. H., and Briggs, M. 1970. Virus-like particles in serum of patients with Australia-antigen-associated hepatitis, Lancet **1:**695.

Debre, R., and Celers, J., eds. 1970. Clinical virology: the evaluation and management of human viral infections, Philadelphia, W. B. Saunders Co.

Dienstag, J. L., Alling, D. W., and Purcell, R. H. 1976. Quantitation of antibody to hepatitis A antigen by immune electron microscopy, Infect. Immun. **13:**1209.

Dodd, K., and Ruchman, I. 1950. Herpes simplex virus not the etiologic agent of recurrent stomatitis, Pediatrics **5:**883.

Dodin, A. 1976. Melioidosis, an Asian disease now a world problem, La Recherche **7:**574.

Dolby, A. E. 1969. Recurrent aphthous ulceration: effect of sera and peripheral blood lymphocytes upon oral epithelial tissue culture cells, Immunology **17:**709.

Douglas, R. G., Jr., and Couch, R. B. 1970. A prospective study of chronic herpes simplex virus infection and recurrent herpes labialis in humans, J. Immunol. **104:**289.

Elek, S. D. 1959. *Staphylococcus pyogenes* and its relation to disease, Edinburgh, E. & S. Livingstone.

Ellison, S. A., Carton, C. A., and Rose, H. M. 1959. Studies of recurrent herpes simplex infections following section of the trigeminal nerve, J. Infect. Dis. **105:**161.

Emmons, C. W., Binford, C. H., and Utz, J. P. 1970. Medical mycology, ed. 2, Philadelphia, Lea & Febiger.

Engel, L. D., and Kenny, G. E. 1970. *Mycoplasma salivarium* in human gingival sulci, J. Periodont. Res. **5:**163.

Ennever, J. 1963. Microbiologic calcification, Ann. N.Y. Acad. Sci. **109:**4.

Ennever, J., Vogel, J., and Takazoe, I. 1968. Calcium binding by a lipid extract of *Bacterionema matruchotii*, Calcif. Tissue Res. **2:**296.

Enright, J. J., Friesell, H. E., and Treschner, M. D. 1932. Studies on the cause and nature of dental caries, J. Dent. Res. **12:**759.

Epker, B. N., and Via, W. F., Jr. 1969. Oral and perioral manifestations of leprosy: report of a case, Oral Surg. **28:**342.

Ericsson, H. M., and Sherris, J. C. 1971. Antibiotic sensitivity testing: report of an international collaborative study, Acta Pathol. Microbiol. Scand. [Suppl.] **217:**3.

Erlichman, M. C., and Trieger, N. 1978. Aspergillus infection in a patient receiving immunosuppressive drugs, J. Oral. Surg. **36:**978.

Evans, F. O., Jr., et al. 1975. Sinusitis of the maxillary antrum, N. Engl. J. Med. **293:**735.

Everts, E. C. 1970. Cervicofacial actinomycosis, Arch. Otolaryngol. **92:**468.

Faillo, P. S., Sube, H. P., and Anderson, N. H. 1959. Mucormycosis of the paranasal sinuses and the maxilla, Oral Surg. **12**:304.

Farber, J. E., Friedland, E., and Jacobs, W. F. 1940. Tuberculosis of the tongue, Am. Rev. Tuberc. **42**:766.

Farmer, E. D. 1954. Serological subdivisions among Lancefield group H streptococci, J. Gen. Microbiol. **11**:131.

Faucett, R. L., and Miller, H. C. 1948. Stomatitis in infants caused by *B. mucosus capsulatus*, Pediatrics **1**:458.

Fawaz, K. A., et al. 1975. Repetitive maternal-fetal transmission of fatal hepatitis B, N. Engl. J. Med. **293**:1357.

Feingold, M., and Gellis, S. S. 1965. Cellulitis due to *Haemophilus influenzae* type b, N. Engl. J. Med. **272**:788.

Feinstone, S. M., Kapikian, A. Z., and Purcell, R. H. 1973. Hepatitis A: detection by immune electron microscopy of a viruslike antigen associated with acute illness, Science **182**:1026.

Feldman, R. E., and Schiff, E. R. 1975. Hepatitis in dental professionals, J.A.M.A. **232**:1228.

Fenner, F., and White, D. O. 1976. Medical virology, ed. 2, New York, Academic Press, Inc.

Fetter, B. F., Klintworth, G. K., and Hendry, W. S. 1967. Mycoses of the central nervous system, Baltimore, The Williams & Wilkins Co.

Finegold, S. M., Martin, W. J., and Scott, E. G. 1978. Bailey and Scott's Diagnostic Microbiology, ed. 5, St. Louis, The C. V. Mosby Co.

Finegold, S. M., et al. 1972. Scope monograph on anaerobic infections, Kalamazoo, Mich., The Upjohn Co.

Fiumara, N. J., and Lessell, S. 1970. Manifestations of late congenital syphilis, Arch. Dermatol. **102**:78.

Foley, T. F., Dines, D. E., and Dolan, C. T. 1971. Pulmonary actinomycosis, Minn. Med. **54**:593.

Fox, H., Purcell, R. H., and Chanock, R. M. 1969. Characterization of a newly identified Mycoplasma (*Mycoplasma orale* type 3) from the human oropharynx, J. Bacteriol. **98**:36.

Fox, J., and Isenberg, H. D. 1967. Antibiotic resistance of microorganisms isolated from root canals, Oral Surg. **23**:230.

Francis, T. C. 1970. Recurrent aphthous stomatitis and Behçet's disease: a review, Oral Surg. **30**:476.

Frauenfelder, D., and Schwartz, A. W. 1967. Coccidioidomycosis involving head and neck. Plast. Reconstr. Surg. **39**:549.

Garibaldi, R. A., et al. 1972. Hospital-acquired serum hepatitis: report of an outbreak, J.A.M.A. **219**:1577.

Gartenberg, G., et al. 1978. Hospital-acquired mucormycosis (*Rhizopus rhizopodiformis*) of skin and subcutaneous tissue: epidemiology, mycology and treatment, N. Engl. J. Med. **299**:1115.

Georg, L. K. 1970. Diagnostic procedures for the isolation and identification of the etiological agents of actinomycosis. In Proc. Int. Symp. Mycoses, Washington, D.C., World Health Organization, p. 71.

Georg, L. K. 1974. The agents of human actinomycosis. In Balows, A., et al., eds.: Anaerobic bacteria: role in disease, Springfield, Ill., Charles C Thomas, Publisher, p. 237.

Georg, L. K., and Brown, J. M. 1967. *Rothia*, gen. nov. an aerobic genus of the family *Actinomycetaceae*, Int. J. Syst. Bacteriol. **17**:79.

Georg, L. K., and Coleman, C. M. 1970. Comparative pathogenicity of various *Actinomyces* species. In Prauser, H., ed.: The actinomycetales, Jena, VEB Gustav Fischer Verlag, p. 35.

Gerin, J. L. 1976. Hepatitis: the search for viral and sub-viral antigens. In Fractions, No. 1, Palo Alto, Spinco Division of Beckman Instruments, Inc.

Germaine, G. R., and Schachtele, C. F. 1976. *Streptococcus mutans* dextransucrase: mode of interaction with high-molecular-weight dextran and role in cellular aggregation, Infect. Immun. **13**:365.

Gibbons, R. J. 1972. Ecology and cariogenic potential of oral streptococci. In Wannamaker, L. W., and Matsen, J. M., eds.: Streptococci and streptococcal diseases, New York, Academic Press, Inc., p. 371.

Gibbons, R. J., and Banghart, S. 1967. Synthesis of extracellular dextran by cariogenic bacteria and its presence in human plaque, Arch. Oral Biol. **12**:11.

Gibbons, R. J., and Nygaard, M. 1968. Synthesis of insoluble dextran and its significance in the formation of gelatinous deposits by plaque-forming streptococci, Arch. Oral Biol. **13**:1249.

Gibbons, R. J., and Nygaard, M. 1970. Interbacterial aggregation of plaque bacteria, Arch. Oral Biol. **15**:1397.

Gibbons, R. J., and van Houte, J. 1973. On the formation of dental plaques, J. Periodontol. **44**:347.

Gibbons, R. J., and van Houte, J. 1975. Bacterial adherence in oral microbial ecology, Annu. Rev. Microbiol. **29**:19.

Gibbons, R. J., van Houte, J., and Liljemark, W. F. 1972. Parameters that effect the adherence of *Streptococcus salivarius* to oral epithelial surfaces, J. Dent. Res. **51**:424.

Gibbons, R. J., et al. 1963. The microbiota of the gingival crevice area of man - II, Arch. Oral Biol. **8**:281.

Gibbons, R. J., et al. 1964. Studies on the predominant cultivable microbiota of dental plaque, Arch. Oral Biol. **9**:365.

Gibbons, R. J., et al. 1974. Interdental localization of *Streptococcus mutans* as related to dental caries experience, Infect. Immun. **9**:481.

Gilmour, M. N. 1961. The classification of organisms termed *Leptotrichia (Leptothrix) buccalis*. II. Reproduction of *Bacterionema matruchotii*, Bacteriol. Rev. **25**:142.

Gilmour, M. N., and Beck, P. A. 1961. The classification of organisms termed *Leptotrichia (Leptothrix) buccalis*. III. Growth and biochemical characteristics of *Bacterionema matruchotii*, Bacteriol. Rev. **25**:152.

Gilmour, M. N., Howell, A., Jr., and Bibby, B. G. 1961. The classification of organisms termed *Leptotrichia (Leptothrix) buccalis*. I. Review of the literature and proposed separation into *Leptotrichia buccalis* (Trevisan, 1879) and *Bacterionema* gen nov., *B. matruchotii* (Mendel, 1919) comb. nov., Bacteriol. Rev. **25**:131.

Glassman, A. B., and Simpson, J. S. 1975. *Eikenella corrodens:* a clinical problem, J. Am. Dent. Assoc. **91:**1237.

Gocke, D. J., and Kavey, N. B. 1969. Hepatitis antigen—correlation with disease and infectivity of blood-donors, Lancet **1:**1055.

Goffinet, D. R., Glatstein, E. J., and Merigan, T. C. 1972. Herpes zoster-varicella infections and lymphoma, Ann. Intern. Med. **76:**235.

Gold, O. Jordan, H. V., and van Houte, J. 1975. The prevalence of enterococci in the human mouth and their pathogenicity in animal models, Arch. Oral Biol. **20:**473.

Goldberg, M. H. 1966. Postoperative oral infection with *Pseudomonas aeruginosa*, J. Oral Surg. **24:**334.

Goldberg, M. H. 1968. Gram-negative bacteremia after dental extraction, J. Oral Surg. **26:**180.

Gordon, D. F., Jr. 1967. Reisolation of *Staphylococcus salivarius* from the human oral cavity, J. Bacteriol. **94:**1281.

Gordon, D. F., Jr., and Gibbons, R. J. 1966. Studies on the predominant cultivable microorganisms from the human tongue, Arch. Oral Biol. **11:**627.

Gordon, D. F., Jr., and Jong, B. B. 1968. Indigenous flora from human saliva, Appl. Microbiol. **16:**428.

Gottlieb, D. S., and Miller, L. H. 1971. *Entamoeba gingivalis* in periodontal disease, J. Periodontol. **42:**412.

Grady, G. F., and Lee, V. A. 1975. Hepatitis B immune globulin—prevention of hepatitis from accidental exposure among medical personnel, N. Engl. J. Med. **293:**1067.

Graykowski, E. A., et al. 1966. Recurrent aphthous stomatitis: clinical, therapeutic, histopathologic, and hypersensitivity aspects, J.A.M.A. **196:**637.

Grayston, J. T., Foy, H. M., and Kenny, G. E. 1959. The epidemiology of Mycoplasma infections of the human respiratory tract. In Hayflick, L., ed.: The Mycoplasmatales and L-phase of bacteria, New York, Appleton-Century-Crofts, p. 651.

Green, M., and Fousek, M. D. 1957. *Hemophilus influenzae* type B cellulitis, Pediatrics **19:**80.

Green, W. H., Goldberg, H. I., and Wohl, G. T. 1967. Mucormycosis infection of the craniofacial structures, Am. J. Roentgenol. Radium Ther. Nucl. Med. **101:**802.

Griffin, J. W. 1963. Fluorescent antibody study of herpes simplex virus lesions and recurrent aphthae, Oral Surg. **16:**945.

Guggenheim, B. 1968. Streptococci of dental plaques, Caries Res. **2:**147.

Guggenheim, B., and Newbrun, E. 1969. Extracellular glucosyl transferase activity of an HS strain of *Streptococcus mutans*, Helv. Odontol. Acta **13:**84.

Hadi, A. W., and Russell, C. 1968. Quantitative estimations of fusiforms in saliva from normal individuals and cases of acute ulcerative gingivitis, Arch. Oral Biol. **13:**1371.

Hadi, A. W., and Russell, C. 1969. Fusiforms in gingival material: quantitative estimations from normal individuals and cases of periodontal disease, Br. Dent. J. **126:**82.

Hambrick, G. W., Jr., Cox, R. P., and Senior, J. R. 1962. Primary herpes simplex infection of fingers of medical personnel, Arch. Dermatol. **85:**583.

Handelman, S. L., and Mills, J. R. 1965. Enumeration of selected salivary groups, J. Dent. Res. **44:**1343.

Hardie, J. M., and Bowden, G. H. 1974. The normal microbial flora of the mouth. In Skinner, F. A., and Carr, J. G., ed.: The normal microbial flora of man, New York, Academic Press, Inc., p. 47.

Hartley, J. H., and Schatten, W. E. 1973. Cervicofacial actinomycosis, Plast. Reconstr. Surg. **51:**44.

Hecht, D. W., and Work, W. P. 1970. Surgery for nonneoplastic parotid disease, Arch. Otolaryngol. **92:**463.

Heitman, K. L., and Brasher, W. J. 1971. Oral infection due to Klebsiella pneumonia microorganism: case report, J. Periodontol. **42:**552.

Hertz, J. 1960. Actinomycosis: borderline cases, J. Int. Coll. Surg. **34:**148.

Hoffman, M. A., and Finberg, L. 1955. Pseudomonas infections in infants associated with high-humidity environments, J. Pediatr. **46:**626.

Hofstad, T., and Kristoffersen, T. 1970. Chemical composition of endotoxin from oral Veillonella, Acta Pathol. Microbiol. Scand. [B] **78:**760.

Holdeman, L. V., and Moore, W. E. C. 1974. Genus *Eubacterium*. In Buchanan, R. E., and Gibbons, N. E., ed.: Bergey's manual of determinative bacteriology, ed. 8, Baltimore, 1974, The Williams & Wilkins Co., p. 641.

Holdeman, L. V., Cato, E. P., and Moore, W. E. C. 1977. Anaerobe laboratory manual, ed. 4, Blacksburg, Va., The Virginia Polytechnic Institute and State University Anaerobe Laboratory.

Holm. P. 1950. Studies on the aetiology of human actinomycosis, Acta Pathol. Microbiol. Scand. **27:**736.

Hoofnagle, J. H., Gerety, R. J., and Barker, L. F. 1973. Antibody to hepatitis-B-virus core in man, Lancet **2:**869.

Hoofnagle, J. H., et al. 1974. Antibody to hepatitis B core antigen—a sensitive indicator of hepatitis B virus replication, N. Engl. J. Med. **290:**1336.

Howell, A., Jr. 1963. A filamentous microorganism isolated from periodontal plaque in hamsters. I. Isolation, morphology and general cultural characteristics, Sabouraudia **3:**81.

Howell, A., Jr., and Pine, L. 1961. The classification of organisms termed *Leptotrichia (Leptothrix) buccalis*. IV. Physiological and biochemical characteristics of *Bacterionema matruchotii*, Bacteriol. Rev. **25:**162.

Hudson, R. 1957. *Neisseria pharyngis* bacteriaemia in a patient with subacute bacterial endocarditis, J. Clin. Pathol. **10:**195.

Hunter, G. C., and Westrick, C. M. 1957. Cervicofacial abscesses by *Actinomyces*, Oral Surg. **10:**793.

Hurst, V., and Fenderson, A. 1969. Establishment of *Bacteroides melaninogenicus* as a component of the anaerobic bacterial flora, Bacteriol. Proc. 1969, Abstract M229, p. 103.

Hutter, R. V. P. 1959. Phycomycetous infection (mucormycosis) in cancer patients: a complication of therapy, Cancer **12:**330.

Ikeda, T., Isoda, A., and Iidako, T. 1964. A study on staphylococci isolated from the acute suppurative diseases in the oral area with reference to their comparative pathogenicity, J. Nihon Univ. Sch. Dent. **6:**88.

Ikeda, T., and Sandham, H. J. 1971. Prevalence of *Streptococcus mutans* on various tooth surfaces in Negro children, Arch. Oral Biol. **16**:1237.

Jansen, G. T., Dillaha, C. J., and Honeycutt, W. M. 1963. Candida cheilitis, Arch. Dermatol. **88**:325.

Jawetz, E., Melnick, J. L., and Adelberg, E. A. 1976. Review of medical microbiology, ed. 12, Los Altos, Calif., Lange Medical Publications.

Jordon, H. V., and Keyes, P. H. 1964. Aerobic, grampositive filamentous bacteria as etiologic agents of experimental periodontal disease in hamsters, Arch. Oral Biol. **9**:401.

Jordon, H. V., Keyes, P. H., and Bellack, S. 1972. Periodontal lesions in hamsters and gnotobiotic rats infected with actinomyces of human origin, J. Periodont. Res. **7**:21.

Jordon, H. V., Keyes, P. H., and Lim, S. 1969. Plaque formation and implantation of *Odontomyces viscosus* in hamsters fed different carbohydrates, J. Dent. Res. **48**:824.

Kantz, W. E., and Henry, C. A. 1974. Isolation and classification of anaerobic bacteria from intact pulp chambers of non-vital teeth in man, Arch. Oral Biol. **19**:91.

Kaplan, P. M., et al. 1973. DNA polymerase associated with human hepatitis B antigen, J. Virol. **12**:995.

Kapsimalis, P., and Garrington, G. E. 1968. Actinomycosis of periapical tissues, Oral Surg. **26**:374.

Katz, H. L., 1941. Tuberculosis of the tongue, Q. Bull. Sea View Hosp. **6**:239.

Kelstrup, J. 1966. The incidence of *Bacteroides melaninogenicus* in human gingival sulci, and its prevalence in adult bronchopulmonary infection. Periodontics **4**:14.

Kenny, G. E. 1974. Mycoplasma. In Lennette, E. H., Spaulding, E. H., and Truant, J. P., eds.: Manual of clinical microbiology, ed. 2, Washington, D.C., American Society for Microbiology, p. 333.

Kesel, R. G., et al. 1958. Further studies on lactobacillus counts after elimination of carious lesions, J. Dent. Res. **37**:50.

Kirner, A., et al. 1969. Die bakteriologischen Befunde aus den Submandibulären Abszessen, Dtsch. Stomatol. **19**:434.

Klyhn, K. M., and Gorrill, R. H. 1967. Studies on the virulence of hospital strains of *Pseudomonas aeruginosa*, J. Gen. Microbiol. **47**:227.

Knighton, H. T. 1962. Relative constancy of specific bacteriophage patterns of staphylococci isolated from oral and nasal areas, J. Dent. Res. **41**:701.

Kofoid, C. A. 1929. The protozoa of the human mouth, J. Parasitol. **15**:151.

Krugman, S., and Ward, R. 1973. Infectious diseases of children and adults, St. Louis. The C. V. Mosby Co.

Krugman, S., Friedman, H., and Lattimer, C. 1975. Viral hepatitis, type A: identification by specific complement fixation and immune adherence tests, N. Engl. J. Med. **292**:1141.

Krugman, S., Giles, J. P., and Hammond, J. 1967. Infectious hepatitis: evidence for two distinctive clinical, epidemiological, and immunological types of infection, J.A.M.A. **200**:365.

Krugman, S., et al. 1974. Viral hepatitis, type B— DNA polymerase activity and antibody to hepatitis B core antigen, N. Engl. J. Med. **290**:1331.

Lancefield, R. C. 1933. A serological differentiation of human and other groups of hemolytic streptococci, J. Exp. Med. **57**:571.

Landau, J. W., and Newcomer, V. D. 1963. Acute cerebral phycomycosis (mucormycosis), J. Pediatr. **61**:363.

Leach, S. A., et al. 1972. Some factors affecting the metabolism of fructan by human oral flora, Arch. Oral Biol. **17**:137.

Leake, D., and Leake, R. 1970. Neonatal suppurative parotitis, Pediatrics **46**:203.

Le Bouvier, G. L., and McCollum, R. W. 1970. Australia (hepatitis-associated) antigen: physicochemical and immunological characteristics, Adv. Virus Res. **16**:357.

Lee, Y. H., et al. 1973. T-mycoplasmas in nongonococcal urethritis—a reappraisal, Clin. Res. **21**:605.

Lehner, T. 1969. Characterization of mucosal antibodies in recurrent aphthous ulceration and Behçet's syndrome, Arch. Oral Biol. **14**:843.

Lehner, T. 1972a. Cell-mediated immune responses in oral disease: a review, J. Oral Pathol. **1**:39.

Lehner, T. 1972b. Immunologic aspects of recurrent oral ulcers, Oral Surg. **33**:80.

Lehner, T. 1977. Progress report: oral ulceration and Behçet's syndrome, Gut **18**:491.

Lennette, E. H., and Magoffin, R. L. 1973. Virologic and immunologic aspects of major oral ulcerations, J. Am. Dent. Assoc. **87**:1055.

Lennette, E. H., and Schmidt, N. J., eds. 1969. Diagnostic procedures for viral and rickettsial infections, ed. 4, New York, American Public Health Association, Inc.

Lennette, E. H., Melnick, J. L., and Magoffin, R. L. 1974. Clinical virology: introduction to methods. In Lennette, E. H., Spaulding, E. H., and Truant, J. P., eds.: Manual of clinical microbiology, ed. 2, Washington, D.C., American Society for Microbiology, p. 667.

Lennette, E. H., Spaulding, E. H., and Truant, J. P., eds. 1974. Manual of clinical microbiology, ed. 2, Washington, D.C., American Society for Microbiology.

Levin, M. L., et al. 1974. Hepatitis B transmission by dentists, J.A.M.A. **228**:1139.

Levy, B. M. 1945. Oral manifestations of histoplasmosis, J. Am. Dent. Assoc. **32**:215.

Limongelli, W. A., et al. 1975. Successful treatment of mucocutaneous mucormycosis after dental extractions in a patient with uncontrolled diabetes, J. Oral Surg. **33**:705.

Lindgren, K. M., Douglas, G. R., and Couch, R. B. 1968. Significance of herpesvirus hominis in respiratory secretions of man, N. Engl. J. Med. **278**:517.

Littleton, N. W., Kahehashi, S., and Fitzgerald, R. J. 1970. Recovery of specific "caries-inducing" streptococci from carious lesions in the teeth of children, Arch. Oral Biol. **15**:461.

Locatcher-Khorazo, D., and Seegal, B. C. 1972. Microbiology of the eye, St. Louis, The C. V. Mosby Co.

Löe, H., Theilade, E., and Jensen, S. B. 1965. Experimental gingivitis in man, J. Periodontol. **36**:177.

Loesche W. J. 1974. Dental infections. In Balows,

A., et al., eds.: Anaerobic bacteria; role in disease, Springfield, Ill. Charles C Thomas, Publisher, p. 409.

Loesche, W. J., Socransky, S. S., and Gibbons, R. J. 1964. *Bacteroides oralis,* proposed new species isolated from the oral cavity of man, J. Bacteriol. **88**:1329.

Loesche, W. J., et al. 1975. Association of *Streptococcus mutans* with human dental decay, Infect. Immun. **11**:1252.

Losli, E. J., and Lindsey, R. H. 1963. Fatal systemic diseases from dental sepsis: report of two cases, Oral Surg. **16**:366.

MacFarlane, T. W., and Helnarska, S. J. 1976. The microbiology of angular cheilitis, Br. Dent. J. **140**:403.

Macotela-Ruiz, E., and Gonzalez-Angulo, A. 1966. Electron microscope studies of granules of *Nocardia brasiliensis* in man, Sabouraudia **5**:92.

Magnius, L. O. 1975. Characterization of a new antigen-antibody system associated with hepatitis B, Clin. Exp. Immunol. **20**:209.

Magnius, L. O., and Espmark, J. A. 1972. New specificities in Australia antigen positive sera distinct from Le Bouvier determinants, J. Immunol. **109**:1017.

Magnius, L. O., et al. 1975. A new antigen-antibody system: clinical significance in long-term carriers of hepatitis B surface antigen, J.A.M.A. **231**:356.

Magoffin, R. L., Jackson, E. W., and Lennette, E. H. 1961. Vesicular stomatitis and exanthem—a syndrome associated with coxsackie virus, type A16, J.A.M.A. **175**:441.

Marsik, F. J., and Parisi, J. T. 1973 Significance of *Staphylococcus epidermidis* in the clinical laboratory, Appl. Microbiol. **25**:11.

Martin, W. J. 1974. Anaerobic cocci. In Lennette, E. H., Spaulding, E. H., and Truant, J. P., eds.: Manual of clinical microbiology, ed. 2, Washington, D.C., American Society for Microbiology, p. 381.

Mashberg, A., Carroll, M. A., and Morrissey, J. B. 1970. Gram-negative infections of the oral cavity and associated structures: report of two cases, J. Oral Surg. **28**:376.

McAuliffe, V. J., Purcell, R. H., and LeBouvier, G. L. 1976. e: a third hepatitis B antigen? N. Engl. J. Med. **294**:779.

McCabe, M. M., and Smith, E. E. 1975. Relationship between cell-bound dextransucrase and the agglutination of *Streptococcus mutans,* Infect. Immun. **12**:512.

McCarthy, C., Snyder, M. L., and Parker, R. B. 1965. The indigenous oral flora of man. I. The newborn to the one-year-old infant, Arch. Oral Biol. **10**:61.

McCormack, W. M., et al. 1973. The genital mycoplasmas, N. Engl. J. Med. **288**:78.

McNamara, M. J., et al. 1967. A study of the bacteriologic patterns of hospital infections, Ann. Intern. Med. **66**:480.

Medak, H., et al. 1971. Cytopathologic study as an aid to the diagnosis of vesicular dermatoses, Oral Surg. **32**:204.

Melish, M. E., and Glasgow, L. A. 1970. The staphylococcal scalded-skin syndrome: development of an experimental model, N. Engl. J. Med. **282**:1114.

Melish, M. E., Glasgow, L. A., and Turner, M. D. 1972. The staphylococcal scalded-skin syndrome: isolation and partial characterization of the exfoliative toxin, J. Infect. Dis. **125**:129.

Mergenhagen, S. E. 1960. Endotoxic properties of oral bacteria as revealed by the local Shwartzman reaction, J. Dent. Res. **39**:267.

Mergenhagen, S. E., and Varah, E. 1963. Serologically specific lipopolysaccharides from oral Veillonella, Arch. Oral Biol. **8**:31.

Mergenhagen, S. E., Hampp, E. G., and Scherp, H. W. 1961. Preparation and biological activites of endotoxins from oral bacteria, J. Infect. Dis. **108**:304.

Mergenhagen, S. E., Zipkin, I., and Varah, E. 1962. Immunological and chemical studies on an oral Veillonella endotoxin, J. Immunol. **88**:482.

Merigan, T. C. 1974. Host defenses against viral disease, N. Engl. J. Med. **290**:323.

Merselis, J. G., Jr., Kaye, D., and Hook, E. W. 1964. Disseminated herpes zoster: a report of 17 cases, Arch. Intern. Med. **113**:679.

Metzger, A. L. 1970. Gonococcal arthritis complicating gonorrheal pharyngitis, Ann. Intern. Med. **73**:267.

Meyer, I., and Shklar, G. 1967. The oral manifestations of acquired syphilis: a study of eighty-one cases, Oral Surg. **23**:45.

Mihm, M. C. 1971. Hand-foot-and-mouth disease. In Fitzpatrick, T. B., ed.: Dermatology in general medicine, New York, McGraw-Hill Book Co.

Miller, W. J., et al. 1975. Specific immune adherence assay for human hepatitis A antibody: application to diagnostic and epidemiologic investigations, Proc. Soc. Exp. Biol. Med. **149**:254.

Mink, J. R. and Winter, G. B. 1970. Hand, foot, and mouth disease, J. Dent. Child. **37**:519.

Moore, W. E. C., and Holdeman, L. V. 1974. Genus *Propionibacterium.* In Buchanan, R. E., and Gibbons, N. E., eds.: Bergey's manual of determinative bacteriology, ed. 8, Baltimore, The Williams & Wilkins Co. p. 633.

Moritsugu, Y., et al. 1976. Purification of hepatitis A antigen from feces and detection of antigen and antibody by immune adherence hemagglutination, Infect. Immun. **13**:898.

Morris, E. O. 1954a. The bacteriology of the oral cavity. IV. (A) *Micrococcus,* (B) *Neisseria* and (C) *Veillonella,* Br. Dent. J. **96**:259.

Morris, E. O. 1954b. The bacteriology of the oral cavity. VI. Fusiformis, Bacillus, Bacterium and Haemophilus. General conclusions, Br. Dent. J. **97**:283.

Morton, H. E., et al. 1951. Isolation of pleuropneumonia-like organisms from human saliva: a newly detected member of the oral flora, J. Dent. Res. **30**:415.

Mosley, J. W., and White, E. 1975. Viral hepatitis as an occupational hazard of dentists, J. Am. Dent. Assoc. **90**:992.

Mosley, J. W., et al. 1975. Hepatitis B virus infection in dentists, N. Engl. J. Med. **293**:729.

Myrvik, Q. N., Pearsall, N. N., and Weiser, R. S. 1974. Fundamentals of medical bacteriology and mycology for students of medicine and related sciences, Philadelphia, Lee & Febiger.

Nahmias, A. J., and Roizman, B. 1973a. Infection with herpes-simplex viruses 1 and 2 (first of three parts), N. Engl. J. Med. **289**:667.

Nahmias, A. J., and Roizman, B. 1973b. Infection with herpes-simplex viruses 1 and 2 (second of three parts), N. Engl. J. Med. **289**:719.

Nahmias, A. J., and Roizman, B. 1973c. Infection with herpes-simplex viruses 1 and 2 (third of three parts), N. Engl. J. Med. **289**:781.

Nally, F. F., and Ross, I. H. 1971. Herpes zoster of the oral and facial structures: report of five cases and discussion, Oral Surg. **32**:221.

Newman, C. W., and Rosenbaum, D. 1962. Oral cryptococcus, J. Periodontol. **33**:266.

Newman, H. N., and McKay, G. S. 1973. An unusual microbial configuration in human dental plaque, Microbios **8**:117.

Nielsen, J. O., Dietrichson, O., and Juhl, E. 1974. Incidence and meaning of the "e" determinant among hepatitis-B-antigen positive patients with acute and chronic liver diseases, Lancet **2**:913.

Nielsen, J. O., LeBouvier, G. L., and The Copenhagen Hepatitis Acute Program. 1973. Subtypes of Australia antigen among patients and health carriers in Copenhagen: a relation between the subtypes and the degree of liver damage in acute viral hepatitis, N. Engl. J. Med. **288**:1257.

Nolte, W. A., ed. 1973. Oral microbiology, ed. 2, St. Louis, The C. V. Mosby Co., p. 81.

Nugent, G. R., and Chow, S. M. 1973. Treatment of labial herpes, J.A.M.A.. **224**:132.

Okada, K., et al. 1976. e antigen and anti-e in the serum of asymptomatic carrier mothers as indicators of positive and negative transmission of hepatitis B virus to their infants, N. Engl. J. Med. **294**:746.

Olson, J. A., et al. 1976. Levamisole: a new treatment for recurrent aphthous stomatitis, Oral Surg. **41**:588.

Onisi, M. 1949. Study on the actinomyces isolated from the deeper layers of carious dentine, Shikazaku Zasehi **6**:273.

Oppenheim, J. J., and Francis, T. C. 1970. The role of delayed hypersensitivity in immunological processes and its relationship to aphthous stomatitis, J. Periodontol. **41**:205.

Oven, J., Kirsten, R., and Bulow, P. 1969. Changing staphylococci and staphylococcal infections, N. Engl. J. Med. **281**:627.

Owen, O. W. 1949. A study of bacterial counts (lactobacilli) in saliva related to orthodontic appliances, Am. J. Orthod. **35**:672.

Pasricha, J. S., Nayyar, K. C., and Pasricha, A. 1973. A new method for treatment of herpes simplex, Arch. Dermatol. **107**:775.

Pheils, M. T., Reid, D. J., and Ross, C. F. 1964. Abdominal actinomycosis, Br. J. Surg. **51**:345.

Pike, E. B., et al. 1962. The taxonomy of micrococci and Neisseriae of oral origin, Arch. Oral Biol. **7**:715.

Pine, L., and Hardin, H. 1959. *Actinomyces israelii*, a cause of lacrimal canaliculitis in man, J. Bacteriol. **78**:164.

Prather, J. R., et al. 1970. Actinomycosis of the thorax—diagnosis and treatment, Ann. Thorac. Surg. **9**:307.

Prier, J. E., Bartola, J., and Friedman, H. 1976. Modern methods in medical microbiology: systems and trends, Baltimore, University Park Press.

Prince, A. M. 1968. An antigen detected in the blood during the incubation period of serum hepatitis, Proc. Natl. Acad. Sci. U.S.A. **60**:814.

Prince, A. M., et al. 1975. Hepatitis B "immune" globulin: effectiveness in prevention of dialysis-associated hepatitis, N. Engl. J. Med. **293**:1063.

Provost, P. J., and Hilleman, M. R. 1979. Propagation of human hepatitis A virus in cell culture in vitro, Proc. Soc. Exp. Biol. Med. **160**:213.

Provost, P. J., et al. 1975a. A specific complement-fixation test for human hepatitis A employing CR326 virus antigen: diagnosis and epidemiology, Proc. Soc. Exp. Biol. Med. **148**:962.

Provost, P. J., et al. 1975b. Physical, chemical and morphologic dimensions of human hepatitis A virus strain CR326, Proc. Soc. Exp. Biol. Med. **148**:532.

Pumper, R. W., and Yamashiroya, H. M. 1975. Essentials of medical virology, Philadelphia, W. B. Saunders Co.

Purcell, R. H., et al. 1976. A microtiter solid-phase radioimmunoassay for hepatitis A antigen and antibody, J. Immunol. **116**:349.

Putman, H. C., Dockerty, M. B., and Waugh, J. M. 1950. Abdominal actinomycosis: an analysis of 122 cases, Surgery **28**:781.

Ranier, A. 1951. Primary laryngeal blastomycosis: a review of the literature and report of a case, Am. J. Clin. Pathol. **21**:444.

Razin, S., Michmann, J., and Shimshoni, Z. 1964. The occurrence of mycoplasma (pleuropneumonia-like organisms, PPLO) in the oral cavity of dentulous and edentulous subjects. J. Dent. Res. **43**:402.

Reade, P. C., and Radden, B. G. 1963. Chronic osteomyelitis of the maxilla associated with a Pseudomonas infection, Br. Dent. J. **115**:246.

Redeker, A. G., et al. 1975. Hepatitis B immune globulin as a prophylactic measure for spouses exposed to acute type B hepatitis, N. Engl. J. Med. **293**:1056.

Reichart, P. 1976. Facial and oral manifestations in leprosy, Oral Surg. **41**:385.

Richardson, R. L., and Jones, M. 1958. A bacteriologic census of human saliva, J. Dent. Res. **37**:697.

Rippon, J. W. 1974. Medical mycology: the pathogenic fungi and the pathogenic actinomycetes, Philadelphia, W. B. Saunders Co.

Ritz, H. L. 1967. Microbial population shifts in developing human dental plaque, Arch. Oral Biol. **12**:1561.

Ritz, H. L. 1969. Fluorescent antibody staining of *Neisseria, Streptococcus,* and *Veillonella* in frozen sections of human dental plaque, Arch. Oral Biol. **14**:1073.

Rizzo, A. A., and Mergenhagen, S. E. 1964. Histopathologic effects of endotoxin injected into rabbit oral mucosa, Arch. Oral Biol. **9**:659.

Robinson, C. R., and Rhodes, A. J. 1961. Vesicular exanthem and stomatitis: report of an epidemic due to coxsackie virus group A, type 16, N. Engl. J. Med. **265**:1104.

Roed-Petersen, B., Renstrup, G., and Pindborg, J. J. 1970. Candida in oral leukoplakias: a histologic and exfoliative cytologic study, Scand. J. Dent. Res. **78**:323.

Rogosa, M. 1956. A selective medium for the isolation and enumeration of the Veillonella from the oral cavity, J. Bacteriol. **72**:533.

Rogosa, M. 1964. The genus *Veillonella*. I. General cultural, ecological and biochemical considerations, J. Bacteriol. **87**:162.

Rogosa, M. 1974a. Genus III. *Bifidobacterium*. In Buchanan, R. E., and Gibbons, N. E., eds.: Bergey's manual of determinative bacteriology, ed. 8, Baltimore, The Williams & Wilkins Co., p. 669.

Rogosa, M. 1974b. Genus I. *Peptococcus*. In Buchanan, R. E., and Gibbons, N. E., eds.: Bergey's manual of determinative bacteriology, ed. 8, Baltimore, The Williams & Wilkins Co., p. 518.

Rogosa, M. 1974c. Genus II. *Peptostreptococcus*. In Buchanan, R. E., and Gibbons, N. E., eds.: Bergey's manual of determinative bacteriology, ed. 8, Baltimore, The Williams & Wilkins Co., p. 522.

Rosan, B. 1973. Antigens of *Streptococcus sanguis*, Infect. Immun. **7**:205.

Rosan, B., and Hammond, B. F. 1974. Extracellular polysaccharides of *Actinomyces viscosus*, Infect. Immun. **10**:304.

Rosato, F. E., Rosato, E. F., and Plotkin, S. A. 1970. Herpetic paronychia—an occupational hazard of medical personnel, N. Engl. J. Med. **283**:804.

Rose, N. R., and Friedman, H., eds. 1976. Manual of clinical immunology, Washington, D.C., American Society for Microbiology.

Rose, S. S. 1954. A clinical and radiological survey of 192 cases of recurrent swellings of the salivary glands, Ann. R. Coll. Surg. Engl. **15**:374.

Ross, P. W. 1971. Beta-haemolytic streptococci in saliva, J. Hyg. **69**:347.

Ross, S., et al. 1974. Staphylococcal susceptibility to penicillin G: the changing pattern among community strains, J.A.M.A. **229**:1075.

Rustigian, R., et al. 1966. Studies on latent infection of skin and oral mucosa in individuals with recurrent herpes simplex, J. Invest. Dermatol. **47**:218.

Sabin, A. B. 1975. Misery of recurrent herpes: what to do? N. Engl. J. Med. **293**:986.

Sabiston, C. G., Jr., Grigsby, B. A., and Sagerstrom, N. 1976. Bacterial study of pyogenic infections of dental origin, Oral Surg. **41**:430.

Sakamaki, S. T., and Bahn, A. N. 1968. Effect of orthodontic banding on localized oral lactobacilli, J. Dent. Res. **47**:275.

Sawyer, S. J., MacDonald, J. B., and Gibbons, R. J. 1962. Biochemical characteristics of *Bacteroides melaninogenicus*—a study of thirty-one strains, Arch. Oral Biol. **7**:685.

Scardovi, V., et al. 1971. Deoxyribonucleic acid homology relationships among species of the genus *Bifidobacterium*, Int. J. Syst. Bacteriol. **21**(4):276.

Schimpff, S., et al., 1972. Varicella-zoster infections in patients with cancer, Ann. Intern. Med. **76**:241.

Schmidt, H., Hjørting-Hansen, E., and Philipsen, H. P. 1961. Gonococcal stomatitis, Acta Derm. Venereol. (Stockh.) **41**:324.

Schmidt, N. J., Lennette, E. H., and Magoffin, R. L. 1969. Immunological relationship between herpes simplex and varicella-zoster viruses demonstrated by complement-fixation, neutralization and fluorescent antibody tests, J. Gen. Virol. **4**:321.

Schmidt, N. J., et al. 1965. Immunofluorescent staining in the laboratory diagnosis of varicella-zoster virus infections, J. Lab. Clin. Med. **66**:403.

Schmitt, J. A. 1971. Epidemiological investigations of oral *Candida albicans*, Mycopathol. Mycol. Appl. **43**:65.

Sherman, J. M. 1937. The streptococci, Bacteriol. Rev. **1**:3.

Shklair, I. L., and Mazzarella, M. A. 1961. Effects of full-mouth extraction on oral microbiota, Dent. Prog. **1**:275.

Shklair, I. L., Keene, H. J., and Cullen, P. 1974. The distribution of *Streptococcus mutans* on the teeth of two groups of naval recruits, Arch. Oral Biol. **19**:199.

Shklair, I. L., Keene, H. J., and Simonson, L. G. 1972. Distribution and frequency of *Streptococcus mutans* in caries-active individuals, J. Dent. Res. **51**:882.

Shklair, I. L., Losse, F. L., and Bahn, A. N. 1963. The isolation and incidence of *Pseudomonas aeruginosa* from human saliva, Bacteriol. Proc. 1963, p. 71, Abstract M68.

Shklair, I. L., et al. 1956. Preliminary report on the effect of complete mouth rehabilitation on oral lactobacillus counts, J. Am. Dent. Assoc. **53**:155.

Shklair, I. L., et al. 1962. Isolation and incidence of pleuropneumoniae-like organisms from the human oral cavity, J. Bacteriol. **83**:785.

Shklar, G. 1971. Oral reflections of infectious diseases (first of two parts), Postgrad. Med. **49**:87.

Sims, W. 1970a. Oral haemophili, J. Gen. Microbiol. **3**:615.

Sims, W. 1970b. The interpretation and use of Snyder tests and lactobacillus counts, J. Am. Dent. Assoc. **80**:1315.

Slack, G. L. 1953. The bacteriology of infected root canals and *in vitro* penicillin sensitivity, Br. Dent. J. **95**:211.

Slack, J. 1942. The source of infection of actinomycosis, J. Bacteriol. **43**:193.

Slack, J. M., and Gerencser, M. A. 1975. Actinomyces, filamentous bacteria: biology and pathogenicity, Minneapolis, Burgess Publishing Co.

Slack, J. M., Landfried, S., and Gerencser, M. A. 1971. Identification of *Actinomyces* and related bacteria in dental calculus by the fluorescent antibody technique, J. Dent. Res. **50**:78.

Slade, P. R., Slesser, B. V., and Southgate, J. 1973. Thoracic actinomycosis, Thorax **28**:73.

Smibert, R. M. 1974. Genus III. *Treponema*. In Buchanan, R. E., and Gibbons, N. E., eds.: Bergey's manual of determinative bacteriology, ed. 8, Baltimore, The Williams & Wilkins Co., p. 175.

Smith, I. W., Peutherer, J. F., and MacCallum, F. O. 1967. The incidence of herpesvirus hominis antibody in the population, J. Hyg. (Camb.) **65**:395.

Snyder, M. L., Church, D. H., and Rickles, N. H. 1969. Primary herpes infection of right second finger, Oral Surg. **27**:598.

Snyder, M. L., et al. 1962. Evaluation of laboratory

tests for estimation of caries activity, J. Am. Dent. Assoc. **65**:30.

Snyder, M. L., et al. 1963. Evaluation of laboratory tests for the estimation of caries activity: correlation with specific surfaces, Arch. Oral Biol. **8**:541.

Snyderman, R. 1973. Immunological mechanisms of periodontal tissue destruction, J. Am. Dent. Assoc. **87**:1020.

Socransky, S. S., and Manganiello, S. D. 1971. The oral microbiota of man from birth to senility, J. Periodontal. **42**:485.

Socransky, S. S., Hubersak, C., and Propas, D. 1970. Induction of periodontal destruction in gnotobiotic rats by a human oral strain of *Actinomyces naeslundii*, Arch. Oral Biol. **15**:993.

Socransky, S. S., et al. 1963. The microbiota of the gingival crevice area of man. I. Total microscopic and viable counts and counts of specific organisms, Arch. Oral Biol. **8**:275.

Spier, W. A., Mitchener, J. W., and Galloway, R. F. 1971. Primary pulmonary botryomycosis, Chest **60**:92.

Spiers, W. 1971. Classification systems of the Bacteroides group, Med. Lab. Technol. **28**:360.

Steigman, A. J., Lipton, M. M., and Braspennickx, H. 1962. Acute lymphonodular pharyngitis: a newly described condition due to coxsackie A virus, J. Pediatr. **61**:331.

Sternberg, S., Hoffman, C., and Zweitler, B. M. 1951. Stomatitis and diarrhea in infants caused by Bacillus mucosus capsulatus, J. Pediatr. **38**:509.

Stevens, C. E., et al. 1975. Vertical transmission of hepatitis B antigen in Taiwan, N. Engl. J. Med. **292**:771.

Stiff, R. H. 1963. Histoplasmosis: report of a case, Oral Surg. **16**:140.

Street, C. M., Goldner, M., and LeRiche, W. H. 1976. Epidemiology of dental caries in relation to *Streptococcus mutans* on tooth surfaces in 5-year-old children, Arch. Oral Biol. **21**:273.

Sutter, V. L., Hurst, V., and Landucci, A. O. J. 1966. Pseudomonads in human saliva, J. Dent. Res. **45**:1800.

Sutter, V. L., Vargo, V. L., and Finegold, S. M. 1975. Wadsworth anaerobic bacteriology manual, ed. 2, Los Angeles, The Regents of the University of California.

Syed, S. A., et al. 1975. Predominant cultivable flora isolated from human root surface caries plaque, Infect. Immun. **11**:727.

Szmuness, W., et al. 1973. Familial clustering of hepatitis B infection, N. Engl. J. Med. **289**:1162.

Takazoe, I., Vogel, J., and Ennever, J. 1970. Calcium hydroxyapatite nucleation by lipid extract of *Bacterionema matruchotii*, J. Dent. Res. **49**:395.

Taplin, J., and Goldsworthy, N. E. 1958. A study of 225 strains of *Staphylococcus* isolated from the mouth, Aust. J. Exp. Biol. Med. Sci. **36**:289.

Taylor, C. G., et al. 1969. Mucormycosis (phycomycosis) involving the maxilla: report of a case with survival, Oral Surg. **27**:806.

Taylor-Robinson, D., et al. 1964. A newly identified oral mycoplasma *(M. orale)* and its relationship to other human mycoplasmas, Am. J. Hyg. **80**:135.

Topazian, R. G. 1966. Rhinosporidiosis of the parotid duct, Br. J. Oral Surg. **4**:12.

Trumbull, M. L., and Greiner, D. J. 1951. Homologous serum jaundice: an occupational hazard to medical personnel, J.A.M.A. **145**:965.

van Houte, J., Gibbons, R. J., and Banghart, S. B. 1970. Adherence as a determinant of the presence of *Streptococcus salivarius* and *Streptococcus sanguis* on the tooth surface, Arch. Oral Biol. **15**:1025.

van Houte, J., Gibbons, R. J., and Pulkkinen, A. J. 1971. Adherence as an ecological determinant for streptococci in the human mouth, Arch. Oral Biol. **16**:1131.

van Houte, J., Gibbons, R. J., and Pulkkinen, A. J. 1972. Ecology of human oral lactobacilli, Infect. Immun. **6**:723.

van Palenstein Helderman, W. H. 1975. Total viable count and differential count of vibrio (campylobacter) sputorum, fusobacterium nucleatum, bacteroides ochroceus and veillonella in the inflamed and non inflamed human gingival crevice, J. Periodont. Res. **10**:294.

Villarejos, V. M., et al. 1974. Role of saliva, urine and feces in the transmission of type B hepatitis, N. Engl. J. Med. **291**:1375.

Waldvogel, F. A., Medoff, G., and Swartz, M. N. 1970a. Osteomyelitis: a review of clinical features, therapeutic considerations and unusual aspects (first of three parts), N. Engl. J. Med. **282**:198.

Waldvogel, F. A., Medoff, G., and Swartz, M. N. 1970b. Osteomyelitis: a review of clinical features, therapeutic considerations and unusual aspects (second of three parts), N. Engl. J. Med. **282**:260.

Waldvogel, F. A., Medoff, G., and Swartz, M. N. 1970c. Osteomyelitis: a review of clinical features, therapeutic considerations and unusual aspects (third of three parts), N. Engl. J. Med. **282**:316.

Wantland, W. W., and Lauer, D. 1970. Correlation of some oral hygiene variables with age, sex, and the incidence of oral protozoa, J. Dent. Res. **49**:293.

Wantland, W. W., and Wantland, E. M. 1960. Incidence, ecology, and reproduction or oral protozoa, J. Dent. Res. **39**:863.

Wantland, W. W., Wantland, E. M., and Winquist, D. L. 1963. Collection, identification, and cultivation of oral protozoa, J. Dent. Res. **42**:1234.

Wantland, W. W., et al. 1958. Studies on human mouth protozoa, J. Dent. Res. **37**:949.

Ward, R., et al. 1972. Hepatitis B antigen in saliva and mouth washings, Lancet **2**:726.

Weed, L. A., and Parkhill, E. M. 1948. The diagnosis of histoplasmosis in ulcerative disease of the mouth and pharynx, Am. J. Clin. Pathol. **18**:130.

Wentworth, B. B. 1963. Bacteriophage typing of the staphylococci, Bacteriol. Rev. **27**:253.

Werner, H., Neuhaus, F., and Hussels, H. 1971. A biochemical study of fusiform anaerobes, Med. Microbiol. Immunol. **157**:10.

Werner, H., Pulverer, G., and Reichertz, C. 1971. The biochemical properties and antibiotic susceptibility of *Bacteroides melaninogenicus*, Med. Microbiol. Immunol. **157**:3.

Whitley, R. J., et al., eds. and the collaborative study group. 1976. Adenine arabinoside therapy of herpes zoster in the immunosuppressed, NIAID collaborative antiviral study, N. Engl. J. Med. **294:**1193.

White, J. C., and Niven, C. F., Jr. 1946. Streptococcus S.B.E.: a streptococcus associated with subacute bacterial endocarditis, J. Bacteriol. **51:**717.

Wiesner, P. J., et al. 1973. Clinical spectrum of pharyngeal gonococcal infection, N. Engl. J. Med. **288:**181.

Williams, N. B., et al. 1950. A study of the simultaneous occurrence of enterococci, lactobacilli, and yeasts in saliva from human beings, J. Dent. Res. **29:**563.

Williams, R. E. O. 1956. *Streptococcus salivarius* (vel hominis) and its relation to Lancefield's group K, J. Pathol. Bacteriol. **72:**15.

Winkelmann, R. K., and Perry, H. O. 1959. Herpes zoster in children, J.A.M.A. **171:**876.

Winkler, K. C., and van Amerongen, J. 1959. Bacteriologic results from 4,000 root canal cultures, Oral Surg. **12:**857.

Witorsch, P., and Utz, J. P. 1968. North American blastomycosis: a study of 40 patients, Medicine. **47:**169.

Youmans, G. P., Paterson, P. Y., and Sommers, H. M. 1975. The biologic and clinical basis of infectious diseases, Philadelphia, W. B. Saunders Co.

CHAPTER 5

Pharmacology

Judith C. Kusek

The administration of a drug can produce three types of effects: (1) placebo effects; (2) therapeutic effects; and (3) adverse effects, which include side effects, toxic effects, and hypersensitivity (allergic) reactions. Placebo effects and drug allergy will not be discussed here. Therapeutic effects, side effects, and toxic effects are produced by interaction of the drug with its tissue-bound receptors, and the intensity of these effects is directly dependent on the concentration of the drug at its receptors.

There are very few examples of direct application of a drug to its receptor, and it is usual to administer the drug at a distant site. Following administration, the drug is subject to various physiochemical and enzymatic processes, that is, absorption, distribution (including redistribution), biotransformation, and excretion. The dynamic equilibrium between these processes determines the quantity of drug available at any given time for interaction with its receptors and thus governs the time course and intensity of the concentration-dependent drug effects.

The primary objective of this chapter is to discuss certain aspects of these basic processes and some factors that alter these processes. This chapter is not intended to be a comprehensive review of the entire scope of pharmacology or to include everything that might be pertinent to the use of drugs in the practice of oral and maxillofacial surgery. It is anticipated that the reader has had some previous exposure to pharmacology, and thus some material is only briefly reviewed; other subjects are covered in more detail. For in-depth discussions of the therapeutic uses of drugs and the basic principles governing drug actions the reader is referred to standard comprehensive texts (DiPalma, 1965; Goldstein, Aronow, and Kalman, 1974; Goodman and Gilman, 1975; La Du, Mandel, and Way, 1971).

BASIC PROCESSES GOVERNING THE DISPOSITION OF DRUGS IN THE BODY

Movement of drugs across biologic membranes

The processes of absorption, distribution, and excretion of drugs are dependent on the movement of drugs across biologic membranes. Drugs cross membranes by two mechanisms: (1) passive diffusion and (2) active transport.

Passive diffusion

Several models have been proposed for biologic membranes: the unit membrane (Robertson, 1960), the protein crystal model (Vanderkooi and Green, 1970), and the fluid mosaic model (Singer and Nicolson, 1972). These models differ in the proposed structural relationship of the two principal components of membranes: proteins and phospholipids. However, a common feature in most currently accepted models is that the lipid phase, which accounts for approximately 40% to 50% of the dry weight of plasma membranes, exists in a bilayer arrangement as originally proposed by Gorter and Grendel (1925).

The passive diffusion of most drugs

appears to occur through the lipid phase of the membrane. Thus one of the important factors governing the rate of diffusion is the lipid solubility of the compound (oil/water partition coefficient). The greater the lipid solubility, the faster the rate of passive diffusion across a membrane. Most drugs are weak acids or weak bases (exceptions are nonionized drugs, such as inhalation anesthetics, and totally ionized compounds, such as quaternary amines) and at the normal pH of the extracellular fluid they exist in both ionized and nonionized forms. The ionized form is more polar and consequently more soluble in polar solvents such as water, while the nonionized form possesses considerably greater lipid solubility. Since the ionized and nonionized forms differ in lipid solubility, the overall rate of diffusion of most drugs will also depend on their degree of ionization. The degree of ionization is a function of the

pH of the solution and the ionization constant of the drug, and it can be calculated from the Henderson-Hasselbalch equation.

The ionization of a weak acid is given in the equation at the top of Fig. 5-1. In the case of a weak acid, an increase in hydrogen ion concentration (acidification of the solution) shifts the equilibrium to the left, that is, decreases the amount of the drug in the ionized form. Alkalinization of the solution (decreasing the H^+ concentration) shifts the equilibrium to the right, resulting in more drug in the ionized form.

Alkalinization of the urine is commonly used to increase the rate of renal excretion of weak acids, for example, barbiturates, salicylates, and so on. The rationale is based on altering the ionization of the drug; alkalinization of the urine increases the proportion of the drug in the ionized form. This form, being less lipid-soluble

$$HA \; \underset{-H^+}{\overset{+H^+}{\rightleftharpoons}} \; H^+ + A^-$$

A. Distribution at equal pH

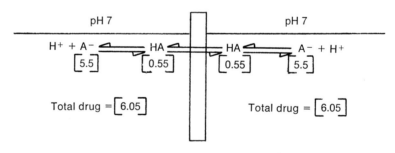

B. Distribution at unequal pH

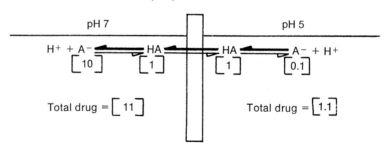

Fig. 5-1. Distribution of weak acid (pK_a 6) across biologic membrane. Numbers in brackets represent concentration of each drug species within compartment.

than the nonionized form, is not as readily reabsorbed from the urine via passive diffusion across the tubular epithelium; thus a greater percentage of the drug is excreted.

The total distribution of weak acids and bases at equilibrium is also a function of the degree of ionization of the drug. The theoretic distribution of a weak acid across a semipermeable membrane is given in Fig. 5-1. Example A illustrates the distribution when the pH of the two compartments is equal. The membrane-permeable form of the drug (nonionized form) distributes equally across the membrane. Since the degree of ionization is a function of pH and the pH of the two compartments is equal, the concentration of the ionized form is also equal.

If the pH of the right compartment is lowered to 5 (example B), the degree of ionization of the drug in that compartment will change, shifting to the formation of the nonionized form. Since the nonionized form is permeable to the membrane, it will diffuse down its con-

centration gradient, across the membrane into the left compartment. The pH of the left compartment (7) favors ionization of the drug. Therefore the nonionized drug that diffused across the membrane will ionize. This process will continue until the concentration of the nonionized (membrane-permeable) form is again equal on both sides of the membrane. However, at equilibrium the concentration of the ionized drug in the left compartment will be greater than that in the right compartment. The unequal distribution of the ionized drug is attributable to its lack of permeability across the membrane and the difference in pH of the two compartments. Thus the ionized form is trapped in the left compartment, resulting in an increase in the concentration of total drug in that compartment at the expense of the total drug in the right compartment.

Fig. 5-2 illustrates the distribution of a weak base. When the hydrogen ion concentrations of the two compartments are equal (example A), both the ionized and

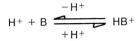

A. Distribution at equal pH

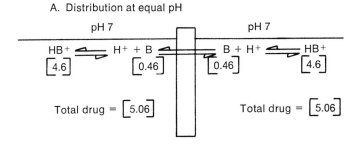

B. Distribution at unequal pH

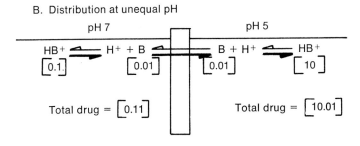

Fig. 5-2. Distribution of weak base (pK_a 8) across biologic membrane.

nonionized forms are equally distributed. However, in the case of a weak base, reducing the pH of the right compartment will favor formation of the ionized drug at the expense of the nonionized form. This will allow nonionized drug from the left compartment to move across the membrane, down its concentration gradient. Once in the right compartment the drug will ionize because of the higher H^+ concentration. Again the process will continue until the concentrations of the membrane-permeable, nonionized form in the two compartments are equal. However, in this case the ionized form is trapped in the right compartment.

A relevant example of the influence of pH on the distribution of a drug across a biologic membrane is the distribution of a local anesthetic (a weak base) across the myelin sheath of a nerve axon (Fig. 5-3). The presence of infection or inflammation surrounding the nerve sheath may cause a decrease in the pH of this compartment, resulting in an increase in the ionized form of the local anesthetic and trapping the drug outside of the nerve sheath. Thus the concentration of the drug adjacent to the nerve membrane is re-duced, and this will greatly decrease the effectiveness of the local anesthetic.

Another example of the effect of pH and the extent of ionization on drug distribution and intensity of drug effects is the distribution of drugs across the blood-brain barrier. Although capillary epithelium does not limit the distribution of free drug, it is probable that the glial cells surrounding the central vasculature function as the blood-brain barrier, limiting the diffusion of ionized compounds and drugs of low lipid solubility. Thus one would predict that alterations in blood pH caused by changes in blood P_{CO_2} would affect the distribution of CNS-active drugs. Respiratory acidosis produced by elevation of P_{CO_2} should decrease the ionization of weak acids and thus facilitate passage across the blood-brain barrier, while alkalosis produced by bicarbonate infusion or hyperventilation should produce the opposite effect. These predicted effects have been confirmed in experimental studies. Acidosis was found to increase the amount of phenobarbital in the brain of dogs, and alkalosis decreased drug content and reduced the degree of

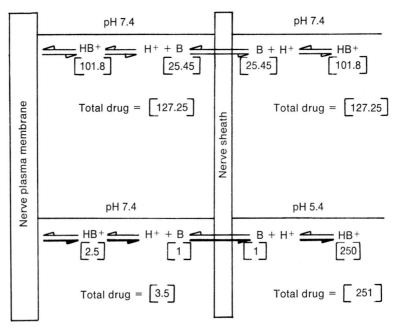

Fig. 5-3. Distribution of lidocaine (pK_a 7.8) across nerve sheath.

CNS depression (Waddell and Butler, 1957). Acidosis also increased salicylate levels in the cat brain (Goldberg, Barlow, and Roth, 1961).

Quaternary amines (for example, neuromuscular blocking agents, such as *d*-tubocurarine, succinylcholine, gallamine, or pancuronium; ganglionic blocking agents, such as hexamethonium or chlorisondamine; and synthetic antimuscarinic agents [substitutes for belladonna alkaloids], such as oxyphenonium or propantheline) are completely ionized at blood pH's compatible with life. Therefore they do not cross the blood-brain barrier following administration of ordinary doses, and they are virtually devoid of CNS side effects.

Active transport

Active transport is a more specific process that requires energy and is capable of forming and transporting drugs against a concentration gradient. It is a process thought to involve "carriers"—membrane components capable of binding a drug at one surface of the membrane, moving across the membrane as a drug-carrier complex, and releasing the drug at the opposite surface. Three general types of transport systems have been identified: anionic, cationic, and nonionized. Each exhibits charge specificity, that is, anionic transport systems transport only ionized anionic substances (drugs or endogenous compounds). Similarly charged substances may compete with each other for transport, if they both possess high affinity for the carrier. Active transport systems have been identified in the renal tubular epithelium and the epithelium of hepatocytes, and these systems function in renal and biliary excretion of drugs. For examples of drug interactions caused by competition for transport, see the section on "Excretion."

Absorption

Absorption refers to the movement of a drug from its site of administration into the general circulation. It is dependent on: (1) the physiochemical properties of the drug, (2) the pharmaceutic properties of the drug preparation, and (3) the biologic properties of the site of administration.

Absorption from the gastrointestinal tract

Absorption of drugs from the gastrointestinal tract follows the general principles that affect the passive diffusion of drugs across biologic membranes. The nonionized form of the drug is absorbed. Thus one series of factors in absorption is the lipid solubility and ionization constant of the drug and the pH of the environment. Highly polar compounds that are predominantly ionized at any pH (for example, quaternary amines) are poorly absorbed after oral administration. A weak base would be almost totally ionized at gastric pH and therefore not absorbed from the stomach. In the more alkaline environment of the intestine, a weak base would be only partially ionized and thus more readily absorbed. A weak acid would not be ionized to any appreciable extent at gastric pH and, given sufficient time, would be completely absorbed from the stomach. This difference in gastric absorption of weak acids and bases has been confirmed in human studies (Hogben et al., 1957).

However, other factors limit the absorption of drugs from the stomach. The most important factor is the relative area of the absorptive surface of the stomach compared to that of the small intestine. Since the surface area of the small intestine is considerably greater, intestinal absorption of both acids and bases is favored, even though the rate of diffusion of weak acids per unit area is faster in the stomach. It has also been observed that the intestinal absorption of weak acids was greater than would be predicted by the pH of the intestinal contents (Hogben et al., 1959). The authors hypothesized that a slightly acidic zone (pH of about 5.3) exists adjacent to the mucosal border of the intestine and that this zone determines the effective pH governing absorption rather than the pH of the intestinal contents.

Since the absorption of most drugs occurs in the proximal portion of the intestine, the rate at which the drug arrives in the duodenum (that is, the rate of gastric emptying) also affects the rate of absorption. Delaying gastric emptying will decrease the rate of drug absorption. Food delays gastric emptying, and this is one of the factors that decreases the absorption of drugs administered with a meal (Kojima, Smith, and Doluisio, 1971). Aluminum hydroxide, an antacid, also slows gastric emptying and decreases absorption. Consequently, the desired response to some rapidly absorbed drugs (for example, pentobarbital, sulfadiazine, and so forth) is reduced by aluminum hydroxide (Hurwitz and Sheehan, 1971).

Oral administration of dilute solutions of drugs increases their rates of absorption and produces higher blood levels than administration of concentrated drug solutions. This effect is probably attributable to the fact that larger volumes of a dilute solution are administered, and the increase in fluid volume increases both the rate of gastric emptying and the extent of exposure to the intestinal surface (Borowitz et al., 1971). By extrapolation, the quantity of fluid ingested with a solid drug preparation would be an important factor in both the dissolution of the preparation and the presentation of the drug to its site of absorption.

Another factor limiting intestinal absorption is the formation of drug complexes that reduce absorption by decreasing the amount of free drug available for passive diffusion. Drugs may interact with food to form nonabsorbable drug complexes. Drugs may also form insoluble chelates with multivalent cations. For example, the absorption of tetracyclines is reduced by chelation with Ca^{++}, Mg^{++}, Al^{+++}, or Fe^{++} present in milk, antacids, or iron preparations.

Drug absorption is also affected by the bioavailability of the drug from the administered pharmaceutic preparation. Solid drug preparations must disintegrate and dissolve in the gastrointestinal juices prior to absorption. Two examples of altered absorption of drugs caused by changes in bioavailability are aspirin and tetracyclines. The rate of dissolution of aspirin tablets is directly proportional to the rate of absorption and to the plasma concentrations that are achieved following oral administration (Leonards, 1963). The dissolution of solid tetracycline preparations is favored by low gastric pH. Elevation of the gastric pH by concurrent administration of sodium bicarbonate inhibits dissolution of solid tetracycline preparations and decreases the total amount of absorbed drug (Barr, Adir, and Garrettson, 1971). The authors also suggested that other conditions that increase gastric pH (for example, achlorhydria, which is common in elderly patients) may also decrease the clinical efficacy of orally administered solid tetracycline preparations. The absorption of liquid tetracycline preparations was not affected by changes in gastric pH.

The effectiveness of oral administration of drugs is also limited by "first-pass metabolism." After diffusion through the intestinal mucosa, drugs are absorbed into the portal circulation, which delivers the drug directly to the liver where it is subject to metabolism. The faster the rate of hepatic metabolism, the more pronounced the effect of "first-pass metabolism" on decreasing the peripheral blood levels of the drug. A good example of the principle is the oral administration of lidocaine as an antiarrhythmic agent. Hepatic metabolism of lidocaine is quite rapid, and, although the drug is readily absorbed from the gastrointestinal tract, therapeutic blood levels cannot be obtained because it is cleared from the blood during the first pass through the liver. Two other drugs that are susceptible to "first-pass metabolism" (although to a lesser degree than lidocaine) are the analgesics propoxyphene and pentazocine. It has been suggested that variations in the extent of first-pass metabolism contribute to the large variations in the plasma concentrations and the clinical effects of these analgesics following oral administration (Ehrnebo, Boreus, and Lonroth, 1977; Verebely and Inturrisi, 1974; Wilson, Atwood, and Shand, 1976).

Other factors affecting gastrointestinal absorption include: (1) intestinal motility, which determines the length of time the drug is in the intestine, and the degree of mixing of the intestinal contents, which affects the exposure of the drug to the absorptive mucosal surface; (2) destruction of drugs by gastric acid or digestive enzymes, or metabolism of drugs by the bacterial flora of the intestine; and (3) irritation of gastrointestinal mucosa, which may cause vomiting or diarrhea and consequent loss of the drug.

The oral route of administration is the most convenient and simplest method of drug administration from a technical point of view, but it is the most complex route from a pharmacologic perspective. Because of the numerous factors influencing gastrointestinal absorption, oral administration is associated with the greatest variability in human drug levels. Both the total amount of drug absorbed and the rate of absorption can be affected. Slowing the rate of absorption will delay the onset of drug action and may result in failure to achieve therapeutic drug levels for those drugs with rapid rates of elimination.

Absorption from the oral cavity

The oral mucosa is a highly vascular, nonkeratinized structure. Absorption of drugs across intact oral mucosa occurs by passive diffusion and is dependent on the lipid solubility and degree of ionization of the compounds. Nitroglycerin is an example of a nonionized lipid-soluble drug that is rapidly absorbed following sublingual administration. In general, drugs that are absorbed across the intestinal mucosa will probably be absorbed from the mouth. Several toxic antibiotics (for example, nystatin, vancomycin, and bacitracin) are not absorbed by intact oral mucosa and therefore are of value for topical administration in the mouth. However, if the oral epithelium is broken, they are rapidly absorbed because of the rich submucosal vasculature, and topical application to denuded mucosa may produce systemic toxicity.

Absorption from submucosal, subcutaneous, and intramuscular sites

Submucosal, subcutaneous, and intramuscular administration usually result in complete and fairly predictable drug absorption; the only exceptions occur with irritating drugs that may cause local tissue damage at the site of injection. The process of absorption via these routes is less complex because the movement of the drug across an epithelial barrier is avoided. The only structure the drug must cross is the capillary wall. Since the capillary epithelium is a very "porous" membrane, diffusion across this structure is usually not the rate-limiting step in absorption. Two important factors that determine the rate of absorption from submucosal, subcutaneous, and intramuscular sites are the vascularity or rate of perfusion of the site of injection and the aqueous solubility of the preparation.

The rate of systemic absorption of local anesthetics may be altered by changing the rate of blood flow at the site of injection. Most local anesthetics cause vasodilatation and thus locally increase blood flow. The extent of vasodilatation varies among this class of drugs, and the rate of absorption was found to be directly related to the degree of drug-induced vasodilatation. Addition of vasoconstrictors reduced the rate of absorption, but the magnitude of the reduction was dependent on the vasodilating potency of the local anesthetic (that is, the greater the anesthetic-induced vasodilatation, the more pronounced the effect of the vasoconstrictor) (Braid and Scott, 1965). The rate of absorption of local anesthetics is important because it determines: (1) the time course of appearance of the drug in the blood, making it a factor in systemic toxicity, and (2) the rate of disappearance of the drug from its site of injection, making it a factor in the duration of axonal blockage.

A drug must dissolve in the aqueous extracellular fluid before it can diffuse across the capillary epithelium. Thus the rate of absorption may be slowed by decreasing the water solubility of the preparation. Repository preparations of penicillin G are sparingly soluble salts of penicillin that are slowly absorbed over long periods of time. Relatively constant plasma concentrations can thus be maintained without the necessity for frequent injections.

Intravenous administration

Intravenous administration delivers the drug directly into the circulation, and the process of absorption is totally bypassed. The rate of injection is important, and rapid intravenous administration should be avoided. Many drugs (in particular, organic bases such as narcotic analgesics, *d*-tubocurarine, and atropine) can precipitate peripheral vascular collapse with rapid intravenous injection. It has been postulated that this effect may be due to extensive release of histamine from mast cells when they are exposed to high concentrations of drug prior to dilution of the injected bolus by the blood.

Distribution

Drugs are distributed as both "free" drug in the body water and "sequestered" drug (that is, bound to plasma or tissue proteins or in solution in the body lipid). The distribution of a drug is important because it can affect: (1) the pharmacologic activity of the drug, since only free drug can interact with its receptors, (2) the rate of elimination, (3) the potential for toxicity, and (4) the onset and duration of activity.

Protein binding

Drugs bind to both tissue proteins and plasma proteins. Tissue proteins represent a potentially larger reservoir for drug binding than do plasma proteins; however, human experimentation on tissue binding is limited and much of the research has been directed toward investigating plasma protein binding. Drug binding is usually a reversible, concentration-dependent process, as depicted below:

$$\text{Free drug} + \text{Protein} \overset{k}{\rightleftharpoons} \text{Drug} \cdot \text{Protein}$$

As the free drug concentration changes, the drug can rapidly associate or dissociate from the protein. The affinity of different drugs for binding varies, and thus the percentage of drug binding or fractional binding is an individual characteristic of each drug.

Extensive binding to plasma proteins in the absence of tissue binding tends to confine the drug within the vascular compartment and to limit its diffusion into peripheral tissues. Capillary membranes are not readily permeable to plasma proteins, and therefore only free, unbound drug may leave the vascular space. Antibiotics are an example of this pattern of distribution. Antibiotics bind to plasma proteins, but the extent of binding varies widely even within a single class of drugs. For example, penicillin binding ranges between 22.5% for ampicillin and 95% to 98% for the isoxazolyl penicillins; tetracyclines range between 35% bound oxytetracycline and 93% bound doxycycline (Kunin, 1967; Kunin et al., 1973). The highly bound antibiotics display high blood levels, but the distribution into interstitial fluid or across biologic membranes (for example, penetration into synovial fluid) is proportional to the plasma concentration of free drug and not total drug levels (Howell, Sutherland, and Robinson, 1972; Tan et al., 1972). Thus high blood levels of total drug may be misleading, since only free drug reaches its site of action. This does not imply that highly bound antibiotics are ineffective in antimicrobial therapy, since the clinical efficacy of an antimicrobial agent depends on both the concentration and the potency of the drug. However, one should differentiate between blood or plasma levels of total drug and plasma levels of free drug.

Binding to plasma proteins may also effect the rate of elimination and consequently the duration of action of drugs. Binding reduces the amount of drug available for glomerular filtration, because only free drug is filtered (Fig. 5-4). Reduction in the rate of renal excretion prolongs the half-life of the drug and decreases the frequency of administration needed to maintain a therapeutic blood level. The tetracyclines are an example of this principle. The tetracyclines with more extensive binding (for example, methacycline and minocycline) exhibit slower renal clearance than the lesser bound derivatives (for example, tetracycline and oxytetracycline). Most penicillins, on the other hand, are eliminated primarily by tubular secretion (an active

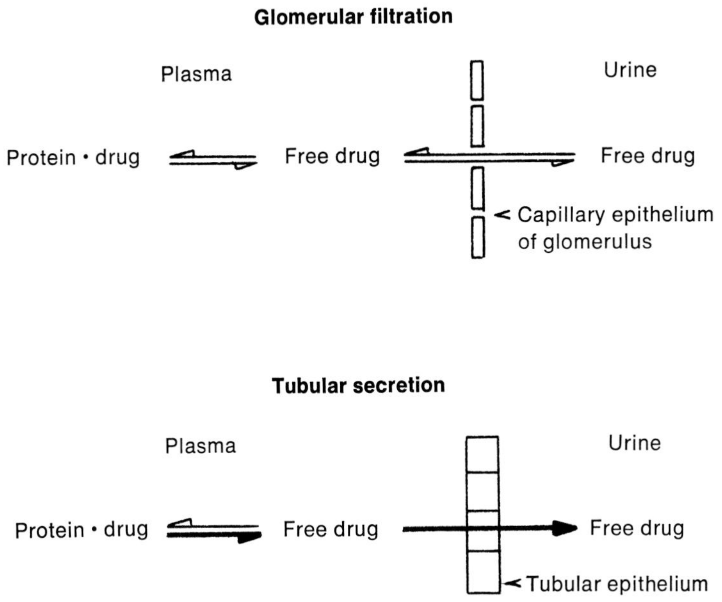

Glomerular filtration

Tubular secretion

Fig. 5-4. Effects of protein binding on excretion of drugs via glomerular filtration or tubular secretion.

transport process). Tubular secretion is a rapid, one-way transport system and is capable of transporting the drug against a concentration gradient. As free drug is removed from the plasma, the bound drug can dissociate from the binding protein and becomes available for secretion into the urine. Thus tubular secretion can virtually clear the plasma of drug in a single pass and is not appreciably affected by protein binding. Consequently, most penicillins are rapidly excreted regardless of their fractional binding.

Drugs may also compete with each other for binding to plasma proteins. Displacement of bound drug may increase the potential for toxicity and is one mechanism of drug interaction. It is generally accepted that reductions in binding become an important consideration only when the amount bound exceeds 80% of the total drug. With highly bound drugs, a small change in the percentage of drug bound will have a proportionately greater effect on free drug concentrations. For example, a 5% reduction of binding, from 95% to 90%, will produce a doubling of free drug, from 5% to 10%, while total displacement of all bound

drug is required to double the free drug concentration for a drug that is 50% bound.

Coumarin anticoagulants and phenytoin are two examples of highly bound drugs. Coumarin derivatives may be displaced from binding sites by a number of acidic drugs (Sellers and Koch-Weser, 1971); of these, phenylbutazone produces consistent and significant clinical prolongation of prothrombin times (Udall, 1969). Aspirin and acetaminophen had no effect on prothrombin time in coumarin-treated patients (Udall, 1969), but salicylates may alter coagulation by inhibiting platelet function. The binding of phenytoin is reduced by phenylbutazone and salicylates (Lunde et al., 1970). Displacement of phenytoin can lead to toxic effects such as ataxia, vertigo, and other cerebellar symptoms.

The intensification of drug action caused by displacement of bound drug may be a transient effect. Increasing the free drug concentration may also lead to more rapid elimination of the drug and a faster decline in plasma drug levels. Thus the half-life of a drug may be shortened and the duration of action reduced.

Disease states may also alter protein binding. Severe renal dysfunction is associated with both a reduction in total plasma proteins and structural alterations in the proteins that can affect their ability to bind drugs. Thus the binding of a number of anionic drugs is reduced during renal failure and uremia (Boobis, 1977; Ehrnebo and Odar-Cederlof, 1975; Reidenberg and Affrime, 1973; Shoeman, Benjamin, and Azarnoff, 1973).

Lipid storage

The distribution or redistribution of drugs to body lipids depends on the oil/water partition coefficient of the drug, the rates of regional perfusion of the tissues, and the lipid composition of the tissues. Highly lipid-soluble substances such as general anesthetics will localize in lipid-rich tissues. Methoxyflurane, for example, accumulates in adipose tissue during administration, and the concentration in fat continues to rise for several hours after administration is discontinued. This suggests continued redistribution of the drug from blood and other tissues into fat. The rate of disappearance from adipose tissue is very slow, and considerable amounts of methoxyflurane have been detected in fat 40 hours after anesthesia (Chenoweth et al., 1962).

Fat-soluble vitamins (vitamins A, D, E, and K) are also stored in adipose tissue. Consequently, these vitamins display a potential for hypervitaminosis or vitamin toxicity, if large amounts are ingested for long periods of time (for example, the current fad of "megavitamin therapy"). Water-soluble vitamins are less likely to cause vitamin toxicity, because they are easily excreted and do not accumulate in the body.

Metabolism

Metabolism or biotransformation usually produces two results: (1) it converts the compound to a more readily excreted form, and (2) it alters the pharmacologic activity of the drug. Excretion is enhanced by decreasing lipid solubility. Highly lipid-soluble substances are extensively reabsorbed into the circulation from the tubular urine. Many of the reactions involved in drug metabolism decrease the lipid solubility of the compounds and thus reduce reabsorption and facilitate excretion.

The pharmacologic activity of most drug metabolites is less than the parent compounds. However, some drugs are metabolized to more toxic compounds (for example, halogenated anesthetics and polycyclic hydrocarbons), and some drugs are administered as inactive precursors that require biotransformation to achieve pharmacologic activity (for example, hetacillin, a biologically inactive penicillin that is hydrolyzed to yield ampicillin).

Drugs are metabolized by four basic types of reactions: oxidation, reduction, hydrolysis, and conjugation.

Oxidation

Oxidation is the most common mode of drug metabolism. Most oxidative reactions of drugs are catalyzed by the mixed-function oxidase (MFO) system, which is present in greatest quantity in the liver and present to a lesser extent in other tissues (for example, kidney and adrenal cortex). MFO is an electron transport system located primarily in the membranes of the smooth endoplasmic reticulum. Cytochrome P-450 functions as the terminal oxidase of this electron transport system, and the P-450 content appears to correlate with the drug-metabolizing activity of the tissue.

An important characteristic of MFO is its inducibility. Chronic administration of any of a large number of drugs induces the synthesis of MFO, causing proliferation of the endoplasmic reticulum and an increase in cytochrome P-450 content. The consequent increase in MFO activity accelerates the metabolism of both the inducer and other MFO substrates (for review, see Remmer, 1972). Several hundred commonly prescribed drugs are capable of inducing MFO in laboratory animals (for review, see Conney, 1967), but for induction to be clinically important the drug should induce MFO in humans at concentrations normally achieved during therapy. Furthermore, the accelerated metabolism should decrease the clinical effectiveness of either the inducer or other substrates. Unfortunately, the clinical therapeutic effects of many drugs are difficult to measure quantitatively, and genetic variations in both the basal rate of drug metabolism among humans (Davies and Thorgeirsson, 1971; Vesell, 1972) and the extent of stimulation of drug metabolism in response to an inducer (Vesell and Page, 1969) make induction difficult to assess clinically. Thus it is not possible to predict the precise degree of induction, the degree of drug interaction owing to induction, or the clinical significance of a given degree of induction in a particular individual. However, one should be aware of, and consider the potential for, stimulated drug metabolism and monitor more rigorously those patients whose history of medications suggests the possibility of MFO induction.

Some examples of documented inducers in humans are barbiturates, glutethimide, phenytoin, griseofulvin, antipyrine, phenylbutazone, meprobamate, and rifampin. Phenobarbital, amobarbital, secobarbital, glutethimide, and antipyrine have been shown to accelerate the metabolism of warfarin and to change the degree of anticoagulant control (Breckenridge and Orme, 1971). The cardiac glycoside, digitoxin, is metabolized by MFO, and administration of phenobarbital (Jelliffe and Blankenhorn, 1966), phenylbutazone, or phenytoin (Solomon et al., 1971) produces clinical evidence of accelerated digitoxin metabolism. Phenobarbital also increased the rate of hydroxylation of corticosteroids and caused a deterioration of the clinical condition of steroid-treated asthmatics (Brooks et al., 1972). Phenobarbital and phenytoin, either alone or in combination, appear to increase the rate of inactivation of vitamin D_3 and its biologically active metabolites and consequently they cause a decrease in plasma calcium concentrations (Hahn et al., 1972). This result appears to explain the increased incidence of osteomalacia and rickets in epileptics receiving anticonvulsant therapy (Richens and Rowe, 1970).

Cigarette smoke contains many polycyclic hydrocarbons that induce a specific type of MFO activity termed "benzpyrene hydroxylase." Smokers appear to metabolize phenacetin via benzpyrene hydroxylase at a faster rate then nonsmokers (Pantuck et al., 1974), Benzpyrene hydroxylase is also important in the production of carcinogenic intermediates during the metabolism of a variety of polycyclic hydrocarbons, and induction of benzpyrene hydroxylase increases the carcinogenicity of these compounds. In addition, smoking may affect the clinical efficacy of some analgesics. Propoxyphene and pentazocine were found to be less effective among heavy smokers (Keeri-Szanto and Pomeroy, 1971; Miller, 1977). Whether these effects can be attributed to accelerated metabolism or to other factors has yet to be resolved.

Chronic inhalation of subanesthetic concentrations of halogenated anesthetics produced signs of MFO induction in laboratory animals (Ross and Cardell, 1978; Van Dyke, 1966). This result has been corroborated in humans. Anesthesiologists who are chronically exposed to low concentrations of anesthetics metabolized halothane at accelerated rates compared to nonexposed persons (Cascorbi, Blake, and Helrich, 1970). In animal studies induction of MFO by phenobarbital increased the rate of metabolism of halogenated anesthetics (Van Dyke, 1966), increased the nephrotoxicity of methoxyflurane (Cousins et al., 1974), increased the hepato-renal-pulmonary toxicity of fluroxene (Munson et al., 1975), and increased the hepatotoxicity of halothane (Reynolds and Moslen, 1977). The question of whether induction of MFO can increase the clinical toxicity of halogenated anesthetics in humans has yet to be answered.

Another characteristic of MFO is its lack of substance specificity. The system oxidizes many structurally diverse molecules, both foreign compounds (drugs) and endogenous substances (steroid hormones, vitamins, and other lipids). The large number of substrates increases the probability that any two drugs may compete with each other for metabolism.

Although many combinations of drugs competitively inhibit metabolism in laboratory experiments, the results of clinical studies suggest that the occurrence of competitive inhibition of drug metabolism during human therapy is much more limited. Competitive inhibition is usually not seen because the therapeutic plasma concentrations of most drugs are usually below the K_m (concentration necessary for half-maximal activity) of the drug-metabolizing systems, and the rates of metabolism are well below the maximum capacity of the system. Thus inhibition of metabolism is less common than induction. However, a few examples of proposed toxicity owing to accumulation of drug secondary to inhibition of metabolism can be found. Toxic hypoglycemic collapse has been reported in tolbutamide-treated maturity-onset diabetics after administration of therapeutic doses of sulfonamides, chloramphenicol, or phenylbutazone, and phenytoin toxicity (vertigo, anorexia, and ataxia) was observed following use of sulfonamides and phenylbutazone (Skovsted et al., 1974). One of the most widely used group of drugs is oral contraceptives, which are steroid hormones metabolized by MFO. Evidence of reduction in the rates of metabolism of antipyrine (Carter et al., 1974; O'Malley, Stevenson, and Crooks, 1972), meperidine and promazine (Crawford and Rudofsky, 1966), and vitamin D_3 (Carter et al., 1975) has been found in women taking oral contraceptives. The impairment in drug metabolism seen during oral contraceptive therapy is probably of little consequence following acute administration of the second drug, but prolonged use could produce cumulative effects.

The rate of hepatic blood flow is a factor in the clearance of drugs that are rapidly metabolized. If the rate of hepatic metabolism is high enough to metabolize all or a very large percentage of the drug as it passes through the liver, then a change in the rate of delivery of drug to the liver will change the rate of disappearance of drug from the peripheral circulation (that is, hepatic blood flow would be the rate-limiting factor in total body metabolism of the drug). Patients with decreased hepatic perfusion caused by congestive heart failure exhibited slower metabolism of lidocaine and abnormally high plasma levels of the drug (Thompson, Rowland, and Melmon, 1971). Halothane prolonged the half-life of lidocaine, pentobarbital, and ketamine and increased their duration of action. This effect of halothane appears to be caused by three mechanisms: (1) decreased hepatic blood flow, (2) alterations in the patterns of regional blood flow and thus altered drug distributions, and (3) acute inhibition of MFO activity (Burney and DiFazio, 1976; Pearson, Bogan, and Sanford, 1973; White et al., 1976).

Age-related changes occur in MFO activity and are an important factor in the sensitivity of the newborn infants to drugs. Although direct administration of drugs to a neonate is not common in dental practice, the fetus and neonate may be indirectly exposed to drugs via maternal routes, since most drugs cross the placenta and many drugs are excreted in the milk of nursing mothers. The neonate is capable of MFO-mediated drug oxidations, but generally the rate of metabolism is much slower than that of children or adults (for review, see Horning et al., 1975). The half-life of drugs that are eliminated solely by hepatic metabolism also appears to be prolonged in older patients, suggesting a decreased rate of metabolism with aging (O'Malley, Crooks, and Duke, 1971).

An important drug oxidation that is not mediated via MFO is alcohol metabolism. A soluble enzyme, alcohol dehydrogenase, catalyzes the oxidation of ethyl alcohol to acetaldehyde. Acetaldehyde is oxidized to acetate by another soluble enzyme, aldehyde dehydrogenase.

Reduction

Under ordinary conditions reduction does not play a prominent role in the metabolism of most commonly prescribed drugs in humans. Reduction of ketone groups to the corresponding alcohols is important in steroid metabolism and results in enhanced glucocorticoid activity (that is, reduction of cortisone to hydrocortisone and reduction of prednisone to prednisolone).

During hypoxia, the reductive metabolism of halothane is favored and results in the formation of large amounts of highly reactive metabolites that covalently bind to various cellular constitutents (Widger, Gandolfi, and Van Dyke, 1976). Such metabolites are likely to possess greater potential for toxicity than those formed during the more common oxidative metabolism of halothane.

Hydrolysis

Esters (for example, procaine and succinylcholine) are metabolized to inactive compounds by pseudocholinesterase (butyrylcholinesterase), an enzyme that hydrolytically cleaves ester bonds. There is a general tendency for pseudocholinesterase activity to decrease with age, but the clinical significance of this effect is questionable (Shanor et al., 1961). Of greater importance is the decrease in pseudocholinesterase activity seen in subacute and chronic liver disease. In these cases the rates of hydrolysis of procaine and succinylcholine were decreased, and the duration of apnea following succinylcholine was three times longer than in patients without liver disease (Foldes et al., 1956). Severe depression of pseudocholinesterase activity has also been observed in: (1) cases of subclinical toxicity from organophosphorus insecticides attributable to occupational exposure (Barnes and Davies, 1951); (2) severe anemia, malnutrition, and cachexia (Foldes and Rhodes, 1953); and (3) uremic patients (Reidenberg, James, and Dring, 1972).

Substrates can also compete with each other for metabolism by pseudocholinesterase. Procaine inhibits the metabolism of succinylcholine and prolongs its duration of action (Foldes et al., 1953). This effect is most important following either intentional or inadvertent intravascular administration of procaine (Salgado, 1961).

Amides (for example, N-dealkylated metabolites of lidocaine) are hydrolyzed to inactive metabolites by amidases (see section on "Local anesthetics").

Conjugation

In humans, drugs are conjugated with carbohydrates (glucuronic acid), amino acids (glycine or glutamine), sulfate, or acetate. Conjugation with glucuronic acid accounts for the majority of conjugated metabolites. Hydroxyl and carboxyl groups constitute the most important target groups for glucuronide conjugation, and therefore oxidation of a drug (that is, production of target groups) is generally followed by conjugation. The enzymes catalyzing glucuronide conjugation, glucuronyl transferases, are found in the endoplasmic reticulum of tissues, primarily the liver, and are induced simultaneously with MFO induction.

Sulfate conjugation of hydroxyl groups is catalyzed by soluble enzymes, the sulfotransferases, and is limited by the availability of cysteine, which serves as the sulfate donor. As stated previously, drug metabolism systems that are saturated (that is, functioning at maximal capacity) at therapeutic drug concentrations are susceptible to competitive inhibition. Since the sulfate pool is limited, competitive inhibition is observed. Coadministration of acetaminophen, which is metabolized primarily by sulfate conjugation, and salicylate, which is a substrate for glycine, glucuronic acid, and sulfate conjugation, decreased the rate of conjugation of acetaminophen (Levy, 1971).

The major metabolite of aspirin is the glycine conjugate, and this pathway is also limited at therapeutic plasma concentrations. Thus the half-life of salicylate in man is prolonged as the dose of the drug is increased because of the limited rate of glycine conjugation (Levy, Vogel, and Amsel, 1969). The plasma concentration of salicylate after a given dose varies widely between individuals and appears to be attributable to differences in the rate of glycine conjugation (Gupta, Sarkissian, and Paulus, 1975). Less than one fourth of a dose of aspirin is metabolized by conjugation with glucuronic acid, and concurrent administration of aspirin has no apparent effect on the rate of glucuronidation of therapeutic doses of morphine (Brunk, Delle, and Wilson, 1973).

Excretion
Renal excretion

The kidney excretes drugs by two mechanisms: glomerular filtration and tubular secretion. The amount of drug filtered by the glomerulus is a function of the free drug concentration and the glomerular filtration rate. Filtration is essentially a process of simple physical diffusion of plasma across the relatively "porous" membrane of the glomerulus and is facilitated by the pressure drop across the membrane (the hydrostatic pressure within the glomerular capsule is less than that of the blood in the glomerular capillaries). Thus the primary glomerular filtrate has essentially the same composition as plasma with the exclusion of (1) high molecular weight substances such as plasma proteins that are relatively impermeable to the glomerular membrane, and (2) substances (for example, drugs and hormones) that are bound to plasma proteins. Protein binding will therefore reduce the fraction of the drug that is filtered, reducing the rate of excretion and prolonging the half-life of the drug.

The concentration of the drug in the primary filtrate is similar to that of the free drug in the plasma. However, as water is reabsorbed from the tubular urine, the urinary concentration of the drug increases, producing a concentration gradient favoring reabsorption via passive diffusion across the membranes of the tubular epithelium. Reabsorption is dependent on the lipid solubility and degree of ionization of the drug. As mentioned previously, the reabsorption of acids may be reduced by alkalinization of the urine. The reabsorption of bases (for example, analgesics such as methadone, meperidine, and ethoheptazine) is decreased by acidification of the urine, which increases the degree of ionization of these compounds (Asatoor et al., 1963; Baselt and Casarett, 1972).

The reabsorption of highly lipid-soluble compounds may also be modified by decreasing the reabsorption of water from the urine. Massive osmotic diuresis reduces reabsorption by decreasing the concentration gradient across the tubular epithelium.

Tubular secretion of drugs is accomplished by high-velocity, active-transport systems capable of transporting substances against a concentration gradient. Tubular secretion is a more efficient mechanism of drug excretion than glomerular filtration and is not significantly affected by reversible binding of drugs to plasma proteins. The velocity of active transport by the proximal tubule is considerably faster than the rate of delivery of blood to the transport site. Thus as free drug is removed, bound drug dissociates from the plasma proteins and becomes available for transport. Consequently, all drug, both free and bound, can be removed during a single pass through the kidneys. Glomerular filtration, on the other hand, can remove only 20% to 25% of the unbound drug during a single pass.

Two separate renal transport systems exist—one for anionic substances, the other for cations. Compounds of similar charge may compete with each other for transport. Penicillin is excreted by the anionic transport system, and its plasma half-life can be prolonged by concurrent administration of other anionic drugs that are also substrates for transport (for example, probenecid, phenylbutazone, indomethacin, aspirin, and sulfaphenazole) (Kampman et al., 1972).

Most common forms of renal disease (glomerulonephritis and nephrosclerosis) alter both glomerular filtration and tubular secretion. The vascular architecture of the kidney is such that the glomerular capillaries converge to form the efferent arteriole, which then supplies the capillary vasculature of the tubules. Thus any decrease in glomerular blood flow also decreases the tubular blood supply. Kampman and co-workers (1972) studied the relationship between the plasma half-life of penicillin and renal function as indicated by endogenous creatinine clearance rates. A strong correlation was found between the extent of prolongation of the half-life of penicillin and the deterioration of renal function. An age-related relationship was also observed; penicillin half-life was approximately five times longer in a population of elderly patients (average age, 71 years) compared to a group with a mean age of 31 years. The age-related effect was presumably attributable to age-related changes in renal function.

Biliary excretion

The hepatocytes lining the canaliculi produce the primary biliary secretion. Separate active-transport systems appear to be present for anions, cations, and nonionized compounds, and similarly charged substances may compete for transport. As with renal tubular secretion, binding to plasma proteins has little effect on the rate of biliary secretion.

Bile is secreted into the duodenum through the papilla of Vater. If the lipid solubility and degree of ionization of the excreted compound are favorable, it may be reabsorbed. Various antibiotics are excreted in the bile and partially reabsorbed; this enterohepatic recycling serves to prolong the plasma half-life of the drug. Quaternary ammonium compounds (for example, *d*-tubocurarine) are also secreted into the bile. However, they are completely ionized and thus are not reabsorbed but are completely excreted in the feces.

Chronic phenobarbital pretreatment was shown to increase biliary transport and bile flow in laboratory animals (Klaassen and Plaa, 1968; Levine, 1978). Drug interactions involving enhanced biliary excretion have not been extensively studied in humans. However, it has been reported that phenobarbital, phenytoin, and carbamazepine (an anticonvulsant used in the treatment of trigeminal neuralgia) all shortened the half-life of doxycycline. The authors attributed this result to induced hepatic drug metabolism (Neuvonen and Penttila, 1974; Penttila et al., 1974). However, other factors may also be involved, such as increased biliary excretion or altered protein binding and consequent increases in renal excretion.

Salivary excretion

Drugs also appear in the saliva via passive diffusion of the unbound, nonionized drug from the plasma. Although salivary secretion is not a major route of elimination of drugs, it is clinically significant since salivary drug concentrations are being considered for use as a convenient clinical index to monitor plasma drug levels. Strong correlations between the concentrations of unbound drug in human plasma and saliva have been reported for barbiturates, acetaminophen, digoxin, theophylline, salicylic acid, tolbutamide, and phenytoin.

The following antibiotics have also been detected in human saliva: tetracyclines (Kraus, Casey, and Johnson, 1951), streptomycin, penicillin G (Bender, Pressman, and Tashman, 1953), and clindamycin (Quayle and Whitmarsh, 1972). It has been suggested that the concentration of antibiotic in saliva may be an important factor in treating bacterial salivary gland infections, since the most common route of bacterial invasion is retrograde movement from the oral cavity through the secretory ducts. Unfortunately, there have been no systematic investigations of the factors affecting the concentration of free antibiotic in human saliva. However, since secretion of drugs into the saliva occurs via passive diffusion, it is likely that the following factors would affect salivary antibiotic concentrations: (1) the extent of protein binding, (2) the pH of the saliva, and (3) the rate of saliva production. The ideal antibiotic for treating salivary gland infections should produce a high concentration of free antibiotic in the saliva; therefore it should not be extensively bound to plasma proteins or to proteins and glycoproteins in the saliva and should not chelate with the Ca^{++} of the saliva. Also, the antibiotic should possess antibacterial activity at the pH of the saliva and should not be inactivated by purulent exudates that may be present. It is likely that the pH of the saliva changes as it traverses the ductal system, since bicarbonate is secreted into saliva in the ducts and would act to alkalinize the saliva. A change in pH could affect antibacterial activity of the drug and could affect the partitioning of the antibiotic between the saliva and the plasma because of passive diffusion across the ductal epithelium. The flow rate of the saliva may also be an important factor, since parasympathetic stimulation may affect ductal permeability and may directly stimulate bicarbonate secretion. Both of these factors would affect partitioning of the antibiotic across the ductal epithelium. Diffusion across the ductal epithelium could also be affected by chronic ductal inflammation and proliferation of connective tissue, which usually accompany chronic infections. Lastly, obstruction of the secretory ducts and the consequent interference with saliva formation owing to pressure and atrophy of the acini could affect the distribution of the antibiotic within the gland and ductal system, and thus the antibiotic might not reach its site of action. The problem of the salivary disposition of antibiotics in the treatment of salivary gland infections is one that demonstrates the applicability of the basic principles of pharmacology to dental practice.

SPECIFIC CLASSES OF DRUGS
Local anesthetics

Local anesthetics are compounds that reversibly block the development of action potentials in electrically excitable membranes. Although the mechanism of action of these drugs has yet to be established with total certainty, one well-accepted hypothesis is that the drug molecule binds to the plasma membrane causing a swelling or expansion (Fig. 5-5). Membrane expansion leads to a disordering of the components of the membrane including the Na^+-conductance channels, which are responsible for the rapid influx of Na^+ during the spike of the action potential. This disordering of the membrane blocks regenerative Na^+ influx and the consequent development and conduction of action potentials (for review, see Seeman, 1972).

Both the therapeutic effect, blockade of axonal conduction, and the systemic toxic effects can be attributed to the same mechanism, since local anesthetics can affect all excitable membranes. Depression of inhibitory pathways in the central nervous system could result in the convulsant activity seen after systemic administration. Toxic doses produce cardiovascular collapse attributable to: (1) depression of central cardiovascular centers, (2) direct depression of myocardial excitability, and (3) direct relaxation of

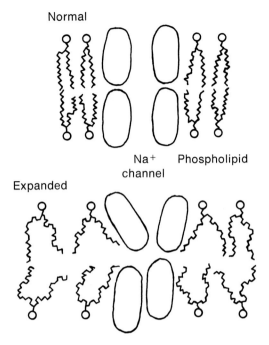

Normal

Na^+ Phospholipid
channel

Expanded

Fig. 5-5. Schematic representation of anesthetic-induced membrane expansion. Central globular structures represent sodium channel and peripheral structures are phospholipids.

vascular smooth muscle. Lethality is usually caused by respiratory arrest via direct depression of central respiratory centers.

Clinically useful local anesthetics can be divided into three groups based on their chemical structures: (1) esters (prototype—procaine), (2) amides (prototype—lidocaine), (3) antihistamines (prototype—phenothiazine derivatives). Since the use of antihistamines as local anesthetics is limited and generally restricted to patients allergic to both esters and amides, this group will not be discussed here (see Chapter 18).

The esters and amides differ in their pattern of metabolism. Procaine (ester) is rapidly hydrolyzed to pharmacologically inactive metabolites by esterases. In man, the bulk of the drug is hydrolyzed in the plasma by pseudocholinesterase, but metabolism may also occur in the liver, kidney, brain, and skeletal muscle (Brodie, Papper, and Mark, 1950; Kalow, 1952).

Lidocaine (amide) is primarily metabolized in the liver via a multistep pathway (Fig. 5-6). The initial reaction, N-de-eth-

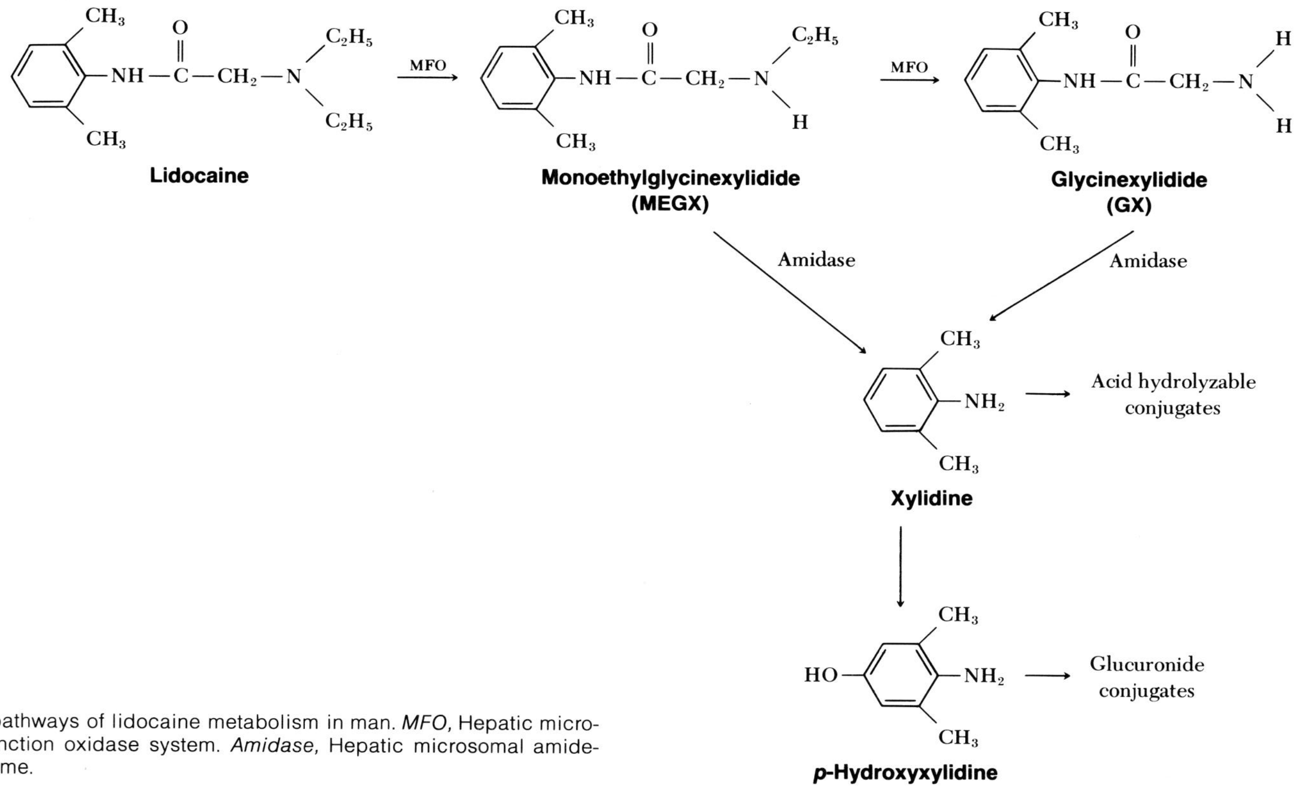

Fig. 5-6. Major pathways of lidocaine metabolism in man. *MFO,* Hepatic microsomal, mixed function oxidase system. *Amidase,* Hepatic microsomal amide-hydrolyzing enzyme.

ylation catalyzed by the hepatic microsomal mixed-function oxidase system (MFO), converts lidocaine, a tertiary amine, to a secondary amine. The metabolite, monoethylglycinexylidide (MEGX) is pharmacologically active and exhibits many of the adverse systemic effects of the parent compound, such as CNS and cardiovascular toxicity. MEGX may be further de-ethylated to glycinexylidide (GX), a metabolite that potentiates the convulsant actions of both MEGX and lidocaine. MEGX and GX are hydrolyzed to inactive metabolites by a hepatic microsomal amidase. Thus lidocaine metabolism is not synonymous with inactivation or detoxification, and the metabolites MEGX and GX, which have a longer half-life than lidocaine, may contribute to lidocaine toxicity (Blumer, Strong, and Atkinson, 1973; Difazio and Brown, 1972; Hollunger, 1960a,b,c; Keenaghan and Boyes, 1972; Strong, Parker, and Atkinson, 1973; Strong et al., 1975).

The rate of systemic absorption of both groups of local anesthetics depends on the vascularity or the rate of perfusion of the injection site. Decreasing the blood flow at the site of injection can significantly reduce the rate of systemic absorption following injection into highly vascular areas such as the oral cavity. Thus the incorporation of a vasoconstrictor can retard systemic absorption. Once absorbed, these lipid-soluble drugs are distributed to all tissues. Following intravascular injection, initially high concentrations are found in those organs receiving the greatest portion of the cardiac output, that is, the best-perfused tissues (brain, liver, and kidney), and, subsequently, the drug redistributes to less well-perfused tissues (adipose tissue and skeletal muscle).

The metabolites of the local anesthetics are eventually excreted in the urine. Approximately 2% of a dose of procaine is found unchanged in the urine, and approximately 10% or less of a dose of lidocaine is excreted as the unmetabolized drug. Lidocaine metabolites are also excreted into bile and, subsequently, reabsorbed by the intestine. This enterohepatic recycling probably contributes to the prolonged half-life of lidocaine metabolites.

General anesthetics

General anesthetics can be divided into two broad categories: (1) inhalation anesthetics, including gases and volatile liquids that vaporize readily at room temperature, and (2) intravenous anesthetics, including ultrashort-acting barbiturates and nonbarbiturates that produce dissociative states.

Inhalation anesthetics

Several basic theories have been proposed as the mechanism of action of the inhalation anesthetics: the lipid theory of Meyer and Overton, the structured water or clathrate theory of Pauling, the microtubule disruption theory, and various theories involving changes in energy metabolism. One feature common to all of these theories is that the anesthetic produces a generalized electrical stabilization of CNS excitability that is not due to specific receptor interaction. Although a mechanism not involving classic drug-receptor interactions appears to explain best the effects of inhalation anesthetics, intravenous anesthetics probably exert their action via specific receptors located in specific areas of the CNS.

The lipid theory is the most widely accepted theory of inhalation anesthesia and is based on the interaction of anesthetics with the lipid component of the membranes of CNS neurons. Meyer and Overton originally observed a correlation between the oil/water partition coefficient (lipid solubility) and the potency of various inhalation anesthetics. They postulated that to obtain a given degree of anesthesia the same number of molecules of anesthetic interact with the lipid of the cells regardless of the anesthetic used. The relationship between potency and lipid solubility has been confirmed by directly measuring the adsorption of anesthetics to cell membranes.

Another method of comparing potencies suitable for clinical application is the determination of the minimum alveolar concentration (MAC) required to prevent gross muscle movement during a standardized surgical incision in 50% of a population. A strong inverse relationship was found between the lipid solubilities of gaseous anesthetics and their MAC values (Saidman et al., 1967). Potent anesthetics had high lipid solubility and required low alveolar concentrations, while anesthetics of low potency (low lipid solubility) required high alveolar concentrations to achieve surgical anesthesia.

Nitrous oxide is an example of a low-potency anesthetic, and it has been estimated that alveolar concentrations of 100% to 110% (that is, 10% greater than the total lung capacity at standard pressures) would be required for surgical anesthesia. Thus nitrous oxide is not potent enough to be used alone for surgical anesthesia. It is frequently used in combination with other anesthetics because it produces few adverse reactions at concentrations less than 65%, that is, minimal cardiovascular or respiratory effects and no effects on skeletal muscle tone. It has the advantage of producing potent analgesic actions even at subanesthetic concentrations. Nitrous oxide produces little, if any, toxic effect on the liver or kidneys, and this lack of toxicity may be related to its lack of metabolism in the body.

The halogenated anesthetics (halothane, methoxyflurane, and so on) are extensively metabolized, and metabolism has been implicated in the hepatic and renal toxicity of these drugs in man. Methoxyflurane and halothane are metabolized in the liver by a pathway involving the mixed-function oxidase system (MFO) (Van Dyke, 1966; Van Dyke and Chenoweth, 1965). Non-MFO enzymes may also play a role in metabolism of these agents, but the precise mode of involvement has yet to be determined (Van Dyke and Wineman, 1971). In man, an estimated 12% to 20% of the total dose of halothane was biotransformed (Rehder et al., 1967). The major urinary metabolites—chloride, bromide, and trifluoroacetic acid—in concentrations found during or after anesthesia were not toxic to humans. Thus it has been postulated that unstable intermediary metabolites, capable of reacting with tissue components, are formed during metabolism (Stier, 1968) and are responsible for the hepatotoxicity (postoperative hepatitis and hepatic necrosis) of halothane. The observation that urinary metabolites can be detected as late as 13 days after halothane administration (Rehder et al., 1967) also suggests reaction with tissue components. Although methoxyflurane exhibits less potential for hepatotoxicity than halothane, hepatic metabolism has been postulated to be an etiologic factor in methoxyflurane-induced liver disease.

The relationship between methoxyflurane metabolism and nephrotoxicity is much clearer. About 65% to 75% of a therapeutic dose of methoxyflurane is metabolized by humans and, because of the extensive tissue storage of the drug, biotransformation and elimination are prolonged, continuing for 9 to 12 days following administration (Holaday, Rudofsky, and Treuhaft, 1970; Yoshimura, Holaday, and Fiserova-Bergerova, 1976). The following reactions are involved: oxidative dechlorination, O-demethylation, and defluorination (for complete metabolic pathway, see Mazze, Trudell, and Cousins, 1971). The inorganic fluoride generated during metabolism is probably the chief factor responsible for the polyuria, hypernatremia, histopathologic changes such as mitochondrial swelling and lysis, and other aspects of nephrotoxicity (Mazze, Cousins, and Kosek, 1972, 1973; Mazze, Shue, and Jackson, 1971). The rate of methoxyflurane metabolism and the generation of inorganic fluoride are accelerated by MFO induction (for instance, chronic phenobarbital pretreatment) and result in enhanced nephrotoxicity (Mazze, Hitt, and Cousins, 1974). It is interesting to note that, although halothane also contains fluoride, inorganic fluoride is not liberated during normal oxidative metabolism, and halothane is not ordinarily nephrotoxic.

Recent epidemiologic studies indicate that operating-room personnel tend to have higher rates of miscarriages and birth defects and an increased incidence of malignancies. A relationship to chronic exposure to trace concentrations of anesthetics has been postulated, but as yet, not proven (for reviews of the teratogenicity and carcinogenicity of anesthetic gases see Corbett, 1976; Ferstandig, 1978).

Adverse effects of the halogenated anesthetics that are not related to metabolism include: sensitization of the heart to catecholamine-induced arrhythmias; respiratory depression, which tends to be more intense with methoxyflurane than halothane; and cardiovascular depression, which is more severe with halothane than methoxyflurane. Halothane also produces profound changes in the regional blood flow to various tissues and thereby affects the distribution and elimination of other drugs.

The halogenated anesthetics are highly lipid-soluble and thus are very potent anesthetics. However, lipid solubility also contributes to their extensive storage in peripheral tissues (methoxyflurane greater than halothane). The high degree of peripheral distribution of methoxyflurane contributes to the prolonged induction and recovery associated with this anesthetic.

Intravenous anesthetics

Ultrashort-acting barbiturates (for example, thiopental, methohexital) are frequently used for induction of anesthesia or as the principle anesthetic for short surgical procedures. The pharmacology of these agents and other barbiturates is discussed in the section on "Sedatives, hypnotics, and tranquilizers."

Inhalation and intravenous anesthetics probably differ in their sites and mechanisms of action, and thus these two groups of anesthetics produce significantly different signs and stages of anesthesia. Ketamine is an excellent example of an anesthetic that does not conform to the classic stages of anesthesia originally described for ether. Ketamine produces a unique type of anesthesia (dissociative anesthesia) consisting of profound analgesia and an immobilized state but without the loss of many protective reflexes (for example, laryngeal, pharyngeal, and corneal reflexes). During anesthesia, tendon reflexes are hyperactive and skeletal muscle tone is increased; it is especially evident in the head and neck area and may include jaw clenching. Cardiovascular stimulation (tachycardia and increases in systolic and diastolic blood pressure) is seen at both anesthetic and subanesthetic doses. Recovery is usually accompanied by psychic disturbances (for example, mood changes, disorientation, or hallucinations), which some adult patients find to be unpleasant or frightening (Domino, Chodoff, and Corssen, 1965). It has been reported that children are less prone to experience undesirable psychic disturbances or to exhibit significant elevations of blood pressure (Elliott et al., 1976).

Premedication with sedatives and tranquilizers (for example, secobarbital or diazepam) can be used to reduce emergence hallucinations. However, these two drugs also prolong recovery time and lengthen the plasma half-life of ketamine in man. Animal studies suggest that secobarbital and diazepam reduce the rate of hepatic metabolism of ketamine, and this mechanism probably contributes to the prolonged duration of action of ketamine (Lo and Cumming, 1975).

Ketamine is metabolized by hepatic MFO to a variety of metabolites. The principle metabolite is formed by N-demethylation and possesses qualitatively similar pharmacologic actions but with about one-third the potency of ketamine (Chang and Glazko, 1972; Chang et al., 1970; Cohen and Trevor, 1974). Further metabolism essentially inactivates the compound.

Ketamine is highly lipid-soluble, and its rapid onset and short duration of action following intravenous administration are caused by rapid initial distribution to the brain and subsequent redistribution to other tissues (for example, skin, muscle, and liver with possible enterohepatic recycling). Thus metabolism plays only a little role in the initial return to consciousness. However, metabolism is a major determinant of total recovery and the duration of the postanesthetic effects (for example, analgesia and psychic disturbances). The rate of metabolism of ketamine and its N-demethylated metabolite is accelerated by MFO induction and results in an accelerated rate of postanesthetic recovery (Cohen et al., 1973; Marietta et al., 1976). Ketamine is also effective following intramuscular injection, but the injection can be painful and a dose three to five times that of the intravenous dose is needed. Furthermore, the onset of anesthesia is slower and recovery is prolonged following intramuscular administration.

Analgesics

Analgesics can be divided into two groups based on their site of action: (1) peripherally acting analgesics; pyrazolone derivatives (phenylbutazone and aminopyrine), indomethacin, fenamic acid derivatives (mefenamic acid), and salicylates and (2) centrally acting analgesics; the opiates and opiate-like analgesics, and the dissociative analgesics. To understand the mechanism of action of these drugs, one must also understand the mechanism of pain transmission.

The investigation of pain and its alleviation by analgesics is difficult, because pain is a complex, multicomponent phenomenon. Pain itself cannot be measured, because it is probably not a specific sensory modality associated with a graded response to a specific stimulus of varying intensity as are sight, hearing, and so on. Pain is most likely an interpretation of, and a psychologic reaction to, multisensory stimulation. Since many factors are involved in the production of pain, many sites of intervention exist that can modify the pain response. The events and anatomic structures involved in pain will be reviewed and the mechanism of action of analgesics will be discussed in the context of this overview.

The initial event in the generation of pain is the elaboration of endogenous substances that act as chemical mediators or modulators of pain. These substances are thought to interact with free nerve endings (pain receptors) and produce depolarization of the nerve endings and propagation of action potentials (pain signals). These signals are transmitted to the spinal cord via two types of nerve fibers, slowly conducting C fibers and faster-conducting A-delta fibers. Both types of fibers synapse in the spinal cord, and the pain signals are transmitted to the brain.

Two major pathways appear to be involved in the central events associated with pain. The classic pain pathway (thalamic-cortical pathway) transmits pain signals to the thalamus (ventral posterolateral nuclei), which acts as a relay for transmission of the signals to the somatosensory areas of the cortex. This direct pathway is primarily involved in the recognition and somatic localization of pain. The subcortical pain pathway is a more diffuse, multisynaptic pathway that communicates with many subcortical structures, such as the reticular-activating system, which is involved in arousal and maintenance of wakefulness, and the limbic system, which is involved in primitive emotional and effective reactions (for example, reward-punishment, aversion, and rage). The subcortical pathway probably functions in arousal and general awareness of pain and affective reactions to pain (for reviews of pain pathways see: Crue, 1975; Domino, 1968; Hassler, 1968).

This is a highly simplified view of the sequence of events in the genesis of pain. It should be recognized that free nerve endings, nerve fibers, and central pathways are not specific for pain; they also transmit information regarding other sensory stimuli. The mechanisms of deciphering the various types of information from the periphery are still largely speculative. Furthermore, there are numerous feedback systems that can modify the transmission of pain signals. One controversial theory (Melzack and Wall, 1965) postulates that the spinal cord contains "gating" mechanisms that function to integrate the information arriving from the periphery and to modulate the transmission of signals from the periphery to the brain. The "gate" opens and closes, permitting or inhibiting the transmission of pain signals, depending on the quality and quantity of other concurrent sensory stimuli. For example, rubbing an injured area or applying pressure frequently decreases the intensity of the pain.

The systems described previously all function in the ascending (periphery to CNS) transmission of pain signals. Recent research has identified a descending pain-inhibitory system that appears to modulate the transmission of pain signals in the ascending system (Liebeskind and Paul, 1977; Mayer and Price, 1976). The descending pain-inhibitory system appears to utilize a series of endogenous peptides with opiate-like activity as one of its neurotransmitters. The peptides are collectively termed "endorphins," and it has been postulated that the endorphins function physiologically to suppress pain (Frederickson and Norris, 1976; Goldstein, 1976).

Peripherally acting analgesics

The probable mechanism of action of this group of drugs is interference with some of the peripheral pain mediators and modulators (Lim, 1968, 1970). Numerous substances have been identified that either directly stimulate free nerve endings or sensitize free nerve endings to other forms of stimulation. Two such groups of substances are the plasma kinins and the prostaglandins. Both the kinins and the prostaglandins function as local or tissue hormones, that is, they are rapidly synthesized and rapidly degraded in localized areas, and only small amounts enter the general circulation. The plasma kinins are a group of short-chained polypeptides that are the most potent pain mediators thus far discovered. Their synthesis is initiated by events occurring during tissue injury (for review of synthesis and actions of kinins, see: Rocha e Silva, 1970; Sander and Huggins, 1972; Wilhelm, 1971). The prostaglandins are a group of fatty acid derivatives that function as peripheral pain modulators. They potentiate the algesic actions of the kinins, prevent development of tachyphylaxis to the kinins, and in general produce a hyperalgesic state in which normally nonpainful mechanical or chemical stimuli produce a pain response. In addition, intermediates in the synthesis of prostaglandins have pain-producing properties and may play a more direct role in acute pain (Ferreira, 1972).

Virtually all tissues of the human body synthesize prostaglandins from unsaturated free fatty acids with a chain length of 20 carbons, such as arachidonic acid (Fig. 5-7). Since most arachidonic acid is incor-

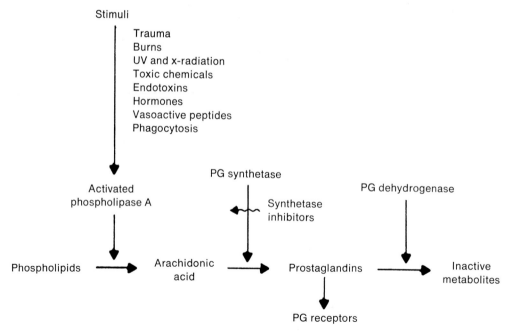

Fig. 5-7. Biosynthesis (release) and degradation of prostaglandins and site of action of non-narcotic analgesics.

porated into the phospholipids of cell membranes, it must be liberated by the action of phospholipase A. Phospholipase A is normally present in an inactive form but can be activated by a variety of physiologic and pathologic stimuli. Once liberated, arachidonic acid is rapidly converted to prostaglandins by a multienzyme system, prostaglandin synthetase. Synthetase activity can be inhibited by the peripherally acting analgesics, and it is postulated that this mechanism is responsible for their analgesic action (for review of synthesis and other actions of prostaglandins, see: Cuthbert, 1973; Ferreira and Vane, 1974; Ramwell and Pharris, 1972).

In addition to the kinins and the prostaglandins, biogenic amines are also capable of producing pain. Thus the release of serotonin from platelets during clotting and the release of histamine from mast cells may contribute to the stimulation of free nerve endings. Increases in extracellular K^+ and H^+ can elicit pain, and local release of K^+ from damaged cells and local acidosis associated with inflammatory reactions or local ischemia may also play a role in pain. Other effects of tissue damage and infections that have been implicated in pain are leakage of acidic metabolic intermediates (citrate, lactate, and so on), release of phospholipids, and hypertonicity of extracellular fluids.

It is clear that the peripheral initiation of pain is produced by a multiplicity of substances. Furthermore, various types of pain may be caused by different combinations of these substances along with physical factors (pressure, temperature, and so on). Interference with only one or a limited number of the components of peripheral initiation cannot be expected to produce total or universal analgesia, and those pain signals that escape peripheral inhibition will be perceived and will also produce an emotional reaction. Consequently, the peripherally acting analgesics commonly used in dental practice tend to possess low analgesic potency.

Inhibition of prostaglandin synthesis has been implicated in other therapeutic effects and side effects of the peripherally acting analgesics. For example, prostaglandins appear to be one of the chemical mediators of the inflammatory process. Thus inhibition of prostaglandin synthesis also contributes to the anti-inflammatory effects of this group of drugs. Hypothalamic synthesis of prostaglandins also has been implicated in the production of fever and the prostaglandin synthetase of the hypothalamus is one of the most sensitive of all tissue synthetases to inhibition by aspirin. This effect correlates well with the clinical efficacy of aspirin as an antipyretic. Gastrointestinal irritation, ulceration, and gastric bleeding are other side effects of aspirin, indomethacin, and phenylbutazone. It has been postulated that inhibition of prostaglandin production in the gastrointestinal tract predisposes to local mucosal damage by stimulating gastric acid production and by reducing mucosal blood flow.

Because of the limited use in dentistry of the other drugs in this group, only the salicylates will be reviewed here. Salicylates are usually administered orally, and one of the rate-limiting factors in absorption of solid preparations appears to be the dissolution rate of the tablet. Addition of an antacid to the tablets increases the rate of dissolution and slightly increases the rate of absorption. Aspirin solutions are absorbed considerably faster than solid preparations with or without antacids (Truitt and Morgan, 1964).

Aspirin, the acetic acid ester of salicylic acid, is rapidly hydrolyzed by plasma and tissue esterases to salicylic acid. Under normal conditions, the bulk of a dose of aspirin circulates as salicylic acid, which is metabolized primarily by conjugation with glycine, glucuronic acid, or sulfate. Both salicylic acid and its conjugates are excreted in the urine. Under normal circumstances, most of the unmetabolized salicylic acid is reabsorbed, and little free salicylate is excreted. The rate of excretion of salicylic acid can be increased by alkalinization of the urine, which reduces reabsorption of the drug in the proximal tubule. Conjugates are not reabsorbed, and therefore their excretion is not pH dependent.

Although aspirin is not bound to plasma proteins to any great extent, salicylic acid is highly bound and may be displaced from its binding sites by other anions. Aspirin may also acetylate plasma proteins and thus may alter the binding of other drugs (Chignell and Starkweather, 1971).

Centrally acting analgesics

Centrally acting analgesics include opiates (morphine and codeine), opiate derivatives (methadone and meperidine and its derivatives, diphenoxylate and fentanyl), and opiate-like drugs with lower abuse potential (propoxyphene, ethoheptazine, and pentazocine). Although the exact sites and mechanisms of analgesia are not certain, it is clear that these drugs produce their analgesic actions by affecting the CNS and not by peripheral actions.

Intracerebral microinjections of morphine have been used to identify the sites of action of the centrally acting analgesics. Morphine appears to elevate the pain threshold following application to only a few specific areas (for example, periaqueductal gray matter and certain portions of the reticular formation); application to other areas of the brain fails to alter the pain threshold (Yaksh and Rudy, 1978). High-affinity, stereo-specific opiate-binding substances (receptors) have been identified in the brain, and there is a fairly good correlation between the localization of the opiate receptors and the areas sensitive to morphine microinjection. Furthermore, these same areas contain high concentrations of enkephalin, a specific endorphin with high affinity for the opiate receptors. Thus the centrally acting analgesics may activate the descending pain-inhibitory system and thereby alter pain thresholds (Simon and Hiller, 1978; Snyder and Simantov, 1977; Terenius, 1978). However, it is a well-recognized clinical phenomenon that the narcotic analgesics alter the emotional reaction to pain and cause an indifference or detachment from the pain rather than a true blockade of pain perception or recognition. Thus other sites of action must also play a role in opiate-induced analgesia. One such area may be the limbic system, which contains high levels of opiate receptors and high concentrations of enkephalins.

Morphine is a naturally occurring product in opium with potent analgesic activity that is administered parenterally. The principal pathway of metabolism is glucuronide conjugation, but a small fraction is metabolized via oxidative reactions. Free drug and metabolites are excreted by renal (filtration and tubular secretion) and biliary routes. The conjugates are hydrolyzed in the intestine to yield the parent compound, which may be reabsorbed; the remainder (about 10% of the dose) is found in the feces. Tolerance to analgesic activity and dependence liability are two factors that limit the use of morphine.

Codeine, the methyl ether of morphine, is metabolized by three principal pathways: (1) O-demethylation to morphine, (2) N-demethylation to norcodeine, and (3) conjugation with glucuronic acid. The generation of morphine may contribute to codeine analgesia. Codeine is not as potent as morphine, but it has lower dependence potential than morphine.

Meperidine exhibits a potency between those of codeine and morphine. Dependence liability is high, although it may be slightly less than that of morphine. It is available for both oral and parenteral administration. Metabolism is via hydrolysis, N-dealkylation, and glucuronic conjugation. The N-dealkylated metabolite possesses some pharmacologic activity and, although it less readily crosses the blood-brain barrier, high doses can produce convulsions.

Fentanyl is an extremely potent analgesic; estimates of its potency range between 80 and 200 times that of morphine. It has a rapid onset and short duration of action and is usually used in combination with a tranquilizer such as droperidol to produce neuroleptanalgesia or neuroleptanesthesia. Fentanyl is highly lipid-soluble, and this factor is the primary determinant of its duration of action. Following parenteral administration, it is rapidly redistributed from the CNS to poorly perfused lipid-rich tissues. The principal metabolic pathway is hepatic N-dealkylation followed by a series of uncharacterized reactions, and in humans the rate of metabolism and the final clearance from the body is very slow (Schleimer et al., 1978). Eight hours after administration only 20% of the dose was recovered in the urine, and urinary excretion of metabolites was detected as late as 4 days after administration (Hess, Stiebler, and Herz, 1972).

Propoxyphene (dextro isomer) is a weak analgesic, structurally related to methadone but with low-dependence liability. It is usually administered orally but is also well absorbed following parenteral administration. Metabolism is primarily via hepatic N-dealkylation.

Pentazocine is a weak narcotic antagonist with analgesic activity in man. If administered to a narcotic addict, it will precipitate withdrawal. In general, narcotic-antagonist analgesics have less abuse potential than narcotic-agonists, and dependence and withdrawal are qualitatively different, with withdrawal symptoms less severe. Pentazocine has weak hallucinogenic activity and may produce dysphoria in some patients. It is well-absorbed both orally and parenterally and is eliminated mainly by hepatic oxidative metabolism to alcoholic derivatives, which may be further oxidized to acids. A small fraction is converted to glucuronide and about 10% is excreted unchanged in the urine.

Ketamine produces profound analgesia at both anesthetic and subanesthetic doses. The mechanisms of ketamine-induced analgesia are even more speculative than those of morphine, but activation of the limbic system may be involved. It is also possible that limbic activation may contribute to the amnestic effect of ketamine.

Sedatives, hypnotics, and tranquilizers

Most sedative-hypnotic agents fall into the barbiturate group. Barbiturates are usually classified according to their duration of action: long-acting, phenobarbital; intermediate-acting, amobarbital; short-acting, secobarbital and pentobarbital;

ultrashort-acting, methohexital and thiopental. However, many factors affect the duration of action and, since the mechanisms of termination of action are different for the different groups of barbiturates, the duration of action may be affected differently for different drugs. Also, one should define the specific action being referred to in "duration of action." The ultrashort-acting barbiturates remain in the body long after recovery from anesthesia and may exert nonanesthetic actions until they are eliminated.

Barbiturates produce "CNS depression," which may range from sedation to sleep, anesthesia, or death. The reticular-activating system is one area of the brain that is readily depressed by barbiturates and probably plays a role in their mechanism of action. However, a single site of action is probably too simplistic a view, and other central structures are most likely involved.

Barbiturates are well-absorbed following oral and parenteral administration. However, subcutaneous administration should be avoided because of the possibility of tissue necrosis at the site of injection.

One of the factors affecting the onset and duration of action of the barbiturates is their lipid solubility. In general, lipid solubility increases from the long-acting to the ultrashort-acting barbiturates. The rate of penetration of the blood-brain barrier is directly proportional to the lipid solubility. Thus, following intravenous administration, ultrashort-acting barbiturates rapidly enter the brain, and the time to onset of action is short, while long-acting barbiturates slowly cross the blood-brain barrier causing a significant lag between injection and the onset of action. The difference in speed of onset is an important consideration in selection of a barbiturate for the termination of a convulsion or for induction of anesthesia.

The termination of action of the ultrashort-acting barbiturates following intravenous administration is accomplished by redistribution. Intravenous administration produces high blood levels of the drug resulting in comparably high CNS levels, but as the blood concentration falls, owing to uptake of the drug by peripheral tissues, the drug leaves the CNS and the central actions are terminated.

Barbiturates are metabolized primarily by hepatic mixed-function oxidases (MFO), but they differ in their rate and pattern of metabolism and pattern of elimination. Phenobarbital is slowly metabolized primarily by hepatic hydroxylation of the phenyl group. Under normal conditions, about 10% to 30% of phenobarbital is excreted unchanged in the urine. However, alkalinization of the urine may increase the rate of excretion of unmetabolized phenobarbital. Secobarbital is more rapidly, and almost totally, metabolized, and little unmetabolized drug is excreted in the urine. Therefore alkalinization of the urine has little effect on the rate of secobarbital elimination. The two principal metabolites of secobarbital are formed by oxidation of the side chains, and termination of action is primarily by metabolism. The ultrashort-acting barbiturates are metabolized by side-chain hydroxylation at rates similar to that of secobarbital. Metabolism plays little role in the termination of anesthetic action, but final elimination is dependent on metabolism.

The nonbarbiturate sedative-hypnotic agents include: (1) compounds that are structurally similar to the barbiturates, glutethimide and methyprylon, (2) methaqualone, (3) ethchlorvynol, and (4) chloral hydrate. As sedative-hypnotic agents, they have little, if any, distinct advantage over the barbiturates, and all exhibit abuse and dependence liability. Methaqualone, ethchlorvynol, and chloral hydrate possess some anticonvulsant and muscle-relaxant activity.

Tranquilizers are generally divided into two groups: the major tranquilizers or antipsychotic drugs and the minor tranquilizers or antianxiety agents. Antipsychotic drugs include phenothiazines, thioxanthenes, and butyrophenones. Of these drugs, only droperidol, a butyrophenone, will be discussed here.

Droperidol is usually used in combination with the short-acting narcotic analgesic fentanyl. It is a potent sedative with a long duration of action (greater than 4 hours) and causes decreased motor activity and indifference to the surrounding environment. Droperidol appears to potentiate the analgesic effects of narcotics and nitrous oxide. However, it also potentiates the respiratory depressant action of narcotics. Like other butyrophenones, it has considerable α-adrenergic blocking activity, which may result in postural hypotension, and it produces extrapyramidal effects such as parkinsonian-like symptoms, dyskinesia, and acute dystonia. The major pathway of butyrophenone metabolism is hepatic N-dealkylation and glycine conjugation (Soudijn, Van Wijngaarden, and Allervijn, 1967). Metabolites are excreted into the bile and urine; little unmetabolized drug is excreted. (For an extensive review of the clinical aspects of neuroleptanesthesia, see Oyama, 1973.)

Antianxiety agents are the most widely used group of drugs in this country and include meprobamate and its derivatives and the benzodiazepines (diazepam, oxazepam, and chlordiazepoxide). The benzodiazepines are metabolized to pharmacologically active compounds that contribute to the effects of these drugs. The metabolites also tend to have longer half-lives than the parent compounds; thus the metabolites prolong the duration of action. Diazepam is metabolized by hepatic MFO to oxazepam, a compound with effective antianxiety and anticonvulsant properties. Although these compounds are usually administered orally for their antianxiety effects, intravenous diazepam is now one of the drugs of choice for termination of convulsions and is effective for both status epilepticus and local anesthetic-induced convulsions. Diazepam is highly lipid-soluble, and the initial high brain concentrations achieved after intravenous administration are followed by redistribution to other tissues. The principle metabolite, oxazepam, is further metabolized by glucuronide conjugation, and the conjugate is excreted in the urine.

Antimicrobial drugs

Antimicrobial drugs are one of the few classes of drugs that effectively treat the etiology of a condition and not simply the symptoms of the disease. Therapy of microbial infections is based on the use of drugs that are selectively toxic to the invading microorganism and nontoxic or relatively nontoxic to the host. Selectivity usually arises from structural or biochemical differences between the microbial cell and the cells of the host.

Inhibitors of bacterial cell wall synthesis

A drug-induced alteration in the bacterial cell wall is an excellent example of selective toxicity. The cell wall is a structure not found in mammalian cells but is essential for bacterial viability, enabling bacteria to maintain internal osmotic pressures that are much greater than their external environment (plasma or interstitial fluid). Synthesis of defective cell walls may result in bacterial lysis or other lethal conditions. All inhibitors of cell wall synthesis tend to be bactericidal and are most effective against actively dividing bacteria, since the rate of synthesis of the cell wall is greatest during the growth phase. If growth and cell division are inhibited by bacteriostatic agents (for example, tetracyclines), the inhibitors of cell wall synthesis cannot exert their bactericidal action.

Inhibitors of bacterial cell wall synthesis may be divided into two groups: (1) drugs in which host toxicity limits their systemic use and thus are most frequently used as topical antibiotics—this group includes bacitracin, vancomycin, and ristocetin; and (2) systemically useful antibiotics—the β-lactam antibiotics, which are the penicillins, cephalosporins, and cephamycins. Only the β-lactam antibiotics will be discussed here.

Absorption of penicillins following oral administration varies widely. Benzyl penicillin is chemically unstable at acid pH and is inactivated by gastric acid. The extent of inactivation depends on the length of exposure to the acidic environment. Food delays gastric emptying and may decrease absorption via acid inactivation of the drug. Phenoxymethylpenicillin and phenethicillin exhibit greater acid stability and more reliable gastrointestinal absorption.

Two types of preparations are available for parenteral administration: (1) soluble salts (Na^+ or K^+ salts), which possess high water solubility, are rapidly absorbed, and may be administered by any parenteral route; and (2) insoluble salts ("repository" preparations—procaine and benzathine penicillins), which possess low water solubility, are slowly but continuously absorbed from the site of injection, and are not suitable for intravenous administration. Topical administration of penicillins should be avoided because of the high incidence of sensitization and hypersensitivity reactions associated with such use.

Penicillins are not uniformly distributed in the body. Under normal circumstances they do not readily cross the blood-brain barrier, and the distribution to other tissues is a function of the extent of binding to plasma proteins (see section on "Distribution"). Penicillins are not readily metabolized and are excreted unchanged. The only exceptions are the ampicillin derivatives, hetacillin and pivampicillin, which are hydrolyzed in the body to ampicillin, the compound that is responsible for the antibacterial activity of these drugs.

Most penicillins are rapidly excreted by active tubular secretion, and excretion is competitively inhibited in the presence of other drugs that are also substrates of the anionic transport system (for example, probenecid). The isoxazolyl penicillins (oxacillin, cloxacillin, dicloxacillin) are excreted by both renal tubular secretion and hepatic biliary excretion. Biliary excretion is the primary route of elimination of nafcillin (approximately 90%), and some enterohepatic recirculation occurs and contributes to the longer half-life of this drug.

The penicillins are the least toxic antibiotic available. However, they are the most allergenic, and hypersensitivity constitutes the only absolute contraindication to their use in treating penicillin-sensitive infections.

The basic chemical structure of all β-lactam antibiotics consists of two-ring structures, one of which is a β-lactam ring that may be hydrolyzed by a group of bacterial enzymes, β-lactamases (Fig. 5-8). Hydrolysis of the β-lactam ring destroys antibacterial activity and is one mechanism responsible for bacterial resistance to the β-lactam antibiotics. Penicillins susceptible to β-lactamase inactivation include: (1) some narrow-spectrum penicillins—benzylpenicillin, phenoxymethylpenicillin, phenethicillin; and (2) the extended-spectrum ("broad"-spectrum) penicillins—ampicillin, carbenicillin, and their derivatives. The β-lactamase–resistant penicillins are narrow-spectrum agents and include methicillin, nafcillin, and the isoxazolyl penicillins. Bacterial resistance to the β-lactamase–resistant antibiotics also develops and is probably due to alterations in the permeability of the bacterial cell wall to the drug, resulting in the inability of the drug to reach its site of action. Because of the development of bacterial resistance, the β-lactamase–resistant antibiotics should be reserved for treatment of serious infections caused by β-lactamase–producing bacteria.

Cephalosporins are broad-spectrum β-lactam antibiotics that are somewhat more widely distributed than penicillins. Cephalexin and cephaloglycin are the only acid-stable cephalosporins suitable for oral administration. Most cephalosporins are excreted by renal tubular secretion; an exception is cefazolin, which is eliminated primarily by glomerular filtration. The cephalosporins are more toxic than the penicillins. Therefore they should not be used as substitutes for penicillins in treatment of penicillin-sensitive infections. They are somewhat less allergenic than the penicillins, but some cases of cross-hypersensitivity between cephalosporins and penicillins have been reported.

The cephamycins are another group of β-lactam antibiotics that are currently undergoing clinical trials.

Drugs affecting cell membrane permeability

Two classes of antibiotics increase cell membrane permeability: (1) polypeptide

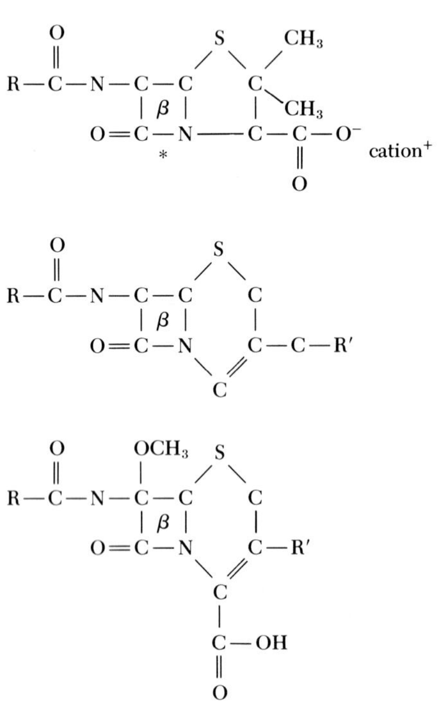

Penicillins

Cephalosporins

Cephamycins

Fig. 5-8. Chemical structures of β-lactam antibiotics. β identifies β-lactam ring; *identifies site of hydrolysis of β-lactam ring by penicillinase and other β-lactamases. R and R′ represent side chain substitutes that modify some actions of compounds.

antibiotics—polymyxins, gramicidins, and tyrocidine; and (2) polyene antibiotics—amphotericins, nystatin, and candicidin. Since the cell membranes of microbial and mammalian cells are quite similar, these antibiotics exhibit a low degree of selectivity and are toxic to the host upon systemic administration. Thus these drugs are predominantly used for topical application.

The polyene antibiotics increase membrane permeability by binding to membrane steroids. Bacterial cell membranes are devoid of steroids; thus the polyenes are not antibacterial. Membranes of mammalian cells and fungal cells contain steroids, and therefore the polyenes are effective antifungal agents. Polyenes are not absorbed from the gastrointestinal tract or from intact oral mucosa, and thus they may be used to treat fungal superinfections of the alimentary canal.

Inhibitors of protein synthesis

The selectivity of antibiotics that inhibit protein synthesis is attributable to the structural differences that exist between bacterial and mammalian ribosomes. Mammalian ribosomes are 80s particles that dissociate into 60s and 40s subunits and have approximately equal amounts of protein and RNA. Bacterial ribosomes are 70s particles consisting of 50s and 30s subunits, and the ratio of protein to RNA is about two to three. Inhibitors of bacterial protein synthesis include tetracyclines, chloramphenicol, lincomycin and clindamycin, macrolide antibiotics, and aminoglycoside antibiotics.

Tetracyclines are broad-spectrum antibiotics that reversibly bind to bacterial ribosomes at normal therapeutic concentrations. If the drug concentration is reduced, the drug will dissociate from the ribosomes, and the bacteria may resume growth. Thus the tetracyclines are bacteriostatic agents at blood levels that would be expected following routine oral administration. Absorption from the gastrointestinal tract is adequate but not complete and may be further reduced by formation of nonabsorbable chelates with metal ions (for example,

Fe^{++}, Mg^{++}, Mn^{++}, Ca^{++}, or Al^{+++}). Intramuscular administration usually causes local irritation and unpredictable absorption.

Tetracyclines are distributed throughout the body and are deposited in calcifying tissues owing to chelation with calcium. Tetracyclines also cross the placenta and are deposited in fetal bone and teeth. Excretion is via two routes, renal glomerular filtration and hepatic biliary excretion. The rate of filtration is inversely proportional to the extent of plasma protein binding, and thus highly bound tetracyclines are primarily excreted into the bile. Some reabsorption occurs in the intestine following biliary excretion, but, since intestinal absorption is poor, some of the drug also appears in the feces. Relatively high concentrations of the tetracyclines are found in the milk of nursing mothers, and this can be a source of inadvertent drug administration to the infant.

The tetracyclines exhibit a greater incidence of undesirable side effects and toxic reactions when compared to the β-lactam antibiotics. Adverse reactions include: (1) an antianabolic effect, which is due to a small amount of inhibition of protein synthesis in the host cells and which leads to a negative nitrogen balance with increased excretion of nitrogenous compounds in the urine. In an otherwise healthy individual the antianabolic effect is of little or no consequence. However, in patients with impaired renal function tetracyclines can cause azotemia and acidosis, and therefore their use in such patients is not recommended. The degree of inhibition of protein synthesis in the host is concentration dependent and the topical application of high concentrations of tetracyclines will delay wound healing. (2) Hepatotoxicity with fatty infiltration of the liver and jaundice may occur in patients receiving large doses of tetracyclines. The highest incidence of hepatotoxicity occurs during pregnancy and fatalities have been reported. (3) Tetracyclines are deposited in the teeth and bones of the fetus and infant owing to their ability to chelate with calcium. Such accumulation of tetracyclines leads to possible teratogenic effects if administered early in pregnancy, a reversible decrease in the rate of bone growth, and a discoloration of the teeth and enamel hypoplasia. (4) Hematologic changes may also occur. Prolonged prothrombin time and delayed coagulation have been attributed to various mechanisms including alterations in the microbial flora of the gut with a consequent decrease in vitamin K synthesis, changes in the plasma lipoproteins, and chelation of plasma calcium. A few cases of thrombocytopenia and leukocytosis have also been reported following long-term tetracycline therapy. (5) Photosensitivity (that is, an increased sensitivity of the skin to the burning effect of sunlight) may develop following administration of any of the tetracyclines but is more frequent with demeclocycline and oxytetracycline. (6) Tetracyclines may cause gastrointestinal irritation with nausea, vomiting, diarrhea, epigastric distress, and so on. Concurrent ingestion of antacids should be avoided because of chelation of the tetracycline with the antacid. If administration of antacids is necessary, ingestion of the drugs should be at different times. (7) Hypersensitivity reactions may also develop, but allergy to tetracyclines is less common than that to penicillin. Cross-hypersensitivity exists between all tetracyclines.

Chloramphenicol, a broad-spectrum antibiotic, reversibly binds to bacterial ribosomes, producing a bacteriostatic effect. It is well-absorbed, both orally and parenterally, and is well distributed throughout the body. Metabolism is primarily via conjugation with glucuronic acid, and the inactive glucuronide is excreted by the kidneys along with a small fraction of unmetabolized drug. Serious adverse reactions (for example, bone marrow depression, aplastic anemia) limit the use of this drug.

Lincomycin and its derivative, clindamycin, are narrow-spectrum antibiotics that are effective against some, but not all, anaerobic bacteria (for example, some types of bacteroides and anaerobic streptococcus). Lincomycin is only partially absorbed from the gastrointestinal tract,

while clindamycin is more completely absorbed. Both drugs are well absorbed via all parenteral routes of administration. Both drugs are well distributed throughout the body, and high concentrations are found in bone. Therefore these antibiotics are among the drugs of choice for treating chronic osteomyelitis. Clindamycin is extensively metabolized by N-dealkylation and sulfoxidation presumably catalyzed by hepatic mixed-function oxidases, and the metabolites are excreted in the urine and bile. Lincomycin is not metabolized to any great extent and is excreted primarily by the hepatic biliary route. Gastrointestinal toxicity to lincomycin and clindamycin ranges from simple gastrointestinal irritation with diarrhea to pseudomembranous colitis (Smart et al., 1976). Diarrhea and colitis may develop during drug therapy or up to several weeks after termination. The FDA has suggested that the use of lincomycin and clindamycin be reserved for serious infections in which the use of less toxic antibiotics is inappropriate.

The macrolides are a group of structurally related antibiotics that include erythromycin, spiramycin, and oleandomycin. They are narrow-spectrum antibiotics that reversibly bind to bacterial ribosomes. Erythromycin is only moderately stable in acid, and prolonged exposure to gastric acid, as a result of delayed gastric emptying, reduces the absorption of active drug. Erythromycin estolate possesses greater acid stability and is better absorbed following oral administration. However, the estolate has no antibacterial activity and must be hydrolyzed to yield erythromycin.

Erythromycin is eliminated primarily by biliary excretion. Preexisting liver disease or any impairment in hepatic function can lead to diminished rates of elimination and consequent accumulation of the drug. A history of hepatic disease constitutes an absolute contraindication to the use of the estolate ester since this form of erythromycin has been associated with a relatively high incidence of cholestatic jaundice. The incidence of toxic and serious hypersensitivity reactions among other erythromycin preparations is low.

Streptomycin, gentamicin, kanamycin, and neomycin constitute the aminoglycoside antibiotics. Toxicity and rapid development of bacterial resistance limit the use of this group of antibiotics to the treatment of serious gram-negative bacterial infections. Streptomycin is bactericidal at high concentrations and is one of the few antibiotics that does not antagonize the antibacterial action of the penicillins.

Drugs affecting intermediary metabolism

The sulfonamides are a group of antibacterial agents that are structurally similar to para-aminobenzoic acid (PABA) and compete with PABA in the bacterial synthesis of dihydrofolic acid (Figs. 5-9 and 5-10) Mammalian cells utilize preformed dietary folate, and thus the folic acid metabolism of the host is not affected. Sulfadiazine is a prototype of this group. It is well absorbed following oral administration and is distributed throughout the body, including diffusion across the blood-brain barrier, which results in therapeutic drug levels in the CNS. Metabolism is principally via hepatic N-acetylation, and although the metabolite exhibits no antibacterial activity, it retains some of the toxic properties of the parent compound. Both the metabolite and the unmetabolized drug are excreted by the kidneys. Most sulfonamides are poorly soluble in aqueous media and may precipitate out of the urine during concentration of the urine in the distal tubules and collecting ducts.

Sulfanilamide

PABA

Tetrahydrofolic acid

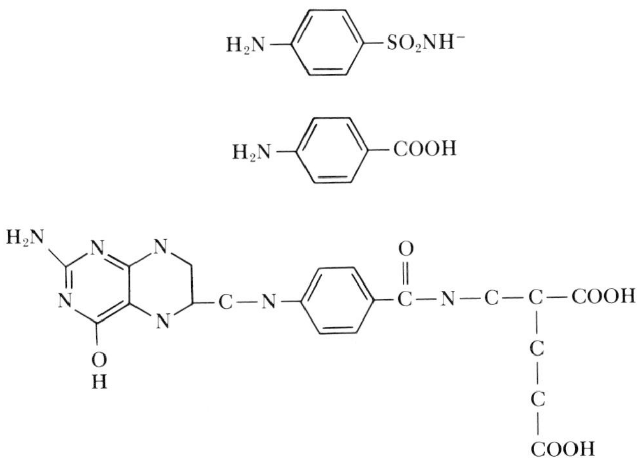

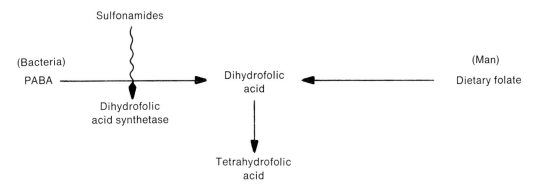

Fig. 5-9. Structural relationships between sulfonamides, para-aminobenzoic acid, and folic acid.

Fig. 5-10. Bacterial and human folate metabolism and site of action of sulfonamides.

Deposition of precipitates in the kidneys and ureters may lead to irritation, obstruction, and renal damage. Renal and hematopoietic toxicity, hypersensitivity reactions, and fairly rapid development of bacterial resistance limit the use of this class of antimicrobial agents.

Factors in antimicrobial therapy

The clinical course of an infection is determined by the balance between the natural resistance of the host and the maintenance of therapeutic levels of an appropriate antimicrobial drug, and the microorganism, its virulence, and sensitivity to antimicrobial agents. The resistance of the host is an important factor during therapy with both bacteriostatic and bactericidal drugs. Host resistance is determined by: (1) local factors, for example, trauma, clot retention, wound closure, and surgical interventions (drainage, débridement, and closure of sinus tracts or fistulas); and (2) systemic factors, for example, electrolyte and nutritional status, hematologic and immunologic status (leukemia, agranulocytosis, immunosuppressants and cytotoxic drugs are all associated with reduced host resistance), and hormonal balance (excess corticosteroids or uncontrolled diabetes also reduce host resistance).

The development of bacterial resistance (that is, a decrease in the sensitivity of a microorganism to a particular antimicrobial agent) is a continual problem in antimicrobial therapy. The most common mechanism of development of resistance is selection. The sensitivity of a strain of microorganisms to an antimicrobial agent is characterized by a normal distribution ranging from very sensitive to relatively insensitive. The inappropriate use of an antimicrobial drug will eliminate the sensitive portion of the population, allowing the relatively insensitive (resistant) microorganisms to predominate. To retard the appearance of resistance by selection, it is important to maintain sufficient drug levels for an adequate period of time, thus allowing the host defense mechanisms to eliminate the relatively insensitive members of the population. The duration of drug therapy should be long enough to eradicate the invading pathogen completely but not so long as to induce toxic effects or superinfections.

REFERENCES

Asatoor, A. M. 1963. The excretion of pethidine and its derivatives, Br. J. Pharmacol. **20:**285.

Barnes, J. M., and Davies, D. R. 1951. Blood cholinesterase levels in workers exposed to organophosphorus insecticides, Br. Med. J. **2:**816.

Barr, W. H., Adir, J., and Garrettson, L. 1971. Decrease of tetracycline absorption in man by sodium bicarbonate, Clin. Pharmacol. Ther. **12:**779.

Baselt, R. C., and Casarett, L. J. 1972. Urinary excretion of methadone in man. Clin. Pharmacol. Ther. **13:**64.

Bender, I. B., Pressman, R. S., and Tashman, S. G. 1953. Studies on excretion of antibiotics in human saliva. I. Penicillin and streptomycin, J. Am. Dent. Assoc. **46:**164.

Blumer, J., Strong, J. M., and Atkinson, A. J. 1973. The convulsant potency of lidocaine and its N-dealkylated metabolites, J. Pharmacol. Exp. Ther. **186:**31.

Boobis, S. W. 1977. Alterations of plasma albumin in relation to decreased drug binding in uremia. Clin. Pharmacol. Ther. **22:**147.

Borowitz, J. L., et al. 1971. Mechanism of enhanced drug effects produced by dilution of the oral dose, Toxicol, Appl. Pharmacol. **19:**164.

Braid, D. P., and Scott, D. B. 1965. The systemic absorption of local analgesic drugs, Br. J. Anaesth. **37:**394.

Breckenridge, A., and Orme, M. 1971. Clinical implications of enzyme induction, Ann. N. Y. Acad. Sci. **179:**421.

Brodie, B. B., Papper, E. M., and Mark, L. C. 1950. Fate of procaine in man and properties of its metabolite diethylaminoethanol, Curr. Res. Anesth. Analg. **20:**29.

Brooks, S. M., et al. 1972. Adverse effects of phenobarbital on corticosteroid metabolism in patients with bronchial asthma, N. Engl. J. Med. **286:**1125.

Brunk, S. F., Delle, M., and Wilson, W. R. 1973. Morphine metabolism in man: effect of aspirin, Clin. Pharmacol. Ther. **15:**283.

Burney, R. G., and DiFazio, C. A. 1976. Hepatic clearance of lidocaine during N_2O anesthesia in dogs, Anesth. Analg. **55:**322.

Carter, D. E., et al. 1975. Effect of oral contraceptives on plasma clearance, Clin. Pharmacol. Ther. **18:**700.

Carter, D. E., et al. 1974. Effect of oral contraceptives on drug metabolism, Clin. Pharmacol. Ther. **15:**22.

Cascorbi, H. F., Blake, D. A., and Helrich, M. 1970. Differences in biotransformation of halothane in man, Anesthesiology **32:**119.

Chang, T., et al. 1970. Metabolic disposition of tritium-labelled ketamine (Ketalar®; Cl-581) in normal human subjects, Clin. Res. **18:**597.

Chang, T., and Glazko, A. J. 1972. A gas chromatographic assay for ketamine in human plasma, Anesthesiology **36:**401.

Chenoweth, M. B., et al. 1962. Blood and tissue levels of ether, chloroform, halothane, and methoxyflurane in dogs, Anesthesiology **23**:101.

Chignell, C. F., and Starkweather, D. K. 1971. Optical studies of drug-protein complexes. V. The interation of phenylbutazone, flufenamic acid, and dicoumarol with acetylsalicylic acid-treated human serum albumin, Mol. Pharmacol. **7**:229.

Cohen, M. L., et al. 1973. Distribution in the brain and metabolism of ketamine in the rat after intravenous administration, Anesthesiology **39**:370.

Cohen, M. L., and Trevor, A. J. 1974. On the cerebral accumulation of ketamine and the relationship between metabolism of the drug and its pharmacologic effects, J. Pharmacol. Exp. Ther. **189**:351.

Conney, A. H. 1967. Pharmacological implications of microsomal enzyme induction, Pharmacol. Rev. **19**:317.

Corbett, T. H. 1976. Cancer and congenital anomalies associated with anesthetics, Ann. N. Y. Acad. Sci. **271**:58.

Cousins, M. J., et al. 1974. The etiology of methoxyflurane toxicity, J. Pharmacol. Exp. Ther. **190**:530.

Crawford, J. S., and Rudofsky, S. 1966. Some alterations in the pattern of drug metabolism associated with pregnancy, oral contraceptives, and the newly born, Br. J. Anaesth. **38**:446.

Crue, B. L. 1975. Pain research and treatment, New York, Academic Press, Inc.

Cuthbert, M. F., ed. 1973. The prostaglandins: pharmacologic and therapeutic advances, Philadelphia, J. B. Lippincott Co.

Davies, D. S., and Thorgeirsson, S. S. 1971. Mechanism of hepatic drug oxidation and its relationship to individual differences in rates of oxidation in man, Ann. N. Y. Acad. Sci. **179**:411.

Difazio, C. A., and Brown, R. E. 1972. Lidocaine metabolism in normal and phenobarbital-pretreated dogs, Anesthesiology **36**:238.

DiPalma, J. R., ed. 1965. Drill's pharmacology in medicine, ed 3., New York, McGraw-Hill Book Co.

Domino, E. F. 1968. Effects of narcotic analgesics on sensory input, activating system and motor output. In Wikler, A., ed.: The addictive states, Baltimore, The Williams & Wilkins Co.

Domino, E. F., Chodoff, P., and Corssen, G. 1965. Pharmacologic effects of Cl-581, a new dissociative anesthetic, in man, Clin. Pharmacol. Ther. **6**:279.

Ehrnebo, M., and Odar-Cederlof, I. 1975. Binding of amobarbital, pentobarbital and diphenylhydantoin to blood cell and plasma proteins in healthy volunteers and uraemic patients, Eur. J. Clin. Pharmacol. **8**:445.

Ehrnebo, M., Boreus, L. O., and Lonroth, U. 1977. Bioavailability and first-pass metabolism of oral pentazocine in man, Clin. Pharmacol. Ther. **22**:888.

Elliot, E., et al. 1976. Ketamine anesthesia for medical procedures in children, Arch. Dis. Child. **51**:56.

Ferreira, S. H. 1972. Prostaglandins, aspirin-like drugs, and analgesia. Nature [New Biol.]**240**:200.

Ferreira, S. H., and Vane, J. R. 1974. New aspects of the mode of action of nonsteroid anti-inflammatory drugs, Annu. Rev. Pharmacol. **14**:57.

Ferstandig, L. L. 1978. Trace concentrations of anesthetic gases: a critical review of their disease potential. Anesth. Analg. **57**:328.

Foldes, F. F., and Rhodes, D. H., Jr. 1953. The role of plasma cholinesterase in anesthesiology, Anesth. Analg. **32**:305.

Foldes, F. F., et al. 1953. Substrate competition between procaine and succinylcholine diiodide for plasma cholinesterase, Science **117**:383.

Foldes, F. F., et al. 1956. Comparison of the respiratory effects of suxamethonium and suxethonium in man, Anesthesiology **17**:559.

Frederickson, R. C., and Norris, F. H. 1976. Enkephalin-induced depression of single neurons in brain areas with opiate receptors — antagonism by naloxone, Science **194**:440.

Goldberg, M. A., Barlow, C. F., and Roth, L. J. 1961. The effects of carbon dioxide on the entry and accumulation of drugs in the central nervous system, J. Pharmacol. Exp. Ther. **131**:308.

Goldstein, A. 1976. Opioid peptides (endorphins) in pituitary and brain, Science **193**:1081.

Goldstein, A., Aronow, L., and Kalman, S. M. 1974. Principles of drug action: the basis of pharmacology, ed 2., New York, John Wiley & Sons.

Goodman, L. S., and Gilman, A., eds. 1975. The pharmacologic basis of therapeutics, ed 5., New York, Macmillan, Inc.

Gorter, E., and Grendel, F. 1925. On biomolecular layers of lipoids on the chromocytes of the blood, J. Exp. Med. **41**:439.

Gupta, N., Sarkissian, E., and Paulus, H. E. 1975. Correlation of plateau of serum salicylate level with rate of salicylate metabolism, Clin. Pharmacol. Ther. **18**:350.

Hahn, T. J., et al. 1972. Effect of chronic anticonvulsant therapy on serum 25-hydroxycalciferol levels in adults, N. Engl. J. Med **287**:900.

Hassler, R. 1968. Interrelationship of cortical and subcortical pain systems. In Lim, R. K. S., Armstrong, D., and Pardo, E. G., eds.: Pharmacology of pain, New York, Pergamon Press.

Hess, R., Stiebler, G., and Herz, A. 1972. Pharmacokinetics of fentanyl in man and the rabbit. Eur. J. Clin. Pharmacol. **4**:137.

Hogben, C. A. M., et al. 1957. Absorption of drugs from the stomach. II. The human, J. Pharmacol. Exp. Ther. **120**:540.

Hogben, C. A. M., et al. 1959. On the mechanism of intestinal absorption of drugs, J. Pharmacol. Exp. Ther. **125**:275.

Holaday, D. A., Rudofsky, S., and Treuhaft, P. S. 1970. The metabolic degradation of methoxyflurane in man. Anesthesiology **33**:579.

Hollunger, G. 1960a. On the metabolism of lidocaine. I. The properties of the enzyme system responsible for the oxidative metabolism of lidocaine, Acta Pharmacol. Toxicol. **17**:356.

Hollunger, G. 1960b. On the metabolism of lidocaine. II. The biotransformation of lidocaine, Acta Pharmacol. Toxicol. **17**:365.

Hollunger, G. 1960c. Some characteristics of an amide-hydrolyzing microsomal enzyme before and after its solubilization, Acta Pharmacol. Toxicol. **17**:384.

Horning, M. G., et al. 1975. Drug metabolism in the human neonate, Life Sci. **16**:651.

Howell, A., Sutherland, R., and Rolinson, G. N. 1972. Effect of protein binding on levels of ampicillin and cloxacillin in synovial fluid, Clin. Pharmacol. Ther. **13**:724.

Hurwitz, A., and Sheehan, M. B. 1971. The effects of antacids on the absorption of orally administered pentobarbital in the rat, J. Pharmacol. Exp. Ther. **179**:124.

Jelliffe, R. W., and Blankenhorn, D. H. 1966. Effect of phenobarbital on digitoxin metabolism, Clin. Res. **14**:160.

Kalow, W. 1952. Hydrolysis of local anesthetics by human serum cholinesterase, J. Pharmacol. Exp. Ther. **104**:122.

Kampman, J., et al. 1972. Effect of some drugs on penicillin half-life in blood. Clin. Pharmacol. Ther. **13**:516.

Keenaghan, J. B., and Boyes, R. N. 1972. The tissue distribution, metabolism and excretion of lidocaine in rats, guinea pigs, dogs and man. J. Pharmacol. Exp. Ther. **180**:454.

Keeri-Szanto, M., and Pomeroy, J. R. 1971. Atmospheric pollution and pentazocine metabolism, Lancet **1**:947.

Klaassen, C. D., and Plaa, G. L. 1968. Studies on the mechanism of phenobarbital enhanced sulfobromophthalein disappearance, J. Pharmacol. Exp. Ther. **161**:361.

Kojima, S., Smith, R. B., and Doluisio, J. T. 1971. Drug absorption. V. Influence of food on oral absorption of phenobarbital in rats, J. Pharm. Sci. **60**:1639.

Kraus, F. W., Casey, D. W., and Johnson, V. 1951. Aureomycin and terramycin in human saliva, Proc. Soc. Exp. Biol. Med. **78**:554.

Kunin, C. M. 1967. Clinical significance of protein binding of the penicillins, Ann. N. Y. Acad. Sci. **145**:282.

Kunin, C. M., et al. 1973. Influence of binding on the pharmacologic activity of antibiotics, Ann. N. Y. Acad. sci. **226**:214.

LaDu, B. N., Mandel, H. G., and Way, E. L., eds. 1971. Fundamentals of drug metabolism and drug disposition, Baltimore, The Williams & Wilkins Co.

Leonards, J. R. 1963. The influence of solubility on the rate of gastrointestinal absorption of aspirin, Clin. Pharmacol. Ther. **4**:476.

Levine, W. G. 1978. Biliary excretion of drugs and other xenobiotics, Annu. Rev. Pharmacol. Toxicol. **18**:81.

Levy, G. 1971. Drug biotransformation interactions in man: non-narcotic analgesics, Ann. N. Y. Acad. Sci. **179**:32.

Levy, G., Vogel, A. W., and Amsel, L. P. 1969. Capacity-limited salicylurate formation during prolonged administration of aspirin to healthy human subjects, J. Pharm. Sci. **58**:503.

Liebeskind, J. C., and Paul, L. A. 1977. Psychological and physiological mechanism of pain, Annu. Rev. Psychol. **28**:41.

Lim, R. K. S. 1968. Neuropharmacology of pain and analgesia. In Lim, R. K. S., Armstrong, D., and Pardo, E. G., eds.: Pharmacology of pain, New York, Pergamon Press.

Lim, R. K. S. 1970, Pain, Annu. Rev. Physiol. **32**:269.

Lo, J. N., and Cumming, J. F. 1975. Interaction between sedative premedicants and ketamine in man and in isolated perfused rat livers. Anesthesiology **43**:307.

Lunde, P. K. M., et al. 1970. Plasma protein binding of diphenylhydantoin in man, interaction with other drugs and the effect of temperature and plasma dilution, Clin. Pharmacol. Ther. **11**:846.

Marietta, M. P., et al. 1976. Biodisposition of ketamine in the rat self-induction of metabolism, J. Pharmacol. Exp. Ther. **196**:536.

Mayer, D. J., and Price, D. D. 1976. Central nervous systems mechanisms of analgesia. Pain **2**:379.

Mazze, R. I., Shue, G. L., and Jackson, S. H. 1971. Renal dysfunction associated with methoxyflurane anesthesia: a randomized prospective clinical evaluation, J. A. M. A. **216**:278.

Mazze, R. I., Trudell, J. R., and Cousins, M. J. 1971. Methoxyflurane metabolism and renal dysfunction: clinical correlation in man, Anesthesiology **35**:247.

Mazze, R. I., Cousins, M. J., and Kosek, J. C. 1972. Dose-related methoxyflurane nephrotoxicity in rats: a biochemical and pathological correlation, Anesthesiology **36**:571.

Mazze, R. I., Cousins, M. J., and Kosek, J. C. 1973. Strain differences in metabolism and susceptibility to the nephrotoxic effects of methoxyflurane in rats, J. Pharmacol. Exp. Ther. **184**:481.

Mazze, R. I., Hitt, B. A., and Cousins, M. J. 1974. Effect of enzyme induction with phenobarbital on the in vivo and in vitro defluorination of isoflurane and methoxyflurane, J. Pharmacol. Exp. Ther. **190**:523.

Melzack, P., and Wall, P. D. 1965. Pain mechanisms: a new theory, Science **150**:971.

Miller, R. R. 1977. Effects of smoking on drug action, Clin. Pharmacol. Ther. **22**:749.

Munson, E. S., et al. 1975. Fluroxene toxicity induced by phenobarbital, Clin. Pharmacol. Ther. **18**:687.

Neuvonen, P. J., and Penttila, O. 1974. Interaction between doxycycline and barbiturates, Br. Med. J. **1**:535.

O'Malley, K., Crooks, J., and Duke, E. 1971. Effect of age and sex on human drug metabolism, Br. Med. J. **3**:607.

O'Malley, K., Stevenson, I. H., and Crooks, J. 1972. Impairment of human drug metabolism by oral contraceptive steroids, Clin. Pharmacol. Ther. **13**:552.

Oyama, T., ed. 1973. Neuroleptanesthesia. Int. Anesthesiol. Clin., vol. 11, no. 3, Fall.

Pantuck, E. J., et al. 1974. Effect of cigarette smoking on phenacetin metabolism, Clin. Pharmacol. Ther. **15**:9.

Pearson, G. R., Bogan, J. A., and Sanford, J. 1973. An increase in the half-life of pentobarbitone with the administration of halothane in sheep, Br. J. Anaesth. **45**:586.

Penttila, O., et al. 1974. Interaction between doxycycline and some antiepileptic drugs, Br. Med. J. **2**:470.

Quayle, A. A., and Whitmarsh, V. B. 1972. Mixed salivary levels of clindamycin following single dose oral administration, Br. J. Oral Surg. **10**:24.

Ramwell, P. W., and Pharris, B. B. 1972. Prostaglandins in cellular biology, New York, Plenum Press.

Rehder, K., et al. 1967. Halothane biotransformation in man: a quantitative study, Anesthesiology **28**:711.

Reidenberg, M. M., James, M., and Dring, L. G. 1972. The rate of procaine hydrolysis in serum of normal subjects and diseased patients, Clin. Pharmacol. Ther. **13**:279.

Reidenberg, M. M., and Affrime, M. 1973. Influence of disease on binding of drugs to plasma proteins, Ann. N. Y. Acad. Sci. **226**:115.

Remmer, H. 1972. Induction of drug metabolizing enzyme system in the liver, Eur. J. Clin. Pharmacol. **5**:116.

Reynolds, E. S., and Moslen, M. T. 1977. Halothane hepatotoxicity: enhancement by polychlorinated biphenyl pretreatment, Anesthesiology **47**:19.

Richens, A., and Rowe, D. J. F. 1970. Disturbance of calcium metabolism by anticonvulsant drugs, Br. Med. J. **4**:73.

Robertson, J. D. 1960. The molecular structure and contact relationship of cell membranes, Prog. Biophys. Chem. **10**:343.

Rocha e Silva, M. 1970. Kinin hormones, Springfield, Ill., Charles C Thomas, Publisher.

Ross, W. T., and Cardell, R. R. 1978. Proliferation of smooth endoplasmic reticulum and induction of microsomal drug-metabolizing enzymes after ether or halothane, Anesthesiology **48**:325.

Saidman, L. J., et al. 1967. Minimum alveolar concentrations of methoxyflurene, halothane, ether and cyclopropane in man: correlation with theories of anesthesia. Anesthesiology **28**:994.

Salgado, A. S. 1961. Potentiation of succinylcholine by procaine, Anesthesiology **22**:897.

Sander, G. E., and Huggins, C. G. 1972. Vasoactive peptides, Annu. Rev. Pharmacol. **12**:227.

Schleimer, R., et al. 1978. Pharmacokinetics of fentanyl as determined by radioimmunoassay, Clin. Pharmacol. Ther. **23**:188.

Seeman, P. 1972. The membrane actions of anesthetics and tranquilizers, Pharmacol. Rev. **24**:583.

Sellers, E. M., and Koch-Weser, J. 1971. Kinetics and clinical importance of displacement of warfarin from albumin by acidic drugs, Ann. N. Y. Acad. Sci. **179**:213.

Shanor, S. P., et al. 1961. The influence of age and sex on human plasma and red cell cholinesterase, Am. J. Med. Sci. **242**:357.

Shoeman, D. W., Benjamin, D. M., and Azarnoff, D. L. 1973. The alteration of plasma proteins in uremia as reflected in the ability to bind dephenylhydantoin, Ann. N. Y. Acad. Sci. **226**:127.

Simon, E. J., and Hiller, J. M. 1978. Opiate receptors, Annu. Rev. Pharmacol. **18**:371.

Singer, S. J., and Nicolson, G. L. 1972. The fluid mosaic model of the structure of cell membranes, Science **175**:720.

Skovsted, L., et al. 1974. Inhibition of drug metabolism in man. In Morselli, P. L., Garattini, S., and

Cohen, S. N., eds. Drug interations, New York, Raven Press.

Smart, R. F., et al. 1976. Severe pseudomembranous colitis after lincomycin and clindomycin, Br. J. Surg. **63**:25.

Snyder, S. H., and Simantov, R. 1977. The opiate receptor and opioid peptides. J. Neurochem. **28**:13.

Solomon, H. M., et al. 1971. Interactions between digitoxin and other drugs in vitro and in vivo, Ann. N. Y. Acad. Sci. **179**:362.

Soudijn, W., Van Wijngaarden, I., and Allewijn, F. 1967. Distribution, excretion, and metabolism of neuroleptics of the butyrophenone type, Eur. J. Pharmacol. **1**:47.

Stier, A. 1968. The biotransformation of halothane, Anesthesiology **29**:388.

Strong, J. M., Parker, M., and Atkinson, A. J. 1973. Identification of glycinexylidide in patients treated with intravenous lidocaine, Clin. Pharmacol. Ther. **14**:67.

Strong, J. M., et al. 1975. Pharmacological activity, metabolism, and pharmacokinetics of glycinexylidide, Clin. Pharmacol. Ther. **17**:184.

Tan, J. S., et al. 1972. A method for measurement of antibiotics in human interstitial fluid, J. Infect. Dis. **126**:492.

Terenius, L. 1978. Endogenous peptides and analgesia, Annu. Rev. Pharmacol. Toxicol. **18**:189.

Thompson P. D., Rowland, M., and Melmon, K. L. 1971. The influence of heart failure, liver disease, and renal failure on the disposition of lidocaine in man, Am. Heart J. **82**:417.

Truitt, E. B., and Morgan, A. M. 1964. Gastrointestinal factors in aspirin absorption, J. Pharm. Sci. **53**:129.

Tucker, W. K., et al. 1973. Hepatorenal toxicity following fluroxene anesthesia, Anesthesiology **39**:104.

Udall, J. A. 1969. Drug interference with warfarin, Am. J. Cardiol. **23**:143.

Vanderkooi, G., and Green, D. E. 1970. Biological membrane structure. I. The protein crystal model for membranes, Proc. Nat. Acad. Sci. **66**:615.

Van Dyke, R. A. 1966. Metabolism of volatile anesthetics. III. Induction of microsomal dechlorinating and ether-cleaving enzymes, J. Pharmacol. Exp. Ther. **154**:364.

Van Dyke, R. A., and Chenoweth, M. B. 1965. The metabolism of volatile anesthetics. II. In vitro metabolism of methoxyflurane and halothane in rat liver slices and cell fractions, Biochem. Pharmacol. **14**:603.

Van Dyke, R. A., and Wineman, C. G. 1971. Enzymatic dechlorination: dechlorination of chloroethanes and propanes in vitro, Biochem. Pharmacol. **20**:463.

Verebely, K., and Inturrisi, C. E. 1974. Disposition of propoxyphene and norpropoxyphene in man after a single oral dose, Clin. Pharmacol. Ther. **15**:302.

Vesell, E. S. 1972. Pharmacogenetics, Pharmacology Society Symposium, Fed. Proc. **31**:1253.

Vesell, E. S., and Page, J. G. 1969. Genetic control of phenobarbital induced shortening of plasma antipyrine half-lives in man, J. Clin. Invest. **48:** 2202.

Waddell, W. J., and Butler, T. C. 1957. The distribution and excretion of phenobarbital, J. Clin. Invest. **36:**1217.

White, P. F., et al. 1976. Effects of halothane anesthesia on the biodisposition of ketamine in rats, J. Pharmacol. Exp. Ther. **196:**545.

Widger, L. A., Gandolfi, A. J., and Van Dyke, R. A. 1976. Hypoxia and halothane metabolism *in vivo:* release of inorganic fluoride and halothane metabolite binding to cellular constituents, Anesthesiology **44:**197.

Wilhelm, D. L. 1971. Kinins in human disease, Annu. Rev. Med. **22:**63.

Wilson, J. T., Atwood, G. F., and Shand, D. G. 1976. Disposition of propoxyphene and propranolol in children, Clin. Pharmacol. Ther. **19:**264.

Yaksh, T. L., and Rudy, T. A. 1978. Narcotic analgetics: CNS sites and mechanism of action as revealed by intracerebral injection techniques, Pain **4:**299.

Yoshimura, N., Holaday, D. A., and Fiserova-Bergerova, V. 1976. Metabolism of methoxyflurane in man, Anesthesiology **44:**372.

CHAPTER 6

Immunobiology

Fred G. Emmings

From a science primarily concerned with resistance to infection, immunology has grown to embrace the knowledge fundamental to the solution of a broad range of human biologic problems. This includes transfusion of blood, transplantation of tissues, diagnosis of many diseases, and understanding the pathogenesis of numerous disorders that have previously been only poorly understood. Every surgical endeavor affects or is affected by immunobiologic mechanisms. Therefore, a clear understanding of immunobiologic principles is essential to the intelligent practice of modern oral and maxillofacial surgery.

Preservation of the species is frequently dependent on the recognition of foreign material and the activation of mechanisms to resist the harmful effects of those substances. These protective mechanisms can be divided into two categories: (1) nonspecific resistance or inflammation, which is genetically determined, and (2) specific or adaptive resistance, which has its roots in the genetic composition of the host but also depends to a large extent on environmental influences such as previous contact with a foreign substance. It is important to remember that these two categories of defense mechanisms, inflammation and immunity, are intimately interrelated at many important functional interfaces. The events that characterize both cellular and humoral immune responses profoundly influence the process of inflammation and vice versa.

INFLAMMATION
Vascular phase

The inflammatory response consists of two phases, vascular and cellular. Whatever the nature or intensity of the insult, there is first a vascular response, which reaches a peak in 5 to 10 minutes. This response takes place in the terminal arterioles, capillaries, postcapillary venules, and arteriovenous shunts at the terminus of the vascular bed and is mediated by vasoactive substances such as histamine that are released from tissue mast cells lying in close proximity to these vessels. Histamine directly causes constriction of postvenular sphincters and indirectly mediates dilation of arterioles in the vicinity by local sensory nerve stimulation acting through an antidromic reflex arc. Histamine also causes the endothelial cells of venules to become more spherical, resulting in gaps between the membranes of neighboring cells. Other mediators called "kinins" are split from serum protein substrates (kininogens) by enzymes (kininogenases or kallikreins). One of these, bradykinin, acts much like histamine. The kinins in general are the most potent known contractors of venular endothelial cells.

Constriction of venular sphincters and dilation of arterioles result in decreased blood flow with stasis, hypoxia, acidosis, and increased capillary and venular hydrostatic pressures. The elevated local intravascular pressure and disrupted endothelial intercellular junctions result in transudation of plasma into the peri-

215

vascular space. Loss of fluid to the extra-vascular space results in hemoconcentration, increased blood viscosity, and further decrease in flow rate. Early transudation across the wall of the venule characterizes a short phase of the vascular response immediately following the initial, hyperemic phase.

Included in the extravasated plasma proteins is Hageman factor (XII), which can be activated by contact with a number of different molecular surfaces including antigen-antibody complexes, collagen, and basement membrane. Several fragments of activated Hageman factor have enzymatic activity that includes: (1) activation of plasma thromboplastin antecedent factor (XI); (2) the conversion, in the presence of a cofactor, of plasminogen to plasmin, which is further capable of activating complement components to generate their wide variety of phlogistic fragments; and (3) conversion of kininogenase from its precursor, which in turn increases the liberation of kinins resulting in increased vascular permeability. Activated Hageman factor is a key substance in that it represents an intersection of four systems important in host response to injury: (1) blood clotting, (2) fibrinolysis, (3) complement activation, and (4) kinin liberation (Fig. 6-1).

Cellular phase

Changes in vasomotor tone and permeability are closely followed by events involving the cellular elements of inflammation. The normal balance of forces tending to repel blood cells from the endothelium is altered in a way that promotes adherence. Following adherence, leukocytes migrate through the

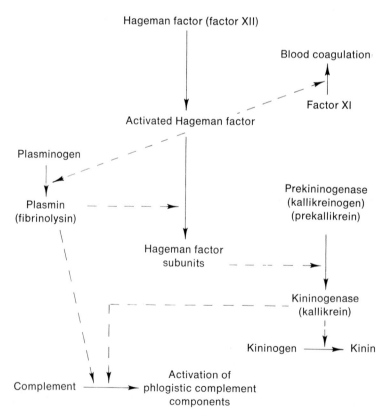

Fig. 6-1. Role of Hageman factor in interrelationship of clotting, kinin, fibrinolysis, and complement systems. (From Bach, F. H., and Good, R. A. 1972. Clinical immunology, vol. 1, New York, Academic Press, Inc.)

vessel wall into the area of injury. The dynamics of the vascular and cellular phases relative to one another are largely dependent on the nature, intensity, and chronicity of the injury and their interrelationships are often indistinct. Polymorphonuclear leukocytes, predominantly neutrophils, and mononuclear phagocytes are the most common cell types found in areas of acute inflammation. The variable histologic characteristics of delayed hypersensitivity and chronic inflammatory reactions may largely be explained by different blends of the chemical mediators involved. The mechanisms responsible for accumulation in a lesion of either bone-marrow derived (B) or thymus-dependent (T) lymphocytes are not fully understood. It has been demonstrated that T-cells undergo blastogenesis and division on contact with antigen and that B-cells bind firmly to specific antigens via receptors on their surfaces. Whether these mechanisms play a role in the immobilization of lymphocytes at sites of injury is not clear. Plasma cells are found late in the development of the inflammatory lesion and may represent the differentiated progeny of lymphoblasts that migrated to the area prior to cell division.

Many other substances have been shown to be important in mediating the events characteristic of inflammation (Weissman, 1974) (Table 6-1). Lymphokines are released from sensitized lymphocytes following exposure to the sensitizing antigen. These are of special importance in cell-mediated, delayed hypersensitivity reactions. Among the lymphokines are factors that can influence macrophages, are chemotactic for several types of leukocytes, and can induce proliferation of lymphocytes. Two factors affecting macrophages, migration inhibition factor (MIF) and macrophage activating factor (MAF), inhibit the migration of macrophages and activate cellular phagocytic mechanisms. Prostaglandins, a ubiquitous series of lipids, exhibit a wide range of effects on blood vessels and smooth muscle but their role is yet largely undefined. Enzymes are also released from lysosomes found in the cytoplasm of leukocytes. These may directly cause tissue damage or act indirectly by generating chemotactic factors from appropriate substrates.

Control of inflammation

There are a multitude of internal and external factors that alter the nonspecific

Table 6-1. Mediators of inflammation*

Agent	Chemical nature	Origin
Histamine, serotonin	Amine (stored)	Basophil, mast cell, platelets
Slow reacting substance of anaphylaxis (SRS-A)	Acid lipid	Leukocyte
Kinins	Polypeptides (split products)	Plasma substrate
Prostaglandins	Acid lipids (newly synthesized)	Ubiquitous intracellular precursors
Plasmin	Protease (split product)	Plasma substrate (liver)
Hageman factor (activated)	Protease	
Complement	Plasma proteins and split products	Reticuloendothelial cells, liver
Lysosomal enzymes	Intracellular proteins (stored)	PMN's, macrophages, mast cells
Lymphokines	Intracellular proteins (newly synthesized)	Stimulated lymphocytes

*From Weissman, G. 1974. Mediators of inflammation, New York, by permission of Plenum Press.

host response and change the course of the inflammatory process (Table 6-2). Genetic constitution determines the synthesis of all body constituents, and differences in susceptibility to certain diseases have been associated with specific genotypes. Racial and individual differences have been shown such as the high susceptibility to tuberculosis of the American Indian and black races compared with Caucasians. The primary immunologic deficiency diseases represent failures of lymphoid function and are genetically determined. Among these are the agammaglobulinemias, ataxia telangiectasia, and DiGeorge's syndrome. Some defects, such as fatal granulomatosis of childhood, are characterized by profoundly altered inflammatory responses.

Many endocrine hormones can exert an influence on the course of inflammation. Deficiencies in growth hormone and thyroid hormone have been associated with a reduction in resistance to infection. Administration of testosterone to recently adrenalectomized and gonadectomized animals causes an abnormality in neutrophil function that can be corrected by estrogen administration. The adrenal corticosteroids exercise the most pervading influence on host defenses of any of the hormones. Corticosteroid therapy affects not only nonspecific responses but immune responses as well. Steroids inhibit adherence of blood cells to endothelium, migration of cells into the perivascular space, and lysosomal digestion of phagocytized materials (Claman, 1972; Fauve, 1970; Mandell, Rubin, and Hook, 1970; Thompson and Van Furth, 1970). Cellular immune mechanisms are compromised by steroid-induced lymphopenia. Patients taking steroids are extremely susceptible to infection, falling prey to microorganisms normally not pathogenic. Secondary infections are common, and severe viral infections are often contract-

Table 6-2. Modifiers of inflammation*

Agent, treatment or disease	Effect on development of an inflammatory lesion and delivery of phagocyte	Effect on reticuloendothelial system	Effect on neutrophil function
Shock	↓ †	? †	N †
Vasopressors	↓	?	?
Foreign bodies	↓	N	N
Glucocorticoids	↓	↑ or ↓ †	↓
Estrogens	?	↑	N
Acute starvation	?	?	N
Multiple vitamin depletion	↓	?	?
Prematurity	↓	↓	↓
Old age	↓	N or ↓	N
X-irradiation	↓	↓	N or ↓
Nitrogen mustard	↓	↓	N
Anticomplement agents	↓	↓	↓
Diabetes	N or ↓	?	N or ↓
Burn injuries	↓	N or ↓	↓
Cancer	N or ↓	↑, N or ↓	N or ↓
Uremia	↓	?	N
Infection	N or ↓	Usually ↑	N
Alcohol intoxication	↓	?	N
Endotoxin	↓ or N	↑ or ↓	?
Pertussis vaccine	↓ or N	↑	?
BCG infection	?	↑	?
Zymosan, restim	?	↑	?
Fever	↑	N or ↑	N

*From Alexander, J., and Good, R. 1970. Immunobiology for surgeons, Philadelphia, by permission of W. B. Saunders Co.
†Symbols: ↑, increased or stimulated; ↓, decreased or depressed; N, no effect; ?, unknown or insufficiently evaluated.

ed owing largely to the defect in cellular immunity.

Pharmacologic agents are often used for control of inflammation. Besides corticosteroids these include salicylates, phenylbutazone, and indomethacin. In general, their mechanisms of anti-inflammatory action are only poorly understood, but they share several distinguishing features that may contribute to their observed effects. They are capable of inhibiting the actions of the inflammatory cells by: (1) direct inhibition of enzyme systems; they are also capable of combining with proteins other than enzymes to form stable complexes less susceptible to enzymatic degradation; for example, stabilization of complement components results in decreased generation of mediators of inflammation; (2) interference with energy metabolism; and (3) decreasing phagocytosis and motility. This last effect probably results from stabilization of the cell membranes by combination of the drug with membrane proteins. The same mechanism is responsible for an increase in stability of lysosomal membranes preventing release of their contents. These drugs are also capable of suppressing the synthesis and release of several mediators of inflammation such as the prostaglandins. There is a growing body of evidence (Vane, 1976) that inhibition of prostaglandin synthesis is the primary mechanism of therapeutic action of aspirin and aspirin-like compounds. This includes their anti-inflammatory, analgesic, and antipyretic effects.

Other drugs also have effects on the inflammatory response. The primary influence of antimetabolites and alkylating agents used for cancer therapy is through reduction of lymphocyte participation. Heparin and related compounds exhibit anticomplementary effects. Vasopressors suppress early hyperemia and thereby the subsequent development of the inflammatory lesion. All of these agents in some way interfere with the normal course of events characterizing inflammation and render the host more susceptible to infection.

Augmentation of nonspecific immunity may occur under the influence of a num-

ber of stimulators. Tuberculin stimulates phagocytosis, and intracellular killing of phagocytized material is increased because of elevated concentrations of lysosomal enzymes. The injection of tuberculin causes localization of immunocompetent cells at that site. The increase in immune responsiveness that results is thought to be partly responsible for the reported antitumor effect of tuberculin injections. Endotoxins are capable of increasing the number of circulating neutrophils, elevating serum titers of opsonizing antibody, and increasing rates of phagocytosis and intracellular killing in mononuclear phagocytes.

Elevated central body temperature, or fever, often accompanies infectious diseases or conditions that produce extensive tissue death. Although some bacterial products are known to elevate body temperature directly, infection and necrosis result in the lysis of many leukocytes that release substances demonstrated to be pyrogenic. Fever has been associated with increased efficiency of host protective functions but the mechanism of this effect is not known.

Cyclic changes in numbers of circulating neutrophils were demonstrated many years ago, but more recently transient changes in neutrophil function, that is, chemotaxis and phagocytosis, have also been reported. Suppressed neutrophil function alters the response to infectious agents resulting in increased susceptibility and tissue destruction. Currently it is hypothesized (Cianciola et al., 1977) that the etiology of idiopathic juvenile periodontitis (periodontosis) is at least partly attributable to diminished resistance to certain bacteria resulting from impaired neutrophil function.

Shock and other hypotensive states reduce tissue perfusion and greatly slow the development of the inflammatory lesion. Susceptibility to infection is increased because of the reduced number of leukocytes transported to the site of injury.

Diabetes mellitus appears to have little effect on inflammation except for a small reduction in intracellular bacteriolysis and for major alterations at those sites where circulation has been indirectly impaired by the disease. Uremic patients have been found more susceptible to bacterial infection. This appears to result from a general multilevel depression of all host defense mechanisms. Ethanol intoxication leads to a transient reduction of migration of phagocytic cells to the site of injury, thereby increasing susceptibility to infection.

Unless a malignancy directly involves the tissues producing inflammatory cells, no alterations in the course of inflammation are evident until late in the disease. Premature infants demonstrate multiple defects in resistance mechanisms of all types accompanied by increased susceptibility to infection. Neutrophil function, in particular, is severely impaired. Both general anesthesia and surgical insult adversely affect the inflammatory response. Exposure to ether anesthesia resulted in increasing interference with complement activity in animals up to 7 days following administration. Anesthetic agents (Bruce and Koepke, 1966) and surgical stress both appear to suppress granulopoiesis in the rat. Bruce (1973) showed a halothane inhibition of phagocytosis by neutrophils in the mouse that lasted only as long as the agent was administered. In subsequent studies 1% halothane was administered for 6 hours following injection of a challenge dose of Salmonella. Depression of neutrophil phagocytosis by halothane was associated with increased proliferation of the challenge organisms and more rapid death. Neutrophil function was not altered by either hypothermia or thiopental sedation.

IMMUNITY (Eisen, 1974; Fudenberg et al., 1976)

In contrast to inflammation, specific immunity implies an adaptive response to an antigenic determinant that results in the synthesis of proteins capable of reacting specifically with the determinant. Specific immunity is also characterized by the acquisition of immunologic memory evoking a secondary, or anamnestic, response on subsequent exposure to the antigen. Specific immunity is

found fully developed in vertebrates only.

Initially, immune responses were of interest to investigators only because of their capacity to protect against infectious diseases. However, specific responses can be induced to a seemingly limitless array of substances including the host's own body constituents, allografts, drugs, pollens, and many other noninfectious materials. Thus, there is now a great deal of interest in the pathologic effects mediated by the immune response as well as its protective functions. In fact, all special areas of clinical practice must be concerned with this protean adaptive response to understand the pathogenesis and prophylaxis of many diseases.

A fairly new, but quickly growing, body of evidence supports the notion that the immune response to specific antigens is under direct genetic control. In experimental animals and man there is evidence that these immune response (IR) genes are closely linked to the major histocompatibility complex. Statistically significant associations have been made between particular HLA genotypes and a variety of diseases including chronic active hepatitis, dermatitis herpetiformis, systemic lupus erythematosus and acute lymphocytic leukemia. The mechanisms by which these genes affect the immune response, susceptibility, or pathogenesis remain unresolved.

When an antigenic stimulus is presented to the lymphoid system, one or more of several types of responses can be elicited. The type of response is dependent on many factors including the chemical and physical nature of the antigen and the quantity and the route of its administration. These responses are divided into two general categories: the humoral, or antibody, response and the cellular, or delayed hypersensitivity, response.

Humoral immunity

Antigens are substances that are capable of stimulating the synthesis of antibodies that will react specifically with the stimulating antigen. Antigens are composed of one or more determinants, which are portions of the three-dimensional chemical structure of the antigen. Immunologic specificity is directly defined by these antigenic determinants. Antibodies are serum proteins synthesized in response to an antigen and capable of reacting specifically with an antigenic determinant. Antibodies are synthesized by cells derived from the bone marrow (perhaps via the gut-associated lymphoid tissue) and are designated B-cells. Antibodies belong to the group of serum proteins called γ-globulins and are referred to as immunoglobulins (Ig). There are five classes of immunoglobulins (Fig. 6-2) composed of heavy (H) and light (L) polypeptide chains.

Antibodies can perform protective functions by neutralizing or eliminating harmful antigens. Specific combination of the antibody molecule with antigen is dictated by the three-dimensional arrangement of amino acid sequences of adjacent H and L chain segments comprising the combining sites. The structure of these sites "fits," chemically and physically, the antigenic determinant to which it is directed. Combining sites are part of the Fab portion of the molecule (Fig. 6-2). Another portion of the Ig molecule is composed of segments of H chain whose chemical structure is relatively constant within an Ig class. The Fc portions contain the structures determining complement fixation, skin fixation, placental transfer, sensitization of mast cells, and Ig class.

It has been amply demonstrated that different classes of Ig mediate different biologic functions (Table 6-3). This intimate relationship of structure to function is important in understanding the operation of the immune system. IgE has been shown to be the class involved in the pathogenesis of immediate hypersensitivity reactions. Its cytophilic property, important to its role in allergic reactions, is conferred on IgE by the structure of its H chain. The beneficial biologic function of IgE has not been elucidated.

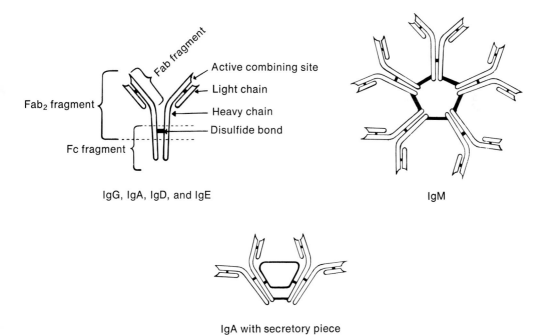

Fig. 6-2. Structures of five classes of immunoglobulins. Basic structural unit of all classes contains two heavy and two light polypeptide chains. IgA monomer is found primarily in serum, while dimer is the predominant immunoglobulin found in external secretions. Fragments referred to are obtained by digestion with proteolytic enzymes. (From Alexander, J., and Good, R. 1970. Immunobiology for surgeons, Philadelphia, W. B. Saunders Co.)

Table 6-3. Relationship of immunoglobulin structure and function

Property	IgG	IgA Serum	IgA Secretory	IgM	IgD	IgE*
Chemical						
Average concentration in normal serum (mg/ml)	13.4	3.9		1	0.03	0.0001
Molecular weight (X10^{-3})	150	160	370	900	180	197
Approximate sedimentation coefficient (S)	7	7	11	19	7	8
Biologic						
Earliest antibody detected in primary immune responses				+		
Predominant antibody in most late responses	+					
Secreted on mucous surfaces	±†	±†	+	±‡	?	±
Crosses placenta	+	−	−	−	−	−
Complement fixation	+	−	±§	+	−	−
Fix to homologous skin and mast cells for anaphylaxis	?	−	−	−	−	+
Bonds to macrophages (cytophilic)	+			+		

*Also called reagin.
†In inflammatory conditions

‡Often found in cases of selective IgA deficiency.
§By alternate pathway.

Secretory IgA is the predominant Ig in secretions from exocrine glands (for example, saliva, colostrum, tears) and is thought to provide the host with an important first line of defense (Tomasi, 1976). Secretory IgA contains two Ig molecules the size of serum IgA and, in addition, two extra polypeptide chains called secretory component (SC) and joining (J) chains. One of the functions of these two chains is to stabilize the dimer ensuring its functional integrity in environments that can inhibit antibody activity. A secretory immune response is most efficiently induced by a local stimulus that gives rise to a local response. Antibodies are synthesized in immunocompetent cells found in the parenchyma of glands or in the lamina propria underlying mucosal surfaces. Local immunization has been demonstrated to be effective in the prevention of diseases caused by viruses (poliovirus—Sabin vaccine) and bacteria, particularly those organisms that depend on adherence to tissue surfaces to cause disease. The secretory IgA molecule is particularly well suited to function on mucous surfaces such as the gastrointestinal tract, since it is the most resistant of all immunoglobulins to proteolytic digestion and is uniquely located to provide the initial protection against invading pathogens.

Complement (Lepow, 1971)

The complement system consists of a series of 11 distinct protein components found in plasma in an inactive form. This system serves primarily to augment, or amplify, the effects of antigen-antibody interactions. When activated, either by antigen-antibody complexes or by some other mechanism, the resultant products help facilitate immune adherence, phagocytosis, intracellular killing of bacteria, chemotaxis, cytolysis, and the release of vasoactive substances (Fig. 6-3). In addition to the classic pathway, the complement cascade may be initiated at C3 without involving C1, C4, and C2. Various initiators, for example, endotoxin and aggregated Ig, react with the properdin system in this "alternate pathway." Activated complement components are important in both inflammation and specific immunity. The interrelationship of the complement and kinin systems was illustrated in Fig. 6-1. Hereditary deficiencies of the complement system have been described in man (Table 6-4). While some of these have been associated with clinical disease, none have been clearly

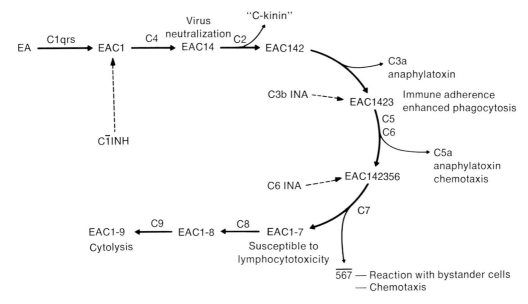

Fig. 6-3. Classic pathway of complement activation. *E,* Erythrocytes; *A,* antibody to erythrocytes; *C,* complement. Numbers represent different components; lower case letters represent subunits of components; *INH* and *INA* are designated control proteins. (From Spragg, J., and Gigli, I. 1975. In Mathieu, A., and Kahan, B. D. Immunologic aspects of anesthetic and surgical practice, New York, Grune & Stratton, Inc.)

Table 6-4. Hereditary complement deficiencies*

Deficiency	Associated clinical disease
C'1 esterase inhibitor	Hereditary angioneurotic edema
C'1q	Lymphopenic agammaglobulinemia
C'2	None
C'3 (probably a deficiency of inhibitor of C'3 inactivation)	Recurrent pulmonary and respiratory infection

*From Alexander, J., and Good, R. 1970. Immunobiology for surgeons, Philadelphia, by permission of W. B. Saunders Co.

correlated with an increased susceptibility to bacterial infection except the rare individual with depressed serum levels of C3 and C5. Some pharmacologic agents such as anti-inflammatory drugs and general anesthetics exhibit anticomplementary activity. Although the primary effect of the C system is protective, it can also cause tissue damage in conjunction with otherwise benign antigen-antibody complexes (Gigli and Austen, 1971; Lepow, 1972).

Effects of anesthesia and surgery

Studies examining the effects of surgery and/or general anesthesia on the humoral immune response are difficult to control. Responses are affected by possible previous contact with the immunogen, the general health of the subjects, pharmacologic agents used for premedication and anesthesia, and the character of the surgical procedure. Sheep erythrocytes (SRBC) are often used as a test antigen, since they are potent immunogens and there are several sensitive assays for detecting antibody to SRBC. One of these, the hemolytic plaque assay (Jerne et al., 1976), quantifies cells synthesizing antibodies by counting the clear regions of hemolysis around antibody-producing cells dispersed in an agar suspension of SRBC. Using this method it was shown (Kesztyus, Szilagyi, and Gyulai, 1954) that daily administration of long-acting barbiturates over several days depressed antibody synthesis. Rats exposed to N_2O

or 0.5% halothane 1 week after immunization with SRBC showed depressed numbers of plaque-forming cells compared with unanesthetized rats (Wingard, Lang, and Humphrey, 1967). Lower levels of serum antibodies were found in the halothane-treated rats. Dye exclusion tests (Humphrey, Wingard, and Lang, 1969) demonstrated no difference in viable immunocompetent cells between anesthetized and control animals, ruling out a cytotoxic effect of the anesthetic agents. In a later study, animals were anesthetized with ether and subjected to amputation of a limb 1 week after immunization with SRBC. No reduction in agglutinating antibody titers or in hemolytic plaques was found in the recovering rats. A more general method for measuring the responsiveness of the humoral immune system is to measure the proliferative capacity of the antibody-synthesizing B-cells. This can be done using nonspecific stimulators of cell division called mitogens, (such as pokeweed mitogen [PWM] or streptolysin-O [SLO]), which are known to stimulate blastogenesis in B-cells. All anesthetic agents depressed blastogenesis when circulating lymphocytes were tested (Jubert et al., 1973) 2 hours after induction of anesthesia. Ether depressed blastogenesis more than did halothane, and significant reduction still existed up to 10 postoperative days. These results can be interpreted to demonstrate interference by anesthetic agents in either the binding of mitogen to the cell, recognition of the mitogen, cell division, or a combination of these effects. Blood loss greater than 500 ml resulted in significant depression of blastogenic responses to two mitogens capable of stimulating both B- and T-cells.

The evidence concerning the effects of general anesthetics on the humoral immune response points to interference with efferent and central portions of the antibody response including antigen recognition, differentiation, proliferation, and initial antibody synthesis. However, there is not enough information to clearly delineate the specific effects of anesthetic agents on the primary immune response.

Detection and measurement of immune reactions: immunodiagnosis
(Rose and Bigazzi, 1973)

Two characteristic properties of immune reactions, sensitivity and specificity, make them very powerful tools for the diagnosis of disease. The older term "serodiagnosis" has been supplanted by immunodiagnosis because of the increased importance of the use of reactions of the cell-mediated variety.

Two fundamental varieties of antibody-mediated immunodiagnostic procedures are used: (1) antibodies with known specificity are used to determine the identity, distribution, or quantity of unknown or known antigens and (2) characterized antigens are used to determine either the presence and/or levels of unknown or known antibodies. Some of the more common tests used today and their respective sensitivities are listed in Table 6-5.

Precipitin reactions. Most antibodies are capable of combining with their antigens and precipitating them from solution. This is largely a function of the divalent (two combining sites) structure of the antibody molecule and depends on the presence of a macromolecular antigen with more than one antigenic determinant on its surface. Antibodies cross-

Table 6-5. Relative sensitivity of some immunodiagnostic procedures (expressed in milligrams antibody nitrogen—mg Ab N)*

Test	Mg, Ab N/ml, or test
Precipitin reactions	3-20
Immunoelectrophoresis	3-20
Double diffusion in agar gel	0.2-1.0
Complement fixation	0.01-0.1
Radial immunodiffusion	0.008-0.025
Bacterial agglutination	0.01
Hemolysis	0.001-0.03
Passive hemagglutination	0.005
Passive cutaneous anaphylaxis	0.003
Antitoxin neutralization	0.003
Antigen-combining globulin technique (Farr)	0.0001-0.001
Radioimmunoassay	0.0001-0.001
Virus neutralization	0.00001-0.0001
Bactericidal test	0.00001-0.0001

*From Alexander, J., and Good, R. 1970. Immunobiology for surgeons, Philadelphia, by permission of W. B. Saunders Co.

link antigen molecules to form large insoluble lattice networks. Excess antibody or excess antigen will result in incomplete precipitation of the reactants. Quantitative precipitation has been used for many years and is still the most dependable general method for determining antibody concentrations. Clinically, however, this reaction is now seldom used. Other types of precipitin reactions, such as the capillary tube precipitin test, are used to identify small quantities of biologic materials such as blood or semen. Precipitation in agar gel is largely used to qualitatively compare antigens for the presence of cross-reacting components. Opposing circular wells are cut in agar gel. Some are filled with solutions containing antigens, while antibodies are applied to opposite wells. These reactants diffuse through the gel toward each other and a precipitin band forms in the gel where they reach equivalent concen-

trations. Two examples of the clinical use of double diffusion in agar gel are to detect fetoprotein and hepatitis-associated antigen (HAA). In immunoelectrophoresis (Fig. 6-4) complex antigen mixtures are applied to agar gel and first separated on the basis of their electrophoretic mobility. Application of antiserum to a trough paralleling the line of electrophoretic migration results in precipitin bands forming between the line and the trough. Using immunoelectrophoresis, over 30 different antigens have been identified in human serum. Homogeneity of the serum proteins associated with plasma cell dyscrasias (for example, myelomas, macroglobulinemia) is often confirmed by this technique.

Radial immunodiffusion is accomplished in a layer of agar gel in which an antiserum specific for a single antigen has been incorporated. Wells are cut in the agar and the addition of antigen to the

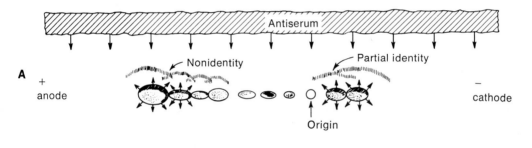

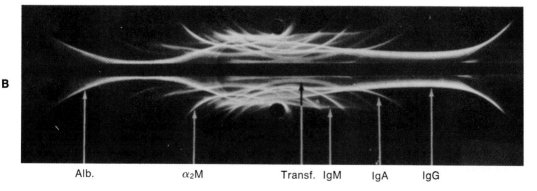

Fig. 6-4. Immunoelectrophoresis. **A,** Mixture of antigens is placed in well (origin) cut in layer of agar gel on glass slide. Electric current is applied to gel causing antigens to migrate to distance from origin dictated by their electrophoretic mobility. Antiserum is then added to trough and antigens and antibodies diffuse toward each other, each antigen-antibody precipitate forming single band. **B,** Human serum placed at origin; trough contains antiserum to whole human serum. (From Williams, C. 1974. In Eisen, H. N. Immunology, New York, Harper & Row, Publishers, Inc.)

well results in a ring of precipitation around it. The area of the ring is directly proportional to antigen concentration. A standard curve is established using known concentrations of antigen, which then allows quantitation of antigen in unknown solutions. This technique has proved diagnostically effective in measuring concentrations of serum proteins such as immunoglobulins in immune-deficiency diseases, haptoglobin in hemolytic anemia, and antitrypsin in chronic obstructive lung disease.

C-reactive protein appears in the blood of humans exposed to acute infection or suffering from inflammatory conditions accompanied by necrosis, for example, rheumatoid arthritis. It is probably a product of the necrotic process. Antiserum to C-reactive protein is prepared by the injection into rabbits of C substance, a polysaccharide obtained from pneumococcus. These antisera can then be used in precipitin tests to quantitate C-reactive protein in human serum.

The sensitivity of precipitin reactions is relatively low but can be increased by the use of special stains or by autoradiography using radiolabeled antigen or antibody.

Agglutination reactions. Agglutination reactions are similar to precipitation reactions except that antibody reacts with an insoluble, particulate antigen instead of a soluble molecule. These reactions are widely used to identify dissociated suspensions of cells such as strains of bacteria or erythrocyte types. Clumping of particles occurs when specific antibody is added in the presence of appropriate concentrations of salts.

Indirect or "passive" agglutination methods have been developed in which particulate carriers are sensitized by attaching soluble antigen molecules to their surfaces. The sensitized particles can then be agglutinated by antibodies to the sensitizing antigen. These techniques are considered very sensitive since the large size of the particle, with only a thin exterior coating of antigen, serves to amplify the reaction. Human erythrocytes (usually type O Rh-negative) or inert particles such as latex or bentonite are used as particulate carriers. Using the hemagglutination reaction, sensitized red blood cells are used as the carrier to detect antibodies to γ-globulins (rheumatoid factor), to penicillin, or to bacterial polysaccharides. Protein antigens usually will not adhere to the erythrocyte surface unless either the cell surface is modified, for example, with tannic acid, or the protein is chemically linked to the cell surface with agents such as bisdiazotized benzidine.

The Coombs, or antiglobulin, test is used to detect incomplete or "blocking" antibodies. These antibodies engage in a different type of blocking than that involved in enhancement of allograft survival. They bind to antigens on the cell surface but agglutination does not occur. Incomplete antibodies are often found in human sera containing antibodies to Rh antigens. For the Coombs test, antisera to human Ig are produced in other species. When these antisera are added to cells coated with incomplete antibody, agglutination occurs. Agglutination following addition of antiglobulin antibodies constitutes a positive Coombs reaction.

Hepatitis. The passive hemagglutination technique has been recently employed in the detection of hepatitis-associated antigen (HAA) and antibodies. Two percent of patients receiving 1 to 3 units of whole blood develop clinical hepatitis, while 50% of those receiving massive transfusions are afflicted. The association of hepatitis B surface antigen (Australia antigen; HB_sAg; HAA) (Table 6-6) with viral, type B (serum) hepatitis generated the development of methods for screening out one group of infected donors. However, insufficient sensitivity of the detection assays and the existence of etiologic agents of hepatitis other than type B virus (HBV) has limited the success of the screening procedure to a 25% reduction in posttransfusion hepatitis using blood from paid, screened donors. Current knowledge suggests that cytomegalovirus, Epstein-Barr virus, and hepatitis A virus (HAV, infectious hepatitis virus) all may be implicated in the etiology of non-B hepatitis. Development of screening techniques for antigens and antibodies associated with these agents is presently underway, and a radioimmunoassay for detection of HAV was recently reported by Hollinger and coworkers (1975). Still the most effective method for preventing posttransfusion hepatitis is the exclusive use of blood from voluntary donors and the use of frozen blood fractions.

Detection of hepatitis B surface antigen in the serum can be carried out by many methods (Table 6-7). Inhibition of passive hemagglutination combines the advantages of high sensitivity, speed, low cost, and use of only small amounts of reactants, and it has been widely used for epidemiologic studies of hepatitis B infection. A preparation of hepatitis B immune globulin (HBIG) has recently been licensed by the FDA for use in individuals accidentally exposed (needle prick, oral ingestion) to material containing HB_sAg. The hepatitis attack rate was reduced in HBIG recipients for several months after incidences of single acute exposure.

Table 6-6. Nomenclature of hepatitis antigens and antibodies*

Type	Description	Name	Abbreviation	Corresponding antibody (abbreviation)
B	22 nm spherical, filamentous forms, coat of Dane particle	Hepatitis B surface antigen	HB_s Ag	Anti-HB_s
	Core of Dane particle	Hepatitis B core antigen	HB_c Ag	Anti-HB_c
	Subtype of HB_s Ag			
	Group reactive	a	/a	anti- /a
	Type specific	d,y,w,r	/d,y,w,r	anti- /d,y,w,r
	Example	Surface antigen with group antigen a, d, and w subtype specificities	HB_s Ag/adw	anti-HB_s/adw
A	27-nm viruslike antigen	Hepatitis A antigen	HA Ag	anti-HA

*From Purcell, R. H. In Mathieu, A., and Kahan, B. D. 1975. Immunologic aspects of anesthetic and surgical practice, New York, by permission of Grune & Stratton, Inc.

Table 6-7. Techniques for measuring hepatitis antigens and antibodies*

Technique	Sensitivity		Ease of performance	Relative cost†	Time required for completion (hours)
	Antigen	Antibody			
Hepatitis, type B					
Immunodiffusion	Insensitive	Insensitive	Simple	Inexpensive	24-72
Counter-electrophoresis	Moderate	Moderate	Simple	Moderate	2.0
Complement fixation	Moderate	Moderate	Moderate	Inexpensive	2-24
Immune adherence	Sensitive	Moderate	Moderate	Inexpensive	2.0
Latex agglutination	Moderate	Moderate	Simple	Inexpensive	0.1-0.2
Agglutination-flocculation	Sensitive	—	Moderate	Inexpensive	0.5-1.0
Charcoal particle agglutination	Moderate	Moderate	Simple	Inexpensive	0.2-1
Passive hemagglutination	Moderate	Sensitive	Moderate	Inexpensive	2.0
Reversed passive hemagglutination	Sensitive	—	Moderate	Inexpensive	2.0-4.0
Radioimmunoassay	Sensitive	Sensitive	Moderate to complex	Expensive	4-120
Immune electron microscopy	Sensitive	Moderate	Complex	Expensive	2.0-4.0
Immunofluorescence	Moderate	Moderate	Complex	Moderate	2.0-4.0
Hepatitis, type A					
Immune electron microscopy	Sensitive	Moderate to sensitive	Complex	Expensive	2.0-4.0

*From Purcell, R. H. In Mathieu, A., and Kahan, B. D. 1975. Immunological aspects of anesthetic and surgical practice, New York, by permission of Grune & Stratton, Inc.
†Relative costs estimated for noncommercial reagents; use of commercial test kits will significantly increase the cost per test.

Blood typing. Another application of agglutination tests, the determination of blood groups, played an essential role in the development of modern surgery. Transfusion is simply the transplantation of a tissue consisting of a suspension of cells in serum. However, transplantation of blood is more routinely successful than other tissues because histocompatibility antigens are not expressed on erythrocyte membranes. Four major blood group phenotypes, A, B, O, and AB, are found in humans. Red blood cell surface antigens A, B, and AB are expressed on the surface of cells of the corresponding phenotype, while type O cells exhibit the antigen designated H. The sera of individuals with type A, B, or O blood contain antibodies against the B, A, or both antigens, respectively. Routine blood typing consists of: (1) testing erythrocytes to determine presence or absence of membrane antigens A, B, and Rh_oD, (2) testing serum for presence or absence of expected antibodies (isoagglutinins), and (3) further serum testing for presence or absence of unexpected antibodies. The chemical structures of the different blood group isoantigens have been characterized as similar oligosaccharides with terminal immunodominant sugars unique for each group (type). Subgroups of the major types are known to exist but seldom (1% of samples) present problems in the interpretation of hemagglutination tests. There are many Rh antigens (C, D, E, c, and e), but Rh-positive or Rh-negative implies the presence or absence of D antigen and should therefore always be reported Rh_oD positive or negative. Rh antigens do not appear to be carbohydrates. The only antigens for which donors and recipients need be routinely examined are A, B, and Rh_oD. In an emergency, blood typed by these criteria can be administered according to the scheme outlined in Fig. 6-5 without cross-matching.

Blood group determinations should always be carried out by test tube centrifugation when the equipment is available in preference to the older slide tests because: (1) there is less evaporation and drying of the reagents, (2) results can be

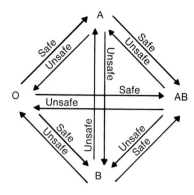

Fig. 6-5. In an emergency typed, but unmatched, blood may be administered as shown. (From Alexander, J., and Good, R. 1970. Immunobiology for surgeons, Philadelphia, W. B. Saunders Co.)

obtained more quickly, (3) sensitivity is increased by bringing the cells into close proximity in the bottom of the tube, and (4) the technique can be easily scaled up to increase the number of specimens tested. Red cells used in blood group determinations must first be washed to remove any of their own plasma, anticoagulants, or soluble ABO blood group substances, which are found in patients with positive secretor status. All of these substances are capable of causing misinterpretation of the test results.

Following the selection of blood for transfusion on the basis of ABO RH_oD typing, a major cross match should be carried out between the erythrocytes of the donor and the serum of the recipient. To provide optimum conditions for the identification of antibodies that have stringent reaction requirements or are present in low concentrations, the compatibility tests are performed at: (1) room temperature, (2) 37°C in a solution containing a high-protein concentration, and (3) 37°C augmented with antiglobulin reagents (Coombs' test). These tests identify antibodies in the recipient serum to donor erythrocyte antigens. Agglutination in the major cross match precludes use of the donor blood.

Minor cross-matching (donor serum with recipient cells) is less important but, to eliminate the possibility of any serious acute transfusion reactions, should be carried out routinely. When blood is needed for elective procedures it should always be typed and fully cross matched.

Most whole blood to be used for transfusion is preserved with ACD solution, which permits storage at 4°C up to 21 days. After 24 hours of storage factor V, AHG activity, neutrophils, and platelets are largely destroyed. Packed erythrocytes are often used when there is known sensitivity to leukocyte antigens or when sensitization or volume overload must be avoided. Platelets prepared from the buffy coat can be infused for the treatment of thrombocytopenia. Fresh frozen plasma and commercial concentrates of cryoprecipitates, can be utilized in the treatment of coagulation disorders.

Hemolytic transfusion reactions are almost entirely the product of human error. They must be treated immediately and the infusion stopped. Allergic reactions and fever can also signal host reaction to transfused blood containing either sensitizing IgE antibody, products of bacterial metabolism, or antibodies induced by previous transfusions. Infection can complicate transfusion, and most bacteria that can grow in blood stored at 4°C belong to the pseudomonas or coliform groups. The transmission of viral hepatitis via donor blood is, as mentioned previously, a serious problem.

Cellular immunity

Immune reactions that can be conferred on a naive host by the transfer of sensitized lymphocytes devoid of their serum are referred to as cell-mediated immune (CMI) responses. Cellular immune response is illustrated by the many types of delayed hypersensitivity reactions including transplant rejection. CMI reactions play an especially important role in protection against viral infections but are also of importance in defense against bacterial infections and neoplastic disease. Some allergies and autoimmune diseases are also mediated by sensitized lymphocytes. Like the humoral immune response, cell-mediated immunity plays an important role in initiating and maintaining inflammatory responses (Cohen, 1976). These biologic functions are largely mediated by vasoactive and chemotactic substances and lymphokines released from stimulated lymphocytes.

Essentially all antigens that can stimulate an antibody response can also induce a cellular response. An immune response involves differentiation of host reactivities into two types: (1) humoral, characterized by antibody synthesis in a population of immunocytes derived from bone marrow (B-cells), and (2) cellular, characterized by sensitization of immunocytes also originating in the bone marrow but differentiated under the influence of the thymus (T-cells) and capable of performing effector functions without intermediary antibody (Fig. 6-6). Some antigens, such as tuberculin, viruses, fungi, and histocompatibility antigens, are capable of stimulating cellular responses more efficiently than humoral responses. Antigen processing by macrophages appears to be a more important step in the evolution of cellular than humoral responses.

The delayed-type hypersensitivity (DTH) reaction is a series of events that characterizes the biologic manifestations of CMI responses. Intradermal injection of an antigen to which an individual has been sensitized will result in an indurated, erythematous wheal reaching maximum size in 24 to 48 hours and regressing slowly over a few days. This lesion provides evidence that a state of cellular immunity exists, and the delayed nature of its clinical development distinguishes it from the antibody-mediated immediate hypersensitivity reactions. The early lesion shows a histologically typical inflammatory neutrophilic infiltrate followed by the characteristic "mononuclear" infiltrate at 48 to 72 hours.

In vivo tests

The easiest and most definitive techniques for evaluating cellular immunity are the in vivo tests classically illustrated by intradermal injection of small amounts of antigen. The intensity of the response can usually be directly correlated with the level of host sensitivity. However, interference with development of the reactive lesion either by blocking antibody (see below) or hypofunctional lymphocytes, occasionally observed in asso-

Cell-mediated immunity

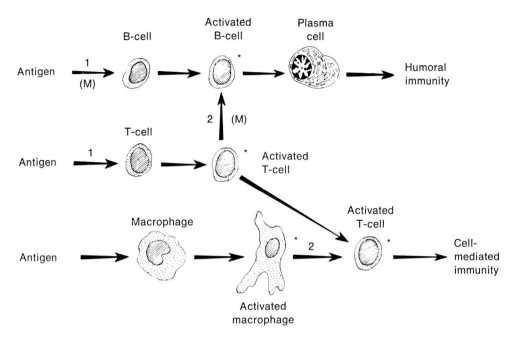

Fig. 6-6. Interrelationships of cellular and humoral immune responses. One and two represent primary and secondary antigenic stimulation. In humoral immunity, antigen (possibly processed by macrophage, *M* primes B-cells and T-cells. Activated T-cells may potentiate differentiation of B-cells into antibody-synthesizing plasma cells. In cellular immunity, antigen activates macrophages as well as priming T-cells, and macrophages potentiate activation of T-cell. (From Tom, B. H. 1975. In Mathieu, A., and Kahan, B. D. Immunologic aspects of anesthetic and surgical practice, New York, Grune & Stratton, Inc.)

ciation with some acute and chronic diseases, can cause erroneous interpretations. Evidence of previous contact with microbial antigens (for example, Mantoux test for tuberculosis) can be gained in this way. CMI function can be evaluated in individuals with suspected anergy by first sensitizing and then skin testing with chemical allergens such as dinitrochlorobenzene or picrylated albumin. A battery of antigens to which most of the population has been naturally sensitized (purified protein derivative — PPD; streptokinase-streptodornase — SK-SD) can also be used to test CMI function.

In vitro tests

The binding of antigen to specific receptor sites on sensitized T-cells stimulates transformation and proliferation of these cells with the elaboration of biolog-

ically important substances. Many of these substances and their biologic functions, while important in the in vivo development of a delayed-type hypersensitivity (DTH) response, can also be assayed by in vitro tests yielding information that can be correlated with the level of the cell-mediated immune sensitivity of the host. One of the functions, cell-mediated cytolysis, occurs when lymphocytes sensitized to antigens from a given source are added to a culture of cells taken from the same source. The exact mechanism of target cell destruction is not known, but examination of cell-free supernatants from antigen-stimulated lymphocytes has yielded two substances that cause cell damage. These have been designated lymphotoxin (LT) and cloning inhibitory factor (CIF). The relationship between cell-mediated cytolysis,

X Antigenic site

◊ Antibody molecule (IgG)

c' Complement

A Cytolysis

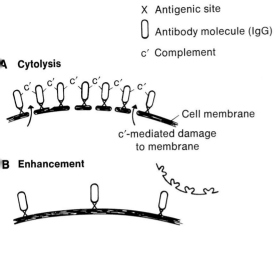

Cell membrane

c'-mediated damage
to membrane

B Enhancement

C Cell-mediated damage

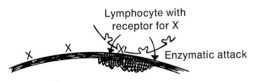

Lymphocyte with
receptor for X

Enzymatic attack

Fig. 6-7. A, Complement mediates damage to cell membrane. **B,** Antibody blocks surface antigen preventing damage mediated by sensitized lymphocyte as illustrated in **C.** Density of antigens on surface of cell plays important role in determining fate of cell. (From Alexander, J., and Good, R. 1970. Immunobiology for surgeons, Philadelphia, W. B. Saunders Co.)

antibody-mediated cytolysis, and cell surface-antigen density illustrates an important immunobiologic concept (Fig. 6-7). The masking of foreign antigens from the host's recognition and disposal system by blocking antibody results in the persistence of the antigen in the host. This can have a beneficial effect, as in the enhancement of allografts and in desensitization to certain allergens, or a deleterious effect if the masked antigens are on the surface of neoplastic cells. In vitro tests of cellular cytotoxicity in the absence of complement are used as indicators to predict the efficiency of in vivo CMI functions such as rejection of grafts and the killing of tumor cells.

Another important in vitro correlate of in vivo cell-mediated immunity is lymphocyte transformation. The binding of specific antigen to the surface of sensi-

tized lymphocytes results in transformation to lymphoblasts, large pyroninophilic cells containing a double complement of DNA, and subsequent division of the cell. Transformation (blastogenesis) can be conveniently assayed by measuring the incorporation of radiolabeled nucleic acids (for example, ^{3}H-thymidine) into the DNA of the transforming cells. Besides specific antigens, lymphocyte transformation can be stimulated by nonspecific mitogens obtained from plants (phytohemagglutinin, pokeweed mitogen). The ability of lymphocytes to transform in the presence of a nonspecific stimulus shows a direct correlation with an individual's ability to mount CMI responses. Testing peripheral lymphocytes in vitro with a battery of mitogens thus allows evaluation of the general reactivity of the cellular immune system. Soluble factors released by stimulated lymphocytes have been demonstrated to recruit nonsensitized lymphocytes in culture to transform and undergo clonal proliferation. Two of these are blastogenic factor (BF) and lymphocyte-transforming factor (LTF). However, most of the large number of lymphoblasts that can be seen in a stimulated culture have been shown to be descended from very few cells through repeated division.

Another soluble substance, transfer factor (TF), acts as an initiator of specific immunologic activity rather than as an effector substance. TF extracted from the lymphocytes of sensitized individuals is a small dialyzable molecule. Administration to nonsensitized recipients induces a new clone of specifically active lymphocytes that responds to the sensitizing antigen by transformation and lymphokine production. Intracutaneous injection of the recipient with the antigen induces a typical DTH response. The use of TF to augment responses in CMI-deficient patients is presently under study. Because of its size TF is not immunogenic. Therefore its repeated administration will not result in untoward hypersensitivity reactions, so that it cannot be quickly eliminated by immune mechanisms.

Nonimmune lymphocytes also will transform in the presence of allogeneic cells. Transformation in a mixed culture consisting of allotypically dissimilar lymphocytes is called a mixed lymphocyte reaction (MLR). One-way MLR is performed by blocking proliferation of one of the two populations of cells by irradiation or mitomycin C. This is an exquisitely sensitive test for dissimilarities in cell surface antigens and appears to be of value in the matching of graft donors and recipients (see "Transplantation," "Lymphocyte reactions"). However, the correlation between HL-A compatibility, MLR reactivity and graft rejection has not been completely clarified.

A third class of in vitro systems providing a means of assessing in vivo cellular immunity requires the measurement of the effect on other cells of factors released by stimulated lymphocytes. When a mixture of sensitized lymphocytes and macrophages is taken up in a capillary tube and the tube laid on an agar bed, the macrophages migrate from the end of the tube forming a fan-shaped pattern. However, migration is inhibited when the sensitizing antigen is added to the cell suspension. Inhibition of migration in vitro is antigen specific and correlates with a positive DTH reaction in vivo. Inhibition appears to be mediated by a protein of 70,000 molecular weight, which is synthesized by lymphocytes and has been named migration inhibitory factor (MIF). The MIF assay has also been adapted to show minor differences in cell surface antigens.

Another phenomenon that has been observed and attributed to a factor produced by lymphocytes is aggregation of macrophages. It has been postulated that macrophage aggregating factor (MAF) may not be a separate substance but that aggregation may be simply attributable to cell-bound MIF. Another factor designated MAF, macrophage activating factor, stimulates increased rates of phagocytosis and intracellular digestion of microorganisms in vitro. Osteoclast activating factor (OAF), leukotactic factor, and skin reactive factors (SRF) are all activities that have been recently demonstrated and for which mediator substances have been postulated. It is neither clear whether a unique factor exists for each of these activities nor whether all of these activities play an important role in in vivo events.

MIF assays are being used to evaluate CMI reactivity in anergic patients and skin test negative patients, sensitivity in patients with drug allergies who cannot be subjected to in vivo testing, and potential reactivity to donor tissue in transplant recipients. Immunosuppressive drugs interfere with MIF activity precluding its use during antirejection chemotherapy. Some of the preceding categories of in vitro tests are being widely used to characterize cell-mediated immunity in laboratory experiments, but use in humans has not reached its predicted potential. Correlation of in vitro test results with the in vivo status of a patient faces many critical theoretical and technical dilemmas. They are being used more widely, however, and valuable information can be obtained by the simultaneous employment of several independent assays, the collective results of which reflect a more reliable picture of in vivo states than using a single diagnostic technique.

Role in host defense

Cell-mediated immunity plays an important role in host defense. Patients with primary immunologic deficiencies (Swiss-type agammaglobulinemia, DiGeorge's syndrome, Wiskott-Aldrich syndrome, Nezelof's syndrome) often face early death because of susceptibility to viral infections, some bacterial infections, fungus infections, and malignancies of lymphoid tissues. Generalized malignancy (for example, Hodgkin's disease) is often accompanied by anergy. Active sensitization with dinitrochlorobenzene is used to screen for patients with metastatic disease, since they are frequently unable to develop a CMI reaction. Some microorganisms cause infections (for example, leprosy, candidiasis, tuberculosis) accompanied by anergy specific for the infecting agent. This nonreactivity appears to be associated with a serum-blocking factor and allows the disease to progress unchecked. This results in the deterioration of the host via a cycle of dependent succeeding steps: increased antigen replication, increased synthesis of blocking antibody, further suppression of protective CMI response, and subsequent increase in antigen replication. Immunologic reconstitution by implantation of cells or tissues and the treatment of nonresponsive patients with transfer factor from the lymphocytes of convalescent patients are being attempted with some success in an effort to solve these problems.

TRANSPLANTATION (Najarian and Simmons, 1974; Russell and Winn, 1970)

Reports of successfully transplanted limbs and organs appeared very early in recorded medical history, but the state of the necessary knowledge and skills in those times made it highly unlikely that these stories were true. The problems that must be overcome to ensure the success of a transplant can be conveniently divided into two major categories, technical and immunobiologic. The first category includes acquisition of the graft from a suitable donor, its preparation and storage, and its final installation in the recipient in such a way that will ensure its functional success and survival. Some examples of organs and tissues for which the technical feasibility has been established in experimental animals and man are skin, blood, kidney, heart, liver, bone marrow, bone, and teeth. Some problems, such as the physioanatomic requirements for nerve regeneration, remain unsolved and stand as major obstacles to the routine use of some transplant procedures.

No real progress in organ transplantation was made until the early 1900's when Carrell and Guthrie reported their successful technique for anastomosing blood vessels. There followed in quick succession the solutions to many of the technical problems that plagued early efforts. Although these early workers suspected that an immunologic reaction was responsible for failure and rejection, it remained for Medawar and his co-workers to provide the initial proof. The evidence collected since then, demon-strating beyond doubt that rejection is mediated by immune mechanisms, includes: (1) a second graft from the same donor is rejected much more quickly than the first (second-set rejection); (2) second grafts are rejected in an accelerated manner whether they are implanted at the same site as the first or at a distant site, which shows the systemic nature of the response; (3) there is a dose-dependent response in which, other things being equal, larger grafts incite a more intense response than smaller ones; and (4) antibodies specific for and/or lymphocytes sensitized to the donor tissue are found in recipients who have recently rejected their grafts.

The general immunobiologic phenomena that influence the transplantation of tissue will be summarized below. Tooth transplantation will be covered elsewhere in this text (see Volume 2).

Immunobiology of transplantation (Billingham and Silvers, 1971)

Recognition of "foreignness" of a graft by the host immune system depends on antigens called transplantation or histocompatibility antigens found in the graft but absent from host cell membranes. Little and co-workers developed the technology that led to the identification of the chromosomal region called the major histocompatibility complex (MHC) responsible for production of the major histocompatibility antigens. The MHC in the mouse is called the H-2 region, while in man the MHC is identified as the HLA region. The HLA region is the only major histocompatibility complex that has been found in man except for the ABO blood grouping system, which also has a profound effect on graft survival. The HLA region has been divided into four loci, three of which (SD loci) control the production of cell surface antigens detectable by serologic methods (for example, cytotoxicity tests). The other (LD) locus controls synthesis of cell surface antigens that can only be observed in lymphocyte reactions (for example, mixed lymphocyte reactions (MLR), cell-mediated cytotoxicity). These findings provided the rationale for the present use of blood typing, microtoxicity testing, and MLR in histocompatibility matching. Use of these techniques has dramatically improved the prognosis of graft survival in man. The HLA region has been shown to control the determination of cell surface structures of importance in a wide array of biologic phenomena including cell-cell interactions, immune responsiveness, and susceptibility to disease (Bach and van Rood, 1976). Histocompatibility antigens are associated with the lipoprotein fraction of the plasma membrane and most of the evidence characterizes them as glycoproteins.

Transplantation terminology has changed over the past few years (Table 6-8). Tissues grafted from one place to another in the same individual are called "autografts" and those grafted from one identical twin to another are termed "isografts." These involve no difference in genotype between donor and recipient so that no foreign antigens confront the host's immune system. Autografts and isografts are routinely and permanently successful. The genotypes of different individuals within the same species differ by the presence of one of many possible alleles of a gene at a given locus. For this reason, grafts between individuals of the same species are now called allografts instead of homografts. Transplantation procedures in which the genotype of the donor is different from the host by one allele at a single locus can result in rejection of the graft. Antigenic differences, reflecting allelic differences, can be detected by histocompatibility tests and donor tissue antigens can be matched closely enough to host antigens

that the allograft will not be quickly rejected. A graft exchanged between individuals of two different species involves genetic differences so great that transplantation antigens must either be removed from the graft or altered. These transplants are now called "xenografts" after the Greek "xeno," meaning foreign, in preference to the older term "heterograft."

Rejection phenomenon

Even when careful pretransplantation histocompatibility matching is carried out, a majority of recipients of organ allografts suffer one or more rejection crises. These reactions vary in intensity and some can be modified by immunosuppressive therapy. Three basic types of rejection have been outlined, differing from one another in time of occurrence and the mechanisms involved. Frequently more than one type occurs simultaneously at the same graft site.

"Hyperacute (acute humoral, immediate) rejection" occurs within minutes or a few hours of graft revascularization. This type of rejection is especially important where major vascular anastomoses are established between graft and host. It is most often a consequence of a blood group incompatibility or the result of previous sensitization of the recipient by an environmental antigen eliciting antibodies that cross-react with donor histocompatibility antigens. These antibodies, already in the serum at the time of transplantation, attach to the endothelium of the small blood vessels of the graft. Complement is fixed by these antigen-antibody complexes, and polymorphonuclear

Table 6-8. Transplantation nomenclature*

Graft	Adjective	Old term	Donor-host relationship
Autograft	Autogeneic (auto-self)	Same	Same individual
Isograft	Isogeneic (iso-same)	Same	Identical twins, inbred strains
Allograft	Allogeneic (allo-other)	Homograft	Same species
Xenograft	Xenogeneic (xeno-foreign)	Heterograft	Different species

*By permission of The American Academy of Periodontology, Chicago, 1974.

(PMN) leukocytes adhere to the complex layer. The endothelium is destroyed by substances released through complement activation or from the PMN leukocytes. Platelets adhere to the denuded surface, and intravascular thrombosis occurs culminating in the death of the graft. Reactions of this type can be prevented by using appropriate typing and matching techniques prior to transplantation to ensure the absence of antibodies to donor antigens in the recipient's serum.

Organ transplants from related donors to recipients unmodified by immunosuppressive therapy usually undergo a functional crisis within 6 to 10 days of transplantation. This "acute rejection" can be modified by immunosuppressive therapy but may occur at any time, even years later, depending on the level of therapy, host response, stresses suffered by the patient, and the rate of graft adaptation or development of tolerance to the graft. The lesion of acute rejection is characterized by increasing infiltrates of mononuclear cells, particularly around small and medium blood vessels. Although antibodies have been shown to play a role in acute rejection, cellular immunity appears to be of primary importance. Thrombosis and the killing of target cells by sensitized T-cells result in graft destruction. Episodes of acute rejection can sometimes be reversed by appropriate immunosuppressive therapy.

"Chronic (late) rejection" occurs in patients with allogeneic transplants who have been receiving prolonged immunosuppressive treatment. Although this type of reaction has a cellular immune mechanism, only moderate infiltration of mononuclear cells is seen. Subintimal thickening and endothelial proliferation result in narrowing of the lumina of blood vessels. Signs and symptoms of slow progressive renal failure are seen in the case of kidney allografts. Fully developed chronic rejection, like hyperacute rejection, is rarely reversible.

Typing and matching of tissues

There are several in vivo and in vitro methods for histocompatibility testing. The degree of genetic polymorphism in human populations is so great that a perfect match is practically impossible. A perfect allograft match would be one in which the recipient's immune system could detect no foreign antigens on the donor tissues. The best that can be hoped for is the most perfect match possible, or available, at the time the transplant is needed. The success of this approach is best illustrated by the extensive experience obtained in renal allografting. Of all the testing procedures available, besides ABO matching, only leukocyte typing and the mixed lymphocyte culture test appear to be of practical clinical value. It is best if results from both tests can be evaluated together, but for practical reasons this is not always possible.

Serologic methods

Among the variety of serologic techniques, lymphocyte cytotoxicity tests are the most used. Cells are reacted with each of the antisera in the panel, with the later addition of complement and trypan blue. If the serum contains complement-fixing antibody to an antigen on the lymphocyte, the cell membrane will be damaged and the dye will stain the cytoplasm. Lymphocytes from the recipient and many donors are tested in this way and their reactions to the antisera compared. Using panels of many carefully characterized allotyping antisera, over 50 different leukocyte (histocompatibility) antigens have been recognized.

Lymphocyte reactions

When antigens are added to cultures of lymphocytes with surface receptors for the antigen, the lymphocytes will be stimulated to transformation and division. During replication the cells will take up radioactive DNA precursors and the measurement of radioactivity incorporated can be taken as an index of the intensity of the reaction to the antigen. In two-way mixed lymphocyte cultures (MLC), donor and recipient lymphocytes are placed in culture together for about 1 week after which tritiated thymidine is added and incorporated radioactivity measured. However, since lymphocytes from both sources stimulate each other, artificially high counts are obtained. If the donor's lymphocytes are prevented from dividing by some method prior to culture (one-way MLC), then only lymphocytes from the recipient will incorporate the labeled DNA precursor and a more accurate measure of compatibility is obtained. Good correlation has been found between lack of reactivity in one-way MLC and the length of skin graft survival. In rats, rejection will sometimes occur in spite of a negative one-way MLC test, but in these cases the in vitro compatibility tests prove to be at least a predictor of prolonged skin allograft survival when used in conjunction with immunosuppressive therapy. Other lymphocyte reactions are used for histocompatibility testing but, at present, only to a limited extent.

Immunosuppression

The continued successful function of a transplant frequently depends on suppression of the host's rejection response. Immunosuppression, however, introduces a concomitant reduction in the efficiency of the recipient's protective immune mechanisms so that management of a suppressed patient requires extremely fine adjustment of the therapeutic regimen. Radiation, steroids, azathioprine, and antilymphocyte globulin are some of the agents used in immunosuppressive therapy.

Bone and tooth transplantation

The allografts most commonly used in the practice of oral and maxillofacial surgery are teeth and bone. There can be no doubt that hard tissues share with soft tissues the same histocompatibility antigens, although they may be less concentrated and/or better disguised in hard tissues. These properties of hard tissues have led some authors to conclude that compatibility requirements for hard tissues are less than for soft tissues. It has also generated the impression that denaturing conditions, such as freezing and freeze-drying, render hard tissues immunobiologically inert. Most of these studies, however, used only clinical behavior of the initial graft as the criterion

for success and did not assess sensitization of the host to donor antigens. Whenever careful assessment of sensitization by immunologic methods has been included, it has been shown that host response to hard tissues was qualitatively, if not quantitatively, similar to soft tissues (Emmings, 1978). Prior sensitization to alloantigens, which increases the likelihood of hyperacute rejection of lifesaving grafts or of transfusion reactions, must be considered part of the cost of every allograft procedure. Methods of despeciation, such as chemical extraction, have been used to reduce allograft antigenicity with varying degrees of success. In summary, it is essential that any proposed allograft procedure be carefully evaluated by immunologic, clinical, and histologic criteria over extended intervals to determine that the benefits actually exceed the risks.

IMMUNOPATHOLOGY (Beers and Bassett, 1976; Beutner et al., 1973; Criep, 1976; Miescher, 1976; Sell, 1975)

Allergy and hypersensitivity are the general terms used to describe the destructive effects of immune reactions. Altered host reactivity resulting from prior contact (for example, idiosyncratic reactions to pharmacologic agents, anaphylactoid reactions resulting from the release of endogenous pharmacologic mediators, and environmental adaptations in response to stress) cannot always be classified as allergic reactions.

The pathogenesis of allergic reactions may be simply viewed as variations of the inflammatory response. Allergic reactions tend to involve more than one organ system and to manifest a similar appearance from system to system. Therefore the traditional classification of disease by organ systems is not particularly helpful in understanding immunopathology. Two methods of classification, either by immune mechanism (Table 6-9) or by source of antigen and origin of response (Table 6-10), provide frameworks for discussion and understanding. In addition, Gell and Coombs (1968) suggested a simple classification for allergic reactions that is commonly used: type I — anaphy-

Table 6-9. Characteristics of the six types of hypersensitivity reactions*

	Antibody-mediated reactions				Cell-mediated reactions	
		Hematologic reaction	Early inflammatory reactions		Late inflammatory reactions	
	Neutralization or inactivation	Cytotoxic or cytolytic	Atopic or anaphylactic	Arthus (toxic complex)	Delayed	Granulomatous
Gell and Coombs classification:		II	I	III	IV	
Clinical state	Deficiencies, resistance to replacement therapy	Hemolysis, leukopenia, thrombocytopenia	Urticaria, hay fever, asthma	Serum sickness, glomerulonephritis	Tuberculosis, bacterial hypersensitivities, contact dermatitis	Tuberculosis, fungi, chronic granuloma
Sensitizing antigens	Hormones, clotting factors	Blood cells, drugs, haptens	Pollens, dander, haptens	Soluble proteins, carbohydrates, haptens	Bacteria, fungi, viruses, proteins, haptens	Insoluble antigens
Antibody	Serum	Serum, complement-fixing, IgG, IgM	Serum, skin-fixing, nonprecipitable, IgE	Serum, precipitable, IgG, complement-fixing	Cellular	?Cellular
Transfer skin reactions	Sera, cells	Sera, cells	Sera, cells; wheal and flare: 5–15 min max; fade 1–2 hr	Sera, cells; Arthus: 6 hr max, fade 24 hr	Cells only Delayed: 24–48 hr max; nothing at 6 hr	Cells only Delayed: weeks
Pathology Primary	Inactivation of biologically active molecules	Cell lysis by complement	Release of pharmacologically active substances	Perivascular poly infiltration	Perivascular and diffuse round-cell infiltration	Epithelioid cell, giant cell, granuloma
Secondary	Metabolic or clotting abnormalities owing to loss of active agents	Anemia, jaundice, hemosiderosis, infection, bleeding	Edema, smooth muscle contraction, eosinophilia	Thrombosis, fibrinoid necrosis	Parenchymal destruction associated with cellular infiltrate (necrosis)	Tissue replacement and destruction with granulomas

*Modified from Sell, S. 1975. Immunology: immunopathology and immunity, Hagerstown, by permission Harper & Row, Publishers, Inc.

Table 6-10. Classification of allergic diseases according to source of antigen and origin of response*

I. *Endogenous* immune response to *endogenous* antigens
  A. Circulating antibody
    1. Autoallergic hematologic diseases
    2. Antibodies to tissue antigens in human diseases
  B. Cellular (delayed) sensitivity
    1. Experimental autoallergic diseases
    2. Human counterparts of experimental autoallergic diseases
II. *Endogenous* immune response to *exogenous* antigens
  A. Circulating antibody
    1. Anaphylactic-type reactions
    2. Atopic reactions
    3. Arthus reactions
  B. Cellular (delayed) sensitivity
    1. Tuberculin reaction
  C. Granulomatous hypersensitivity
    1. Berylliosis
III. *Exogenous* immune response to *endogenous* antigens
  A. Transfer of maternal antibody to fetus
    1. Erythroblastosis fetalis
    2. Neonatal leukopenia; thrombocytopenia
    3. Neonatal myasthenia gravis
  B. Experimental transfer of antibodies
    1. Masugi nephritis
  C. Experimental transfer of cells
    1. Graft-vs-host reaction
IV. *Exogenous* immune response to *exogenous* antigens
  A. Experimental transfer of antibodies and antigens
    1. Passive anaphylaxis (Prausnitz-Küstner reaction)
    2. Passive Arthus reaction
  B. Experimental transfer of cells and antigens
    1. Tuberculin reaction
    2. Contact dermatitis
V. *Endogenous* immune response to *complex* antigens (hapten-protein)
  A. Circulating antibody
    1. Drug-induced blood dyscrasias
    2. Drug-induced lupus erythematosus
  B. Cellular sensitivity
    1. Contact dermatitis

*Modified from lecture notes of Frank J. Dixon, M.D. From Sell, S. 1975. Immunology, immunopathology and immunity, Hagerstown, by permission Harper & Row, Publishers, Inc.

lactic reactions, type II—cytotoxic reactions, type III—immune complex reactions, and type IV—delayed or cell-mediated reactions.

Neutralization or inactivation of biologically active molecules

Antibodies directed to hormones, enzymes, or other mediators of biologic functions can combine with their target substances, resulting in either inactivation of the substance or an increase in its rate of elimination from the body. Inactivation depends either on directly blocking the specific site of biologic reactivity or on altering the tertiary structure of the molecule to indirectly render the site inactive.

Neutralization or inactivation by antibodies has been implicated in either the etiology, resistance to therapy, or secondary symptoms of several diseases. Insulin resistance has been correlated with a serum protein neutralizer (Pope, 1966). Insulin combined with its antibody is biologically inert but is also protected from insulinase degradation in the liver so that its half-life is essentially that of the associated antibody (Yalow and Berson, 1957). However, no correlation has been demonstrated between antibody concentrations and insulin requirements. Skin reactions (Paley and Tunbridge, 1952) and anaphylactic shock (Yasuna, 1940) may occur on administration of insulin to sensitive patients.

Antibodies to antihemophilic globulin (AHG) are often detectable in the serum of hemophiliacs. The infusion of donor AHG into hemophiliacs who are genetically deficient in this protein results in the identification of AHG as a foreign substance by the recipient's immune system. Humoral antibodies have been associated with pernicious anemia (anti-intrinsic factor) (Roitt and Doniach, 1976), Graves's disease (long-acting thyroid stimulator) (Doniach and Roitt, 1976), and myasthenia gravis (Rule and Genkins, 1976).

Cytotoxic reactions

Death or lysis of a cell results when humoral antibody reacts with a component of the cell membrane or with an antigen that has become attached to the cell membrane. The subsequent activation of the complement system by the antigen-antibody complex on the cell surface alters the cell membrane. Functional alterations can result in osmotic disequilibrium or opsonization, which is followed by cell death.

Immune destruction of blood and vas-

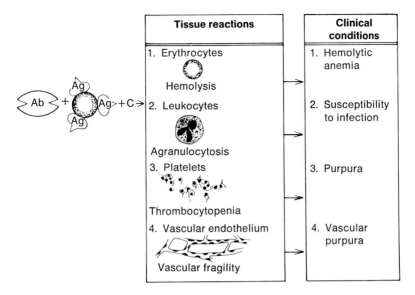

Tissue reactions	Clinical conditions
1. Erythrocytes Hemolysis	1. Hemolytic anemia
2. Leukocytes Agranulocytosis	2. Susceptibility to infection
3. Platelets Thrombocytopenia	3. Purpura
4. Vascular endothelium Vascular fragility	4. Vascular purpura

Fig. 6-8. Cytotoxic or cytolytic reactions. Humoral antibody reacts with cells that have direct contact with serum. Complement is fixed and activated by antigen-antibody complex, causing membrane damage and cell death. Cell destruction results in signs and symptoms associated with disease. (From Sell, S. 1975. Immunology, immunopathology and immunity, ed. 2, Hagerstown, Harper & Row, Publishers, Inc.)

cular cells is classified as immunohematologic disease (Fig. 6-8). Hemolytic anemias accompanying transfusion reactions and erythroblastosis fetalis (anti-RhD) have been discussed previously. Another group of hemolytic anemias is caused by the production of antibodies to antigens on the individual's own erythrocytes (Miescher, 1976). The cause of these autoallergic disorders is unclear, but the presence of humoral autoantibodies to erythrocyte membrane antigens is usually demonstrated by the Coombs test (see p. 226). Two types of autoimmune hemolytic anemia have been identified on the basis of the temperature at which the antibodies can combine with antigen: (1) warm type in which antibodies can combine at 37°C is most often associated with collagen disease or lymphocytic leukemia, and (2) cold type in which antibodies can only combine at exposed body surfaces (below 37°C) most often is not disabling.

Penicillin can combine with erythrocytes to stimulate an immune response to the drug. In this case the red blood cell acts as a carrier and later as the target cell for the immune response. Erythrocyte

destruction stops when the drug is withdrawn. The combination of alpha-methyldopa with erythrocyte membranes induces changes in red cells that render them immunogenic. Antibodies can then react with these altered cells in the absence of the drug. The allergic reactions to erythrocytes just described can also occur with polymorphonuclear leukocytes.

Thrombocytopenia can result from increased destruction of platelets mediated by antibodies (Miescher, 1976). Antiplatelet antibodies can be detected in the serum of about 60% of patients with purpura and some other hemorrhagic symptoms. Antibodies may be induced as a result of an autoallergic response, as a response to a drug or infectious agent adherent to platelets, and by transplacental maternal immunization with fetal antigens. Anaphylactoid purpura results from destruction of vascular endothelium mediated by an allergic reaction.

Anaphylactic reactions (Becker and Austen, 1976)

The term "anaphylactic reactions" is generally reserved for acute cutaneous reactions (wheal and flare) and for systemic shock. Antigens capable of sensitizing an individual and later stimulating anaphylactic reactions are called "allergens." Antibodies induced by allergens that also mediate anaphylactic reactions are termed "reagins." Most reagins are found in the IgE immunoglobulin class and their reaginic activity is dependent on their ability to bind to the membranes of many cells including skin, mast cells, and basophils. This property is termed "skin fixing" because detection of these antibodies commonly depends on injecting small amounts of antigen into the skin. In some cases antibody can be detected at a skin site 45 days after its injection at that site, attesting to the strength of the binding mechanism. IgE molecules bind to cell membranes by their Fc regions, leaving their combining sites free to react with antigen. The number of IgE molecules on the surface of a cell varies between 10 to 40×10^3, and the concentration of bound antibody is probably directly related to the sensitivity of the cell to allergen.

When allergen combines with reagin on the mast cell membrane, pharmacologically active substances are released from the cells. These substances include histamine, serotonin, heparin, bradykinin, and slow-reacting substance. These agents are released either by fusion of cytoplasmic granules (lysosomes) with the cell membrane or by lysis of the cell membrane. The former, called "degranulation," does not result in cell death. Degranulation is associated with significant metabolic changes in the cell marked by decreased cellular concentrations of cyclic AMP (Orange and Austen, 1971). These observations help to explain part of the pathogenesis of anaphylactic reactions.

The effect of released mediators on their target tissues results in the clinical manifestations of the anaphylactic reaction: bronchospasm, hypotension, tachycardia, edema, and urticaria. The type of reaction depends on the dose, type, and route of administration of the antigen, the relative excitability of the various target tissues, and the general sensitivity of the individual. Sensitivity may be affected by numerous conditions including genetic constitution and environmental factors. The severity of the reaction depends largely on quantities of antigen and antibody, antibody affinity, excitability of the target tissue, sensitivity of the mast cells, and the concomitant effects of the autonomic nervous system. The treatment of an allergic individual on exposure to the specific allergen is directed to the amelioration of these factors.

Patients at special risk of anaphylasis are those who have a genetic disposition to respond to environmental antigens by synthesizing reaginic antibodies (atopic individuals). Their histories are filled with periodic bouts of eczema, rhinitis, bronchial asthma, or urticaria. The chronically ill who have had contact with many drugs are also at great risk. A meticulous history is essential to prevent these reactions. Diagnostic tests can also be performed in conjunction with an allergist; however, a severe allergic reaction can result from a very small dose of allergen in a highly sensitive individual. The patch test, intradermal skin test, and Prausnitz-Küstner test are the most commonly used in vivo diagnostic procedures. Skin tests are performed directly on the subject, while in the last test serum suspected to contain antibody is injected intradermally into a monkey and 24 hours later the antigen is injected at the same site. In either type of test an immediate wheal and flare is considered positive. In vitro tests, such as basophil degranulation, are seldom used.

Some of the more common agents used by the oral and maxillofacial surgeon that have been implicated in anaphylactic reactions are penicillin, barbiturates, sedatives, narcotics, and local anesthetics. Penicillin may induce several different types of allergic reactions, and reported incidence of allergy varies from 0.7% to 10%. Barbiturates account for more rashes than any other drug, partly because of their wide use, and about 20 cases of anaphylactic reactions have been reported. The incidence of allergic reaction to local anesthetics is indeterminable; in most reported incidents it is impossible to establish whether the reaction has been caused by an allergy, intravenous injection, or an idiosyncratic response. Hypersensitivity appears to be most common with the ester group of local anesthetics, although their chemical structure induces some cross-reactive antibodies that can react with either ester or amide groups. There also appears to be cross-reactivity between the esters and methylparaben, a bacteriostatic agent used in some local anesthetics. Skin testing (Aldreti and Johnson, 1969) can be carried out in the event of a believable history of allergy to local anesthetics. A reliable diagnostic procedure would include testing for sensitivity to the agent, the preservative, a placebo, and a chemically unrelated agent.

Anaphylactic reactions are much more easily prevented than treated. A detailed description of the treatment of anaphylaxis appears elsewhere in this text (see Chapter 15). In general, therapy is directed to the modulation of the cellular events just described and is summarized in Table 6-11.

Immune complex reactions

Immune complex reactions may be caused by the interaction of antibodies with antigens that are either integral components of cells or are found free in the body fluids. They are dependent on the formation of antigen-antibody complexes in the presence of a slight antigen excess. Within tissue spaces these complexes form microprecipitates in and around small vessels causing local cell damage. The "antigen excess irritant" complexes are formed with antibodies of almost any immunoglobulin class. The principal requirement seems to be the formation of microprecipitates in tissues, since nonprecipitating antibodies appear to be ineffective.

The classic reaction of this type is the Arthus reaction. Inflammation, hemorrhage, and subsequent necrosis characterize the experimentally induced lesions in the skin and similar changes may be found in other tissues. The Arthus reaction, unlike anaphylaxis, is not inhibited by antihistamines, and it appears that the release of pharmacologically active mediators is not important for the tissue changes. Tissue damage is a consequence of the liberation of lysosomal enzymes from the polymorphonuclear (PMN) leukocytes. Activation of the complement system is involved in the chemotactic attraction of PMN leukocytes to the area. The suggested sequence of events in the Arthus reaction is the following: (1) antigen-antibody aggregates form in and around the walls of small blood vessels; (2) components of complement are fixed and a leukotactic response is initiated; (3) PMN leukocytes surround and ingest the complexes and subsequently release lysosomal enzymes, causing focal necrosis of the blood vessel wall and other inflammatory changes. Serum sickness, glomerulonephritis, collagen diseases, some skin diseases, and amyloidosis are examples of pathologic conditions involving this type of reaction. Glomerulonephritis may be caused by deposition in the kidney of immune complexes formed elsewhere, by reaction of antibodies directly with kidney tissue antigens, or by activation of complement via the alternate pathway. Those diseases that most concern the oral and maxillofacial surgeon are briefly discussed as follows.

Table 6-11. Biologic basis for treatment of anaphylactic reactions*

Vasopressors: increase adenylcyclase activity; increase concentration of 3'5' cAMP; inhibit release of histamine, SRS-A (for example, epinephrine, isoproterenol)

Methylxanthines: competitive inhibitors of phosphodiesterase, which catalyzes catabolism of 3'5' cAMP; inhibit release of histamine and SRS-A

Antihistamines: compete with histamine for some tissue receptors (bronchial or intestinal smooth muscle)

Steroids: thought to enhance the action of epinephrine on adenylcyclase; interfere with histamine release

*Mathieu, A, and Kahan, B. D. 1975. Immunologic aspects of anesthetic and surgical practice, New York, by permission of Grune & Stratton, Inc.

Collagen diseases (Sell, 1975, p. 189)

Collagen diseases are disorders of connective tissue that are characterized by their clinical and morphologic similarity to immunologic reactions. The characteristic lesion is fibrinoid necrosis marked by fragmentation of collagen and exhibiting necrotic, structureless areas containing large numbers of eosinophils. Most of the lesions accompanying collagen diseases appear to be caused by immune complex mechanisms; however, evidence for the participation of toxic immune complexes does not exist for all of the diseases in this category.

Polyarteritis nodosa (PAN). Inflammation of the small arteries results in thrombosis and the formation of multiple focal infarcts affecting any organ in the body. Clinical manifestations include weakness, fever, muscle cramps, hepatomegaly, polyneuritis, anemia, and renal insufficiency. Eosinophilia is commonly associated with the disease. Muscle biopsy frequently provides a definitive diagnosis. There is a great deal of evidence implicating hypersensitivity in the etiology of polyarteritis, with bacterial and viral antigens, drugs, parasite antigens, and foreign sera the primary suspect allergens. The association between PAN and hepatitis has long been recognized, and Australia antigen has been demonstrated by Gocke and co-workers (1970) in about 40% of those patients with biopsy-proven PAN.

Several types of polyarteritis have been described, usually related to the portion of the body affected by the disease. Wegener's granulomatosis (Miescher, 1976, p. 1020), of which lethal midline granuloma is thought to be one form, is characterized by a granulomatous angiitis of the respiratory tract. Gingival lesions have also been reported. Cogan's syndrome may produce deafness and blindness. Hypersensitivity angiitis sometimes occurs as a reaction to a drug (Miescher, 1976, p. 1017). Arteritis may occur in the major vessels (aorta, carotid, temporal) with the symptoms related to the anatomic location of the inflammatory process.

Treatment with corticosteroids signifi-cantly improves the prognosis, but only half of those afflicted with polyarteritis nodosa survive longer than 5 years (Trohnert and Sheps, 1967). Recently the addition of immunosuppressive therapy to the anti-inflammatory drugs has produced improved results. Less severe, localized episodes of arteritis respond well to short-term steroid therapy.

Systemic lupus erythematosus (Miescher, 1976, p. 963). Systemic lupus erythematosus (SLE) is a complex syndrome occurring primarily in women of childbearing age. Evidence suggests a familial predisposition in the etiology of SLE (Leonhard, 1957). It appears to be caused by autoantibodies directed primarily to antigens within the nucleus or on the nuclear membranes. Several investigators have suggested that loss of suppressor T-cells may be important in the pathogenesis of SLE. Severity of the disease ranges from only myalgia and malaise to a fatal form including nephritis, polyarthritis, CNS symptoms, rash, and high fever. Lesions in the various organs have been attributed to vascular deposition of immune complexes (Brentjens et al., 1977). The clinical course is marked by wide swings from spontaneous remission to acute exacerbation. The disease has been shown to occur clinically and experimentally following administration of penicillin and hydralazine, but it can also be virus-induced and exacerbated during conditions causing tissue necrosis. Drug-induced LE syndrome differs from SLE in that the former is usually arrested on withdrawal of the drug.

Several reports (Bain, 1960; Dubois and Tuffanelli, 1964) demonstrate the association of Mikulicz's and Sjögren's syndromes with SLE. One patient (Romero, Nesbitt, and Ichinose, 1977) developed Mikulicz's disease 2 years prior to the onset of SLE. Onset was charactericized by a further substantial enlargement of the salivary glands. This and other findings suggest a common autoimmune etiology. An acidic nuclear protein that reacts with serum taken either from patients with SLE or from patients with Sjögren's syndrome has been isolated (Akizuki, Powers, and Holman, 1977).

In the past, identification of the LE cell in the blood was the diagnostic finding of primary value. LE cells are formed when PMN leukocytes phagocytize nuclear material coated with antibody (Fig. 6-9). The important addition of immunofluorescent staining to the diagnostic armamentarium has largely replaced the LE cell test except as a rapid screening technique. Several staining patterns have been differentiated on the basis of the specific allergen involved. A solid phase radioimmunoassay was recently reported (Smith, Harrington, and Gehle, 1977), which is a more sensitive assay for the detection of circulating autoantibodies in patients with SLE.

Other serologic abnormalities often appear concomitantly with antinuclear antibody. These include hypergammaglobulinemia, positive Coombs' and Wassermann tests, antibodies to clotting factors, thyroglobulin, hypocomplementemia, and anticytoplasmic antibodies. These antibodies are probably responsible for the lesions of SLE that are histologically consistent with immune complex disease.

Treatment of SLE is designed to reduce inflammation and to decrease serum concentrations of pathogenic antibodies. To this end steroids and immunosuppressive agents, sometimes in combination, are administered. Suppressor T-cell activity has been induced in cells taken from SLE patients by incubation with thymosin or thymic epithelium, suggesting that thymic manipulation may be useful in the therapy of SLE (Horowitz et al., 1977).

Rheumatic fever (Read and Zabriskie, 1976). Rheumatic fever is an acute disease characterized by polyarthritis, carditis, and subcutaneous nodules. It sometimes appears as a sequel to group A streptococcal infections. Streptococcal antigens, cardiac muscle, and heart valve glycoproteins share some antigenic determinants. Cross-reacting antibodies appear in the serum of patients with rheumatic fever and cellular responses have also been detected. It is thought that these antibodies may react with the myocardium, resulting in typical fibrinoid necrotic lesions characteristic of rheumatic fever and immune complex disease in general. There is some evidence that responsiveness to these

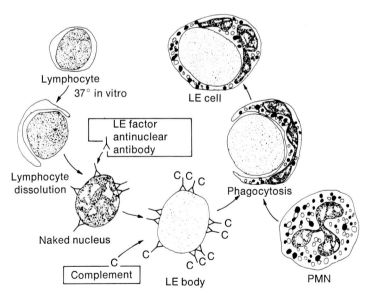

Fig. 6-9. Formation of LE cell. Lymphocytes break up releasing their nuclei, which become coated with antibody. Coated nuclei are phagocytosed. (From Sell, S. 1975. Immunology, immunopathology and immunity, ed. 2, Hagerstown, Harper & Row, Publishers, Inc.)

streptococcal cross-reacting antigens and susceptibility to the disease may be associated with a specific HLA haplotype. The correlation between infection with the organism and the sequence of pathologic events resulting in the disease is still not clear.

During the acute phase a positive C-reactive protein test can be observed. Elevated serum titers of antibody to streptolysin can also be detected. Awareness of the pathogenesis, prompt diagnosis, and prevention by antibiotic therapy (Kaplan et al., 1977) have significantly reduced the incidence of cardiac sequelae to rheumatic fever.

Rheumatoid arthritis (RA) (Lightfoot and Christian, 1976). Rheumatoid arthritis (RA) is a chronic, progressive, symmetric inflammatory disease in which autoallergic toxic complexes have been implicated as an important etiologic agent. Most joints can be afflicted, and chronic inflammation progresses to a destructive granulomatous process (pannus) that destroys the articular surfaces. The temporomandibular joint is involved in approximately 50% of those individuals with rheumatoid arthritis. Although the etiology remains obscure, the evidence supports the role of the immune response in the pathogenesis of rheumatoid arthritis.

Rheumatoid factor (RF) is found in the serum of 60% to 90% of patients with rheumatoid arthritis. It is most often an IgM antibody (IgM$_{RF}$) synthesized in response to altered autogenous IgG. RF can also be an IgG antibody (IgG$_{RF}$) to altered IgG (or IgG-IgG$_{RF}$) complexes. Because of the complement-fixing properties of IgG, it may play an important role in the pathogenesis of RA. RF does not initiate RA, rather it serves to amplify the inflammatory process. Besides denatured autogenous IgG, RF has also been shown to react with xenogeneic and allogeneic immunoglobulins. RF can be detected using the sheep agglutination reaction and typed by immunoglobulin class using a technique involving treatment with mercaptoethanol (Riera et al., 1977). Its concentration in the serum seems to correlate with the severity,

prognosis, and occurrence of rheumatoid nodules. Serositis, peripheral neuropathy, vasculitis, and myocarditis are associated with the arthritis. These may result from the circulating toxic complexes of RF and altered IgG. Synovial fluid from arthritic joints contains immune complexes, PMN leukocytes, lowered concentrations of complement components, and elevated levels of B$_2$-microglobulin. Neutrophil chemotaxis and phagocytosis have both been found to be depressed in patients with RA (Corberand et al., 1977; Mowat and Baum, 1971). Lymphocytes can also be found in large numbers in synovial fluid and tissues suggesting a possible role for cell-mediated immunity in the etiology of rheumatoid arthritis.

Determination of RF, C-reactive protein levels, erythrocyte sedimentation rate, examination of synovial fluid, and radiographs are important diagnostic aids. Treatment is directed at controlling pain and inflammation. Salicylates and low doses of steroids are most commonly used (Fremont-Smith and Bayles, 1965). Gold therapy has been used for many years and has been associated with oral ulcerations. The mechanism of this side effect has not been elucidated.

Scleroderma (systemic sclerosis) (Shulman, 1976). Scleroderma is a chronic disease characterized by sclerotic thickening of the dermis and diffuse fibrosis of many organs including the gastrointestinal tract. It occurs in women twice as often as men and most frequently between the ages of 30 and 50. Earliest signs of disease include Raynaud's phenomenon and stiffness and swelling of the fingers. The esophagus is the most common site of visceral involvement and this occurs early in the course of the disease generating complaints of difficulty in swallowing, sour eructations, or substernal discomfort. These symptoms are caused by impaired esophageal peristalsis secondary to submucosal fibrosis. In one study, intraoral and panoramic radiographs revealed abnormally thickened periodontal ligaments in 37% of patients with scleroderma, while 18% demonstrated some resorption of the mandibular angle and coronoid process (White et al., 1977). Atrophy in the mandible and other bones associated with scleroderma is thought to be caused by pressure or ischemia. Sixteen of thirty-one patients with scleroderma showed labial salivary gland biopsies consistent with Sjögren's syndrome. Intralobular fibrosis was probably a direct manifestation of scleroderma (Fressinger, 1975).

Corticosteroid therapy has not been effective in the treatment of scleroderma. Low molecular weight dextran, penicillamine, and immunosuppression are being evaluated but no conclusions can yet be drawn.

Skin diseases (Beutner et al. 1973; Beutner, Jordan, and Chorzelski, 1976)

A number of dermatologic conditions are thought to be caused by antibody-mediated allergic reactions, and many of them are manifested in the oral cavity. Some skin immunopathology is caused by the direct action of antibodies on target cells in the skin, while other diseases depend on the presence of cellular infiltrates to fully develop.

Pemphigus vulgaris. Pemphigus is a progressive skin disease characterized by severe vesiculation and acantholysis. The initial lesions usually occur on the trunk, although the primary site of involvement is often the oral mucous membrane. The intraepidermal fluid-filled blebs result from separation of the upper layers from the basal layer. Acantholytic cells (Tzanck cells) found in the vesicular fluid are diagnostic but not pathognomonic. IgG and IgM autoantibodies to intracellular substances found in the epithelium are thought to be important in the pathogenesis of the disease. Disruption of the epidermal layers by prevesicular edema allows the epithelium to be easily rubbed from apparently normal skin surfaces. This is called Nikolsky's sign, and it can also be demonstrated on the oral mucosa. Immunofluorescence is used to demonstrate deposition of antibodies in the intercellular areas and provides a reliable diagnostic test. Determination of relative concentrations of intercellular antibody by immunoflu-

orescent staining recently has been used as an index for the adjustment of corticosteroid therapy. Complement deposits are found in areas around blebs, and the entire complement sequence is activated in the vesicular fluid. Identification of all the components of immune complex reactions at the site of the lesion substantiates the role of antiepithelial antibodies in the etiology. Corticosteroids sometimes induce remission of the disease, and antibiotics are administered for complicating secondary infections.

Benign mucous membrane pemphigoid (bullous pemphigoid). The highest incidence of benign mucous membrane pemphigoid (BP) occurs over 50 years of age, and women appear to be affected more often than men. Serum IgG and IgE antiepidermal autoantibodies are found in most of those afflicted. These antibodies have been shown by immunofluorescence to be directed against antigens in the basement membrane. Therefore separation and bulla formation occur between the basal layer and the dermis in contrast to the intradermal bullae of pemphigus. The bullae are thick walled and do not break easily and acantholytic cells are not present in biopsies. BP is often accompanied by blood and tissue eosinophilia. Some authorities feel that bullous pemphigoid is a variant of dermatitis herpetiformis (DH) rather than synonymous with benign mucous membrane pemphigoid (Jablonska et al., 1976). BP is difficult to differentiate from either dermatitis herpetiformis or erythema multiforme on the basis of clinical or histologic findings, but immunofluorescent staining can usually distinguish BP. BP and DH also differ in that DH responds to treatment with sulfapyridine or sulfones and BP does not. For these and other reasons separation of DH and BP as unrelated diseases appears to be justified. Forman and Nally (1977) reported a possible variant of bullous pemphigoid occurring primarily on the gingiva.

Erythema multiforme. The occurrence of this disease has been associated with the use of certain drugs, with some infectious diseases, and with the simultaneous presence of certain malignancies

(Bóhatka and Alföldy, 1977; DiFabio and Lee, 1979). The pathogenesis of the disease is still unclear. It usually occurs 10 to 20 days following exposure to the etiologic agent. If a drug, withdrawal results in remission and subsequent reexposure causes recurrence with lesions appearing after only a few hours. The dermal, oral, genital, and conjunctival lesions may occur in several combinations characterizing different syndromes, for example, Behçet's and Stevens-Johnson syndromes. Early lesions are characterized by an extensive lymphocytic infiltrate in the dermis or submucosa. Histologic findings are consistent with a nonspecific vasculitis. Circulating autoantibodies have not been found, nor has it been possible to demonstrate the components of a cytotoxic reaction at the site of the lesion. Therefore it has been suggested that erythema multiforme is a type of immune complex disease. Steroids are often used in treating this disease, with antibiotics to control secondary infections (Sell, 1975, p. 201).

Amyloidosis (Missmahl, 1976)

Immunopathologic mechanisms of both the humoral and cellular type probably play an essential role in the pathogenesis of amyloidosis. Amyloid is a mixture of proteins, glycoproteins, polysaccharides, and probably lipids that stains with Congo red. This stain is considered specific for linear polysaccharides, hence the name amyloid (starchlike). Amyloid is deposited extracellularly in association with many conditions including genetic syndromes, collagen diseases, chronic infections, and malignancies such as myelomas and Hodgkin's disease. Primary amyloidosis, for which no predisposing condition can be found, comprises another category of amyloid diseases. The etiology is unknown, but the tendency for the disease to occur in association with chronic antigenic insult suggests that excessive stimulation of the reticuloendothelial system is involved. Polypeptide chains showing primary structural homology with immunoglobulin light chains have been identified in amyloid deposits associated with primary amyloidosis and myeloma. This finding has prompted the suggestion that excessive production or diminished catabolism of Ig results in amyloid deposition. Fiber structures similar to those found in amyloid have been produced in vitro by proteolytic digestion of Ig light chains. Experimental amyloidosis has been induced by chronic injection of casein (Jaffé, 1926) or bacterial products (Howes et al., 1963).

Oral manifestations of primary and secondary amyloidosis may include macroglossia, mucosal petechiae and ecchymosis, hemorrhagic bullae, macular lesions, and dry mouth. Localized lesions have been reported on the palate (Timosca and Garilita, 1977), tongue, and in the parotid gland. Biopsy of oral lesions and/or clinically normal gingiva may be preferable to rectal biopsy in the diagnosis of amyloidosis (Schwartz and Olson, 1975).

Delayed hypersensitivity reactions
(Remold and David, 1976)

Delayed hypersensitivity reactions are initiated on the recognition of antigens by lymphocytes that have been specifically modified by previous contact with that antigen. These lymphocytes display on their surface membranes antibody-like receptors that mediate responses to that antigen. The response usually involves the release from the modified lymphocytes of factors that recruit other mononuclear cells. Thus most cells involved at the site of a delayed type hypersensitivity (DTH) response are not specifically sensitized to the antigen. The reaction of specifically sensitized cells with antigen results in damage to normal tissue along with antigen inactivation and disposal. The clinical appearance of DTH reactions depends on the location of the antigen. Mechanisms of cellular immune reactions were discussed previously.

Delayed skin reaction (Sell, 1975, p. 218)

The prototype skin reaction can be induced by the injection of PPD (purified protein derivative) or OT (old tuberculin) into the skin. Erythema, induration, and swelling begin in a sensitive individual after a delay of 4 to 6 hours and reach maximum intensity at 24 to 48 hours. A cellular infiltrate dominated by mononuclear cells can be observed in the dermis.

Contact allergy

Contact allergies occur in the mucous membranes as well as the skin (Sell, 1975, p. 220). The most common allergens in contact stomatitis (stomatitis venenata) are found in toothpastes, cosmetics, dental materials, and therapeutic agents. Allergens are usually fat-soluble haptens capable of combining with proteins in skin and mucosa to form a complete antigen. Repeated exposure to sufficient concentrations of the allergen results in sensitization. The reaction is first noticeable by 24 hours and reaches maximum intensity by 48 to 72 hours. Erythema, induration, and vesiculation characterize the clinical appearance of the lesion. The epidermis or submucosa is infiltrated with lymphocytes and histiocytes, and intraepidermal edema and cell death are evident microscopically. Microabscess (bleb) formation occurs, and active allergen can be found in the bleb fluid that is capable of spreading the reaction on rupture. Resolution and healing may take as long as 2 weeks. Therapy consists of topical steroid application and symptomatic treatment. In the oral cavity identification and withdrawal of the substance containing the allergen is often the only practical and necessary treatment.

Allergic stomatitis was reported (Schriver et al., 1976) in a patient whose jaws had been immobilized using stainless steel wire fixation following a fracture. Skin tests revealed hypersensitivity to nickel. Following replacement of the wires with Mersilene sutures the symptoms subsided.

Viral infections

Cell-mediated immunity plays an important role in protection against viral infections. In some reactions host cells infected with virus are destroyed. Measles, choriomeningitis, viral encephalitis, and viral hepatitis are examples of diseases in which host cell destruction is an aspect of the disease process. The mechanism of the destructive process often involves an autoallergic response.

Autoimmune diseases (Sell, 1975, p. 244)

Autoallergies are characterized by an immune response to endogenous antigens, which results in damage to host tissues. Criteria for classification as an autoimmune disease were suggested by Witebsky and Milgrom and include these requirements: (1) antibody or immunocompetent cells that react specifically with antigens of the target organ; (2) localization of the specific antigen within the target organ; (3) immunization of experimental animals with the antigen must elicit an immune response; (4) the response must be followed by the disease in the experimental animal; and (5) the disease can be transferred to a normal animal by serum and/or cells from a diseased animal.

Most autoallergic diseases exhibit a delayed type of immune response. In general, there is seldom correlation between serum antibody levels and autoimmune disease. Conversely, delayed skin reactions are usually associated with autoimmune disease. Modes of immunization that favor the induction of delayed hypersensitivity most successfully produce autoimmune disease in experimental animals, and the histologic appearance is comparable to that of a delayed reaction. Antibody is capable of causing damage only when antigens are accessible. Therefore, autoimmune destruction of solid tissues is rarely passively transferred in serum from a diseased to a normal animal. Passive transfer of cells, however, has often been demonstrated to confer the disease on the recipient.

The cause of autoimmunization is still unknown but it seems clear that no single mechanism can explain all of the autoimmune diseases. There are four major theories proposed (Sell, 1975, p. 257): (1) Autoantigens are unavailable to the immune system during embryogenesis so that the host is not tolerant of them. On later release of these antigens to the circulation, the immune system recognizes them as foreign. (2) Endogenous tissue substances altered by infection or chemicals are recognized as foreign by the host. Tolerance to the native substance is broken, resulting in an immune response to that tissue component. (3) Immunocompetent cells that are capable of reacting with endogenous antigens are normally present in all individuals. Autoallergic phenomena result when these cells, for some unknown reason, lose control and recognize endogenous antigens as foreign. (4) Suppressor T-cells may act to prevent responses to endogenous antigens. When suppressor cell function is impaired, as with age, higher incidence of autoimmune disease should result. In fact, certain autoimmune diseases develop with high frequency when immune function is deficient for any reason such as aging.

Infection has been implicated in the induction of autoimmune diseases. Both viral and bacterial infections cause tissue damage, which results in alteration of endogenous antigens. Some renal diseases and many vascular and tissue lesions have been associated with viral agents. Antibodies that cross react with human heart tissue have been found in the serum of patients convalescing from infections with group A streptococci. These antibodies are thought to play a role in the etiology of subacute bacterial endocarditis.

Acquired hemolytic anemia, idiopathic thrombocytopenic purpura, encephalomyelitis, glomerulonephritis, thyroiditis, multiple sclerosis, lupus erythematosus, orchitis, and sialadentitis are some of the diseases considered to exhibit autoimmune phenomena. Sjögren's syndrome is often associated with connective tissue diseases (for example, systemic lupus erythematosus, rheumatoid arthritis), and the histologic appearance of the salivary glands suggests immunopathology. Antibodies to salivary gland tissues have been detected. However, there is some evidence that this antibody may function to block the cellular response and reduce the intensity of the disease (Anderson et al., 1973).

Sjögren's syndrome (Bloch, 1976). Sjögren's syndrome (SS) is a complex disease linking benign lymphoid hyperplasia with collagen disease and malignant lymphoma (Anderson and Talal, 1972). Autoimmune processes, vitamin deficiency, and endocrine dysfunction have been suggested in the etiology of Sjögren's syndrome.

The syndrome is characterized by at least two of three components: (1) keratoconjunctivitis sicca, (2) xerostomia, and (3) rheumatoid arthritis. Two types of Sjögren's syndrome have been observed. One type exhibits the sicca complex along with a connective tissue disorder, while in the second only the sicca complex can be found. If only the parotid gland is involved, the disorder is called Mikulicz's syndrome. Symptoms attributable to dry eyes and mouth are first noticed, and the diagnosis is substantiated by use of Schirmer's test for tear formation and fluorescein dye to reveal nonvital corneal epithelium. Increased levels of serum antinuclear antibody and LE cells are often found. One half of patients with the syndrome report salivary gland enlargement. Recently, salivary scintigraphy with sodium pertechnetate has been used more frequently to evaluate salivary gland function (see Chapter 11). Antibodies that cross react with salivary gland duct cells and pancreatic duct cells have been demonstrated (Ludwig et al., 1977) in the serum of patients with Sjögren's syndrome and rheumatoid arthritis.

Granulomatous reactions

Many similarities exist between delayed hypersensitivity reactions and granulomatous reactions. However, for histologic reasons, some authors prefer to separate granulomatous reactions from the type IV reactions. These lesions are characterized by the arrangement of epithelioid cells into tubercles or granulomas. The reaction has been characterized as an immune response to poorly soluble substances. Bacterial products, metal salts, and suture materials are among the many causative agents. Reactions develop after delays of weeks or months, and many diseases show varying proportions of both granulomatous reaction and vasculitis. Tuberculosis, leprosy, berylliosis, sarcoidosis, and Wegener's granulomatosis are all examples of this type of reaction.

Wegener's granulomatosis (Miescher, 1976, p. 1020)

Granulomatous arteritis, glomerulonephritis, and sinusitis are all components of Wegener's granulomatosis. Granulomas are most often found in the lungs, spleen, and nasal or oral cavity. Some authors have felt it to be a variant of polyarteritis nodosa or a hypersensitivity angiitis. Oral lesions are rarely the earliest signs of the disease. The lesions contain scattered giant cells and vasculitis is routinely observable. Elevated serum IgE levels have been found in patients with Wegener's granulomatosis (Conn et al., 1976). Possible roles in its etiology have been suggested for certain infectious agents, suppressor T-cells, or immune complexes. The disease is usually fatal but recently immunosuppressive agents have been shown to be of value (Fauci and Wolff, 1973).

Sarcoidosis (Boeck's sarcoid)

The lesions of this disease are indistinguishable from tuberculosis and may be found to involve most sites including the mouth. Prevalence of sarcoidosis is much higher in the Eastern than Western United States. Familial studies suggest a hereditary predisposition, and it occurs more frequently in blacks. Subcutaneous injection of extracts of diseased human lymph nodes (Kveim test) results in the induction of a cutaneous granuloma in affected individuals 3 to 4 weeks following injection. The Kveim test and biopsy are the most useful methods for establishing the diagnosis. Oral lesions in tissues other than salivary glands are rare. They can resemble herpetic lesions and appear as either fluid-filled blebs or solid nodules. Salivary gland involvement in association with sarcoidosis has been well documented and gland function can be severely impaired (Beeley and Chisholm, 1976). Uveoparotid fever is considered a form of sarcoidosis. An etiologic

agent has not been identified. However, impaired T-cell function was recently found to be associated with sarcoidosis (Greer and Sanger, 1977) and may provide a clue to its cause.

Miscellaneous pathology

Many pathologic processes exhibit components of more than one type of allergic reaction. The pathogenesis of these destructive processes may be accounted for by different mechanisms in different individuals, different mechanisms at different times during the course of the disease, or several mechanisms operating simultaneously. Those conditions previously discussed exhibit at least an identifiable reaction primarily accountable for the disease. In those listed below the dominant mechanism either has not been defined or multiple mechanisms have been described that preclude classification in the preceding categories.

Bone resorption

There exist many possible mechanisms that can account for bone resorption. Among the allergic reactions, immune complexes in the presence of complement stimulates the release of ^{45}Ca from fetal rat bone in an in vitro system (Hausmann, 1974). Using a similar experimental system, a soluble factor (osteoclast activating factor — OAF) (Horton et al., 1972) and prostaglandins (Klein and Raisz, 1970) have both been shown to stimulate bone resorption. These mechanisms have been proposed to account for part of the bone loss associated with periodontitis. It has also been demonstrated (Harris et al., 1973) that enucleated dental cyst tissues synthesize prostaglandin-like material. These tissues were cultured and the culture media were found to cause significant bone resorption in an in vitro system. Resorption was inhibited by a prostaglandin antagonist. This evidence suggests that prostaglandins may also contribute to bone resorption that accompanies dental cysts. In addition, mononuclear cells were shown to release a soluble factor (Dayer, Robinson, and Krane, 1977) that stimulates the synthesis of prostaglandin E_2 by cultured rheumatoid synovial cells. This finding suggests another mechanism by which bone resorption can be stimulated by inflammation.

Some recent reports (Kuntz and Genco, 1974; Pulver, Taubman, and Smith, 1978; Toller, 1971) present evidence that antibody-mediated allergic reactions may play a role in the pathogenesis of pulpal and periapical pathology. These findings suggest that periapical bone resorption associated with cysts or granulomas may result in part from these immune mechanisms.

Lichen planus

Lichen planus has been diagnosed in association with several diseases having allergic etiologies. Tissue fixed IgG and IgM antibodies have been demonstrated in oral lesions by immunofluorescent staining. Antinuclear and anticytoplasmic antibodies were demonstrated (Goldstein, 1977) by indirect immunofluorescent staining of normal human skin. Preliminary evidence also suggests participation of the cellular immune response in the pathogenesis of lichen planus. Emotional stress has often been considered an important element in the induction of lichen planus, which may explain its association with some other diseases.

REFERENCES

Akizuki, M., Powers, R., Jr., and Holman, H. A. 1977. Soluble acidic protein of the cell nucleus which reacts with serum from patients with systemic lupus erythematosus and Sjögren's syndrome, J. Clin. Invest. **59:**264.

Aldreti, J. A., and Johnson, D. A. 1969. Allergy to local anesthetics, J.A.M.A. **207:**356.

°Alexander, J. W., and Good, R. A. 1970. Immunobiology for surgeons, Philadelphia, W. B. Saunders Co.

Anderson, L. G., and Talal, N. 1972. The spectrum of benign to malignant lymphoproliferation in Sjögren's syndrome, Clin. Exp. Immunol. **9:**199.

Anderson, L. G., et al. 1973. Cellular-versus-humoral autoimmune responses to salivary gland in Sjögren's syndrome, Clin. Exp. Immunol. **13:**335.

Bach, F. H., and van Rood, J. J. 1976. The major histocompatibility complex—genetics and biology (Parts I to III), N. Engl. J. Med. **295:**806; 872; 927.

°Bach, F. H., and Good, R. A. 1972. Clinical immunobiology, vol II, New York, Academic Press, Inc.

°Bach, F. H., and Good, R. A. 1974. Clinical immunobiology, vol II, New York, Academic Press, Inc.

Bain, G. O. 1960. The pathology of Mikulicz-Sjögren disease in relation to disseminated lupus erythematosus, Can. Med. Assoc. J. **82:**143.

Becker, E. L., and Austen, K. F. 1976. Anaphylaxis. In Miescher, P. A., and Müller-Eberhard, H. J., ed.: Textbook of immunopathology, vol. II, New York, Grune and Stratton, Inc., p. 117.

Beeley, J. A., and Chisholm, D. M. 1976. Sarcoidosis with salivary gland involvement: biochemical studies on parotid saliva, J. Lab. Clin. Med. **88:**276.

Beers, R. F., Jr., and Bassett, E. G. 1976. The role of immunological factors in infectious allergic and autoimmune processes, New York, Raven Press.

Beutner, E. H., Jordan, R. E., and Chorzelski, T. P. 1976. Autosensitization in pemphigus, bullous pemphigoid and other chronic bullous diseases. In Miescher, P. A., and Müller-Eberhard, H. J., eds.: Textbook of immunopathology, vol II, New York, Grune & Stratton, Inc., p. 931.

Beutner, E. H., et al. 1973. Immunopathology of the skin labeled antibody studies, Stroudsburg, Pa., Dowden, Hutchinson & Ross.

°Billingham, R., and Silvers, W. 1971. The immunobiology of transplantation, Englewood Cliffs, N. J., Prentice-Hall, Inc.

Bloch, K. J. 1976. Sjögrens syndrome. In Miescher, P. A., and Muller-Eberhard, H. J., eds.: Textbook of immunopathology, vol II, New York, Grune & Stratton, Inc., p. 1037.

Bohátka, L., and Alföldy, G. 1977. Oral manifestations in the paraneoplastic syndrome, Oral Surg. **44:**684.

Brentjens, J., et al. 1977. Disseminated immune deposits in lupus erythematosus, Arthritis Rheum. **20:**962.

Bruce, D., and Koepke, J. 1966. Changes in the rat associated with halothane anesthesia, Anesthesiology **27:**811.

Bruce, D. L. 1973. Acute and chronic anaesthetic actions on leukocytes, Can. Anaesth. Soc. J. **20:**55.

Cianciola, L. J. et al. 1977. Defective polymorphonuclear leukocyte function in a human periodontal disease, Nature **265:**445.

Claman, H. N. 1972. Corticosteroids and lymphoid cells, N. Engl. J. Med. **287:**388.

°Cluff, L. E., and Johnson, J. E. 1972. Clinical concepts of infectious diseases, Baltimore, The Williams & Wilkins Co.

Cohen, S. 1976. Cell mediated immunity and the inflammatory system, Hum. Pathol. **7:**249.

Conn, D. L., et al. 1976. Raised serum immunoglobulin E in Wegener's granulomatosis, Ann. Rheum. Dis. **35:**377.

Corberand, J., et al. 1977. Neutrophil function in rheumatoid arthritis, Scand. J. Rheumatol. **6:**49.

°Criep, L. H. 1976. Allergy and clinical immunology, New York, Grune & Stratton, Inc.

Dayer, J. J., Robinson, D. R., and Krane, S. M. 1977. Prostaglandin formation by rheumatoid synovial cells, J. Exp. Med. **145:**1399.

DiFabio, V. L., and Lee, J. C. 1979. Stevens-Johnson syndrome associated with malignant lymphoma, personal communication.

°General reference texts.

Doniach, D., and Roitt, I. M. 1976. Autoimmune thyroid disease. In Miescher, P. A., and Müller-Eberhard, H. J., eds.: Textbook of immunopathology, vol. II, New York, Grune & Stratton, Inc., p. 723.

Dubois, E. L., and Tuffanelli, D. L. 1964. Clinical manifestations of systemic lupus erythematosus, J.A.M.A. 190:104.

*Eisen, H. N. 1974. Immunology, Hagerstown, Pa., Harper & Row, Publishers, Inc.

Emmings, F. G. 1978. The fundamentals of transplantation immunobiology and the transplantation of teeth and bone. In Shaw, J., et al., eds.: Textbook of oral biology, Philadelphia, W. B. Saunders Co.

Fauci, A. S., and Wolff, S. M. 1973. Wegener's granulomatosis: studies in eighteen patients and a review of the literature, Medicine 52:535.

Fauve, R. M. 1970. The effect of corticosteroids on some functions of macrophages. In van Furth, R., ed.: Mononuclear phagocytes, Oxford, Blackwell, Scientific Publications, Ltd.

Forman, L., and Nally, F. 1977. Oral non-dystrophic bullous eruption mainly limited to the gingivae: a mechano bullous response, Br. J. Dermatol. 96:111.

Fremont-Smith, K., and Bayles, T. B. 1965. Salicylate therapy in rheumatoid arthritis, J.A.M.A. 192:1133.

Fressinger, J. N., 1975. Rapports entre la sclerodermic et le syndrome de Sjögren, Nouve. Presse. Med. 4:3177.

Frohnert, P. P., and Sheps, S. G. 1967. Long-term follow-up study of periarteritis nodosa, Am. J. Med. 43:8.

*Fudenberg, H. H., et al. 1976. Basic and clinical immunology, Los Altos, Lange Medical Publications.

Gell, P. G. H., and Coombs, R. R. A. 1968. eds.: Clinical aspects of immunology, ed. 2, Philadelphia, F. A. Davis Co.

Gigli, I., and Austen, K. F. 1971. Phylogeny and function of the complement system, Annu. Rev. Microbiol. 25:309.

Gocke, D. J., et al. 1970. Association between polyarteritis and Australia antigen, Lancet 2:1149.

Goldstein, B. H. 1977. Is lichen planus an immunologic disease? Annual Scientific Session, American Society of Oral Surgeons, Sept. 23-28.

Greer, R. O., Jr., and Sanger, R. G. 1977. Primary intraoral sarcoidosis, J. Oral Surg. 35:507.

Harris, M., et al. 1973. Prostaglandin production and bone resorption by dental cysts, Nature 245:213.

Hausmann, E. 1974. Potential pathways for bone resorption in human periodontal disease, J. Periodontal. 45(5,11):338.

Hollinger, F. B., et al. 1975. Detection of hepatitis A viral antigen by radioimmunoassay, J. Immunol. 115:1464.

Horowitz, S., et al. 1977. Induction of suppressor T cells in systemic lupus erythematosus by thymosin and cultured thymic epithelium, Science 197:999.

Horton, J. E., et al. 1972. Bone resorbing activity in supernatant fluid from cultured human peripheral blood leukocytes, Science 177:793.

Howes, E. L., Jr., et al. 1963. A model of amyloidosis, Arthritis Rheum. 6:278.

Humphrey, L. J., Wingard, D., and Lang, R. 1969. Effect of surgery and anesthesia on the immunologic responsiveness of the rat. Surgery 65:946.

Jablonska, S., et al. 1976. Dermatitis herpetiformis and bullous pemphigoid, Arch. Dermatol. 112:45.

Jaffé, R. H. 1926. Amyloidosis produced by injections of proteins, Arch. Pathol. Lab. Med. 1:25.

Jerne, N. K., et al. 1976. The agar-plaque technique for recognizing individual antibody forming cells. In Williams, C. A., and Chase, M. W., eds.: Methods in immunology and immunochemistry, vol. IV., New York, Academic Press, Inc.

Jubert, A. V., et al. 1973. Effects of surgery, anesthesia and intraoperative blood loss on immunocompetence, J. Surg. Res. 15:399.

Kaplan, E. L., et al. 1977. Prevention of bacterial endocarditis, Circulation 56:139A.

Kesztyus, L., Szilagyi, T., and Gyulai, F. 1954. Nervensystem und immunitat, Acta Microbiol. 1:359.

Klein, D. C., and Raisz, L. G. 1970. Prostaglandins: stimulation of bone resorption in tissue culture, Endocrinology 86:1436.

Kuntz, D., and Genco, R. J. 1974. Localization of immunoglobulin and complement in persistent periapical lesions, J. Dent. Res. 53(special issue):215.

Leonhard, T. 1957. Familial hypergammaglobulinemia and systemic lupus erythematosus, Lancet 2:1200.

Lepow, I. H. 1972. Biologically active fragments of complement. In Amos, D. B., ed.: Progress in immunology, New York, Academic Press, Inc.

Lightfoot, R. W., and Christian, C. L. 1976. Rheumatoid arthritis. In Miescher, P. A., and Müller-Eberhard, H. J. eds.: Textbook of immunopathology, vol. II, New York, Grune & Stratton, Inc., p. 1025.

Ludwig, H., et al. 1977. Antibodies to pancreatic duct cells in Sjögrens syndrome and rheumatoid arthritis, Gut 18:311.

Mandell, G. L., Rubin, W., and Hook, E. W. 1970. The effect of an NADH oxidase inhibitor (hydrocortisone) on polymorphonuclear leukocyte bactericidal activity, J. Clin. Invest. 49:138.

Mathieu, A., and Kahan, B. D. 1975. Immunological aspects of anesthetic and surgical practice, New York, Grune & Stratton, Inc.

*Miescher, P. A., and Dayer, J. M. 1976. Autoimmune hemolytic anemias. In Miescher, P. A., and Müller-Eberhard, H. J. eds.: Textbook of immunopathology, vol. II, New York, Grune & Stratton, Inc., p. 649.

Miescher, P. A., and Müller-Eberhard, H. J. 1976. Textbook of immunopathology, New York, Grune & Stratton, Inc.

Missmahl, H. P. 1976. Amyloidosis. In Miescher, P. A., and Müller-Eberhard, H. J. eds.: Textbook of immunopathology, vol. II, New York, Grune & Stratton, Inc., p. 607.

Mowat, A. G., and Baum, J. 1971. Chemotaxis of polymorphonuclear leukocytes from patients with rheumatoid arthritis, J. Clin. Invest. 50:2541.

°Najarian, J. S., and Simmons, R. L. 1974. Transplantation, Philadelphia, Lea & Febiger.

°Neter, E., and Milgrom, F. 1974. The immune system and infectious diseases; Fourth International Convocation on Immunology, Buffalo, N.Y., S. Karger.

Orange, R. P., and Austen, K. F. 1971. Chemical mediators of immediate hypersensitivity, Hosp. Pract. **6**:79.

Paley, R. G., and Tunbridge, R. E. 1952. Dermal reactions to insulin therapy, Diabetes **1**:22.

Pope, C. G. 1966. The immunology of insulin, Adv. Immunol. **5**:209.

Pulver, W. H., Taubman, M. A., and Smith, D. J. 1977. Immune components in normal and inflamed dental pulp, Arch. Oral Biol. **22**:103.

Pulver, W. H., Taubman, M. A., and Smith, D. J. 1978. Immune components in human dental periapical lesions, Arch. Oral Biol. **23**:435.

Read, S. E., and Zabriskie, J. B. 1976. Immunological concepts in rheumatic fever pathogenesis. In Miescher, P. A., and Müller-Eberhard, H. J. eds.: Textbook of immunopathology, vol. II, New York, Grune & Stratton, Inc., p. 471.

Remold, H., and David, J. R. 1976. Cellular or delayed hypersensitivity. In Miescher, P. A., and Müller-Eberhard, H. J. eds.: Textbook of immunopathology, vol. II, New York, Grune & Stratton, Inc., p. 157.

Riera, C. M., et al. 1977. A simple method for detection of IgG rheumatoid factor, J. Immunol. Methods **15**:223.

Roitt, I. M., and Doniach, D. 1976. Gastric autoimmunity. In Miescher, P. A., and Müller-Eberhard, H. J., eds.: Textbook of immunopathology, vol. II, New York, Grune & Stratton, Inc., p. 737.

Romero, R. W., Nesbitt, L. T., and Ichinose, H. 1977. Mikulicz disease and subsequent lupus erythematosus development, J.A.M.A. **237**:2507.

°Rose, N. R., and Bigazzi, P. E. 1973. Methods in immunodiagnosis, New York, John Wiley & Sons.

°Rose, N. R., and Friedman, H. 1976. Manual of clinical immunology, Washington, D.C., American Society of Microbiology.

Rule, A. H., and Genkins, G. 1976. Myasthenia gravis (muscles). In Miescher, P. A. and Müller-Eberhard, H. J. eds.: Textbook of immunopathology, vol. II, New York, Grune & Stratton, Inc., p. 841.

Russell, P. S., and Winn, H. J. 1970. Transplantation, N. Engl. J. Med. **282**(14):786; **282**(15):848; **282**(16):896.

°Schmidtke, J. R., and Ferguson, R. M. 1977. Immunology for the practicing physician, New York, Plenum Publishing Corp.

Schriver, W. R., et al. 1976. Allergic response to stainless steel wire, Oral Surg. **42**:578.

Schwartz, H. C., and Olson, D. J. 1975. Amyloidosis: a rational approach to diagnosis by intraoral biopsy, Oral Surg. **39**:837.

°Sell, S. 1975. Immunology, immunopathology and immunity, New York, Harper & Row, Publishers, Inc.

Shulman, L. E. 1976. Scleroderma (systemic sclerosis). In Miescher, P. A., and Müller-Eberhard, H. J. eds.: Textbook of immunopathology, vol. II, New York, Grune & Stratton, Inc., p. 1007.

Smith, K. O., Harrington, J. T., and Gehle, W. D. 1977. A solid phase radioimmunoassay for detection of serum autoantibodies in systemic lupus erythematosus, J. Immunol. Methods **15**:17.

°Taylor, O. 1975. Immunology in medical practice, London, W. B. Saunders Co., Ltd.

Thompson, J., and van Furth, R. 1970. The effect of glucocorticosteroids on the kinetics of monocytes and peritoneal macrophages. In van Furth, R., ed.: Mononuclear phagocytes, Oxford, Blackwell, Scientific Publications, Ltd.

Timosca, G., and Garilita, L. 1977. Primary localized amyloidosis of the palate, Oral Surg. **44**:76.

Toller, P. A. 1971. Immunological factors in cysts of the jaws, Proc. R. Soc. Med. **64**:555.

Tomasi, T. B., Jr. 1976. The immune system of secretions, Englewood Cliffs, N.J., Prentice-Hall, Inc.

Vane, J. R. 1976. The mode of action of aspirin and similar compounds, J. Allergy Clin. Immunol. **58**:691.

Weissman, G. 1974. Mediators of inflammation, New York, Plenum Press, Inc.

White, S. C., et al. 1977. Oral radiographic changes in patients with progressive systemic sclerosis (scleroderma), J.A.D.A. **94**:1178.

Wingard, D., Lang, R., and Humphrey, L. 1967. Effect of anesthesia on immunity, J. Surg. Res. **1**:430.

Yalow, R. S., and Berson, S. A. 1957. Apparent inhibition of liver insulinase activity by serum and serum fractions containing insulin-binding antibody, J. Clin. Invest. **36**:648.

Yasuna, E. 1940. Generalized allergic reactions to insulin, J. Allergy **12**:295.

PART TWO

PRINCIPLES OF ORAL AND MAXILLOFACIAL SURGERY

CHAPTER 7

General principles and techniques of surgery

David S. Evaskus

Good surgical care begins with the application and integration of basic sciences such as anatomy, biochemistry, histology, microbiology, pathology, pharmacology, and physiology to the management of the ill or diseased patient. Clinically, this takes the form of the evaluation process, presurgical preparations, intraoperative management, techniques of asepsis, craft of surgery, and postoperative care. While some of these topics are covered in detail elsewhere in this book (see Chapters 9, 10, 12, and 16), the basic principles will be presented here.

PRESURGICAL EVALUATION

The first step in presurgical evaluation is the recognition of existing medical conditions. For example, a history of hepatitis B, uncontrolled diabetes mellitus, pseudocholinesterase deficiency, or sickle cell anemia may alter the usual approach to the patient's surgical problem. The recognition of nutritional deficiency states is also important, and preoperative dietary supplements may be indicated in elective situations. Some patients may also require prophylactic medication before surgery. This is true, for example, in patients with a history of rheumatic heart disease who will require prophylactic antibiotics and those with adrenal hypofunction who will need to have steroids administered (see Chapters 9 and 16). Some patients will already be on medications such as insulin or anti-

coagulants, and the route, time schedule, or dosage may require adjustment (see Chapter 9). In the patient with a medical problem, consultation with a physician is often indicated to confirm the diagnosis and establish a proper plan for management.

Certain disease states such as asthma or epilepsy can be aggravated by psychologic or physical stress. Patients with a history of hypertension, angina pectoris, myocardial infarction, or cerebrovascular accident may also be susceptible to the ill effects of stress. Sedation with appropriate agents may help allay the stress of surgery and prevent complications. Patients with medical problems may also require changes in surgical technique, special consideration of fluid and blood replacement, and variations in anesthetic procedure.

A consideration of the patient's medical status also helps in the anticipation of complications. For example, individuals with anemia or agammaglobulinemia or those taking immunosuppressive drugs may have increased susceptibility to infection and delayed healing. Patients with a history of alcoholism, recent ingestion of large doses of aspirin, or hypertension may have prolonged bleeding. When complications are anticipated, the proper measures can be taken to prevent them or at least to lessen their severity.

The evaluation should begin with the medical history (see Chapter 12). The depth to which the practitioner goes in the evaluation process is based on the complexity of the presenting problem and the past medical history. It is important to learn and understand the full process, however, so that when indicated this procedure can be carried out efficiently. The ability to appropriately abbreviate the evaluation procedure will occur as the practitioner gains experience.

A history questionnaire, which the patient completes or which is completed with the aid of a nurse, is commonly used in office practice. When used properly, the questionnaire becomes a timesaving adjunct to the history taking process. However, it is only an adjunct, and depending on it as the sole means of obtaining the history can be dangerous. Besides negatively affecting the doctor-patient relationship, relying solely on the questionnaire fails to expose those patients who are misrepresenting the truth. For example, a patient may feel offended by the impersonal nature of the form and react by being less than complete in answering the questions. Other patients may feel that personnel other than the doctor will have access to the form, and therefore they may be reluctant to report certain problems that they consider intimate. Still others may not understand the wording or the intent of the questions and therefore may answer them incorrectly. Many of these deficits are easily remedied in the personal interview by the doctor, who can detect hesitancies in the manner or voice of the patient or who can readily clarify what information is being sought. Following the medical history, the evaluation process continues with the physical examination, the differential diagnosis, laboratory tests including radiographs, the diagnosis, and finally the treatment plan.

PRESURGICAL PREPARATION
General considerations

It would be desirable to have every patient who is to undergo a surgical procedure in optimum health. However, this state does not exist in the majority of patients. The tolerance of the surgical procedure, the postoperative course, the in-cidence of complications, and the quality and rate of healing can all be positively or negatively affected by the health of the patient. Therefore it becomes the goal of the surgeon to maximize the physical condition of the patient prior to surgery. For example, a patient with a history of alcoholism and nutritional deficiency may require vitamin K to prevent bleeding because of a lack of the vitamin K–dependent coagulation factors II, VII, IX, and X. Multiple vitamins including thiamine may also be needed, and, if the patient has a protein deficiency, a high protein diet may be instituted preoperatively to aid wound healing and body defenses. The specifics of a disease state will dictate the appropriate corrective action (see Chapters 9 and 16).

Prophylactic medications

Medications are given prophylactically to prevent anticipated complications that arise with some degree of predictability. Certain indications for the use of drugs in this manner are well documented, and others remain empiric and unsubstantiated. Besides the use of sedative agents to minimize stress, the two most frequently used types of drugs for prophylaxis are antibiotics and corticosteroids.

Doubtless, antibiotics are overprescribed, particularly for self-limiting infections, for inflammatory processes without infection, and in situations where removal of the primary etiology would eliminate the infection. However, certain specific indications for the use of prophylactic antibiotics do exist; perhaps the most common one is for patients with certain pathologic cardiac conditions.

Subacute bacterial endocarditis is a serious complication of heart disease carrying a high degree of morbidity and mortality (Kaplan et al., 1977). This type of infection occurs most often in patients with congenital or acquired structural abnormalities of the heart or great vessels. Any bloodletting procedure, including dental treatment but not including the shedding of deciduous teeth or the adjustment of orthodontic bands, is associated with a transitory bacteremia. These bacteria may lodge on damaged or abnormal valve leaflets, such as are found in rheumatic or congenital heart disease, or on a congenitally abnormal endocardium, causing an endocarditis or endarteritis (Everett and Hirschmann, 1977; Finland, 1972). Antibiotic prophylaxis is recommended for patients with most forms of congenital heart disease (ventricular septal defect, tetralogy of Fallot, aortic stenosis, pulmonary stenosis, complex cyanotic heart disease, patent ductus arteriosus, systemic to pulmonary artery shunts), idiopathic hypertrophic subaortic stenosis, mitral valve prolapse syndrome with mitral insufficiency (some controversy exists for the necessity of antibiotics in this condition), rheumatic or other acquired valvular heart disease, and prosthetic heart valves (Durack and Petersdorf, 1973; Durack, Starkebaum, and Petersdorf, 1977; Pelletier, Durack, and Petersdorf, 1975; Sande et al., 1969, 1972; Sipes, Thompson, and Hook, 1977). This does not include uncomplicated secundum atrial septal defects. The prophylaxis regimen for these problems can be found in Chapters 9 and 16.

Other indications for the use of preoperative prophylactic antibiotics may include patients with compound fractures; those who are immunologically suppressed, as in agammaglobulinemia or from taking immunosuppressants; or those on long-term corticosteroids. Controversy exists over the use of prophylactic antibiotics for patients with hip prostheses (Benson and Hughes, 1975; Cruess et al., 1975; Downes, 1977; Langdon, 1977; Rubin, Salvati, and Lewis, 1976; Wilson, Salvati, and Blumenfeld, 1975). The need for prophylactic antibiotics in diabetics also has not been proved. However, it is advisable in the severe form, or for those who frequently contract infections or whose disease is often out of control. The antibiotic dosage and frequency in these situations is empiric, but the antibiotic chosen should probably be one that is effective against the normal oral flora, such as penicillin or erythromycin. For patients who have a history of poststreptococcal glomerulonephritis, no prophylaxis is recommended, as the efficacy of this procedure in preventing further renal damage has not been established.

Corticosteroids may have to be administered prophylactically under certain circumstances. These agents contribute to water and salt balance, are involved in the maintenance of capillary integrity, and maintain control over precapillary sphincters, among other functions. A deficiency of corticosteroids in the stressed patient results in a precipitous drop in blood pressure because of pooling of blood in capillary beds and increased vessel permeability. In patients who have adrenal insufficiency, prophylactic use of corticosteroids prior to surgery is important to prevent a possibly fatal episode. Patients with adrenal insufficiency include those who have been taking corticosteroids for longer than 2 weeks or those who have been on long-term steroid therapy and have discontinued it within the last year. In these patients, adrenal atrophy attributable to the lack of stimulation by ACTH has started to take place, and therefore the adrenal cortex will not respond normally to stress.

Banks (1970) studied normal cortisol excretion in patients undergoing oral surgery ranging from extractions to major oral surgical procedures under hypotensive general anesthesia. He found that during the minor procedures, plasma cortisol was not different from control levels but that 4 to 7 hours postoperatively the plasma level did rise abruptly and then returned to normal at 24 hours. A similar pattern was seen with major oral surgical procedures. Interestingly, the degree of postoperative rise was suppressed in patients who routinely received a narcotic analgesic 1 hour postoperatively. This lends support to the theory that at least a portion of the rise is a stress response to postoperative discomfort. When these results are compared with those cited for major general surgical operations, a marked difference is observed. In the latter, a marked rise in cortisol is generally seen during the operative procedure, and the blood level remains elevated for longer than 36 hours (Cope, 1966; Estep et al., 1963; Mattingly and Tyler, 1965).

In general, oral and maxillofacial surgery patients who are deficient in endogenous steroids should have prophylactic steroids administered preoperatively, intraoperatively, and postoperatively. A full-spectrum corticosteroid such as hydrocortisone should be used instead of one that has primarily glucocorticoid activity such as dexamethasone, methylprednisolone, or triamcinolone. A further discussion of this subject can be found in Chapters 9 and 16.

Corticosteroids are also given prophylactically to limit postoperative edema. This has revolutionized procedures such as the sagittal split osteotomy in which the postoperative period was previously filled with concern over edema potentially obstructing the airway. With prophylactic steroids, patients now often leave the hospital 24 to 36 hours following this procedure.

Those steroids exhibiting the greatest amount of glucocorticoid activity are also the most potent anti-inflammatory agents and are therefore preferable to the full-spectrum type when prevention of edema is the primary objective. These may be administered in large doses in the immediate postoperative period (2 to 3 days) without affecting wound healing, body defenses against infection, or adrenal function. The adrenal cortex will undergo suppression during the duration of the therapy, but no atrophy will take place in such a short time. Following cessation of the steroids, even without gradual dose reduction, the adrenal cortex will begin normal function immediately. A further discussion of this topic can be found in Chapter 9.

PREPARATION OF THE SURGEON AND PATIENT FOR SURGERY

A discussion of surgical dress, scrubbing, gowning, gloving, and surgical site preparation, including draping, may be found in Chapter 10.

SURGICAL TECHNIQUE

Skin incisions

Skin tension was first noted by Dupuytren in 1834. When confronted with the corpse of a man who had stabbed himself with an awl, Dupuytren observed that the wounds were elliptical instead of round. Other early researchers such as Filhos (1833), Eschricht (1837), Malgaigne (1838), and Voight (1857), studied this phenomenon. In 1861 K. Langer, a Viennese professor of anatomy, studied incisions and puncture wounds in cadavers. The results were published as a schematic representation of the lines of greatest normal skin tension for all regions of the body (Fig. 7-1). In 1907 Kocher, the renowned Swiss surgeon, set forth the principle that surgical incisions should be made along these Langer lines of normal skin tension; in this manner the skin would be closed under the least amount of tension and the resulting scar would be minimal. Rubin (1948), Kraissl (1951), and Bulacio Nunez (1974) have challenged Langer's original concepts and have provided new maps of skin tension. Langer's lines tend to run parallel with skin creases, which generally are perpendicular to the action of the underlying muscles. The action of these muscles would tend to pull an incision apart. In these newer studies many of the lines are perpendicular to Langer's lines, particularly in the head and neck region. Despite this, skin incisions are still generally placed within skin creases to hide the scar.

Fig. 7-2 illustrates the location of some of the commonly used extraoral incisions in oral and maxillofacial surgery. The submandibular incision is used for surgery of the body and angle of the mandible as well as the submandibular gland. If the incision is extended posteriorly, then the ramus and condylar process are also accessible. The incision line usually tucks beneath the mandible in thin or young people. In obese persons the scar line is more noticeable. The Risdon incision is used for surgery of the mandibular angle and ramus area (Risdon, 1934). It is a slightly curved incision, and the subsequent scar is apparent but not unsightly. With both the Risdon and submandibular incisions, care must be taken to avoid injury to the marginal mandibular branch of the facial nerve.

The retromandibular incision provides

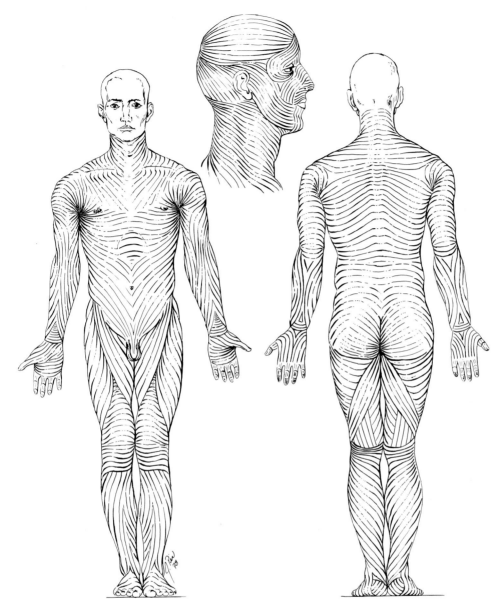

Fig. 7-1. Langer's lines. It was Langer's theory that these lines represented skin tension, an idea that has since been disproved. Underlying muscle action generally runs perpendicular to these lines, which causes skin creases when muscles contract. In areas where scar formation may be unsightly, incisions are generally made parallel to Langer's lines so that the scar will be hidden within natural skin folds.

access to the ramus, angle, and condylar process. In the young, reconstruction of the temporomandibular joint for agenesis or ankylosis can be accomplished through this approach. The incision affords the advantage of avoiding the branches of the facial nerve, facial artery, and vein. The scar line is usually imperceptible and can be totally hidden with longer hair styles.

The preauricular incision is made within the skin crease anterior to the ear. It affords access to the temporomandibular joint. Facial nerve weakness, usu-

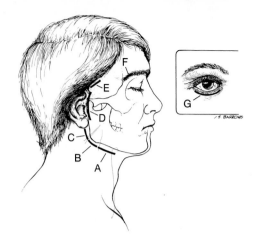

Fig. 7-2. Commonly used skin incisions. *A*, Submandibular, *B*, Risdon, *C*, retromandibular, *D*, preauricular, *E*, Gillies, *F*, brow, *G*, lid.

ally involving the temporal or zygomatic branches, may sometimes accompany surgery in this area. Generally this is caused by stretching the skin flap and is of a temporary nature. The scar line is almost invisible.

The Gillies approach is used for reduction of a fractured zygoma or zygomatic arch. It is made within the hairline, and when the hair regrows it is completely hidden. The brow incision is made without shaving the hair. It provides access to the lateral bony orbit and the zygomaticofrontal suture. This area heals readily, and the scar is hidden within the brow. The lid incision gives access to the inferior bony orbit and the zygomaticomaxillary suture. While the scar is almost undetectable, contraction can produce ectropion.

When planning the incision, the surgeon may elect first to draw the incision line on the skin. To be certain of the location of the skin creases and underlying anatomic structures, the patient's head and neck should be in a straight-forward, unstrained posture so that these landmarks will not be contorted. On long incisions some surgeons crosshatch the skin perpendicular to the incision line to facilitate accurate wound edge approximation at the end of surgery.

Whenever an incision is made, the blade should be held perpendicular to the epithelial surface and not obliquely, which will result in a bias cut. The knife should be passed in one stroke over the predetermined length of the incision to avoid causing irregularities in the wound edges. The skin should be slightly tensed by finger pressure to produce uniform resistance to the passage of the blade and a predictable depth of penetration.

When operating in vascular areas, the surgeon may decide to modify the incision technique to reduce bleeding. For example, electrosurgery may be used instead of a scalpel. A thorough discussion of this technique can be found on p. 285. Another method, used more commonly, is the injection of a vasoconstricting solution into the area prior to making the incision. Because local anesthetic solutions containing a vasoconstrictor such as epinephrine are readily available, these are often used for this purpose. Otherwise, a solution of 1:100,000 epinephrine can be prepared by mixing 0.1 ml of 1:1000 epinephrine with 9.9 ml of sterile isotonic saline solution. The solution should be used that day, as this dilute concentration of epinephrine is very unstable without preservatives.

In patients undergoing general anesthesia with a halogenated hydrocarbon inhalation agent such as halothane or enflurane (Ethrane), the concomitant use of epinephrine can produce ventricular arrhythmias (Millar, Gilbert, and Brindle, 1958; Raventos, 1956; Rosen and Roe, 1963). This complication appears to be dose related (Rosen and Roe, 1963), and therefore it is prudent to use minimum amounts of epinephrine in these patients. A study by Siegel, Vistnes, and Iverson (1973) demonstrated no significant difference in the degree and duration of hemostasis using epinephrine solutions of 1:100,000, 1:400,000, and 1:800,000. Egbert and Fosburg (1962) felt that 1:200,000 solutions were optimal, and Munchow and Denson (1964) observed effective hemostasis with solutions of 1:1,000,000. Therefore it would seem unnecessary to use solutions more concentrated than 1:100,000 for hemo-

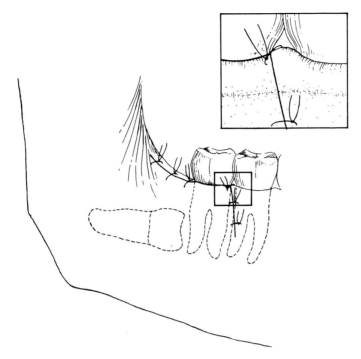

Fig. 7-3. Mucosal incisions. Location of incision is dictated by access. Incision around teeth is within gingival sulcus. Margins of flap are away from surgical site so that undisturbed tissue can support and provide rapid revascularization of flap. Gingival papilla is left intact (Insert). Releasing incision is used to reduce tension on flap and gain access.

stasis. Such dilute solutions are reliable and lessen the danger of cardiac problems. A waiting period of at least 5 minutes following the injection is necessary for the epinephrine to act fully. It should be pointed out that with this technique the possibility of postoperative bleeding exists from vessels that did not bleed at the time of surgery because of the effect of the vasoconstrictor.

Mucosal incisions and flaps

Because intraoral scars are not visible, the placement of incisions and flaps in this region is determined mainly by convenience, access, and avoidance of damage to nerves and blood vessels. The incisions should not be made over the operative site but rather in the adjacent, undisturbed areas, so that the flap will be supported by normal tissue and the potential for rapid revascularization is preserved (Fig. 7-3). The incisions should also be placed so that major nerves are not transected unless necessary. The maintenance of an adequate blood supply is of prime importance. This is accomplished by incising parallel to major vessels, minimizing the number of side cuts, and having the base of the flap as wide as or wider than the apex. Incisions should not be made in an area of thinned mucosa like that found over an exostosis or other bony prominence because the blood supply is reduced, suturing is difficult, and the rate of dehiscence is high. When developing flaps around teeth, the incisions should be made in the gingival crevice. It is also important to maintain the integrity of the interdental papillae and not to include them with the flap (Fig. 7-3) because of the difficulty in precisely reapproximating them.

An envelope flap is one that is developed from a simple straight incision. If access is not adequate, the surgeon may extend the length of the incision or make a releasing incision. The releasing incision is usually made at about a 45-degree angle from the direction of the parent incision. Generally, releasing incisions should be avoided if an envelope flap will provide adequate access. As previously mentioned, releasing incisions reduce blood supply to the flap and cause added discomfort. If possible, the releasing incision should not be made at a sharp angle to the primary incision but instead curve gradually from it.

If the flap is to include both mucosa and periosteum, the incision should be made directly to bone with one cut, and it should be elevated in one piece without tearing the periosteum. After the necessary surgery, clotted blood should be expressed from beneath the flap to lessen the possibility of infection and permit tissue fluid to penetrate more readily.

Tissue dissection

After the skin incision has been made, the subcutaneous tissues must be divided. Care must be exercised to identify underlying neurovascular structures. Obviously, a thorough knowledge of the surgical anatomy of the area is a prerequisite. The surgeon should be well acquainted with the location of the major arteries, veins, nerves, ducts, fascial planes, and muscles, and their relationship to each other (see Chapter 1). Because of the extensive collateral circulation of the head and neck, arteries and veins can usually be transected without endangering the blood supply to an area. Before transection, the vessel should be isolated by blunt dissection, clamped both proximal and distal to the division site, and then severed. The two clamped ends are then tied to prevent blood loss. A resorbable suture such as chromic gut is sufficient for veins and small arteries. The proximal ends of large arteries should be tied with a nonresorbable suture, and because of good collateral circulation, it may sometimes be necessary to use the same type of suture material for the distal end as well. Some surgeons prefer to place double sutures around the proximal end of large arteries.

The control of oozing from smaller vessels may be accomplished by electrocoagulation. This may be done by touching the bleeding areas directly with the electrode or by clamping the bleeding vessel with a hemostat or forceps and then applying the electrode to the instrument. The current will be transmitted to the tissue through the instrument and produce coagulation. The hemostat must not touch any other surface, such as the skin or mucosa, or a burn will result at the contact point.

Structures thought to be nerves should be either isolated by blunt dissection or avoided by changing the plane of dissection. Generally, nerves should not be cut because of resulting numbness or paralysis. Division of the cervical branch of the facial nerve is sometimes necessary to gain access to the mandible, but the actions of the denervated muscle, the platysma, are not missed. However, the marginal mandibular branch must be preserved. An electrostimulator should be used to determine if the isolated structure is neural. If the structure is a motor nerve, the innervated muscles will contract when it is stimulated. Mechanical stimulation, such as grasping the structure with a hemostat, is an inferior method and may result in temporary or even permanent damage to the nerve.

When dissecting through multiple tissue layers, the site of incision through each layer should be in a different place than the preceding one. By varying these sites, the final line of wound contraction and scarring will not be in a single direction, and skin dimpling and scar inversion will be minimized. Also, each layer should be undermined as the dissection progresses so that tension-free closure of identifiable layers is ensured.

Wound closure

Closure of the wound is one of the most important aspects of the operation, and yet it is frequently one that is given the least attention. It should be remembered that the most common cause of postoperative infections is poor surgical technique, usually related to devitalized tissue remaining in the wound or inadequate closure. In the process of closure the surgeon has the opportunity to scrutinize the previous surgery and compensate for any inadequacies. All osseous and soft tissue with severely compromised blood supply should be removed. Hemostasis must be obtained before each layer is closed, and each layer should be identified before closure to ensure correct apposition. Tension should be checked at each level and further undermining done if necessary. The subcutaneous layers should be adapted with absorbable material using interrupted sutures to minimize the amount of foreign body placed in the wound. These sutures will help obliterate dead space where accumulation of blood or other tissue fluids could prevent direct apposition of tissues and provide an environment favorable for bacterial growth. They also distribute the tension of wound closure over a larger volume of tissue. These sutures should not touch the skin sutures, since this would provide a channel of deep invasion by bacteria. The loose ends of the sutures are generally trimmed to the knot to minimize the amount of foreign material. Therefore the knots should be securely tied, as any slippage will result in untying. If a subcuticular suture is used, the knots should be inverted away from the skin surface. An absorbable 4-0 suture material is generally used for this purpose. The skin incision can be sutured with fine monofilament nonabsorbable material (5-0, 6-0) or taped if subcuticular sutures have been placed and there is minimal tension on the wound margins.

SUTURING

Needles

Proper suturing begins with an understanding of the physical and biologic properties of both the needle and the suture material. Needles are made of either stainless steel or carbon steel and are manufactured in two basic shapes, straight and curved.

The straight needle can be obtained with either a tapered or a cutting configuration. The former is circular or oblong in cross section and tapers gradually to a point. The cutting needle is triangular in cross section, and the points of the trian-

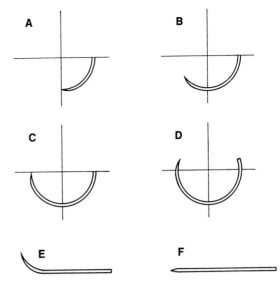

Fig. 7-4. Needles. **A,** ¼ circle, **B,** ⅜ circle, **C,** ½ circle **D,** ¾ circle **E,** straight with curved end, **F,** straight.

gle represent blades that are finely sharpened to permit passage through keratinized tissue. The straight cutting needle is used for skin closure in places with adequate access, such as the abdominal, thoracic, or iliac regions. In oral and maxillofacial surgery these needles are most often used for the passage of circumzygomatic or circummandibular wires.

The curved needle is generally used for both skin and mucous membrane surgery. It is manufactured with varying curvatures, such as the ¼, ⅜, ½, and ⅝ circle (Fig. 7-4). The thickness of the needle and the radius of curvature differ somewhat among manufacturers, as there are no industry standards. The needles generally come in either tapered or cutting types. The cutting needles are further categorized as conventional or reverse cutting; the conventional cutting needle has one of its three cutting edges along the internal curvature of the needle, while the reverse cutting needle has a flat internal surface (Fig. 7-5). The reverse cutting needle is the more popular. Manufacturers have also modified these basic shapes, for example, by making a five-edged cutting needle or by making a

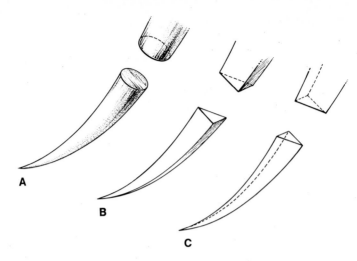

Fig. 7-5. Needles in cross-section. **A,** Tapered, **B,** cutting, **C,** reverse cutting.

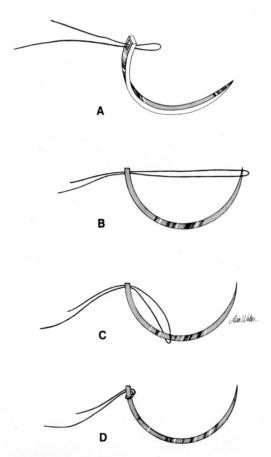

Fig. 7-6. Tying suture on an eyed needle. **A,** Loop of suture material is inserted through eye; **B,** loop is placed over tip of needle; **C,** loop is drawn backwards over needle; **D,** final result.

tapered needle that is elliptical instead of round. The tapered needle is generally used for closing mesenchymal layers such as muscle or fascia that are soft and easily penetrable. The cutting needle is used for keratinized mucosa, skin, or subcuticular layers where the tissue is difficult to penetrate.

Needles also vary in their attachments for the suture material. In the swaged needle the suture material is inserted into the hollow end during manufacture and the metal is compressed around it. The needle is not reusable. The eyed needle is designed to be reused, and the suture material is tied to the needle (Fig. 7-6). Since the eye is necessarily larger than the diameter of the suture, these needles do produce a slightly larger hole in the tissue than the swaged needle. Also available is a split-eye needle, which facilitates the threading and release of the suture and is used where interrupted sutures are placed in rapid succession or when all the sutures are placed along an incision before being tied. There is no doubt that the swaged needle has working qualities superior to the eyed needles, but its cost can be about ten times greater.

Suture materials (see also chapter 8)

The basic purpose of a suture is to hold severed tissues in close approximation until the healing process provides the wound with sufficient strength to withstand stress without the need for mechanical support. An ideal suture material would have adequate strength, good handling and knot tying characteristics, and would be sterilizable and evoke little tissue reaction.

Sutures are sized such that No. 3 is the largest and 7-0 is the smallest in general use. The more zeroes in the number, the smaller the diameter of the strand. Sutures of 5-0 or 6-0 are generally used for skin closure in the head and neck, while 3-0 and 4-0 are used intraorally. Sutures may be broadly categorized into two groups, absorbable and nonabsorbable.

ABSORBABLE SUTURES
Gut

Gut is the oldest known absorbable suture material. According to Katz and Turner (1970), Galen referred to gut suture as early as 175 A.D. Although often erroneously referred to as catgut, it is derived from sheep intestinal submucosa or bovine intestinal serosa. The origin of the word catgut is the Arabic "kitstring" or "kitgut," meaning the string of a dancing master's fiddle, which was also made of animal intestine. Over the years "kit" was confused with kitten or cat, and the misuse of the term was propagated. Although classified as a monofilament, plain gut suture viewed microscopically is composed of several plies that have been twisted slightly and then machine ground and polished to yield a smooth surface that is monofilamentous in appearance (Fig. 7-7). Grinding and polishing provide uniformity of diameter but also produce weak spots and tearing of fibrils, which result in fraying and breakage during use (Rhoads, Hottenstein, and Hudson, 1937). Because of its manner of manufacture and differences in the basic biologic source, gut is the most variable suture material in terms of tensile strength and absorbability (Gaskin and Childers, 1963; Rhoads, Hottenstein, and Hudson, 1937). As shown by Herrmann (1971), gut has the smallest tensile strength of any of the commonly used suture materials. Because it is an

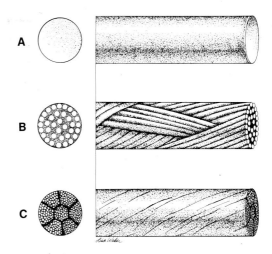

Fig. 7-7. Suture material in cross section. **A,** Monofilament; **B,** braided; **C,** gut.

organic material and highly susceptible to enzymatic degradation, it is packaged in isopropyl alcohol as a preservative, which also serves to condition or soften it. The suture absorbs the alcohol, causing it to swell and increase in diameter. The alcohol is combustible and is also irritating to tissue; it should be removed by a quick rinse in saline prior to use (Van Winkle, 1974). The suture should not be soaked, however, as Perey and Watier (1975) have shown that gut loses from 20% to 30% of its tensile strength when soaked in saline solution for 2 hours. This rapid loss in tensile strength is also seen in vivo, as shown by Mead and Ochsner (1940), Postlethwait and co-workers (1959), and Katz and Turner (1970). After 2 weeks of implantation, only 20% of the original tensile strength is present.

Gut suture is absorbed by proteolytic degradation and phagocytosis. This is accompanied by considerable inflammation and tissue reaction, as shown by Postlethwait and co-workers (1959, 1975); Postlethwait (1969, 1970a); Localio, Casale, and Hinton (1943); and Jenkins and colleagues (1942). When implanted abdominally in rabbits, total absorption of the suture material takes from 40 to 60 days (Katz and Turner, 1970). When placed intraorally through mucosal surfaces, the sutures generally are gone in 3 to 5 days, but because of the nature of the material this is variable (Wallace, Maxwell, and Cavalaris, 1970).

Plain gut is somewhat more difficult to use than other suture materials, as it is stiff and has insecure knot-holding characteristics when wet (Herrmann, 1971).

Chromic gut is plain gut that has been tanned with a solution of chromium salts prior to being spun, ground, and polished. The chromium salts act as a cross-linking agent and increase the tensile strength of the material and its resistance to absorption by the body (Edlich et al., 1973). Chromic gut has essentially the same physical and biologic properties as plain gut except for its slightly increased strength, prolonged rate of absorption, and lesser stimulation of tissue reaction. According to Van Winkle and Hastings (1972), chromic gut sutures may remain 80 days when implanted but according to Wallace, Maxwell, and Cavalaris (1970), most are degraded by 7 days when used intraorally. Again, there is much variability in the suture material and the tissue reaction to it.

Collagen

Reconstituted collagen sutures are obtained by grinding the native collagen of deep flexor tendons of cattle, which is then acidified to form a gel and extruded into a neutralizing dehydration bath. While this material was touted as having more uniform physical characteristics than gut, Truhlsen and Fitzpatrick (1964) have shown that it undergoes premature absorption. Reconstituted collagen sutures are not widely used.

Polyglycolic acid and polyglactin 910

Polyglycolic acid and polyglactin 910 differ significantly from other suture materials in that they are resorbed by hydrolysis. Since they are synthetic polymers, they produce very little tissue reaction. Polyglycolic acid is hydroxyacetic acid, which, in the presence of heat and a catalyst, is converted to a high molecular weight, linear chain polymer. The suture material is manufactured by orienting

these filaments by means of stretching and braiding (Fig. 7-7). Polyglactin 910 is a copolymer of glycolide and lactide, which are derived from hydroxyacetic and lactic acid, respectively. These two suture materials, when braided, are the strongest of the absorbable materials. According to Dardik, Dardik, and Laufman (1971), metabolic studies utilizing ^{14}C showed that the metabolites of polyglycolic acid are used as food substances via the citric acid cycle and produce energy, carbon dioxide, and water. Other studies by Herrmann, Kelly, and Higgins (1970), Maxwell (1969), Morgan (1969), Katz and Turner (1970), Wallace, Maxwell, and Cavalaris (1970), and Perey and Watier (1975) have shown the material to be well tolerated when implanted or used intraorally. Wallace, Maxwell, and Cavalaris (1970) have shown that the material will last in excess of 14 days when used intraorally, while Van Winkel and Hastings (1972) have shown that the suture may remain for 4 months when implanted. Edlich and co-workers (1973) have shown a reduction in bacterial counts in cultures of *Staphylococcus aureus* exposed to glycolic acid buffered to pH 7.4. They postulated that the degradation products of polyglycolic acid may destroy bacteria in the wound and thereby minimize tissue reaction. Postlethwait (1970b) reported that implanted polyglycolic acid sutures lose tensile strength significantly more rapidly than chromic gut sutures and that no residual tensile strength was seen after 28 days of implantation. Conn and colleagues (1974), Craig and colleagues (1975), and Salthouse and Matlaga (1976) have studied the tissue reaction to polyglactin 910 and found it well tolerated. One advantage was its quicker dissolution (80 days) when implanted (Salthouse and Matlaga, 1976) as compared with polyglycolic acid. Wallace, Maxwell, and Cavalaris (1970) have shown that polyglycolic acid sutures remain in the mouth too long to be used as an absorbable suture but can be used as a nonabsorbable suture and removed in 5 to 7 days. Another problem is the difficulty in tying this suture material. The material does not

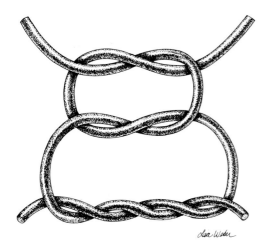

Fig. 7-8. Suggested knot for polyglycolic acid, polyglactin 910, and synthetic suture materials. First tie involves three throws of material. This is followed by two ties in opposite directions, which provide square knot over first tie.

slide easily on itself, making tying difficult. The manufacturer recommends wetting the material with saline solution to facilitate tying. A knot such as used for the synthetic suture materials (Fig. 7-8) is recommended to prevent loosening of the tie. These suture materials are useful in the subcuticular area, but their expense limits routine use in situations where nonabsorbable sutures are indicated.

NONABSORBABLE SUTURES

Silk

Although classed as a nonabsorbable suture, silk is an organic substance that undergoes slow proteolysis when implanted (Douglas, 1949). Before it was recognized that silk was not a true nonabsorbable suture, several disastrous results involving suture line rupture around vascular prostheses and dislodgment of artificial heart valves occurred because of degradation of the silk sutures. Silk will lose most of its tensile strength after 1 year of implantation and usually disappears after 2 years.

Silk is the most popular suture material for intraoral use. It is braided, which gives it excellent handling characteristics; it produces a moderate tissue response; it does not irritate adjacent mucous membrane; and it is inexpensive. Postlethwait (1970a) and Van Winkle and co-workers (1975) have shown that silk initially produces more tissue reaction in terms of the amount of inflammation than synthetic nonabsorbable sutures, but the reaction at 7 days is only slightly greater than that seen with other materials. According to Herrmann (1971), silk has one of the lowest tensile strengths among suture materials, ranking just above gut and collagen, and in terms of knot-holding ability it ranks the lowest of all the commonly used suture materials. Therefore at least three ties should be used for each knot.

Nylon

Nylon can be obtained in braided or monofilament forms. In its monofilament form it is the most popular skin suture material (Fig. 7-7). Madsen (1953), Sewell (1966), Postlethwait (1970a), Postlethwait and co-workers (1975), Salthouse and Matlaga (1975), Van Winkle and Hastings (1972), and Van Winkle and co-workers (1975) have studied the tissue reaction to implanted nylon suture and found that it was minimal. Edlich and co-workers (1973) have shown that in vitro the degradation products of nylon, adipic acid, and 1,6 hexanediamine, even when buffered to pH 7.4, cause a marked reduction in counts of *Staphylococcus aureus* in culture. They postulated that this antibacterial activity may account in part for the good tissue response.

Nylon, like other synthetic polymeric materials, possesses the property of "memory." This memory is actually the built-in orientation of the polymer produced by extruding and stretching during the manufacture of the filament. When tied, the suture tends to "remember" that it was originally a straight fiber and knots slip and untie. Accordingly, some surgeons facetiously say that they tie one knot for every day they desire the suture to remain in place. Generally, multiple square knots are necessary to maintain the tie. Herrmann (1971) has shown that nylon has good tensile strength but ranks below that of steel, Dacron, and polyglycolic acid. Because of its stiffness, the large knot required, and a tendency to tear through nonkeratinized tissue, nylon is not frequently used intraorally.

Cotton and linen

Cotton suture is made from noncontinuous natural fibers of cotton, which are combined into yarns and then twisted into plies. Following the report by Mead and Ochsner (1940), cotton became popular during World War II when silk was relatively unavailable. While its strength is similar to silk, its handling characteristics are inferior. Tissue reaction, as shown by Postlethwait (1970a), is similar. Linen is somewhat stronger than cotton but otherwise has similar characteristics. Neither of these materials has been widely used in recent years.

Metal

Stainless steel or tantalum sutures are either monofilament or braided. They are the strongest and produce the most secure knot of any suture materials (Herrmann, 1971). Tissue tolerance is good but is less than that found with nylon, Dacron, or polypropylene (Edlich et al., 1973). Metallic material may undergo degradation through corrosion, resulting in transfer of ions from the suture to the tissue. Although this degradation process is slow, tissue reaction to these ions can occur. The physical properties of the metallic suture may also negatively affect tissue reaction. Metallic sutures are stiff and do not conform to the suture pathway during host movement. The resultant irritation may produce tissue damage and increased susceptibility to infection. These materials are sometimes used in scar revision in keloid-forming patients, but in oral and maxillofacial surgery they are generally used for suspension of splints or arch bars and not as a suture material.

Dacron polyester, polypropylene, polyethylene, Teflon-coated or -impregnated Dacron polyester, silicone-coated Dacron polyester

Dacron polyester, Teflon-coated or -impregnated Dacron polyester, and silicone-coated Dacron polyester are braided suture materials. This class of synthetics exhibits the greatest tensile strength and knot holding ability of the nonmetallic suture materials (Herrmann, 1971). The tissue reaction is minimal and is unaffected by the presence of an inert coating or impregnation with silicone or Teflon (Edlich et al., 1973; Van Winkle and Hastings, 1972; Varma et al., 1974). Difficulties that were encountered in handling multifilament Dacron sutures led to the development of coated Dacron sutures. The surface of a Dacron suture has a high coefficient of friction, which interferes with the ties being slipped into place. The inert coating enables the surgeon to tie more easily. A modified method for tying these sutures can be found in Fig. 7-8. Edlich and colleagues (1973) showed that these inert coatings were very irregular. While it would seem that the coating would eliminate or minimize tissue fluid absorption by the material and reduce the rate of infection, no difference in the infection rate was found in comparing coated and uncoated sutures.

TISSUE REACTION TO SUTURES

The initial body response to sutures is almost identical in the first 4 to 7 days, regardless of the suture material (Edlich and co-workers, 1973; Schoen, 1976). The damage done to the tissue by the needle evokes a significant inflammatory response even without the presence of suture material (Madsen, 1953). The early response is a generalized acute aseptic inflammation, involving primarily polymorphonuclear leukocytes. After a few days, mononuclear cells, fibroblasts, and histiocytes (tissue macrophages) become evident (Schoen, 1976). Capillary formation occurs at the end of this initial phase (Sewell, 1966).

After 4 to 7 days the response is related more to the type of suture material. For example, plain gut elicits an intense response with macrophages and polymorphonuclear leukocytes predominating (Jenkins et al., 1942; Postlethwait et al., 1959), while the nonabsorbable materials show a less intense, relatively acellular histologic pattern (Postlethwait, 1969). If the suture material leads to mucosal or skin surfaces, epithelial cells will begin tracking down the suture pathway at 5 to 7 days (Van Winkle et al., 1975; Wallace, Maxwell, and Cavalaris, 1970). The longer the suture remains, the deeper the epithelial invasion of the underlying tissue. When the suture is removed, an epithelial tract remains. These cells may eventually disappear or remain to form keratin and epithelial inclusion cysts. The epithelial pathway may also cause the site of the suture to be visible and the typical "railroad track" scar results.

The development of surgical infections is greatly enhanced by the presence of a suture in a contaminated wound. In human volunteers, Elek and Conen (1957) noted that an injection of 10^6 *Staphylococcus pyogenes* was required to produce a purulent clinical infection. Under identical conditions, except for the inclusion of a single silk suture, the necessary amount of bacteria was reduced to 100 cocci. The presence of the suture thus increased the susceptibility to infection by a factor of 10,000 times. The use of monofilament sutures rather than braided sutures has been advocated to reduce the potential for infection. It has been suggested that multifilament sutures provide a haven for bacteria, which can penetrate the interstices of the suture—places that are too small to admit granulocytes and macrophages. Indeed, Alexander, Kaplan, and Altemeier (1967) have shown an increased incidence of infection with *Staphylococcus aureus* implanted subcutaneously with braided materials containing six knots compared with monofilament suture material under similar conditions. However, nonknotted braided and unbraided suture material showed no difference in the incidence of infection in a study by Edlich and colleagues (1973). It was their contention that knots tended to exaggerate the physical differences between the braided and unbraided material.

Although certain monofilament materials such as nylon or polypropylene provide good protection against infection partially because of their acceptability by tissue (Edlich et al., 1973; Varma et al., 1974), other factors must be considered when dealing with an already infected wound. Studies have shown that plain gut is superior to chromic gut in infected wounds, despite the fact that there is greater tissue tolerance to chromic gut suture (Edlich et al., 1973). The proposed explanation of this phenomenon is that the plain gut suture disappears faster than the chromic gut suture, and once rid of the foreign material the body defenses are allowed to concentrate on the infection. Edlich et al. (1973) also found that the infection rate was much higher in the presence of contamination plus even the least tissue reactive suture material when compared to the same situation without a suture. Therefore sutures should generally not be used in the presence of an infection, and they should be removed if an infection becomes evident.

All sutures passing through the mucous membrane or skin provide a "wick" down which bacteria can gain access to the underlying tissues (Postlethwait et al., 1959; Lilly, 1968; Lilly et al., 1968). Because of this and the downward growth of epithelial tissue, the sutures should be removed as early as possible consistent with adequate healing. Generally, sutures should be removed after 3 to 5 days on skin of the head and neck, 5 to 7 days intraorally, 5 to 10 days in other sites, and longer for areas subjected to considerable stress, such as over joints or the iliac crest, or in areas of slower healing, such as the palms or soles. Freshly incised and sutured tissue has only 25% of the original tensile strength of the tissue before incision (Botsford, 1941). The tissue strength of the wound at 10 days may be only 10% of the original strength. Approximately 3 weeks of healing is required for the wound to strengthen to 25% of the original tensile strength. Therefore cutaneous wounds should be supported with sterile tape following suture removal. It should be noted that Capendale and Sereda (1965) reported a 16.7% incidence of infection in skin wounds closed with suture and no infection in wounds closed with tape.

PRINCIPLES OF SUTURING

1. The needle holder should grasp the needle at approximately ¾ of the distance from the point. The suture end of the needle is the weakest area because either it is hollow, as in the case of a swaged needle, or it contains the eye. Grasping the suture end will result in at least a bent needle, if not a broken one.

2. The needle should enter the tissue perpendicular to the surface (Fig. 7-9). If the needle pierces the tissue obliquely, a tear may develop.

3. The needle should be passed through the tissue following the curve of the needle. Treating a curved needle (Fig. 7-9) as a straight needle, for example, will result in tissue tearing.

4. The suture should be placed at an equal distance (2 to 3 mm) from the incision on both sides and at an equal depth. This principle can be modified in cases where the tissue edges to be sutured are at different levels; then passage of the suture closer to the edge of the lower side and farther from the edge of the higher side will tend to approximate the levels (Pick, 1941). Another method involves passage of the suture at an equal distance from the wound margins on both sides (May, 1971) but deeper into the tissue on the lower side and more superficially on the higher side. These techniques are pictured in Fig. 7-10.

5. If one tissue side is free (as with a flap) and the other fixed, the needle should be passed from the free to the fixed side.

6. If one tissue side is thinner than the other, then the needle should be passed from the thinner to the thicker side.

7. If one tissue plane is deeper than the other, then the needle should be passed from the deeper to the superficial side.

8. The distance that the needle is passed into the tissue should be greater than the distance from the tissue edge. This will ensure a degree of tissue eversion (Fig. 7-9). Some degree of tissue eversion is desirable in anticipation of scar contracture.

9. The tissues should not be closed under tension, since they will either tear or necrose around the suture. If tension is present, the tissue layer should be undermined to relieve it (Fig. 7-11).

10. The suture should be tied so the tissue is merely approximated, not blanched.

11. The knot should not be placed over the incision line.

12. Sutures should be placed approximately 3 to 4 mm apart. The closeness of the sutures depends on the anticipated tension across the suture line. Closer spaced sutures are indicated in areas of underlying muscular activity such as the tongue or in other areas of increased tension.

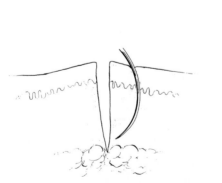 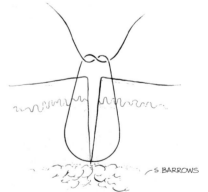

Fig. 7-9. Needle passage through tissue. Needle should enter perpendicular to epithelium and pass through tissue along curvature of needle. Distance from incision to point of needle penetration should be less than depth to which needle penetrates to cause eversion of wound margins when suture is tied. Suture should be equal distance and equal depth from wound margin on both sides.

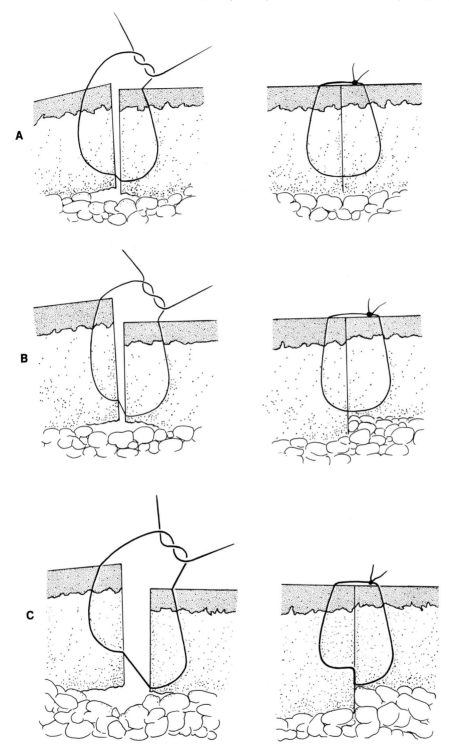

Fig. 7-10. Techniques of leveling tissue edges. **A,** When tissue edges are of equal thickness but one side is elevated, tying knot on depressed side will tend to reapproximate edges. **B,** When tissues are of unequal thickness, passage of needle further from incision on thinner side will tend to even edges. **C,** When tissues are of unequal thickness, deeper penetration of needle in thinner tissue will tend to even edges.

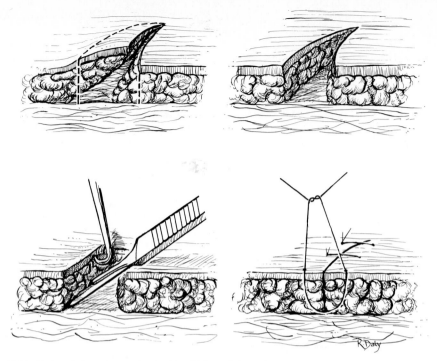

Fig. 7-11. Undermining of wound margins. Oblique injury may result in loss of tissue vitality. When this tissue is excised, it may leave defect that cannot be closed without tension. Undermining tissue margins, either sharply or bluntly, will result in closure that is tension-free.

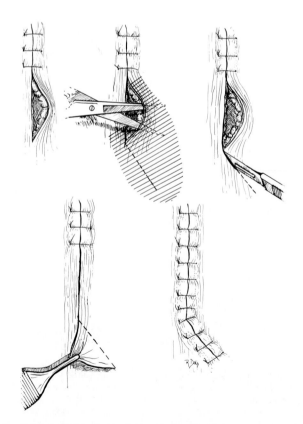

Fig. 7-12. Eliminating "dog-ear" at end of incision. After undermining excess tissue, incision is made at approximately 30 degrees to parent incision directed toward undermined side. Extra tissue is pulled over incision and the appropriate amount is excised. Incision is then closed in normal manner.

13. Occasionally, extra tissue may be present on one side of the incision and cause a "dog-ear" to be formed in the final phase of wound closure. Simply extending the length of the incision to hide the excess will produce an unsatisfactory result. A technique to deal with this problem is illustrated in Fig. 7-12. Other techniques to deal with this have been proposed by Converse (1975).

KNOT TYING

The surgeon may use either the instrument tie (Fig. 7-13) or the one- or two-hand tie (Fig. 7-14). The instrument tie is more convenient in closed areas such as the mouth but can be used in open areas as well. Therefore mastery of this technique is recommended.

Square knot

The basic knot is the square knot, which is illustrated in Fig. 7-15. Although only two ties are illustrated, it is prudent to provide at least three ties for surface knots. Certain types of suture material such as nylon, polypropylene, polyglycolic acid, and gut may require more ties.

Surgeon's knot

Because of the double throw, the surgeon's knot offers the advantage of reducing slippage of the first tie, while the second tie is put in place. This is particularly useful in confined or difficult to reach places where the first tie would ordinarily be loosened in the process of producing the second tie. A third tie

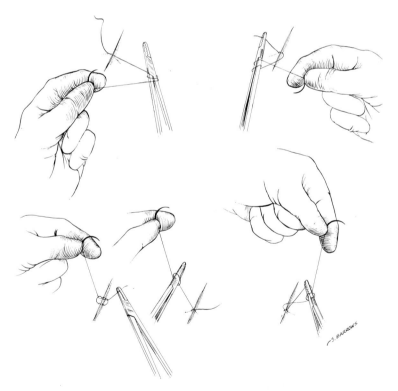

Fig. 7-13. Instrument tie. Following passage of needle through tissue, suture material is wrapped around needle holder. Needle holder grasps end of suture and suture is tied. Suture is then wrapped around needle holder in opposite direction, suture is grasped, and final tie is made resulting in knot (surgeon's knot is illustrated).

One-hand tie

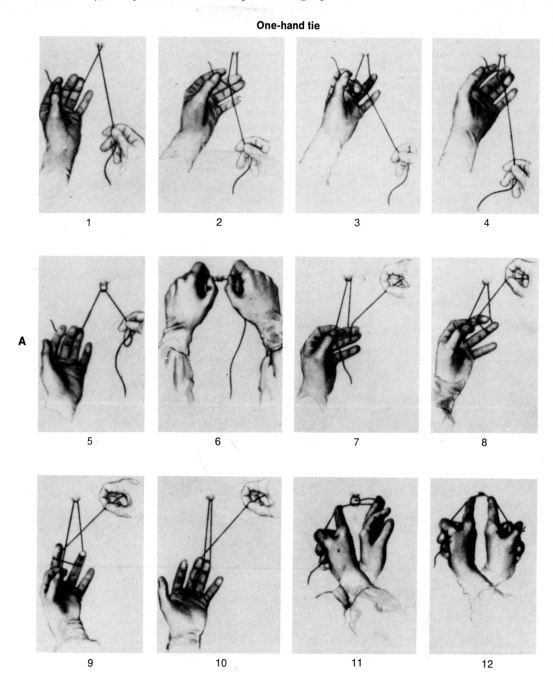

A

Fig. 7-14. A, One-handed tie. Step 1: Suture has one end longer than the other. Left hand grasps shorter end, which is crossed under longer end held in right hand. Step 2: Long end is crossed over fingers, creating loop. Steps 3 to 6: Middle finger is used to bring short end back through loop, and then tie is tightened. Step 7: Long end of suture being held by right hand is curled around fourth finger of left hand. Steps 8 and 9: Middle finger is used to create loop with long end, which lies beneath short end. Steps 10 to 12: Third and fourth fingers grasp shorter suture end and bring it back through loop making tie that, when tightened, will create square knot. Note that hands are crossed to perform this last step.

Two-hand knot tie
(after Partipilo)

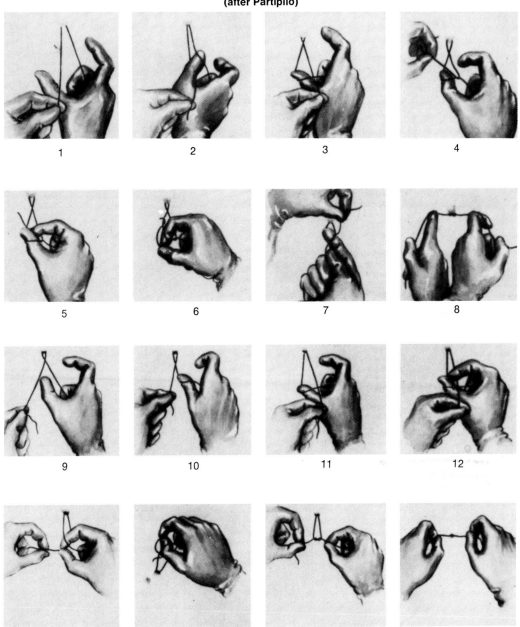

B

Fig. 7-14, cont'd. B, Two-handed tie. Step 1: Left hand holds short suture end. Spool of suture material or longer end is held in right hand. Steps 2 and 3: Thumb engages longer suture end and pulls it over short end, creating loop. Steps 4 to 6: Short end is crossed over loop and then guided through it by second finger of right hand. Short end is released by left hand during this maneuver. Steps 7 and 8: Short end is regained by left hand and tie tightened to place with hands crossed. Step 9: Long end, held in right hand, is crossed beneath short end. Steps 10 to 12: Long end is curled around thumb and thumb extended beneath short suture end to create loop. Step 13: While loop is maintained by second finger, thumb slips from loop to grasp short end between it and second finger. Steps 14 to 16: Short end is directed through loop by thumb. Tie is then tightened with hands in uncrossed position, creating square knot. In either one- or two-handed techniques, additional ties may be required, depending on suture material, to ensure stable knot. (Courtesy Ethicon, Inc., Sommerville, N.J.)

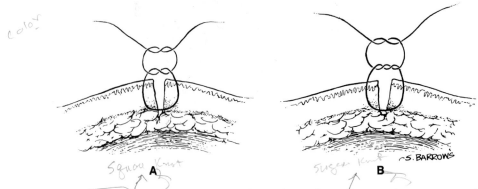

Fig. 7-15. Square knot and surgeon's knot. **A,** Square knot is formed by wrapping suture around needle holder once in opposite directions between ties. **B,** Surgeon's knot is formed by two throws of suture around needle holder on first tie and then one throw in opposite direction on second tie.

squared on the surgeon's knot is usually made for security (Fig. 7-15). This method is modified for use with polyglycolic acid and synthetic sutures (Fig. 7-8).

Granny knot

This knot involves a tie in one direction followed by a single tie in the same direction as the first. This will allow the knot to be slipped to place and provide initial holding similar to the surgeon's knot. However, a third tie squared on the second must be made to hold the knot permanently.

SUTURE METHODS

Interrupted suture

The interrupted suture (Fig. 7-16) is the most commonly used. Its advantages are that it is strong and that successive sutures can be placed in a manner to fit the individual requirements of the situation. Each suture is independent of the next, and the distance between each suture and between the sutures and the incision line can be easily varied. The loosening of one suture will not produce loosening of any of the other sutures. A degree of eversion of the incision can be produced by ensuring that the depth of the bite is greater than the distance from the suture to the wound edge (Fig. 7-9). Should the wound become infected, removal of a few selected sutures may be satisfactory treatment. For a strong closure or in areas of tension, this technique is preferred over the continuous suture.

Continuous suture

The continuous suture provides a rapid technique for closure (Fig. 7-17). Another advantage of the continuous suture is the even distribution of tension over the entire suture line. If the tissues should swell in one area, as for example with the formation of a hematoma, the remaining sutured area can provide a degree of slack that will help relieve the pressure. The continuous suture also provides a more watertight closure (Shoen, 1976), which is important in intraoral bone grafting. It should not be used in areas of existing tension.

Locking continuous suture

This suture technique offers two advantages over the simple continuous technique (Fig. 7-18). First, the suture will align itself perpendicularly to the incision. Second, the locking feature prevents continuous tightening of the suture as wound closure progresses. However, care must be exercised not to tighten the individual lock excessively, since this can produce tissue necrosis. Also, the locking feature may prevent adjustment of tension over the suture line as tissue swelling occurs.

Mattress suture

The main purpose of mattress sutures is to provide more tissue eversion than occurs with simple interrupted sutures. They also may be used in areas where wound contraction could cause dehiscence or broad scar formation. These are

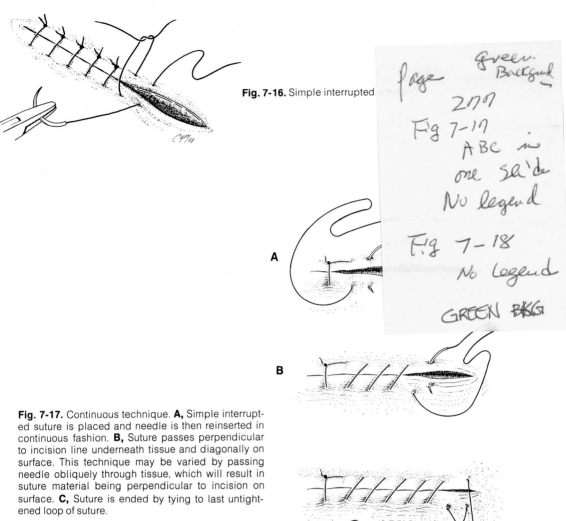

Fig. 7-16. Simple interrupted

A

B

Fig. 7-17. Continuous technique. **A,** Simple interrupted suture is placed and needle is then reinserted in continuous fashion. **B,** Suture passes perpendicular to incision line underneath tissue and diagonally on surface. This technique may be varied by passing needle obliquely through tissue, which will result in suture material being perpendicular to incision on surface. **C,** Suture is ended by tying to last untightened loop of suture.

C

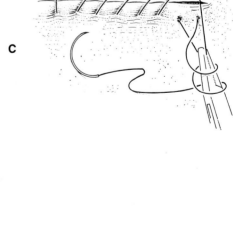

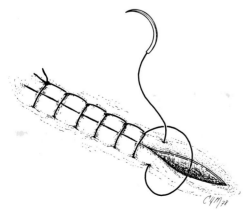

Fig. 7-18. Continuous locking technique. Suture is passed perpendicular to incision line and degree of locking is provided by withdrawing suture through its own loop. This suture technique is begun and ended identically to continuous technique (Fig. 7-17).

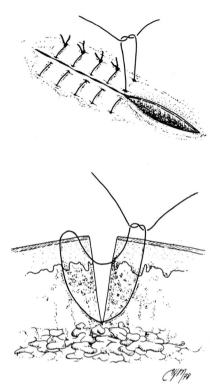

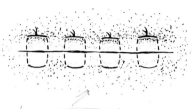

Fig. 7-20. Horizontal mattress technique. Placement of these sutures may compromise blood supply to flap edge on both sides of incision.

Fig. 7-19. Vertical mattress technique. Needle is passed close to incision line on both sides and then engages tissue deep to first pass when returning toward original side.

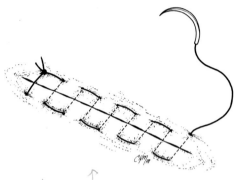

Fig. 7-21. Continuous horizontal mattress technique. A great deal of tissue eversion can be accomplished with this technique without endangering blood supply to edges of incision.

generally skin surfaces such as the abdomen or hip and not the head and neck, although some surgeons do use the vertical mattress suture in neck closures. The vertical mattress suture offers the advantage of running parallel to the blood supply to the edge of the flap and therefore not interfering with healing (Fig. 7-19).

The interrupted horizontal mattress suture (Fig. 7-20) produces broad contact of the wound margins and is useful where such a condition is needed. However, it suffers from the disadvantage of constricting the blood supply to the edges of the incision. If improperly used, this can cause necrosis and dehiscence. The continuous horizontal mattress suture (Fig. 7-21) does limit the blood supply to the flap edge. but only minimally, and does not interfere with wound healing. It is a technique often used after in-

traoral bone grafting, as the eversion and continuity provide a very watertight closure.

Figure-of-8 suture

The figure-of-8 suture (Fig. 7-22) is used over extraction sites, where it provides some protection to the surgical area as well as adaptation of the gingival papillae around the adjacent teeth.

Subcuticular suture

An absorbable 4-0 suture material is generally used for closure of the subcuticular layer. If individual subcuticular sutures are placed, they should be buried with the knot inverted (Fig. 7-23). A continuous subcuticular suture, as popularized by Halsted (1893), may be used with no knots by having the ends exit a short distance from the wound and taping them

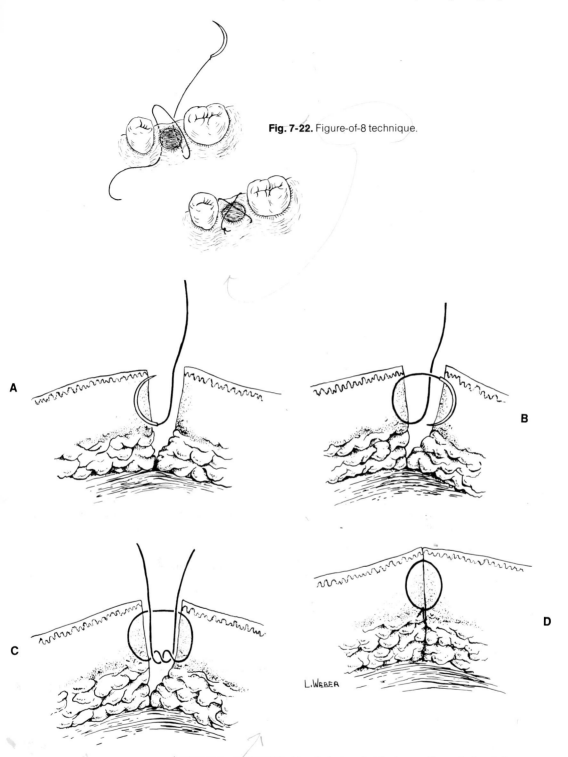

Fig. 7-22. Figure-of-8 technique.

Fig. 7-23. Knot inversion in subcuticular sutures. **A,** Needle is inserted in deeper tissue first and directed toward surface. **B,** Needle is inserted in opposite side going from superficial to deep tissue. **C,** Square knot is tied in usual manner. **D,** Suture ends are cut short to minimize amount of material that is buried. Knot will be inverted within tissue.

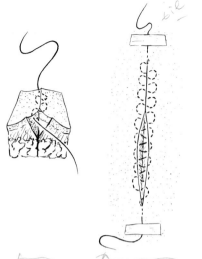

Fig. 7-24. Continuous subcuticular technique. Needle penetrates skin ahead of incision and exits within wound. Needle is then inserted on opposite sides of incision in continuous fashion. At end of incision, suture is brought out at distance from wound. By pulling both ends of suture, incision is closed. Suture ends are taped to skin.

to the skin (Fig. 7-24). In this technique a thicker nonabsorbable (3-0) suture is used. Free passage of the suture along the incision to facilitate subsequent removal is ensured by pulling the ends after placement. The wound may be further supported by sterile tape across the incision. A continuous subcuticular suture may be left for 7 to 10 days and removed by untaping both ends and pulling in one direction.

SUTURE REMOVAL

When sutures are removed, the suture should be grasped with an instrument and elevated above the epithelial surface. A scissors should be used to transect one side of the loop as close to the epithelial surface as possible. In this way a minimal amount of the portion of the suture that was exposed to the outside environment and has become laden with debris and bacteria will be dragged through the tissue.

DRAINS AND PACKING

Drains are used to help prevent the formation of hematomas or seromas within soft or hard tissue dead spaces that may subsequently become infected. A pressure dressing is often a more effective way to eliminate this problem in soft tissue, but there are areas where a pressure dressing cannot be applied. The most popular drain material is rubber, as it is both smooth and relatively nonporous. The drain should be sutured to an outside surface to prevent it from accidentally being removed or from disappearing within the wound. Tying a knot in a drain to accomplish this is inadvisable, since it blocks drainage and does not prevent slippage into the wound. In uncontaminated intraosseous defects, the formation of a hematoma should be considered favorable toward the process of bony healing. Should the area become infected, either a small section of the original incision or a separate incision can be used for drainage.

Drains are also used to provide an exit for purulence to an outside surface. Making cuts in a tubular drain is an anachronism from the days when antibiotics were flushed through the drain and allowed to seep into an abscess cavity. This practice of using antibiotics topically has been almost totally abandoned except for a few specific instances. Notching the drain does not enhance drainage and may serve to weaken it so that it separates inside the wound at the time of removal.

Packing of a wound is done to obliterate dead space or to permit healing by secondary intention. It may be used following the removal of a tumor or odontogenic keratocyst where there may be recurrence. In this manner the whole surgical area can be watched while it heals, and any abnormal tissue may be quickly noticed and easily biopsied. Packing may also be done to apply topical medications to a surgical wound, as in the treatment of localized osteitis. Iodoform gauze is a common material used for packing, and it may be impregnated with an antibiotic ointment, eugenol, balsam of Peru, or other medicaments as necessary.

DRESSINGS

A dressing may provide wound coverage and support, pressure to an area to

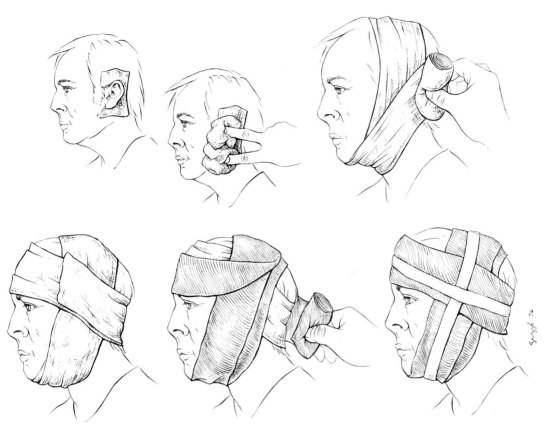

Fig. 7-25. Pressure dressing to ramus area. Ear pad is fashioned to prevent compression of auricle, and fluffed gauze is placed over area to receive pressure. Gauze bandage is placed over this, taking care not to obstruct airway. Bandage may be turned as it is passed beneath chin to minimize amount of gauze in this area (not pictured). This wrap may be followed by a bias-cut stockinette bandage, which is placed firmly but not too tightly.

prevent hematoma formation, or temporary support to facial fractures. It is generally recommended that freshly sutured wounds have coverage for the first 24 to 48 hours. The dressing material should be sterile and have properties such that adherence to the wound does not take place. If the dressing material is taped to the skin, nonallergenic paper tape is superior to cloth tape for this purpose.

A pressure dressing is usually placed for 48 to 72 hours to limit swelling and prevent hematoma formation. The dressing may be removed before this time to permit wound observation but should be promptly replaced. Fig. 7-25 demonstrates the placement of a dressing designed to apply pressure over the ramus or preauricular areas. The padding for the ears is placed first, followed by fluffed

gauze over the area to receive the pressure. The first wrap is gauze, which is placed firmly but passively over the head. The second wrap is bias-cut stockinette, which is elastic and can produce great pressure. This is only slightly tensed as it is wrapped around the head. If swelling develops, the stockinette will become more tense and exert more inward pressure.

A dressing useful for placing pressure over the anterior maxilla is shown in Fig. 7-26. An eye patch is placed over the eye and a piece of gauze over the other eye. Fluffed gauze is placed over the area to receive the pressure. A wrap of gauze is made around the head and below the occiput, and the gauze over the eye is tied to expose it.

A pressure dressing over the chin can

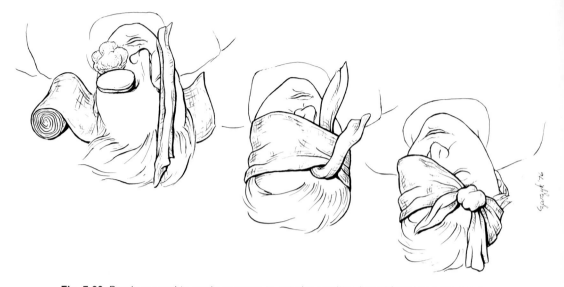

Fig. 7-26. Bandage used to apply pressure to anterior maxilla viewed from head of operating room table. With patient in supine position, fluffed gauze is placed over area to receive pressure, eye patch is placed over adjacent eye, and gauze strip is placed over opposite eye. Area is wrapped with gauze bandage and then strip is tied to elevate dressing from eye on opposite side.

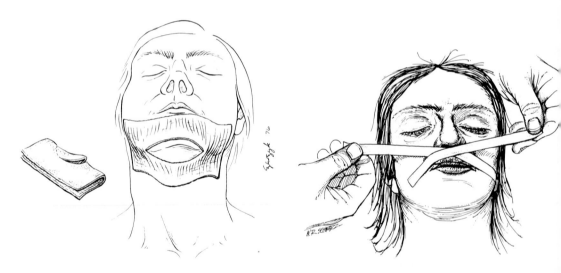

Fig. 7-27. Pressure applied with self-adhesive elastic bandage.

Fig. 7-28. Pressure applied with tape placed over gauze.

be placed following procedures like vestibuloplasty or subapical osteotomy (Fig. 7-27). An adhesive elastic bandage with a semicircular piece removed is used. This allows space for the point of the chin to protrude without pressure. Pressure on this area can cause necrosis

of the skin. Pressure over the anterior maxilla or mandible may also be applied by using two pieces of tape crisscrossed over fluffed gauze placed on the area that is expected to swell (Fig. 7-28).

The Barton bandage is used to support a fractured mandible (Fig. 7-29). This is

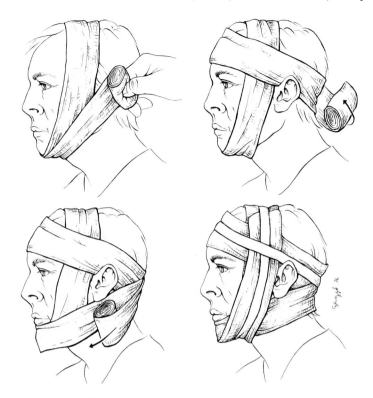

Fig. 7-29. Barton bandage. This bandage is used for support and must be firmly applied with non-elastic materials. Posterior portion must be applied under occiput or bandage will loosen and slip off.

usually a temporary measure that can be done quickly in the emergency room to provide some relief for the patient until a more definitive treatment can be administered.

ELECTROSURGERY
History

Cusel, a Russian, was the first to apply electricity to surgical excision when in 1847 he attempted to destroy a neoplasm with electrical current (Valobra and Fiandesio, 1968). In France in 1893, d'Arsonval published his study on tissue reaction to radio frequency currents. It was not until 1925 that the concept of electrothermy was introduced into the American literature when Ward reported the destruction of malignancies with this method. Other pioneers, such as Cushing and Bovie, were responsible for the re-

finement in equipment and increasing the popularity of this technique (Walter, 1972).

Definitions (Jackson, 1970)

Medical diathermy. Using two electrodes, an alternating current may be passed through the body with no effects other than the production of heat. The current must be of sufficiently high frequency to avoid nervous or muscular response. The heat produced is solely the result of the resistance offered by the tissue to the passage of the current. When one electrode is large (dispersive) and the other small (active), the current is no longer evenly dispersed. This results in a concentration of current at the smaller electrode, and the effects are dehydration, warming of the area, coagulation, or tissue destruction by heat depending on the type, the size and frequency of the current, the size of the active electrode, and the duration of application. Most surgical applications of electricity make use of this principle.

Electrodesiccation (electrofulguration). In this technique a high-frequency alternating current of high voltage and low amperage is used. The oscillations of the current are dampened such that the intensity of the voltage rapidly diminishes with each oscillation followed by a gap when the voltage declines to zero. Only one electrode is used, and desiccation is produced when it is placed in contact with the tissue. If the electrode is held away from the tissue, a spark will jump from the electrode to the tissue resulting in a superficial burn, or carbonization. This process is called fulguration. Both of these techniques were popular in the earlier days of electrosurgery but are rarely used today.

Electrocoagulation. Two electrodes, one active and one dispersive, are used with a high-frequency damped alternating current with lower amperage and voltage than that used for electrodesiccation. The resultant heat at the active electrode promotes coagulation within severed vessels, but more importantly for hemostasis, it burns and seals the edges of these vessels. This method does produce localized necrosis and inflammation (Feldman et al., 1970).

Electrosurgery. Two electrodes, one active and one dispersive, use a high-frequency alternating current that is either undamped and rectified, producing a pure cutting effect, or moderately damped and rectified, producing a blend of cutting and coagulation. Most electrosurgical machines use this blend. The disadvantage of electrosurgery causing increased tissue necrosis may be outweighed by less bleeding in the surgical field. Feldman and co-workers (1970) believe that electrocoagulated nerve ends give less postoperative pain.

Electrocautery. In this technique a low voltage, high-amperage current is passed through a wire that becomes heated. The heated wire is applied to the tissue to produce burning. This technique does not use the principle of diathermy. The term electrocautery is often misapplied to electrocoagulation.

Tissue effects

Early researchers disagreed on the tissue effects of electrosurgery. In some studies tissue healing was found not to differ significantly following electrosurgical or scalpel surgery (Burgess, 1933; Edwards and Dunphy, 1958; Eisenmann, Malone, and Kusek, 1970; Ellis, 1933; Klug, 1966; Lampert, 1970; Malone and Manning, 1968; Malone et al., 1969; Mock, 1935; Oringer, 1969). Other investigators found that electrosurgery produced delayed healing, tissue slough, and infection (Glickman and Imber, 1970; Jackson and Jackson, 1958; Lawrenson and Stephens, 1970; Orban, 1944; Pope et al., 1968; Poswillo, 1971; Smity, 1964). One reason for the differing results was the use of varying instrumentation in these studies. Before 1970, it was not generally realized that a difference in tissue response to the application of rectified versus unrectified currents existed. Feldman and co-workers (1970), Eisenmann and co-workers (1970), and Oringer (1976) have pointed out that rectified current produces less tissue damage than unrectified current. This discovery, however, has not eliminated the controversy. Eisenmann and co-workers (1970) reported no difference in pain, wound texture, inflammation, or cellular definition using a fully rectified cutting electrosurgical unit versus the scalpel. Sozio, Riley, and Shklar (1976) found different results including delayed healing, suppuration, cellular necrosis, and a foreign body reaction in underlying tissues. These differing results ·may be related to varying surgical techniques as discussed by Oringer (1976).

Techniques

The initial process begins with the placement of the dispersive electrode. This electrode should have broad body contact as close to the operating site as possible. The complications of improper placement will be elaborated in the following section.

If electrosurgery is used, the unit ideally should be one with a fully rectified wave (Oringer, 1976). When setting the machine, it is more prudent to err by setting the current a little too high than a little too low (Feldman et al., 1970). With the current too high, a small amount of searing of the margins may result. If the current is too low, the surgical electrode will produce tissue shredding and delayed healing.

The active electrode should be passed through the tissue as quickly and precisely as possible in a brush stroke movement with no pressure (Friedman, 1973). A continuous rapid movement is important because delay in one area will cause tissue burning. Allowing time between each stroke will allow the heat to dissipate and produce less damage. Oringer (1976) recommends that the tissue not be stretched when cutting but allowed to remain at normal tension. The active electrode must not come in contact with periosteum or bone (Glickman and Imber, 1970), although this has been disputed by Malone and co-workers (1969) and Oringer (1969).

Electrosurgery has been used for retraction of gingival tissues (Klug, 1966; Malone and Manning, 1968; Ogus, 1942; Oringer, 1960; Podshady, 1968; Saghirian, 1940), in periodontics (Lampert, 1970; Malone, 1969; Oringer, 1969), in endodontics for canal sterilization (Feldman et al., 1970; Oringer, 1962; Shomberg and Malone, 1969), for desensitization of exposed cementum (Shomberg and Malone, 1969), for removal of lesions (Smity, 1964), and in making incisions in vascular areas, as in LeFort I osteotomies.

When used as a coagulation device, it is better to err by adjusting the machine on the low side of the current setting, as this can always be increased. Too high a setting will result in a large area of necrosis and slough. The electrode may be applied directly or indirectly (via a hemostat or forceps) to the bleeding tissue. If the hemorrhage is brisk, the blood will dissipate the heat around the active electrode and the searing effect of the current will not occur. In this case the field must be temporarily dried by aspiration or pressure, or the bleeding vessel may be grasped with a hemostat to first stop the bleeding. In the latter instance the active electrode is applied to the hemostat, thus converting it to the active electrode, and coagulation will occur in tissues that are grasped. The surgeon must be careful to wear intact rubber gloves or he may be inadvertently shocked.

Complications

Explosion of volatile anesthetic gases, burns at sites remote from the surgery, ignition of dry sponges in the mouth, burning of the endotracheal tube, ventricular fibrillation, and electrocution are all complications that have been reported resulting from the use of faulty electrical equipment or the inappropriate use of good electrical equipment in the operating room (Arnow et al., 1969; Bruner, 1967; Dobbie, 1969; Hopps, 1968; Hungerbuhler, Swope, and Reves, 1974; Stanley, 1971; Taylor and Desmond, 1970; Walter, 1969; Walter, 1972). All that is necessary to burn, shock, or electrocute a patient is a source of electricity attached to the patient and a sink or ground that will allow the electricity to leave the patient and complete the circuit. As little as 0.1 amps current at 60 cycles per second can produce ventricular fibrillation (Arbeit, Parker, and Rubin, 1972). Patients in the operating room of a modern hospital are surrounded by a variety of monitoring devices attached to and entering their bodies. Electrocardiogram leads; temperature probes; stethoscopes; urinary catheters; endotracheal tubes; intravenous, intra-arterial, and central venous pressure lines; and grounding leads are among the equipment that provides a pathway by which electricity may travel to or from the patient. Faulty electrical equipment with poorly maintained plugs, sockets, switches, or line cords is usually the source of aberrant electricity in the operating room (Taylor and Desmond, 1970). However, if the patient is not attached to a grounding source, there is no danger.

All of the operating room electrical monitoring devices, as well as the operating table, are grounded to avoid the buildup of static electricity. When these devices are attached to the patient, they become a potential grounding mechanism for the patient as well. While normal dry skin provides an electrical resistance of 100,000 ohms, wet skin has 10,000 ohms of resistance, and cleaned skin with electrode jelly applied has only 1,000 ohms of resistance (Dobbie, 1969). Therefore the body leads of a cardiac monitor with improper impedance to electrosurgical frequencies can provide a ground for the passage of electricity. Wet drapes or a blood soaked gauze can provide a bridge between the patient and the operating room table, and a ground can be established in this manner.

To avoid shocking the patient, it is important to have electrical equipment in good repair. This also includes having electrical outlets fitted with an adequate ground. The patient should remain ungrounded. The electrosurgery or coagulation groundplate, which is actually a dispersion electrode, must have broad soft tissue contact and be as close to the operating site as possible. The further this plate is from the active electrode, the more electrical energy must be used to accomplish the same surgical effect. When attaching monitoring electrodes, saline sponges or jellies that dry should not be used, as the contact will narrow over time and create a potential burning situation. All equipment in the office and operating room, including the operating table or chair, should be grounded to avoid static charge. By using these simple principles, the potential of shock to the patient will be greatly reduced.

CRYOSURGERY
History

Cryosurgery involves the application of cold to tissue to freeze and destroy it. Almost 300 years ago Robert Boyle observed that the freezing of tissue produced necrosis (Parks, 1957). In 1777 Spallanzani showed that supercooling (rapid cooling to a temperature below the freezing point before freezing takes place) was less destructive to living organisms than slow freezing. More recent

investigators demonstrated that when tissue is frozen and thawed, some cells can survive (Leibo et al., 1970; Mazur et al., 1969; Rapatz, Sullivan, and Luyet, 1968). Moreover, certain cell types have differing susceptibilities to the effects of freezing (Asahina, 1967; Luyet and Gehenia, 1940; Meryman, 1966; Parks, 1957; Rey, 1959; Smith, 1961; Wolstenholme and O'Connor, 1970). In general, less cellular tissues like sclera or scar tissue are less susceptible to necrosis from freezing. Lower temperatures are also required to produce necrosis in vascular and connective tissues than in epithelial tissues. Other factors that influence the amount of tissue damage are the rate of cooling, the final temperature reached, the time spent in the frozen state, the rate of thawing, and the medium in which these take place. These discoveries have lead to the study of the long-term preservation by freezing of blood and its components, sperm, body organs, and other tissues. This science is labelled cryobiology. The search for ways to preserve cells for long periods at low temperatures uncovered many principles of cellular injury that were then applied by those interested in cryosurgery.

Effects of freezing

The events that are involved in cellular necrosis during freezing are as follows:
1. Formation of extracellular ice
2. Concentration of extracellular solutes
3. Decrease in intracellular water
4. Cell shrinkage
5. Concentration of intracellular solutes
6. Cell membrane damage
7. Formation of intracellular ice

The composition of the interior of cells is greatly different from that of the extracellular fluids. During slow cooling, freezing almost invariably begins in the extracellular areas where the ice crystals can grow unencumbered (Asahina, 1967). As a result of ice formation, the solvent, water, is removed from the extracellular fluid, causing a high extracellular solute concentration. Intracellular water then leaves the cell under increased osmotic pressure and cellular shrinkage occurs, as well as an increase in the intracellular solute concentration (Farrant, 1971; Meryman, 1968). This may in itself be sufficient to cause cellular necrosis. Cell membrane damage may also occur and be responsible for the intracellular sodium influx following thawing and the resultant cellular swelling and lysis (Farrant, 1971). If the freezing process is accomplished rapidly, intracellular ice is formed, which may result in direct mechanical injury to cellular structures, including the cell membrane (Rapatz, Nath, and Luyet, 1963). The rate at which the tissue is thawed is also crucial to the amount of damage done (Meryman, 1967; Smith, 1961). Both fast and slow thawing can produce cellular damage, but the mechanisms involved in these phenomena are not clear.

When a cryoprobe is inserted into tissue, freezing progresses concentrically outward producing an ice ball with distinct margins (Holden, 1975). Within the ice ball, a temperature gradient exists between the area adjacent to the probe, which is the coldest, and the exterior surface of the ice ball, which is the warmest. In the tissue surrounding the ice ball, a temperature gradient exists for approximately 6 to 8 mm, beyond which the tissue temperature is normal. A histologic transitional zone of 1 to 2 mm surrounds the ice ball, but the cells in this zone will survive (Poswillo, 1971).

Following thawing, cellular damage is characterized by pyknotic nuclei and edematous cytoplasm, and a demarcation of the frozen margin from the normal tissue is evident (Walder, 1971). Within 1 hour, the tissue shows fragmentation and vascular stasis. This is followed over the next few days by inflammatory cell infiltration, resorption of the necrotic tissue, and then fibrous tissue ingrowth. Skin and mucous membrane generally heal with minimal scar formation (Cooper, 1971).

A promising aspect of cryosurgery involves autoimmunity. In certain situations the body will produce antibodies against tissue that has undergone freezing (Cahan, 1965, 1967; Cooper, 1963;

Cooper et al., 1962; Shulman, 1967, 1968, 1969). The advantages of stimulating autoantibody production against cancer cells are obvious, and this application is undergoing careful investigation.

Clinical applications

Cryosurgery has been used for a variety of clinical conditions, including brain tumors (Cooper and Stellar, 1963); Parkinson's disease (Waltz et al., 1966); epilepsy (Mullen et al., 1967); vascular anomalies including hemangiomas (Cooper, Samra, and Yaghami, 1968); cataracts (Henderson, 1971; Walder, Haspar, and Meyer, 1970; Worthen and Brubaker, 1968) and other ocular problems (Kelman, 1966); premalignant lesions (Sako, Marchette, and Hayes, 1969); mucous membrane tumors and other neoplasms (Cahan, 1971; Cooper, 1965; Emmings, Koepf, and Gage, 1967; Emmings et al., 1966; Gage, 1968; Gage and Emmings, 1966; Smith and Weaver, 1976; Zacarion, 1968); intraosseous tumors (Emmings et al., 1966; Gage et al., 1965, 1966; Gage and Emmings, 1966) ameloblastoma (Marciani et al., 1977); giant cell lesions (Marcove, Leyden, and Huvos, 1972); and aneurysmal bone cysts (Marcove, 1971; Marcove and Miller, 1969).

Several types of cryosurgery units are available. The most expensive type utilizes liquid nitrogen to freeze the surgical site through an insulated probe. Liquid nitrogen can be used to achieve temperatures of $-196°$ C. Other refrigerant media are carbon dioxide, nitrous oxide, and Freon. These may reach temperatures of $-20°$ C to $-89°$ C depending on the apparatus (Barron, 1971). Obviously, the time necessary for the probe to be in contact with the tissue to be destroyed depends on the minimum temperature reached as well as the size of the lesion and the type of tissue.

According to Poswillo (1971), most tissues freeze at $-2.2°$ C. However, Cahan (1965) recommends using a temperature of at least $-20°$ C to ensure necrosis. Generally, 4 to 5 minutes of freezing at $-80°$ C will result in sufficient tissue necrosis to eradicate most intraoral mucosal lesions. At this time, the necessary extent of surgical freezing is largely a clinical decision not based on calculation. Therefore inaccuracies exist in which more or less tissue is frozen than is necessary. If the tumor lies deep in the tissue, the tissue may be incised, the tumor exposed, and the cryoprobe applied directly to the tumor. An interesting observation is that once frozen, the tissue is more susceptible to the lethal effects of cryosurgery on successive freezes (Fraser and Gill, 1967). Gill, Fraser, and Carter (1968) have determined that repetitive freezing five to seven times will maximize the volume of tissue necrosis. One of the clinical disadvantages of cryosurgery is the lack of a specimen for microscopic examination. Therefore many surgeons perform an incisional biopsy to obtain such a specimen just prior to using the cryosurgery.

While ablation of vascular tumors may be the most useful application of cryosurgery, some problems remain with this technique. Following thawing, the tissue that was frozen undergoes slough, and underlying vessels may be exposed. Rarely, these may undergo spontaneous rupture even several days following surgery (Hoki, 1971; von Leden, 1971). If accessible, the bleeding vessels may be treated with cryosurgery.

Cryosurgery probably would be used more often today if it were not for the expense and bulkiness of the equipment. As technology advances and the units become more compact, portable, and less expensive, cryosurgery may become a more routine surgical technique.

REFERENCES

Alexander, J. W., Kaplan, J. Z., and Altemeier, W. A. 1967. Role of suture materials in the development of wound infection, Ann. Surg. **165**:192.

Arbeit, S. R., Parker, B., and Rubin, I. L. 1972. Controlling the electrocution hazard in the hospital, J.A.M.A. **220**:1581.

Arnow, S., et al. 1969. Ventricular fibrillation associated with an electrically operated bed, New Engl. J. Med. **281**:31.

Asahina, E., 1967. Cellular injury and resistance in freezing organisms, Hokkaido University, Sapporo, The Institute of Low Temperature Science.

Banks, P. 1970. The adreno-cortical response to oral surgery, Br. J. Oral Surg. **8**:32.

Barron, R. F. 1971. Cryoinstrumentation. In von Leden, H., and Cahan, W. G., eds.: Cryogenics in surgery, Flushing, N. Y., Medical Examination Publishing Co.

Benson, M. K. D., and Hughes, S. P. F. 1975. Infection following total hip replacement in a general hospital without special orthopedic facilities, Acta Orthop. Scand. **46**:968.

Botsford, T. W. 1941. The tensile strength of sutured skin wounds during healing. Surg. Gynecol. Obstet. **72**:690.

Bruner, J. M. 1967. Hazards of electrical apparatus, Anesthesiology **28**:396.

Bulacio Nunez, A. W. 1974. A new theory regarding the lines of skin tension, Plast. Reconstr. Surg. **53**:663.

Burgess, A. H. 1933. Electrosurgery, Lancet **2**:1411.

Cahan, W. G. 1965. Cryosurgery of malignant and benign tumors, Fed. Proc. **24**:5241.

Cahan, W. G. 1967. Cryosurgery of malignant and benign tumors, J. St. Barnabas Medical Center, **4**:285.

Cahan, W. G. 1971. Cryosurgery: the management of massive recurrent cancer. In von Leden, H., and Cahan, W. G., eds.: Cryogenics in surgery, Flushing, N. Y., Medical Examination Publishing Co.

Carpendale, M. T. F., and Sereda, W. 1965. The role of percutaneous suture in surgical wound infection, Surgery **58**:672.

Conn, J., Jr., et al. 1974. Vicryl (polyglactin 910) synthetic absorbable sutures, Am. J. Surg. **128**:19.

Converse, J. M. 1975. Surgical treatment of facial injuries, Baltimore, The Williams & Wilkins Co., vol. 1.

Cooper, I. S. 1963. Cryogenic surgery, New Engl. J. Med. **268**:743.

Cooper, I. S. 1965. Cryogenic surgery for cancer, Fed. Proc. **24**:S237.

Cooper, I. S. 1971. Cryogenic surgery, In von Leden, H., and Cahan, W. G., eds.: Cryogenics in surgery, Flushing, N. Y., Medical Examination Publishing Co.

Cooper, I. S., and Stellar, S. 1963. Cryogenic freezing of brain tumors for excision or destruction in situ, J. Neurosurg. **20**:921.

Cooper, I. S., Samra, K., and Yaghami, M. 1968. Intra-arterial approach to internal carotid aneurysms, J. Am. Geriatr. Soc. **16**:363.

Cooper, I. S., et al. 1962. Cryogenic congelation and necrosis of cancer, J. Am. Geriatr. Soc. **10**:289.

Craig, P. H., et al. 1975. A biologic comparison of polyglactin 910 and polyglycolic acid synthetic absorbable sutures, Surg. Gynecol. Obstet. **141**:1.

Cruess, R. L., Bickel, W. S., and von Kessler, K. L. C. 1975. Infections in total hips secondary to a primary source elsewhere, Clin. Orthop. **106**:99.

Dardik, H., Dardik, I., and Laufman, H. 1971. Clinical use of polyglycolic acid polymer as a new absorbable synthetic suture, Am. J. Surg. **121**:656.

d'Arsonval, M. A. 1893. Production des courants de haute frequence et de grande intensite; leurs effets physiologiques, C. R. Soc. Biol. **45**:122.

Dobbie, A. K. 1969. Electrical aspects of surgical diathermy, Biomed. Eng. (London) **4**:206.

Douglas, D. M. 1949. Tensile strength of sutures.

II. Loss when implanted in living tissue, Lancet **2:**499.

Downes, E. M. 1977. Late infection after total hip replacement, J. Bone Joint Surg. **59B:**42.

Dupuytren, J. F., 1834. Traite theorique et practique des blessure par Armes de guerre, Paris, J. B. Bailliere, vol. 1.

Durack, D. T., and Petersdorf, R. G. 1973. Chemotherapy of experimental streptococcal endocarditis. 1. Comparison of commonly recommended prophylactic regimens, J. Clin. Invest. **52:**592.

Durack, D. T., Starkebaum, M. K., and Petersdorf, R. G., 1977. Chemotherapy of experimental streptococcal endocarditis. VI. Prevention of enterococcal endocarditis, J. Lab. Clin. Med. **90:**171.

Edwards, L. C. and Dunphy, J. E. 1958. Wound healing, New Engl. J. Med. **259:**224.

Egbert, L. D., and Fosburg, R. G. 1962. Reduction of bleeding by the addition of vasoconstrictor drugs to local anesthetics, Ann. Surg. **155:**20.

Eisenmann, D., Malone, W. F., and Kusek, J. 1970. Electron microscopic evaluation of electrosurgery, Oral Surg. **29:**660.

Edlich, R. F., et al. 1973. Physical and chemical configuration of sutures in the development of surgical infection, Ann. Surg. **177:**679.

Elek, S. D., and Conen, P. E. 1957. The virulence of *Staphylococcus pyogenes* for man. A study of the problems of wound infection, Br. J. Exp. Pathol. **38:**573.

Ellis, J. D. 1933. Electrosurgical incisions, Arch. Surg. **26:**981.

Emmings, F. G., Koepf, S. W., and Gage, A. A. 1967. Cryotherapy for benign lesions of the oral cavity, J. Oral Surg. **25:**320.

Emmings, F. G., et al. 1966. Freezing the mandible without excision, J. Oral Surg. **24:**145.

Eschricht. 1837. In Bulacio Nunez, A. W. 1974. A new theory regarding the lines of skin tension, Plast. Reconstr. Surg. **53:**663.

Everett, E. D., and Hirschmann, J. V. 1977. Transient bacteremia and endocarditis prophylaxis, Medicine **56:**61.

Farrant, J. 1971. Cryobiology: the basis for cryosurgery. In von Leden, H., and Cahan, W. G., eds.: Cryogenics in surgery, Flushing, N. Y., Medical Examination Publishing Co.

Feldman, G., et al. 1970. Electrosurgery: endodontic applications, N. Y. State Dent. J. **36:**605.

Filhos. 1833. In Bulacio Nunez, A. W. 1974. A new theory regarding the lines of skin tension, Plast Reconstr. Surg. **53:**663.

Finland, M. 1972. Current problems in infective endocarditis, Mod. Concepts Cardiovasc. Dis. **41:**53.

Fraser, J., and Gill, W. 1967. Observations on ultrafrozen tissue, Br. J. Surg. **54:**770.

Friedman, J. 1973. The technical aspects of electrosurgery, Oral Surg. **36:**177.

Gage, A. A. 1968. Cryotherapy for oral cancer, J. A. M. A. **204:**565.

Gage, A. A., and Emmings, F. 1966. Treatment of human tumors by freezing, Cryobiology **2:**14.

Gage, A. A., et al. 1965. Freezing bone without excision: an experimental study of bone cell destruction and regrowth, J. A. M. A. **192:**558.

Gage, A. A., et al. 1966. Freezing bone without excision, J. A. M. A. **196:**770.

Gaskin, E. R., and Childers, M. D., Jr. 1963. Increased granuloma formation from absorbable sutures, J. A. M. A. **185**(3):212.

Gill, W., Fraser, J., and Carter, D. C. 1968. Repeated freeze-thaw cycles in cryosurgery, Nature **219** (5152):410.

Glickman, I., and Imber, L. R. 1970. Comparison of gingival resection with electrosurgery and periodontal knives: a biometric and histologic study, J. Periodont. **41:**142.

Halsted, W. S. 1893. The radical cure of inguinal hernia in the male, Bull. Johns Hopkins Hosp. **4:**17.

Henderson, R. L. 1971. Cryosurgical treatment of hemangiomas, Arch. Otolaryngol. **93:**511.

Herrmann, J. B. 1971. Tensile strength and knot security of surgical suture materials, Am. Surg. **37:**209.

Herrmann, J. B., Kelly, R. J., and Higgins, G. A. 1970. Polyglycolic acid sutures: laboratory and clinical evaluation of a new absorbable suture material, Arch. Surg. **100:**486.

Hoki, A. 1971. Problems of cryosurgery in head and neck diseases. In Haschek, H., ed.: Latest developments in cryosurgery, Vienna, Verlag der Weiner Medizinischen Akademie.

Holden, H. B., ed. 1975. Practical cryosurgery, Chicago, Year Book Medical Publishers, Inc.

Hopps, J. A. 1968. Electric shock hazard in hospitals, Can. Med. Assoc. J. **98:**1002.

Hungerbuhler, R. F., Swope, J. P., and Reves, J. G. 1974. Ventricular fibrillation associated with use of electrocautery, J. A. M. A. **230:**432.

Jackson, R. 1970. Basic principles of electrosurgery: a review, Can. J. Surg. **13:**354.

Jackson, D., and Jackson, D., Jr. 1958. Results of electrosurgical radical mastectomy with routine skin grafts and postoperative X-ray therapy, Cancer **11:**18.

Jenkins, H. P., et al. 1942. Absorption of surgical gut (catgut): III. Duration in the tissues after loss of tensile strength, Arch. Surg. **45:**74.

Kaplan, E. L., et al. 1977. Prevention of bacterial endocarditis, Circulation **56:**139a.

Katz, A. R., and Turner, R. J. 1970. Evaluation of tensile and absorption properties of polyglycolic acid sutures, Surg. Gynecol. Obstet. **131:**701.

Kelman, C. D. 1966. Atlas of cryosurgical techniques in ophthalmology, St. Louis, The C. V. Mosby Co.

Klug, R. G. 1966. Gingival tissue regeneration following electrical retraction, J. Prosthet. Dent. **16:**955.

Kocher, T. 1907. Chirurgische—Operationslehre. Jena, Verlag. Von Gustav Fisher.

Kraissl, C. 1951. The selection of appropriate lines for elective surgical incision, Plast. Reconstr. Surg. **8:**1.

Lampert, S. H. 1970. Combined electrosurgery and gingival retraction, J. Prosthet. Dent. **23:**164.

Langdon, J. D. 1977. Late infection after total hip replacement, Br. Med. J. **2**(6085):517.

Langer, K. 1861. Ueber die Spaltbarkeit der Cutis,

Sitzungsb. d., k. Akad. d. Wissensch. Mathnaturw. Cl. **43**:233.

Lawrenson, K. B., and Stephens, F. O. 1970. The use of electrocutting and electrocoagulation in surgery, Aust. N.Z. J. Surg. **39**:417.

Leibo, S. P., et al. 1970. Effects of freezing on marrow stem cell suspensions, Cryobiology **6**:315.

Lilly, G. E. 1968. Reaction of oral tissues to suture materials, Oral Surg. **26**:128.

Lilly, G. E., et al. 1968. Reaction of oral tissues to suture materials, Oral Surg. **26**:592.

Localio, S. A., Casale, W., and Hinton, J. W. 1943. Wound healing: experimental and statistical study, Surg. Gynecol. Obstet. **77**:376.

Luyet, B. J., and Gehenia, P. M. 1940. Life and death at low temperatures. Normandy, Mo., Biodynamica.

Madsen, E. T. 1953. An experimental and clinical evaluation of surgical suture materials, Surg. Gynecol. Obstet. **97**:73.

Malgaigne, J. F. 1838. Traite d'anatomie chirurgicale et de chirurgie experimentale, Paris, J. B. Bailliere.

Malone, W. F., and Manning, J. L. 1968. Electrosurgery in restorative dentistry, J. Prosthet. Dent. **22**:555.

Marciani, R. D., et al. 1977. Cryotherapy in the treatment of ameloblastoma of the mandible: report of cases, J. Oral Surg. **35**:289.

Marcove, R. C. 1971. Cryosurgery in orthopedic surgery. In von Leden, H., and Cahan, W. G., eds.: Cryogenics in surgery, Flushing, N. Y. Medical Examination Publishing Co.

Marcove, R. C., and Miller, T. R. 1969. The treatment of primary and metastatic localized bone tumors by cryosurgery, Surg. Clin. North Am. **49**(2):421.

Marcove, R. C., Leyden, J. P., and Huvos, A. G. 1972. Giant cell tumors of bone treated by cryosurgery. In Haschek, H., ed.: Latest developments in cryosurgery, Vienna, Verlag der Weiner Medizinischen Akademie.

Maxwell, G. R. 1969. Polyglycolic acid suture for oral surgery: a clinical and histologic study, Thesis, Ohio State University.

May, H. 1971. Plastic and reconstructive surgery, Philadelphia. F. A. Davis Co.

Mazur, P., et al. 1969. Survival of hamster tissue culture cells after freezing and thawing, Cryobiology **6**:1.

Mead, W. H., and Ochsner, A. 1940. The relative value of catgut, silk, linen, and cotton as suture materials, Surgery **7**:485.

Meryman, H. T., ed. 1966. Cryobiology, London, Academic Press.

Meryman, H. T. 1967. The relationship between dehydration and freezing injury in the human erythrocyte. In Asahina, E., ed.: Cellular injury and resistence in freezing organisms, Hokkaido University, Sapporo, The Institute of Low Temperature Science.

Meryman, H. T. 1968. Modified model for the mechanism of freezing injury in erythrocytes, Nature **218**:333.

Millar, R. A., Gilbert, R. G. B., and Brindle, G. F.

1958. Ventricular tachycardia during halothane anesthesia, Anaesthesia **13**:164.

Mock, H. E. 1935. Electrosurgery, J.A.M.A. **104**:2341.

Morgan, M. N. 1969. New synthetic absorbable suture material, Br. Med. J. **2**:308.

Mullen, S., et al. 1967. Thalamic lesions for the control of epilepsy, Arch. Neurol. **6**:277.

Munchow, O. B., and Denson, J. S. 1964. The effect of various vasoconstrictors on the blood vessels of the human skin, Surgery **56**:989.

Ogus, W. I. 1942. Electrosurgery in dentistry, Dent. Dig. **48**:411.

Orban, B. 1944. Tissue healing following electrocoagulation of gingiva, J. Periodontol. **15**:17.

Oringer, M. J. 1960. Fundamentals of electrosurgery, J. Oral Surg. **18**:39.

Oringer, M. J. 1962. Electrosurgery in dentistry, Philadelphia, W. B. Saunders Co.

Oringer, M. J. 1969. Electrosurgery for definite conservative modern periodontal therapy, Dent. Clin. North Am. **13**:53.

Oringer, M. J. 1976. Reason and remedy for conflicting reports on comparative effects of steel scalpel and electrosurgical cutting on gingival tissues and alveolar bone, J. Am. Dent. Assoc. **92**:850.

Parks, A. S. 1957. Introductory remarks to a discussion on viability of mammalian cells and tissues after freezing, Proc. R. Soc. **147B**:424.

Pelletier, L. L., Jr., Durack, D. T., and Petersdorf, R. G. 1975. Chemotherapy of experimental streptococcus endocarditis. IV. Further observations on prophylaxis, J. Clin. Invest. **56**:319.

Perey, B., and Watier, A. 1975. Effect of human tissues on the breaking strength of catgut and polyglycolic acid sutures, Chirurgia Gastroenterol. **9**:87.

Podshadley, A. G. 1968. Electrosurgical procedures in crown and bridge restorations, J. Am. Dent. Assoc. **77**:1321.

Pick, J. F. 1949. Surgery of repair, Philadelphia, J. B. Lippincott Co.

Pope, J. W., et al. 1968. Effects of electrosurgery on wound healing in dogs, Periodontology **6**:30.

Postlethwait, R. W. 1969. In Dunphy, J. E., and Van Winkle, H. W., Jr., eds.: Repair and regeneration, New York, McGraw-Hill Book Co.

Postlethwait, R. W. 1970a. Long-term study of nonabsorbable sutures, Ann. Surg. **171**:892.

Postlethwait, R. W. 1970b. Polyglycolic acid surgical suture, Arch. Surg. **101**:489.

Postlethwait, R. W., Willigan, D. A., and Ulin, A. W. 1975. Human tissue reaction to sutures; Ann. Surg. **181**:144.

Postlethwait, R. W., et al. 1959. Wound healing: II. An evaluation of surgical suture material, Surg. Gynecol. Obstet. **108**:555.

Poswillo, D. E. 1971. Cryosurgery and electrosurgery compared in the treatment of experimentally induced oral carcinoma, Br. Dent. J. **131**:347.

Rapatz, G., Nath, J., and Luyet, B. 1963. Electron microscope study of erythrocytes in rapidly frozen mammalian blood, Biodynamica **9**:83.

Rapatz, G., Sullivan, J. J., and Luyet, B. 1968. Preservation of erythrocytes in blood containing various cryoprotective agents, frozen at various rates and brought to a given final temperature, Cryobiology 5:18.

Raventos, J. 1956. The action of fluothane—a new volatile anesthetic, Br. J. Pharmacol. 11:394.

Rey, L. 1959. Conservation de la vie par le foid, Paris, Hermann.

Rhoads, J. E., Hottenstein, H. F., and Hudson, I. F. 1937. The decline in strength of catgut after exposure to living tissues, Arch. Surg. 34:377.

Risdon, F. 1934. Ankylosis of the temporomandibular joint, J. Am. Dent. Assoc. 21:1933.

Rosen, M. D., and Roe, R. B. 1963. Adrenaline infiltration during halothane anesthesia: a report of two cases of cardiac arrest, Br. J. Anesth. 35:51.

Rubin, L. 1948. Langer's lines and facial scars, Plast. Reconstr. Surg. 3:147.

Rubin, R., Salvati, E. A., and Lewis, R. 1976. Infected total hip replacement after dental procedures, Oral Surg. 41:18.

Saghirian, L. M. 1940. Electrosurgery in the mouth, Dent. Dig. 46:20.

Sako, E., Marchette, F. C., and Hayes, R. L. 1969. Evaluation of cryosurgery in the treatment of intra-oral leukoplakia, J. Cryosurg. 2:239.

Salthouse, T. N., and Matlaga, B. F. 1975. Significance of cellular enzyme activity at nonabsorbable suture implant sites, J. Surg. Res. 19:127.

Salthouse, T. N., and Matlaga, B. F. 1976. Polyglactin 910 suture absorption and the role of cellular enzymes, Surg. Gynecol. Obstet. 142:544.

Sande, M. A., et al. 1969. Bacteremia associated with cardiac catheterization, N. Engl. J. Med. 281:1104.

Sande, M. A., et al. 1972. Sustained bacteremia in patients with prosthetic cardiac valves, N. Engl. J. Med. 286:1067.

Schoen, F. J. 1976. Surgical sutures, New Phys. 25:40.

Sewell, I. A. 1966. The microvascular responses induced by materials used in operative surgery, Br. J. Surg. 53:712.

Shomberg, F., and Malone, W. F. 1969. Electrosurgical sterilization, Bull. Am. Acad. Gen. Dent. March:43.

Shulman, S. 1967. Cryosurgery and cryo-immunology, Bull. Millard Fillmore Hospital 14:87.

Shulman, S. 1968. Cryoimmunology: the production of antibody by the freezing of tissue. In Rand, R. W., Rinfret, A. P., and von Leden, H., eds.: Cryosurgery, Springfield, Ill., Charles C Thomas Publisher.

Shulman, S. 1969. Cryosurgery and autoimmunization, J. Cryosurg. 2:84.

Siegel, R. J., Vistnes, L. M., and Iverson, R. E. 1973. Effective hemostasis with less epinephrine, Plast. Reconstr. Surg. 51:129.

Sipes, J. N., Thompson, R. L., and Hook, E. W. 1977. Prophylaxis of infective endocarditis: a re-evaluation, Ann. Rev. Med. 28:371.

Smith, A. U. 1961. Biological effects of freezing and supercooling, London, Edward Arnold.

Smith, D. B., and Weaver, A. W. 1976. Cryosurgery for oral cancer—a six year retrospective study, J. Oral Surg. 34:245.

Smity, J. 1964. Clinical study of inflammatory papillary hyperplasia, J. Prosthet. Dent. 14:1034.

Sozio, R. B., Riley, E. J., and Shklar, G. 1976. A controlled study of electrosurgical currents and wound healing, Oral Surg. 41:709.

Spallanzani, L. 1777. Opuscules de Physique Trans J. Senebier, Geneva, B. Chirol, vol. 1.

Taylor, K. W., and Desmond, J. 1970. Electrical hazards in the operating room with special reference to electrosurgery, Can. J. Surg. 13:362.

Truhlsen, S. M., and Fitzpatrick, J. 1964. A new collagen suture: tissue reaction and absorption, Invest. Ophthalmol. 3:470.

Valobra, G. N., and Fiandesio, D. 1968. Storia breve dell'elettrocaustica e diatermocaustica, Minerva Med. 59:829.

Van Winkle, W., Jr. 1974. Catgut sutures should have isopropyl alcohol preservative removed before use, (Editorial,) J.A.M.A. 230:1063.

Van Winkle, W., Jr., and Hastings, J. C. 1972. Considerations in the choice of suture materials for various tissues, Surg. Gynecol. Obstet. 135:113.

Van Winkle, W., Jr., et al. 1975. Effect of suture materials on healing skin wounds, Surg. Gynecol. Obstet. 140:7.

Varma, S., et al. 1974. Comparison of seven suture materials in infected wounds, J. Surg. Res. 17:165.

Voight. 1857. In Bulacio Nunez, A. W. 1974. A new theory regarding the lines of skin tension, Plast Reconstr. Surg. 53:663.

von Leden, H. 1971. Cryosurgery of the head and neck. In von Leden, H., and Cahan, W. G., eds: Cryogenics in surgery, Flushing, N. Y., Medical Examination Publishing Co.

Walder, H. A. D. 1971. Experimental cryosurgery. In von Leden, H., and Cahan, W. G., eds.: Cryogenics in surgery, Flushing, N. Y., Medical Examination Publishing Co.

Walder, H., Haspar, H., and Meyer, E. 1970. Application of cryotherapy to cerebral vascular anomalies, Psychol. Neurol. Neurochir. 73:471.

Wallace, W. R., Maxwell, G. R., and Cavalaris, C. J. 1970. Comparison of polyglycolic acid suture to black silk, chromic and plain catgut in human oral tissues, J. Oral Surg. 28:739.

Walter, C. W. 1969. Safe electric environment in hospital, Bull Am. Coll. Surg. 54:177.

Walter, C. W. 1972. The knowledge and skills of electrosurgery, Surg. Gynecol. Obstet. 134:484.

Waltz, J. M., et al. 1966. Cryothalamectomy for Parkinson's disease, Neurology 16:994.

Ward, G. E. 1925. Value of electrothermic methods in the treatment of malignancy, J.A.M.A. 84:660.

Wilson, P. D., Salvati, E. A., and Blumenfeld, E. L. 1975. The problem of infection in total prosthetic arthroplasty of the hip, Surg. Clin. North Am. 55(6):1431.

Wolstenholme, G. E. W., and O'Connor, M., (eds.) 1970. The frozen cell, London, Ciba Foundation Symposium, Churchill Livingstone.

Worthen, D. M., and Brubaker, R. F. 1968. An evaluation of cataract extraction, Arch. Ophthamol. 79:8.

Zacarian, S. A. 1968. Cryosurgery in dermatologic disorders and in the treatment of skin cancer, J. Cryosurg. 1:70.

CHAPTER 8

Biomaterials

Frederick J. Schoen

Developments in biomaterials over the last decade have contributed to dramatic advances in the overall therapeutic armamantarium of the oral and maxillofacial surgeon. Significant applications have included implanted artificial teeth and tooth roots, endosseous and subperiosteal implants for dentures, soft tissue and alveolar ridge augmentation, and prosthetic reconstruction of the mandible, temporomandibular joints, and orbital floor. The purpose of this chapter is to provide an introduction to the biomaterials employed in surgery of the jaws and adjacent tissues. While predominant attention is paid to those biomaterials most applicable to the reconstructive and cosmetic surgery of the face and oral tissues, biomaterials used as adjuncts to surgical wound management are also discussed.

In order to reliably perform their desired function, biomaterials must have stable properties in the physiologic environment and must not cause adverse biologic effects on the host. For reconstructive applications, the selected materials must possess sufficient strength to withstand cyclic masticatory and other potentially severe forces. Alloplastic materials must be capable of fabrication and sterilization by conventional techniques and must resist corrosion and dissolution in the oral tissues. All implanted materials, regardless of application, must not evoke severe local or systemic inflammatory or immunologic reactions. They must not support the growth of bacteria or other microbes. Certainly, tumor induction also must not be a long-term result of implantation. The materials and the techniques employed in their fabrication and utilization must be economically feasible. For special applications, adhesion to natural tissues, wear resistance, or intentional and controlled dissolution may be desirable.

Although most implants yield a long-term clinically acceptable result, the current rate of prosthetic reconstruction failures is considerable. Many failures may be attributed to structural failure or corrosion of biomaterials, wound dehiscence, local tissue inflammatory reactions, or infection. Therefore a discussion of some basic principles related to biomaterials, including properties and tissue interactions, is presented in an effort to provide a rational basis for the use of such materials and to facilitate more effective communication among biomaterials specialists and oral and maxillofacial surgeons. A description of specific reconstructive biomaterials, both alloplastic and biologically derived, is included to define the scope of clinically available and experimentally promising systems. Finally, the applied science of sutures, tissue adhesives, and other hemostatic agents is presented to promote a more sophisticated selection of these surgical adjuncts.

GENERAL PRINCIPLES IN THE USE OF BIOMATERIALS

The functional permanence of an implanted device depends on the effect of the physiologic environment on the properties of the implant and on the local and systemic histocompatibility of the im-

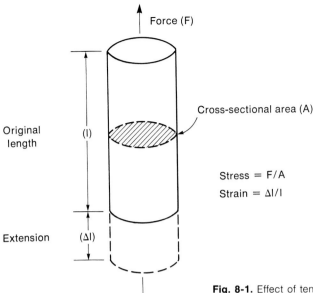

Force (F)

Cross-sectional area (A)

Original
length ......(l)

Stress = F/A

Strain = Δl/l

Extension ......(Δl)

Fig. 8-1. Effect of tensile force, *F*, acting on uniform rod of cross-sectional area, *A*, of length, *l*, showing extension of rod Δ*l*.

planted biomaterial. Thus two aspects of implant performance, often called functionality and compatibility, must be considered in assessing biomaterial suitability. Although dysfunction and tissue pathology may be synergistic in certain instances of implant failure, the more usual occurrence is material failure with no evidence of tissue intolerance or rejection of suitably functional implants adjacent to pathologic tissue in a symptomatic patient. These two aspects of implant performance, materials properties and tissue reaction, are considered below.

Properties of implant materials

Traditionally, selection of biomaterials was based solely on bulk property specifications. It has since become recognized that reduction of problems associated with the interfacial reaction of host tissues and fluids also requires consideration of the surface behavior of materials. Thus both bulk and surface behavioral aspects of materials are of pertinence to the oral and maxillofacial surgeon.

Mechanical properties

The most important bulk properties of implant biomaterials are those that deter-

mine the response to mechanical loading.

Stress/strain behavior. Consider a simple cylinder of a material of cross-sectional area, A, and length, l, to which a force, F, is applied, as in Fig. 8-1. Such a load is a tensile force, since it is acting to extend the rod. The ability of the material to resist the applied force is predominantly dependent on the strength of the atomic bonding within its structure.

Conditions within the material are described by two basic quantities: stress and strain. These parameters relate the applied force and resultant overall deformation to the situation existing at any point within the specimen. For example, stress describes the force acting at each point in the material. Mathematically:

$$\text{Stress} = \frac{\text{Force (F)}}{\text{Cross-sectional area (A)}}$$

Thus, while force is measured in pounds, kilograms, or newtons (N),* the units of stress are pounds per square inch (psi),

---

*1 newton = 22.48 pounds weight; 1 MN (meganewton) = 10^6 newtons; 1 GN (giganewton) = 10^9 newtons.

kilograms per square centimeter, or newtons per square meter (N/m²). The stress produced in the rod in Fig. 8-1 is a tensile stress.

Application of the tensile force just described results in a pulling apart of the atoms seen in the overall specimen as an increase in length, Δl. Since each atom is separated from its adjacent atom by a distance dependent on the applied force, the total extension (deformation) depends on the length of the specimen and is greater for a longer specimen (more atomic bonds to stretch). Strain is the parameter that expresses the extent of stretching of the atomic bonds within the material. Hence:

$$\text{Strain} = \frac{\text{Extension } (\Delta l)}{\text{Original length (l)}}$$

Strain is a dimensionless term, since both numerator and denominator are measures of length.

Pure tensile stresses are rarely encountered in oral and maxillofacial surgery. Most applications of force encountered in practice produce a combination of stresses in the material. For example, bending forces produce both tensile stresses, as described above, and compressive stresses, where the atoms are being pushed together. In a bar subjected to bending the atoms on the convex surface are under tension, while atoms on the concave surface are in compression.

When a material is subjected to a small tensile load, the atoms are pulled slightly apart. On release of the load, the atoms return to their normal positions. If the load is increased, the atoms move further from their normal, or equilibrium, sites but again return when the load is released. Such behavior, exhibited to some extent by all materials, is referred to as elasticity; that is, the material returns to its original shape, and deformation disappears when the applied load is removed.

Each material has a point beyond which, when stretched, the atoms are pulled so far from their equilibrium positions that return to these sites on release of the applied load is not possible; that is, some bonds are broken, and permanent displacement of atoms from their equilib-

rium sites occurs. Such deformation is called plasticity, and the shape of the specimen is permanently altered. When the deformation is so severe that many bonds are broken, the material may fracture.

Data on the mechanical properties of materials are obtained from a test in which a standardized cylindric specimen (similar to that shown in Fig. 8-1) is subjected to an increasing tensile load until it fractures. The quantities stress and strain allow comparison of the mechanical properties of different materials independent of the configuration of the specimen used to determine them.

As the test specimen is loaded, deformation occurs. Stress and strain are calculated as previously discussed from the applied load and resultant deformation, respectively. It is conventional to plot stress on the vertical and strain on the horizontal axis as illustrated in Fig. 8-2. During initial stretching, the bonds between the atoms of the material behave as simple mechanical springs, and the relationship between stress and strain is a straight line. The slope of this line is called the modulus of elasticity and is a measure of the stiffness of the material, that is, the ease of stretching the bonds between the atoms. The behavior is linear almost up to the elastic limit, the point where deformation is no longer reversible and permanent stretching results. At slightly less stress than the elastic limit, deviation from linearity occurs. A material stressed to this point will spring back to its original dimensions on release of the applied load. This is true at all levels of stress up to the elastic limit.

When a material reaches its limit of elastic deformation, it will deform plastically (permanently). Once plastic deformation begins, the strain appears to increase faster than the stress, as seen in Fig. 8-3. Since the elastic limit is difficult to determine experimentally, the quantity known as the yield stress is used to describe the elastic-plastic transition (that is, the change from reversible to irreversible behavior). This is usually specified as the stress at which a given amount of plastic strain is achieved

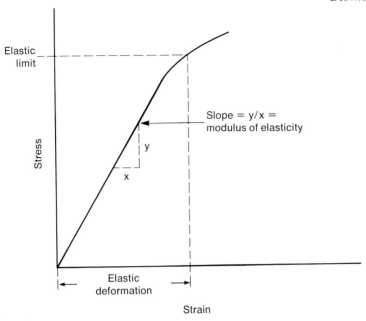

Fig. 8-2. Relationship between stress and strain for initial deformation of a material. Up to elastic limit, material will recover its initial dimensions when load is removed. Slope of linear portion of stress/strain curve is modulus of elasticity and reflects stiffness of material.

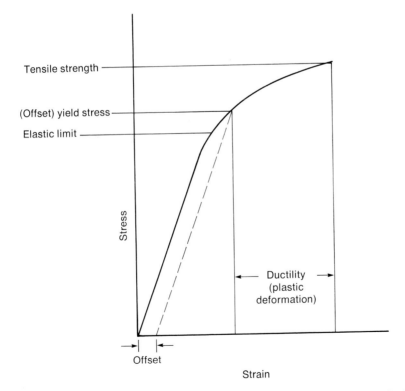

Fig. 8-3. Entire stress/strain relationship for a material, emphasizing features beyond limit of elastic deformation. Offset yield stress approximates elastic limit and is readily determined. Tensile strength is maximum stress achieved before material fractures. Ductility is total amount of permanent deformation in material at fracture.

(the offset) and is determined by drawing a line parallel to the linear portion of the curve at the offset strain and noting where it intersects the curve. The yield stress, determined in this manner, is called the offset yield stress and the value of the offset is affixed to it. Usually the offset is selected as 0.2%. These data are provided by materials manufacturers in product information. Although the yield stress is slightly higher than the elastic limit, it is a reasonable approximation of the level of stress at which permanent deformation occurs. The strain taking place after yield is called plastic strain. It is important to note that the functional form of the prosthetic device may be irrevocably altered when yield has occurred, even though the material has not yet fractured.

If loading is continued, the applied load and the resultant stress increase. The tensile strength or ultimate tensile strength (UTS) is the maximum load achieved divided by the original cross-sectional area of the specimen. The ultimate tensile strength is a measure of the maximum tensile stress the material can withstand. Thus, for certain applications such as those where device failure depends on material fracture, the ultimate tensile strength may represent important data used for comparison of suitable materials.

Ductility is the amount of plastic strain that has occurred when a material fractures. Thus a ductile material (a material with a large amount of ductility) has the ability to undergo substantial plastic deformation prior to fracture.

A material fracturing without the presence of appreciable plastic deformation (low ductility) is said to be brittle. The stress/strain relationship for a brittle material compared with that for a material having substantial ductility is shown in Fig. 8-4. While comparison of ductile materials utilizes the parameters yield strength, tensile strength, and ductility, comparison of the mechanical properties

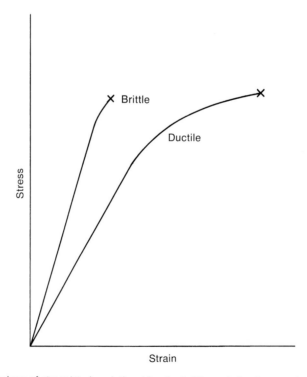

Fig. 8-4. Comparison of stress/strain relationships for brittle and ductile materials. Brittle material shows little if any plastic deformation prior to fracture.

of brittle materials occurs by either the flexural strength (the fracture stress determined in a bending test), the fracture strain, or the total area under the stress/strain curve (strain energy to fracture). Ceramics and carbons characteristically exhibit brittle behavior, while metals and polymers exhibit variable amounts of ductility. The modulus of elasticity is also generally an important quantity for comparison of materials. Fig. 8-5 illustrates representative stress/strain curves for various types of materials encountered.

Hardness. Hardness is a term generally used to express the resistance of a material to indentation and/or scratching of its surface. Although in actuality it is the result of interaction of a variety of mechanical properties including modulus of elasticity, elastic limit, ductility, and resistance to cutting, hardness often provides a rapid and reliable general comparison of the mechanical properties of materials. Indentation hardness is measured as the amount of deformation produced in a specimen surface by a standard indentor when a specified force is applied.

Fatigue. Failure of materials under repeated stresses is called fatigue. This is a problem of particular importance to the oral and maxillofacial surgeon in that the majority of prosthetic materials are subjected to cyclic masticatory loading. In this regard, it is important to note that fatigue failure is a problem not only of material selection but also of device design and fabrication.

Fatigue failure requires the initiation and propagation of a crack. Initiation occurs where the local stresses are sufficient to cause a small amount of plastic deformation, for example, at a concentration of stress. The crack is then capable of being propagated in minute increments by cyclic stressing until the remaining cross-sectional area free of cracking is no longer capable of supporting the applied load. Device failure then occurs. Stress concentrations promoting fatigue failure may result from internal defects, such as pores, or from errors in design or fabrication that produce sharp reentrant corners or surface cracks.

If cyclic stresses of various levels are applied to a laboratory specimen of a material and the number of cycles necessary for failure at a given stress level is recorded, then curves such as those

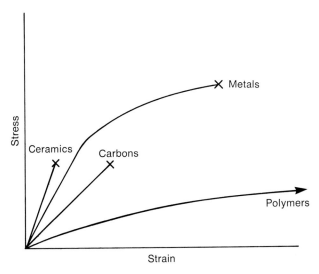

Fig. 8-5. Comparison of various types of mechanical behavior exhibited by classes of materials of interest.

shown in Fig. 8-6 are generated. Most materials show a behavior as represented by curve A, in which failure occurs after many cycles of stress even at comparatively low levels of loading. Some materials, however, notably ferrous (iron-base) alloys of which stainless steel is an example, show a limit of stress below which fatigue failure does not occur even at very large numbers of stress cycles. Such behavior is illustrated by curve B. The stress below which failure does not result is called the endurance limit, and is usually approximately one half of the fracture stress as measured in a tensile test. Most nonferrous alloys (such as cobalt-chrome and titanium alloys) behave in a manner illustrated by curve A, in which case fatigue behavior is quantified as the stress that leads to failure in an arbitrary number of cycles such as 10^7. This value of stress may in some cases be less than 25% of the ultimate tensile strength measured in a tensile test. Since the mechanism producing fatigue failure requires some degree of plastic deformation, brittle materials generally show almost no tendency toward fatigue failure (a completely flat curve) as illustrated by

curve C. Structural damage in these materials is not cumulative; only if the stress generated is higher than that causing failure in a simple tensile test does the material fracture. Many cases of stress-bearing surgical implants that failed owing to fatigue have appeared in the literature. As will be discussed in a later section, the presence of repeated stressing in a corrosive environment may accelerate processes promoting failure.

Chemical deterioration of materials

Corrosion of metals. Metals exposed to the atmosphere absorb oxygen or other available elements to satisfy the bonding requirements of the surface atoms. Such a reaction is physical in nature and readily reversible. Corrosion, or chemical interaction between a metal and its environment, results in transformation of the metal from the elemental to the ionized (oxidized) state, usually as an oxide, sulfide, or chloride. The production of an oxidized material similar to that found in nature results in a stable, not readily altered, structure. Ceramics are examples of such structures.

When the environment is a solution,

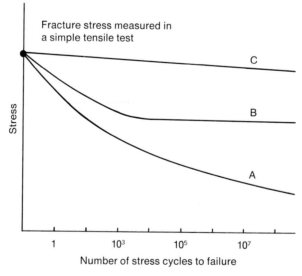

Fig. 8-6. Behavior of materials when subjected to repetitive loading. Curve *A* is characteristic of most metallic materials: failure after cyclic stressing occurs even at loads much smaller than the fracture stress. Materials such as stainless steel exhibit behavior as illustrated by curve *B*: there is a level of stress, the endurance limit, below which fatigue failure does not occur. Ceramics and carbons, on the other hand, show almost no tendency toward cumulative fatigue damage. Their behavior is represented by curve *C*.

the tendency toward oxidation is expressed by the ease with which the metal atoms ionize, go into solution, and release free electrons. The tendency for oxidation varies for different metals (electrodes) and for different solutions (electrolytes) and may be measured as the electrical potential difference between the particular metal and solution at equilibrium relative to a standard (the electrode potential). A listing of metals in order of their propensity to corrode in a specific environment is the electrochemical series. It has often been assumed that the corrosion behavior of metals in vivo may be predicted from the electrochemical series for metals in seawater.

Contemporary implant metals obtain corrosion resistance from the presence of a thin adherent oxide film. Since further corrosion requires the diffusion of metal ions through the oxide layer outward to freshly adsorbed oxygen and/or the diffusion of oxygen atoms through the oxide film to the metal surface, the oxide layer is generally self-limiting in extent. Protection from corrosion by such a film is called passivity.

The protective ability of the oxide film depends on the ease with which regener-ation of the film occurs when disturbed. Rapid self-healing (reoxidation of the denuded areas) is mandatory for permanence of corrosion protection in surgical appliances. The metals aluminum, titanium, chromium, and tantalum form good, protective, thin oxide films; the latter accounts for corrosion protection in current surgical implant alloys. Titanium and its alloys have a protective layer of TiO_2, while the chromium-containing alloys, stainless steel, and cobalt-chromium alloys obtain corrosion resistance through the formation of a chromium oxide film. Other metals, such as iron, form various oxides, but these are not stable since they are easily disrupted and regenerate poorly. The presence of stable oxide films is dependent on a variety of factors, including the pH and the oxygen tension of the environment. Thus the acidic environment created locally by sepsis may decrease the stability of certain oxides and thereby potentiate corrosion.

If two dissimilar metals are placed in a solution, each will develop its own characteristic potential. If the two metals are joined together by a metallic conductor as in Fig. 8-7, electrons will flow through the conductor from the metal with the

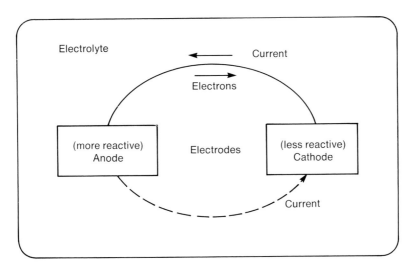

Fig. 8-7. Schematic diagram illustrating flow of electric current generated when two dissimilar metals (electrodes) are placed in solution (electrolyte) and connected by electrical conductor. More reactive electrode (anode) dissolves (corrodes). It is important to understand that two electrodes may be slightly different components of single device or may actually be different regions of same metal with slightly different composition or metallurgic condition.

greater number of free electrons (more reactive or anodic) to the other metal (less reactive or cathodic), thereby creating an electrical current. Since there must be a counter flow of positive ions in the opposite direction through the electrolyte, a continuous electrical current results. Such an electrical couple defines the electrochemical cell that is, in essence, a battery. Metals and alloys in aqueous environments corrode according to this process.

Although the mechanism of corrosion just described is for distinctly different metals, any condition producing areas of differing potential in a single piece of metal, such as local mechanical working or precipitation of a second phase, will also lead to corrosion. Similarly, areas of metal protected from solution exchange, such as in the space between a bone plate and its screws, may become anodic to the bulk of the material since the local electrolyte composition will be different. Such corrosion caused by stagnant solution in shielded areas is called crevice corrosion. The lack of oxygen exchange in these areas may decrease the ability of the oxide film to reform when abraded, thereby altering the electrode potential and rendering this region anodic to the remaining surface.

It is obvious that two different metallic materials (such as stainless steel and a cobalt-chromium alloy) should not be used as components in a single device, since this automatically generates an electrochemical cell as a result of their differing potentials. However, it is also important to note that even combinations of the same material in different conditions or with slightly different compositions, such as wrought and cast cobalt-chromium alloy, can lead to corrosion-related failure.

The synergistic action of mechanical factors and corrosion is of extreme importance and can cause failure even when the individual influences themselves are insufficient. The most important varieties of these combined effects are fretting, stress corrosion cracking, corrosion fatigue, and intergranular corrosion.

Fretting is a mechanism of corrosion resulting from the relatively slight motion of two metal surfaces, thereby disrupting the protective oxide film and causing localized corrosion and tearing out of small pieces of metal.

The simultaneous application of stress and a corrosive atmosphere may lead to stress corrosion cracking. Although direct mechanical loading during service is the most obvious cause of this phenomenon, residual stresses from fabrication may be contributory. Fatigue failure may also occur at a reduced number of cycles or a reduced level of stress in a corrosive medium.

Intergranular corrosion results from preferential corrosion of the metal at the interfaces between its crystals (grains) called the grain boundaries. During solidification or heat treatments, precipitation of new phases at the grain boundaries may occur. This can lead to the depletion near the grain boundaries of elements that formerly enhanced the corrosion resistance. Corrosion deep in the metal along such boundaries may occur, greatly weakening the metal and thereby allowing potentially catastrophic failure at minimal stresses.

Clinical case histories illustrating these various failure mechanisms have been reviewed (Byrne, Lovasko, and Laskin, 1973; Dumbleton and Miller, 1975).

Polymer degradation. Polymers are high molecular weight materials composed of long chains of repeating units, usually with a carbon-to-carbon bonded backbone. The silicones with a —Si—O—Si— backbone are exceptions. The chemistry of the repeat unit, or monomer, and the extent of cross-linking among chains determine in large measure the physical and chemical properties of the polymer. Susceptibility of the polymer to chemical degradation is dependent on the strength of the atomic bonding in the molecule and the proximity of weaker bonds to the surface. Effects caused by the spatial arrangement of atoms may hide various chemical bonds and thus protect these bonds from degradation.

Although the exact mechanisms of chemical disintegration of polymers are speculative, hydrolytic reactions, oxidation-reduction reactions, and reactions involving free radicals are probably involved. Degradation may also occur by decarboxylation and addition to and cleavage of double bonds (Bischoff, 1972). Attack may be random, or it may act to selectively separate individual monomer units.

Polyesters (Dacron), polyester-type urethanes, and polyamides (nylon) have bonds that are easily hydrolyzed and suffer mechanical property deterioration in vivo (Williams and Roaf, 1973). When breakdown is dependent on hydrolytic mechanisms, the relative hydrophilic nature of the polymer partially determines its stability.

Polyethylene, with a backbone of only carbon-to-carbon bonds, should not be vulnerable to hydrolytic or oxidation-reduction reactions. Yet slow loss of strength does take place (Levine, 1968) and probably involves the cleavage of carbon-to-carbon bonds, perhaps caused by free radical interactions. Silicone rubber, poly (methyl methacrylate), and polytetrafluoroethylene (Teflon) generally show minimal changes of mechanical properties in vivo.

Degradation may also occur by the leaching out of plasticizers, catalysts, antioxidants, and other additives. Such products are potentially toxic to the tissues. Thus the limitation to use only implants of polymers designated as "medical grade" is emphasized.

Ceramic dissolution. Ceramics are highly stable products of oxidation reactions. Although high-density implant ceramics such as alumina (Al_2O_3) are exceedingly inert in the physiologic environment, porous alumina (Frakes, Brown, and Kenner, 1974) and other porous ceramics such as calcium aluminate, calcium phosphate, and zirconia may show substantial reductions in their mechanical strength after long-term implantation (Hench and Ethridge, 1975). Even oxide ceramics, usually outstanding in their chemical stability, can undergo surface and grain boundary attack in an aqueous environment. Studies on the physical chemistry of glass surfaces have indicated a wide spectrum of activity depending on composition and processing variables (Hench and Clark, 1978). Controlled rate surface reactions have been used to advantage in the development of bioglass and bioglass-ceramics for stimulating osseous mineralization (Clark, Hench, and Paschall, 1976).

Host reactions to implanted biomaterials

Surgical implantation of a biomaterial, prosthesis, or medical device leads to a variety of sequelae, some of which are potentially harmful to the host. Complications may result indirectly from the surgical procedure or directly from the implant itself. Surgery and implant may each have local and distant or systemic effects. The various effects of surgery and implants are often superimposed. The following is a list of the major recognized local and systemic biomaterials/tissue interactions in soft and hard tissues.

Local
 Inflammation and fibrous encapsulation
 Infection
 Tumorigenesis
 Necrosis
 Mechanical effects
Distant (systemic)
 Migration of the biomaterial
 Hypersensitivity
 Immunologic inhibition
 Accumulation of toxic elements

For reviews of inflammation and surgical wound healing the reader is referred elsewhere: soft tissue (Ross, 1969) and hard tissue (Ham, 1974; Hench and Ethridge, 1975).

Local tissue reactions

Inflammation and fibrous encapsulation. The initial result of placement of a biomaterial in the tissues is acute inflammation, a physiologic response to injury. That this reaction results from aseptic surgery need not be discussed here; that it can result from nontraumatic biomaterials implantation is not as fully appreciated (Schoen, 1978). The histologic appearance of the acute inflammatory response does not depend on the specific nature of the injurious agent (for example, chemical, mechanical, circulatory, infectious). Nevertheless, the outcome of acute inflammation is in part dependent on the etiologic agent. The reaction may resolve if the noxious stimulus is removed and damaged tissue is regenerated (as in certain epithelia or bone); it may repair by scar formation if the damaged tissue cannot regenerate (as in muscle, nerve, or some types of connective tissue); or it may go on to a chronic inflammatory response if the injurious agent persists. An intermediate level of reaction incorporating repair and chronic inflammation is fibrous encapsulation. This is the characteristic late reaction around a surgically implanted biomaterial. The implant is surrounded by a thin, mostly avascular, layer of fibrous tissue, with variable amounts of inflammatory cell infiltrate. The capsule serves to isolate the implant from the host. If near a body or organ surface, frank extrusion may occur.

An example of the response to a relatively inert surgical implant is illustrated in Fig. 8-8. In most clinical situations, the histologic appearance shown is a favorable outcome. There is a relatively thin fibrous tissue capsule (composed of collagen and fibroblasts), with a fine capillary network at its junction with normal tissue and virtually no inflammatory cell infiltrate. The fibrous layer is partly caused by the surgery of implantation, and its thickness is dependent on technique. The surface of the capsule adjacent to the implant is not epithelialized. If the implant is removed, collapse and obliteration of the defect usually occur (Thompson, 1973).

If tissue irritation and/or damage continues, chronic inflammation results. In chronic inflammation, histologic examination reveals macrophages, lymphocytes, fibroblasts, collagen, and possibly necrotic tissue and other inflammatory cells. There is variability in form and degree depending somewhat on the nature of the inciting agent. Fig. 8-9 shows the histologic appearance of the tissue surrounding an implant inducing diffuse chronic inflammation with enhanced

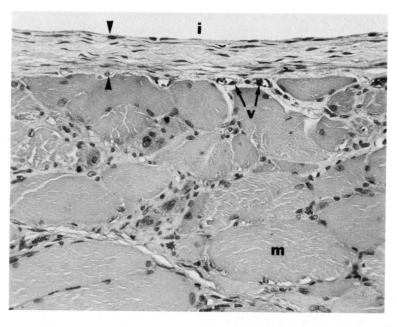

Fig. 8-8. Tissue reaction to biocompatible material, *i*, in form of cylinder 4 mm diameter by 40 mm length surgically implanted into rabbit muscle 6 weeks previously. Limits of thin and discrete fibrous capsule are marked by arrowheads. Note absence of significant inflammatory cell infiltrate and presence of fine vascularity, *v*, at capsule/muscle interface. Muscle fiber is identified, *m*. Hematoxylin and eosin. Light photomicrograph; original magnification × 250.

fibrosis. Compared to that illustrated in Fig. 8-8, the reaction is considerably more intense and involves a greater volume of tissue.

Chronic inflammation may be diffuse, as shown in Fig. 8-9, or granulomatous. The basic structural feature of granulomatous inflammation is the granuloma—a collection of mononuclear inflammatory cells organized around a nidus of poorly soluble and/or toxic irritant. The most prominent functional cell type in the foreign body granuloma is the macrophage, although other cells including lymphocytes may be present in fewer numbers. Macrophages, derived from bone marrow cells (Spector and Ryan, 1970), attempt to phagocytose the material, but degradation may be difficult and/or incomplete. The foreign body giant cell, often prominent in granulomatous inflammation, is derived from the local fusion of macrophages (Mariano and Spector, 1974). The presence of such cells, indicative of the inability to dispose of a highly irritating substance, is generally considered to be evidence of a severe reaction. Granulomatous inflammation in response to an implanted Dacron mesh is illustrated in Fig. 8-10.

The specific histologic appearance of the tissue surrounding a given implant depends on a variety of host, implant, and technical factors, some of which are listed below.

Implant factors
  Composition (chemistry, crystal structure, ?additives, ?cytotoxicity, ?hypersensitivity)
  Surface characteristics (roughness, porosity, electrical charge, hydrophobicity)
  Configuration (size, shape)
  Mechanical aspects (stiffness, relative tissue/implant movement)

Host factors
  Species
  Age
  Site of implantation
  Immunologic status

Technical factors
  Surgery of implantation (extent of tissue damage, size of surgical defect, ?hematoma, ?contamination)
  Duration of implantation

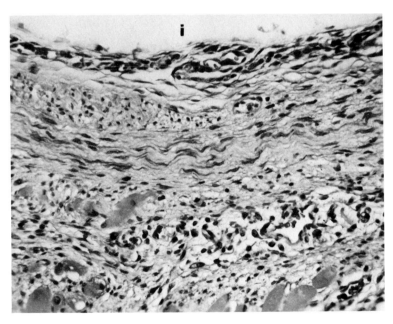

Fig. 8-9. Untoward tissue reaction to poorly tolerated biomaterial, *i*, in experiment identical to that described in Fig. 8-8. There is intense mononuclear inflammatory cell infiltrate throughout ill-defined fibrous capsule. Volume of tissue involved is considerable. Hematoxylin and eosin. Light photomicrograph; original magnification × 250.

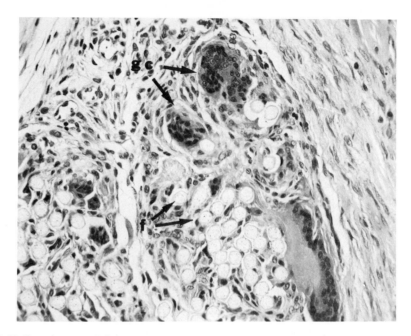

Fig. 8-10. Granulomatous inflammatory response to surgically implanted mesh biomaterial in experiment identical to that described in Fig. 8-8. Individual fibers in mesh are identified, *f.* Several foreign body giant cells, *gc,* are also identified. Hematoxylin and eosin. Light photomicrograph; original magnification × 250.

Although this list has been determined by experimentation (many reported studies), many of these factors have considerable clinical significance as well. A detailed discussion of some aspects of the problem has been published (Coleman, King, and Andrade, 1974). Those factors discussed below require additional consideration.

The physical and chemical characteristics of the material are of primary importance in determining tissue response. Composition, including the presence of contaminants, and surface configuration must be ascertained. Fabrication history, especially that influencing degradation and corrosion behavior, may have a major effect on in vivo response. The physical form of the material influences results; for example, sharp corners may induce substantially more response than flat surfaces (Wood, Kaminski, and Oglesby, 1970).

The site of implantation is a major determining factor in the tissue reaction to a biomaterial and its time evolution. Tissue vascularity and movement are impor-

tant features in this regard, as well as the more obvious physiologic differences between hard and soft tissue. Thus the site employed for preclinical biomaterials testing should approximate as closely as possible the intended site of application. In addition, tests of duration less than that required for physiologic wound healing are confusing and meaningless in comparison of materials.

Although there is recent recognition that endogenous factors, such as tumor bearing by the host, may depress the inflammatory response to foreign bodies (Normann and Schardt, 1978), intentional pharmacologic manipulation of the host's response to biomaterial implants by clinical anti-inflammatory agents has not been attempted.

Infection. In most cases it is possible to distinguish the histologic appearance of inflammatory reactions caused by infectious agents from those resulting from sterile foreign bodies. However, if an infection produces an extremely mild inflammation, differentiation may be difficult. Thus low-grade infection must be ruled out before implicating the implant biomaterial in the case of an untoward tissue reaction. In all cases, when an implant is removed at surgery, swabs of the implant site should be submitted for culture. Infection remains the major cause of clinical failure of orthopedic prosthetic joint reconstructions (Harris, 1977). Gram-positive organisms, particularly *Staphylococcus aureus*, are the most common pathogens cultured (Fitzgerald et al., 1977).

The presence of a foreign body increases tissue susceptibility to infection. An implant may reduce, by a factor as much as 10^4, the number of pathogenic bacteria necessary to elicit a clinical infection (Elek and Conen, 1957). Therefore eradication of an established infection at an implant site generally requires removal of the biomaterial.

Although there are probably many mechanisms by which foreign bodies potentiate infection, the most important seem to be related to:

1. The presence of extra inflammatory fluids and hematomata as bacterial nutrients over those present in a normal wound
2. The compromise of tissue vascularity as a result of surgical manipulation and the pressure created by the implant
3. The presence of spaces and crevices in the implant large enough to harbor bacteria, but not of sufficient size to allow appropriate utilization of host defenses such as leukocytes
4. Direct inhibitory or cytotoxic effects of the biomaterial on cells or humoral mechanisms mediating inflammation and healing

Tumorigenesis. Almost any solid material implanted into rodents will induce neoplastic growth, with induction periods of approximately 1 to 2 years. Although it was initially thought that the chemical nature of the implant was highly important, tumor formation is now considered to be primarily dependent on the physical features of the implant (providing that the implant does not contain direct chemical carcinogens).

Most of the experimental tumors are sarcomas of several types; however, this may be due to the fact that most surgical implants are placed into connective tissue. The subject of foreign body tumorigenesis has been recently reviewed (Brand et al., 1976). Experimental tumors in mice appear to arise from preneoplastic cells in the fibrous capsule that must migrate to and contact the implant surface for the development of clinical tumors. The preneoplastic cell is thought to be the pericyte, a multipotential cell in the tissues surrounding blood vessels. The density of preneoplastic cells has been estimated to be 1 per 220 mm². Implants inducing sustained tissue inflammatory activity appear to reduce tumor incidence (Ferguson, 1978).

There are few reports of tumors related to therapeutic implants in humans. This may be a result of a relatively long induction period required for malignant transformation in man. Nevertheless, a bone sarcoma at the site of a stainless steel plate and screw device and a hemangioendothelioma of bone after implantation of a stainless steel plate and screws have been reported (Duke and Fischer, 1972; McDougall, 1956). In each case, implantation was of approximately 30 years duration, and the components were of mixed composition leading to severe corrosion.

Necrosis and mechanical effects. Implanted polymeric material may cause local tissue necrosis owing to leachable additives. An example of this is the leaching of cytotoxic organotin compounds from certain commercial poly (vinyl chloride) preparations. Although polymerized acrylic cement (poly [methyl methacrylate]) is a biocompatible material, setting of this material in vivo results in extensive direct soft and hard tissue damage. This effect appears to be due primarily to the high polymerization temperature and secondarily to the cytotoxicity of nonpolymerizing monomer (Feith, 1975).

All implanted biomaterials and prosthetic devices may exert mechanical effects on the surrounding tissue because their elastic properties usually differ from those of soft tissue or bone. The implications of elastic mismatch and its potential for bone resorption have been addressed (Katz and Mow, 1973). In soft tissue, increased inflammation and fibrous capsule thickness are the usual consequences of mechanical irritation. Implants also may exert pressure on vital structures such as nerves, blood vessels, and lymphatics.

Distant and systemic effects

There is recent evidence that there may be distant or systemic effects of a biomaterial. Several general types of reactions have been recognized: transport of materials or a material's constituents to sites remote from the implant and induced aberrations in the host's specific and nonspecific immunologic systems.

Silicone particles were found in the axillary lymph nodes 5 years after insertion of a silicone finger joint prosthesis (Christie, Weinberger, and Dietrich, 1977) and 10 years after mammary augmentation with a silicone gel-filled bag prosthesis (Hausner, Schoen, and Pierson, 1978). It is thus clear that insoluble particles may be transported through the lymphatics by cellular mechanisms. Experimental studies utilizing metals and ceramics have also shown evidence of lymphatic transport of materials by macrophages.

Although external contact hypersensitivity to metals causing dermatitis is well established, dermatitis resulting from implanted metallic materials has been only recently recognized. Pruritis and urticaria have been reported after insertion of a Vitallium device (McKenzie, Aitken, and Ridsill-Smith, 1967). A stainless steel orthopedic implant was shown to be responsible for severe eczematous dermatitis (Barranco and Solaman, 1972). In both cases, patch testing for nickel, a well-known cause of metal contact reactions, was positive. The criteria and tests available for determination of the specific metal causing an allergic reaction and preimplantation patch test procedures have been described (Fisher, 1973). Recently, it has been suggested that loosening of total joint prostheses is attributable to sensitivity to the metallic components (Elves et al., 1975), although this has not been supported by other studies (Brown et al., 1977). Local inhibition of the immune response may be a result of implantation. Methyl methacrylate has been shown in vitro to depress components of cellular (polymorphonuclear and lymphocytic) immunity and serum activity against microbes (Panush and Petty, 1978; Petty, 1978; Petty and Caldwell, 1977).

RECONSTRUCTIVE BIOMATERIALS

A wide variety of materials have been utilized in prosthetic reconstruction of the jaws and face. Many of these materials are described below. No attempt is made to dictate selection or describe manipulation for specific applications. Supplementary data may be found in the text by Williams and Roaf (1973). For more clinical detail, the reader is referred to an excellent paper by Irby (1974) and to the other contributors to this text.

Alloplastic biomaterials
Metals

The comparatively high strength and high ductility, and the ease of fabrication of metals, have rendered this class of materials the traditional choice for implanted stress-bearing human prosthetic appliances. As the need for significant corrosion resistance was recognized even in early attempts to implant materials, repair of the supporting members of the human body was initially carried out with the noble metals (for example, gold and platinum). Since then, a wide variety of metals and their alloys have been used as surgical implants. Detailed historic accounts of the use of and problems associated with metallic surgical implants have been published (Bechtol et al., 1959; Brettle, 1970; Ludwigson, 1964).

There are presently three primary families of metals that are used for structural surgical implants: stainless steels, cobalt-chromium alloys, and titanium and its alloys. Representative alloy compositions are given in Table 8-1. Each of these metals systems is discussed in detail below. Tantalum has also achieved some clinical success, predominantly in the form of wires and mesh but occasionally

Table 8-1. Representative compositions of surgical implant alloys*

	Fe	Ni	Cr	Co	Mo	W	Ti	Al	V
Stainless steel (316)	Bal†	12	17		2.5				
Cobalt-chromium alloy (cast)		2.5	27.5	Bal†	6.0				
Cobalt-chromium alloy (wrought)		10	20	Bal†		15			
Titanium							99+		
Titanium alloy (Ti-6Al-4V)							Bal†	6	4

*Concentrations are expressed in weight percent.
†Bal = balance.

in bulk form. Although only incomplete characterization of this metal has been carried out, the application of tantalum to oral and maxillofacial surgery is considered briefly.

Stainless steels. Although early steels for surgical implants were of a variety of compositions, only stainless steels containing 17% to 20% chromium and 10% to 14% nickel are presently used. These compositions, designated as austenitic for the stable homogeneous corrosion-resistant phase (austenite) comprising the structure, may be recognized as the only major class of steels that is not magnetic. Austenitic stainless steels have the best corrosion resistance of the various stainless steel types, and although they have a lower strength than the martensitic and ferritic types, their high ductility reduces the likelihood of mechanical failure. A brief discussion of the physical metallurgy of stainless steels is recommended for interested readers (Phillips, 1973; Williams and Roaf, 1973).

Since the corrosion resistance of stainless steels is a result of the protective surface layer of chromium oxide, compositions containing less than 17% to 18% chromium do not possess the necessary corrosion resistance. Nickel, in amounts of 10% to 14%, allows retention of the austenitic phase at room temperature. The most favorable compositions also contain approximately 2% to 4% molybdenum to enhance the resistance to corrosion in chloride-containing environments. Surgical stainless steels possess a low carbon content that reduces problems associated with embrittlement and

susceptibility to intergranular corrosion (sensitization). Intergranular corrosion may result from precipitation of chromium carbides at the grain boundaries and the local depletion of chromium in these areas. The appropriate compositions are designated as AISI (American Iron and Steel Institute) 316L and 317. Although it is possible to cast stainless steel components directly, the mechanical properties of stainless steel castings are poor and thus surgical stainless steels are utilized in wrought (worked) form.

Surgical stainless steels cannot be appreciably strengthened by heat treatment. The alloys are, however, capable of significant work hardening, leading to increased yield and ultimate tensile and fatigue strengths, although there is a concurrent loss in ductility. Subsequent annealing (heating to allow relief of internal stresses) lowers strength and partially restores ductility. Representative mechanical properties of these structures, as well as the other alloys to be discussed, are given in Table 8-2. It is seen that the ultimate tensile strength and ductility of annealed stainless steels are reasonably high, but the yield strength is low. In the hardened variety, restricted ductility is evident.

The main advantages of stainless steel for surgical implants relate to the favorable economics of availability and fabrication. In vitro and in vivo corrosion resistance of stainless steels is generally not as good as that of either titanium and its alloys or the cobalt-base alloys. Cold worked stainless steel is especially prone to stress corrosion cracking.

Like the corrosion behavior, experi-

Table 8-2. Representative properties of metallic surgical implants*

Metal/alloy	Density (gm/cm³)	Yield strength (10³ psi [MN/m²])	Tensile strength (10³ psi [MN/m²])	Modulus of elasticity, (10⁶ psi [GN/m²])	Ductility (percent elongation)
316L Stainless steel (annealed)	8.0	35 (241)	85 (586)	28.0 (193)	55
316L Stainless steel (work hardened)	8.0	115 (793)	140 (965)	29.0 (200)	8
Co-28Cr-6Mo-C (cast)	8.3	75 (517)	105 (724)	33.4 (230)	10
Co-20Cr-15W-10Ni-C (wrought)	8.4	60 (414)	146 (1007)	36.3 (250)	39
Titanium	4.5	60 (414)	75 (517)	17.4 (120)	18
Ti-6Al-4V	4.4	115 (791)	125 (862)	18.1 (125)	10
Tantalum	16.6	27.4 (189)	43.6 (301)	27.6 (190)	40

*Data in this table are adapted from numerous sources (1 MN/m² = 144 psi).

mental and clinical tissue response to stainless steel implants has been generally inferior to that exhibited to the titanium or cobalt-chromium alloys when comparative studies are performed. Detailed comparison of the corrosion resistance and tissue compatibility of the commonly utilized surgical implant alloys appears in a later section of this chapter (p. 310).

Cobalt-chromium alloys. Although none of the currently available implant alloys completely meets the necessary requirements, cast cobalt-chromium alloys have attained the widest clinical usage, having been used for approximately four decades in stress-bearing orthopedic implants. In general, the alloys have quite adequate mechanical properties except that their ductility is relatively low (Table 8-2). These alloys are strengthened predominantly by carbide precipitates and thus significant property alteration by conventional heat treatment procedures is not possible. Since this class of alloys is the only major group that is easily cast, it is the one presently used in the fabrication of "individualized" appliances, such as subperiosteal implants. In addition, cobalt-chromium alloys generally possess high-abrasion resistance, which has made them a favorite choice for two-component orthopedic joint replacements.

Cast cobalt-chromium alloys, such as surgical Vitallium, have an approximate basic composition Co-28Cr-6Mo-C (28% chromium + 6% molybdenum + small amounts of carbon in a cobalt base). Although the orthopedic alloy contains only 0.35C maximum, dental casting alloys allow a slightly higher carbon content for facilitation of casting. The alloys Nobilium and Haynes Stellite (HS) 21 have a similar composition. Related casting alloys with some of the cobalt replaced by nickel (20% to 40%), such as Ticonium, have been introduced.

Wrought cobalt-chromium alloys such as Haynes Stellite (HS) 25 and wrought Vitallium with the basic composition Co-20Cr-15W-10Ni-C are available and are used to fabricate certain implants. In general, the corrosion resistance of cast alloys is superior to that of the wrought alloys. Recently, high-temperature mechanical processing techniques have been developed to fabricate wrought components from Co-Cr-Mo-C alloys, without the loss in corrosion resistance usually associated with mechanical working of the structure (Hollander and Wulff, 1975). The more uniform and finer distribution of carbides achieved by thermomechanical processing also accounts for a favorable change in the mechanical properties.

In vitro and in vivo corrosion resistance of these alloys is generally excellent. Occasional reports of corrosion-related failure have appeared, however, that seem to be related to either design errors leading to stress corrosion and/or corrosion fatigue or compositional variations within a single device, such as a wrought fixation plate used with cast screws (Cohen and Wulff, 1972).

Related wrought alloys MP35 (Co-20Cr-15Ni-10Mo) and Elgiloy (40Co-20Cr-15Ni-7Mo-Fe) have also been shown to have acceptable mechanical properties and corrosion resistance for implant application (Younkin, 1974). The alloy MP35N is strengthened by work hardening and aging (causing precipitation of a second phase by heating) and has excellent fatigue behavior and corrosion resistance. Initial in vivo compatibility studies have been encouraging (Escalas et al, 1975). Although the alloy is castable, its cast properties are inferior to those of other cast cobalt-chromium alloys.

Additional improvements in mechanical properties, including ductility, without concurrent sacrifice in corrosion resistance and biocompatibility may be forthcoming in cobalt-base alloys with virtual elimination of carbon and modest additions of certain alloying elements such as tantalum (Mohammed and Asgar, 1973).

Titanium and its alloys. Because of the difficulty of casting titanium in air, special vacuum casting methods are employed, and the resultant "commercially pure titanium" contains controlled additions of oxygen and nitrogen. Therefore the metal and its alloys are used in wrought form. Since cold working not only improves strength but also severely limits ductility, the metal and its alloys are generally annealed after device fabrication. Properties of titanium in this condition are similar to those of annealed stainless steel, except that the elastic modulus is very much less (Table 8-2). In addition, titanium has a much lower density than stainless steel.

Alloys of titanium have recently been introduced; the most widely considered for implant purposes has been an alloy containing 6% aluminum, and 4% vanadium, which has enhanced mechanical properties relative to the pure metal. As seen in Table 8-2, the modulus of elasticity of Ti-6A1-4V is similar to that of pure titanium, but the strength properties are improved. There is, however, a certain loss in ductility. An additional important property of Ti-6A1-4V is that its fatigue limit is significantly greater than that of any other currently available surgical implant material (80,000 psi [551 MN/m²] at 10^7 cycles [Bardos, 1974]).

In vitro corrosion resistance of titanium and its alloys is extremely favorable. Animal tests and clinical trials demonstrate excellent corrosion resistance and tissue compatibility of these materials. A disadvantageous property of titanium and its alloys is the propensity to galling (tearing out of metal particles) when used as a bearing surface. This has resulted in limited use of titanium in various types of joint replacement.

Recently there have been attempts to nitride (induce a high concentration of nitrogen in) the surface of titanium alloy implants in order to improve the wear characteristics. The nitrided layer imparts a gold-colored appearance and provides a convenient identification of the alloy, precluding the dangers associated with mixing alloys. Biocompatibility data on the nitrided alloy have not as yet appeared in the literature.

Tantalum. Tantalum is a very dense high-melting transition metal, which, when essentially pure, can be readily fabricated into a wide variety of shapes and maintains a relatively high corrosion resistance by virtue of a stable oxide film. Although many clinical studies have appeared in the literature, characterization of this metal has been less extensive than that of the metals previously considered. The basic mechanical properties are summarized in Table 8-2. Although the elastic modulus is relatively high, the yield strength and tensile strength are relatively low. Improvement in strength occurs on cold working, but the mechanical properties have generally been considered unsuitable for stress-bearing applications. Nevertheless, the material has found application in oral and maxillofacial surgery in the form of clips, plates, and in wire mesh or foil. Tantalum gauze has been used to build up knife-edge alveolar ridges, and a perforated plate has been used to fabricate a subperiosteal implant by swaging onto a model made during the operation (Thoma, 1969). Perforated tantalum plates have performed adequately in mandibular reconstruction (Hinds et al., 1963). Thin tantalum foil has been used in temporomandibular joint arthroplasty (Goodsell, 1968).

Comparison of surgical implant metals: corrosion and tissue reaction. Corrosion rates of most industrial metals may be determined directly by weight-loss measurements. However, for special corrosion-resistant alloys, such as those for surgical implants where corrosion rates are exceedingly low, these methods are not practical, and sophisticated electrical techniques were necessarily developed (Jones and Greene, 1966). The most useful of these methods for prediction of in vivo corrosion behavior are anodic polarization methods (Fontana and Greene, 1967).

The anodic polarization technique has been used to assess the relative corrosion resistance of several metallic implant materials in vitro (Cahoon et al, 1973; Hoar and Mears, 1966; Mueller and Greener, 1970). Chloride-containing solutions were used in an effort to simulate the physiologic environment. While stainless steel, cobalt-chromium alloy, and titanium all exhibited spontaneous passivation (formation of the protective oxide layer), subsequent breakdown of the film occurred readily for the stainless steel and later for the cobalt-chromium alloy. Titanium remained passive throughout the tests. Stainless steel was found to undergo pitting corrosion, which did not occur with the other metals under the test conditions. Solution deaeration and mechanical working caused more rapid passive breakdown of the stainless steel (Cahoon et al., 1973; Mueller and Greener, 1970). Thus titanium appears to be the most corrosion resistant of the common surgical implant alloys in vitro. Although certain titanium alloys such as Ti-6Al-4V have enhanced corrosion resistance (Hoar and Mears, 1966), these same alloys may have greater susceptibility to stress corrosion cracking. Reported instances of clinical failures caused by corrosion have generally been linked to poor device design, poor fabrication, and/or poor selection of materials (Cohen and Wulff, 1972; Pugh, Jaffe, and Jaffe, 1975; Rose, Schiller, and Radin, 1972; Scales, Winter, and Shirley, 1961).

In studies of large numbers of implants removed after prolonged use, stainless steel devices generally show, at best, moderate uniform corrosion (Hughes and Jordan, 1972; Laing, 1973; Williams and Meachim, 1974). Susceptibility is particularly high in crevices and narrow spaces between device components, owing to the difficulty of maintenance of the passivating oxide film in these regions of diminished fluid exchange. Cobalt-chromium alloy implants show little generalized corrosion. While excellent corrosion resistance of titanium has been demonstrated in vivo, accumulation of titanium in the tissues surrounding the implant appears to be a common occurrence (Laing, 1973; Lemons, 1975).

The cellular tissue reaction seen around cobalt-chromium alloys is generally less than that seen around stainless steel implants; tissue reaction to titanium in the absence of wear is minimal (Laing, 1973). The presence of titanium in the tissues mentioned previously appears to be inconsequential and, as yet, is lacking explanation. Although recent detailed histologic studies are scarce, tantalum appears to be clinically well tolerated (Goldberg et al., 1976; Thoma, 1969).

Polymers

Polymers are generally the class of materials of choice for nonstress-bearing soft tissue reconstruction. They have also found application in hard tissue sites under certain circumstances.

Until recently the results associated with polymeric implant materials were inconsistent owing to the use of incompletely characterized industrial materials. It has since become clear that the chemical stability and tissue reactivity of such materials are extremely sensitive to the presence of additives such as catalysts, plasticizers, antioxidants, and residual monomer. Presently used implant polymers are specifically prepared for biomedical application under controlled conditions.

Polymers differ from other types of materials in their mechanical properties. In general, polymers exhibit much lower strength and modulus of elasticity and much higher ductility than other materials. For a particular polymer, as the average molecular weight and/or degree of cross-linking of the polymer chains increase, the strength and modulus of elasticity increase while the ductility decreases. Table 8-3 shows representative mechanical properties for some polymers of interest in oral and maxillofacial surgery.

Polymers exhibit viscoelastic mechanical behavior, that is, there is a time-dependent component of deformation superimposed on the purely elastic deformation even at fairly low stresses. The faster the rate of application of stress, the stronger the material appears. Thus, under relatively low stress, deformation of polymers may continue over long periods of time. The importance of this phenomenon lies in the possibility of slowly manifested dimensional changes (cold flow) of polymers. It is also important to note that some polymers show mechanical properties that are sensitive to stress concentrations. Thus proper device design may increase functional permanence.

Although most polymers used as reconstructive biomaterials are organic and nondegradable in nature (polyethylene, poly [methyl methacrylate], and polyurethane), inorganic chain structures (silicones) have been used as well as certain forms of rapidly degradable chain structures (polyglycolic acid, polylactic acid).

Silicones. Silicone rubber is based on the polymer polydimethylsiloxane, a relatively low molecular weight silicon-oxygen chain polymer with terminal hydroxyl groups (Braley, 1970). Medical grade silicone elastomer, Silastic, may be heat vulcanized to form ready made specific implants, or it may be used in a two-component room-temperature–vulcanizing (RTV) system. Vulcanizing involves the establishment of cross-links between the separate polymer chains.

Medical grade silicone rubbers contain fillers and vulcanizing agents, but they do not contain the wide variety of additives used in industrial processing. The three commonly used medical grade heat-vulcanized silicone rubbers are Silastic 370, 372, and 373, which cover the hardness range of soft to medium to hard. Available in the raw state for custom fabrication of implants, they are known as MDX 4-4514, MDX 4-4515, and MDX 4-4516, respectively. Silastic 382 is the most widely used medical grade RTV. Representative mechanical properties of the silicones are given in Table 8-3.

Silicones are highly resistant to chemical and environmental attack, although the early silicones used in cardiovascular

Table 8-3. Representative properties of implant polymers*

Polymer	Density (gm/cm³)	Tensile strength (10³ psi [MN/m²])	Modulus of elasticity (10⁶ psi [GN/m²])	Elongation at fracture (percent)
Silicone rubber (RTV)	1.13	0.4 (2.8)	<0.0015 (<0.01)	160
Silicone rubber (heat cured)	1.14	1.2 (8.3)	0.0015 (0.01)	450
Poly (methyl methacrylate) (heat cured)	1.2	10.2 (70)	0.435 (3)	5
Polyethylene (low density)	0.92	2.2 (15)	0.02 (0.14)	600
Polyethylene (high molecular weight)	0.94	5.4 (37)	0.1 (0.69)	400
Polytetrafluoroethylene	2.2	2.9 (20)	0.072 (0.5)	400

*Data in this table are adapted from numerous sources (1 MN/m² = 144 psi).

devices exhibited a tendency to absorb lipids in vivo (Hylen, 1971). Alterations in manufacture have apparently eliminated this problem. The material elicits a minimal tissue inflammatory reaction and is reported to be noncarcinogenic and nonallergenic (Mullison, 1966). Fabrication in a wide variety of configurations is feasible at relatively low cost. The main disadvantage of the silicones is their poor mechanical properties, especially the tear resistance, even with substantial additions of filler to the polymer. Applications have included soft tissue and alveolar ridge augmentation, interposition after temporomandibular joint arthroplasty, and other nonstressed or very lightly stressed prosthetic reconstructions.

Methyl methacrylate. Acrylic polymers have been used for intraoral splints, removable dentures, and artificial teeth for many years. Although a number of investigators have implanted acrylic roots or teeth with limited success, the self-supporting acrylic tooth replica implant introduced by Hodosh appears to be the most practical (Hodosh, 1959; Hodosh, Shklar, and Povar, 1970). The material for these implants, presently incorporating porosity for tissue ingrowth and stabilization, is heat-cured in a gypsum mold. Most other applications have used a self-cured resin.

For either thermally or chemically (self) activated cure, powdered prepolymerized methyl methacrylate is mixed with liquid monomer in the ratio of approximately 2:1 by weight. The polymerization process begins with the production of free radicals by decomposition of an initiator, usually benzoyl peroxide. This occurs either by thermal activation or, in the case of a self- or cold-curing material, by chemical reaction of the initiator with an accelerator. The reaction is exothermic and autocatalytic. Residual monomer is generally less than 1% in a heat-cured material and approximately 3% to 5% in the chemically cured material (Smith, 1971). Histocompatibility in the cured state is favorable (Hodosh, Shklar, and Povar, 1972).

Methyl methacrylate has been used as a bone substitute in alveolar ridge reconstruction (Thoma, 1969). In this and related applications, the material is chemically cured on a model of the mandible. Other applications of methyl methacrylate utilize in-situ polymerization and have included the fixation of dental and orthopedic implants (Smith, 1973; Zarb, Melcher, and Smith, 1972), the primary treatment of avulsive wounds of the mandible, stabilization of mobile segments in surgical orthodontics, support of the mandible after partial resection, restoration of mandibular defects created by surgery for malignancies, and stabilization of comminuted fractures (Worley, 1973). It has also been used after temporomandibular joint arthroplasty (Kameros and Himmelforb, 1975).

For in-situ polymerization the plastic dough is packed in the desired space and formed to the appropriate shape. The reaction reaches near completion in about 6 to 7 minutes. Local temperature elevations during polymerization may reach 70° C at the bone/methacrylate interface in clinical total hip arthroplasty (Meyer, Lautenschlager, and Moore, 1973). Necrosis of the adjacent bone is caused by the polymerization heat and unreacted monomer (Feith, 1975). The nonviable bone, which functions similarly to a bone graft, may require several years for replacement by viable bone (Willert, Ludwig, and Semlitsch, 1974). A thin layer of fibrous tissue appears to separate acrylic from bone in numerous histologic studies after long-term implantation (Charnley, 1964; Laing, 1973; Willert, Ludwig, and Semlitsch, 1974; Worley, 1973; Yaman et al., 1973). However, the reaction appears otherwise benign. The fibrous connective tissue may cause nonunion or pseudarthrosis in certain cases, as new bone does not form in areas in direct contact with acrylic (Yablon, 1976). The use of high pressure during the packing of acrylic in bony defects is to be avoided, since this may be responsible for cardiovascular collapse occasionally seen in total hip replacement (Cohen and Smith, 1971). Such effects are probably related to unreacted monomer gaining access to the circulation. The cardiovascular and respiratory effects of methyl methacrylate monomer are currently under investigation (Wong et al., 1977).

Methyl methacrylate is clear, hard, rigid, and brittle but relatively strong (Table 8-3). Cured resins may be carved with burs and polished to a high gloss. The material is degraded only slowly in vivo. Resistance to impact and fatigue fracture are poor. Residual monomer may act as a plasticizer, reducing strength and stiffness (Smith, 1962). The 3% to 5% residual monomer thus accounts for the fact that the cold-cured material exhibits 60% to 75% of the strength of heat-cured material (Smith, 1974). The strength may be further reduced by approximately 2% water absorption, which can also lead to a form of stress-corrosion failure. Antibiotic-loaded acrylic cement may be efficacious in reducing infection after toal joint replacement (Welch, 1978) without impairing mechanical properties.

Polyethylene. Polyethylene may be considered the simplest polymer with the repeating unit ($-CH_2-$). The variety of properties attainable with this material depend on the molecular weight and the degree of crystallization. The low-density variety, produced by the polymerization of ethylene gas under high pressure, has a lower molecular weight and degree of crystallinity; thus it is more flexible. High-density polyethylene, which is stiffer and has superior mechanical properties owing to a much higher molecular weight and a greater degree of crystallinity, is obtained by a low-pressure polymerization process. The polyethylenes are weaker and more flexible than most other polymeric materials of interest (Table 8-3). Some polyethylenes deform slowly over time at low loads even at ambient or body temperatures, thus exhibiting a property known as cold flow. Furthermore, the material may be susceptible to stress cracking, and slight chemical deterioration of polyethylene may occur in the body environment.

Ultra-high–density polyethylene has especially good wear properties bearing against metals and good tissue acceptance and chemical stability. Therefore this variant has been widely used in the total hip joint replacement. Skull implants custom fabricated from ultra-high–density polyethylene have had favorable results (Polisar and Cook, 1973).

Polypropylene is somewhat similar to polyethylene in structure and properties except that it is somewhat less subject to in vivo degradation, and the mechanical properties, especially the fatigue life, are superior. Although the material has been used extensively in surgical sutures, use in reconstructive applications has been limited.

Both polyethylene and polypropylene are easily fabricated by injection molding, extrusion, and blow molding

Polytetrafluoroethylene. Polytetrafluoroethylene (PTFE, Teflon, Fluon) is a polymer of extreme chemical inertness and tissue compatibility. Use in bulk form has been limited as a result of vastly inferior mechanical properties (Table 8-3). In spite of a low coefficient of friction, wear properties in prosthetic joints are poor (Charnley, 1963). Soft tissue prostheses are usually manufactured more easily from silicone rubber. Although PTFE is usually a thermoplastic polymer, injection molding is difficult, so that processing is usually by means of a technique using the heating of powders to cause fusion. Production of complex shapes by this method is time consuming and expensive. Widespread use has not occurred as a result of these limitations.

Polymer sponges and foams. As a result of the poor mechanical properties of the foams themselves, these materials have not been successful in stress-bearing applications. Rather, they are used where tissue ingrowth is intended for stabilization of a prosthesis (strong substrate covered with foam) or tissue augmentation where tissue acceptance is the primary requirement.

Polyvinyl alcohol sponge (Ivalon) has been used for ridge augmentation in humans (Cranin, 1970; Topazian et al., 1971). Although satisfactory in hard tissue after infiltration, the main objection to the use of Ivalon as a soft tissue replacement is its tendency toward shrinkage and loss of resiliency owing to fibrous tissue invasion (Schwartz and Erich, 1960).

An acrylate-amide sponge implant has been used to repair alveolar bone defects in primates (Henefer, McFall, and Hauschild, 1968). A well-vascularized fibrous tissue infiltrated the implant, with some forming areas of new bone. Contact with medullary bone appears to be essential for generation of new bone with polymer foam implants (Amler, Johnson, and Bevelander, 1958).

Biodegradable polymers. Polylactic acid (PLA) is a well-tolerated material that is hydrolyzed in vivo (Brady et al., 1973; Cutright, Beasley, and Perez, 1971; Cutright, Hunsuck, and Beasley, 1971; Cutright et al., 1974). Degradation of plates and screws used for fixation of mandibular fractures in dogs was demonstrated at 8 to 12 weeks (Getter and Cutright, 1972), and the fractures appeared well healed. At 40 weeks, virtually complete disappearance of the prosthesis was demonstrated. Bone replaced the PLA screws. Polylactic acid has also been considered as an experimental suture material (Cutright and Hunsuck, 1971; Cutright, Beasley, and Perez, 1971; Cutright, Hunsuck, and Beasley, 1971). By varying the proportions in a copolymer of polylactic acid to polyglycolic acid, a related hydrolyzable polymer used extensively in surgical sutures, resorption times may be varied from less than 100 days to greater than 220 days (Cutright et al., 1974).

Ceramics

Ceramics are compounds of metallic and nonmetallic elements whose structures are held together by strong ionic and/or covalent bonding. In general, such materials are crystalline, with long-range order to the structure. Examples of crystalline ceramics are oxides such as alumina (Al_2O_3) or metal salts such as calcium phosphate $(Ca_3[PO_4]_2)$. Some ceramics, however, have short-range atomic order only; these materials are noncrystalline and are known as glasses. Glasses containing nucleated crystalline phases are known as glass-ceramics.

The mechanical behavior of ceramics is characteristically brittle. Sensitivity to stress concentrations renders ceramics stronger in compression than in tension (usually by a factor of approximately 5 to 1). Despite this brittle behavior and some difficulty in fabrication, ceramics are attractive implant biomaterials as a result of extreme chemical inertness and tissue compatibility. Certain structures such as the bioglass-ceramic and biodegradable ceramics are unique in their controlled reactivity with the physiologic environment as a result of large concentrations of calcium and phosphorus ions.

Porous ceramics. The use of plaster of paris as an osseous replacement dates approximately to the end of the nineteenth century. More recently, it was found that such implants were well tolerated by the surrounding tissues and that osseous regeneration occurred in association with resorption of the plaster, although the material itself did not stimulate osteogenesis (Peltier et al., 1957). Applications have included the filling of mandibular fracture defects (Calhoun, Greene, and Blackledge, 1965), mandibular ridge augmentation, and the obliteration of other bony defects (Bahn, 1966). In these studies, plaster implants compared favorably with autogenous bone. However, variable and incomplete resorption and poor mechanical properties have prevented plaster implants from achieving widespread use.

As plaster of paris could not withstand the stresses imposed on its use in large osseous defects, strengthening by filling with epoxy resin was attempted. Absorption, however, did not occur, and nonunion resulted with a severe chronic inflammatory response (Gourley and Arnold, 1960). Subsequently, a 48% porous aluminate ceramic impregnated with epoxy resins (Cerosium) was used for experimental osseous replacement (Smith, 1963). Although this particular material has not achieved clinical success, the concept stimulated considerable research into porous ceramics as well as porous metals and polymers for various osseous reconstruction applications.

Although Cerosium had 48% bulk porosity, the average pore size is approximately 18 μm in diameter, small compared to the size of a single osteon. Thus tissue adherence is along the external surface only. The possibility of obtaining osseous ingrowth into porous ceramics was subsequently investigated (Hulbert et al., 1970; Klawitter and Hulbert, 1971). It was found that porous $CaO \cdot Al_2O_3$ ceramics were well tolerated and that significant ingrowth of bone would occur if the size of pores and pore interconnections exceeded approximately 100 to 150 μm in diameter. Smaller pore sizes 10 to 40 μm lead to fibrous tissue ingrowth only. The concept of porous inert ceramics has since been investigated extensively, with representative applications being those of alumina endosseous implants (Klawitter et al., 1977) and calcium aluminate for alveolar ridge augmentation (Hammer et al., 1973; Topazian et al., 1971). It is important to realize, however, that the introduction of porosity in ceramic materials generally causes a massive deterioration in mechanical properties (Table 8-4).

Bioglass-ceramic. Glass and glass-ceramic materials that achieve a direct chemical bond at the interface of the material and bone through control of surface reactivity have been developed over the last 5 years. These materials, based on the system $45SiO_2$-$24.5CaO$-$24.5Na_2O$-$6P_2O_5$, release calcium and phosphorus ions in vivo and induce the precipitation of hydroxyapatite crystals in an oriented collagen matrix at the interface (Clark, Hench, and Paschall, 1976; Hench, 1973). It is possible that the additional feature of silicon accumulation at the interface may be an integral factor in the interfacial bond stability (Carlisle, 1970). The mineralized bone/ceramic interface maintains considerable strength; after 4 weeks, the femur into which the biomaterial is implanted fractures before the interface or the bioglass-ceramic under torsional loads (Hench et al., 1975).

It is interesting that the addition of fluorine to the formulation decreases the surface reactivity and promotes fibrous encapsulation in osseous tissue (Clark, Hench, and Paschall, 1976). Thus, by adjusting compositions, it is possible to achieve a spectrum of surface responses. Bioglass and bioglass-ceramics suffer from the mechanical property limitations of ceramic materials in general (Table 8-4). However, it is unnecessary to use these materials in the porous condition to achieve stabilization. Since the favorable reactions are limited to the surface of the materials, they may be applied as a coating to high-strength substrates such as highly dense alumina. Techniques have been developed for this purpose (Hench et al., 1975).

Although bioglass and bioglass-ceramics have not as yet achieved clinical utilization, experimental work in progress includes modified tooth root dental implants (Stanley et al., 1976) and mandibular ridge augmentation.

Resorbable bioceramics. Recent studies of porous calcium aluminate ($12CaO \cdot 7Al_2O_3$) (Hentrich et al., 1971) and tricalcium phosphate (Getter et al., 1972; Levin et al., 1974; Levin, Getter, and Cutright, 1975) implants in bone show that they undergo controlled resorption, are well tolerated by the tissues, and are replaced by bone (Cutright et al., 1972; Getter et al., 1972; Hentrich et al., 1971). After several months, de-

Table 8-4. Representative properties of bioceramics*

Ceramic	Density (gm/cm³)	Flexural strength (10³ psi [MN/m²])	Modulus of elasticity (10⁶ psi [GN/m²])
Alumina (Al_2O_3)	3.9 (99%)	40.0 (276)	50 (345)
	3.3 (85%)	16.8 (116)	34 (235)
	2.5 (65%)	7.9 (54)	19 (131)
Bioglass	3.0	12.0 (83)	6 (41)

*Data in this table are adapted from numerous sources (1 MN/m² = 144 psi)

pending on the size of the implant and the site of implantation, the implants are no longer visible in the tissues. It is possible that these materials actively participate in the process of bone regeneration through the contribution of calcium and phosphorus ions to the advancing bone front. Experimental periodontal defects have been filled with biodegradable tricalcium phosphate ceramic with apparent good success (Levin et al., 1974).

Carbons

Carbonaceous materials have shown recent promise in stress-bearing implants. Useful materials possess a poorly crystalline structure resembling that of graphite, with substantial interplanar and intercrystallite cross-linking, rendering suitable strength properties for certain structural applications. In addition, biocarbons are extremely resistant to corrosion and chemical attack.

Vitreous (glassy) carbons result from the controlled and complete carbonization of certain polymers preformed in the desired bulk configuration. Approximately 20% to 40% shrinkage occurs during the carbonization process, in which all other elements are volatilized. Both the external surface after carbonization and fracture surfaces resemble those of glass, thus leading to the description vitreous or glassy (Cowlard and Lewis, 1967). Although the material maintains a flexural strength of approximately 25,000 psi (Table 8-5), brittle mechanical behavior

and stress concentration sensitivity are exhibited.

Originally used in components of cardiovascular prostheses, low-temperature–isotropic (LTI) pyrolytic carbons (Pyrolite carbons) have recently demonstrated promise as dental implants. These carbons are fabricated in a fluidized bed deposition process at temperatures of the order of 1000° C from a hydrocarbon-containing gaseous environment. For this process a suitable preformed substrate, usually a high-strength graphite, must be provided onto which the carbon is deposited. The process has been described in detail by Bokros and co-workers (1973). The high densities achieved with this process (1.8 to 2 gm/cm³) are due to a droplet deposition mechanism. Optimal properties are obtained when silicon is codeposited with the carbon in amounts approximately 10% to 15% by weight. The high density and silicon alloying account for the attainment of flexural strengths of the order of 75,000 psi and a strain energy to fracture that is approximately seven times that of the vitreous carbons that have densities of 1.5 to 1.6 gm/cm³ (Kaae, 1972).

An interesting property of both vitreous and LTI pyrolytic carbons is their lack of susceptibility to fatigue degradation (Shim, 1974). This is in contrast to the previously described behavior exhibited by metals. In addition, as seen in Table 8-5, the modulus of elasticity of the carbons is in the range of that reported for bone; this may be a useful feature for certain applications.

Carbons have been shown to possess favorable histocompatibility in both hard and soft tissue (Belton et al., 1973; Kenner et al., 1975; Markle, Grenoble, and Melrose, 1975). Vitreous carbons have shown initial success in a modified tooth root endosseous implant configuration (Dumas and Myers, 1974), while the LTI pyrolytic carbons are showing promise as blade-vent endosseous implants (Haubold, 1977).

Composites

Desirable properties are achieved in composites through the use of a stiff and

Table 8-5. Representative properties of biocarbons*

	Vitreous carbon	LTI pyrolytic carbon
Density (gm/cm³)	1.47	1.85
Flexural strength (10³ psi [MN/m²])	25 (172)	75 (517)
Modulus of elasticity (10⁶ psi [GN/m²])	3.4 (23.4)	4.0 (27.6)
Strain at fracture (percent)	1.0	1.9
Strain energy to fracture (in-lb/in³ [m-MN/m³])	90 (0.62)	700 (4.8)

*Data in this table are adapted from numerous sources (1 MN/m² = 144 psi).

strong second phase dispersed in a tough but usually weak matrix. Bonding between the dispersed and matrix phases is necessary for the attainment of optimal properties, and although the strength of the composite is usually increased with increasing volume fractions of the dispersed phase, the structure must be carefully designed. Natural hard tissues, such as enamel, dentin, and bone, are composite materials of organic and inorganic components.

Polytetrafluoroethylene/glassy carbon composite. Proplast is a 70% to 90% porous spongy composite of glassy carbon fibers in a polytetrafluoroethylene (Teflon) matrix (Homsy, Kent, and Hinds, 1973). Rapid ingrowth of fibrous tissue subsequent to implantation is fostered by a pore size range of 100 to 500 μm. The low-modulus, fibrous, tissue-filled implant is purported to allow smooth shear stress transfer between the implant and the surrounding tissues. The elastic modulus and ultimate tensile strength of Proplast are 580 psi (4 MN/m^2) and 145 psi (1 MN/m^2), respectively. No distinct yield stress is exhibited.

Although normally applied as a coating to a metallic substrate such as for endosseous blade-vent implants or temporomandibular joint prostheses (Hinds, Homsy, and Kent, 1974), bulk material has been used in mandibular alveolar ridge augmentation and facial contour reconstruction (Kent, Homsy, and Hinds, 1975). Large coated implants and bulk implants have not achieved widespread success owing to problems associated with sepsis and wound dehiscence. Small implants, especially those employed for facial contour restoration, have yielded somewhat more favorable results.

Reinforced acrylics. In the belief that the high stiffness of previously available rigid internal fixation plates overprotects bone from beneficial functional stresses during healing and leads to cortical osteopenia beneath the plate, a graphite-fiber reinforced methyl methacrylate internal fixation plate was developed (Woo et al., 1974). Such a plate has a modulus of elasticity approximately that of bone,

with a relatively high fracture strength. The plates have exhibited good histocompatibility and improved bony healing characteristics in canine long bone experiments (Akeson et al., 1975).

Dental composite resins. Composite structures of ceramic particles embedded in an organic polymer matrix have been employed for some time as esthetic dental restorative resins. Recently, these have been applied in oral surgery as bonding agents for fixation of orthodontic bands and brackets for intermaxillary fixation without circumdental wiring (Booth, 1976; Iranpour, 1974). Advantages are said to be the lack of injury to the gingival tissues and periodontium and minimal patient discomfort.

Biologically derived materials

Bone

As the subject of bone grafting is extensively covered elsewhere in this text, no attempt has been made to provide additional treatment of this topic here. However, there are two aspects of the use of bone as a biomaterial that merit discussion in this section. First, the behavior of bone is that of a multiphase composite material, and its structure and properties should be understood by the oral and maxillofacial surgeon. Second, since alloplastic trays and microporous filters for shaping and confining the bone are sometimes used in grafting procedures, some aspects of their use should also be considered.

Biomechanical aspects of bone. Bone is a complex multiphase material containing inorganic as well as organic components. Collagen, the protein comprising the major portion of the extracellular matrix of bone, is present in the form of long, highly oriented fibers. Other extracellular components are mainly protein mucopolysaccharides and lipids. The continuous fibers of collagen are densely packed and are infused with bone mineral, which consists of small crystals of hydroxyapatite and amorphous calcium phosphate. The detailed structure and biomechanical properties of bone have been reviewed in detail by Katz and Mow (1973).

Although the mechanical properties of human long bones have been extensively measured and analyzed (Curry, 1970; Reilly and Burstein, 1974), mandibular bone has not received adequate attention. Reasonable values that are representative for long-bone cortex are an elastic modulus of about 2.2×10^6 psi (15 GN/m^2) and an ultimate tensile strength of 18,900 psi (130 MN/m^2). The elastic modulus and ultimate tensile strength of mandibular alveolar bone are often considered to approximate those of human cranial bone, 1.5×10^6 psi (12.3 GN/m^2) and 11,500 psi (79 MN/m^2), respectively (measured by McElhaney et al., 1970). It is important to note that bone, as well as most other biologic materials, exhibits viscoelastic deformation behavior; that is, the mechanical properties depend on the rate of loading. Both the elastic modulus and the strength will increase with increasing rates of deformation.

An exciting and potentially important area of interest relates to the interrelationship between mechanical deformation and bioelectrical phenomena in bone (Bassett, 1968; Spadaro, 1977). When electrodes are implanted in bone with a small direct current of 3 to 4 μA established for 21 days, increased osteogenesis is observed around the cathode (Bassett, Pawluk, and Becker, 1964). Such electrical enhancement of bone healing in man has been demonstrated in long bones (Becker, Spadaro, and Marino, 1977; Lavine et al., 1972) and in the healing of jaw fractures (Masuriek and Eriksson, 1977). Since techniques have recently been developed for the noninvasive application of pulsed electronic fields to accelerate bone repair (Bassett, Pawluk, and Pilla, 1974), it appears that this may become a clinically applicable technique in the treatment of fractures and other pathologic conditions involving osteogenesis. It is intriguing to note that the electromagnetic fields used in the above studies produce voltages in the bone of a magnitude equivalent to that produced by physiologic deformation.

Adjuncts in bone grafting. The technique of autogenous particulate cancellous bone and marrow grafting, developed by Boyne and others, uses an alloplastic mesh implant to contain and shape the graft. A tissue-compatible membrane filter further contains the graft, while inhibiting the growth of fibrous tissue between the individual graft particles (Boyne, 1974a). The technique has been used for a wide variety of applications, including reconstruction of segmental mandibular defects (Boyne, 1969, 1970; Leake, 1974a,b; Marble et al., 1970; Nahum and Boyne, 1972), treatment of fracture nonunions (Boyne, 1974a), and alveolar ridge augmentation (Boyne, 1974b; Leake, 1974a).

While some investigators have used a metal mesh tray for graft stabilization (Boyne, 1969, 1970; Marble et al., 1970; Nahum and Boyne, 1972), others have recently utilized both Dacron supported (Leake, 1974a,b; Leake and Habal, 1975) and unsupported polyether urethane elastomer (Rappoport and Leake, 1973). The polymer implant is said to provide for more esthetic bone contours. An additional advantage in certain situations may be its radiolucency.

Nylon-backed cellulose acetate filter material (Millipore) has been used in bone grafting as a lining material within the trays. A pore size of approximately 0.5 μm (Marble et al., 1970) assures entrapment of all cells with osteogenic potential, prevents ingress of fibrous tissue to the graft site from the surrounding soft-tissues and allows ample nutrition of the graft by extracellular fluid exchange. However, some question as to the importance of using such a filter in these grafts has recently been raised (White et al., 1974).

Nonosseous biologic implants

Collagen. Collagen is the major connective tissue protein in animals, comprising approximately 25% of the total body protein in vertebrates. Complete degradation of collagen at controlled rates may be obtained in biologic environments. While a wide variety of studies have utilized collagen in extracorporeal situations, such as in dialysis membranes or as corneal grafts, studies using collagen as a reconstructive bioma-terial have been limited. An excellent review of the structure, properties, and clinical applications of collagen has been published (Chvapil, Kronenthal, and Van Winkle, 1973). Collagen sponges and gels have been found to be especially valuable in bone healing (Cucin et al., 1972). The extent of aldehyde cross-link-ing achieved by pretreatment controls the rate of degradation (White et al., 1973).

Denatured animal collagen in sponge form (Gelfoam) has been advocated for obliteration of bone cavities created, for example, by removal of mandibular cysts. Thoma (1969) has discussed in detail the techniques for utilization of this material. The use of Gelfoam instead of auto-genous bone eliminates the need for an additional operation required for har-vesting of graft material. If impregnated with blood, it is said to be osteogenic, and ossification occurs throughout the mesh. Postoperative bleeding is effec-tively controlled, and antibiotics may be added. The use of synthetic absorbable sponges in this application is not recom-mended.

It has been suggested that collagen might be used as a biodegradable matrix for containing particulate cancellous bone and marrow grafts for mandibular reconstruction without resorting to either permanent alloplasts or two-stage pro-cedures (Kramer, 1971; Riley and Leake, 1976).

Fibrin. Recently, interest has been generated in the use of heat-treated anti-genically modified bovine fibrin in tissue reconstruction. As with collagen, degra-dation rates may be altered by variations in aldehyde cross-linking, and the break-down products are easily metabolized (Torok et al., 1975) while the implant site is invaded by host tissue. Extraction sites filled with a coagulum of fibrin powder, autogenous blood, thrombin, and antibi-otics in anticoagulated patients show immediate hemostasis and excellent healing (Kovacs, Toth, and Kerenyi, 1976). This technique has been suggest-ed for other mandibular defects such as sites of enucleated cysts.

MATERIALS FOR TISSUE JOINING AND HEMOSTASIS

Techniques such as suturing or the use of clips or tissue cements must hold the tissues in close approximation until the healing process provides the wound with sufficient strength to withstand stress without mechanical support. Maximal healing will occur if the tissue-joining and hemostatic techniques evoke mini-mal local tissue reaction during the time in contact with the tissues.

Sutures

Available materials

Sutures may be temporary (absorbable) or permanent unless intentionally re-moved from the tissues (nonabsorbable). The specific available materials are out-lined in Table 8-6. Absorbable sutures are degraded in vivo by enzymatic and phagocytic mechanisms and/or hydroly-sis and thus over time diminish in strength and disappear from the tis-sues.

The speed of absorption of a suture is roughly proportional to the vascularity of the surrounding tissues. Thus absorption of plain surgical gut (sheep intestinal submucosa or beef intestinal serosa) placed subcutaneously is more rapid than that approximating fascia.

Phagocytic degradation, such as occurs

Table 8-6. Sutures available for oral and maxillofacial surgery

Biologically derived materials	Synthetic materials
Absorbable	
Plain surgical gut (catgut)	Polyglycolic acid (Dexon*)
Chromic catgut	Polyglactin 910 (Vicryl†)
Nonabsorbable	
Silk	Nylon‡
Cotton	Dacron‡ (Mersilene†)
	Polypropylene (Prolene†)
	Stainless steel
	Tantalum
	Titanium

Trademarks: Suture materials.
*Davis & Geck, American Cyanamid Co., Pearl River, N.Y.
†Ethicon, Inc., Somerville, N.J.
‡DuPont, Wilmington, Del.

with the biologically derived absorbable sutures (plain surgical gut, chromic catgut, and collagen) is usually accompanied by considerable tissue reaction. The formation of exudative fluids and their dissection along tissue planes may delay the healing process and possibly potentiate infection. The newer synthetic absorbable suture materials, polyglycolic acid (Dexon) and polyglactin 910 (Vicryl), appear to be degraded primarily by hydrolytic mechanisms (Craig et al., 1975), and there is minimal cellular inflammatory reaction. The subject of synthetic absorbable sutures has recently been reviewed (Laufman and Rubel, 1977).

Nonabsorbable suture materials may be natural products, such as silk or cotton, synthetic polymers, such as nylon, polypropylene, or Dacron polyester, or metallic materials, such as stainless steel, tantalum, or titanium.

Tissue response to sutures

The initial histologic response to sutures, as with other implanted materials, is primarily of an acute inflammatory nature, and is caused by the passage of the needle, and less so by the presence of a foreign body (Van Winkle and Hastings, 1972). Subsequent to the phase of generalized aseptic inflammation, plain surgical gut elicits an intense response with macrophages predominating and the return of polymorphonuclear cells. Chromic catgut causes a more moderate reaction. The nonabsorbable sutures ultimately show a mild, relatively acellular, histologic response. Differences in the amount of inflammation caused by the various nonabsorbable sutures are usually not significant, although the natural fibers such as cotton and silk generally induce slightly more reaction than the synthetics (Postlethwait, Willigan, and Ulin, 1975; Postlethwait et al., 1959).

Development of surgical infections is greatly enhanced by the presence of a suture in a contaminated wound. A wound closed with sutures requires fewer pathogenic bacteria to cause gross infection than one left open or closed with tape. Potentiation of infection correlates with the degree of inflammatory response to specific suture materials (Edlich et al., 1973).

Eradication of infection in the presence of a persistent foreign body is extremely difficult, so that local infection usually necessitates removal of the sutures. Since percutaneous sutures provide an avenue for bacteria to enter a wound, it is desirable to remove them as early as possible, consistent with adequate healing.

No single material or technique fulfills all the needs of patient and surgeon in all situations. Although there is considerable variation in use, the most frequently employed suture material for closure of intraoral incisions is black braided silk, since intraoral suturing requires a soft material, nonirritating to the tongue. Recently, it has been shown that the newer synthetic absorbable sutures may represent an alternative to not only silk but also to plain and chromic gut in the oral tissues. Human clinical trials have indicated that polyglycolic acid handled as easily as silk suture and evoked a milder tissue response than silk, plain surgical gut, and chromic gut (Lilly, 1972; Wallace, Maxwell, and Cavalaris, 1970).

Tissue adhesives

Surgical adhesives based on the epoxy resins, the polyurethanes, and the cyanoacrylates, as well as other polymer systems have been considered for clinical use (Cooper and Falb,1968). The epoxy resins give high bond strengths but apparently form bonds at a rate too low for practical application. Polyurethanes, produced by reactions between isocyanates and polyesters, although yielding good bond strengths in dry systems, exhibit adverse bonding behavior in the presence of moisture. The rapid setting of the cyanoacrylate systems produced by the polymerization of a monomer, and the minor effects of moisture on this reaction, have made this the most widely investigated system.

Numerous experimental studies have shown that the strength of cyanoacrylate-bonded wounds is not very different from that of sutured wounds (Katz and Woodward, 1970; Sussman et al., 1966). Other studies, however, have indicated long-term superiority of sutured wounds (Houston et al., 1969). Cyanoacrylate polymers degrade completely in vivo through hydrolytic mechanisms, producing formaldehyde and an alkyl cyanoacetate (Leonard, 1968). Removal of breakdown products occurs entirely by normal excretory routes.

The alkyl-2 cyanoacrylates are a series of polymers that are essentially of the same structure except that the nature of the alkyl radical differs: the homologous series being polymethyl-, ethyl-, propyl-, butyl-, isobutyl-, and so on. In general, the lower in the homologous series, the more rapid the rate of resorption. The methyl-2 cyanoacrylate monomer has been shown to cause severe tissue reaction (Woodward et al., 1965,) but the butyl, isobutyl, ethyl, propyl, hexyl, heptyl, and octyl homologues are better in this respect (Bhaskar and Cutright, 1969; Bhaskar, Frisch, and Margetis, 1967). Although the cyanoacrylates are hemostatic and bacteriostatic, use in the oral cavity should be limited to surface applications, since removal from deep tissues does not appear to be complete (Bhaskar and Frisch, 1968).

The subject of tissue adhesives in dentistry, including current clinical applications, has been reviewed by Bhaskar (1972). Advantages of the use of these materials are the immediate cementation of opposing tissue surfaces, immediate permanent hemostasis, and local phagocytosis with minimal inflammation. Bhaskar describes the use of isobutyl cyanoacrylate as a surface dressing after soft tissue surgery of the oral cavity. Healing areas were indistinguishable from those where silk sutures were employed. After dental extractions, the application of cyanoacrylates as a surface dressing on the blood-filled socket prevents secondary inflammation, reduces edema, and promotes healing. Pulp capping with these materials produces immediate hemostasis, subsequent secondary dentin formation, and retained pulpal vitality. Tissue adhesives have also been used as a surgical dressing over free mucosal grafts. Complete desquamation of the dressing occurs with superior healing of the tissues.

Other hemostatic biomaterials

The most widely used of the commercially available materials are gelatin foam (Gelfoam), oxidized cellulose (Oxycel), and oxidized regenerated cellulose (Surgicel). These materials function partially by transmitting pressure against the wound surfaces and partially by providing a scaffold on which the clot can organize.

Gelfoam is manufactured from denatured animal skin collagen. Although having no intrinsic thrombogenic action, Gelfoam can be used as an absorbable carrier for thrombin. Its main activity relates to the large surface area of contact and its weight when saturated with blood (more than 10 times that in the dry state). Premoistening with Ringer's solution or thrombin assures the removal of air from the interstices. The material is absorbed in a relatively short period of time and replaced by connective tissue. Little tissue reaction is seen during removal.

In contrast, the altered cellulose materials, Oxycel and Surgicel, will react chemically with blood to form an artificial clot. They should be applied dry. Degradation occurs over a period of a few weeks. In contaminated wounds the material should be removed by forceps or gentle irrigation prior to closure. Moreover, whenever possible, removal is also recommended in noninfected cases as soon as bleeding is controlled. Although they are nontoxic and relatively inert, these materials are to be used judiciously since they are excellent culture media and require phagocytosis for removal.

REFERENCES

Akeson, W. H., et al. 1975. Quantitative histological evaluation of early fracture healing of cortical bones immobilized by stainless steel and composite plates, Calcif. Tissue Res. 19:27.

Amler, M. H., Johnson, P. L., and Bevelander, G. 1958. Bone regeneration following grafts with polyvinyl plastic sponge, Oral Surg. 11:654.

Bahn, S. L. 1966. Plaster: A bone substitute, Oral Surg. 21:672.

Bardos, D. I. 1974. An evaluation of Ti-6A1-4V alloy

for orthopedic application, J. Bone Joint Surg. **56A:**847.

Barranco, V. P., and Soloman, H. 1972. Eczematous dermatitis from nickel, J. Am. Dent. Assoc. **220:** 1244.

Bassett, C. A. L. 1968. Biologic significance of piezoelectricity, Calcif. Tissue Res. **1:**252.

Bassett, C. A. L., Pawluk, R. J., and Becker, R. O. 1964. Effects of electrical currents in-vivo, Nature **204:**652.

Bassett, C. A. L., Pawluk, R. J., and Pilla, A. A. 1974. Acceleration of fracture repair by electromagnetic fields: a surgically noninvasive method, Ann. N.Y. Acad. Sci. **238:**242.

Bechtol, C. O., Ferguson, A. B., and Laing, P. G. 1959. Metals and engineering in bone and joint surgery, Baltimore, The Williams & Wilkins Co.

Becker, R. O., Spadaro, J. A., and Marino, A. A. 1977. Clinical experiences with low intensity direct current stimulation of bone growth, Clin. Orthop. **124:**75.

Belton, D., et al. 1973. An evaluation of VC 1800 as a soft tissue replacement material, Biomater. Med. Devices Artif. Organs **1:**563.

Bhaskar, S. N. 1972. Tissue adhesives in dentistry: a review, J. Can. Dent. Assoc. **38:**337.

Bhaskar, S. N., and Cutright, D. E. 1969. Healing of skin wounds with butyl cyanoacrylate; adhesives in would healing, J. Dent. Res. **48:**294.

Bhaskar, S. N., and Frisch, J. 1968. Use of cyanoacrylate adhesives in dentistry, J. Am. Dent. Assoc. **77:**831.

Bhaskar, S. N., Frisch, J., and Margetis, P. M. 1967. Tissue response of rat tongue to hexyl, heptyl, and octyl cyanoacrylate, Oral Surg. **24:**137.

Bischoff, F. 1972. Organic polymer biocompatibility and toxicology, Clin. Chem. **18:**869.

Bokros, J. C., LaGrange, L. D., and Schoen, F. J. 1973. Control of structure of carbon for use in bioengineering, Chem. Phys. Carbon **9:**103.

Booth, D. F. 1976. Use of direct bonding materials for fixation and stabilization in correction of facial deformities, J. Oral Surg. **34:**142.

Boyne, P. J. 1969. Restoration of osseous defects in maxillofacial casualties, J. Am. Dent. Assoc. **78:**767.

Boyne, P. J. 1970. Autogenous cancellous bone and marrow transplants, Clin. Orthop. **73:**199.

Boyne, P. J. 1974a. Osseous grafts and implants in the restoration of large oral defects, J. Periodontol. **45:**378.

Boyne, P. J. 1974b. Restoration of deficient edentulous ridges by bone grafting and the use of subperiosteal metal implants, Int. J. Oral Surg. **3:**378.

Brady, J. M., et al. 1973. Resorption rate, route of elimination, and ultrastructure of the implant site of polylactic acid in the abdominal wall of the rat, J. Biomed. Mater. Res. **7:**155.

Braley, S. A. 1970. The chemistry and properties of the medical grade silicones, J. Macromol. Sci. Chem. **A4:**529.

Brand, K. G., Johnson, K. H., and Buoen, L. C. 1976. Foreign body tumorigenesis, CRC Crit. Rev. Toxicol. **4:**973.

Brettle, J. 1970. A survey of the literature on metallic surgical implants, Injury **2:**26.

Brown, G. C., et al. 1977. Sensitivity to metal as a possible cause of sterile loosening after cobalt-chromium total hip replacement arthroplasty, J. Bone Joint Surg. (Am.) **59A:**164.

Byrne, J. E., Lovasko, J. H., and Laskin, D. M. 1973. Corrosion of metal fracture fixation appliances, J. Oral Surg. **31:**639.

Cahoon, J. R., Chaturevdi, M. C., and Tennese, W. W. 1973. Corrosion studies on metallic implant materials, Med. Instrum. **7:**131.

Calhoun, N. R., Greene, G. W., and Blackledge, G. T. 1965. Plaster: a bone substitute in the mandible of dogs, J. Dent. Res. **44:**940.

Carlisle, E. M. 1970. Silicon: a possible factor in bone calcification, Science **167:**279.

Charnley, J. 1963. Tissue reactions to polytetrafluoroethylene, Lancet **2:**1379.

Charnley, J. 1964. The bonding of prostheses to bone by cement, J. Bone Joint Surg. **46B:**518.

Christie, A. J., Weinberger, K. A., and Dietrich, M. 1977. Silicone lymphadenopathy and synovitis: complications of silicone elastomer finger joint prosthesis, J.A.M.A. **237:**1463.

Chvapil, M., Kronenthal, R. L., and Van Winkle, W. 1973. Medical and surgical applications of collagen, Int. Rev. Connect. Tissue Res. **6:**1.

Clark, A. E., Hench, L. L., and Paschall, H. A. 1976. The influence of surface chemistry on implant interface histology: a theoretical basis for implant materials selection, J. Biomed. Mater. Res. **10:**161.

Cohen, C. A., and Smith, T. C. 1971. The intraoperative hazard of acrylic bone cement, Anesthesiology **35:**547.

Cohen, J., and Wulff, J. 1972. Clinical failure caused by corrosion of a Vitallium plate, J. Bone Joint Surg. **54A:**617.

Coleman, D. L., King, R. N., and Andrade, J. D. 1974. The foreign body reaction: a chronic inflammatory response, J. Biomed. Mater. Res. **8:**199.

Cooper, C. W., and Falb, R. D. 1968. Surgical adhesives, Ann. N.Y. Acad. Sci. **146:**214.

Cowlard, F., and Lewis, J. C. 1967. Vitreous carbon—a new form of carbon, J. Mater. Sci. **2:**507.

Craig, P. H., et al. 1975. A biologic comparison of polyglactin 910 and polyglycolic acid synthetic absorbable sutures, Surg. Gynecol. Obstet. **141:**1.

Cranin, A. N. 1970. Polyvinyl resin sponge implants in rebuilding atrophic ridges: a new surgical approach. In Cranin, A. N., editor: Oral implantology, Springfield, Ill., Charles C Thomas, Publisher, p. 314.

Cucin, R. L., et al. 1972. The effect of reconstituted collagen gels on the healing of experimental bony defects: a preliminary report, J. Surg. Res. **12:**318.

Currey, J. D. 1970. The mechanical properties of bone, Clin. Orthop. **73:**210.

Cutright, D. E., and Hunsuck, E. E. 1971. Tissue reaction to the biodegradable polylactic acid suture, Oral Surg. **31:**134.

Cutright, D. E., Beasley, J. D., and Perez, B. 1971. Histologic comparison of polylactic and polyglycolic acid sutures, Oral Surg. **32:**165.

Cutright, D. E., Hunsuck, E. E., and Beasley, J. D. 1971. Fracture reduction using a biodegradable material, polylactic acid, J. Oral Surg. **29:**383.

Cutright, D. E., et al. 1972. Reaction of bone to tricalcium phosphate ceramic pellets, Oral Surg. **33**:850.

Cutright, D. E., et al. 1974. Degradation rates of polymers and copolymers of polylactic and polyglycolic acids, Oral Surg. **37**:142.

Duke, V. E., and Fisher, D. E. 1972. Hemangioendothelioma of the leg following metallic fixation of the tibia, Cancer **30**:1260.

Dumas, M., and Myers, H. M. 1974. The vitreous carbon tooth root replacement system: a surgical discipline, Int. J. Oral Surg. **3**:273.

Dumbleton, J. H., and Miller, E. H. 1975. Failures of metallic orthopedic implants. In Boyer, H. E., editor: Failure analysis and prevention: metals handbook, ed. 8, vol. 10, ASM, Metals Park, Ohio, p. 571.

Edlich, R. F., et al. 1973. Physical and chemical configuration of sutures in the development of surgical infection, Ann. Surg. **177**:697.

Elek, S. D., and Conen, P. E. 1957. The virulence of Staphylococcus pyogenes for man: a study of the problems of wound infection, Br. J. Exp. Pathol. **38**:573.

Elves, M. W., et al. 1975. Incidence of metal sensitivity in patients with total joint replacement, Br. Med. J. **4**:376.

Escalas, F., et al. 1975. Corrosion resistant, high strength alloy for orthopedic surgical implants: bioassay results, J. Biomed. Mater. Res. **9**:303.

Feith, R. 1975. Side effects of acrylic cement implanted into bone, Acta Orthop. Scand. (Suppl.) **161**:5.

Ferguson, D. J. 1978. Cellular attachment to implanted foreign bodies in relation to tumorigenesis, Cancer Res. **37**:4367.

Fisher, A. A. 1973. Contact dermatitis, Philadelphia, Lea & Febiger.

Fitzgerald, R. H., et al. 1977. Deep sepsis following total hip arthroplasty, J. Bone Joint Surg. **59A**:847.

Fontana, M. G., and Greene, N. D. 1967. Corrosion engineering, New York, McGraw-Hill Book Co.

Frakes, J. T., Brown, S. C., and Kenner, G. H. 1974. Delayed failure and aging of porous alumina in water and physiological media, J. Am. Ceram. Soc. **53**:183.

Getter, L., and Cutright, D. E. 1972. Fracture fixation using biodegradable material, J. Oral Surg. **30**:344.

Getter, L., et al. 1972. Three biodegradable calcium phosphate slurry implants in bone, J. Oral Surg. **30**:363.

Goldberg, S. J., et al. 1976. A fractured mandible, from initial operation to removal of tantalum mesh, Oral Surg. **41**:32.

Goodsell, J. 1968. Tantalum in temporomandibular joint arthroplasty, J. Oral Surg. **16**:517.

Gourley, I. M., and Arnold, J. P. 1960. The experimental replacement of segmental defects in bone with a plaster of Paris epoxy resin mixture, Am. J. Vet. Res. **21**:1119.

Ham, A. W. 1974. Histology, Philadelphia, J. B. Lippincott Co.

Hammer, W. B., et al. 1973. Alveolar ridge augmentation with ceramics, J. Dent. Res. **52**:356.

Harris, W. H. 1977. Total joint replacement, N. Engl. J. Med. **297**:650.

Haubold, A. 1977. Carbon in prosthetics, Ann. N.Y. Acad. Sci. **283**:383.

Hausner, R. J., Schoen, F. J., and Pierson, K. K. 1978. Foreign body reaction to silicone gel in axillary lymph nodes after an augmentation mammaplasty, Plast. Reconstr. Surg. **62**:381.

Hench, L. L. 1973. Ceramics, glasses and composites in medicine, Med. Instrum. **7**:136.

Hench, L. L., and Clark, D. E. 1978. Physical chemistry of glass surfaces, J. Noncryst. Solids **28**:83.

Hench, L. L., and Ethridge, E. C. 1975. Biomaterials: the interface problem. In Brown, J. H. U., and Dickson, J. F., editors: Advances in biomedical engineering, New York, Academic Press, Inc., vol. 5, p. 35.

Hench, L. L., et al. 1975. Interfacial behavior of ceramic implants. In Biomaterials, National Bureau of Standards Special Publication No. 415, p. 19.

Henefer, E. P., McFall, T. A., and Hauschild, D. C. 1968. Acrylate-amide sponge for repair of alveolar bone defects, J. Oral Surg. **26**:577.

Hentrich, R. L., et al. 1971. An evaluation of inert and resorbable ceramics for future clinical orthopedic applications, J. Biomed. Mater. Res. **5**:25.

Hinds, E. C., Homsy, C. A., and Kent, J. N. 1974. Use of a biocompatible interface for binding tissues and prostheses in temporomandibular joint surgery, Oral Surg. **38**:512.

Hinds, E. C., et al. 1963. Use of tantalum trays in mandibular surgery, Plast. Reconstr. Surg. **32**:439.

Hoar, T. P., and Mears, D. C. 1966. Corrosion resistant alloys in chloride solutions: materials for surgical implants, Proc. R. Soc. Lond. (Phys.) **A294**:456.

Hodosh, M. 1959. A new concept in implant dentistry with a preliminary report of four cases, R.I. Med. J. **42**:253.

Hodosh, M., Shklar, G., and Povar, M. 1970. Current status of the polymer tooth concept, Dent. Clin. North Am. **14**:103.

Hodosh, M., Shklar, G., and Povar, M. 1972. The totally self-supporting tooth replica polymer implant, Oral Surg. **33**:1022.

Hollander, R., and Wulff, J. 1975. New technology for mechanical property improvement of cast Co-Cr-Mo-C surgical implants, J. Biomed. Mater. Res. **9**:367.

Homsy, C. A., Kent, J. N., and Hinds, E. C. 1973. Materials for oral implantation: biological and functional criteria, J. Am. Dent. Assoc. **86**:817.

Houston, S., et al. 1969. The effect of α-cyanoacrylate on wound healing, J. Biomed. Mater. Res. **3**:281.

Hughes, A. N., and Jordan, B. A. 1972. Metallurgical observations on some metallic surgical implants which failed in-vivo, J. Biomed. Mater. Res. **6**:33.

Hulbert, S. F., et al. 1970. Potential of ceramic materials as permanently implantable skeletal prostheses, J. Biomed. Mater. Res. **4**:433.

Hunsuck, E. E. 1973. Resorption rate, route of elimination, and ultrastructure of the implant site of polylactic acid in the abdominal wall of the rat, J. Biomed. Mater. Res. **7**:155.

Hylen, J. C. 1971. Durability of prosthetic heart valves, Am. Heart J. **81**:299.

Iranpour, B. 1974. Application of enamel adhesives in oral surgery, Int. J. Oral Surg. **3**:233.

Irby, W. B. 1974. Techniques for application of alloplastic materials in reconstructive or corrective surgery of the jaws. In Irby, W. B., editor. Current advances in oral surgery, St. Louis, The C. V. Mosby Co., p. 155.

Jones, D. A., and Greene, N. D. 1966. Electrochemical measurement at low corrosion rates, Corrosion **22**:198.

Kaae, J. L. 1972. The mechanical properties of glassy and isotropic pyrolytic carbons, J. Biomed. Mater. Res. **6**:279.

Kamerons, J., and Himmelfarb, R. 1975. Treatment of TMJ ankylosis with methyl methacrylate interpositional arthroplasty, J. Oral Surg. **33**:282.

Katz, A. R., and Woodward, S. C. 1970. Test systems for evaluation of cyanoacrylate tissue adhesives, J. Biomed. Mater. Res. **4**:487.

Katz, J. L., and Mow, V. C. 1973. Mechanical and structural criteria for orthopedic implants, Biomater. Med. Devices Artif. Organs **1**:575.

Kenner, G. H., et al. 1975. Biocompatibility and static fatigue behavior of glassy carbon, J. Biomed. Mater. Res. **9**:111.

Kent, J. N., Homsy, C. A., and Hinds, E. C. 1975. Proplast in dental facial reconstruction, Oral Surg. **39**:347.

Klawitter, J. J., and Hulbert, S. F. 1971. Application of porous ceramics for the attachment of load bearing internal orthopedic applications, J. Biomed. Mater. Res. Symp. No. **2**:161.

Klawitter, J. J., et al. 1977. An evaluation of porous alumina ceramic dental implants, J. Dent. Res. **56**:768.

Kovacs, B., Toth, K., and Kerenyi, G. 1976. Post-extraction hemostasis during coumarin anticoagulant therapy with a locally applied coagulation-active substance, Int. J. Oral Surg. **5**:3.

Kramer, H. S. Preliminary studies on the clinical application of antigenically altered collagen as a biomaterial in oral surgery, International Conference on Oral Surgery, Amsterdam, May 1971, p. 223.

Laing, P. G. 1973. Compatibility of biomaterials, Orthop. Clin. North Am. **4**:249.

Laufman, H., and Rubel, T. 1977. Synthetic absorbable sutures, Surg. Gynecol. Obstet. **145**:597.

Lavine, L. S., et al. 1972. Electric enhancement of bone healing, Science **175**:1118.

Leake, D. L. 1974a. An interim report on osseous contour reconstruction using alloplastic materials and particulate bone grafting, Int. J. Oral Surg. **3**:386.

Leake, D. L. 1974b. Dacron/urethane composite: a new biomaterial for osseous contour reconstruction, J. Prosthet. Dent. **32**:182.

Leake, D. L., and Habal, M. B. 1975. Osteoneogenesis: a new method for facial reconstruction, J. Surg. Res. **18**:331.

Lemons, J. E. 1975. Investigations on the response of primate and rabbit marrow, bone, and soft tissues to porous titanium implants, J. Dent. Res. **54**:B166.

Leonard, F. 1968. The N-alkyl alpha cyanoacrylate tissue adhesives, Ann. N.Y. Acad. Sci. **146**:203.

Levin, M. P., Getter, L., and Cutright, D. E. 1975. A comparison of iliac marrow and biodegradable ceramic in periodontal defects, J. Biomed. Mater. Res. **9**:183.

Levin, M. P., et al. 1974. Healing of periodontal defects with ceramic implants, J. Clin. Periodontol. **1**:197.

Levine, S. N. 1968. Survey of biomedical materials and some relevant problems, Ann. N.Y. Acad. Sci. **146**:3.

Lilly, G. E. 1972. Reaction of oral tissues to suture materials, Oral Surg. **33**:152.

Ludwigson, D. C. 1964. Today's prosthetic metals, J. Metals **16**:226.

Marble, H., et al. 1970. Grafts of cancellous bone and marrow for restoration of avulsion defects of the mandible, J. Oral Surg. **28**:138.

Mariano, M., and Spector, W. C. 1974. The formation and properties of macrophage polykaryons (inflammatory giant cells), J. Pathol. **113**:1.

Markle, D. H., Grenoble, D. E., and Melrose, R. J. 1975. Histologic evaluation of vitreous carbon implants in occlusion in dogs, Biomater. Med. Devices Artif. Organs **3**:97.

Masureik, L., and Eriksson, C. 1977. Preliminary evaluation of the effect of small electrical currents on the healing of jaw fractures, Clin. Orthop. **124**:84.

McDougall, A. 1956. Malignant tumor at site of bone plating, J. Bone Joint Surg. **38B**:709.

McElhaney, J. H., et al. 1970. Mechanical properties of cranial bone, J. Biomech. **3**:495.

McKenzie, A. W., Aitken, C. V. E., and Ridsill-Smith, R. 1967. Urticaria after insertion of a Smith-Peterson nail, Br. Med. J. **4**:36.

Meyer, P. R., Lautenschlager, E. P., and Moore, B. K. 1973. On the setting properties of acrylic bone cement, J. Bone Joint Surg. **55A**:149.

Mohammed, H., and Asgar, K. 1973. A new dental superalloy system. II. Mechanical properties, J. Dent. Res. **52**:145.

Mueller, H. J., and Greener, E. H. 1970. Polarization studies of surgical materials in Ringer's solution, J. Biomed. Mater. Res. **4**:29.

Mullison, E. G. 1966. Current status of silicones in plastic surgery, Arch. Otolaryngol. **83**:59.

Nahum, A. M., and Boyne, P. J. 1972. Restoration of the mandible following partial resection, Trans. Am. Acad. Ophthalmol. Otolaryngol. **76**:957.

Normann, S. J., and Schardt, M. 1978. A cancer related macrophage dysfunction in inflamed tissues, J. Reticuloendothel. Soc. **24**:147.

Panush, R. S., and Petty, W. 1978. Inhibition of human lymphocyte responses by methylmethacrylate, Clin. Orthop. **134**:356.

Peltier, L. J., et al. 1957. The use of plaster to fill defects in bone, Ann. Surg. **146**:61.

Petty, W. 1978. The effect of methyl methacrylate on bacterial phagocytosis and killing by human polymorphonuclear leukocytes, J. Bone Joint Surg. **60A**:752.

Petty, W., and Caldwell, J. R. 1977. The effect of methylmethacrylate on complement activity, Clin. Orthop. **128**:354.

Phillips, R. W. 1973. Skinner's science of dental materials, ed. 7, Philadelphia, W. B. Saunders Co.

Polisar, R. S., and Cook, A. W. 1973. Use of polyethylene in cranial implants, J. Prosthet. Dent. **29**:310.

Postlethwait, R. W., Willigan, D. A., and Ulin, A. W. 1975. Human tissue reaction to sutures, Ann. Surg. **181**:144.

Postlethwait, R. W., et al. 1959. Wound healing. II. An evaluation of surgical suture material, Surg. Gynecol. Obstet. **108**:555.

Pugh, J., Jaffe, W. L., and Jaffe, F. 1975. Corrosion failure in stainless steel implants, Surg. Gynecol. Obstet. **141**:199.

Rappoport, M., and Leake, D. L. 1973. Current experiments in polymeric mandibular implants for bone induction, Br. J. Oral Surg. **10**:326.

Reilly, D. T., and Burstein, A. H. 1974. The mechanical properties of cortical bone, J. Bone Joint Surg. **56A**:1001.

Riley, R. W., and Leake, D. L. 1976. Cancellous bone grafting with collagen stents, Int. J. Oral Surg. **5**:29.

Rose, R. M., Schiller, A. L., and Radin, E. L. 1972. Corrosion-accelerated mechanical failure of a Vitallium nail-plate, J. Bone Joint Surg. **54A**:854.

Ross, R. 1969. Wound healing, Sci. Am. **220**:40.

Scales, J. T., Winter, G. D., and Shirley, H. T. 1961. Corrosion of orthopedic implants, Br. Med. J. **2**:478.

Schoen, F. J. 1978. Foreign body/tissue reactions: injected micro-particles. In Proceedings of the 52nd Colloid and Surface Science Symposium, Knoxville, Tenn., June 12-14, p. 63. (abstract.)

Schwartz, A. W., and Erich, J. B. 1960. Experimental study of polyvinyl formal (Ivalon) sponge as a substitute for tissue, Plast. Reconstr. Surg. **25**:1.

Shim, H. S. 1974. The behavior of isotropic pyrolytic carbons under cyclic loading, Biomater. Med. Devices Artif. Organs **2**:55.

Smith, D. C. 1962. Recent developments and prospects in dental polymers, J. Prosthet. Dent. **12**:1066.

Smith, D. C. 1971. Medical and dental applications of cements, J. Biomed. Mater. Res. Symp. No. **1**:189.

Smith, D. C. 1973. Lutes, glues, cements and adhesives in medicine and dentistry, Biomed. Eng. **8**:108.

Smith, D. C. 1974. Materials used for construction and fixation of implants, Oral Sci. Rev. **5**:23.

Smith, L. 1963. Ceramic-plastic material as a bone substitute, Arch. Surg. **87**:653.

Spadaro, J. A. 1977. Electrically stimulated bone growth in animals and man: review of the literature, Clin. Orthop. **122**:325.

Spector, W. G., and Ryan, G. B. 1970. The mononuclear phagocyte in inflammation. In Van Furth, R., ed.: Mononuclear phagocytes, Philadelphia, F. A. Davis Co., p. 219.

Stanley, H. R., et al. 1976. The implantation of natural tooth form bioglasses in baboons, Oral Surg. **42**:339.

Sussman, M. D., et al. 1966. Strength of glued incisional wounds, J. Surg. Res. **6**:228.

Thoma, K. H. 1969. Oral surgery, ed. 5, St. Louis, The C. V. Mosby Co.

Thompson, H. G. 1973. The fate of the pseudosheath pocket around silicone implants, Plast. Reconstr. Surg. **51**:667.

Topazian, R. G., et al. 1971. Use of alloplastics for ridge augmentation, J. Oral Surg. **29**:792.

Torok, B., et al. 1975. Resorption of ^{125}I labeled fibrin Bioplast from the dorsal muscle of rats, Biomater. Med. Devices Artif. Organs **3**:205.

Van Winkle, W., and Hastings, J. C. 1972. Considerations in the choice of suture material for various tissues, Surg. Gynecol. Obstet. **135**:113.

Wallace, W. R., Maxwell, G. R., and Cavalaris, C. J. 1970. Comparison of polyglycolic acid suture to black silk, chromic, and plain catgut in human oral tissues, J. Oral Surg. **28**:739.

Welch, A. 1978. Antibiotics in acrylic bone cement: in-vitro studies, J. Biomed. Mater. Res. **12**:679.

White, M. J., et al. 1973. Collagen films: effect of cross-linking on physical and biological properties, Biomater. Med. Devices Artif. Organs **1**:703.

White, R. D., et al. 1974. Experimental study of cellulose acetate-lined and unlined metal trays in mandibular bone grafting, J. Oral Surg. **32**:897.

Willert, H. G., Ludwig, J., and Semlitsch, M. 1974. Reaction of bone to methacrylate after hip arthroplasty: a long-term gross, light microscopic and scanning microscopic study, J. Bone Joint Surg. **56A**:1368.

Williams, D. F., and Meachim, G. 1974. A combined metallurgical and histological study of tissue-prosthesis interactions in orthopedic patients, J. Biomed. Mater. Res. Symp. No. **5**:1.

Williams, D. F. and Roaf, R. 1973. Implants in surgery, London, W. B. Saunders Co., Ltd.

Wong, K. C., et al. 1977. Cardiovascular effects of total hip placement in man: with observations on the effects of methylmethacrylate on the isolated rabbit heart, Clin. Pharmacol. Ther. **21**:709.

Woo, S. L-Y., et al. 1974. Potential applications of graphite fiber and methyl methacrylate resin composites as internal fixation plates, J. Biomed. Mater. Res. **8**:321.

Wood, N. K., Kaminski, E. J., and Oglesby, R. J. 1970. The significance of implant shape in experimental testing of biological materials: disc vs. rod, J. Biomed. Mater. Res. **4**:1.

Woodward, S. C., et al. 1965. Histotoxicity of cyanoacrylate tissue adhesives in the rat, Ann. Surg. **162**:113.

Worley, R. D. 1973. The experimental use of poly (methyl methacrylate) implants in mandibular defects, J. Oral Surg. **31**:170.

Yablon, I. G. 1976. The effect of methyl methacrylate on fracture healing, Clin. Orthop. **114**:358.

Yaman, P., et al. 1973. Self-setting acrylic as an immobilizing agent in mandibular fractures: a histologic study, Oral Surg. **36**:459.

Younkin, C. N. 1974. Multiphase MP35N alloy for medical implants, J. Biomed. Mater. Res. Symp. No. **5**:219.

Zarb, G. A., Melcher, A. H., and Smith, D. C. 1972. Cementation of dental implants: rationale and preliminary observations, J. Can. Dent. Assoc. **38**:328.

CHAPTER 9

General care of the surgical patient

R. Bruce Donoff

The oral and maxillofacial surgeon must know both the physical and emotional status of his patient; this information is as significant for apparently healthy patients undergoing simple exodontia with local anesthesia as it is for hospitalized and medically compromised patients with complex surgical problems. Careful history taking is the method by which crucial data are gathered for evaluation. For patients with a serious medical illness who may have a poor understanding of their problems, obtaining a list of medications being taken is often very helpful. An index of suspicion based on sound medical knowledge is of greatest importance in patient evaluation. Appropriate consultation with and participation by the patient's physician may be necessary in some situations. For each patient, the oral and maxillofacial surgeon must ask himself two basic questions: (1) What is the precise nature of the patient's disease? (2) What features of his general condition are likely to influence the course of the surgical procedure? More extensive history and physical examination, additional laboratory studies, and further consultations are required when the answers to these questions are incomplete.

PREOPERATIVE EVALUATION

Preoperative evaluation is the process of defining those features of a patient's general condition that may affect the course of surgery adversely. These include extremes of age, contracted blood volume, debilitation and malnutrition, dehydration and electrolyte imbalance, decreased cardiac reserve, diminished pulmonary reserve, renal insufficiency, hepatic insufficiency, endocrine dysfunction, infection, and coagulation defects.

Renal status

The clinical manifestations of renal insufficiency are changes in hydration, electrolyte concentration, acid-base balance, and calcium and phosphorus levels. Patients with inadequate renal function represent increased risk for surgical procedures primarily when general anesthesia is required or when oral intake will be affected. Patients with occult obstructive uropathy may develop signs of urinary retention postoperatively; patients with chronic infection are prone to development of sepsis. Severe fluid and electrolyte imbalance may be present.

It is axiomatic that anyone suspected of having renal disease or insufficiency should be evaluated to provide a precise diagnosis of the urinary tract disorder. In general, the patient with renal disease is aware of his malady. A random urinalysis for specific gravity, pH, glucose, protein, acetone, occult blood, bacteria, and casts is an excellent screening method in the relatively young individual with no personal or family history of renal disease or in the patient with unsuspected disease.

The specific gravity should be above 1.015 and the pH 6 or less, reflecting the ability of the kidneys to concentrate urine and to excrete acid. If the specific gravity is low, the first voided morning specimen should be checked; it should have a specific gravity above 1.020. Measurement of serum creatinine or the blood urea nitrogen (BUN) should be carried out if the specific gravity is low or if the urine is alkaline or contains protein, blood cells, or casts. The BUN, however, must be evaluated with care; a high protein diet, massive erythrocyte destruction, or blood in the gastrointestinal tract may cause its elevation. The serum creatinine, which is not subject to variations caused by changes in protein intake, is therefore a more reliable measure of renal function in surgical patients.

Cardiac status

The most frequent high-risk situation encountered by the oral and maxillofacial surgeon is that of treating a patient, either ambulatory or hospitalized, with decreased cardiac reserve. In the ambulatory situation, the surgeon must choose between local anesthesia, local anesthesia with sedation, or general anesthesia. Cardiac impairment, per se, is not a contraindication to a properly administered general anesthetic. Similarly, for the hospitalized patient, a well-regulated general anesthesia may be more appropriate than multiple manipulations with local anesthesia. The oral and maxillofacial surgeon must have the ability to make sound clinical judgments based on medical knowledge and, where indicated, on the results of consultation with the patient's physician. Patients with recent myocardial infarction, severe angina pectoris, congestive heart failure, uncontrolled cardiac arrhythmia, and extensive aortic valvular disease constitute especially bad surgical risks.

A careful history and physical examination are the most important means for preoperative assessment of a patient's cardiac status. A past history of rheumatic fever signals potential valvular disease. Myocardial or coronary artery disease is strongly suggested by a past or current history of the use of digitalis, diuretics, nitroglycerin, or propranolol, or complaints of such symptoms as decreased exercise tolerance, progressive shortness of breath, dyspnea on exertion, orthopnea, peripheral edema, chest pain, episodes of syncope, or palpitations. Historic data that raise suspicion of cardiac illness in an allegedly healthy patient must be followed by proper physical examination. For patients over 40 years of age or in patients of any age with suspected heart disease, screening should involve a routine chest radiograph and an electrocardiogram. The chest film can provide evidence of cardiac enlargement, pulmonary congestion, and valvular heart disease; the electrocardiogram can furnish information on heart rate, rhythm, premature beats, conduction blocks, arrhythmias, ischemic change patterns, cardiomegaly, myocardial infarction, electrolyte abnormalities, and digitalis effects. Management of patients with diminished cardiac reserve must begin with determination of their capacity to tolerate the indicated oral surgery, whether major or minor. Prophylactic methods to prevent subacute bacterial endocarditis in patients with valvular heart disease must be employed (see p. 330). Management of patients with coronary artery disease is discussed on p. 332.

Pulmonary status

The patient with decreased pulmonary reserve may present a significant surgical risk. The predominant sign of respiratory insufficiency is dyspnea on exertion. History of cigarette smoking, tuberculosis, chronic bronchitis, asthma, or emphysema must be noted. Physical signs include increased anteroposterior chest diameter, clubbing, of the fingers, and cyanosis. The most important point of the oral and maxillofacial surgeon's evaluation is to ascertain restricted ventilation that may impair the patient's ability to tolerate general anesthesia. Although there are several simple tests of pulmonary function — the cough test to identify patients with chronic bronchitis and the match test to identify those with diminished vital capacity — nothing can replace the history and physical examination in evaluation of these patients. Routine chest radiographs may show evidence of parenchymal lung disease, emphysema, or pulmonary fibrosis. It is imperative to identify chronic respiratory insufficiency in combination with an acute respiratory infection. Generally, the patient with chronic obstructive pulmonary disease should be considered a poor risk for outpatient general anesthesia. As a group, patients with asthma, bronchitis, and chronic restrictive or obstructive pulmonary disease are best managed with local anesthesia for outpatient procedures.

The hospitalized patient with chronic or productive cough, but normal pulmonary function tests, should be prepared for elective general anesthesia in ways that can reduce the postoperative complications of atelectasis and infection. Use of tobacco and other respiratory tract irritants should be stopped. Preoperatively, intermittent positive pressure devices or blow bottles can be used and deep breathing and coughing exercises taught. The use of iodides or guaiacol derivatives, together with adequate hydration, will help liquify tracheobronchial secretions and facilitate their removal. Bronchodilators such as aminophylline often cause tachycardia and should be used with some caution; theophylline (Elixophyllin) has less cardiac effect. After a sputum specimen has been obtained for culture and antibiotic sensitivity testing, patients with chronic purulent sputa or those with asthma secondary to chronic bronchitis may benefit from a preoperative course of antibiotics. The patient with asthma may undergo a general anesthetic after careful preparation. Clinical sense dictates that generous use be made of consultants in such situations.

SPECIFIC MANAGEMENT PROBLEMS
Patients with diabetes

Most well-controlled patients with diabetes mellitus present no great management problem for either ambulatory or inpatient oral and maxillofacial surgery, although established odontogenic infection often requires more aggressive care in the diabetic and may also alter glucose tolerance. It is the necessary modifications in food and fluid intake during operative periods that raise significant management questions.

The oral and maxillofacial surgeon should have little difficulty in evaluating the state of a patient's diabetes, although consultation with the physician should also be sought. It is important to know whether onset was juvenile or adult; whether control is by diet alone, oral hypoglycemic drugs, single-dose long-acting insulin, or long-acting and short-acting insulin; whether the patient has episodes of hypoglycemia manifested as insulin shock; whether the patient has ever been in diabetic coma; whether the patient tests his urine regularly and with what results; and whether any complications of diabetes are present.

It is a basic rule that the diabetic on insulin must have carbohydrate to cover the insulin. Since the use of general anesthesia will change the patient's balance, albeit briefly, it will require alterations in his management. The stress of anesthesia causes increased glucose intolerance. Since hypoglycemia is a more hazardous condition than hyperglycemia, all methods of management, for either the ambulatory or the hospitalized patient, are promulgated on attempts to prevent hypoglycemia. The patient having a single extraction with local anesthesia should be treated soon after mealtime, preferably in the morning, regardless of the method by which his diabetes is controlled. Some source of glucose must be available to treat hypoglycemia. Ambulatory patients undergoing a general anesthetic and requested not to eat or drink prior to the procedure may require the following modifications: If they are taking oral hypoglycemics twice a day, the prior evening's dose as well as the morning dose is omitted. They are treated early in the morning. As soon as oral intake is reestablished, they should eat and take their morning dose of medication and thereafter return to their normal regimen. Patients taking a single morning dose of long-acting insulin may take half their dose before coming to the office even though they have not eaten. After the procedure, as soon as adequate oral intake is reestablished, the remaining daily dose of insulin should be taken. Patients taking both long-acting and regular insulin may halve each in similar fashion. Patients taking multiple doses of different types of insulin usually represent less well-controlled patients and, although the basic management decisions apply, consultation with the physician is a must. Hospitalization may be indicated.

Hospitalization of the oral surgical patient with diabetes mellitus permits closer monitoring of blood glucose levels and the provision of continuous glucose via intravenous infusion. For the adequately controlled diabetic, whose control is by diet alone or NPH or lente insulin, surgery should be done early in the day. Intravenous 5% or 10% glucose in water is administered and half the usual dose of long-acting insulin is given at the time the infusion is begun. On completion of the procedure, the remaining half of the insulin is given; glucose infusion is continued. Oral fluids and foods are given as soon as the patient's condition permits, and urine sugar and ketones are checked every 4 hours. Strict control of hyperglycemia and glucosuria is not necessary, although the use of a "sliding scale" for determining insulin administration is beneficial. Thus, 4+ or 3+ glucosuria would be covered by an additional 10 or 5 units of crystalline or short-acting insulin, respectively. Additional insulin is added for the presence of ketosis. The well-controlled diabetic usually returns to his preoperative regimen rather quickly unless there is marked limitation of oral intake, as might occur with intermaxillary fixation. The sliding scale regimen is continued in such cases.

There is no reason other than an emergency to operate on a poorly controlled diabetic. Preoperative regulation should be obtained first. The difficulties and subtleties of each individual's diabetes, in terms of renal threshold and of peculiarities of insulin sensitivity, make medical consultation very important. Even in the emergency situation, some history is usually obtainable. Again, the use of an intravenous glucose infusion and sliding-scale insulin coverage is recommended. (See also Chapter 16.)

Patients taking anticoagulants

Systemic anticoagulation is used in a variety of cardiovascular diseases. Patients receive therapeutic systemic anticoagulants for atrial fibrillation with mitral stenosis, phlebitis with risk of thromboembolism, thrombotic cerebral vascular accidents, transient ischemic attacks, prosthetic heart valves, and sometimes following a myocardial infarction complicated by heart failure. Agents used include heparin (antithrombin in action; used for rapid anticoagulation and measured by the partial thromboplastin time); warfarin sodium (Coumadin) (a depressant of synthesis of factors II, VII, IX, and X; used for long-term anticoagulation and measured by the prothrombin time); and aspirin (used for long-term anticoagulation and measured by the clotting time).

The majority of ambulatory patients requiring oral surgery may need little or no adjustment in their anticoagulation regimen. For example, a patient who takes 5 mg of warfarin sodium daily and whose prothrombin time (PT) is 19 seconds with a control of 12 seconds usually requires no adjustment in anticoagulation for a simple, single extraction. Suturing, pressure packs, and attention to measures that will protect the clot usually give satisfactory results. However, the alteration of an anticoagulation regimen may become necessary with increased magnitude of surgery or if the medical risk would be substantially increased by the decreased level of coagulation. There is little evidence to contraindicate the reduction in PT from 19 to 15 seconds by omission of one or two doses of warfarin sodium in most patients requiring oral surgery in the office. This is not applicable, however, in the patient with phlebitis and recent pulmonary emboli; it applies to the patient with a prosthetic heart valve or stroke who has been on long-term anticoagulation. The rebound phenomenon when anticoagulation is withdrawn does not appear to have clinical significance.

In patients where the risk of decreased anticoagulation may be significant and where surgery is necessary, hospitalization should be considered. Rapid, controllable anticoagulation with heparin or low molecular weight dextran can be used in this setting.

Patients susceptible to endocarditis

There is general agreement that the following patients should receive prophylactic antibiotics: (1) patients with heart murmur of rheumatic or calcific etiology, including those with click murmur syndrome; (2) patients with graft-repaired atrial and ventricular septal defects; (3) all patients with congenital defects except repaired patent ductus arteriosus and nongraft-repaired atrial septal defects; and (4) patients with prosthetic heart valves (Table 9-1). There is no evidence to suggest that patients who have had coronary artery bypass graft procedures require prophylaxis against endocarditis.

Although a number of acceptable protocols exist, basic treatment preferably includes administration of a bactericidal antibiotic, so that adequate levels are present at the time of bacteremia, and careful avoidance of a premature administration that might lead to development of resistant organisms. The oral flora may be changed within 48 hours of penicillin prophylaxis; thus it is advisable to start antibiotics on the day of surgery rather than the day before an extraction. In the nonallergic patient penicillin is the drug of choice. Table 9-1 contains the recommended regimens of the American Heart Association for prophylaxis prior to surgery, and Table 9-2 provides the details of these regimens.

Daily, low doses of penicillin, for example, 400,000 U per day by mouth, are often taken to prevent a recurrence of rheumatic fever. The streptococci suppressed by this dose of penicillin, which probably does not alter the oral flora significantly, cause rheumatic fever but not systemic bacterial endocarditis. Thus increased doses of penicillin have a major place in the prophylactic management of this group of patients, who should be treated by the same regimen as anyone else who is at risk for systemic bacterial endocarditis.

The ambulatory patient with a prosthetic heart valve replacement is now fairly common. It is appropriate to consider if prophylaxis for endocarditis in this group differs from the usual regimen. Unfortunately, the situation is unclear. There is some evidence that staphylococcal endocarditis is more common than streptococcal endocarditis in patients with a prosthetic valve. Although an oral source of these bacteria has not been es-

Table 9-1. Prophylaxis for dental and surgical procedures of the upper respiratory tract*

	All dental procedures that are likely to result in gingival bleeding†	Surgery or instrumentation of the respiratory tract‡
Most congenital heart disease;§ rheumatic or other acquired valvular heart disease; idiopathic hypertrophic subaortic stenosis; mitral valve prolapse syndrome with mitral insufficiency‖	Regimen A or B	Regimen A or B
Prosthetic heart valves¶	Regimen B	Regimen B

*From American Heart Association. 1977. Circulation **56**:139A. By permission of the American Heart Association, Inc.
†Does not include shedding of deciduous teeth; does not include simple adjustment of orthodontic appliances.
‡Tonsillectomy, adenoidectomy, bronchoscopy, and other surgical procedures of the upper respiratory tract involving disruption of the respiratory mucosa.
§Ventricular septal defect, tetralogy of Fallot, aortic stenosis, pulmonic stenosis, complex cyanotic heart disease, patent ductus arteriosus, or systemic to pulmonary artery shunts. Does *not* include uncomplicated secundum atrial septal defect.
‖Although cases of infective endocarditis in patients with mitral valve prolapse syndrome have been documented, the incidence appears to be relatively low and the necessity for prophylaxis in all of these patients has not yet been established.
¶Some patients with a prosthetic heart valve in whom a high level of oral health is being maintained may be offered oral antibiotic prophylaxis for routine dental procedures except the following: parenteral antibiotics are recommended for patients with prosthetic valves who require extensive dental procedures, especially extractions, or oral or gingival surgical procedures.

tablished, some cardiologists suggest that in patients undergoing oral surgery, in addition to penicillin prophylaxis, intramuscular oxacillin or oral cloxacillin be used. Because of its effectiveness against staphylococci, a suitable single drug regimen would be erythromycin, 500 mg q.i.d., the day before surgery, the day of surgery, and the day after surgery. The American Heart Association recommends that streptomycin be used with penicillin for prophylaxis of patients with prosthetic heart valves in place. In the allergic patient intravenous vancomycin is recommended. These suggestions are based on a rabbit model of endocarditis and the possibility of staphylococcal endocarditis in these patients. It is obvious that recommendations vary so greatly that the oral and maxillofacial surgeon must make this decision in consultation with the patient's cardiologist.

Table 9-2. Antibiotic prophylaxis*

Regimen A (penicillin)	Regimen B (penicillin plus streptomycin)
Parenteral-oral combined	**Parenteral-oral combined**
Adults: Aqueous crystalline penicillin G (1,000,000 units intramuscularly) mixed with procaine penicillin G (600,000 units intramuscularly). Give 30 minutes-1 hour prior to procedure, then give penicillin V (formerly called phenoxymethyl penicillin), 500 mg orally, every 6 hours for 8 doses.†	Adults: Aqueous crystalline penicillin G (1,000,000 units intramuscularly) mixed with procaine penicillin G (600,000 units intramuscularly) plus streptomycin (1 gm intramuscularly). Give 30 minutes-1 hour prior to the procedure, then penicillin V 500 mg orally every 6 hours for 8 doses.†
Children:‡ Aqueous crystalline penicillin G (30,000 units/kg intramuscularly) mixed with procaine penicillin G (600,000 units intramuscularly). Timing of doses for children is the same as for adults. For children less than 60 pounds, the dose of penicillin V is 250 mg orally every 6 hours for 8 doses.†	Children:‡ Aqueous crystalline penicillin G (30,000 units/kg intramuscularly) mixed with procaine penicillin G (600,000 units intramuscularly) plus streptomycin (20 mg/kg intramuscularly). Timing of doses for children is the same as for adults. For children less than 60 pounds, the recommended oral dose of penicillin V is 250 mg every 6 hours for 8 doses.†
Oral§	
Adults: Penicillin V (2.0 gm orally 30 minutes-1 hour prior to the procedure, then 500 mg orally every 6 hours for 8 doses.)†	*For patients allergic to penicillin:*
Children:‡ Penicillin V (2.0 gm orally 30 minutes-1 hour prior to procedure, then 500 mg orally every 6 hours for 8 doses.† For children less than 60 pounds, use 1.0 gm orally 30 minutes-1 hour prior to the procedure, then 250 mg orally every 6 hours for 8 doses.)†	Adults: Vancomycin (1 gm intravenously over 30 minutes to 1 hour). Start initial vancomycin infusion ½-1 hour prior to procedure; then erythromycin, 500 mg orally, every 6 hours for 8 doses.†
For patients allergic to penicillin:	Children:‡ Vancomycin (20 mg/kg intravenously over 30 minutes-1 hour.)‖ Timing of doses for children is same as for adults.
Use either vancomycin (see Regimen B) or use:	Erythromycin dose is 10 mg/kg every 6 hour for 8 doses.†
Adults: Erythromycin (1.0 gm orally 1½-2 hours prior to the procedure, then 500 mg orally every 6 hours for 8 doses.)	
Children: Erythromycin (20 mg/kg orally 1½-2 hours prior to the procedure, then 10 mg/kg every 6 hours for 8 doses.)	

*From American Heart Association. 1977. Circulation **56**:139A. By permission of the American Heart Association, Inc.
†In unusual circumstances or in the case of delayed healing, it may be prudent to provide additional doses of antibiotics, even though available data suggest that bacteremia rarely persists longer than 15 minutes after the procedure. The physician or dentist may also choose to use the parenteral route of administration for all of the doses in selected situations.
‡Doses for children should not exceed recommendations for adults for a single dose or for a 24-hour period.
§In those patients receiving continuous oral penicillin for secondary prevention of rheumatic fever, alpha-hemolytic streptococci, which are relatively resistant to penicillin, are occasionally found in the oral cavity. While it is likely that the doses of penicillin recommended in regimen A are sufficient to control these organisms, the physician or dentist may choose one of the suggestions in regimen B or oral erythromycin.
‖For vancomycin the total dose for children should not exceed 44 mg/kg/24 hours.

Patients with coronary artery disease

Certain management questions exist for the oral and maxillofacial surgeon treating patients with coronary artery disease. Although major elective procedures are not undertaken in these high-risk patients, they nevertheless often require minor and even major oral and maxillofacial surgery. History of myocardial infarction carries an increased morbidity and mortality in patients undergoing general anesthesia; if surgery is within 3 weeks of a fresh myocardial infarction, 100% of these patients will extend their infarct and 25% will die of their disease. In contrast, 6 months after a myocardial infarct, there is no difference in mortality experience with general anesthesia, provided there is either no angina or only minimal exertional angina and no congestive heart failure. The situation is ambiguous during the 6 months following infarction; one would not routinely undertake a full-mouth extraction under general anesthesia at 3 months, although an extraction for the relief of pain and anxiety could be carried out with proper precautions.

In general, current management of the patient with coronary artery disease has changed. Hypertension and tachyarrhythmias, which increase cardiac work, are thought to be more detrimental in this group of patients than are hypotension and bradycardia. Consequently, the relief of anxiety, either by preoperative oral or intravenous sedation techniques, has a significant place in management. In some situations, a patient with moderate angina pectoris requiring a full mouth extraction may be placed under less risk with a well-controlled general anesthetic than with local anesthesia. The oral and maxillofacial surgeon is frequently in the best position to accurately judge the extent of the stress. If this information is conveyed to the physician, joint decisions in the patient's best interests can be made.

Specific decisions regarding medications may often arise. All antiarrhythmic drugs are cardiac depressants, as are the arrhythmias themselves. However, antiarrhythmic drugs do not arbitrarily require discontinuation. In the cardiac patient taking digitalis, diuretics, and potassium supplements who is judged to be in sufficient condition to tolerate a general anesthetic, the lack of a single dose of the medications is not clinically significant when he is requested not to take food or liquids prior to the procedure.

Electrolytes must be checked prior to general anesthesia; hypokalemia resulting from diuretic action is potentially lethal. Discontinuation of propranolol remains controversial. Although there is no conclusive evidence to suggest that it is detrimental to a patient undergoing general anesthesia, there are data now available suggesting a rebound in coronary insufficiency following abrupt withdrawal of propranolol in the patient with angina pectoris.

Patients taking steroids

A patient's ability to withstand stress depends on the ability of the adrenal glands to adequately increase the output of hydrocortisone. Although the area is clouded in anecdotal tradition, certain principles remain significant. The normal adrenal cortices produce about 20 mg of hydrocortisone daily. A patient receiving steroids, or who has received steroids for 2 or more weeks within the last 6 to 12 months, must be considered to have a variable degree of functional adrenocortical suppression. These patients will need a source of exogenous glucocorticoid during stressful periods; this prevents hypoglycemia, hypotension, and shock. A basic tenet of practice is that short-term excess of glucocorticoids is relatively harmless, whereas short-term deficiency during stress can be fatal. The review of this subject by Axelrod (1976) is highly recommended.

The following schedule is widely used and is designed to provide adequate steroid during the stress of operation and recovery (see also Chapter 11). Because there is some evidence that intramuscular cortisone acetate is not well absorbed (Fariss, B. L., et al., 1978), the schedule uses cortisone hemisuccinate to replace the intramuscular doses of cortisone acetate in older regimens. Twelve hours preoperatively 100 mg of cortisone hemisuccinate is given intramuscularly. The day of surgery 100 mg of cortisone hemisuccinate is given intramuscularly with the other preoperative medicines. During the procedure, 100 mg of cortisone hemisuccinate is given by IV drip. Postoperatively, cortisone hemisuccinate is given intramuscularly, 50 mg every 6 hours the first day, 50 mg every 8 hours the second day, 25 mg every 6 hours the third day, 25 mg every 8 hours the fourth day, and 12.5 mg every 6 hours the fifth day. For patients previously taking daily steroids the tapering dose can be stopped at the equivalent therapeutic level. Also, oral steroid of equivalent doses may be given in place of injections in patients able to take medications by mouth. Obviously, the clinical status of the patient —the presence of fever, pain, hypotension, or electrolyte imbalance—will result in variations of postoperative management. These suggestions are employed when a general anesthetic is administered and are subject to modification.

Banks (1970) has studied steroid requirements in the oral surgical patient and noted that standard steroid coverage protocols are based on the stress of a laparotomy under general anesthesia. Based on evaluation of plasma cortisol levels in suppressed patients, he suggests that 50 mg of cortisone acetate, both pre- and postoperatively, is adequate coverage for an osteotomy performed under general anesthesia. These data should not be applied clinically in patients having extensive surgery, because adrenal crisis, although uncommon, can be fatal. On the other hand, excess short-term steroid administration is harmless.

Banks' recommendations can be considered in managing the ambulatory patient undergoing less complex procedures, either with local or general anesthesia. Even this is somewhat arbitrary, however, since the overall stress of a procedure may be greater for the patient given only a local anesthetic, even though he is free of the pharmacologic influences of anesthetic drugs. Thus for the patient thought to have functional adrenal suppression and who is scheduled for limited oral surgery under local anesthesia, doubling the daily dose the night before surgery and on the day of surgery is suggested. If a general anesthetic is to be used, and the patient has not eaten, doubling of the oral dose the night before and the day of surgery, combined with 50 mg of cortisone hemisuccinate one-half hour before the procedure, is recommended. A maintenance regimen can be resumed the next day, since the amount of steroid given prophylactically is not sufficient to cause withdrawal symptoms. It should also be noted that the question of steroid coverage is sufficiently empirical to warrant consultation with the patient's physician before surgery is performed.

GENERAL PREOPERATIVE PREPARATION

This phase of patient care is designed to prepare the patient for the operation, relieve discomfort and anxiety, and facilitate the induction of general anesthesia.

Routine orders

Routine orders for the hospitalized patient represent a standard method of conveying what the surgeon wants done for the patient. Although such orders vary from institution to institution and patient to patient, they are designed to combine the basics of laboratory investigation with preparation of the patient for operation. For the oral surgical patient undergoing an elective procedure, routine orders include the following.

Diagnosis. The diagnosis immediately alerts the hospital staff to the kind of care the patient may need and potential complications he may encounter.

Diet. The selection of a diet for the majority of patients having elective oral and maxillofacial surgery will be normal in content and consistency. Patients with heart disease may need a salt-restricted diet; diabetics may have calorie restrictions and specific carbohydrate needs.

Activity. Maximum activity within the bounds of the patient's condition should be allowed.

Vital signs. A preoperative record of the pulse, blood pressure, and respiration must be made. This information is of the utmost importance in the case of intra- or postoperative complications.

Sedation. The patient should have a restful night before surgery. An order for the use of a short-acting barbiturate, flurazepam (Dalmane) or chloral hydrate, should be included in case it is needed.

Medications. A patient may be taking medications for the surgical problem itself or for other medical reasons (that is, cardiac drugs, hypoglycemic agents, antihypertensive agents, thyroid drugs, steroids, antibiotics, tranquilizers, anticonvulsants, antacids, and anticholinergics). Unless contraindicated, these should be continued. The use of antihypertensive drugs deserves some comment. Although not common in clinical use at present, reserpine acts by depleting stores of neurotransmitters and is felt by many anesthesiologists to add a risk to general anesthesia. It is, therefore, omitted at least 2 weeks before surgery if this can be done safely. Another antihypertensive agent, methyldopa (Aldomet), may cause orthostatic hypotension. Current opinion holds that such medications should be omitted if orthostatic hypotension is present but not as a routine measure.

Laboratory tests. A complete blood count and urinalysis are routine at most hospitals. Since the availability of rapid blood chemistry determinations, such an expanded workup is now often routine. The patient taking cardiac drugs and diuretics should have electrolytes determined; potassium levels in particular should be checked. A screening prothrombin time or partial thromboplastin time is often part of the preoperative routine. Chest radiographs for all patients, and electrocardiograms for patients over 40 years of age, complete the routine laboratory investigations.

Specific orders

Specific preoperative orders include the following.

Nothing by mouth. The night before surgery, solids are usually discontinued after the evening meal and liquids after bedtime. This ensures time for the patient's stomach to empty, reducing the risk of vomiting and aspiration on induction of anesthesia.

Anesthetic premedication. Drugs to be given prior to an anesthetic are usually ordered by the anesthesiologist. They are prescribed in combination to achieve one or more of the following effects: sedation, tranquility, amnesia, analgesia, reduction in salivary secretions, vagal blockade, the inhibition of nausea and vomiting. Typical orders may consist of 0.4 to 0.6 mg of atropine and 6 mg of morphine given intramuscularly 1 hour before surgery.

Blood and blood products. Blood typing and cross-matching should be ordered for all patients in whom significant blood loss is anticipated.

Preparation of the field. Cutaneous areas of the proposed operative field should be prepared by shaving and thorough washing the night before surgery. Areas of graft harvesting, for example, hip or chest, should be included. There is no evidence that attempts at intraoral sterilization are clinically beneficial, although thorough dental prophylaxis and adequate gingival health are desirable prior to certain orthognathic and other surgical procedures.

Prophylactic antibiotics. The use of prophylactic antibiotics is another area that suffers from lack of documentation. Prophylactic antibiotic use and abuse are frequently discussed without documentation or clinical reasoning. Antibiotic abuse begins when the simplest, most effective, and safest antibiotics are not used. The use of a broad-spectrum antibiotic does not necessarily enhance its prophylactic qualities, and it can lead to complicating superinfections. Selection of the proper antibiotic should be based on a rational consideration of the organism or organisms most often involved in the condition for which prophylaxis is being considered. There is convincing evidence that the overwhelming number of infections seen by oral and maxillofacial surgeons is caused by organisms sensitive to penicillin and erythromycin.

Controversy abounds as to what procedures and which patients require prophylactic antibiotics. As previously noted, the patient with a congenital or acquired heart defect and a potential for vegetative growth should be protected with prophylactic antibiotics, as should patients with severe kidney disease or severe metabolic or hematologic derangements, including uncontrolled diabetes, leukemia, agranulocytosis, aplastic anemia, and immunodeficiencies. Patients receiving antimetabolites, steroids, and other immunosuppressive therapy also should be protected. Prophylactic antibiotics are probably justified in the patient taking daily steroids for whatever reason.

There is ample evidence to support the use of prophylactic antibiotics in the treatment of facial bone fractures that are compounded into the mouth or paranasal sinuses. Kay (1966) has also presented data to suggest that morbidity is reduced when antibiotics are used, along with other local measures, in a combined prophylactic-therapeutic manner prior to removal of a third molar involved with pericoronitis, although Rud (1970) has presented evidence to the contrary. The prophylactic use of antibiotics in intraoral orthognathic and reconstructive procedures is well accepted but not well documented. Prophylaxis in the case of apicoectomies and odontectomies is similarly undocumented and is less universally accepted. The rationale and use of prophylactic antibiotics in other soft tissue wounds, osteoradionecrosis, and bone grafting procedures will be discussed in succeeding chapters.

Steroids. The use of systemic and topical steroids has been advocated for the reduction of edema and certain other undesirable postoperative sequelae, Hooley and Francis (1969) used betamethasone for the reduction of postoperative edema and trismus following difficult third molar surgery; Guernsey and DeChamplain (1971) have reported on the use of dexamethasone to reduce the undesirable edema of the intraoral sagittal ramus split; Hall (1975) reported the use of dexamethasone in vestibuloplasty procedures. It has also been suggested that topical steroids be used to prevent excoriation and ulceration of the lips and corners of the mouth caused by retraction.

The use of steroids in third molar surgery is still debatable. Although not universally accepted, one regimen involves two 0.6 mg tablets of betamethasone the evening before surgery, two tablets q.i.d. the day of surgery, and two tablets q.i.d. postoperatively for a total dose of 24 tablets or 14.4 mg of betamethasone. Hooley, Bradley, and Haines (1971) have shown this regimen to significantly decrease plasma cortisol levels, although in all cases the plasma cortisol level returned to normal within 4 days after cessation of steroid therapy. To eliminate the need for postoperative oral medication, Hooley and Hohl (1974) have advocated intramuscular betamethasone consisting of equal parts of the sodium phosphate and acetate. The phosphate is soluble and rapidly absorbed; the acetate provides sustained action by slow absorption. The regimen consists of two 0.6 mg tablets the evening before surgery, one 0.6 mg tablet the morning of surgery, and 6 mg of betamethasone intramuscularly at the time of surgery. Modification is required for the ambulatory patient undergoing general anesthesia.

Considerable interest is presently focused on the use of high-dose, short-term, systemic steroids for major reconstructive and preprosthetic surgery, where its use can eliminate the need for vacuum drains and bulky constricting pressure dressings, as well as possibly decrease hospitalization time. The original regimen of Guernsey and DeChamplain (1971) consisted of 4 mg dexamethasone the night before surgery, 4 mg b.i.d. the day of surgery, 2 mg b.i.d. on the first postoperative day, and 1 mg on the second and third postoperative days. Modifications include higher dose and shorter term administration. There is evidence suggesting a lack of effect of high-dose, short-term steroids on wound healing, as well as an absence of withdrawal symptoms that would require longer tapering dose regimens. Thus 8 mg dexamethasone intramuscularly the night before surgery and the morning of surgery, followed by 4 mg intramuscularly the first postoperative day, has given excellent results, especially in patients treated by intraoral oblique osteotomy. Hall, Chase, and Payor (1975) advocate 125 mg of methylprednisolone, intramuscularly, with the preoperative medications, 125 mg in the intravenous fluids during surgery, and 20 mg q.i.d. for 24 to 48 hours postoperatively.

It must be kept in mind that systemic steroids are adjunctive and will not prevent sequelae of improper tissue handling or careless surgery. Clinical impressions suggest a greater effect in intraoral vertical osteotomies than in sagittal split osteomies — apparently a function of the surgical procedure itself. Topical steroids similarly appear to be clinically useful in reducing lip excoriations and edema; various types in concentrations up to 1% have been used. There is no evidence that topical steroids used in such a manner will cause adrenal suppression.

Absolute and relative contraindications exist to the use of topical and systemic steroids. These include active, incompletely healed, or healed tuberculosis, ocular herpes simplex, primary glaucoma, and acute psychosis. Relative contraindications include diverticulitis, active or latent peptic ulcer, recent intestinal anastomosis, Cushing's syndrome, thrombophlebitis, osteoporosis, diabetes mellitus, myasthenia gravis, psychotic tendencies, acute and chronic infections (especially varicella and vaccinia), and fungal diseases. The first trimester of pregnancy is also a relative contraindication to the use of corticosteroids. Although clinical judgment may vary, if the surgical trauma appears to warrant use of systemic steroids, the concurrent use of prophylactic antibiotics is indicated.

MAINTENANCE OF FLUID, ELECTROLYTE, AND ACID-BASE BALANCE

Parks (1966) and Shires, Williams, and Brown (1961) provide excellent comprehensive analyses of this subject; discussion here is limited to considerations of the patient undergoing oral and maxillofacial surgical procedures. Intricate electrolyte imbalances seldom occur in such patients, and their fluid and electrolyte problems are usually characterized by the need for only short-term intravenous therapy. A systematic approach to fluid and electrolyte balance rests on knowledge of daily maintenance requirements, losses during treatment, and present or potential imbalances. Two assumptions are made in this discussion — that the patient is of "normal" size and that renal function is adequate.

Fluids

The maintenance of correct water balance is of great importance. In general, water depletion is due either to lack of intake, unreplaced loss, or increased excretion. It can result from such conditions as fever accompanying severe odontogenic infections, fluid loss during a long operative procedure, and persistent postoperative vomiting or diarrhea. Signs of dehydration include thirst, decreased tissue turgor, a severely furrowed tongue, parched lips, postural hypotension and tachycardia. Poor tissue turgor is a reflection of decreased interstitial fluid compartment volume, while changes in blood pressure and pulse are indicators of changes in the circulating blood volume. Meyer (1971), Everett, Meyer, and Allen (1969), Meyer and Allen (1968), and Bergan, Gores, and Wakin (1958) have conducted studies of the changes in fluid balance resulting from loss of blood in multiple extractions and in open and closed fracture reduction. Although such studies often lack adequate control groups, they highlight the importance of adequate fluid therapy to prevent and minimize certain postoperative complications in the oral and maxillofacial surgical patient. The summary of Wang and Waite (1974) shows that adequate intravenous fluid therapy alone, without blood transfusion, is usually sufficient even in major potential blood-losing procedures such as the sagittal split osteotomy.

Urine is the largest source of sensible water loss. An adult surgical patient needs to excrete a solute load of about

450 mOsm daily. Since normal urine has a solute concentration of about 300 mOsm/L, a volume of 1500 ml per day is needed to excrete a load of 450 mOsm. Sensible water loss via the feces is about 50 to 200 ml/day. Insensible water loss, occurring through the lungs and skin, amounts to about 500 ml/m² of body surface, per day, in a basal state. For convenience, the insensible daily water loss in adults is assumed to be 500 to 1000 ml. Total maintenance fluid requirement is, therefore, 2000 to 2500 ml/day. When oral intake is not possible, this must be supplied parenterally (see p. 338).

Blood volume changes owing to the preoperative fast, operative and postoperative blood loss, fever, edema, and inadequate oral intake are easily determined. The use of an intake and output chart also allows comparison of urine output with total fluid intake and serves as a check on fluid balance. Fluid requirements and administration must be reduced in patients with diminished cardiac reserve. Care must be taken in these patients to prevent overhydration, which causes increased cardiac work, either as a result of rapid administration of relatively small volumes or of gross increase in daily load.

Anesthesia and surgery, as well as trauma, represent forms of stress to which the body responds by increased secretion of aldosterone and antidiuretic hormone (ADH). This results in a reduced renal capacity to excrete water or sodium loads and in increased potassium loss—hence the recommendation that water and sodium intake be restricted in postoperative and posttrauma patients. While the patient with head trauma certainly should have his free water intake limited to reduce chances of cerebral edema, much of the activation of ADH and aldosterone secretion is related not only to stress but to preoperative restriction of fluid intake and to inadequate replacement of fluid losses during and after surgery.

The syndrome of inappropriate secretion of antidiuretic hormone is of interest. Water intoxication, serum hypotonicity, and urine hypertonicity originally de-scribed in patients with bronchogenic carcinoma have been reported in patients with head injury and maxillofacial trauma by Davis and Matukas (1976). Diagnosis is important, since the neurologic signs and symptoms, although correctible, mimic those of cerebral deterioration. In addition, diabetes insipidus may be present in a patient with maxillofacial injury. Massive negative fluid balance must be recognized and treated.

In the patient undergoing routine oral surgery, simple fluid replacement is the rule. Duration of need is usually 1 day or less, but may be longer following major procedures that require intermaxillary fixation. To keep the patient in satisfactory volume balance, it is necessary to check urine output, which is usually 1500 ml ± 500 ml/day (60 ± 20 ml/hour) but may decrease following trauma or stress to 750 to 1200 ml per day. Decreased urine output with high urine specific gravity suggests a water deficit. In the absence of hemorrhage, a significantly elevated hematocrit suggests dehydration or, more significantly, a sodium deficit. The most common postoperative problem is a mild hypotension readily corrected by intravenous fluid.

Electrolytes

The interpretation of electrolyte values is discussed in Chapter 14. This information is of particular importance in the patient taking diuretics or digitalis, in the diabetic patient, in the patient with renal disease, and in the patient with maxillofacial trauma requiring extended intravenous therapy. Briefly stated, serum sodium concentration reflects salt concentration in all body compartments. A decrease in serum sodium is most commonly caused by water excess and reflects a need for restriction of electrolyte-free water intake. In the oral and maxillofacial surgical patient, it is rare to see abnormal gastrointestinal losses, losses of extracellular fluid (either externally, as in burns, or internally, as in peritonitis), excessive urine sodium wastage (as in chronic nephritis), or adrenal failure—all causes of hyponatremia that requires administration of sodium-containing fluids. Hyponatremia caused by water excess is often associated with increased urine volume and body weight reflecting the water overload. Nausea, vomiting, and convulsions usually do not appear unless shifts have been rapid or the serum sodium concentration is below 120 mEq/L.

Increased serum sodium concentration is usually caused by either abnormal renal retention of sodium or by increased sodium reabsorption, for example, increased activity of aldosterone. Edema is the main clinical sign and usually appears when 3 or 4 L of excess water are retained.

Potassium is the major intracellular cation. The serum potassium concentration represents only a small fraction of total body-exchangeable potassium and is a reliable but insensitive guide to potassium need. There is an obligatory daily urinary excretion of potassium that continues even in the presence of depletion—unlike sodium, which may be conserved by regulatory mechanisms. The single most important reason for avoiding hypokalemia is the arrhythmias that occur in the patient with frank or borderline digitalis toxicity.

Hyperkalemia is usually associated with renal failure but may also be seen in patients with multiple injuries when intracellular potassium is released by massive tissue destruction, hematoma formation, and red cell destruction. Serum potassium values above 7 mEq/L also may cause severe arrhythmias.

In summary, fluid and electrolyte therapy for the generally healthy adult oral and maxillofacial surgical patient is usually managed easily. A balanced electrolyte solution, such as lactated Ringer's solution, is administered to the patient during surgery. Such solutions contain 130 mEq/L of sodium, 4 mEq/L of potassium, 109 mEq/L of chloride, 28 mEq/L of bicarbonate, and 3 mEq/L of calcium. They are used as a vehicle to administer drugs and to replace the deficits resulting from the preoperative fast. About 1 L of such a solution, followed by 1500 ml of 5% dextrose in water, will meet the patient's daily fluid and electrolyte require-

ments—2500 ml of volume, 30 to 100 mEq of sodium, and 30 to 80 mEq of potassium. Variations include the intraoperative administration of 1 L 5% dextrose in water (D5W), followed by 1 L D5W and 500 ml of 5% dextrose in saline (D5S), which supplies 77 mEq of sodium chloride. If continued intravenous therapy is needed, requirements can be met by 2000 ml of D5W and 500 ml of D5S to which 40 mEq of potassium chloride is added. In addition, such formulation must include consideration of intraoperative blood loss, fever, oral intake, intravenous antibiotic volume and electrolyte content, serum electrolytes, hematocrit, urine output, and, most importantly, the general status of the patient.

Acid-base problems

The oral and maxillofacial surgeon dealing with the hospitalized patient must know when the cardiovascular, respiratory, or metabolic status of his patient requires determination of objective data regarding acid-base balance. The primary laboratory tool used is measurement of arterial blood gases (ABGs). which are of value before, during, and after surgery.

Preoperative assessment of acid-base balance via ABGs is of value in the evaluation of the respiratory status of the patient with chronic lung disease. Certain patients in this group may demonstrate marginal oxygenation or show chronic hypercarbia that can affect both anesthetic and postoperative management. Pulmonary function tests, as well as blood gas data, are of great value in identifying these problems and in properly preparing the patient.

Blood gas measurement provides ready assessment of the adequacy of ventilation via an endotracheal tube in the traumatized patient with intracranial or thoracic injury. Intraoperative ventilatory status may be assessed similarly. The most frequent cause of arrhythmias during induction of general anesthesia is hypercarbia and its resultant acidosis. In addition, the acid-base status of the patient requiring transfusion can be effectively monitored with serial ABGs. Postoperatively, the indications for ABG determination include: (1) acute respiratory distress; (2) acute cardiac events, including arrhythmias; (3) prolonged recovery or acute agitation following general anesthesia; (4) postoperative intubation or assisted ventilation; and (5) uncontrolled postoperative diabetes mellitus. In each instance, clinical judgment—based on appropriate history, physical examination, and radiographs—determines the appropriate use of ABG measurement. Nomograms are available and are helpful in determining the patient's acid-base balance and respiratory status. Rapid evaluation—so important to general patient care—is both possible and practical if the following method is used: Inspired oxygen concentration at the time of blood sampling is known; normal pH is assumed to be 7.40 and normal PCO_2 to be 40 mm Hg. Each 10 mm Hg shift in PCO_2 then accounts for a shift in pH of 0.08. Changes in pH caused either by metabolic alterations or by respiratory compensation will occur slowly unless iatrogenically induced—for example, sodium bicarbonate infusion—while changes owing to primary changes in respiratory function will be evident acutely.

Determination of the efficiency of oxygenation of the blood by alveolar gas exchange depends on knowledge of the amount of oxygen delivered to the alveolus; 80 to 100 mm Hg is the normal range of PO_2 for the patient breathing room air containing 21% oxygen. The "normal" PO_2 varies with age. It is crucial to realize that only at an inspired oxygen concentration of 100% can definitive knowledge of the efficiency of oxygenation be measured.

Acidosis and alkalosis problems may be difficult to diagnose because of the multiple combinations of primary derangement and secondary compensation—for example, metabolic acidosis with respiratory compensation. Again, useful clinical information may be obtained rapidly by following a simplified schema and with a knowledge of the clinical setting. A pH less than 7.40 indicates acidosis; a pH above 7.40 indicates alkalosis. If an acidosis is present and the PCO_2 is greater than 40 mm Hg, a respiratory acidosis exists; if the PCO_2 is less than or equal to 40, the primary derangement is a metabolic acidosis. A similar rationale is used for evaluating an alkalosis. Using the axiom that each 10 mm Hg shift in PCO_2 accounts for a pH shift of 0.08, the extent of combined respiratory and metabolic factors in altered acid-base balance can be assessed. For example, a PCO_2 of 60 mm Hg would be expected to lower the pH by 0.16 to 7.24. If the actual pH was 7.32, then partial metabolic compensation for a respiratory acidosis may be assumed, realizing that metabolic compensation occurs gradually. Similarly, a PCO_2 of 60 mm Hg with a pH of 7.20 may be interpreted as a combined metabolic and respiratory acidosis, since the PCO_2 alone is not sufficient to explain the pH of 7.20.

Acidosis is generally treated by management of the underlying disease. Sodium bicarbonate can be administered in severe cases. Metabolic alkalosis can be controlled with sodium chloride and respiratory alkalosis by rebreathing of expired CO_2 plus use of sedation.

POSTOPERATIVE CARE
Postoperative orders

Routine postoperative orders are designed to provide for the immediate needs of the patient during recovery from the anesthetic and throughout the night of surgery. The procedure performed and any drains present should be noted. Vital signs must be monitored carefully every 15 minutes for the first hour, every half hour thereafter until stable, and finally at least every 4 hours. To prevent pulmonary congestion and vascular stasis, the patient should be encouraged to cough, to breathe deeply, and to ambulate with assistance as soon as possible. Elevation of the head is most comfortable for the patient, prevents pooling of secretions, and makes elimination of blood and saliva easier. Intravenous fluid and electrolyte needs have been discussed earlier (see p. 336). Medications to control pain and nausea should be ordered; intramuscular injections of meperidine (Demerol), 50 to 75 mg, and prochlorperazine dimaleate (Compazine), 5 to 10 mg, are quite satisfactory. When oral intake is possible, oral analgesic medication can eliminate the discomfort of intramuscular injections. If indicated, antibiotics are ordered. Cold packs should be used to minimize swelling, and a suction apparatus should be ordered to help in evacuation of oral secretions. For most patients not in intermaxillary fixation, a full liquid or soft solid diet, as tolerated, may be ordered. Some specific areas of postoperative management merit more thorough consideration.

Control of pain

Postoperative discomfort is usual, but it is the responsibility of the surgeon to minimize actual pain. There are a number of satisfactory analgesics, and choice, based on relative effectiveness, is an individual matter. For anticipated mild pain, acetylsalicylic acid or acetaminophen may be used. For moderate pain, such as following third molar surgery, they may be combined with codeine. Oxycodone has somewhat greater potency. Meperidine (Demerol), administered orally, is usually reserved for more severe pain problems; in hospitalized patients who usually have poor oral intake owing to the magnitude of surgery, intramuscular Demerol, 50 to 75 mg, is quite useful. The adjunctive use of ice is most helpful in cases of painful swelling.

Control of swelling

The use of steroids in the control of postoperative edema has been discussed on p. 335. Their use after more major procedures is generally accepted. The best means of preventing edema following surgical extraction or third molar surgery is the application of cold—a superb modality when used properly—as it constricts capillaries and reduces oozing. The most dramatic clinical application is the use of iced saline sponges following periorbital injury or surgery. Cold should be used intermittently (20 minutes on area and 20 minutes off) during the first 24 to 48 hours. The intermittent application avoids compensatory vasodilation and increase in exudation.

Postoperative swelling is usually caused by a combination of hematoma resulting from hemorrhage and lymphedema resulting from lymphatic exudation. Lip swelling after injudicious retraction is a good example of the latter. Obviously, the first method of controlling swelling is hemostasis, although the nature of most oral and maxillofacial surgical procedures, with concomitant oozing from muscle, precludes complete hemostasis. Pressure, therefore, is the next most useful method to control swelling (see Chapter 7). It is most effective when a firm backing is available—for example, pressure dressing after open reduction of the mandible in which the bone provides the firm backing. It is least useful when it merely contains or directs swelling internally, as in sagittal split or other major intraoral ramus surgery.

When using facial pressure dressings, pads must be placed behind the ears to protect the auricular cartilage. As a matter of consideration for the patient, an Elastoplast or other adhesive dressing should not cover hair-bearing regions. Care must also be taken with any pressure dressing to see that it does not impair the airway or produce major vascular compression.

Drains to prevent or reduce swelling are designed to allow elimination of fluid and are most useful when dependency can be gained. Their use following intraoral dentoalveolar surgery is probably unnecessary. Lack of dependency also impairs the use of intraoral rubber drains following procedures such as sagittal split osteotomy, although the use of external suction drains in place of pressure dressings has been recommended by Moore, Upton, and Frederickson (1975).

The use of enzyme preparations of plant or animal origin (papain, hyaluronidase, trypsin, chymotrypsin) or antihistamines for reduction of postoperative swelling has given variable results and is generally not recommended.

Even with use of the various modalities described above, some swelling may occur. After 48 hours, heat in the form of oral rinses and/or externally applied moist packs is helpful in increasing circulation and reducing this swelling. As with cold applications, heat should be used intermittently (20 minutes on area, 20 minutes off) to avoid producing the reverse hemodynamic effect.

Nutrition

Although only a minority of oral and maxillofacial surgical patients suffer from debilitating diseases, the nutritional status of such patients is highly significant to postoperative recovery and wound healing. Nutritional status is frequently compromised with oral cancer or its possible sequel—osteoradionecrosis, in those with inadequate dentures requiring preprosthetic surgery, and in those with pseudo- or true ankylosis. These patients represent poor operative risks and may benefit from a careful preoperative feeding regimen.

Undernutrition may be defined as the loss of 30% or more of ideal body weight owing to lack of food intake; the oral and maxillofacial surgical patient can rarely be so classified. However, these patients may suffer from malnutrition, that is, improper diet. Principles of adequate nutrition include sufficient carbohydrate to prevent protein catabolism and to maintain a positive nitrogen balance; sufficient protein to provide the building blocks of repair; and adequate vitamins to permit normal metabolic events, wound healing, and coagulation. In extreme situations, preoperative use of intravenous hyperalimentation can be used effectively; certainly hyperalimentation has assumed a routine place in the postoperative management of the patient requiring intravenous feeding for longer than a week.

Patients may receive some feeding via intravenous fluid in the form of 5% dextrose in water, containing 50 gm of glucose (200 calories) per liter; 10% glucose is also available. Preoperatively, calories as well as fluid therapy are important to the nutrition of the trauma patient. Patients who suffer acute anemia should receive a blood transfusion; those with chronic anemias should receive therapy appropriate to the etiology—for example, iron, vitamin B_{12}, or folate.

Postoperatively, most patients can manage a diet that is limited in consistency. However, a single day of minimal nutrition is generally of no consequence if fluid requirements are met. Although usually not needed, carefully arranged liquid diets are available. The patient in intermaxillary fixation is the major exception to this rule and is discussed under "Special problems."

Special problems
Maxillary sinus

Particular attention should be paid to the patient who has undergone a primary maxillary sinus procedure or in whom the sinus is violated secondarily, as in an anterior maxillary osteotomy. These patients are usually on antibiotics for primary infection or for postoperative prophylaxis. The use of phenylephrine (Neo-Synephrine) nasal spray and oral pseudoephedrine (Sudafed) is very helpful in promoting hemostasis and decongestion. Precautions such as avoidance of nose blowing and sneezing with the mouth open, designed to prevent positive pressure in the sinus, should be instituted. In most cases in which the sinus is involved secondarily, there is a "clean" sinus and problems are minimal.

The patient in intermaxillary fixation

Explanations and reassurance as to the normalization of speech and nutrition should be part of the preoperative preparation of the patient. At the end of the procedure, before fixation is applied, the throat packs must be removed, the throat is suctioned, and the tongue is freed from the occlusal table. When significant blood loss has occurred, the evacuation of the stomach via a nasogastric tube and suction helps in reducing postoperative nausea and vomiting; the tube may be left in place for 24 hours when seepage of blood is expected, as in LeFort osteotomies. Immediate postoperative parenteral administration of an antiemetic is also useful in reducing nausea and preventing vomiting. To ensure comfort and prevent aspiration, it is advisable to tape either a scissors or a wire cutter, and a hemostat to the bed for rapid removal of elastic or wire traction in case of vomiting. In some instances a sterile tracheostomy set should also be kept at the bedside during the first 48 hours. The availability of bedside suction is also invaluable and may be used by either the nursing staff or the patient.

The decision as to how long to maintain endotracheal intubation is based on clinical judgment. Adequacy of recovery, as judged by mental status, respiratory pattern, continued bleeding, and tolerance of the endotracheal tube all must be considered. The anesthesiologist should play an active part in this final decision.

It is never necessary to remove anterior teeth or open the bite in order to provide a gap for feeding purposes. There is always adequate space behind the last molars to allow passage of fluid and semi-solid material, even in a mouth with a full complement of teeth. Initially, fluids by flexible straw are well tolerated. The use of an Asepto syringe with rubber catheter or feeding cup may be needed in some patients. Most patients will adapt readily when dietary needs are explained. This can be reinforced by having a dietician instruct each patient in nutritional requirements and how to prepare a varied diet. Frequent and small feedings are advised and the use of a blender is invaluable. There is no substitute for patient ingenuity and determination. Using water, milk, or juices as diluents, almost any food can be blenderized. There is only a small group of patients in whom special measures or devices are needed.

Ritzau (1973) studied 33 patients with jaw fractures and intermaxillary fixation and found that weight loss was a greater possibility than was stable or increased weight. Patients in his study received no organized nutritional instruction, only recommendations to eat liquid and blenderized food. There were no statistically significant correlations between loss of weight and hospital stay or duration of immobilization. The average weight loss was greater for inpatients than outpatients, however, probably reflecting the severity of injury and disability.

Some variation in bowel habits should be expected in patients taking a diet of limited consistency, especially those in whom narcotics are administered concomitantly. There is little need for real concern, and enemas should be avoided, although mild laxatives such as milk of magnesia may be helpful. The one exception is the patient who has undergone removal of iliac bone. Inadvertent violation of the inner cortical plate may traumatize the peritoneum and result in an ileus. Bowel sounds indicative of peristalsis should be present in these patients before permitting oral intake.

Oral hygiene is another matter of concern. In order not to disrupt oral wounds, lavage during the early healing period should be done carefully and mouthwashes with a high alcohol content should be avoided. Use of a soft toothbrush and the Water-Pik gives very satisfactory results during intermaxillary fixation.

POSTOPERATIVE COMPLICATIONS
Fever

Fever is not a disease but a clinical sign; any major surgery can produce low-grade fever for several days. If fever is high (102+), prolonged, or recurrent, the oral and maxillofacial surgeon must determine if the cause is local or systemic, if the fever is of infectious origin, and if the appropriate treatment is to stop drugs, start drugs, or perform more surgery. There are certain clues to look for in any postoperative patient; there are also some particular to the oral and maxillofacial surgical patient. The following is presented as a guide to etiology and differential diagnosis.

Fever during first 24 hours

Malignant hyperthermia. Malignant hyperthermia is seen as catastrophic fever beginning within 2 hours of induction of anesthesia, especially when succinylcholine is part of the anesthetic regimen. An excellent discussion of this subject has been written by Arens and McKinnon (1971) and by Schwartz and Gracia (1975).

Transfusion reactions. Transfusion reactions may be due to immunologic incompatibilities, pyogenic reactions, or contaminated solutions.

Drug hypersensitivity or contamination. Although hypersensitivity is usually a more frequent cause of late fever, contamination through the use of multidose vials is possible.

Atelectasis. Atelectasis is a common cause of postoperative fever and is produced by inadequate pulmonary ventilation or obstruction, usually from inspissated mucus. Patients with chronic bronchitis and emphysema are predisposed to this condition and warrant preoperative preparation as discussed on p. 327. Factors that tend to increase the incidence of postoperative atelectasis include use of narcotics, prolonged postoperative immobilization, pulmonary congestion, and aspiration. A physical examination disclosing moist rales and decreased breath sounds, especially at the lung bases, is diagnostic. Treatment is directed at routine reexpansion of the involved lung by deep breathing, coughing, and the other means outlined earlier. An excellent review of the pathogenesis of atelectatis has been written by Schlenker and Hubay (1973).

Aspiration pneumonia. Direct aspiration of blood, gastric contents, and particulate material may occur inadvertently. Aspiration pneumonia is a different condition than the pneumonitis that results if atelectasis is not diagnosed and treated. The major clinical judgment to be made is whether blood or gastric contents have been aspirated. If blood is aspirated, therapy includes clearing the tracheobronchial tree by nasotracheal suction or aspiration bronchoscopy, adequate oxygenation, and prophylactic use of a broad-spectrum antibiotic. The bacteriology of infection caused by aspiration has been discussed by Bartlett, Gorback, and Finegold (1974). If aspiration of gastric contents is presumed or if solid material is aspirated, immediate treatment should begin. The tracheobronchial tree should be cleared by bronchoscopy; massive lavage is not indicated as it may spread the material. Hydrocortisone, 400 to 800 mg/day should be given intravenously or intramuscularly and continued for 3 to 5 days and then reduced rapidly. Intratracheal steroids—hydrocortisone 50 mg in 5 ml of saline—may be administered via the nasotracheal catheter or via the respirator nebulizer if respiratory support is being used. Careful monitoring of the patient for pulmonary infection and lung abscess is of primary importance. Although experimental studies by Down and co-workers (1974) have failed to support the benefits of lavage and steroids, most centers continue to employ these methods in the clinical situation.

Wound infection. Wound infection is rarely an early cause of fever.

Endocrine dysfunction. The occurrence of endocrine dysfunction is very rare; it includes acute adrenal insufficiency, thyroid storm, and pheochromocytoma.

Fever after the first 24 hours

Anesthesia. The existence of halothane hepatitis is controversial. Features include early fever after multiple exposures, malaise, anorexia, jaundice, and elevated SGOT. The discussion by McPeek, Mathieu, and Guralnick (1974) is suggested.

Transfusion reactions. Occasionally, a blood transfusion can cause fever after 24 hours. This may be due to the introduction of viable bacteria into the patient's bloodstream or from a delayed allergic reaction.

Intravenous complications. Intravenous complications are unusual in an oral and maxillofacial surgery patient, since the need for such therapy is usually short. Causes include contaminated fluids or catheters and infection owing to intravenous cannulae. There may or may not be accompanying phlebitis.

Drug hypersensitivity. Frequently a workup for fever produces no answers and cessation of all drugs not necessary to maintain life becomes an important diagnostic move. Drug fever may occur with any antibiotic, even in the absence of rash and eosinophilia. Cardiac drugs such as procainamide (Pronestyl), quinidine, and propranolol are also often implicated.

Hematoma. Hematoma is usually not a

cause of high fever unless it is massive, as in the retroperitoneal space.

Lung infection. Atelectasis is still common at this time, although pneumonia and pulmonary infarction should be considered in the differential diagnosis.

Urinary tract infection. The surgeon's index of suspicion should be high in patients with a history of recurrent urinary tract infections, presence of cells and organisms on preoperative urinalysis, or symptoms of dysuria or frequency. In patients requiring either temporary or indwelling Foley catheters, bladder infection is a real risk.

Wound infection. Systemic factors predisposing to wound infection include debilitation, diabetes, use of corticosteroids, generalized infections, or previous use of antibiotics. Local factors include necrotic tissue, devascularization, foreign bodies, and hematoma. Most infections after intraoral procedures occur late and are probably caused by superinfection from prolonged antibiotic therapy or by devascularization.

Fat emboli. In the patient with multiple trauma, the syndrome of fever, tachycardia, and respiratory deficit appearing 1 to 2 days after injury should suggest this diagnosis. A review by Miller (1975) is recommended.

• • •

The cause of postoperative fever must be determined in a systematic manner. In evaluating the history, careful attention should be paid to the kind of anesthesia, use of transfusions, duration of intravenous therapy, drugs being used, presence of a urinary catheter, and, of course, to the patient's specific complaints. Careful and complete physical examination is mandatory. Special attention should be given to the wound, the lungs, the urinary tract, the liver, and signs of phlebitis. If appropriate, laboratory aids in the form of chest radiographs, CBC, and liver function tests should be obtained. Appropriate cultures and Gram stains must also be obtained.

Hypotension

Determination of the etiology of decreased postoperative blood pressure is important. For most previously healthy adults, mild hypotension with tachycardia reflects negative fluid balance. Another common cause is overmedication with narcotic analgesics, singly or in combination with sedative drugs, although specific complaints and the possibility of such catastrophic events as myocardial infarction, even in the previously healthy patient, must not be overlooked. The presence of a tachycardia must be noted, since arrhythmias are a leading cause of hypotension. Other causes of tachycardia include CO_2 retention, hypoxia, and fever.

Urinary retention

It is most important to realize that postoperative anuria is usually not synonymous with renal failure or obstruction. In the otherwise healthy patient in whom there is no suspicion of acute renal damage, the most common cause is diminished bladder tone owing to anesthesia, recumbency, and sedation; a conservative approach is indicated. Having made the diagnosis of a full bladder by examination, ambulation and suprapubic hot packs usually help. Catheterization performed in a sterile fashion after a period of more than 12 hours usually corrects the problem.

Follow-up examination

The performance of surgery demands adequate periodic examination during the convalescent period and beyond. Such follow-up provides valuable information as to the accuracy of diagnosis and prognosis. Most importantly, it provides the patient with the assurance of a continuum of care. This is particularly significant in conditions where the recurrence rate may be significant.

REFERENCES

Arens, J. F., and McKinnon, W. M. P. 1971. Malignant hyperthermia during anesthesia, J.A.M.A. **215**:919.

Axelrod, L. 1976. Glucocorticoid therapy, Medicine **55**:39.

Banks, P. 1970. The adrenocortical response to oral surgery, Br. J. Oral Surg. **8**:32.

Bartlett, J. G., Gorback, S. L., and Finegold, S. M. 1974. The bacteriology of aspiration pneumonia, Am. J. Med. **56**:202.

Bergan, R. D., Gores, R. J., and Wakin, K. G. 1959. Fluid balance after multiple dental extractions and alveoplasty, Oral Surg. **12:**929.

Davis, B. P., and Matukas, V. J. 1976. Inappropriate secretion of antidiuretic hormone after cerebral injury, J. Oral Surg. **34:**609.

Down, J. B., et al. 1974. An evaluation of steroid therapy in aspiration pneumonitis, Anesthesiology **40:**129.

Everett, G., Meyer, R., and Allen, G. D. 1969. Blood volume changes associated with surgical fractures of the mandible, J. Oral Surg. **27:**637.

Fariss, B. L., et al. 1978. Comparison of absorption of cortisone acetate and hydrocortisone hemisuccinate, J. Clin. Endocrinol. Metab. **47:**1137.

Guernsey, L. H., and DeChamplain, R. W. 1971. Sequelae and complications of the intraoral sagittal osteotomy in the mandibular rami, Oral Surg. **32:**176.

Hall, H. D. 1971. Vestibuloplasty, mucosal grafts (palatal and buccal), J. Oral Surg. **29:**786.

Hall, H. D., Chase, D. C., and Payor, L. G. 1975. Evaluation and refinement of the intraoral vertical subcondylar osteotomy, J. Oral Surg. **33:**333.

Hooley, J. R., and Francis, F. H. 1969. Betamethasone in traumatic oral surgery, J. Oral Surg. **27:**398.

Hooley, J. R., Bradley, P. B., and Haines, M. P. 1971. Plasma cortisol levels following short-term betamethasone therapy for oral surgical procedures. Transactions of the Fourth International Conference on Oral Surgery, Copenhagen, Munksgaard.

Hooley, J. R., and Hohl, T. H. 1974. Use of steroids in the prevention of some complications after traumatic oral surgery, J. Oral Surg. **32:**864.

Kay, L. W. 1966. Investigation into the nature of pericoronitis, Br. J. Oral Surg. **4:**52.

McPeek, B., Mathieu, A., and Guralnick, W. C. 1974. Fact or fancy—a reasoned view of halothane, J. Oral Surg. **32:**8.

Meyer, R. A. 1971. Blood volume considerations in oral surgery, J. Oral Surg. **29:**617.

Meyer, R., and Allen, G. D. 1968. Blood volume studies in oral surgery. II. Postoperative complications and the state of hydration, J. Oral Surg. **26:**800.

Miller, G. A. 1975. Fat embolism: a comprehensive review, J. Oral Surg. **33:**91.

Moore, J. W., Upton, L. G., and Frederickson, G. C. 1975. Intraoral suction drain for reduction of postoperative edema, J. Oral Surg. **33:**462.

Parks, C. R. 1966. Operative fluid shifts: a review of the literature, Anesth. Analg. **45:**495.

Ritzau, M. 1973. Weight changes in patients with intermaxillary immobilization after jaw fractures, Int. J. Oral Surg. **2:**122.

Rud, J. 1970. Removal of impacted lower third molars with acute pericoronitis and necrotizing gingivitis, Br. J. Oral Surg. **7:**153.

Schlenker, J. D., and Hubay, C. A. 1973. The pathogenesis of postoperative atelectasis: a clinical study, Arch. Surg. **107:**846.

Schwartz, H. C., and Gracia, R. M. 1975. Malignant hyperthermia, J. Oral Surg. **33:**57.

Shires, T., Williams, J., and Brown, F. 1961. Acute change in extracellular fluids associated with major surgical procedures, Ann. Surg. **154:**803.

Wang, J. H., and Waite, D. E. 1974. Evaluation of the surgical procedure of sagittal split osteotomy of the mandibular ramus, Oral Surg. **38:**167.

CHAPTER 10

Sterilization and asepsis

David S. Evaskus

The discovery of the importance of asepsis in the prevention of infection may be the single most important advance in the history of surgery. According to Maki (1976), the concept was advocated decades before bacteria were conclusively implicated in wound suppuration and even before contagion was generally accepted. Wangensteen, Wangensteen, and Klinger (1973) noted that the general principles of asepsis were supported by Ignaz Semmelweis in Europe and Oliver Wendell Holmes in America against bitter opposition. It was not until Joseph Lister's studies on the prevention of wound infection, made between 1865 and 1891, that these principles were accepted. Lister initially applied dilute carbolic acid (phenol) to contaminated wounds and then progressed to its application in all surgical wounds, as well as in the operating room by nebulization of the solution. Further developments in Listerian asepsis occurred rapidly in the 1890's with the advent of steam sterilization, surgical masks, sterile gloves, sterile gowns, sterile drapes, and sterile sponges for the surgical wound.

Despite modern methods of sterilization and the use of aseptic techniques, microorganisms are introduced into surgical sites. Studies by Dillon, Postlethwait, and Bowling (1969), Jepsen (1973), and Krizek and Robson (1975) have implicated bacteria introduced into the operative wound at the time of surgery as the cause of many postoperative infections. A report by the Ad Hoc Committee of the Committee on Trauma, National

Academy of Science (1964) and a study by Cruse and Foord (1973), both of which reviewed over 15,000 surgical cases, emphasized the importance of meticulous surgical technique and asepsis for the prevention of infection. Although it is probable, as suggested by Elek and Conen (1957), that most postoperative infections today result from faulty surgical technique, the importance of disinfection, asepsis, and sterility in minimizing the patient's exposure to pathogenic bacteria cannot be overemphasized.

DEFINITIONS (Patterson, 1932)

antiseptic a chemical that is applied to living tissues such as skin or mucous membrane to reduce the number of microorganisms present through inhibition of their activity or destruction

disinfectant a chemical used on nonvital objects to kill surface vegetative pathogenic organisms, but not necessarily spore forms or viruses

sterilization a process by which all microbial forms are destroyed

Unfortunately, living tissue cannot withstand sterilization by known methods without irrevocable damage or loss of its own vitality. Therefore, while it would be advantageous to have the surgeon, operating room, patient, instruments, nurses, anesthetic equipment, and operating room air sterile, this is not practical by present means. For this reason, each of the preceding is cleaned and treated with antiseptics or disinfectants, or draped, or sterilized by means applicable to that object. These methods will be reviewed in the following sections.

CLEANSING INSTRUMENTS

According to Lawrence and Block (1968), protein and other polymolecular structures, particularly when dry, can serve as a protective covering for microorganisms and prevent penetration of a sterilizing medium. Therefore, to allow penetration by heat or chemicals, surgical instruments must first be scrupulously cleaned of all debris including blood, saliva, and necrotic material.

Time-consuming and careful scrubbing by hand may be necessary to clean certain instruments such as bone burs or bone files, where solid particles are wedged into small crevices. Usually a stiff wire brush will facilitate the cleaning. However, the greatest portion of the cleaning procedure can be managed by ultrasonic cleaning devices. These devices act by converting electrical energy into vibratory sound waves, which then pass through a soap solution containing the instruments to be cleaned (Rubbo and Gardner, 1965). In a process termed "cavitation," microscopic bubbles rapidly form and then collapse on the instrument surfaces, creating a suction that removes the debris.

Soaps and detergents are commonly used to aid in the removal of debris from instruments. Soaps are the salts of fatty acids and detergents are synthetic compounds. The Drug and Therapeutics Bulletin (1966) states that both groups act by reducing surface tension along the instrument surface, allowing emulsification of the contaminants, which can then be removed in the rinsing phase. Soaps possess a very small amount of antibacterial activity, chiefly against some gram-positive organisms. According to Accepted Dental Therapeutics (1975), soaps are only effective at pH 9 or higher, and even in a weakly acidic environment or in one containing the soluble salts of calcium or magnesium, precipitation of the soap will occur. Detergents, however, are compatible with calcium and magnesium ions and maintain their efficacy in neutral or slightly acidic solutions. Some deter-

gents possess bactericidal activity against some specific gram-positive organisms. For example, sodium lauryl sulphate (Dreft) is effective against *Streptococcus pneumoniae*, and this property can be used in the laboratory to identify the organism. However, the spectrum of antibacterial activity of the detergents is too narrow to classify them as disinfectants.

Other fat solvent solutions such as acetone, ether, and xylene are sometimes used in cleaning. These are relatively expensive, caustic to living tissues, and probably less effective in overall cleaning ability than soaps and detergents.

Some disinfectant solutions, such as the aldehyde and the phenolic compounds, are also used in instrument cleaning. These will be discussed fully in the following section. It must be remembered that these solutions should be thoroughly rinsed from the instrument surfaces prior to use because of their toxicity to living tissues.

DISINFECTANTS

Alcohols

Ethanol and isopropyl alcohols are overused as disinfectants. They are more frequently and correctly used as antiseptics (see p. 350). Alcohols possess some antibacterial activity, particularly in the gram-positive spectrum and especially against *Mycobacterium tuberculosis*. They act by denaturing protein. Spores and viruses are generally unaffected by the alcohols. Spaulding (1939) found that to reach maximum effectiveness, the alcohol must have at least a 10-minute contact with the organisms. Solutions of 70% alcohol are thought to be more effective than higher concentrations, because the presence of water speeds the protein denaturation process (Lawrence and Block, 1968). Since they evaporate so quickly, the alcohols do not function as disinfectants when instruments, handpieces, or other equipment are simply wiped with them. They are corrosive to carbon steel, and instruments of this composition should not be soaked in alcoholic solutions. Rubber articles absorb alcohol, and prolonged soaking can cause a reaction when the article subsequently comes in contact with living tissue. Alcohols can dissolve cements holding instruments together, and plastics may harden or swell in their presence.

Aqueous quaternary ammonium compounds

Benzalkonium chloride (Zephiran) is one of the most common aqueous quaternary ammonium compounds and is used both as an antiseptic and as a disinfectant. According to Neugeboren and co-workers (1972), its antibacterial spectrum is similar to the alcohols, being limited largely to gram-positive organisms and some gram-negative organisms. However, it is not effective against spores, viruses, and *Mycobacterium tuberculosis*. Hotchkiss (1946) noted that this molecule is a strong surfactant that increases the permeability of the bacterial wall and permits the escape of phosphorous and nitrogen. It also denatures intracellular protein. Recent reviews and reports by Dixon and co-workers (1976), Kaslow, Mackel, and Mallison (1976), and Frank and Shaffner (1976) have implicated quaternary ammonium compounds contaminated with Pseudomonas, Enterobacter, and other gram-negative organisms with outbreaks of nosocomial infection in different areas of the country. Hospital and office personnel too often assume that liquid disinfectants will sterilize treated objects. However, disinfectants, when used optimally, will merely reduce surface contamination to levels unlikely to be hazardous. Because the effectiveness of these compounds depends on strength, activity, and duration of contact, even this goal may not be reached. Additionally, these solutions may be contaminated with pathogens. Therefore, while disinfectants are valuable tools in reducing contamination, danger exists in overexpansion of their indications for use.

Phenolic compounds

Phenolic compounds are one of the oldest groups of disinfectants, having been used by Joseph Lister in the form of carbolic acid. Phenol itself is toxic to the skin and bone marrow. Substituted phenolic compounds (Amphyl, O-Syl, Staphene, Ves-Phene) have been developed to reduce these side effects, but they are still toxic to living tissues. None of these compounds are sporicidal at room temperature, but they are active against many viruses, fungi, and bacteria (Lawrence and Block, 1968). These compounds are often used for disinfection of walls, floors, and furniture. They may cause damage to some plastics, and they do corrode certain metals, such as brass, aluminum, and carbide steel.

Aldehyde compounds

Aldehyde compounds such as aqueous formaldehyde (formalin) and glutaraldehyde (Cidex) are very effective disinfectants. Formalin is not popular because of its noxious odor and because contact of 18 to 30 hours is necessary for cidal action. Glutaraldehyde will kill vegetative bacteria, spores, fungi, and perhaps all viruses by alkylation on 10-hour contact (Stonehill, Krop, and Borick, 1963). Its effectiveness against the hepatitis viruses is not proven, but the Center for Disease Control now includes it in a list of effective agents against these viruses. Glutaraldehyde is toxic and irritating and therefore is not used on certain surfaces such as furniture, walls, and floors. It may be safely used on metal instruments (for less than 24 hours), rubber, plastics, and porcelain. It is activated by the addition of sodium bicarbonate, but in its activated form it retains potency for only 14 days. Prior to patient exposure, the instruments must be thoroughly rinsed with sterile water or alcohol to remove the compound. Therefore porous objects that come in contact with patients should probably not be disinfected with these compounds because of the difficulty in removing them.

METHODS OF STERILIZATION

Heat is the most common and one of the most effective methods of sterilization. Heat may be transmitted through the air, water, or oil. The temperature reached by these modalities is important when calculating the time necessary for sterilization, but properties such as the penetration ability and the heat of vaporization are also important. For example, at a temperature of 121° C, it takes 2000 times longer to kill *Bacillus subtilis* in dry heat than with steam heat (Lawrence and Block, 1968). This difference is attributable to the greater penetrating ability of moist heat.

Boiling water

Water maintains and conducts heat extremely well. Moist heat kills microorganisms by coagulation of their protein. Boiling water at normal atmospheric pressure will produce a temperature of 100° C. While exposure to this temperature for 10 minutes will kill many bacteria, time periods of up to 24 hours may be necessary to kill bacterial spores, and even this prolonged time will not kill many viruses. For this reason, boiling water is not recommended for sterilization of tissue penetrating instruments.

Steam heat

Saturated steam under pressure is the most effective and practical method of sterilization. At a 15 psi pressure, the temperature of steam can reach 121.5° C. Once the objects to be sterilized reach this temperature, only 10 to 12 minutes are needed to kill all living organisms. Higher temperatures at greater pressures can be obtained, and this will shorten the time necessary for sterilization. For example, at 29.4 psi, a temperature of 134° C can be reached, and 3 minutes is all that is required for sterilization. This process, termed "flash sterilization," has practical use in the operating room where fast sterilization of instruments may be necessary.

The time needed to sterilize a particular item also varies with the amount of material and thickness of the wrap. Perkins (1969) has written a thorough discussion of instrument wrapping technique and the placement of packs within the autoclave. It should be remembered that the killing of microorganisms is not instantaneous but rather follows a logarithmic curve versus time. Usually 20 to 30 minutes are used in autoclave sterilization to provide a margin of safety. Liq-

uids may also be sterilized by autoclave, providing their contents will not be inactivated by the temperatures reached. Rubber and plastic goods may melt or be damaged so that alternative methods may have to be used. To avoid or minimize the corrosive action of the steam on metals, Crawford and Oldenburg (1967) recommend the addition of ammonia to the autoclave. Accepted Dental Therapeutics (1977) recommends dicyclohexylammonium nitrite or cyclohexylamine and decylamine. Bertolotti and Hurst (1978) have found 2% sodium nitrate to be effective.

Oil

Hot oil baths have been used to sterilize metallic instruments. The oil can reach a temperature of 175° C, and after the instruments reach this temperature, 15 minutes of submersion is necessary for sterilization. To ensure the temperature conversion of the instruments, often 1 hour or more of submersion is used. However, oil has poor penetration properties and poor sporicidal activity, presents a fire hazard, and is difficult to remove from instruments such as handpieces without recontamination. It should never be used on hypodermic syringes or needles because of the danger of oil embolization.

Dry heat

The hot air oven may be used to sterilize items that will not be damaged by the high temperatures that are generated. Usually 160° C for 2 hours is necessary to accomplish sterility. The long time period is necessary, according to Kelsey (1969), because of the poor heat conduction by air and the poor penetration properties of dry heat. Dry heat kills by dehydration and oxidation. It does not penetrate grease, oil, and powders, and equipment containing these substances should be sterilized by other means. One proposed advantage of this method is the maintenance of sharp edges on cutting instruments. However, Custer and Coyle (1970) found that carbon steel instruments can lose their hardness during dry heat sterilization.

Another method of dry heat sterilization employs a heat transfer device. Glass beads, molten metal, and salt are media that are used. Temperatures of 220° C can be reached, and submersion of small instruments such as endodontic files may produce sterility in 10 seconds, providing the instrument is clean. Oliet, Sorin, and Brown (1958) reported that temperatures vary in different areas of the sterilizer. To ensure uniform temperatures in these sterilizers, a warm-up time of at least 20 minutes is recommended. Even then, gradients of up to 140° C in salt and glass bead sterilizers have been noted. Grossman (1974) recommends salt media sterilization over the others because the accidental introduction into the root canal of metal or glass clinging to the endodontic instruments could cause blockage.

Gas

Ethylene oxide, a gas at temperatures above 10.8° C, is a highly toxic compound that destroys organisms by alkylation. It is very flammable, but when it is mixed with carbon dioxide or Freon this danger is minimized. It is an excellent sterilizer of articles that are susceptible to damage by heat, but it is highly toxic and will blister living tissues on contact. The time that the gas must be in contact with the material to be sterilized is dependent on temperature, humidity, pressure, and the amount of material. Once exposed to the gas, some objects such as plastic require 1 to 7 days to degas (Roberts and Rendell-Baker, 1972). This process may be hastened by warming the objects during the degasing period.

As noted by McLundie and co-workers (1968), formaldehyde can also be used as a gas sterilization agent, but it is less popular than ethylene oxide because of its odor.

Irradiation

Ionizing radiation, such as x-rays, gamma rays, and high-speed electrons, or nonionizing radiation in the form of ultraviolet light can be used to kill or inactivate microorganisms. Ionizing radiation has great penetrating properties and is commonly used by industry to sterilize disposable materials such as needles, suture material, cannulas, and pharmaceuticals sensitive to heat (Bellamy, 1959). According to the Radiosterilization of Medical Products and Recommended Code of Practice (1967), much more radiation is necessary to kill microorganisms than that which would be lethal to man. However, no residual radiation remains on materials treated in this manner, and it is very effective for heat labile items.

Nonionizing radiation, such as ultraviolet light, is used most commonly to purify air, such as in the operating room. As reported by the International Atomic Energy Agency (1967), the purine and pyrimidine bases of the nucleic acids absorb this light energy causing excitation. Adjacent thymine bases combine covalently to form dimers that prevent unwinding of the DNA helix during replication. The optimal lethal wave length for this type of irradiation is 2650 Angstroms. Although ultraviolet sterilization is effective, it has no penetrating ability and is largely limited in the medical field to air sterilization and the preparation of immunizing antigens by viral or bacterial attenuation.

ANTISEPTICS

To be tolerated by living tissues, antimicrobial chemicals must be less toxic than the disinfectants or agents used for sterilization and as a result they are generally less effective. However, relatively effective agents with good antibacterial activity, notably the iodophor compounds, have been developed and should be used whenever possible.

Alcohols

Alcohols are frequently used for skin antisepsis prior to needle puncture. They are good organic solvents and their benefit is derived primarily from their cleansing action. To be antibacterial, the alcohol must have prolonged contact with the organisms. Its rapid evaporation prevents this contact and eliminates the possibility of chemical buildup on repeated usage. In a study by Price in 1939, alcohol was found effective in a 1-minute scrub compared with the other products available at that time. However, the use of hexachlorophene and iodophor compounds has been shown to be much more effective in reducing the bacterial contamination of skin. Alcohol is sometimes used as a rinse following a surgical scrub, but again its effectiveness lies in its solvent action and not its antibacterial properties. In addition, this technique may suffer the disadvantage of removing the soap solution from the skin, which would ordinarily have remained and retarded the regrowth of resident skin flora during the operation.

Aqueous quaternary ammonium compounds

Benzalkonium chloride (Zephiran) is the aqueous quaternary ammonium compound most commonly used as an antiseptic. Its antimicrobial activity is primarily against gram-positive bacteria. Reliance on it as a sterilizing medium has resulted in many iatrogenic infections. It is well tolerated by living tissues, but because of the narrowness of its activity spectrum, its use is not widespread.

Hexachlorophene

Hexachlorophene compounds have been used for many years for surgical scrubs and preoperative preparation of the surgical site. They are particularly effective against gram-positive organisms. They are less effective against gram-negative organisms and fungi and are not effective against viruses, spores, and *Mycobacterium tuberculosis*. Their popularity was established at a time when gram-positive organisms were held accountable for most infections, but because of the increase in gram-negative infections, the reliance on these antiseptics may be obsolete. When skin is cleansed with any agent, a reduction in surface bacteria is observed. However, bacteria in crevices and follicles will begin multiplying immediately. Studies by Best and coworkers (1950) and Lowbury and Lilly (1960) have shown that repeated scrubs will allow the hexachlorophene to build up on the skin and cause a reduction in the skin bacterial

counts. Harber, Targovnik, and Baer (1967) reported that hexachlorophene solutions are susceptible to bacterial contamination. Smylie, Webster, and Bruce (1959) have shown that hexachlorophene, to be fully effective, must be applied to dry skin because the combination of water and protein will precipitate it. Because of studies linking central nervous system edema with repeated hexachlorophene use, the Federal Drug Administration in 1976 disapproved it as a routine bathing solution in nurseries, where it had been used prophylactically to prevent staphylococcal skin infections. Despite these disadvantages, the hexachlorophene compounds are a valuable surgical preparation solution for patients who are sensitive to iodine.

Iodophor compounds

According to Joress (1962), Close and co-workers (1964), and Crowder and co-workers (1967), the most effective antiseptics are the iodophor compounds. In them, iodine is complexed with organic surface-active agents such as polyvinylpyrrolidone (Betadine, Isodine). Their activity depends on the release of the iodine from the complex. The surface agent is film forming, which prevents the solution from staining clothes or skin. Because of this complexing action, skin sensitivity to the iodine is not a major problem (Boswick, Kissell, and Metzger, 1961). These compounds exhibit an effective activity against most bacteria, spores, viruses, and fungi. While no antiseptic will produce sterility when applied to skin, the compound remaining on the skin will help keep the bacterial count low. Geraci (1963) has shown that the iodophor compounds build up on the skin after successive scrubs and that this provides long-lasting antibacterial activity.

THE HAND SCRUB

The surgeon begins his efforts at aseptic technique with the hand scrub. Wise and co-workers (1959) have shown that 20% to 30% of surgeons' gloves are punctured at the end of an average operation.

Cole and Bernard (1964) have document-ed the outpouring of bacteria from the surgeon's hand into the wound once a puncture in the glove was made. Because the gloves of an oral surgeon are frequently punctured or ripped while working with wire or instruments, clean hands beneath the gloves are imperative. The purposes of the hand scrub are to remove superficial contaminants and loose epithelium and to reduce the bacterial count on the skin. Probably these purposes are largely accomplished by the mechanical action of the brush. However, with the use of the iodophor scrubbing solutions, the effectiveness of the scrub in reducing surface bacterial counts increases to 95% of accessible organisms (Selwyn and Ellis, 1972). Because about 20% of skin bacteria are inaccessible, residing in the follicles, crevices, and lipids of the skin, the residual antiseptic scrub solution also helps keep the surface bacterial count low.

Many techniques of hand scrub have been suggested, but most are empirically based. Before beginning the hand scrub, the nails should be checked for cleanliness. All gross subnail contamination should be removed with the use of a nail cleaner before the scrub continues. The arms are then wetted to several inches above the elbows. The hands are kept elevated above elbow height so that the direction of water flow will be toward the elbows.

Many hospitals use prepackaged disposable scrub brushes already impregnated with soap solutions, as advocated by Bornside and co-workers (1967), and others employ the reusable scrub brush with a soap dispenser. Whichever is used, the scrub begins at the tip of one finger of one hand. The long axis of the finger is then divided into four surfaces and 30 scrub strokes are applied to each surface. After this is done, the interfinger webbing is given 30 strokes and the next finger is begun and so on until the fingers of one hand are completed. Then the ventral, dorsal, and lateral surfaces of the hand are cleaned. The length of the forearm is divided into thirds, and each of the four surfaces is scrubbed progressing by

thirds toward the elbow. The scrub should extend to 2 inches above the elbow. Once one hand and arm are completed, the surgeon then scrubs the other hand and arm in a like manner, beginning at the fingertips and working toward the elbow. When one area is scrubbed it should not be touched again because of the possibility of contamination from an unscrubbed area. Dunphy and Way (1973) recommend that the scrubbing procedure should take approximately 10 minutes. Successive scrubs that day need last only 5 minutes, if no major contamination has been encountered.

After both arms are scrubbed, the brush is discarded and the arms are rinsed of excess soap. Most hospitals have foot or knee pedals for water control, but if the older faucet handles are being used, the surgeon must be careful not to contaminate the scrubbed areas of his arms while turning the water on and off with his elbow. The rinse should be done with elevated arms so that the water will drain from the fingertips progressing down the hands, arms, and finally the elbows. The hands and arms are not rubbed during the rinse, and only the superficial excess soap will be removed in the process. As shown by Dobson and Shulls (1967), the residual soap will provide about 3 hours of antibacterial action for the surgeon's hands.

The surgeon next approaches the scrub nurse for a drying towel. Under certain circumstances, the scrub nurse may not be present, or the drying towel may be placed on a separate stand requiring the surgeon to take the towel. Care should be exercised not to drip on or otherwise contaminate the instruments or other sterile materials. The technique of drying traditionally begins at the fingertips of one hand and progresses down the hand and arm. Then, using the opposite side of the towel, the other hand and arm are dried in a similar manner.

An alternative to hand scrubbing, proposed by Cutright and co-workers (1972), is a device utilizing pulsating water and soap lavage. With this method, the surgeon inserts his hands into the device and they are automatically cleaned in 90 seconds.

GLOVING

There are essentially two types of gloves presterilized for surgical use. The most common type is a clear latex glove. For those who are allergic to latex, there are brown milled rubber gloves. These are thinner than the latex gloves and may provide a better tactile sensation, but they are also more fragile and more frequent glove changes during the operation may be necessary.

Gloving usually begins with the right hand. If the surgeon is assisted by a scrub nurse, the glove will be extended for him to slip his hand into it. Fig. 10-1 demonstrates the donning of gloves when the surgeon is alone. In this case the left hand may be gloved first. The cuff of the glove is turned up, exposing the inner surface of the glove. Using the right hand, the cuff (inner surface) of the left glove is grasped and the glove is pulled on. The right hand glove is then lifted by inserting the fingers of the left glove on the inside (outer surface) of the rolled cuff of the right glove. The right hand is

inserted into the glove and the glove pulled into place.

PREPARATION OF THE SURGICAL SITE

Preparation of the surgical site is important to reduce contamination by the patient's own normal flora as well as resistant bacteria acquired from the hospital environment. The operative site cannot be sterilized by current methods, but the gross cleansing action does significantly reduce the incidence of postoperative infections. All extraoral procedures should be accompanied by a presurgical scrub. A circumoral preparation should precede intraoral procedures to prevent transference of the resident skin flora to the intraoral wound. The same antiseptic solutions are available for skin preparation prior to surgery that are available for the hand scrub. The iodophor compounds are by far the most effective solutions for the skin preparation and, as shown by Prigot and Roc (1962), they do not interfere with wound healing. Hexachlorophene solutions, while less effective, are also good. Again, patient sensitivities may dictate the use of one or another solution or even plain soap.

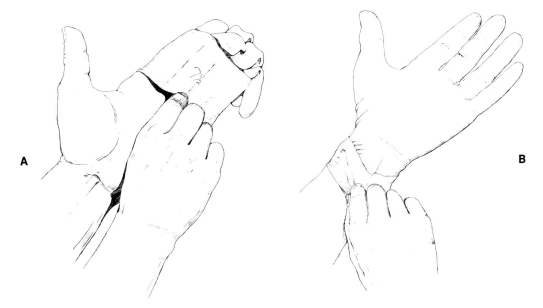

A **B**

Fig. 10-1. A, Right hand grasps inside cuff surface of left glove. **B,** Left glove is pulled into place.
Continued.

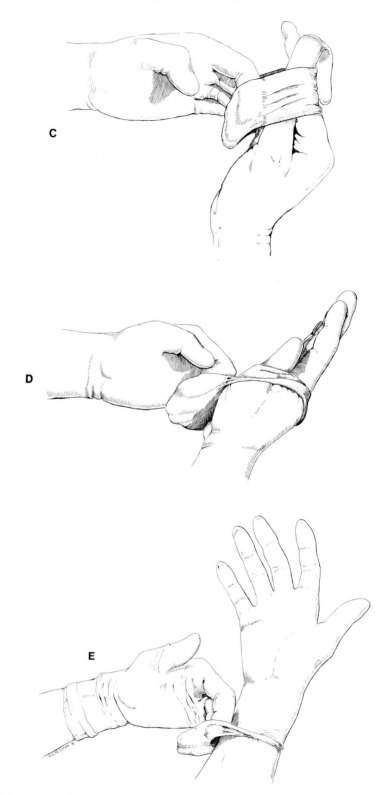

Fig. 10-1, cont'd. C, Gloved fingers of left hand are inserted into cuff (outer surface) of right glove. **D,** Right glove is pulled into place. **E,** Cuff of left glove is unfolded.

Before the preparation, a lubricating ointment should be applied to the patient's eyes and the eyes taped shut. Also, if bleeding in proximity to the ear is anticipated, the external auditory meatus should be gently capped with petroleum jelly–impregnated gauze.

If there is hair in the surgical area, it is generally removed just prior to scrubbing the skin. Shaving the area the night before produces small abrasions on the skin and resident bacteria multiply as a result of the injury. This phenomenon is lessened by decreasing the time interval between the shave and the skin preparation. Some surgeons feel the close shave is unnecessary, and indeed in some surgical sites such as the eyebrow the shave is never done routinely.

The scrub should begin in the center of the area to be prepared and then move outward concentrically, if possible. Preparing the central part first and then successive areas away from the operative site will minimize contamination of the already cleansed region from an unscrubbed one. Once the center has been scrubbed it should not be touched again with the same sponge. The surgeon may choose to scrub the area a second time with a new sterile sponge, but this process must again start in the middle and extend toward the periphery. The skin preparation should take about 5 minutes unless the area is grossly contaminated.

Intraoral preparation before surgery traditionally has not been done because of the improbability of significantly reducing the bacterial count of the mouth. However, studies by Zinner, Jablon, and Saslaw (1961), Jones and co-workers (1970), Scopp and Orvieto (1971), and Cutcher and co-workers (1971) have shown remarkable reduction in bacteremia during tooth extraction following preparation with iodophor or phenol-alcohol mouth rinses. This bacteremia-reducing capability does not seem to be merely a function of the mechanical cleansing action of the rinse, because researchers have found that cetylpyridinium (Huffman et al., 1974) and vancomycin (Bartlett and Howell, 1973) rinses did not reduce the incidence of postextraction bacteremias. While these transient bacteremias may not be of great importance in normal patients, this preparation is very important in patients with histories of rheumatic heart disease, prosthetic heart valves, prosthetic hip replacements and shunts for dialysis, and in patients on immunosuppressive therapy or with other debilitating conditions.

OPERATING ROOM PROCEDURES

The operating room is merely a clean environment in which to do surgery. It is not sterile. The ceiling, walls, and floors are regularly disinfected, especially following a contaminated case. The air may be filtered or flow past an ultraviolet radiation device to reduce bacterial counts. The operating rooms are set away from the hospital by two sets of doors. People are required to remove their street clothes and don scrub suits before entering the operating room area. Masks, gowns, gloves, and special shoes or shoe covers are worn during the operation. The patient and surgical site are draped and isolated. The surgical instruments and related equipment are sterile. All these precautions tend to reduce the chance of wound contamination, but still the operative site is only clean, not sterile.

The scrub suit consists of a pair of pants or skirt and a shirt or blouse, which should be tucked inside. A cap is placed over the hair. If the surgeon has long hair, surgical hoods are available and should be used. A mask is then tied in place over the surgeon's nose and mouth. Conductive shoes should also be worn. These shoes will prevent the buildup of static electricity, which could cause a spark and subsequent explosion involving the volatile inflammable anesthestic gases. The shoes also lessen the chance of patient electrocution. Today the many electrical devices surrounding and attached to the patient in the operating room are potential sources of electrical shock. According to Arbeit, Parker, and Reuben (1972), one tenth of a milliampere of a 60 cycle per second current can produce ventricular fibrillation. By wearing conductive shoes, the surgeon becomes an alternate pathway for aberrant currents. If conduc-

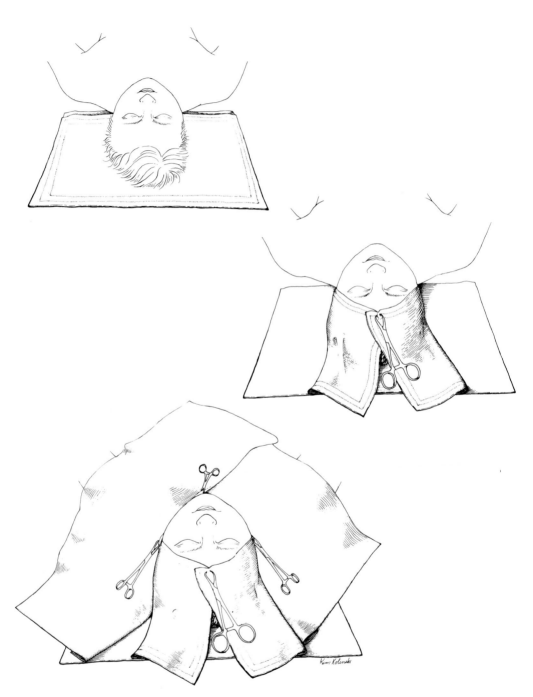

Fig. 10-2. Patient's head is placed on sterile sheet covered by two towels. Towels are used to drape patient's head. Additional towels may then be added to isolate surgical area.

tive shoes are not available, the surgeon must use conductive shoe covers. These have a conductive string that runs along the bottom of the shoe cover and exits at the heel. This string should be tucked inside the surgeon's sock next to the skin to ensure conductivity.

After entering the operating theater and before gowning, personnel should take precautions to avoid contaminating open packs of draping material or instruments. Contact should not be made with any person who is scrubbed and gowned. Once the patient is prepared and draped, only those who are scrubbed, gowned, and gloved may work in the surgical site. The backs of those gowned are considered nonsterile, as are areas below the waist. Therefore one must be careful to keep the arms above the waist when resting and not to back into any sterile areas. Also, one must remember that the mask and surgical cap are not sterile, and these can contaminate any sterile object they touch. Some hospitals have sterilizable handles that may be attached to the light so the surgeon may adjust it, but when these are not available, the light must be adjusted by the operating room personnel not scrubbed for the case.

DRAPING THE PATIENT

The purpose of draping a patient is to isolate the surgical area from other parts of the body that have not been prepared for surgery and also from nonsterile operating room equipment and personnel. A double-layered drape is usually considered necessary for effective isolation. One of the main problems in draping for oral surgery procedures is to effectively isolate the nose and mouth from the surgical field, since these contain a multitude of bacteria and contaminants.

A frequently used type of head drape is illustrated in Fig. 10-2. Its advantage over other types is the presence of a sterile drape around the patient's head, which lies against another sterile drape over the operating table. This will allow the patient's head to be turned from side to side without contamination. To apply this drape without displacing the endotracheal tube, it is suggested that the

anesthesiologist temporarily disconnect the tube from the anesthesia machine so that the patient's head may be lifted and the drape placed beneath. An additional two, three, or four towel drape is then placed over the endotracheal tube and adjacent unscrubbed areas to complete the isolation of the surgical site.

An effective way of isolating the mouth from the surgical site is by using a clear plastic drape with an adhesive side (ViDrape), as illustrated in Fig. 10-3. Raahave (1974) has demonstrated the efficacy of this barrier to bacterial contamination. The adhesive is pressed tightly around the lower face and lower lip, preventing saliva from flowing onto the surgical sites when bilateral extraoral procedures are done and the head is turned from side to side. It also allows entrance to the mouth by simply pulling the drape over as illustrated, and re-isolation of the nose and mouth by returning the drape to its original position. When draping for a minor intraoral procedure, the drape illustrated in Fig. 10-4 may be sufficient.

OFFICE PROCEDURES

The office of the oral and maxillofacial surgeon presents special problems in the maintenance of sterility, particularly for hinged instruments, the dental handpiece, and the storage of anesthetic cartridges. Disposable needles have been used regularly for many years, and their use has significantly reduced the transfer of infection. Sterile disposable gloves are another important method for the reduction of infection and particularly the transfer of hepatitis B between patients and between patient and surgeon.

The storage of anesthetic cartridges is still an unsolved problem. Shannon and Feller (1972) showed that when cartridges were stored in alcohol, the alcohol penetrated them and, when subsequently injected, could potentially cause permanent nerve damage. Heat sterilization does not inactivate local anesthetics (Bridenbaugh and Moore, 1964), but damage can occur to the rubber plunger and its coating within the cartridge.

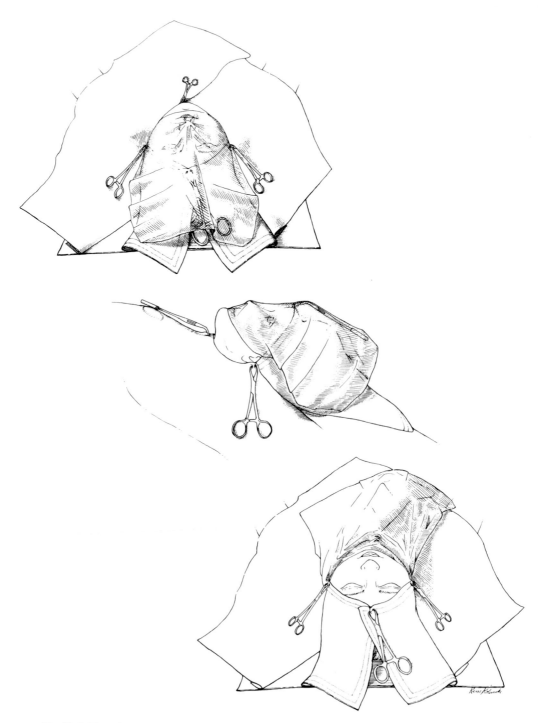

Fig. 10-3. Clear drape is placed with adhesive surface contacting skin just below mouth, which effectively isolates it from surgical site. Mouth or nasal area may be entered by pulling drape forward and then reisolated by returning drape to its original position.

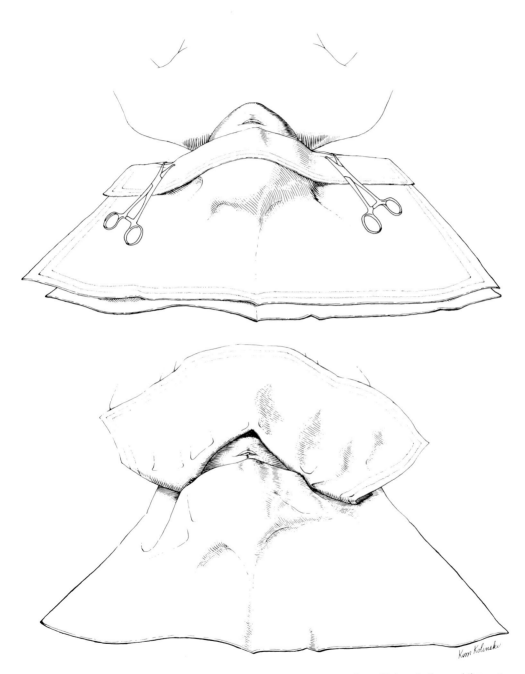

Fig. 10-4. Two towels with edges folded to outside are joined together with towel clips and then unfolded to create opening through which operator may enter oral cavity.

Maintaining sterility of the dental handpiece was recognized by Ham, Patterson, and Healey (1970) as a tremendous problem. During use, saliva, bone debris, bacteria, and other contaminants are sucked into the inner workings of the handpiece. Cleaning of most commercially available handpieces is difficult. Once the handpiece is cleaned, sterilization is still a problem, as only a few marketed handpieces are autoclavable. Autoclaving also increases corrosion and makes subsequent cleaning more difficult. The handpieces must also be lubricated after sterilization and before use, which is an opportunity for contamination. Immersion in boiling oil has been advocated for handpiece sterilization, but the oil that collects in the inner workings of the handpiece is impossible to remove and invariably ends up dripping into the surgical site. Many oral and maxillofacial surgeons rely on disinfectants for preparing their handpieces for surgery, but this is not a laudable practice.

According to Crump (1966), instrument storage is also a problem. In many offices the sterilized instruments are stored in drawers or other containers and in others they are stored in packs or on sterilized trays. The maintenance of sterility between the time of autoclaving and placement in storage, as well as during storage, is paramount.

Many times the oral and maxillofacial surgeon relies on the use of prophylactic antibiotics to prevent postoperative infections when there is really no specific indication. This is a misuse and overutilization of antibiotics, and it can contribute to the development of resistant bacterial strains. It is imperative that surgeons understand that the use of the techniques discussed in this chapter is a much safer and more effective method of reducing postoperative morbidity.

REFERENCES

Accepted dental therapeutics. 1977. Chicago, American Dental Association.

Ad Hoc Committee of the Committee on Trauma, Division of Medical Sciences, National Academy of Science–National Research Council. 1964. Postoperative wound infections: the influence of ultra-violet irradiation of the operating room and of various other factors, Ann. Surg. Suppl. **160**:1.

Arbeit, S. R., Parker, B., and Rubin, I. R. 1972. Controlling the electrocution hazard in the hospital, J.A.M.A. **220**:1581.

Bartlett, R. C., and Howell, R. M. 1973. Topical vancomycin as a deterrent to bacteremias following dental procedures, Oral Surg. **35**:780.

Bellamy, W. D. 1959. In Umbreit, W. W., ed.: Advances in applied microbiology, New York, Academic Press, Inc., p. 49.

Bertolotti, R. L., and Hurst, V., 1978. Inhibition of corrosion during autoclave sterilization of carbon steel dental instruments, J. Am. Dent. Assoc. **97**:628.

Best, R. R., et al. 1950. Effectiveness of soaps containing hexachlorophene for the surgical scrub, Arch. Surg. **61**:869.

Bornside, G. H., et al. 1967. Disposable hexachlorophene impregnated polyurethane scrub brushes, Ann. Surg. **166**:129.

Boswick, J. A., Kissell, E., and Metzger, W. I. 1961. Laboratory and clinical studies of a new presurgical skin antiseptic, J. Abdom. Surg. **3**:157.

Bridenbaugh, L. D., and Moore, D. C. 1964. Does repeated heat sterilization of local anesthetic drugs affect potency? Anesthesiology **25**:372.

Close, A. S., et al. 1964. Preoperative skin preparation with povidone-iodine, Am. J. Surg. **108**:398.

Cole, W., and Bernard, H. 1964. Inadequacies of present methods of surgical skin preparation, Arch. Surg. **89**:215.

Crawford, J. R., and Oldenburg, T. R. 1967. Practical methods of office sterilization and disinfection, J. Oral Med. **22**:133.

Crowder, V. H., et al. 1967. Bacteriological comparison of hexachlorophene and polyvinylpyrrolidone-iodine surgical scrub soaps, Am. Surg. **33**:906.

Crump, M. C. 1966. Cellulose dialysis tubing for the sterile storage of dental instruments, Oral Surg. **22**:658.

Cruse, P. J. E., and Foord, R. 1973. A five year prospective study of 23,649 surgical wounds, Arch. Surg. **107**:206.

Custer, F., and Coyle, T. 1970. Instrument changes during sterilization, J. Dent. Res. **49**:487.

Cutcher, J. L., et al. 1971. Control of bacteremia associated with extraction of teeth, Oral Surg. **31**:602.

Cutright, D. E., et al. 1972. A new method of presurgical hand cleansing, Oral Surg. **33**:162.

Dillon, M. L., Postelthwait, R. W., and Bowling, K. A. 1969. Operative wound cultures and wound infections: a study of 342 patients, Ann. Surg. **170**:1029.

Dixon, R. E., et al. 1976. Aqueous quaternary ammonium antiseptics and disinfectants, J.A.M.A. **236**:2415.

Dobson, T., and Shulls, W. A. 1967. A study of various surgical scrubs by glove counts, Surg. Gynecol. Obstet. **124**:57.

Drug and therapeutics bulletin. 1966. Special soaps and cleansers for the skin, **4**:81.

Dunphy, J. E., and Way, L. W. 1973. Current surgical diagnosis and treatment, Los Altos, Calif., Lange Medical Publications.

Elek, S. D., and Conen, P. E. 1957. The virulence of *Staphylococcus pyogenes* for man: a study of the problems of wound infection, Br. J. Surg. **38**:573.

Frank, W., and Shaffner, W. 1976. Contaminated aqueous benzalkonium chloride, J. A. M. A. **236**:2407.

Geraci, C. L. 1963. New iodine compound for degerming skin surface, Arch. Surg. **87**:560.

Grossman, L. I. 1974. Endodontic practice, Philadelphia, Lea & Febiger.

Ham, J. W., Patterson, S. S., and Healey, H. J. 1970. An evaluation of handpiece sterilization for periapical surgery, J. Oral Surg. **28**:353.

Harber, L. C., Targovnik, S. E., and Baer, R. L. 1967. Contact photosensitivity patterns to halogenated salicylanilides, Arch. Dermatol. **96**:646.

Hotchkiss, R. D. 1946. The nature of the bactericidal action of surface-active agents, Ann. N.Y. Acad. Sci. **46**:479.

Huffman, G. G., et al. 1974. The effects of preoperative rinsing with cetylpyridinium chloride on bacteremia associated with the surgical removal of impacted molars, Oral Surg. **38**:359.

Jepsen, O. B. 1973. Contamination of the wound during operation and postoperative wound infection, Ann. Surg. **177**:178.

Jones, J. C., et al. 1970. Control of bacteremia associated with extraction of teeth, Oral Surg. **30**:454.

Joress, S. M. 1962. A study of disinfection of the skin: a comparison of povidone-iodine with other agents used for surgical scrubs, Ann. Surg. **155**:296.

Kaslow, R. A., Mackel, D. C., and Mallison, G. F. 1976. Nosocomial pseudobacteremia, J.A.M.A. **236**:2407.

Kelsey, J. C. 1969. Sterilization and disinfection: objectives and perspectives, Ann. R. Coll. Surg. Engl. **44**:214.

Krizek, T. J., and Robson, M. C. 1975. Evolution of quantitative bacteriology in wound management, Am. J. Surg. **130**:579.

Lawrence, C. A., and Block, S. S. 1968. Disinfection, sterilization and preservation, Philadelphia, Lea & Febiger.

Lowbury, E. J. L., and Lilly, H. A. 1960. Disinfection of the hands of surgeons and nurses, Br. Med. J. **1**:1445.

Maki, D. G. 1976. Lister revisited: surgical antisepsis and asepsis, N. Engl. J. Med. **294**:1286.

McLundie, A. C. 1968. Sterilisation in general dental practice, Br. Dent. J. **124**:214.

Neugeboren, N., et al. 1972. Control of cross-contamination, J. Am. Dent. Assoc. **85**:123.

Oliet, S., Sorin, S., and Brown, H. 1958. A temperature analysis of thermostatically controlled root canal sterilizers using molten metal, glass beads, or salt, Oral Surg. **11**:37.

Patterson, A. M. 1932. Meaning of "antiseptic," "disinfectant," and related words, Am. J. Public Health **22**:465.

Perkins, J. J. 1969. Principles and methods of sterilization in health sciences, Springfield, Ill., Charles C Thomas, Publisher.

Price, P. B. 1939. Ethyl alcohol as a germicide, Arch. Surg. **38**:528.

Prigot, A., and Roc, S. 1962. An iodophor, alkyl, aryl, polyether alcoholester iodine complex, Am. J. Surg. **103**:589.

Raahave, D. 1974. Aseptic barriers of plastic to prevent bacterial contaminations of operation wounds, Acta Chir. Scand. **140**:603.

Radiosterilization of medical products and recommended code of practice, 1967. Vienna, International Atomic Energy Agency.

Roberts, R. B., and Rendell-Baker, L. 1972. Ethylene oxide sterilization, Anaesthesia **27**:237.

Rubbo, S., and Gardner, J. F. 1965. A review of sterilization and disinfection, London, Lloyd-Luke Medical Books, Ltd.

Scopp, I. W., and Orvieto, L. D. 1971. Gingival degerming by povidone-iodine irrigation: bacteremia reduction in extraction procedures, J. Am. Dent. Assoc. **83**:1294.

Selwyn, S., and Ellis, H. 1972. Skin bacteria and skin disinfection reconsidered, Br. Med. J. **1**:136.

Shannon, I. L., and Feller, R. P. 1972. Contamination of local anesthetic carpules by storage in alcohol, Anesth. Prog. **19**:6.

Smylie, H. G., Webster, C. V., and Bruce, M. L. 1959. "pHisoHex" and safer surgery. Br. Med. J. **2**:606.

Spaulding, E. H. 1939. Chemical sterilization of surgical instruments, Surg. Gynecol. Obstet. **69**:738.

Stonehill, A. A., Krop, S., and Borick, P. M. 1963. Buffered glutaraldehyde—a new chemical sterilizing solution, Am. J. Hosp. Pharm. **20**:458.

Wangensteen, O. H., Wangensteen, S. D., and Klinger, C. F. 1973. Some pre-Listerian post-Listerian antiseptic wound practices and the emergence of asepsis, Surg. Gynecol. Obstet. **137**:677.

Wise, R., et al. 1959. Environmental distribution of *Staphylococcus aureus* in operative suite, Ann. Surg. **149**:30.

Zinner, D. D., Jablon, J. M., and Saslaw, M. S. 1961. Bactericidal properties of povidone-iodine and its effectiveness as an oral antiseptic, Oral Surg. **14**:1377.

CHAPTER 11

Prevention and treatment of medical emergencies

Jerry E. Patterson

Managing the rare emergency situation in the oral and maxillofacial surgery office can be a frightening experience at best; however, this experience can quickly turn into a catastrophe if the doctor and his staff are not adequately prepared. Many emergency problems can be avoided by simple preventive measures, the best of which is an adequate patient history and examination, including vital signs. Knowledge of possible allergies, current medications, and major diseases is invaluable in planning surgery for an individual patient. The medical history should be reviewed periodically if the patient is being seen over a period of time. If after the history and examination any doubt exists about potential problems, the patient's physician should be contacted. The physician's letter or a note concerning the telephone conversation with the physician should be placed in the patient's record. If the patient does exhibit some disease state such as angina pectoris or diabetes, the condition should preferably be stable before elective work is performed.

In some cases, apprehension, fear, or anxiety may contribute to an adverse reaction. Dworkin (1973) showed that the strength of fear 1 hour before routine dental treatment in the office is the same as that prior to general surgery in a hospital setting. Relieving fear and anxiety, whether by reassurance, a calming attitude, good rapport, or drug therapy, may be an important preventive measure.

During any particular procedure, the doctor and his surgical team should closely observe the patient and be alert for the onset of a potential emergency. If an emergency does occur, it is best handled by a doctor and his staff who have practiced as a team in simulated emergencies. This includes the administration of cardiopulmonary resuscitation on appropriate mannequins and the actual handling of drugs and equipment so that all facets of emergency care are familiar to all personnel. A program for preparedness in anesthesia and medical emergency techniques similar to the one sponsored by the Southern California Society of Oral Surgeons is encouraged, as 98% of this program's participants thought the endeavor improved efficiency and dispatch in managing emergencies (Hagen et al., 1971). Courses conforming to American Heart Association standards and recommendations in basic life support (cardiopulmonary resuscitation) and advanced life support are also available and are excellent sources for increasing preparedness for emergencies.

Drugs and equipment should be checked periodically to ensure that the drugs are not outdated and that equipment is functioning properly (Fig. 11-1). Emergency telephone numbers, including those of a rescue squad or ambulance service, the local emergency room, and several neighboring physicians should be placed on the office telephone for ready access.

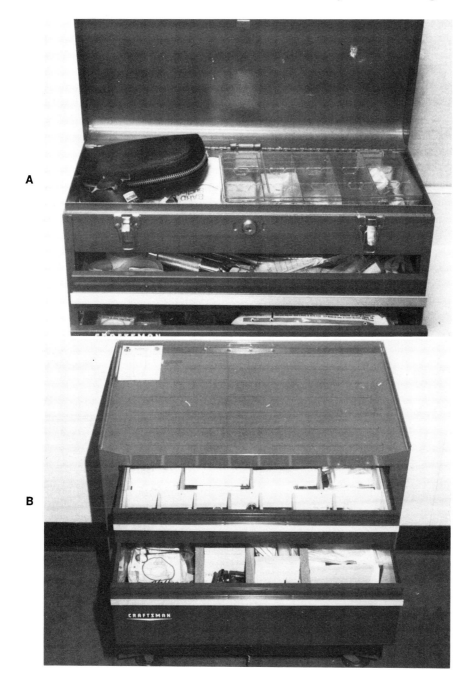

Fig. 11-1. Drugs and equipment should be stored in neat, orderly manner for quick and easy access. Tackle box, **A,** will suffice; however, cart, **B,** will provide for more organized storage.

If in spite of the best preventive measures an emergency situation does arise, appropriate notes should be recorded later in the patient's chart concerning time of onset of the reaction, patient condition, including vital signs, drugs administered, and other therapy rendered.

Commonly used emergency drugs and equipment that should be kept in a readily available place in the office are listed below.

Emergency drugs
A. Oxygen
B. Aromatic ammonia
C. Nitroglycerine tablets 1/200 gr; amyl nitrite (Vaporole)
D. Diphenhydramine HCl (Benadryl) 50 mg/ml
E. Atropine, 0.5 mg/5 ml prefilled syringe or 0.4 mg/ml or 0.5 mg/ml vial
F. Epinephrine (Adrenalin 1:1000 dilution, 1 ml ampule (1 mg), 1:10,000 dilution, 10 ml prefilled syringe (1 mg)
G. Vasopressors
   1. Phenylephrine (Neo-Synephrine), 10 mg/ml
   2. Methoxamine (Vasoxyl), 10 mg/ml or 20 mg/ml
   3. Norepinephrine (Levophed), 0.2%, 4 ml ampule (8 mg)
   4. Ephedrine, 50 mg/ml
   5. Mephentermine (Wyamine), 15 mg/ml
   6. Metaraminol (Aramine), 10 mg/ml
H. Sodium bicarbonate, 7.5%, 50 ml prefilled syringe (44.6 mEq) or 8.4%, 50 ml prefilled syringe (50 mEq)
I. Calcium chloride, 10%, 10 ml prefilled syringe (1 gm)
J. Lidocaine, 1%, 5 ml or 10 ml prefilled syringe (50 mg, 100 mg) or 2%, 5 ml prefilled syringe (100 mg)
K. Isoproterenol, 1 mg ampule
L. Morphine, 8 mg/ml, or 10 mg/ml, or 15 mg/ml
M. Meperidine (Demerol), 50 mg/ml
N. Steroids
   1. Methylprednisolone sodium succinate (Solu-Medrol), 40 mg or 125 mg Mix-O-Vial
   2. Hydrocortisone sodium succinate (Solu-Cortef), 100 mg or 250 mg Mix-O-Vial
O. Procaine (Novocain), 1%
P. Naloxone (Narcan), 0.4 mg/ml
Q. Diazepam (Valium), 5 mg/ml
R. Aminophylline, 250 mg/10 ml ampule
S. Sugar
   1. Sugar cubes or small packages, orange juice
   2. Dextrose, 50%, 50 ml vial
T. Glucagon, 1 mg (1 unit) dry powder with 1 ml diluent
U. Succinylcholine chloride, 20 mg/ml
V. Sterile water for injection, 30 ml vial

Emergency equipment
A. Equipment to administer oxygen
B. Oropharyngeal airways
C. Endotracheal tubes and connectors
D. Laryngoscope and blades
E. Suction catheter
F. Tonsillar suction tip and hose
G. Cricothyroid cannulae
H. Scalpel blades and handle
I. Needles
   1. 22 gauge
   2. 25 gauge
   3. Butterflies, 19 and 21 gauge
   4. Angiocath, 18 and 20 gauge
J. Syringes 1 ml, 5 ml, 10 ml, 50 ml
K. IV fluid (5% D/W; 5% D/S; lactated Ringer's solution) and administration set
L. Tourniquet
M. Stethoscope
N. Sphygmomanometer
O. Hemostats
P. Padded tongue blades
Q. Tape
R. K-Y jelly
S. Alcohol sponges

SYNCOPE
Problem

Syncope, literally meaning "cutting short," "cessation," or "pause" (Wintrobe, 1974) refers to a transient loss of consciousness secondary to cessation or a decrease in cerebral blood flow. Syncope (fainting, vasovagal syncope, vasodepressor syncope) is the most common untoward reaction seen in the dental office (ADA, 1975), with Hannington-Kiff (1969) reporting a 2% incidence of fainting among dental patients. It is perhaps more prevalent in younger people and some evidence tends to support the highest incidence in men under age 35 (Hannington-Kiff, 1969). The most common predisposing factors are fear, anxiety, and pain, but other factors such as grief, sight of blood, physical and mental exhaustion, hot environment, debility, fasting, and minor surgical procedures may also contribute (Chue, 1975b; Des Fourie, 1968). These factors trigger a vasodepressor reaction, with dilation of blood vessels in skeletal muscles being most significant but also occurring in the splanchnic region. A fall in peripheral resistance with decreased venous return to the heart results, leading to a fall in arterial pressure. Vagal reflexes are activated, causing bradycardia, a reduction in the cardiac output, and a further reduction in blood pressure, all leading to decreased cerebral perfusion.

Recognition

Syncope is almost always preceded by a prodrome lasting from seconds to several minutes during which the patient has a feeling of warmth, weakness, possible epigastric discomfort or nausea, and a general sense of "feeling badly." The patient then develops sweating, pallor, coldness of the extremities and dizziness, and there may be a slight increase in pulse and blood pressure. If treatment is promptly instituted, unconsciousness can be averted in many cases; Hannington-Kiff (1969) showed in his series that only 28% of syncopal attacks resulted in unconsciousness. However, without treatment at this stage the eventual outcome is unconsciousness with marked ashen gray pallor, shallow respirations, slow and weak pulse, low blood pressure, and dilated pupils. Sphincter tone is usually maintained and voluntary musculature is relaxed, although it is not unusual to see clonic jerks of the arms and twitching of the face shortly after the patient becomes unconscious (Thorn, 1977). Unconsciousness usually lasts a few seconds to a few minutes, but after recovering consciousness the patient, although mentally clear, may remain somewhat weak and nauseous for a period of time.

Treatment

The mainstay of treatment consists of placing the patient in a supine position with legs elevated to improve venous return to the heart. Tight constricting clothing should be loosened. In all instances a patent airway should be maintained, which may require removing foreign bodies from the mouth, suctioning of excessive salivary secretions, maintaining the lower jaw forward, and inserting an oropharyngeal airway. Although certain authors state that administration of oxygen is necessary only if the patient is cyanotic or dyspneic (Chue, 1975a), routine use of oxygen during syncopal attacks is preferable based on blood gas data showing hypoxemia during syncope (Campbell et al., 1976).

In addition to good arterial oxygen saturation, the patient also needs good perfusion to ensure that oxygenated blood is getting to the various tissues. Therefore vital signs should be checked as soon as possible and used along with clinical judgment in assessing recovery. The fall in blood pressure and pulse is usually transient, but if it remains at a low level for several minutes, further treatment should be instituted. Adjunctive therapy such as inhalation of aromatic spirits of ammonia or cold towels to the forehead may be helpful. If vital signs remain low despite these procedures, and especially if there is bradycardia, atropine (0.4 mg intravenously) should be administered. If hypotension persists despite the absence of bradycardia, the use of a vasopressor such as phenylephrine (Neo-Synephrine) or methoxamine HCl (Vasoxyl), which acts mainly by vasoconstriction, is appropriate. Neo-Synephrine, 2 to 5 mg, subcutaneously or intramuscularly, Neo-Synephrine, 0.2 mg slowly intravenously, or Vasoxyl, 5 mg intravenously or 15 mg intramuscularly should be administered. If at any time respiration or circulation ceases, one must be prepared to support these systems by positive pressure oxygen and cardiac compression (CPR).

Even though vasovagal syncope is the most common cause of "fainting" (Wayne, 1961), when unconsciousness persists longer than 8 to 10 minutes or complete recovery has not occurred in 15 to 20 minutes, one should begin to think of other causes of "fainting" rather than simple syncope. Differential diagnosis of fainting is covered in various publications (Chue, 1975b; Des Fourie, 1968; Friedberg, 1971; Friedberg, 1973; Harrison, 1973; Thorn, 1977; Wright and McIntosh, 1971). After a syncopal episode, the patient should be brought slowly from the supine to the sitting position to avoid recurrence of the problem.

Prevention

As syncope usually occurs in the sitting position, operating on patients in a dental chair in a supine or somewhat reclining position may be preventive in many cases. This is particularly true in patients with a previous history of fainting during dental treatment. Approximately 50% of patients undergoing syncopal attacks during dental appointments report previous episodes of fainting (Hannington-Kiff, 1969). Relieving fear and anxiety, whether by good rapport or sedative drugs, alleviating pain with adequate local anesthesia or general anesthesia as indicated, and reducing other predisposing factors such as sight of blood may also be helpful in preventing syncope. One should observe the patient during the procedure and be aware that the two most frequent times of syncopal attack in the office are during or immediately after injection of local anesthetics and during a surgical procedure. By early recognition, and therefore early treatment, many syncopal attacks may be abated before unconsciousness ensues.

HYPERVENTILATION

Problem

Hyperventilation is simply an increase in alveolar ventilation caused by abnormally rapid and deep breathing. Although hyperventilation may occur in various conditions, such as lesions of the central nervous system and metabolic acidosis, the form most likely to be seen in the office is hyperventilation syndrome caused by a state of anxiety. This is not a common emergency, but reports of hyperventilation during dental treatment (Lemmer, 1968; Naylor, 1959) require that one be knowledgeable of this syndrome.

Hyperventilation syndrome is often precipitated by anxiety, fear, excitement, nervousness, emotional stress, and psychoneurotic reactions, but it may also appear without obvious external cause. Although hyperventilation syndrome may occur in both sexes, it most often appears in women, especially those who are somewhat anxious and nervous (Chue, 1975a; Thorn, 1977).

Hyperventilation results in hypocapnia, a lowering of the $PaCO_2$. Rotsztain and co-workers (1970) showed in 14 healthy patients with a mean resting $PaCO_2$ of 37, that after 2 minutes of hyperventilation the $PaCO_2$ decreased to a mean of 19. Hypocapnia causes a reduc-

tion in cerebral blood flow by as much as one-third; the reduction probably being related to cerebral vasoconstriction (Corbett et al., 1971; Kety and Schmedt, 1946). Whether this reduction in cerebral blood flow actually causes hypoxic damage is debatable (Allen and Morris, 1962; Granholm, 1971; Litwin et al., 1970; Morgan and Ward, 1970; Murrin and Nagarajan, 1974; Riggs et al., 1972; Sugioka and Davis, 1960). However, the decrease in blood flow certainly could be of significance in patients with increased cerebral metabolic requirements, such as when there is fever or when there is already a diminished rate of cerebral perfusion, that is, arterial hypotension, cerebrovascular disease, or advanced age (Alexander et al., 1965). The effects of hypocapnia on the systemic circulation result in an increased blood flow through skeletal muscles (Jung et al., 1971) with a decrease in peripheral resistance, leading to a reduction in blood pressure in most instances (Burnum, 1974; Burnum et al., 1954; Garcia et al., 1971; Little and Smith, 1964). Other authors, however, have reported no significant blood pressure changes with hyperventilation (Kety and Schmedt, 1946).

The hypocapnia is also accompanied by a respiratory alkalosis, with the normal blood pH of 7.4 rising to 7.5 or 7.6 (Harrison, 1973). This respiratory alkalosis favors a decrease in ionized calcium levels (Seamonds et al., 1972), leading to muscular spasms and symptoms suggesting tetany.

Recognition

The patient initially complains of dizziness and difficulty in getting a breath. Cardiovascular symptoms such as palpitations and tightness or mild pain in the chest may appear. The patient may also complain of epigastric discomfort. Numbness, tingling, or paresthesia of the fingers, toes, and lips are commonplace, with muscular twitching, carpopedal spasms, and tetany resulting if hyperventilation does not cease. The patient may develop headache, faintness, fatigue, and even mental confusion and loss of consciousness if no treatment is rendered.

The attack lasts from a few minutes to hours.

Treatment

Treatment consists of placing the patient in a comfortable position and ensuring that a patent airway exists. Often an explanation of the problem, along with calming and reassuring the patient, may suffice to terminate the hyperventilation. If after explanation the patient continues to overbreathe, he should be instructed to breathe slowly and shallowly into a paper bag or Ambu mask and bag at the rate of approximately 10 times per minute. Breathing into a paper bag will increase the carbon dioxide content of the inspired air, tending to reverse the hypocapnia and alkalosis. Normally inspired air contains a carbon dioxide partial pressure of 0.3 mm Hg, but the air inside a paper bag after 15 to 20 breaths has a partial pressure of 43 ± 7 mm Hg (Riley, 1974). After symptoms abate, the patient should continue to breathe room air slowly and shallowly at the rate of 12 to 14 times per minute for 5 to 10 minutes.

Prevention

In prevention of future attacks, explanation of the pathophysiology of this syndrome is helpful. In fact, one may reproduce the signs and symptoms of hyperventilation by having the patient overbreathe for 2 to 3 minutes, or until symptoms begin, to convince him of the etiology of this condition. Reducing anxiety and fear by a calming manner or sedative drugs (Walters and Klein, 1970) may be in order, and careful observation for early recognition will usually allow treatment before symptoms become severe.

ALLERGIC REACTIONS
Problem

An allergic reaction to a drug results from an immunologic response by a patient who has become sensitized to the drug (antigen) through a prior exposure (see Chapter 6). Because drugs are low molecular weight compounds, they act as haptens and join with tissue proteins or polypeptides to become antigens, usually after metabolic degradation (Parker, 1975c).

Allergic reactions can be either cellular (delayed) or humoral (immediate). The cellular reaction is mediated by lymphocytes derived from the thymus gland (T-lymphocytes), which react directly with an antigen. These reactions are exemplified by the tuberculin skin test, many contact allergies, and the allograft rejection phenomenon. The humoral type of allergic reaction is mediated through serum antibodies (immunoglobulins) that are produced by lymphocytes derived from the bone marrow (B-lymphocytes). It is thought that the B-lymphocytes, after interacting with the antigen, differentiate into plasma cells, which then secrete the antibody (Thorn, 1977). The antigen-antibody reaction may cause damage to cells at the site of reaction or release pharmacologically active agents into the circulation. These agents in turn react at secondary sites, which in man usually involve smooth muscle and vascular tissue, causing clinical manifestations such as bronchospasm or vascular collapse. Mediators noted to cause smooth muscle contraction and increased vascular permeability include histamine, slow-reacting substance of anaphylaxis (SRS-A), and bradykinin. Other mediators also have contributory roles in the allergic phenomenon. These include basophil kallikrein of anaphylaxis, prostaglandins, platelet-activating factor (PAF), eosinophil chemotactic factor of anaphylaxis (ECF-A), and neutrophil chemotactic factor of anaphylaxis (NCF-A). Eosinophils are often found in increased numbers in allergic situations, and they appear to release a histaminase and also a phospholipase that can inactivate SRS-A and PAF (Hubscher, 1975; Thorn, 1977).

Humoral allergic responses may vary from a mild skin reaction to anaphylaxis, and although penicillin is the worst drug offender, almost every drug and material used in clinical dentistry and oral surgery has been implicated. This includes reactions to various antibiotics (Booth, 1972; Coates, 1963; Glauda et al., 1975; Hooley and Meyer, 1966), local anesthetics (Road, 1973; Shields, 1972; Wellins, 1969), preservatives in local anesthetics (Aldrete and Johnson, 1969), analgesics

(Phills and Perelmutter, 1974), and general anesthetics (Driggs and O'Day, 1972), as well as materials such as eugenol (Koch et al., 1973), periodontal dressings (Poulsom, 1974), chrome cobalt (Brendlinger and Tarsitano, 1970), mercury in amalgam (Wright, 1971), methyl methacrylate denture material (Danilewicz-Stysiak, 1971; Gote et al., 1972), and orthodontic rubber elastics (Everett and Hice, 1974).

Previous exposure to the drug in question is needed for an allergic response, but this may occur without the patient's awareness. An unnamed, unlabeled drug may have been previously prescribed, or the patient may have received a small amount of the drug in foods. The fact that the patient has taken a certain drug several times before without sequelae does not mean that an allergy to that drug cannot develop at subsequent exposure. The likelihood of this happening with a particular drug increases with duration and number of courses of therapy (Parker, 1975b).

However, persons may also lose their allergy to certain drugs when given an appropriate interval of time without additional exposure (Budd et al., 1964). Allergic reactions to drugs are more common in adults than children and more common with drugs administered parenterally than orally (Parker, 1975b). Atopic or allergic persons (those with asthma, hay fever, allergies to dusts, pollen, foods, drugs, and so forth) may have an increased tendency to develop drug allergies (Thorn, 1977) and an apparent increased susceptibility to anaphylactic reactions (Parker, 1975b).

Recognition

Allergic manifestations may involve skin reactions, drug fever, organ cytotoxicity, serum sickness, or anaphylaxis. This discussion, since it centers around emergencies, will be confined to situations needing acute therapy, namely, cutaneous, respiratory, and circulatory problems.

The most frequent manifestation of drug allergy is skin eruptions that may take any form including urticarial, bullous, erythematous, maculopapular, nodu-lar, edematous, or petechial. These lesions may be mild or severe, localized or diffuse, and can be accompanied by pruritis and edema. Similar lesions may occur on the mucous membranes. Angioneurotic edema (angioedema) may also occur and has a predilection for the facial areas, that is, lips, tongue, and eyelids, as well as the glottis and bronchi. Respiratory problems may consist of allergic rhinitis, edema, bronchospasm, wheezing, dyspnea, cyanosis, or asphyxia. Circulatory reactions run the gamut from pallor and mild hypotension to vascular collapse and irreversible shock (anaphylaxis).

Treatment

The interval between administration of the allergenic drug and appearance of symptoms is important because the shorter the period, the greater the chance of a serious reaction (Barnard, 1970). The patient should be treated as soon as possible.

Cutaneous symptoms

If symptoms are cutaneous and mild, an antihistamine should be prescribed orally. In more severe cases the intramuscular or intravenous route is preferable, using diphenhydramine HCl (Benadryl), 50 mg, or another suitable antihistaminic drug followed by oral tablets, such as Benadryl, 50 mg t.i.d., for several days. If cutaneous symptoms progress and extensive edema is present, epinephrine 1: 1000 (0.1 to 0.3 mg) should be injected subcutaneously or intramuscularly and may be repeated in 10 to 15 minutes if necessary. If the inciting material was injected intramuscularly, the epinephrine may be injected into the same area to help delay absorption of the drug.

Respiratory symptoms

If respiratory symptoms (bronchospasm and wheezing) are the most prominent, epinephrine is the drug of choice. Epinephrine is a bronchodilator and a vasopressor, has an antihistaminic action and interferes with further mediator release (Parker, 1975a). A dosage of 0.3 to 0.5 mg. (0.3 to 0.5 ml) 1: 1000 epinephrine should be given subcutaneously or intramuscularly (deltoid or ventral surface of the tongue) and repeated in 10 to 15 minutes, if necessary. A patent airway should be maintained at all times, oxygen administered, and, when indicated, respiration supported. An antihistaminic drug (that is, Benadryl, 50 mg, intramuscularly or intravenously) can be of some benefit after the preceding measures, and corticosteroids may be helpful after epinephrine and an antihistaminic drug have been given. Hydrocortisone (Solu-Cortef), 100 mg; methylprednisolone (Solu-Medrol), 40 mg; or dexamethasone (Decadron), 8 mg, intramuscularly or intravenously can be used. Steroids may require 1 hour or longer to work and therefore should be used only after epinephrine and antihistamines have been administered. If edema is severe and completely obstructing the glottic area, a cricothyroidotomy may have to be performed (see p. 372).

Circulatory symptoms

Moderate reactions involving the circulatory system may be treated the same as the respiratory symptoms just described. However, if the reaction is truly an anaphylactic shock with sudden cardiovascular collapse, the following regimen should be followed.

1. Place patient in supine position.
2. Maintain airway, breathing, and circulation.
3. Administer epinephrine 1:1000, 0.5 mg intramuscularly.*
4. Administer oxygen.
5. Monitor vital signs — respiration, pulse, blood pressure.
6. Titrate epinephrine, 0.2 to 0.3 mg, intravenously *slowly* if intravenous route is available.
7. Administer intravenous fluid rapidly (lactated Ringer's solution) if possible.

8. Administer antihistamine (Benadryl, 50 mg) intravenously, if possible, or intramuscularly.
9. Administer steroid (Solu-Cortef, 100 mg) intravenously, if possible, or intramuscularly.
10. Support respiration and circulation as required.
11. Put office emergency plan for medical consultation and ambulance into action when deemed advisable.
12. Be prepared to recognize and treat concomitant problems that may arise, that is, vomiting, convulsions, cardiac arrythmias.

Prevention

The single most important item in preventing an allergic reaction is an accurate history of previous allergies or drug reactions. Remember that allergic reactions are more likely to occur in atopic persons. Although the patient's version of an "allergic" episode in the past may represent an exaggeration or misinterpretation of a toxic or psychic reaction, it is best to place some credence in the patient's story until more evidence can be gathered. Persons with documented allergies should have their office or hospital charts so labeled.

One should have a valid indication for using a drug before prescribing it. Patients should be observed for period of time after administration of a drug in the office, especially when penicillin is given intramuscularly. One must remember certain cross-sensitivities and realize that patients allergic to penicillin G may react to other semisynthetic penicillins as well as cephalothins (Keflin). Testing for allergies may be reliable with some drugs, but since testing can be misleading and dangerous, it should be performed by someone competent in that particular area.

AIRWAY OBSTRUCTION BY FOREIGN BODY
Problem

Airway obstruction may be caused by swelling of the neck owing to infection or trauma, tumors growing in the air passages, unconsciousness causing the tongue to fall posteriorly and block the

---

*Note: Dosages of epinephrine used may be modified by severity of reaction, age of patient, cardiac status, and other concurrent medical problems such as hyperthyroidism or hypertension. In using intravenous epinephrine a 1:10,000 dilution may be advantageous, since it allows a more accurate dose determination than when small volumes are given: 0.1 mg (0.1 ml) of 1:1000 epinephrine = 0.1 mg (1 ml) of 1:10,000 epinephrine. Use of epinephrine should be stopped when the pulse rate exceeds 150 or becomes irregular.

pharynx, or foreign bodies at any level along the air passages. In most of these circumstances, one has time to plan airway management, but with complete obstruction from a foreign body an emergency situation arises that requires immediate action.

Airway obstruction may occur in the waiting room owing to food or partial dentures and in the operatory from various oral surgical instruments and materials, teeth, and vomitus. One may also find himself in the position of managing an airway obstruction outside the office situation, that is, in a restaurant with the so-called cafe coronary caused by choking on food. Inhalation of food is now the sixth leading cause of accidental death in the United States (Holen and Dicklor, 1973). Foreign body obstruction or aspiration is more likely to occur when consciousness is reduced, that is, alcohol excess, use of depressant drugs, or disease states (Donaldson et al., 1971).

Recognition

When a foreign body disappears from the oral cavity and there are signs of laryngeal and bronchial irritation, it must be presumed to have passed into the respiratory passage until proved otherwise (McCarthy, 1972). Symptoms may be mild, or patients may cough, gag, choke, or wheeze in attempting to eject the object. If only mild symptoms are present, radiographs of the chest and abdomen should be taken to confirm the location of the foreign body. Patients with foreign bodies located in the trachea or bronchi should be referred immediately for removal by bronchoscopy or thoracotomy if bronchoscopy is unsuccessful. With complete obstruction, the patient may gasp for breath with great effort, show suprasternal and intercostal retraction, and be unable to speak. The chest wall may rise and fall, but this should not be interpreted as air exchange (Thompson, 1975) when one cannot demonstrate the passage of air from the mouth or nose by feeling with the back of the hand or by listening with the ear, or when one cannot make the chest rise with mouth-to-mouth or bag and mask resuscitative efforts. Without treatment the patient shortly becomes cyanotic and collapses.

Treatment

One should have an orderly plan devised for treating airway obstruction beginning with simple nonsurgical treatment and progressing to more complex management, utilizing surgical therapy if necessary. One can try leaning the patient over the chair and pounding firmly on the back with hopes of dislodging the foreign body. Small children may be held upside down by their legs and sharp blows rendered to the back. These treatments may or may not be successful. If unsuccessful, the patient should be laid supine on the floor, or in slight Trendelenburg position if in the dental chair, and with the head to the side and the mouth open, the middle and index fingers should be placed into the pharynx and swept laterally in an attempt to remove the object. Cochrane (1974) states that one half of all obstructions from food particles can be removed by this method. If one has access to a laryngoscope and Magill forceps, these may be tried with care even in the face of some patient resistance. If the airway obstruction is not complete, mouth-to-mouth or bag and mask resuscitation may move enough air around the obstruction to be livesaving.

Another procedure to be considered before surgical intervention is the Heimlich procedure (Heimlich, 1974; Heimlich, 1975; Heimlich et al., 1975). The Heimlich procedure takes advantage of the remaining air within the lungs and by forcefully compressing the lungs, increases the air pressure within the trachea and larynx, thus ejecting the offending bolus like a "cork from a champagne bottle" (Heimlich, 1974).

Heimlich procedure
1. With the rescuer standing behind the victim he wraps his arms around the victim's waist and grasps his fist with his other hand placing the thumb side of the fist against the victim's abdomen (Fig. 11-2). He then exerts a quick upward thrust. This is repeated several times if necessary. When the victim is sitting, the rescuer stands behind the victim's

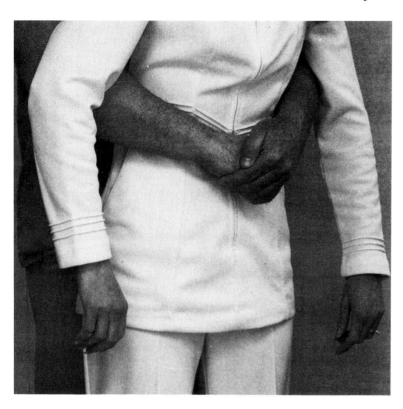

Fig. 11-2. Heimlich procedure: patient standing.

chair and performs the maneuver in the same manner.

2. If the victim is lying on his back, the rescuer faces the victim, knees astride his hips, and with one of his hands on top of the other, places the heel of his bottom hand on the abdomen slightly above the navel and below the rib cage. He presses into the victim's abdomen with a quick upward thrust (Fig. 11-3). This is repeated several times if necessary. With any of the above procedures, suction to remove excess secretions or vomitus may be necessary at any time.

Experimentally, the Heimlich maneuver produces an average air flow rate of 205 L/min and a pressure of 31 mm Hg, expelling an average volume of 0.94 L of air in approximately ¼ sec (Heimlich et al., 1975). Since the introduction of the Heimlich maneuver, hundreds of cases of lives saved utilizing this procedure have

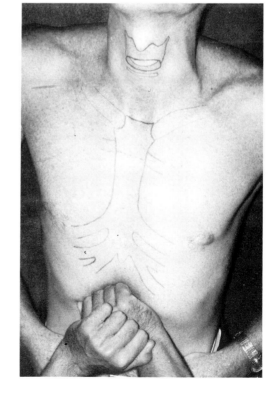

Fig. 11-3. Heimlich procedure: patient lying on back. Pressure is applied inward and upward.

been collected. The procedure has even been successfully self-administered.

If all the preceding procedures have failed, surgical intervention is necessary. Unless in an operating room, puncture of the cricothyroid membrane by cricothyroidotomy or coniotomy is the procedure of choice. The cricothyroid space is located easily by observation and palpation. It is an advantageous area because it has no major nerves or vessels over it and because it is the shortest distance from the skin in gaining access to the laryngotracheal region. The posterior part of the cricoid ring also helps to prevent esophageal puncture. The neck should be moderately hyperextended with the chin and sternal notch in the median plane (Fig. 11-4). The cricothyroid space can be identified by palpating the prominence of the thyroid cartilage (Adam's apple) and carrying the finger inferiorly to the soft depression between the thyroid and cricoid cartilages. In women and children, the thyroid cartilage may not be as prominent, and one may find orientation easier by starting in the sternal notch and moving the finger superiorly until it hits the prominent cricoid cartilage. One should grasp and fix the thyroid cartilage between the thumb and fingers and place the tip of the index finger at the edge of the cricothyroid space (Fig. 11-5). A number of instruments have been used to perform the actual cricothyroid puncture, including scalpel blades, scissors, and specially designed trocars (Tarsitano and Jerman, 1970). As the skin overlying this area is loose and tough, a 1.5 cm skin incision with a scalpel blade, using the index finger as the guide, may facilitate the procedure (Fig. 11-6). One can then use a scissors or a scalpel blade, held to allow no more than ½ to ¾ inch penetration, to effect puncture into the larynx (Fig. 11-7). Direction should be straight posteriorly, remembering the vocal cords are just superior to the puncture site. A hiss of air is usually heard and some coughing may ensue. The opening is spread transversely and maintained by the handle of the scalpel or insertion of a tube or cricothyroid cannula. Care should then be exercised to maintain this airway and ensure passage of air.

Slight bleeding may complicate the

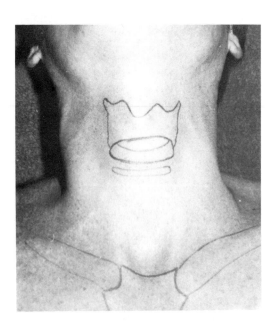

Fig. 11-4. Cricothyroidotomy: neck hyperextended with chin and sternal notch in median plane.

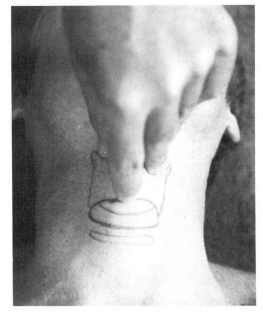

Fig. 11-5. Cricothyroidotomy: thyroid cartilage grasped and index finger at edge of cricothyroid space.

procedure and laryngeal stenosis may occur if the cricothyroid airway is left in place for an extended period. If airway maintenance is required for over 48 hours, a tracheostomy should be considered.

Prevention

Prevention of foreign body obstruction and aspiration involves mainly common sense, utilizing care when dealing with instruments within the oral cavity. A gauze screen protecting the pharynx

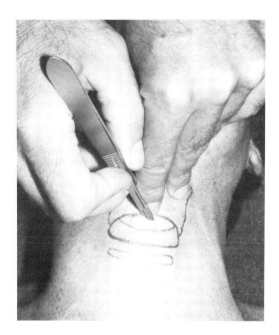

Fig. 11-6. Cricothyroidotomy: scalpel blade in position to incise skin.

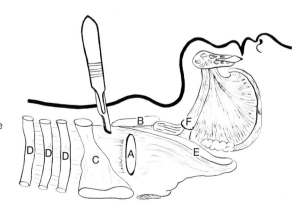

A. Vocal cords
B. Thyroid cartilage
C. Cricoid cartilage
D. Tracheal rings
E. Epiglottic cartilage
F. Hyoid bone

Fig. 11-7. Cricothyroidotomy: tracheal anatomy.

should be used whenever a patient is sedated or is receiving a general anesthetic, or at any time that badly decayed teeth that may fragment are being extracted.

ASTHMA—BRONCHOSPASM

Problem

Bronchospasm is a generalized contraction of the smooth muscles of the bronchi and bronchioles. Outside the realm of general anesthesia, it is most likely to be seen in patients with a history of asthma. Asthma is characterized by increased irritability of the tracheobronchial tree to various stimuli, including allergens, infections, and nonspecific irritants (Tennenbaum, 1974). With an asthmatic attack there is bronchospasm, mucosal edema, and intraluminal secretions, all of which contribute to air flow obstruction (Fig. 11-8).

Recognition

An asthmatic attack may be very mild with few symptoms or present as status asthmaticus, a life-threatening episode initially unresponsive to therapy with hydration and bronchodilators. The narrowed lumens of the bronchi and increased amounts of thick sputum make wheezing a prominent sign. This wheezing may be heard during inspiration as well as expiration. Cough is also a common sign as patients try to clear the mucus from the tracheobronchial tree. Patients may be diaphoretic, anxious, and show labored breathing with use of accessory muscles and intercostal retraction. Subjectively, patients rated airway obstruction symptoms (that is, shortness of breath, wheezing, chest tightness, chest congestion) most common during an asthmatic attack, followed by symptoms of fatigue, panic-fear, and irritability

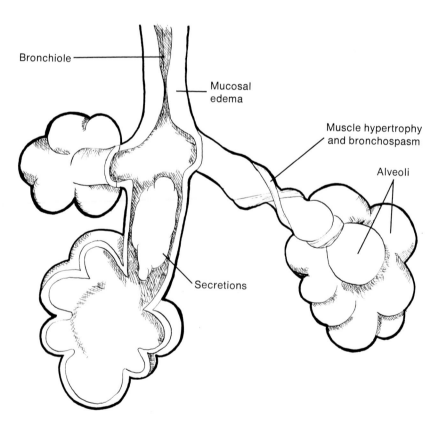

Fig. 11-8. Asthmatic attack: muscle hypertrophy, bronchospasm, mucosal edema, and intraluminal secretions contribute to air flow obstruction.

in that order (Kinsman et al., 1973). With severe airway obstruction, hypoxemia can result with cyanosis and confusion. One must keep in mind that one of the most prominent features, wheezing, is not a reliable guide to the severity of the problem. When air flow is great, turbulence may produce wheezing even though obstruction is minimal; when obstruction is severe or the patient is greatly fatigued so that maximal effort produces little air flow, wheezing may be absent (Franklin, 1974).

Treatment

Treatment of bronchospasm caused by an asthma attack in the office should consist primarily of bronchodilators supplemented with oxygen and hydration. Often the sitting position is most comfortable and affords the best position for breathing during an asthmatic attack. Oxygen administration, that is, 20% to 30%, is useful, but high concentrations are seldom needed (Franklin, 1974). Patients may have their own medication for an attack, consisting of isoproterenol as an aerosol. If so, this can be tried first. If unavailable, epinephrine, 0.3 to 0.5 mg subcutaneously, should be administered and may be repeated in 15 minutes. It may seem logical to use isoproterenol, a pure beta drug, or even better a drug such as albuterol (salbutamol), which is more specific for the beta$_2$ receptors of the bronchial tree, rather than epinephrine, which has mixed alpha and beta effects. However, epinephrine is highly effective and has been used for over 50 years, and more specific agents have not been evaluated as well in severe asthma (Franklin, 1974).

If little or no change is noted with epinephrine, aminophylline usually brings prompt relief. A loading dose of 5 to 6 mg/kg in 5% D/W can be given intravenously over 15 to 20 minutes, slowing or stopping the injection of aminophylline if pronounced side effects such as nausea, vomiting, tachycardia, or arrhythmias develop. Following the loading dose, 1 mg/kg/hr can be initiated. If the above measures have not terminated the attack, the patient should be accompanied to the

emergency room for further treatment where spirometry, chest radiographs, Gram stains of the sputum, arterial blood gases, and so on are available to aid in management. Corticosteroids may be needed but require several hours to be effective and therefore do not replace bronchodilators in initial office management. Along with bronchodilators, hydration with oral or intravenous fluids may help thin secretions and thus aid in their removal.

Prevention

Certain factors interact in many asthmatics to produce attacks: (1) allergy to external inhaled allergens, that is, pollens, dust, feathers, foods, animal danders; (2) respiratory infections; and (3) psychophysiologic reactions to life stress (Thorn, 1977). Any known allergens, such as feather pillows on a recovery room cart, should be eliminated. Elective surgery should not be scheduled when the patient reports cold, flu, or other respiratory symptoms, and stress should be kept at a minimum. If sedatives are used to reduce stress, mild sedation is preferable. If an asthmatic attack occurs during treatment, deep sedation is contraindicated as the patient needs to exert maximum effort to ensure adequate ventilation (Senior et al., 1975).

Use of narcotics should be avoided in asthmatic patients, if possible, since they constrict smooth muscle, dry secretions, and depress respiration. Atropine and antihistaminic drugs with atropine-like action also tend to dry secretions, which can hinder their removal. Aspirin should probably be avoided in asthmatics as this drug can make the condition worse in certain patients. These patients are usually adults that have a triad of severe asthma, sinusitis, and nasal polyposis (Thorn, 1977). With general anesthesia one expects some increase in intraoperative and postoperative complications (Gold and Hebrick, 1963), but even steroid-dependent asthmatics can undergo surgery and general anesthesia with adequate preoperative preparation (Soo and Patterson, 1974).

If allergy plays some role in a patient's

asthma and the patient has other allergy-related problems such as hay fever, he may be prone to allergic reactions to various drugs. Local anesthesia, however, appears to be safe in this regard, as Gottlieb and Constantine (1967), in performing dental work on 250 children under treatment for intractable asthma, used lidocaine on all patients with no allergic reactions.

A preoperative history of asthma and the severity of the disease, medicines required for treatment, and knowledge as to the degree of control is essential. Whether or not the patient has ever reported to the emergency room for treatment of his asthma may help to determine the severity of the disease.

HYPERTENSIVE EMERGENCY
Problem

Harrison's textbook of medicine states that "when a resting adult has an arterial pressure above 150/90 mm Hg, hypertension may be considered to be present" (Thorn, 1977). Approximately 20% of Americans are afflicted with hypertension, the degree being greater in nonwhite than white populations (Kannel, 1975; Page and Sidd, 1972c; Wintrobe, 1974). Because of this prevalence, the oral and maxillofacial surgeon cannot avoid treating hypertensive patients routinely in his office. Hypertension leads to complications mainly involving the heart, brain, and kidneys, and in a surgical setting problems including the cardiovascular system (angina pectoris, myocardial infarction, arrythmias, acute congestive heart failure) and the cerebrovascular system (strokes) are certainly possible. This is especially true in patients with extremely high blood pressures preoperatively and in those with a history of preexisting complications such as angina pectoris, congestive heart failure, and so forth.

Stress accompanying oral surgical procedures can be responsible for rises in blood pressure and even the stress of sitting in the waiting room has been shown to significantly elevate blood pressures above measurements obtained at basal conditions (Cheraskin and Prasertsuntar-asai, 1957). Other problems in hypertensive patients include the possibility of increased bleeding during surgery (ASOS, 1971), problems related to therapy with antihypertensive medication such as orthostatic hypotension (Page and Sidd, 1972a; Page and Sidd, 1972b), and increased sensitivity to sedatives and epinephrine (ASOS, 1971).

Recognition

The diagnosis of an acute hypertensive episode should be considered when an extremely high elevation of diastolic blood pressure (that is, approximately 120 mm Hg or greater) is detected along with symptoms such as headaches, dizziness, nausea, and vomiting, and signs of visual impairment or other neurologic changes (Curry and Hosten, 1975). Retinal changes such as hemorrhages, exudates, and even papilledema may be present on fundoscopic examination.

Treatment

If during surgery the diastolic blood pressure rises to the range of 120 mm Hg or greater, coupled with the symptoms just mentioned, one should try to lower the blood pressure to the range of 100 to 110 mm Hg in an effort to avoid possible complications. The patient should be allowed to rest in a semisitting position and oxygen should be administered. This alone may be sufficient to lower the blood pressure, but if the pressure remains elevated and symptoms persist, drug therapy may be indicated. A small amount of diazepam (Valium) slowly titrated intravenously has been recommended to reduce stress and thereby reduce blood pressure (Bustad, 1976). A small dose of chlorpromazine (Thorazine) can also be used to lower blood pressure, especially in patients undergoing surgery (Sharpe, 1969). Parenteral antihypertensive medications such as diazoxide (Hyperstat) (Vidt, 1975), methyldopa (Aldomet), or reserpine are potent, accompanied by side effects, and usually require some degree of monitoring; therefore, unless one is very familiar with these drugs, they are best administered in a hospital setting. If rest, oxygen, and a small amount of Valium are not effective in abating symptoms and lowering pressure, it should be considered a serious emergency and the patient should be taken to the emergency room where more accurate assessment is possible and additional therapy can be instituted.

If, because of the hypertensive episode, other complications occur in the office, such as angina pectoris or stroke, they should be handled as described in appropriate sections of this chapter.

Prevention

An accurate history regarding hypertension, antihypertensive medicines, and any hypertension related complications such as congestive heart failure, coronary artery disease, stroke, and kidney problems is essential. If the patient is on medication, one should ascertain the degree of compliance, as hypertensive patients often do not take medications as prescribed. A preoperative blood pressure for diagnostic as well as baseline purposes is mandatory. One should establish an office policy, setting a maximum diastolic blood pressure (for example, 100 mm Hg) above which consultation is obtained before elective surgery is performed. One should be aware of the possibility of orthostatic hypotension when antihypertensive medication is being used, and these patients should be raised slowly from a supine position in the dental chair. It should also be remembered that such patients may be more sensitive to sedatives and sedative drugs should be titrated accordingly. Use of epinephrine containing local anesthetics in hypertensive patients is not contraindicated (Cheraskin and Prasertsuntarasai, 1958a). A maximum of 0.2 mg epinephrine per appointment is permissible (Report N.Y. Heart Assoc., 1955); however, the least amount required should be used, and aspiration is essential to avoid intravascular injection.

Sedation for hypertensive patients should be encouraged to reduce stress, as there is some evidence to indicate that such patients fare better when sedated (Cheraskin and Prasertsuntarasai, 1958b; Cheraskin and Prasertsuntarasai, 1959).

HYPOTENSIVE EMERGENCY
Problem

Hypotension in the oral surgery office may result from a variety of causes ranging from simple syncope to adrenal crisis. One should keep in mind that hypotension is a reduction in blood pressure, whereas with shock peripheral circulatory failure also is present.

Recognition

Hypotension is detected by taking the blood pressure, usually at a time when vital signs appear to be unstable. The pulse may be weak, and bradycardia (pulse less than 60) may exist. With associated shock, the patient may show restlessness, agitation, confusion, nausea, stupor, and coma (Staples, 1973). There is no exact blood pressure figure that denotes hypotension, although a systolic blood pressure less than 80 mm Hg can arbitrarily be used when a normal preoperative systolic pressure was present. However, the amount of systolic pressure drop may be more important than the actual systolic blood pressure. For example, a systolic blood pressure drop from 180 mm Hg to 90 mm Hg may be more significant than a drop from 100 mm Hg to 80 mm Hg.

Treatment

Initial treatment should be supportive; the patient should be placed in a horizontal position with the legs elevated or in Trendelenburg's position, and oxygen should be administered. (Women in late pregnancy should be turned on their side, as the supine position may in fact cause hypotension as the gravid uterus impedes return of blood to the heart by impinging on the inferior vena cava. Patients with cardiac insufficiency and orthopnea should be placed in a semisitting position.) Vital signs should be determined and monitored frequently. An intravenous line should be inserted for fluid and possible drug administration. If the systolic pressure is above 80 mm Hg in a patient with a normal preoperative pressure, one should continue monitoring and supportive therapy while trying to determine the cause of the reaction. Although vasopressors may be indicated with a systolic blood pressure below 80 mm Hg, the amount of blood pressure drop as well as the general condition of the patient are also important factors to consider before vasopressor therapy is instituted.

If the pulse is less than 60, atropine, 0.4 to 0.6 mg, should be given intravenously. With patients receiving phenothiazines or antihypertensive medicines such as reserpine that reduce the body's catecholamine stores, norepinephrine (levarterenol) or phenylephrine (Neo-Synephrine) should be used (ASOS, 1971). As levarterenol must be administered as an intravenous infusion, and since it causes tissue necrosis and slough with extravasation outside the vein, phenylephrine is probably simpler to use. Phenylephrine, 2 to 5 mg subcutaneously or intramuscularly, or phenylephrine, 0.2 mg, given slowly intravenously can be used. Levarterenol, if used, can be administered 2 to 4 mcg/1 min by infusion (4 ml levarterenol in 1000 ml 5% D/W; 1 ml of mixture equals 4 mcg).

If the cause of hypotension is unknown or a myocardial infarction or cerebrovascular accident is suspected, one of the least potent vasopressors, mephentermine (Wyamine), can be used intravenously or intramuscularly. A dosage of 15 mg can be administered for systolic blood pressure between 60 and 80 mm Hg and 30 mg mephentermine for systolic blood pressure below 60 mm Hg.

For other causes of hypotension such as syncope, allergy, or adrenal crisis, treatment is discussed under the section concerning those conditions.

Prevention

An adequate history is essential in prevention of hypotension and is also mandatory to establish the correct diagnosis so that proper treatment can be assured.

ISCHEMIC HEART DISEASE
Problem

Ischemic heart disease, the most common form of adult heart disease in the United States (Herman, 1971), results from an inadequate perfusion of a portion of the myocardium. The etiology of this problem in the vast majority of instances is atherosclerosis of the coronary arteries (Fowler, 1972; Jastar and Cowan, 1973). The resultant ischemia may lead to arrythmias, conduction defects, or cardiac failure, but the majority of patients with ischemic heart disease present with angina pectoris, myocardial infarction, or sudden death. These patients are certainly at an increased risk during oral and maxillofacial surgery treatment.

Recognition

Angina pectoris is a paroxysmal discomfort often described as heaviness, pressure, tightness, choking, or squeezing (Herman, 1971; Thorn, 1977). The pain is characteristically retrosternal but may radiate to the shoulders and arms, particularly on the left. On occasion it may also radiate to the neck and jaw. Typically, the pain is precipitated by physical activity, but it may also be related to emotional upset or stress, exposure to cold, meals, or it can occur spontaneously. It is relieved by rest or nitroglycerin. The pain of myocardial infarction is similar to angina pectoris but is usually more severe and prolonged, not alleviated by rest or nitroglycerine, and other symptoms such as weakness, pallor, nausea, sweating, and restlessness are more often seen (McCarthy, 1972; Thorn, 1977).

Treatment

If an anginal attack occurs during oral surgery treatment, the procedure should be stopped, the patient allowed to rest in a semisitting position, and oxygen administered. A tablet of nitroglycerine, preferably the patient's own medicine, is placed sublingually. If the patient has no nitroglycerine, a 0.03 mg ($\frac{1}{200}$ gr) tablet from the emergency kit should be used. If effective, relief should take place in 45 seconds to 2 minutes (Boedeker and Dauber, 1974; Fowler, 1972). If pain persists, sublingual nitroglycerine can be repeated twice at 5 minute intervals. If the pain is severe, an ampule of amyl nitrate broken under the patient's nose can be tried after the first tablet of nitroglycerine has failed. If effective, amyl nitrate should provide relief in 30 seconds (Boedeker and Dauber, 1974). These drugs reduce myocardial oxygen consumption mainly by systemic vasodilation of venules and arterioles, decreasing venous return and thereby lowering blood pressure, and to a lesser degree by causing coronary dilation (Lesch and Gorlin, 1973; Zelis, et al., 1974). Because these drugs are vasodilators, one may see side effects such as headache, flushing, dizziness, and even syncope (Arora, 1975; Lesch and Gorlin, 1973).

If the patient remains symptomatic after the preceding treatment, one must consider the possibility that the patient is having a myocardial infarction. The office emergency plan must be instituted, the patient's physician notified, and the patient brought to the hospital emergency room. If heart failure develops, corrective measures should be promptly instituted, (see section on "Congestive Heart Failure,"). If pain is severe and unrelenting, meperidine (Demerol), 25 mg, or small amounts of morphine may be given intramuscularly or titrated slowly intravenously, utilizing extreme care if hypotension exists or if the patient has chronic lung disease. Atropine 0.4 to 0.6 mg intravenously or intramuscularly may be given if the heart rate is excessively slow. If hypotension exists, mephentermine (Wyamine) 15 to 30 mg intramuscularly or intravenously can be administered. If respiration or circulation cease, these systems must, of course, be supported by cardiopulmonary resuscitative measures.

Prevention

One should seek a prior history of ischemic heart disease, inquiring about angina pectoris, previous myocardial infarctions, arrythmias, cardiac medications, and cardiovascular symptoms such as shortness of breath, orthopnea, paroxysmal nocturnal dyspnea (PND), and ankle edema. However, since many patients with ischemic heart disease have no positive history or symptoms (Herman, 1971) and because of the high prevalence of ischemic heart disease, certain risk factors may need to be considered in a preoperative history. These are classically hypertension, cigarette smoking, hypercholesterolemia, sex (males more prevalent), age (peak age 55 to 59), obesity, diabetes mellitus, positive family history, and an aggressive, competitive, deadline-conscious personality (Fowler, 1972; Leonard and Heslin, 1971b).

If a history of angina pectoris is elicited, one should inquire as to whether the condition is stable. Stable angina is defined as recurrence of pain that follows predictable precipitating events and has no change in duration, severity, or frequency of attacks, or alteration in response to therapy over a period of several months (Boedeker and Dauber, 1974). With this history, short appointments and sedation should be considered to minimize stress. If the patient is taking nitroglycerin, he should be told to bring his medication with him. One should check to see if the medication is fresh as it often deteriorates over some months' time, especially if not stored properly (Zelis, 1974). Some authors suggest prophylactic premedication with nitroglycerin approximately 5 minutes before initiating treatment (McCarthy, 1972).

As opposed to stable angina, unstable, progressive, or preinfarction angina is characterized by prolonged pain (more than 15 minutes) or by recurring spontaneous attacks of increased severity and frequency in which the pain has a wider or altered radiation (Boedeker and Dauber, 1974). In this instance, elective surgery should be deferred and consultation with the patient's physician obtained.

With a history of recent myocardial infarction, elective surgery should be postponed for at least 6 months. Even though this recommendation is based mainly on statistics concerning varied operations performed under general anesthsia, the reinfarction rate with surgery within 6 months of its occurrence is significant enough to make the recommendation sound (Tarhan et al., 1972).

CONGESTIVE HEART FAILURE
Problem

Congestive heart failure or more simply heart failure may be defined as the "inability of the heart to pump sufficient blood to the body tissues to meet ordinary metabolic demands" (Parmley, 1977).

Heart failure may result from varied etiologies including any form of heart disease. Hypertensive cardiovascular disease is implicated in a significant number of patients with heart failure.

Over and above the underlying cause of heart failure, certain precipitating factors may increase the problem by acutely placing an additional load on myocardial function. These events may include pulmonary embolus, thyrotoxicosis, pregnancy, arrhythmias, myocardial ischemia and infarction, bacterial endocarditis, rheumatic fever or other forms of myocarditis, infection, fever, anemia, hot and humid environment, exposure to cold, and physical and emotional stress (Boedeker and Dauber, 1974; Dack, 1978; Thorn, 1977).

Problems encountered by the oral and maxillofacial surgeon involve development of signs and symptoms of heart failure in patients with underlying heart disease or a change from chronic to acute heart failure (that is, acute pulmonary edema) during surgical treatment.

Recognition

Certain signs and symptoms may dominate, depending on whether there is mainly left or right heart failure, although after a prolonged period of time a combination of right and left heart failure is often seen.

With mainly left heart failure (that is, postmyocardial infarction with impairment of left ventricular function) dyspnea or shortness of breath, orthopnea, paroxysmal nocturnal dyspnea, chronic cough, and possibly bronchospasm usually predominate. Dyspnea occurs when the left ventricle can no longer efficiently pump the amount of blood supplied by the left atrium and pulmonary venous system. This blood then backs up and creates increased pressures in the left atrium, pulmonary veins, and finally in the pulmonary capillaries. If this high pressure exceeds the osmotic pressure of the blood, transudation of fluid will occur

from the pulmonary capillaries into the pulmonary interstitial tissues and eventually into the alveolar spaces (Fig. 11-9). This obviously causes a decreased compliance of the lungs and interferes with alveolar gas exchange resulting in dyspnea. Once normal pulmonary capillary pressures of 5 to 12 mm Hg are exceeded, pulmonary congestion is possible; when

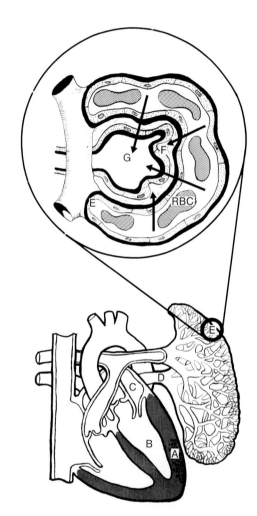

Fig. 11-9. Heart failure: myocardial infarction, *A*, with decrease in myocardial function causes backup of blood and increased pressure in left ventricle, *B*, left atrium, *C*, pulmonary venous system, *D*, and finally pulmonary capillary system, *E*. When this increased pressure exceeds osmotic pressure inside vessels, transudation of fluid from pulmonary capillaries, *E*, into pulmonary interstitial tissues, *F*, and alveolar spaces, *G*, results.

pressures rise to 20 to 30 mm Hg or more, pulmonary edema usually results (Boedeker and Dauber, 1974; Forrester et al., 1976).

Orthopnea, or shortness of breath when lying down, presumably occurs because of increased venous return caused by the alteration in gravitational forces in the recumbent position and because the increased intrathoracic blood volume reduces vital capacity. This ultimately leads to increased pulmonary venous and capillary pressures.

Paroxysmal nocturnal dyspnea (PND) refers to severe shortness of breath awakening the patient from sleep, at which time the patient usually must sit up or get out of bed for relief. Etiologic factors may include augmentation of blood volume owing to reabsorption of edema fluid from dependent parts of the body when lying down. This increased blood volume places an even greater overload on the left ventricle and again increases pulmonary capillary pressures.

Because of the pulmonary congestion, auscultation of the lungs, especially the posterior lung bases, often reveals rales. Pulsus alternans, a regular rhythm with alternating strong and weak pulse beats, may often be detected by sphygmomanometry or in more severe cases by palpation of the peripheral pulse. A pleural effusion, most frequently on the right side, may be noted on physical or radiographic examination because of transudation of fluid into the pleural cavity. Radiographs may also show prominent hilar vascular shadows, and a "fuzzy" shadow may extend from the hilar area into the lungs producing a "butterfly" pattern. Thin horizontal lines (Kerley's B lines), most evident at the lung bases, may also be noted on radiographic examination.

With right heart failure, blood backs up in the systemic venous system and leads to increased jugular venous distention (distended neck veins), positive hepatojugular reflux (increased filling of jugular veins with sustained pressure over the liver), hepatomegaly, and peripheral edema.

With heart failure in general one may see fatigue and weight loss, and examination may reveal tachycardia, a third heart sound, and cardiac enlargement. With acute pulmonary edema an accentuation of these symptoms occurs, and bronchospasm and cyanosis may also appear. There is often frothy pink sputum production, and the chest is filled with rales that can be heard on auscultation.

Treatment

Therapy of heart failure revolves around treatment of the underlying or precipitating causes, reducing the cardiac work load, and controlling excessive fluid retention. Physical and mental rest often result in a significant diuresis, and patients are usually more comfortable with the head of the bed elevated 30 to 45 degrees for rest and sleep. Salt restriction is helpful in managing fluid retention. Digitalis, because of its inotropic effect, increases the efficiency of the failing heart, having its greatest value in low-output heart failure. Diuretics are also important drugs in managing heart failure.

When acute pulmonary edema is present, more aggressive treatment is indicated. The patient should be made comfortable in a sitting or semisitting position to reduce venous return to the right heart and thus reduce pulmonary blood flow and congestion. Oxygen (100%) should be administered, possibly under positive pressure. Oxygen reduces dyspnea, anoxemia, and pulmonary congestion by raising alveolar oxygen concentration; it helps raise arterial oxygen saturation; and when given under positive pressure, intra-alveolar pressure is increased reducing transudation of fluid from the pulmonary capillaries (Dack, 1978; Thorn, 1977).

Morphine given subcutaneously, intramuscularly, or intravenously reduces anxiety, exerts a positive inotropic effect, and, probably most importantly, decreases vascular resistance with pooling of blood in the veins that reduces venous return. It should be given with caution to patients with chronic lung disease or hypotension. Dosages depend on the route of administration and the severity of the problem and may range from 1 to 15 mg.

Rotating tourniquets or even phlebotomy can be employed to decrease intravascular volume by again reducing the venous return. Tourniquets or blood pressure cuffs can be placed on the upper and lower limbs, being applied to constrict venous return without impeding the arterial pulse. The tourniquets should be applied to three of the four limbs and rotated every 15 to 20 minutes (Dack, 1978).

Rapidly acting diuretics such as furosemide (Lasix) and rapidly acting digitalis glycosides are also utilized. If bronchospasm is present, aminophylline is helpful.

If a patient develops acute pulmonary edema in the office, initial therapy with proper positioning, oxygen, rotating tourniquets, and even judicious use of morphine should be instituted as plans are made for transportation to the hospital.

Prevention

Prevention begins with recognition of patients with hypertensive cardiovascular disease or other heart problems that could lead to congestive heart failure or acute pulmonary edema. Careful questioning regarding symptoms (that is, dyspnea, orthopnea, PND) and careful examination noting signs of heart failure if present (that is, distended neck veins, peripheral edema) allow the practitioner to detect poor risk patients. Knowledge of the patient's present medications and his reliability in taking these medications is important as congestive heart failure can be exacerbated by discontinuance of digitalis, diuretics, or antihypertensive drugs. Overmedication with beta blocking drugs, such as propranolol, can also lead to congestive symptoms.

It should be remembered that fever, infection, exposure to cold or hot environments, as well as physical and emotional stresses can worsen heart failure in certain patients. If a patient has an acute ischemic episode in the office, that is, an angina attack or a myocardial infarction, the patient should be observed carefully for development of heart failure. Proper positioning in a semisitting or sitting position may be preventive when working on patients with congestive heart failure or patients at high risk for developing heart failure.

CARDIOPULMONARY ARREST
Problem

Cardiopulmonary arrest (sudden death) is the sudden and unexpected cessation of ventilation and circulation. Although uncommon in the oral surgery office, it does occur. The 1972 ASOS Anesthesia Morbidity and Mortality Survey revealed 11 deaths in 5,250,000 anesthetics (ASOS Committee on Anesthesia, 1974). Causes other than general anesthetic, sedative, or local anesthetic reactions may include asphyxia, myocardial infarction, and allergic reactions to medications, such as antibiotics, administered in the office (Gaum, 1970; Sherman, 1974).

Recognition

Absence of ventilation is detected by the lack of thoracic or abdominal movements, the absence of air movements through the mouth and nose, and the absence of breath sounds. However, one should keep in mind that movements of the thoracic and abdominal areas may be seen without ventilation in cases of upper airway obstruction.

The absence of circulation is detected by the lack of a carotid or femoral pulse, confirmed by manifestations of inadequate cerebral perfusion (dilated pupils, unresponsiveness, comatose state) and inadequate peripheral perfusion (ashen gray color). In infants and children it may be more practical to place the hand gently over the precordium to feel the apical beat rather than feeling for a carotid pulse.

Treatment

Cardiopulmonary resuscitation has been adequately described by various authors (Goldberg, 1974; Moser, 1974; Stein, 1975; Vijay and Schoonmaker, 1975). Basic life support consists of the A-B-C steps of cardiopulmonary resuscitation: maintaining an airway, breathing, and circulation. These steps should be started as quickly as possible, since irreversible brain damage may occur in 4 to 6 minutes or less in the absence of cerebral oxygenation. The most important immediate action is opening the airway. This is easily accomplished by placing one hand behind the victim's neck and lifting it, and the other hand on the forehead, tilting the head backward (Fig. 11-10). This extends the neck and lifts the tongue away from the posterior pharyngeal wall. If this maneuver is unsuccessful in opening the airway, the fingers should be placed behind the angles of the mandible, forcing the jaw forward while keeping the head tilted backward.

If spontaneous breathing does not resume, artificial ventilation must be started immediately. Ideally, this is accomplished with an anesthetic machine or a bag and mask device using atmospheric oxygen (Ambu-Bag). If these are unavailable, mouth-to-mouth or mouth-to-nose ventilation can be used. Insertion of an oropharyngeal airway or endotracheal intubation will assist in maintaining adequate ventilation when using mechanical ventilation. However, they should be used only if the patient is unconscious. Otherwise, they may cause vomiting and laryngospasm. The initial ventilatory effort should be four quick insufflations (full breaths) without allowing time for full lung deflation between breaths. If this ventilatory effort is unsuccessful despite proper technique, a foreign body in the airway should be considered. The mouth is quickly opened and several fingers of one hand are used to sweep through the pharynx and oral cavity to remove any foreign object.

Once patency of the airway is established, ventilation is continued at the rate of once every 5 seconds in adults and

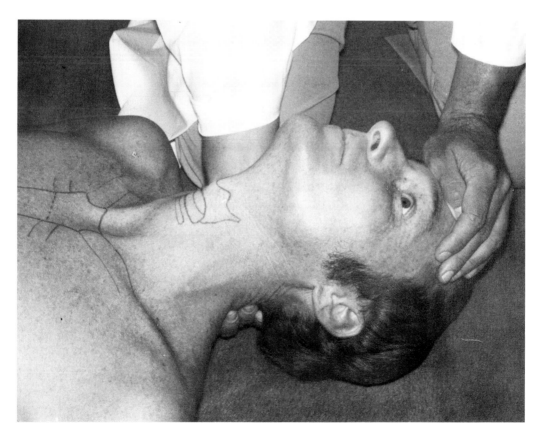

Fig. 11-10. Hyperextension of neck to open airway.

once every 3 seconds for infants and small children. Mouth-to-mouth resuscitation provides 16% to 17% oxygen to the victim. During a cardiopulmonary arrest there is low cardiac output, intrapulmonary shunting, and ventilation perfusion abnormalities leading to hypoxemia, anaerobic metabolism, and metabolic acidosis, which often interfere with the beneficial effect of drugs and defibrillation used in resuscitation efforts. Therefore, supplemental oxygen should be used as soon as possible.

If circulation is absent, artificial circulation by external cardiac massage must be initiated. With the rescuer close to the victim's side, the heel of one hand is placed over the lower half of the sternum, 1 to 1½ inches above the xiphoid process, and the other hand is placed on top of the first one (Fig. 11-11). Care should be taken to keep the hands off the tip of the xiphoid and the fingers off the chest wall, as this technique leads to fewer complications. With the arms straight and the

shoulders over the patient's sternum, pressure is exerted to depress the lower sternum approximately 1½ to 2 inches (Fig. 11-12). This compresses the heart between the lower sternum and spine, producing a pulsatile flow. When properly performed, this results in systolic blood pressure peaks of over 100 mm Hg, but as the diastolic blood pressure is zero, a mean blood pressure of 40 mm Hg is seldom exceeded (Moser, 1974). With one rescuer, a ratio of 15:2 should be maintained with two very quick lung inflations after each 15 chest compressions. The compressions should be at a rate of once each second (60 compressions per minute), with compression and relaxation of equal duration. With two rescuers, one lung inflation should be quickly interposed after each five chest compressions (ratio of 5:1) without any pause in compressions.

In children only the heel of one hand is used for cardiac compression, and with infants only the tips of the middle and

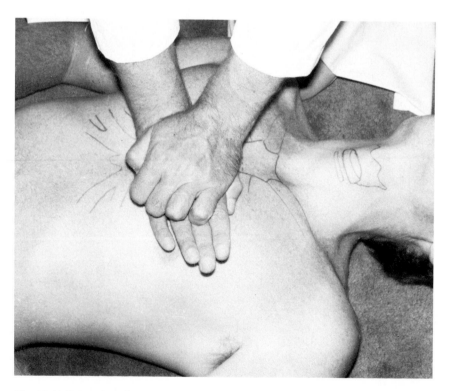

Fig. 11-11. External cardiac massage: correct position of hands over lower half of sternum.

index fingers are used. Pressure should be exerted over the midsternum, as the ventricles in infants and small children lie higher in the chest, and the rate of compression should be 80 to 100 per minute (Moser, 1974).

Checking for effectiveness of the cardiopulmonary resuscitative efforts should be done after the first minute and every few minutes thereafter. This is accomplished by determining if a palpable carotid or femoral pulse results with each compression and observing the pupillary reaction. Pupils that constrict when exposed to light indicate adequate blood flow and oxygenation to the brain.

A precordial thump (a sharp, quick single blow over the midportion of the sternum, hitting with the bottom fleshy part of the fist from 8 to 12 inches over the chest) may be beneficial as the initial step of resuscitation during arrest in monitored patients. (Moser, 1974; Vijay and

Schoonmaker, 1975). This blow generates a small electrical stimulus in the heart and, if given within the first minute after arrest, may reverse ventricular tachycardia or ventricular fibrillation and be effective in restoring a beat in ventricular asystole. There are, however, hazards associated with the precordial thump since in an anoxic heart that is still beating, the electrical stimulus may induce ventricular fibrillation. Therefore, the precordial thump is presently recommended only for arrest in monitored patients. If there is no immediate response to the precordial thump, cardiopulmonary resuscitation should be initiated at once.

Over and above the basic A-B-C's of resuscitation there are certain drugs essential for proper cardiopulmonary resuscitation. After 2 minutes of resuscitative efforts, sodium bicarbonate, 1 mEq/kg, should be given intravenously as a bolus

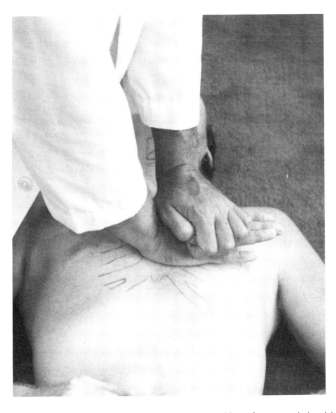

Fig. 11-12. External cardiac massage: correct position of arms and shoulders.

or as a continuous infusion over a 10-minute period to combat metabolic acidosis. The initial dose can be repeated after 10 minutes, and one-half the initial dose every 10 minutes thereafter. This schedule hopefully avoids overmedication causing metabolic alkalosis and hyperosmolality.

Sodium bicarbonate should be used in conjunction with epinephrine, which increases myocardial contractility, elevates perfusion pressure, helps restore electrical activity in asystole, and enhances defibrillation in ventricular fibrillation. It is therefore recommended in all three causes of cardiac arrest: (1) cardiovascular collapse (electromechanical dissociation), (2) ventricular fibrillation, and (3) ventricular standstill (asystole). The dose of epinephrine is 0.5 mg (5 ml of a 1:10,000 solution) intravenously every 5 minutes during resuscitation procedures.

Calcium chloride, like epinephrine, provides a positive ionotropic and chronotropic effect. It is useful when there is electromechanical dissociation and may be useful in asystole and ventricular fibrillation. Dosages are: calcium chloride 2.5 ml to 5 ml of a 10% solution (3.4 to 6.8 mEq calcium) or calcium gluconate 10 ml of a 10% solution (4.8 mEq calcium). Caution should be used in administering calcium to digitalized patients, and calcium should not be used if digitalis toxicity is suspected.

Atropine should be used when there is a sinus bradycardia with a pulse less than 60 beats per minute, especially if the systolic blood pressure is low or when the bradycardia is accompanied by premature ventricular contractions. The recommended dose is 0.5 mg intravenously, repeated at 5-minute intervals (not exceeding 2 mg) until the pulse exceeds 60. Other drugs such as lidocaine, vasoactive drugs, and corticosteroids may also be useful in certain instances but are usually not considered as essential as those discussed.

Defibrillation should be carried out as soon as possible in cases of ventricular fibrillation. One electrode is placed to the right of the sternum, just below the clavicle, and the other is placed just to the left of the cardiac apex and a shock of 400 watt-seconds from a direct current defibrillator is administered (Fig. 11-13).

A complication rate of 20% to 30% is

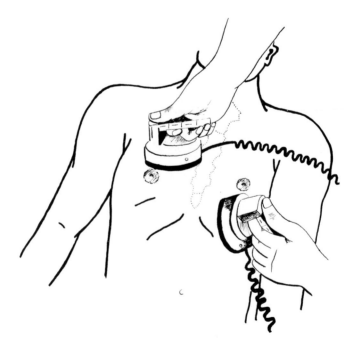

Fig. 11-13. Standard paddle placement for defibrillation.

usual after cardiopulmonary resuscitation, with the most common problems being fracture of the ribs and sternum or separation and fracture of the costochondral junctions. However, other adverse reactions are also possible, such as fat and bone marrow emboli, hemothorax, pneumothorax, hemopericardium, and lacerations of the liver, spleen, and stomach.

Prevention

Prevention begins with a good history, recognizing high-risk patients, and continues with adequate monitoring during procedures. Prompt recognition and treatment may also be preventive in a way, as promptness in treatment helps to assure successful treatment.

DIABETIC EMERGENCIES (INSULIN SHOCK, KETOACIDOSIS)
Problem

There are two major emergency problems facing the oral and maxillofacial surgeon in treating patients with diabetes: insulin shock (hypoglycemia), and ketoacidosis (hyperglycemia). Both conditions are more likely to occur in patients with juvenile-onset diabetes as opposed to adult-onset diabetes, since juvenile-onset diabetes is more difficult to control and is usually insulin-dependent (requires insulin for treatment). Because hypoglycemia can develop quickly, it is seen more frequently than ketoacidosis in an office setting. It occurs when there is inadequate carbohydrate intake in relation to insulin or oral hypoglycemic drug administration. Perhaps the most frequent cause in an oral surgery practice is when the patient receives his normal dose of insulin in the morning but because of anxiety and nervousness prior to the appointment fails to eat adequately and arrives at the office with little carbohydrate intake. This is even more likely to occur when the patient is scheduled for general anesthesia and was told not to eat, but the dose of insulin or other hypoglycemic drug was not adjusted.

Ketoacidosis, on the other hand, usually develops progressively over a period of several days. Omission or reduction of insulin, plus factors that increase the amount of required insulin such as infection, trauma, surgery, pregnancy, and severe emotional stress, is the usual cause (Boedeker and Dauber, 1974).

Recognition

Symptoms of hypoglycemia result from excessive sympathetic activity as well as an inadequate blood glucose supply to the brain; they usually occur when the blood glucose level falls below 40 mg% (Arky and Arone, 1971). Because of sympathetic discharge, the patient may show pallor, sweating, and tremor, and may have apprehension, palpitations, weakness, and hunger. With inadequate cerebral glucose, there may be irritability, confusion, mental depression, headache, and other neurologic abnormalities such as speech and visual disturbances (Chue, 1976; Levine, 1974; Maw, 1975). If no treatment is instituted, convulsions, coma, or even death may ensue. The patient with hypoglycemia is usually not dehydrated and has a normal or slightly elevated blood pressure and pulse.

With diabetic ketoacidosis the patient gives a history of thirst, polyuria, and polydipsia and may have nausea, vomiting, abdominal pain, confusion, and ultimately coma. Because the respiratory system tries to compensate for the metabolic acidosis by eliminating carbon dioxide, rapid deep breathing (Kussmaul's respiration) is usually present. The odor of acetone may appear on the breath. The patient looks ill and, because of the polyuria, is usually dehydrated. There is rapid pulse, decreased blood pressure, decreased skin turgor, dry mouth, and enophthalmus (Leonard and Heslin, 1972).

Treatment

Treatment of hypoglycemia (Chue, 1976; Maw, 1975) is simple if initiated early while the patient is conscious; it consists of administering 10 to 20 gm of glucose or its equivalent orally. This can be accomplished by giving orange juice, sugar in water, sugar cubes, or soda pop. If the patient is unconscious, 20 to 50 ml of 50% glucose should be administered intravenously. If possible, such as in a hospital setting, blood for glucose determination should be obtained just prior to glucose infusion. Relief is usually immediate. If an intravenous line cannot be obtained because of obesity, restlessness, and so forth, 1 mg of glucagon may be administered intramuscularly or subcutaneously and oral sugar given when consciousness ensues. Glucagon works by glycogenolysis, breaking down glycogen in the liver to glucose. Its peak action occurs in 10 to 15 minutes (Boedeker and Dauber, 1974).

The treatment for ketoacidosis (Boedeker and Dauber, 1974; Kidson et al., 1974; Matz, 1974; Page et al., 1974; Semple et al., 1974; Winegrad and Clements, 1971) is complicated and in the best of circumstances is associated with some degree of mortality (Beigelman and Warner, 1973). As treatment involves administration of insulin and fluids, and monitoring electrolytes, vital signs, blood gases, and other parameters, it is best carried out in a hospital. If there is any doubt as to whether hypoglycemia or ketoacidosis exists, glucose should be given. If hypoglycemic, the patient should recover immediately; if ketoacidosis exists, no harm will have been done (Newmark et al., 1975). The patient should be placed supine, made comfortable, and transported to the hospital. If unconscious, a patent airway must be maintained.

Prevention

Questioning should reveal that the patient is a diabetic, whether the diabetic condition is adult or juvenile-onset, and the manner in which the patient is being treated, that is, diet, oral drugs, insulin. One should also determine whether the diabetes is under adequate control by checking for the symptoms listed above, testing the urine for sugar and ketones, or conferring with the patient's physician. Elective surgery should be deferred until good control is obtained. Whether office or hospital procedures are planned, proper preoperative management of the dia-

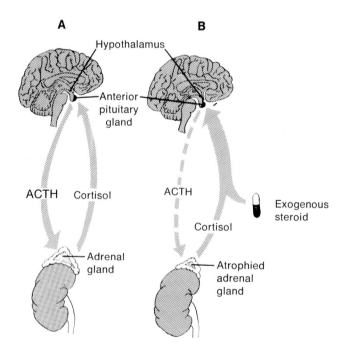

Fig. 11-14. A, Hypothalamic-pituitary-adrenal axis: Cortisol production is under direct control of ACTH secreted by anterior pituitary. Cortisol then exerts negative feedback control on ACTH production. **B,** With exogenous steroid administration, increased cortisol leads to decrease in ACTH production. This in turn results in decrease in endogenous cortisol production with possible adrenal atrophy.

betic is the best preventive measure (see Chapter 9).

ADRENAL INSUFFICIENCY
Problem

Adrenal insufficiency in an oral and maxillofacial surgery practice is most likely to occur with patients taking steroids or those who have previously taken steroid medication. Cortisol production is under the direct control of adrenocorticotropic hormone (ACTH) secreted by the anterior pituitary gland. An increase in ACTH production, as occurs with stress, stimulates an increased production of cortisol; conversely, a fall in ACTH levels is accompanied by a decrease in cortisol production. Because of a feedback mechanism between cortisol and ACTH, administration of exogenous steroids leads to a fall in the production of ACTH, which causes a decrease in endogenous steroid production. This leads to a suppression of the pituitary-adrenal axis and over a period of time can cause adrenal atrophy (Fig. 11-14). Because of this, the patient may not be able to respond normally to the stress of surgery with an increase in cortisol production.

Steroids are required in times of stress, as they promote cardiovascular stability by (1) maintaining normal vascular responses to circulating vasoconstrictor factors, (2) increasing vasomotor tone, and (3) increasing the contractile force of the myocardium (ASOS, 1971; Thorn, 1973). The degree of pituitary-adrenal suppression depends on the amount, duration, and mode of steroid administration. It is not known exactly how large a steroid dose is sufficient to cause suppression problems. Cawson and James (1973) reported a case of adrenal crisis in a dental patient taking 5 mg prednisolone daily, a low dosage of steroid. Therefore, duration of steroid administration may be a more important indicator of suppression of the pituitary-adrenal axis than amount. According to Ney (1971), when exogenous steroids are given for less than 10 days, the pituitary-adrenal axis recovers rapidly and clinical difficulties are generally not encountered. If large amounts of steroids are taken for more than a year,

recovery is much slower and may take as long as 9 months. Condon and Nyhus (1972) state that patients receiving steroids for more than 1 to 2 weeks within a 6- to 12-month period prior to surgery are a potential risk for iatrogenic adrenocortical insufficiency. However, Plumpton and associates (1969b), investigating corticosteroid therapy and surgery, state that adrenocortical suppression is unlikely to occur 2 months after cessation of steroid medication.

It has also been stated that administration of steroids every other day (alternate day therapy), as opposed to daily administration, helps to prevent ACTH suppression. In the final analysis, there seems to be no definitive answer as to who is at risk from acute adrenal insufficiency, and therefore consultation with the patient's physician prior to treatment is indicated. Since there is very little risk with short-term steroid administration, steroids should be given preoperatively if doubt exists about the patient's adrenal status.

Recognition

Adrenal crisis is characterized by anxiousness, severe nausea and vomiting, abdominal pain, cool and clammy skin, lethargy, and hypotension or shock (Boedeker and Dauber, 1974; Broutsas and Seldin, 1972).

Treatment

Initial therapy should involve administration of steroids to increase the circulating adrenocortical hormone level. If the patient is responsive and not in profound shock, 100 to 200 mg of a soluble hydrocortisone preparation added to 1000 ml of 5% D/S allowed to run over 4 hours is often advocated. Along with this, 100 mg of cortisone acetate is given intramuscularly for more sustained action (Boedeker and Dauber, 1974; Thorn, 1977; Thorn and Lauler, 1972). However, if profound shock is present, 100 mg of hydrocortisone sodium succinate (Solu-Cortef) should be given intravenously, increasing the dose to 400 to 500 mg if no response is seen (Boedeker and Dauber, 1974; Cawson and James,

1973). Vasopressors, such as epinephrine (Thorn and Lauler, 1972) or metaraminol bitartrate (Aramine) (Broutsas and Seldin, 1972) may also be useful in conjunction with steroids to combat hypotension. Other supportive therapy should be administered as indicated and the patient should be transported to the hospital for further care.

Prevention

Prevention starts with a good history, asking if the patient has taken steroid or "cortisone" medication. As some patients do not know the name of their medication, one should be aware of the conditions that may be treated with steroids (Strecten and Phil, 1975a). These include disorders such as arthritis, asthma, regional enteritis, ulcerative colitis, some types of hepatitis, pemphigus and other severe dermatoses, and collagen vascular diseases. They are also used to prevent graft rejection, that is, in kidney transplant patients, and in conjunction with other medicines in treating certain malignancies such as lymphosarcoma or lymphocytic leukemia.

If one elicits a history of steroid administration, and if consultation with the patient's physician reveals a possible chance of adrenocortical insufficiency with the stress of surgery, preoperative preparation with steroids should be undertaken. The steroid regimen, however, differs with various authors (see Chapter 9). Strecten and Phil (1975b) recommend increasing oral medication for patients presently taking steroids as follows: (1) mild stress, such as single dental extraction—double daily dose; (2) moderate stress, such as dentoalveolar surgery under local anesthesia or "severe dental extractions"—oral hydrocortisone, 100 mg, or prednisolone, 20 mg daily; (3) severe stress, such as general anesthesia—hydrocortisone, 200 mg, or prednisolone, 40 mg daily. Certain authors (Boedeker and Dauber, 1974; Condon and Nyhus, 1972), however, recommend parenteral administration of steroids, giving cortisone acetate 50 to 100 mg intramuscularly approximately 12 hours prior to surgery and 100 mg of cortisone the morning of surgery. An intravenous infusion of hydrocortisone hemisuccinate or phosphate is begun at surgery and 200 to 300 mg is given during the day of operation. Steroid medication is then tapered postoperatively by reducing the daily dose by 50% until maintenance levels are reached. Others (Banks, 1970; Plumpton et al., 1969a) have argued that cortisone acetate, although recommended for its sustained action, gives minimal raises of plasma cortisol. Plumpton (1969a) recommends hydrocortisone hemisuccinate 100 mg intramuscularly every 6 hours for 3 days beginning with the procedure for major operations; he states that for simple procedures 100 mg hydrocortisone intravenously at the time of induction would probably suffice. Banks (1970) states that the major need for steroids in oral surgery patients is from the commencement of surgery until 24 hours postoperatively. The ASOS Office Anesthesia Manual (1971) has the following recommendations: (1) Patients previously on cortisone for only a few months but presently off cortisone therapy for 6 months with no adverse effects need no supplementation. (2) Patients having received steroids for more than 1 year should be off medication for 1 year before no steroid supplementation is advised. (3) Patients presently on cortisone or having had a recent course of steroids for longer than 1 week should be given 200 mg orally the day before surgery, 100 mg orally postoperatively, 100 mg orally the day after surgery, with return to a regular dose the second day postoperatively.

Since there is such a variety of opinions, it is recommended that the patient's physician be contacted to help determine a suitable steroid regimen.

EPILEPTIC CONVULSION
Problem

The main concern in treating epileptic patients is the possibility of a convulsion or epileptic seizure occurring during treatment. Status epilepticus, two or more major seizures occurring without intervening consciousness, is the most serious possibility, having a mortality incidence of 10% to 20% (Boedeker and Dauber, 1974; Josephson, 1974). Status epilepticus occurs in 3% to 5% of the epileptic population (Josephson, 1974). Idiopathic epilepsy, however, is not the only consideration when convulsions do occur. Convulsions may be seen in relation to infection, fever, neurologic problems (disease, tumor, injury), metabolic imbalances (hypoglycemia, hypocalcemia, hypernatremia, hyponatremia), and toxic reactions to drugs, including local anesthetics (Boedeker and Dauber, 1974; Josephson, 1974; Thorn, 1977).

As most epileptics are on long-term drug therapy, other complications may be related to this therapy. Phenytoin (Dilantin) can occasionally cause bone marrow depression, resulting in reduced numbers of white and red cells in the blood (Leonard and Heslin, 1971a). Evans (1975) also warns of the possibility of Dilantin toxicity (nystagmus, ataxia, tremor, nausea) associated with anesthesia because of the following: (1) Since epileptics are on long-term drug regimens, these drugs may tend to accumulate in the body. (2) Dilantin levels may be raised by certain drugs such as diazepam (Valium), a premedicant to anesthesia, because of enzyme inhibition in which drugs compete for the same metabolic pathways. (3) General anesthesia may also cause general cellular depression and thus retard hepatic degradation of Dilantin.

Recognition

A grand mal epileptic seizure is characterized by a generalized convulsion usually lasting less than 5 minutes. The convulsion is often preceded by prodromal symptoms (aura) that may consist of brief sensory, motor, or psychic sensations. There is loss of consciousness, there may be urinary and fecal incontinence, and one often sees injury from falling or tongue and cheek biting. Respirations may become jerky. The postictal state is usually characterized by drowsiness, headaches, and confusion (Castle and Fishman, 1973; Chue, 1975b; Harrison, 1973; Leonard and Heslin, 1971).

Treatment

Treatment revolves around airway maintenance, patient protection, and termination of convulsions. A patent airway should be maintained and any oral appliances or dental prostheses should be removed immediately. Tight restrictive clothing about the neck should be loosened. Oxygen administration may help protect against hypoxia. If vomiting occurs, the head should be lowered, turned to the side, and the mouth and throat suctioned free of saliva and vomitus. By judiciously restraining the patient, injury during the seizure can be avoided. To prevent tongue biting, a towel or padded tongue blades should be inserted between the teeth, taking care to avoid airway obstruction.

The above treatment often suffices as the convulsion is usually quite brief. If, however, the convulsion has not stopped after several minutes, drug administration (Boedeker and Dauber, 1974; Forman, 1974; Josephson, 1974) may be required to terminate it and thus reduce morbidity and mortality. Diazepam is the initial drug of choice, and in the adult, 5 to 10 mg intravenously (at a rate of 5 mg/min) may be given. In children, 0.25 to 0.50 mg/kg of diazepam should be administered intravenously. The initial dose may be repeated at 10 to 15 minute intervals, but a maximum of 30 mg diazepam should be administered in 1 hour's time. The intramuscular route can be used if an intravenous line cannot be obtained. As small a dose of diazepam as possible should be used to terminate the seizure, as this therapy may add to the postictal depression. The initial dose controls seizure activity in 70% to 90% of patients (Boedeker and Dauber, 1974; Ferngren, 1974); however, recurrence of the seizure is possible.

Succinylcholine, intravenously or intramuscularly, can also be used if one is prepared to adequately support respiration (ASOS, 1971; McCarthy, 1972). For proper follow-up after the seizure, the patient's physician should be notified.

Prevention

An adequate history should alert the clinician to the possibility of complications (since most patients know that they have epilepsy). The degree of control should be ascertained and elective procedures delayed if the patient is not under good control. The medicines taken by the patient should be known by the doctor, and the patient should be asked if he is indeed taking the medicine as prescribed. Juul-Jensen (1968) has shown that often recurrence of seizures is in close association with discontinuance of medication. The doctor should also be aware that infection or fever may precipitate seizures. Adequate sedation or general anesthesia may be beneficial as preventive measures. If a patient has a seizure in the office, he should be taken home by an escort because of the postictal depression.

CEREBROVASCULAR ACCIDENT (STROKE)

Problem

A cerebrovascular accident (CVA), or stroke, is a serious event that, although unlikely, can take place in the office. A CVA can result from thrombosis (over 50%), embolism, or hemorrhage, all of which result in focal brain damage (Kannel et al., 1965; Thorn, 1977). The disease afflicts mainly the older population, with atherosclerosis being an important contributing factor. Vascular malformation, inflammatory disease of the arteries, hematologic disorders, hypertension (Beevers et al., 1973; Lavy et al., 1973; Veterans Administration Study, 1967), hypotension, and drugs such as anticoagulants and oral contraceptives (Collaborative Group Study, 1975) may also be precipitating factors in stroke. (Greer, 1973).

Recognition

The hallmark of a CVA is a sudden onset or change in neurologic function with the specific symptoms depending on the area and extent of brain damage. Weakness, hemiplegia, hemianesthesia, and speech and visual problems may occur (Vroom, 1974). Severe headache is frequent if the CVA is a result of hemorrhage. A change in the level of consciousness is also possible, with overt unconsciousness at the time of the stroke carrying a very serious prognosis (Oxbury et al., 1975).

Treatment

Emergency treatment is mainly supportive. The patient should be kept comfortable. A patent airway should be maintained and oxygen administered if respiratory difficulty develops. Because of the possibility of continued hemorrhage, the head should be kept elevated. The patient should be transported to the hospital for definitive treatment.

Prevention

There may be little a practitioner can do to prevent a stroke, but he should be aware of those patients who are at risk. They include elderly patients, hypertensive patients, and patients with evidence of arteriosclerosis, that is, angina pectoris, myocardial infarction, or peripheral vascular disease. Sedation should be used in these individuals. One should also be aware that in approximately 80% of stroke cases caused by cerebral thrombosis, there are preceding minor signs or transient warning ischemic attacks (Thorn, 1977), and the history and physical examination should be directed toward recognition of this possibility.

REFERENCES

Aldrete, J. A., and Johnson, D. A. 1969. Allergy to local anesthesia, J.A.M.A. **207**:356.

Alexander, S. C., et al. 1965. Cerebral carbohydrate metabolism during hypocarbia in man, Anesthesiology **26**:624.

Allen, G. D., and Morris, L. E. 1962. Central nervous effects of hyperventilation during anesthesia, Br. J. Anaesth. **34**:296.

American Dental Association. 1975. Accepted dental therapeutics, ed. 36, Chicago, American Dental Association.

American Society of Oral Surgeons. 1971. Office anesthesia — emergency self-evaluation manual.

American Society of Oral Surgeons Committee on Anesthesia. 1974. ASOS anesthesia morbidity and mortality survey, J. Oral Surg. **32**:733.

Arky, R. A., and Arone, D. L. 1971. Hypoglycemia in diabetes melitus, Med. Clin. North Am. **55**:919.

Arora, B. K. 1975. Surgical complications of significance in dental practice, J. Can. Dent. Assoc. **41**:281.

Banks, P. 1970. The adreno-cortical response to oral surgery, Br. J. Oral Surg. **8**:32.

Barnard, J. H. 1970. Nonfatal results in third-degree anaphylaxis from *Hymenoptera* stings, J. Allergy Clin. Immunol. **45**:94.

Beevers, D. G., et al. 1973. The influence of antihypertensive treatment over the incidence of cerebral vascular disease, Postgrad. Med. J. **23**:905.

Beigelman, P. M., and Warner, N. E. 1973. Thirty-two fatal cases of severe diabetic ketoacidosis including a case of mucormycosis, Diabetes **22**:847.

Boedeker, E. C., and Dauber, J. H., eds. 1974. Manual of medical therapeutics, ed. 21, Boston, Little, Brown & Co.

Booth, D. F. 1972. Acute anaphylaxis from orally administered penicillin G: report of a case, J. Am. Dent. Assoc. **85**:1367.

Brendlinger, D. L., and Tarsitano, J. J. 1970. Generalized dermatitis due to sensitivity to a chrome cobalt removable partial denture, J. Am. Dent. Assoc. **81**:392.

Broutsas, M. G., and Seldin, R. 1972. Adrenal crisis after tooth extraction in an adrenalectomized patient: report of a case, J. Oral Surg. **30**:301.

Budd, M. A., et al. 1964. Evaluation of intradermal skin tests in penicillin hypersensitivity, J.A.M.A. **190**:203.

Burnum, J. F. 1974. Hyperventilation, J.A.M.A. **229**:521.

Burnum, J. F., et al. 1954. The effect of hypocarbia on arterial blood pressure, Circulation **9**:89.

Bustad, L. 1976. Personal communication.

Campbell, R. L., et al. 1976. Vasovagal response during oral surgery, J. Oral Surg. **34**:698.

Castle, G. F., and Fishman, L. S. 1973. Seizures, Pediatr. Clin. North Am. **20**:819.

Cawson, R. A., and James, J. 1973. Adrenal crisis in a dental patient having systemic corticosteroids, Br. J. Oral Surg. **10**:305.

Cheraskin, E., and Prasertsuntarasai, T. 1957. Use of epinephrine with local anesthesia in hypertensive patients. I. Blood pressure and pulse rate observations in the waiting room, J. Am. Dent. Assoc. **55**:761.

Cheraskin, E., and Prasertsuntarasai, T. 1958a. Use of epinephrine with local anesthesia in hypertensive patients. III. Effects of epinephrine on blood pressure and pulse rate, J. Am. Dent. Assoc. **57**:507.

Cheraskin, E., and Prasertsuntarasai, T. 1958b. Use of epinephrine with local anesthesia in hypertensive patients. II. Effects of sedation on blood pressure and pulse rate in the waiting room, J. Am. Dent. Assoc. **56**:210.

Cheraskin, E., and Prasertsuntarasai, T. 1959. Use of epinephrine with local anesthesia in hypertensive patients. IV. Effect of tooth extraction on blood pressure and pulse rate, J. Am. Dent. Assoc. **58**:61.

Chue, P. W. Y. 1975a. The hyperventilation syndrome: diagnosis and management, Dent. Surv. **51**:31.

Chue, P. W. Y. 1975b. Transient loss of consciousness: common faint or serious symptom? Dent. Surv. **51**:40.

Chue, P. W. Y. 1976. Hypoglycemic attack: causes and treatment, Dent. Surv. **52**:29.

Coates, W. H. 1963. Case of anaphylactic shock following the administration of oral penicillin, case report, Aust. Dent. J. **8**:189.

Cochrane, B. M. 1974. What can we do to reduce deaths from asphyxiation due to choking? Can. Med. Assoc. J. **111**:460.

Collaborative Group for the Study of Stroke in Young Women. 1975. Oral contraceptives and stroke in young women, J.A.M.A. **231**:318.

Condon, R. E., and Nyhus, I. M., eds. 1972. Manual of surgical therapeutics, ed. 2, Boston, Little, Brown & Co.

Corbett, J. L., et al. 1971. Modification of cerebral vasoconstriction with hyperventilation in normal man by thymoxamine, Lancet **2**:461.

Curry, C. L., and Hosten, A. C. 1975. Current treatment of malignant hypertension, J.A.M.A. **232**:1367.

Dack, S. 1978. Acute pulmonary edema, Hosp. Med. **14**:112.

Danilewicz-Stysiak, Z. 1971. Allergy as a cause of denture sore mouth, J. Prosthet. Dent. **25**:16.

Des Fourie. 1968. Vasovagal syncope, J. Dent. Assoc. S. Afr. **23**:244.

Donaldson, O., et al. 1971. Partial dentures as a hazard to the airway, Br. Dent. J. **131**:546.

Driggs, R. L., and O'Day, R. A. 1972. Acute allergic reaction associated with methohexital anesthesia: report of six cases, J. Oral Surg. **30**:906.

Dworkin, S. F. 1973. Psychodynamics of dental emergencies, Dent. Clin. North Am. **17**:403.

Evans, D. E. N. 1975. Anaesthesia and the epileptic patient, Anaesthesia **30**:34.

Everett, F. G., and Hice, T. L. 1974. Contact stomatitis resulting from the use of orthodontic rubber elastics: report of a case, J. Am. Dent. Assoc. **88**:1030.

Ferngren, H. G. 1974. Diazepam treatment for acute convulsions in children, Epilepsia **15**:27.

Forman, P. M. 1974. Therapy of seizures in children, Am. Fam. Physician **10**:144.

Forrester, J. S., et al. 1976. Medical therapy of acute myocardial infarction by application of hemodynamic subsets, N. Engl. J. Med. **295**:1356.

Fowler, N. O. 1972. Clinical diagnosis, Circulation **46**:1079.

Franklin, W. 1974. Treatment of severe asthma, N. Engl. J. Med. **290**:1469.

Friedberg, C. K. 1973. Fainting, causes and cures, Med. Times **101**:41.

Friedberg, C. K. 1971. Syncope: pathological physiology: differential diagnosis and treatment, Mod. Concepts Cardiovasc. Dis. **40**:61.

Garcia, A. C., et al. 1971. Lactate and pyruvate accumulation during hypocapnia, Respir. Physiol. **12**:371.

Gaum, L. I. 1970. Basic steps in cardiopulmonary resuscitation, J. Can. Dent. Assoc. **36**:158.

Glauda, N. M., et al. 1975. Nonfatal anaphylaxis caused by oral penicillin: report of a case, J. Am. Dent. Assoc. **90**:159.

Gold, M. I., and Hebrick, M. 1963. A study of the complications related to anesthesia in asthmatic patients, Anesth. Analg. **42**:283.

Goldberg, A. H. 1974. Cardiopulmonary arrest, N. Engl. J. Med. **290**:381.

Gote, N., et al. 1972. Contact allergy to medicaments and materials used in dentistry (III). Odontol. Revy **23**:197.

Gottlieb, S. J., and Constantine, J. F. 1967. Dental anesthesia with lidocaine hydrochloride for children with intractable asthma and associated allergies, J. Oral Ther. **3**:468.

Granholm, L. 1971. Cerebral effects of hyperventilation, Acta Anaesthesiol. Scand. (Suppl.) **45:**114.

Greer, M. 1973. Management of the patient with acute stroke, Geriatrics **28:**48.

Hagen, J., et al. 1971. A program for preparedness in anesthetic and emergency technique in the oral surgery office, J. Oral Surg. **29:**166.

Hannington-Kiff, J. G. 1969. Fainting and collapse in dental practice, Dent. Pract. **20:**2.

Harrison, J. B. 1973. Faints and spells, Dent. Clin. North Am. **17:**461.

Heimlich, H. J. 1974. Pop goes the café, Emergency Med. p. 154.

Heimlich, H. J. 1975. A life-saving maneuver to prevent food choking, J.A.M.A. **234:**398.

Heimlich, H. J., et al. 1975. Food choking and drowning deaths prevented by external subdiaphragmatic compression, Ann. Thorac. Surg. **20:**188.

Herman, M. U. 1971. The clinical picture of ischemic heart disease, Prog. Cardiovasc. Dis. **14:**321.

Holen, S., and Dicklor, E. H. 1973. Missing teeth and dentures—killers of 2,500 annually, J. D.C. Dent. Soc. **48:**26.

Hooley, J. R., and Meyer, R. 1966. Anaphylactic reaction to oral penicillin: report of a case and review of the literature, Oral Surg. **22:**474.

Hubscher, T. 1975. Role of the eosinophil in the allergic reactions. I. EDI—an eosinophil-derived inhibitor of histamine release, J. Immunol. **114:**1379.

Jastar, J. T., and Cowan, F. F. 1973. Patients at risk, Dent. Clin. North Am. **17:**363.

Josephson, D. A. 1974. Status epilepticus, Am. Fam. Physician **10:**168.

Jung, R. C., et al. 1971. Response of human forearm muscle blood vessels to hyperventilation, Cardiovasc. Res. **5:**347.

Juul-Jensen, P. 1968. Frequency of recurrence after discontinuance of anticonvulsant therapy in patients with epileptic seizures. A new follow-up study after five years, Epilepsia **9:**11.

Kannel, W. B. 1975. Role of blood pressure in cardiovascular disease: the Framingham Study, Angiology **26:**1.

Kannel, W. B., et al. 1965. Vascular disease of the brain—epidemiologic aspects: the Framingham Study, Am. J. Public Health **55:**1355.

Kety, S., and Schmedt, C. F. 1946. The effects of active and passive hyperventilation on cerebral blood flow, cerebral oxygen consumption, cardiac output, and blood pressure of normal young men, J. Clin. Invest. **25:**107.

Kidson, W., et al. 1974. Treatment of severe diabetes mellitus by insulin infusion, Br. Med. J. **2:**691.

Kinsman, R. A., et al. 1973. Subjective symptoms of acute asthma within a heterogenous sample of asthmatics, J. Allergy Clin. Imunol. **52:**284.

Koch, G., et al. 1973. Contact allergy to medicaments and materials used in dentistry (IV), Odontol. Revy **24:**109.

Lavy, S., et al. 1973. Hypertension and diabetes as risk factors in stroke patients, Stroke **4:**751.

Lemmer, J. 1968. Respiratory tetany—an unusual clinical phenomenon, J. Dent. Assoc. S. Afr. **23:**105.

Leonard, M., and Heslin, L. 1972. Diabetes and dentistry, J. Irish Dent. Assoc. **18:**25.

Leonard, M., and Heslin, L. 1971a. The health questionnaire in general dental practice. 6. Epilepsy and fainting, J. Irish Dent. Assoc. **17:**168.

Leonard, M., and Heslin, L. 1971b. The health questionnaire in general dental practice. 4. Coronary artery disease, J. Irish Dent. Assoc. **17:**90.

Lesch, M., and Gorlin, R. 1973. Pharmacological therapy of angina pectoris, Mod. Concepts Cardiovasc. Dis. **42:**5.

Levine, R. 1974. Hypoglycemia, J.A.M.A. **230:**462.

Little, R. C., and Smith, C. W. 1964. Cardiovascular response to acute hypocapnia due to overbreathing, Am. J. Physiol. **206:**1025.

Litwin, M. S., et al. 1970. Metabolic effects of prolonged passive hyperventilation, Surg. Forum **21:**205.

Matz, R. 1974. Diabetic coma: guidelines in therapy, N.Y. State J. Med. **74:**642.

Maw, D. S. J. 1975. The emergency management of diabetes mellitus, Anaesthesia **30:**520.

McCarthy, F. 1972. Emergencies in dental practice, ed 2, Philadelphia, W. B. Saunders Co.

Morgan, P., and Ward, B. 1970. Hyperventilation and changes in the electroencephalogram and electroretinogram, Neurology **20:**1009.

Moser, R. H., ed. 1974. Standards for cardiopulmonary resuscitation (CPR) and emergency cardiac care (ECC), J.A.M.A. (Suppl.) **227.**

Murrin, K. R., and Nagarajan, T. M. 1974. Hyperventilation and psychometric testing, Anaesthesia **29:**50.

Naylor, M. N. 1959. Tetanic symptoms in the dental chair, Br. Dent. J. **106:**146.

Newmark, S. R., et al. 1975. Hyperglycemia and hypoglycemia crisis, J.A.M.A. **231:**185.

Ney, R. L., In Thorn, T. W., ed. 1971. Steroid therapy, New York, Medcom Inc.

Oxbury, J. M., et al. 1975. Predicting the outcome of stroke: acute stage after cerebral infarction, Br. Med. J. **3:**125.

Page, L. B., and Sidd, J. J. 1972a. Medical management of primary hypertension, Part III, N. Engl. J. Med. **287:**1074.

Page, L. B., and Sidd, J. J. 1972b. Medical management of primary hypertension, Part II, N. Engl. J. Med. **287:**1018.

Page, L. B., and Sidd, J. J. 1972c. Medical management of primary hypertension, Part I, N. Engl. J. Med. **287:**960.

Page, M. M., et al. 1974. Treatment of diabetic coma with continuous low dose infusion of insulin, Br. Med. J. **2:**687.

Parker, C. W. 1975a. Drug allergy (third of three parts), N. Engl. J. Med. **292:**957.

Parker, C. W. 1975b. Drug allergy (second of three parts), N. Engl. J. Med. **292:**732.

Parker, C. W. 1975c. Drug allergy (first of three parts), N. Engl. J. Med. **292:**511.

Parmley, W. W. 1977. Axioms on congestive heart failure, Hosp. Med. **13:**44.

Phills, J. A., and Perelmutter, L. 1974. IgE mediated and nonIgE mediated allergic-type reactions to aspirin, Acta Allergol. **29:**474.

Plumpton, F. S., et al. 1969a. Corticosteroid treatment and surgery. 2. The management of steroid cover, Anaesthesia **24**:12.

Plumpton, F. S., et al. 1969b. Corticosteroid treatment and surgery. 1. An investigation of the indications of steroid cover, Anaesthesia **24**:3.

Poulsom, R. C. 1974. An anaphylactoid reaction to periodontal surgical dressing: report of a case, J. Am. Dent. Assoc. **89**:895.

Report of the Special Committee of the New York Heart Association, Inc., on the use of epinephrine in connection with procaine in dental procedures, 1955. J. Am. Dent. Assoc. **50**:108.

Riggs, T. E., et al. 1972. Physiologic effects of passive hyperventilation on oxygen delivery and consumption, Proc. Soc. Exp. Biol. Med. **140**:1414.

Riley, D. J. 1974. The "oily" paper bag and hyperventilation, J.A.M.A. **229**:638.

Road, J. P. 1973. A case of lignocaine hypersensitivity, Br. Dent. J. **135**:411.

Rotsztain, A., et al. 1970. Blood gas changes during voluntary hyperventilation in normal and disease states, Am. Rev. Respir. Dis. **102**:205.

Seamonds, B., et al. 1972. Determination of ionized calcium in serum by use of an ion-selective electrode, Clin. Chem. **18**:155.

Semple, P. F., et al. 1974. Continuous intravenous infusion of small doses of insulin in treatment of diabetic ketoacidosis, Br. Med. J. **2**:694.

Senior, R. M., et al. 1975. Status asthmaticus, J.A.M.A. **231**:1277.

Sharpe, J. C., ed. 1969. Management of medical emergencies, ed. 2, New York, McGraw-Hill Book Co.

Sherman, P. M. 1974. Cardiac arrest with diazepam, J. Oral Surg. **32**:567.

Shields, P. N. 1972. Local anesthetic sensitivity: case report, Aust. Dent. J. **17**:51.

Soo, H. C., and Patterson, R. 1974. Surgery in corticosteroid-dependent asthmatics, J. Allergy Clin. Immunol. **53**:345.

Staples, A. F. 1973. Cardiopulmonary crisis in the dental office, Dent. Clin. North Am. **17**:473.

Stein, R. M. 1975. Cardiopulmonary resuscitation procedures, Med. Times. **103**:64.

Strecten, D. H. P., and Phil, D. 1975a. Corticosteroid therapy. II. Complications and therapeutic indications, J.A.M.A. **232**:1046.

Strecten, D. H. P., and Phil, D. 1975b. Corticosteroid therapy. I. Pharmacological properties and principles of corticosteroid use, J.A.M.A. **232**:944.

Sugioka, K., and Davis, D. A. 1960. Hyperventilation with oxygen: a possible cause of cerebral hypoxemia, Anaesthesiology **21**:135.

Tarhan, S., et al. 1972. Myocardial infarction after general anesthesia, J.A.M.A. **220**:1451.

Tarsitano, J. J., and Jerman, A. C. 1970 Cricothyroidotomy kit, J. Am. Dent. Assoc. **81**:1392.

Tennenbaum, J. I. 1974. Current treatment of status asthmaticus, Am. Fam. Physician **10**:92.

Thompson, D. S. 1975. Emergency airway management, Am. Fam. Physician **11**:146.

Thorn, G. W. 1973. The adrenal cortex: reflections, progress, and speculations, Trans. Assoc. Am. Physicians **86**:65.

Thorn, G. W., and Lauler, D. P. 1972. Clinical therapeutics of adrenal disorders, Am. J. Med. **53**:673.

Thorn, G. W., ed. 1977. Harrison's principles of internal medicine, ed. 8, New York, McGraw-Hill Book Co.

Veterans Administration Cooperative Study Group in Antihypertensive Agents. 1967. Effects of treatment on morbidity in hypertension: results in patients with diastolic blood pressure averaging 115-129 mm Hg, J.A.M.A. **202**:1028.

Vidt, D. G. 1975. Diazoxide for hypertensive crisis, Am. Fam. Physician **11**:128.

Vijay, N.K., and Schoonmaker, F. W. 1975. Cardiopulmonary arrest and resuscitation, Am. Fam. Physician **12**:85.

Vroom, F. Q. 1974. Treatment of stroke: Medical or surgical? Geriatrics **29**:123.

Walters, E., and Klein, J. C. 1970. Precautions before anesthesia for the dental office patient, J. Am. Dent. Assoc. **81**:406.

Wayne, H. H. 1961. Syncope: physiological considerations and an analysis of the clinical characteristics in 510 patients, Am. J. Med. **30**:418.

Wellins, S. L. 1969. Hypersensitivity to lidocaine hydrochloride, Oral Surg. **28**:761.

Winegrad, A. I., and Clements, R. S. 1971. Diabetic ketoacidosis, Med. Clin. North Am. **55**:899.

Wintrobe, M. M., ed. 1974. Harrison's principles of internal medicine, ed. 7, New York, McGraw-Hill Book Co.

Wright, F. A. C. 1971. Allergic reactions to mercury after dental treatment, N.Z. Dent. J. **67**:251.

Wright, K. E., Jr., and McIntosh, H. D. 1971. Syncope: a review of pathophysiological mechanisms, Prog. Cardiovasc. Dis. **13**:580.

Zelis, R., et al. 1974. Current concepts in the drug management of angina pectoris, Cardiovasc. Clin. **6**:239.

PART THREE

EXAMINATION AND DIAGNOSIS

CHAPTER 12

Clinical history and physical examination

Jeffrey L. Laskin

Patients present themselves to the oral and maxillofacial surgeon with a large variety of problems, involving both emergency and elective care. In every case, whether the patient has facial trauma, is in need of orthognathic or preprosthetic management, or is coming to the office for any of the multitude of procedures that are performed by the oral and maxillofacial surgeon, a systematic history should be taken and a careful examination must be performed to define and delineate the clinical problems and help establish a rational treatment plan.

HISTORY TAKING

The history consists of two parts—the history of the presenting complaint (onset and course) and the general history, which provides information about medical, surgical, psychologic, social, occupational, and family background. An inquiry by systems is also part of the general history. The areas covered and the extent of the questions asked in this portion of the history are governed by their relevance to the clinical situation.

It is preferable to begin the history with questioning about the present problem because this permits easier interpretation of the significance of the more general findings. When possible, the patient should be encouraged to provide information in chronologic order. Sufficient time should be devoted to the history, since the information obtained is often equally as important in helping to establish a diagnosis and treatment plan as the physical findings.

Given the opportunity, most patients are eager to discuss the history of their problem and their symptoms. The clinician should guide them through the use of both open and closed-ended questions, allowing patients to freely relate their complaints while still keeping to the subject at hand. "Would you tell me more about the pain?" or "What seems to make the pain worse?" are examples of open-ended questions that give patients a broad area to discuss. Closed-ended questions such as "Is the pain a dull ache?" or "Is the pain worse in the morning?" require a more limited response and help elicit specific information that patients might not ordinarily provide. It is also helpful to ask patients what they think is causing their condition, since this gives valuable insight into their understanding of the problem.

All of the data gathered from the history should be recorded in a logical order, using essentially the same format each time so that information is not inadvertently omitted. As much detail as possible should be included so that even data that initially seem irrelevant will be readily available for review at any time such information may become important.

A general summary of the components of a standard medical history follows.

Identification and general information

Record the patient's complete name, including the maiden name for a married woman. Other data include age, sex, race, occupation, and marital status.

Source of data and qualitive reliability

At times the medical history will not be obtained from the patient because of age or general condition. Occasionally, an interpreter may be necessary for a patient interview in another language. It is important that the source of the data, as well as a qualitative statement of the reliability of the information, be included in the record, especially if the patient's records will be used or reviewed by other than the original interviewer.

Chief complaints

The chief complaints are generally recorded in the patient's own words, but at times medical terminology is used. It is important to record symptoms as the chief complaints rather than the patient's or a prior doctor's diagnosis. All symptoms should be listed in order of importance to the patient. The duration of each symptom should be stated.

History of the present illness

The history of the present illness is the most important part of the patient interview, as it contains the basic historic diagnostic data. Its purpose is to furnish the interviewer with a clear chronologic order of symptoms beginning with the appearance of the initial symptom, the circumstances surrounding the first symptom, and how the patient has been affected by the course of the illness. Past treatments for the condition and results should be noted. It is also customary to include the review of that major system affected by the illness in this section.

Past medical history

The past medical history section contains the information that summarizes the patient's health status prior to the present illness. It can be divided into several sections.

Childhood diseases

Many childhood diseases are not serious and pass without causing any significant sequelae. A few childhood illnesses such as scarlet fever, rheumatic fever, or glomerulonephritis, however, have the potential to cause serious functional and organic impairments. These must be noted to enable the treatment plan of the patient to be modified accordingly. Even the less serious conditions should also be considered since some of the so-called childhood diseases can occur in adults, and knowledge of the patient's history can be important in differential diagnosis.

Adult illnesses

Many medical illnesses have a significant bearing on the total management of surgical cases. Infectious diseases such as tuberculosis and hepatitis, as well as parasitic, fungal, and bacterial infections, may have debilitating or generalized systemic effects that will alter the treatment plan for even minor procedures. Diseases that affect the endocrine system, such as those of the thyroid gland or diabetes mellitus, will modify the patient's response to anesthetic agents and surgical stress and influence postoperative healing and medication. Anemias, coagulation defects, agranulocytosis, and other hematologic disorders will also affect the course of anesthesia and surgery.

Diseases of the respiratory system, such as pneumonia, bronchitis, asthma, and emphysema, as well as such upper respiratory conditions as a deviated nasal septum or chronic allergic rhinitis significantly affect the anesthetic management of the patient. Cardiovascular disorders such as rheumatic heart disease, ischemic heart disease, hypertension, myocardial infarction, cerebral vascular disease, congestive heart failure, angina pectoris, and heart valve surgery also are significant in reducing the patient's tolerance to the stresses of anesthesia and surgery. In addition, many diseases of other body systems, such as the digestive, musculoskeletal, genitourinary, and nervous system, can affect surgical, anesthetic, and drug therapy.

Previous hospitalizations, operations, and anesthetics

A record of a patient's prior hospitalizations can be useful, not only to establish the cause of the hospitalization but in some instances to help obtain historic laboratory and radiographic data. Moreover, future problems in patient care can be anticipated from a knowledge of the patient's response to prior operations and anesthetics.

Accidents or injuries

Not every injury is serious enough to require hospitalization, but the history of such an occurrence may be significant in establishing a diagnosis and appropriate plan of treatment. The type of injury, the date it happened, and any complications should be recorded.

Allergies

Existing allergies and their manifestations, as well as allergic tendencies, are elicited in this section of the past medical history. Many patients mistake side effects of drugs, such as nausea from a narcotic, for drug allergy, and it is important to make this distinction.

Immunization record

Knowledge of the patient's immunization record, especially for tetanus, is essential. This often fatal disease can be easily avoided by the appropriate use of either active or passive immunization, depending on the severity of the injury and the patient's immunization record.

Present and recent medications

There are a large number of drug effects, side effects, and interactions. The patient's present and recent medication history can have important implications in differential diagnosis and determining the course of therapy. Preoperative consultations, alterations in surgical and anesthetic techniques, and special postoperative management may be necessary owing to the use of certain medications such as dicumarol, MAO inhibitors, antihypertensive drugs, and so forth.

Habits

Questions about the use of tobacco, drugs, alcohol, tea, and coffee can elicit information that may not only be significant in relation to the patient's presenting complaint but may also be important in consideration of their general physical condition. Sleeping and eating habits should also be considered.

Social history

Information in the social history is intended to summarize the patient's life with respect to how the environment may be contributing to the disease. It may include questions about the patient's marital history, social and economic status, birthplace, and areas of residency. The regional occurrence of diseases such as histoplasmosis, malaria, and some parasitic diseases, or the high incidence of hepatitis in homosexuals are examples of how information from the social history can be helpful in differential diagnosis.

Family history

The family history involves information about the present state of parents, siblings, and offspring. It includes ages and health status for all living members and age at death and cause for deceased family members. Certain diseases have a familial tendency and others have a hereditary basis.

Review of systems

The review of systems has two main purposes. The first is to detect illness in systems other than those involved in the present illness; the second is to help the patient recall symptoms of the present illness that may have been omitted during other parts of the interview.

Integument

Important symptoms include pruritis or urticaria. These may involve an allergic reaction, a viral infection such as herpes zoster, or idiopathic conditions such as erythema multiforme, psoriasis, or lichen planus. Changes in skin pigmentation or color can occur with Addison's disease, lupus erythematosus, polycythemia, and conditions that produce jaundice or cyanosis. Signs of blood dyscrasias or a coagulation defect can also produce recognizable changes in the skin such as petechial hemorrhages or ecchymosis.

Endocrine system

Fatigue, dry skin, weight gain, hot or cold intolerance, tremors, nervousness, or exophthalmus can suggest thyroid disease. A history of radiation for acne or tonsillitis warrants continued monitoring of the thyroid for tumor development. The well-known triad of polydypsia, polyphagia, and polyuria is indicative of diabetes mellitus.

Head

Important symptoms involving the head include headaches, the location, duration, periodicity, type, and prodromal symptoms of which are used to discriminate the variety and cause. Also important is a history of trauma, dizziness, or episodes of syncope.

Eyes

Visual disturbances are the most common findings. Symptoms such as icterus suggest liver disease; other symptoms include inflammation, ocular pain, or diplopia. Edema of the lower lids may suggest congestive heart disease.

Ears

Important symptoms of the ears include decreased hearing, earache, tinnitus, vertigo, and discharge.

Nose and sinuses

Symptoms involving the nose and sinuses include anosmia, discharge, obstruction, trauma, epistaxis, frequency of colds, and sinusitis.

Jaws

Information about jaw fractures, dislocation, subluxation, pain on opening or closing movements, trismus, and joint noises should be obtained.

Oral cavity

History of dental disease and the patient's attention to these problems are indicative of what may be expected in the future dental management of the patient. Important symptoms include pain, swelling, and hemorrhage. Glossitis may indicate anemia or vitamin deficiency. Taste defects caused by a zinc-poor diet may indicate a potential candidate for impaired healing. Other questions should relate to looseness of teeth, previous extractions or oral surgery, bruxism, mouth breathing, dryness, excessive salivation, ulcerations, odor, and so forth.

Pharynx and larynx

Tumors in the throat can produce symptoms of hoarseness, difficulty in swallowing, and progressive dysphagia. Other symptoms include pain, swelling, and hemorrhage.

Neck

Limitation of motion, swelling, and pain are the major symptoms of diseases involving the neck.

Respiratory system

Important symptoms include dyspnea on exertion, hemoptysis, cough, pain, and wheezing.

Cardiovascular system

Important findings include a history of hypertensive heart disease, angina pectoris, congenital heart disease, rheumatic heart disease, heart failure, and heart murmurs. The ability of a patient to withstand the stresses of surgery and anesthesia are directly related to cardiovascular and respiratory reserve and these parameters must be thoroughly evaluated.

Gastrointestinal system

Significant symptoms include loss of weight, indigestion, epigastric pain, anorexia, hematemesis, change in bowel habits, nausea, vomiting, diarrhea, and blood in the stool.

Genitourinary system

Diseases of the genitourinary system may cause symptoms of polyuria, hematuria, pyuria, dysuria, oliguria, and nocturia. Lumbar pain and urethral discharge may also occur. A history of possible venereal disease should be elicited.

Gynecologic system

Questions should relate to metrorrhagia, gravida, para, abortions, and complications. A discussion about missed menstrual periods may lead to recognition of an unknowingly pregnant patient.

Hematopoietic and lymphatic systems

Symptoms of dysfunction of the hematopoietic and lymphatic systems include anemia, bleeding problems, swollen lymph nodes, petechiae, and purpura.

Orthopedic system

Symptoms such as pain, limitation of motion, and swelling of the joints are present in diseases involving the extremities.

Nervous system

Important symptoms include convulsions, anesthesia and paresthesia, ataxia, paresis or paralysis, tics, and tremors.

Psychiatric status

Findings include a history of psychiatric treatment, insomnia, behavioral changes, nervousness, anxiety, and depression.

PHYSICAL EXAMINATION

Once the complete medical history and review of systems have been completed, the clinician can then proceed with the physical examination. The extent of this examination is guided by the symptoms that were elicited by the prior questioning. A description of the complete examination is beyond the scope of this text; therefore this discussion will be limited to the vital signs and the examination of the facial, cervical, and oral regions. The reader is referred to any standard textbook on physical diagnosis for a description of the procedures involved in the complete physical evaluation of the patient.

To perform the clinical examination, the oral and maxillofacial surgeon must master the techniques of *inspection, palpation, percussion,* and *auscultation.* The clinician must also learn to use mechanical devices such as the ophthalmoscope, otoscope, laryngoscope, and others that can be of assistance in observing areas that cannot be examined more directly.

The actual clinical examination of the patient begins from the first moment of contact between the clinician and the patient. Observations about the patient's physical and emotional status can be made during the initial questioning. Skin condition, facial configuration, eye contact and movements, voice quality, speech habits, and a myriad of other objective as well as subjective qualities are appreciated by the astute clinician before the formal examination begins. During this less formal time the patient may be observed in a more dynamic state than during the set routine of the examining room.

The order of examination is not nearly as important as the establishment of an orderly routine that will minimize errors of omission. Included in the physical examination are the observation and measurement of the patient's vital signs.

Vital signs

The vital signs include blood pressure, pulse, respiration, and temperature. Vital signs relate directly to the physiologic status of the patient and are used for comparison with future observations as well as with physiologic norms.

Blood pressure

Normal blood pressure varies with age, being lowest in the infant and increasing with age. It is most frequently determined by the auscultatory method using a sphygmomanometer placed around the upper arm and a stethoscope placed over the brachial artery. It is usually taken with the patient in a sitting or supine position and frequently the pressures in both arms are compared. The cuff is inflated to over 200 mm Hg, occluding the arterial blood flow, then slowly deflated, while listening with a stethoscope for the vibrations of the pulsing blood.

Initially, there is no sound; the systolic pressure is the reading at which sound first becomes audible. As the cuff is continually deflated and more blood flow is permitted, the sounds become louder. The sounds then become muffled and finally disappear. The reading at which the sounds become muffled is generally regarded as the diastolic pressure, although there is some disagreement as to whether this or the point at which the sound disappears represents the closest approximation to intra-arterial diastolic pressure.

The systolic pressure is the maximum pressure created by the left ventricle, and in the average adult a pressure above 150 mm Hg is generally regarded as systolic hypertension, while a pressure below 90 mm Hg is regarded as systolic hypotension. The diastolic pressure is an indication of the resistance the ventricle must overcome as well as a measure of the lowest constant pressure within the arterial system. In an average adult a pressure above 90 to 100 mm Hg is regarded as diastolic hypertension, while a value below 60 mm Hg is regarded as diastolic hypotension.

The pulse pressure is the difference between the systolic and diastolic values in millimeters of mercury. It is usual for a man to have a greater pulse pressure than a woman. The normal pulse pressure of 30 to 40 mm Hg may be narrowed with tachycardia, aortic stenosis, constrictive pericarditis, or ascites. The pulse pressure may be widened with both systolic and diastolic hypertension, aortic insufficiency, thyrotoxicosis, patent ductus arteriosus, coarctation of the aorta, and during emotional periods. A value called the rate pressure product, which is the heart rate multiplied by the systolic blood pressure, can be of assistance in determining the need for sedation of the patient prior to oral surgical procedures. The normal value is 8,000 to 12,000, and if the value is over 12,000 sedation is advisable.

Pulse

The pulse is a pressure wave traveling through the arterial system. It may be palpated at any accessible artery, but it is most commonly taken at the radial, brachial, or temporal arteries. When pal-pating the artery, the rhythm and quality as well as the rate should be determined. The character and compressibility of the vessel wall are also significant observations. Pulse rate varies with age, being more rapid in the young. In the average adult, a rate of less than 60 per minute is regarded as bradycardia, although this is not uncommon among well-trained athletes, and a rate above 100 per minute is regarded as tachycardia. If irregularities in the rhythm are detected, the cause can be diagnosed with an electrocardiogram.

Respiration

In evaluating respiration, the rate, depth, and rhythm are observed. Respiratory rate varies with age. In the young child the rate may be up to 30 per minute. The rate for the average adult is 14 to 18 per minute.

Temperature

Temperature is generally measured orally or rectally. The oral route is considered the standard and a value of 98.6° F (37° C) is considered normal. Rectal values average ½ to 1 degree higher than oral. In most individuals, there is a daily variance in body temperature, or a diurnal rhythm of several tenths of a degree. The lowest value is usually reached during sleep and the value usually peaks toward the late afternoon or evening.

Facial, cervical, and oral examination

The following discussion organizes the clinical evaluation of the maxillofacial region into a facial, cervical, and oral examination. Although there are many ways in which to organize the examination, the important factor is to develop a specific sequence so that there is an orderly progression and no areas are omitted. It is generally advisable to divide the examination into extraoral and intraoral portions, with the former performed first. It is also a good routine to start the oral examination with the nondental structures and to examine the teeth and gingiva last. The use of a diagram on which to indicate abnormal findings is a valuable adjunct to the written record (Figs. 12-1 and 12-2).

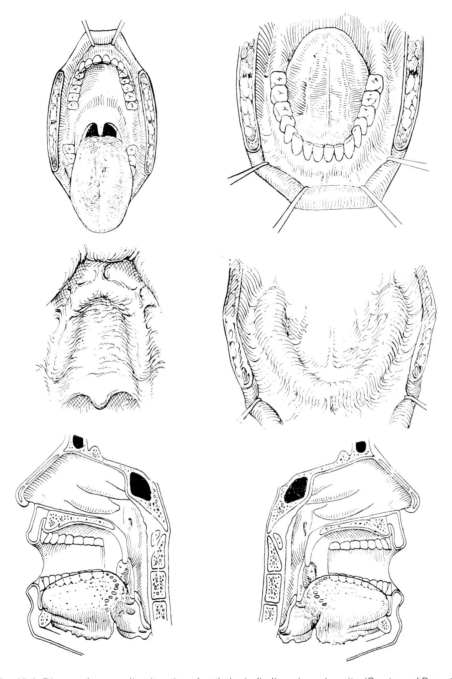

Fig. 12-1. Diagram for recording location of pathologic findings in oral cavity. (Courtesy of Department of Oral Pathology, University of Illinois, College of Dentistry.)

Extraoral examination

The extraoral examination involves the face, parotid and submandibular salivary glands, submandibular and submental lymph nodes, jaws and temporomandib- ular joints, neck and cervical lymph nodes, and the lips and corners of the mouth. The facial examination includes evaluation of the integument for color, temperature, texture, sensory alterations,

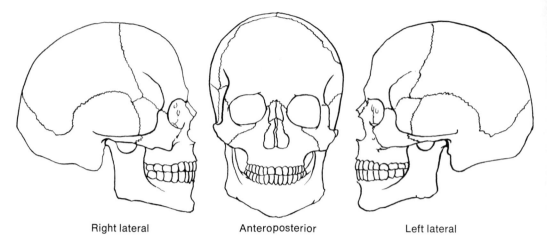

Right lateral   Anteroposterior   Left lateral

Fig. 12-2. Diagram for recording location of pathologic findings in facial skeleton.

lesions, scars, and keloids (Fig. 12-3). Facial symmetry and harmony are also observed. The deeper soft tissues should be palpated for areas of myofascial tenderness, lesions, and swelling. The symmetry of the facial skeleton is determined by palpating both sides simultaneously. Examination of the face should also include the eyes, ears, nose, and sinuses when indicated by the findings from the history. After the general facial examination, the temporomandibular joints are examined for tenderness, crepitation or clicking, and limitation or hypermobility. Auscultation as well as palpation of the joint is useful. Palpation should be done intrameatally as well as from a lateral approach.

Next, the parotid glands are examined for swelling or masses. At the same time, the parotid and posterior auricular lymph nodes are palpated. After this, the regions of the submental, submandibular, and superficial and deep cervical lymph nodes are examined in progressive order (Fig. 12-4). The submandibular salivary glands can also be palpated, but usually complete evaluation of these structures should await the intraoral examination when bimanual palpation can be performed.

After examination of cervical lymph nodes, the neck should be inspected for cysts, swelling, or sinus tracts. The muscles are palpated for tenderness, and the thyroid gland is examined for masses.

The vascular structures should be palpated and auscultated for abnormal pulsations or a bruit. Finally, the bony and cartilaginous structures are examined for tenderness, limitation of motion, dislocations, or fractures.

The lips and corners of the mouth are inspected as the final step in the extraoral examination. This serves as an orderly introduction to the intraoral examination.

Intraoral examination

The intraoral examination includes the mucous membranes of the lips and cheeks, the papillae of the parotid ducts, the floor of the mouth, the sublingual gland and submandibular gland and duct, all surfaces of the tongue, the tonsillar area, the pharynx, hard and soft palate, gingiva and alveolar ridges, and finally the teeth.

The oral examination usually begins with an evaluation of the oral hygiene. The odor of the breath occasionally indicates an underlying systemic condition such as acetone breath of ketonemia from diabetic or starvation acidosis or the smell of ammonia that may occur with uremia. A fetid odor commonly indicates oral infection, but sometimes it can be caused by pyloric obstruction, bronchiectasis, or a lung abscess.

The mucosa of the lips and cheeks is examined for keratosis, leukoedema, inflammatory changes, and neoplastic lesions (Fig. 12-5). The patency of the parot-

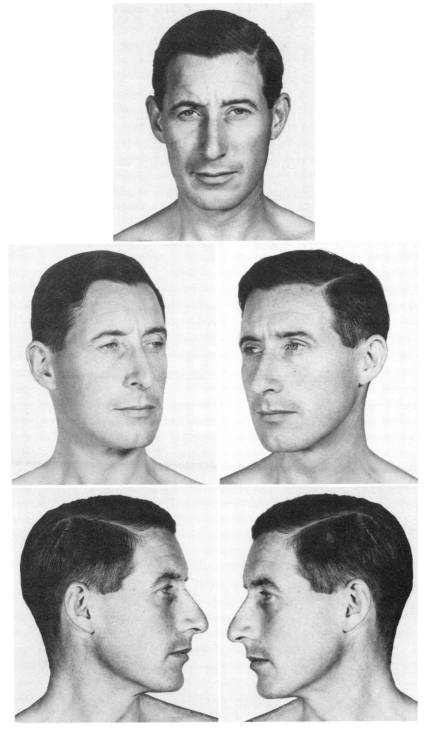

Fig. 12-3. Inspection of head, neck, and face. Patient is observed from frontal, oblique, and lateral views for lesions, abnormal pigmentations, swellings, asymmetries, and pulsations. (Reproduced with permission from Sarnat, B. G., and Schour, I. Essentials of oral and facial cancer, ed. 2. Copyright © 1957 by Year Book Medical Publishers, Inc., Chicago.)

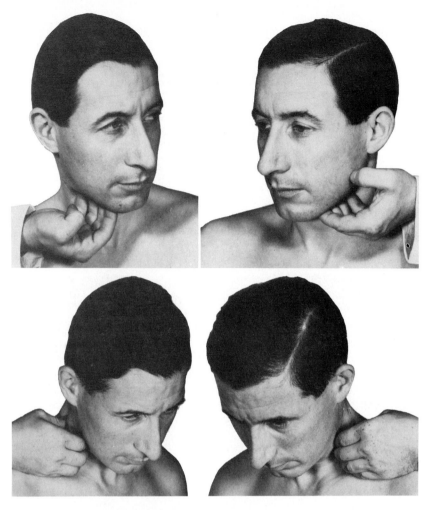

Fig. 12-4. Palpation of submental, submandibular, and cervical regions. Submandibular region is also palpated bimanually during intraoral examination. (Reproduced with permission from Sarnat, B. G., and Schour, I. Essentials of oral and facial cancer, ed. 2. Copyright © 1957 by Year Book Medical Publishers, Inc., Chicago.)

id duct should be determined. The floor of the mouth, sublingual gland, and submandibular gland and duct are then inspected for abnormalities. The floor of the mouth is the second most common intraoral site for carcinomas.

Next, the tongue is examined for size, color, symmetry, masses, and other lesions. The patient should be asked to protrude the tongue and it should be observed for tremor, deviation, or limitation of movement (Fig. 12-6, *A*). Then the tongue is elevated and the ventral surface is examined for swellings and varicosities (Fig. 12-6, *E*). Finally, the tongue is grasped at the tip with a piece of gauze

and pulled forward so that the base and posterolateral aspects can be visualized and palpated (Fig. 12-6, *B, C,* and *D*). The latter areas are common sites for carcinoma of the tongue.

The tonsillar area and pharynx are examined next (Figs. 12-7, *B,* and 12-8). A tongue blade or dental mirror is used to depress the tongue and provide better visualization. Instructing the patient to say "ah" will provide even better exposure of the oropharynx. Visualization of the naso- and hypopharynx are also facilitated by the use of a dental mirror.

After completion of the pharyngeal

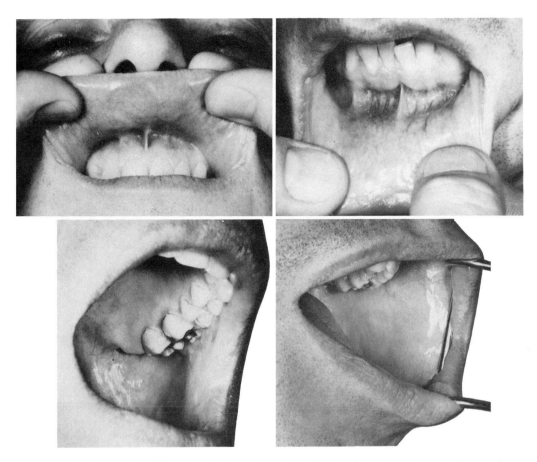

Fig. 12-5. Examination of lips and cheeks. Patency of parotid ducts is determined during this part of examination. (Reproduced with permission from Sarnat, B. G., and Schour, I. Essentials of oral and facial cancer, ed. 2. Copyright © 1957 by Year Book Medical Publishers, Inc., Chicago.)

examination, the hard and soft palates are examined (Fig. 12-7, A). The palate is a common site for several types of lesions. Tumors of salivary gland origin are more common in the soft palate, while epidermoid carcinoma is more common in the hard palate. Pancytopenia frequently induces palatal ulcers owing to the high degree of trauma to the area. Petechiae can appear on the palate in various coagulopathies. The palate is also a frequent site of changes associated with excessive smoking.

The next aspect of the oral examination involves the alveolar ridges and gingiva. The gingival tissues should be observed for changes in color and stippling, periodontal disease, lesions, and spontaneous bleeding. Although gingivitis and periodontitis are the most common causes of

hemorrhage, it can on occasion be an early indicator of a blood dyscrasia such as thrombocytopenia or leukemia.

Lastly, the teeth are examined. Such findings as caries, impactions, malalignment, missing teeth, restorations, and prosthetic replacements should be noted. It is important to examine the teeth in occlusion as well as with the mouth open so that tooth and jaw relationships can be observed.

PROBLEM-ORIENTED MEDICAL RECORD

Weed, in 1969, introduced a new concept for organizing and utilizing the information obtained from the history, physical examination, and laboratory tests. It not only provides an efficient method of record keeping, but it also provides for an effective audit system.

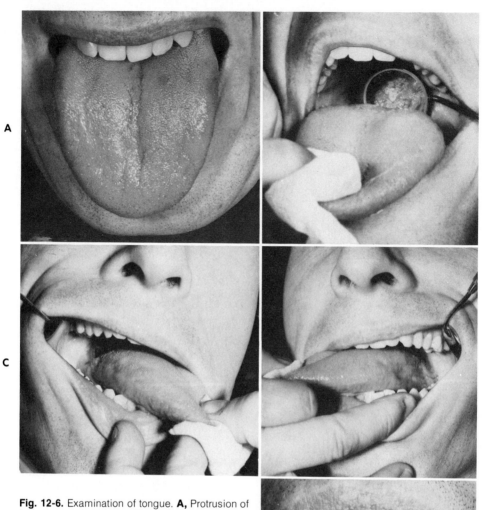

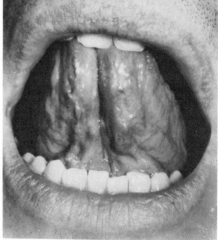

Fig. 12-6. Examination of tongue. **A,** Protrusion of tongue permits observation of dorsal surface. **B,** Posterodorsal surface is examined by grasping tip with gauze, extending tongue, and using a dental mirror. **C** and **D,** While tongue is extended, it can be pulled laterally for inspection and palpation of lateral and posterolateral surfaces. **E,** Elevation of tongue permits examination of ventral surface and floor of mouth. (Reproduced with permission from Sarnat, B. G., and Schour, I. Essentials of oral and facial cancer, ed. 2. Copyright © 1957 by Year Book Medical Publishers, Inc., Chicago.)

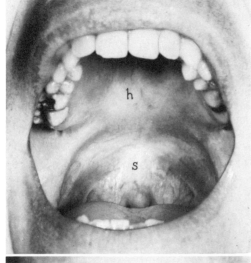

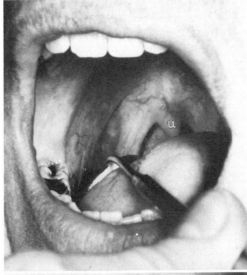

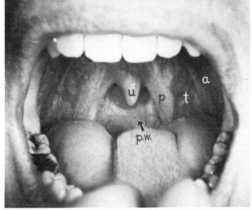

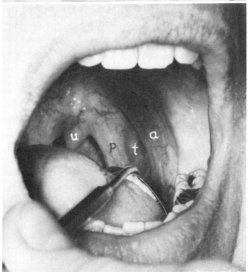

Fig. 12-7. A, Examination of palate (*h*, hard palate; *s*, soft palate). **B,** Depression of tongue permits better visualization of pharynx (*a*, anterior tonsillar pillar; *p*, posterior tonsillar pillar; *pw*, posterior pharyngeal wall; *t*, tonsil; *u*, uvula). (Reproduced with permission from Sarnat, B. G., and Schour, I. Essentials of oral and facial cancer, ed. 2. Copyright © 1957 by Year Book Medical Publishers, Inc., Chicago.)

Fig. 12-8. Examination of tonsillar area (*a*, anterior tonsillar pillar; *p*, posterior tonsillar pillar; *t*, tonsil; *u*, uvula). (Reproduced with permission from Sarnat, B. G., and Schour, I. Essentials of oral and facial cancer, ed. 2. Copyright © 1957 by Year Book Medical Publishers, Inc., Chicago.)

The problem-oriented record has the further advantages of (1) clearly identifying patient problems, (2) promoting problem solving, (3) improving communication among members of the health team by having a table of contents so that data on each identified problem can be easily followed through the record, and (4) expediting computerization of the medical record and evaluation of patient care.

There are four components to the problem-oriented record: a defined data base, a numbered problem list, plans for management of each problem, and progress notes on the follow-up on each problem. By numbering each of the last two entries with the same number assigned in the problem list, the sequence of events can be easily followed in the patient's chart.

Data base

The data base consists of the pertinent information obtained from the history, physical examination, and laboratory data available on admission. Depending on the situation, it may be comprehensive or problem specific. For the dental outpatient and most inpatients admitted for elective surgery, accumulation of a comprehensive data base may not be necessary.

Problem list

All current and past problems reported by the patient or identified by the examining doctor are listed and numbered. A problem is defined as anything that requires management or diagnostic workup. Each item should have a date of entry and date of onset. The problems should also be identified as active (requiring attention) or inactive (a past event or one not requiring attention). The problems are numbered according to order of recognition rather than presumed order of importance. As each problem is subsequently clarified, altered, or resolved, this is indicated opposite the original notation and dated. As new problems arise, they are added to the list and dated accordingly. The complete problem list is placed at the front of the chart and serves as a "table of contents."

Initial plan

A management plan for each active problem is developed and numbered accordingly. It is similarly identified in the progress notes and implemented on the order sheet under the same number. Plans are divided into three categories: those for further data collection to establish a diagnosis, those for specific treatment, and those for patient education about his illness and his part in its management.

Progress notes

Progress notes are numbered and titled to match the numbers assigned to the problems. The mnemonic SOAP is used to describe the sequence of the material included: "S" stands for the subjective statement by the patient; "O" represents the objective findings and pertinent laboratory data; "A" is an assessment by the doctor of what he thinks the findings mean; and "P" are further plans for diagnosis, treatment, and education of the patient and family.

The SOAP concept of organization suggested for the progress notes can be effectively applied in patient management even in those situations where the total problem-oriented medical record is not utilized. For example, it can be used in the evaluation of a patient requiring orthognathic surgery to correct a facial deformity:

Problem No. 1: *Increased vertical facial height* (*"long face"*)
   S: Difficulty in bringing lips together, "gummy" smile, unable to bite some foods
   O: Lip incompetence of 5 mm; total maxillary hyperplasia
   SNA = 80 degrees
   SNB = 71 degrees
   MP-SN = 42 degrees
   N-Gn = 128 mm
   Class II malocclusion
   A: Total maxillary hyperplasia with skeletal class II malocclusion
   P: Le Fort I maxillary osteotomy with superior positioning and autorotation of the mandible
Problem No. 2: *Decreased mandibular length*
   S: "Weak chin"
   O: Soft tissue chin point 1 cm posterior to Gonzalez line
   Go-Pg = 68 mm
   A: Microgenia
   P: Augmentation genioplasty

Such an approach develops an orderly process for analyzing any clinical situation and assures that the necessary data have been accumulated to support the diagnosis and therapeutic solution. It also lessens the possibility of overlooking or neglecting to manage any portion of the patient's total condition.

REFERENCE

Weed, L. L. 1969. Medical records, medical education, and patient care: The problem oriented record as a basic tool, Cleveland, Press of Case Western Reserve University.

CHAPTER 13

Radiographic examination

Alan M. Miller

INTERPRETATION

The face and jaws present unusual difficulties in radiographic examination. To overcome these problems a great many special projections have been devised with which the oral and maxillofacial surgeon should be familiar. In some instances, such as traumatic injury or generalized bone disease, a routine lateral and anteroposterior projection of the entire skull should be made first for orientation. After this, there can be concentration on special regions. If the patient has a localized disease, only the various special projections may be used.

The radiographic examination is of great value in diagnosis. It gives evidence of abnormalities of the anatomic structure of the bones and discloses changes in their architecture and alterations in their radiability. Its diagnostic value, however, is often considerably overestimated because it does not show disease—radiographs only portray the effects of pathologic processes on the bone. If bone is destroyed, the radiability is increased and the process is called osteolytic, whereas the deposit of bone or an increase in calcification decreases the radiability of the affected part, producing a radiopaque condition. If normal cavities in the bone, such as sinuses, are filled with soft uncalcified or calcified tissue or even with fluid, they also become radiopaque. Other findings that have pathologic significance are expansions of the cortex, reactions of the periosteum, and alterations in the tissue adjacent to the lesion.

The radiographic findings also give some indication of the development of the disease. There may be a single defect, or there may be multiple foci, which may or may not show a tendency to coalesce. The lesion may be circumscribed, or it may spread by infiltrating the adjacent tissue. Lesions developing at the surface may expand into the surrounding soft tissues or invade the substance of the underlying bone, whereas central lesions may extend within the bone, break through the cortex, or even penetrate the periosteum.

There are certain radiographic signs considered characteristic of malignancy. These include an indefinite outline of the lesion, invasion of adjacent tissue, breaking through the cortex, involvement of both the inside and outside of a bone, development of additional foci, spreading through and enlargement of nutrient canals, and pathologic fracture. However, such signs are not infallible. Multiple foci, for example, occur in benign giant cell lesions. Suppurative processes, such as alveolar abscesses, break through the bone to the outside. Pathologic fracture occurs in osteomyelitis.

The relationship of lesions to other structures, such as foramina, nerve canals, the roots of the teeth, and the nasal cavity and accessory sinuses, is easily determined by radiographic examination. It should be remembered, however, that radiographs are two-dimensional pictures and that a structure may appear involved by a lesion when actually it lies in front or behind; likewise a highly cal-

413

cified structure, normal or abnormal, may hide a smaller defect. It should also be remembered that what is closer to the x-ray film is sharply defined and what is farther away becomes indistinct or blurred. A perforation in the external cortex of the mandible gives a clear and well-defined picture on an extraoral film, whereas it is likely to be indistinct on an intraoral exposure on a dental film. In many cases exposures from different angles are useful, and often tomographic and stereoscopic films are needed.

Teeth that are affected by caries or periodontal disease may cause pathologic changes in the bone, and bone lesions may sometimes involve otherwise sound teeth. A few characteristics that can be helpful in differential diagnosis should be noted. Dentigerous cysts generally prevent the eruption of the involved teeth, or, if erupted, the teeth are generally displaced and tilted. Tumors are more likely to cause resorption of the teeth without disturbing their position. Local destruction of the lamina dura of the alveolar socket generally occurs at the apex in periapical infections and at the alveolar border in cases of periodontal disease. The lamina dura may be resorbed completely in diseases causing general bone resorption such as hyperparathyroidism. In Paget's disease, resorption of the bone and teeth occurs and there may be repair by deposit of new but altered bone.

Soft tissue lesions may be visualized when they alter the contour of the structure involved (for example, thickening of the periosteum) or because they are made up of tissue that is more radiopaque than that in which they develop. A lipoma, for example, is considerably more radiopaque than the subcutaneous tissue by which it may be surrounded. If there is any calcified tissue in a tumor, it is more radiopaque, and the radiograph at once reveals its presence. The calcified tissue may show a pattern such as the formation of bone trabeculae in an ossifying fibroma; the tissue then is spoken of as being osteogenic. It may also resemble tooth substances, and it is then termed odontogenic. In other instances the mass

may become completely calcified. An example is a calcified organic plug in a gland or its secreting duct, which finally forms a stone.

Contrast media are often employed to bring out features not otherwise recognizable. In the maxilla, cystic cavities may be visualized by injection of a contrast medium to differentiate them from the shadows made by the maxillary sinus. The injection of such substances into glands (sialography) allows visualization of their ducts and acini. Various abnormalities that are an aid in diagnosis may thus be discovered.

A foreign body in some instances may be recognized by the outline of its image. In the instance of calcified tissue, a tooth can be differentiated from a piece of bone such as a sequestrum; even tooth rudiments as seen in an odontoma can be recognized. Other radiopaque substances such as vulcanized rubber, glass, gravel, and metal may have their own characteristics. Foreign bodies of great variety may be found in the maxillary sinuses. Even if only slightly radiopaque, they may be demonstrated easily.

Often a number of projections are required to locate foreign bodies, and unconventional exposures may be needed. Stereoscopic films can be of great value. Stereoscopic technique in dental and maxillary radiography was first described by Ivy (1917). More recently Silva (1956) has enumerated the advantages of stereoradiographic examination, giving a simplified technique. He pointed out its value in localizing impacted and supernumerary teeth, retained roots, and foreign bodies.

Details of interpretation of individual radiographs and specific radiographic signs that help to diagnose disease will be covered in the various chapters dealing with the treatment of specific diseases. This chapter concerns itself principally with the techniques employed for various exposures.

TECHNIQUE
Standard skull examination

The radiographic examination of the entire skull is desirable under certain conditions, especially in traumatic injuries and generalized skeletal disease. The following projections are recommended for a basic survey (Potter, 1975; Stafne, 1975, p. 410-417; Wuehrmann and Manson-Hing, 1977; and Yale and Rosenberg, 1975).

Posteroanterior (Granger) projection

In a posteroanterior projection the patient's forehead and nose are positioned against the film cassette. The central ray is directed to the midline of the skull so that the x-ray beam passes through the canthomeatal plane perpendicular to the film plane (Fig. 13-1).

This view is excellent for evaluating the inner and middle ear because the petrous pyramid can be viewed through the orbits. The resulting projection also shows the frontal bone, frontal sinuses, orbital areas, nasal cavity, and ethmoidal area. The superior aspect of the maxillary sinuses is generally obliterated by the floor of the middle and posterior cranial fossae (Fig. 13-2).

Inclined posteroanterior (Caldwell) projection

The Caldwell view is a 23-degree variation of the Granger view. The head is positioned so the canthomeatal line is perpendicular to the film. The central ray is directed at a 23-degree angle to the canthomeatal line entering the skull about 3 cm above the external occipital protuberance and exiting at the glabella (Fig. 13-3).

This angulation will cause the petrous ridges to be superimposed on the maxillary sinuses, thus allowing for a more accurate examination of the orbits and ethmoid air cells.

Townes projection

The Townes projection is an anterioposterior view. Again the canthomeatal line is perpendicular to the film. The central ray is directed 30 degrees to the canthomeatal line and passes through it at a point between the external auditory canals (Fig. 13-4).

This view is primarily used to observe the occipital area of the skull. The necks

Fig. 13-1. Posteroanterior (Granger) projection.

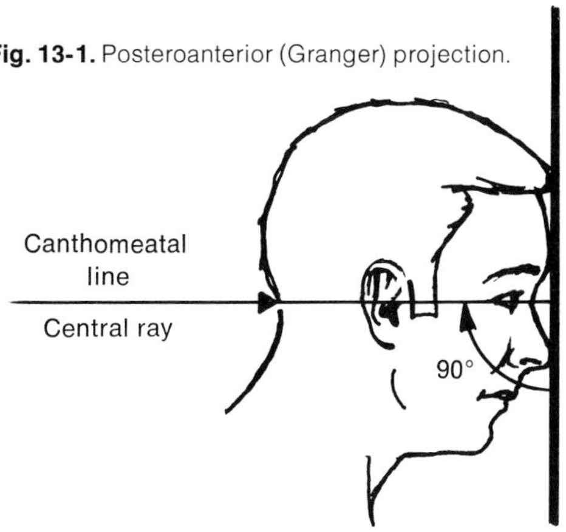

of the condyloid processes can also be viewed; however, panoramic radiography has become the view of choice for evaluating this area of the mandible (see p. 424).

Lateral projection

In lateral projection the head is positioned so that the midsagittal plane is parallel to the film and a line connecting the external auditory meati is perpendicular to the film. The central ray is perpendicular to the midsagittal plane and perpendicular to the plane of the film (Fig. 13-5).

In the standard lateral projection the posterior borders of the mandible are superimposed. The orbits are not superimposed because they are not in line with the central ray, and therefore the orbit farthest from the film is projected forward. Many anatomic structures of the midface are obscured because of superimposition. However, this projection gives a fine view of the calvarium and base of the skull. The shape and depth of the sella turcica may be evaluated, and the soft tissues of the nasopharynx are seen best on lateral view. The posterior wall of the nasopharynx should be concave; a convexity is abnormal. In a child, hypertrophy of the pharyngeal tonsils is usually responsible for the convexity. Both frontal and sphenoidal sinuses can be evaluated. The pterygopalatine fossa and the hard palate can also be readily visualized (Fig. 13-6).

Text continued on p. 420.

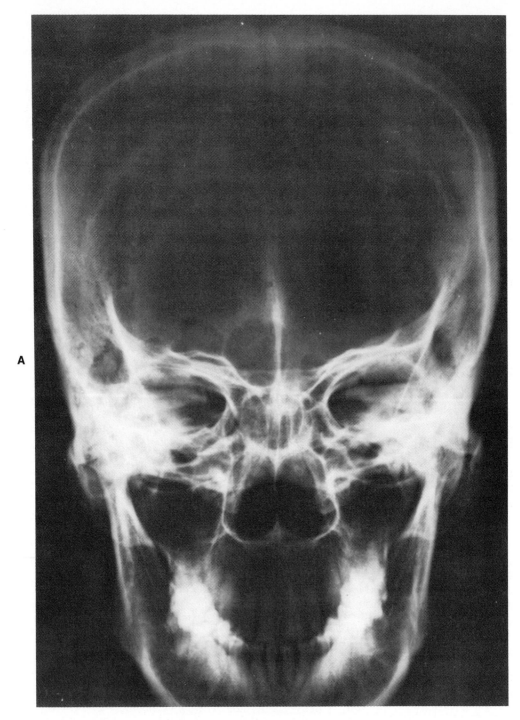

A

Fig. 13-2. For legend see opposite page.

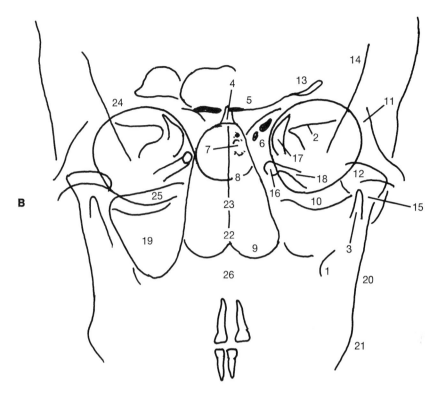

Fig. 13-2. A, Posteroanterior (Granger) exposure and, **B,** labeled line drawing of same radiograph. *1,* Maxillary tuberosity; *2,* petrous pyramid (houses inner ear); *3,* coronoid process; *4,* crista galli; *5,* dorsum sellae; *6,* ethmoid air cells; *7,* sphenoid air cells; *8,* floor of sphenoid sinus; *9,* floor of nasal fossa; *10,* floor of posterior cranial fossa; *11,* frontal process of zygoma; *12,* mandibular condyle; *13,* floor of anterior cranial fossa; *14,* temporal surface greater wing sphenoid (linea innominata); *15,* mandibular neck; *16,* foramen rotundum; *17,* superior orbital fissure; *18,* inferior orbital fissure; *19,* maxillary antrum; *20,* mandibular ramus; *21,* mandibular angle; *22,* anterior nasal spine; *23,* nasal septum; *24,* supraorbital rim; *25,* infraorbital rim; and *26,* anterior maxilla.

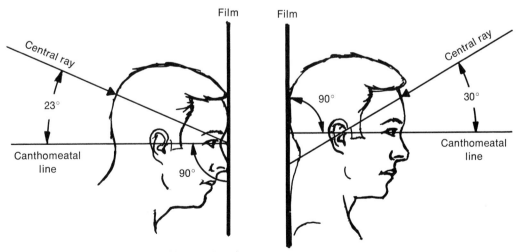

Fig. 13-3. Inclined posteroanterior (Caldwell) projection.

Fig. 13-4. Townes projection.

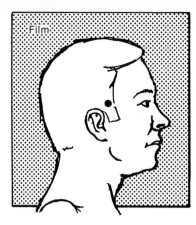

Fig. 13-5. Lateral projection.

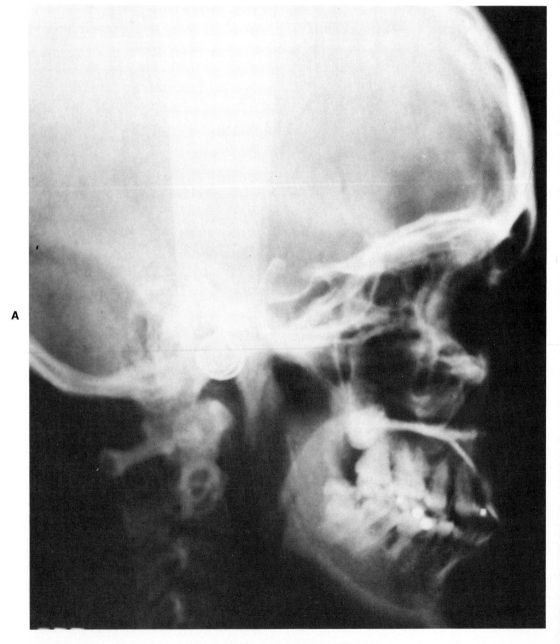

A

Fig. 13-6. For legend see opposite page.

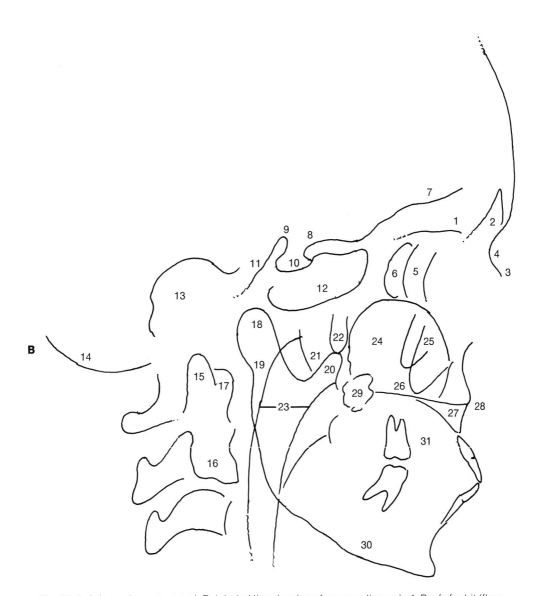

Fig. 13-6. A, Lateral exposure and, **B,** labeled line drawing of same radiograph. *1,* Roof of orbit (floor of anterior cranial fossa); *2,* frontal sinus; *3,* nasal bone; *4,* nasion; *5,* frontal process of zygoma (lateral orbital rim); *6,* ethmoid air cells; *7,* cerebral surface anterior cranial fossa; *8,* anterior clinoid process; *9,* posterior clinoid process; *10,* floor of sella turcica; *11,* clivus; *12,* sphenoid sinus; *13,* mastoid air cells; *14,* floor posterior cranial fossa; *15,* odontoid process; *16,* body of C$_2$; *17,* anterior arch of C$_1$; *18,* mandibular condyle; *19,* mandibular neck; *20,* coronoid process; *21,* pterygoid plate; *22,* pterygo-palatine fossa; *23,* nasopharyngeal soft tissue; *24,* maxillary antrum; *25,* zygomatic recess maxillary antrum; *26,* hard palate; *27,* premaxilla; *28,* anterior nasal spine; *29,* unerupted maxillary third molar; *30,* body of mandible; and *31,* maxilla.

By varying the exposure factors, soft tissues of the midface can be seen on lateral views. These exposures are particularly useful in the preoperative cephalometric workup of candidates for orthognathic surgery. Xerocephalography (Lopez, 1976), which utilizes specialized processing, has gained some popularity for this purpose in recent years owing to the detail and contrast in hard and soft tissues in the resulting film.

Waters projection

To obtain the Waters view the head is extended so that the canthomeatal line forms an angle of 37 degrees with the central ray. The central ray, which is perpendicular to the film, enters the skull 3 cm above the external occipital protuberance and exits through the tip of the nose (Fig. 13-7).

An accurate projection will result in an excellent view of the almost triangular maxillary sinuses. The angles of the mandible are barely contained within the occipital bone, and the anterior edge of the foramen magnum is covered by the inferior border of the mandible.

The Waters view is used to study the maxillary, frontal, and ethmoidal sinuses; if the projection is taken with the mouth

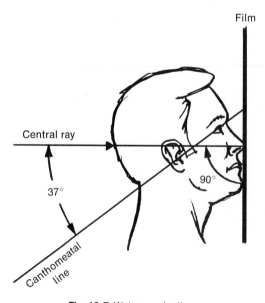

Fig. 13-7. Waters projection.

open, a good view of the sphenoidal sinus may also be achieved. In addition, this projection provides excellent views of the facial bones, zygomatic arches, and orbital floors, and it is used extensively to evaluate traumatic injuries to these areas (Fig. 13-8).

Base (inferior-superior, submental-vertex) projection

The base view is taken with the head positioned so that the canthomeatal line is parallel to the film and perpendicular to the central ray. The central ray enters the skull in the midline between the mandibular angles (Fig. 13-9).

This view is uniquely valuable for visualization of the structures in the base of the skull. Structures such as the middle cranial fossa, sphenoidal sinus, foramen ovale, foramen spinosum, bony eustachian tube, ear ossicles, pterygoid plates, zygomatic arches, lateral wall of the orbit, and lateral wall of the maxillary antrum are all demonstrated in this view.

Facial bone examination

Mandible

Extraoral radiographic views of the mandible are useful for a general survey and are indispensable for the diagnosis of any lesion involving a larger area than can be covered by a dental film. They should be used in all cases of fracture, displaced and malposed teeth, bone infections, cysts, and tumors, especially if extensive and complicated. The four projections that are useful are the two lateral views of the body and ascending ramus, the posteroanterior projection for the symphysis (p. 415), and the projection for the symphysis by means of an occlusal film (p. 428).

Projection for body. In the projection for the body the cassette is placed against the mandible with the head extended backward and the chin up so as to minimize the overshadowing effect of the cervical spine. The lower border of the mandible should be parallel to the long side of the film. The central ray is directed at an angle of 25 degrees from behind and beneath the angle of the opposite side and should extend through the mandibu-

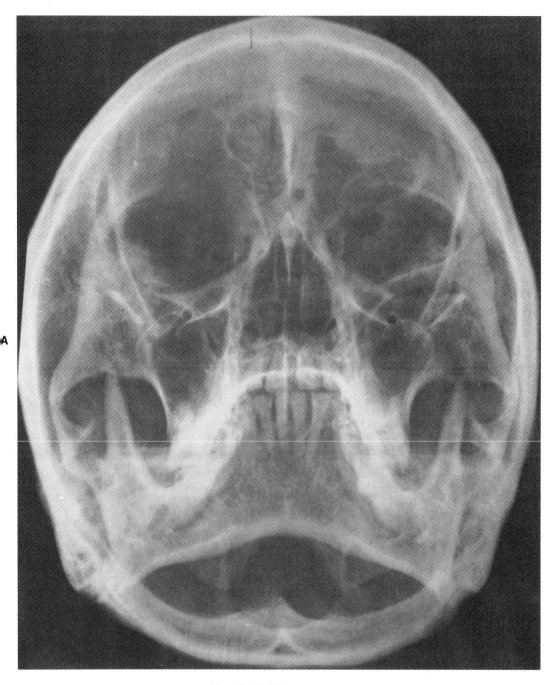

A

Fig. 13-8. A, Waters exposure.

Continued,

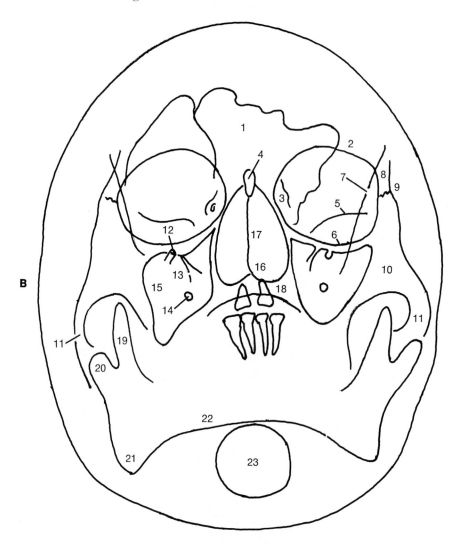

B

Fig. 13-8, cont'd. B, Labeled line drawing of same radiograph. *1,* Frontal sinus; *2,* orbital roof (anterior margin); *3,* ethmoid air cells; *4,* crista galli; *5,* sphenoid ridge (posterior portion orbital roof); *6,* orbital floor (anterior margin); *7,* linea innominata; *8,* zygomatic process of frontal bone; *9,* frontozygomatic suture; *10,* zygoma; *11,* zygomatic arch; *12,* infraorbital foramen; *13,* superior orbital fissure; *14,* foramen rotundum; *15,* maxillary sinus; *16,* anterior nasal spine; *17,* nasal septum; *18,* hard palate; *19,* coronoid process; *20,* mandibular condyle; *21,* mandibular angle; *22,* inferior border mandible; and *23,* foramen magnum.

lar second molar of the side to be radiographed as shown in Fig. 13-10. The exposed film should show the area from the canine to and including the third molar. With an additional angle of 10 degrees toward the chin and rotation of the head so that the chin is in contact with the cassette, the symphysis and the incisors may be shown as in Fig. 13-11.

Projection for ramus. The projection for the ramus is used for fractures, cysts, and tumors that are located in or extend into the ramus from the body of the mandible. In most instances the coronoid process and condyle are easily included. The cassette is placed so that the patient's head rests with the ear in close contact with the film. The chin is extended upward, with the head manipulated forward so that superimposition of the cervical

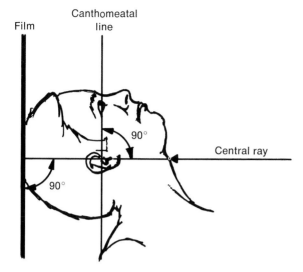

Film

Canthomeatal line

90°

90°

Central ray

Fig. 13-9. Base projection.

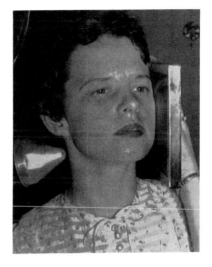

Fig. 13-10. Projection for radiographic examination of body of mandible.

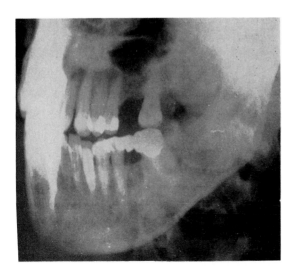

Fig. 13-11. Lateral jaw radiograph showing body of mandible.

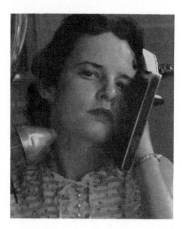

Fig. 13-12. Projection for radiographic examination of ramus.

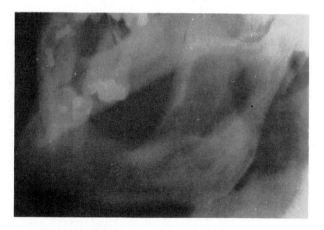

Fig. 13-13. Radiograph showing cyst in ramus.

spine is eliminated. The central ray is directed from underneath the mandible at an angle of 15 degrees above horizontal so as to pass through the third molar on the side to be exposed, as shown in Fig. 13-12. The film will show the molar region, the angle of the jaw, and the entire ramus (Fig. 13-13).

Panoramic radiography

Panoramic radiography is becoming increasingly popular, especially for use in oral and maxillofacial surgery. Its popularity may be attributed to the extensive area visualized on a single film, the relative ease of the procedure, and the small amount of radiation involved. This curved layer radiograph essentially rep-

resents a well-defined outline of most structures of the midface and in many instances can be substituted for a series of films to evaluate trauma or pathology in the mid- and lower facial area (Fig. 13-14). The following references are a helpful guide to both technique and interpretation of panoramic radiography: Blackman, 1960, 1961; Hudson, Kumpula, and Dickson, 1957; Paatero, 1961; Smith, 1974; Takeshi, 1975; Updegrave, 1963, 1966; Wuehrmann and Manson-Hing, 1977.

Occlusal film radiography

The occlusal film is probably the most versatile tool for evaluating the various segments of the jaws. Numerous tech-

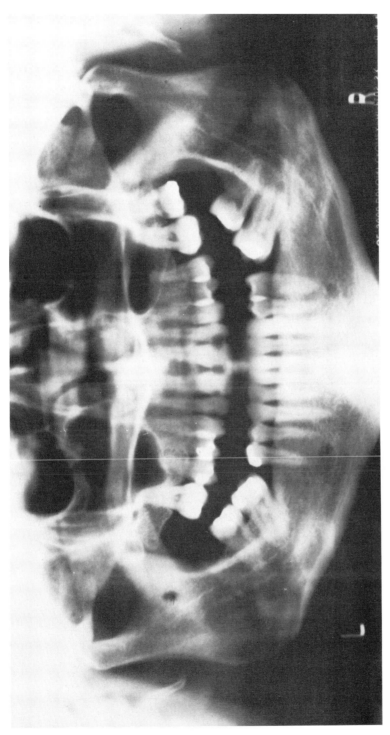

Fig. 13-14. A, Panoramic exposure.

Continued,

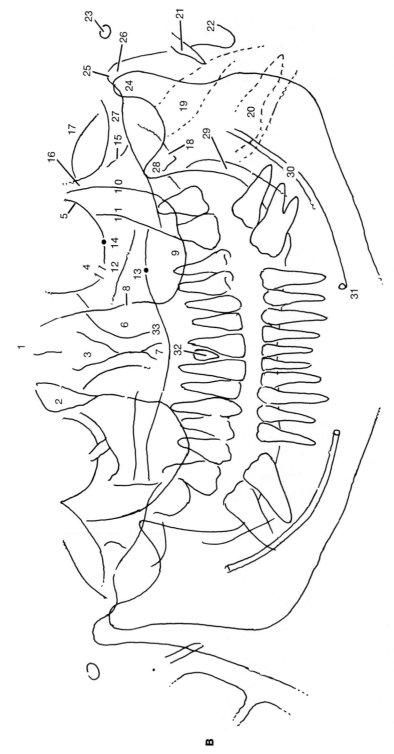

Fig. 13-14, cont'd. B, Labeled line drawing of same radiograph. *1,* Perpendicular plate of ethmoid; *2,* ethmoid air cells; *3,* nasal septum; *4,* inferior orbital fissure; *5,* lateral orbital rim; *6,* inferior nasal concha; *7,* anterior nasal spine; *8,* lateral wall of nasal cavity, medial wall maxillary antrum; *9,* floor of maxillary antrum; *10,* lateral wall maxillary antrum; *11,* zygomatic process of maxilla; *12,* shadow of vomer; *13,* posterior hard palate; *14,* inferior orbital rim, roof of maxillary antrum; *15,* zygomatico-temporal suture line; *16,* frontal process of zygoma; *17,* floor of middle cranial fossa; *18,* lateral pterygoid plate; *19,* air shadow of nasopharynx; *20,* air shadow of oral pharynx; *21,* styloid process; *22,* soft tissue shadow of earlobe; *23,* external auditory meatus; *24,* mandibular condyle; *25,* articular eminence; *26,* articular fossa; *27,* zygomatic arch (zygomatic process temporal bone); *28,* coronoid process; *29,* anterior border ramus and external oblique ridge; *30,* mandibular canal; *31,* mental foramen; *32,* incisive foramen; *33,* anterior aspect of hard palate floor of nasal cavity.

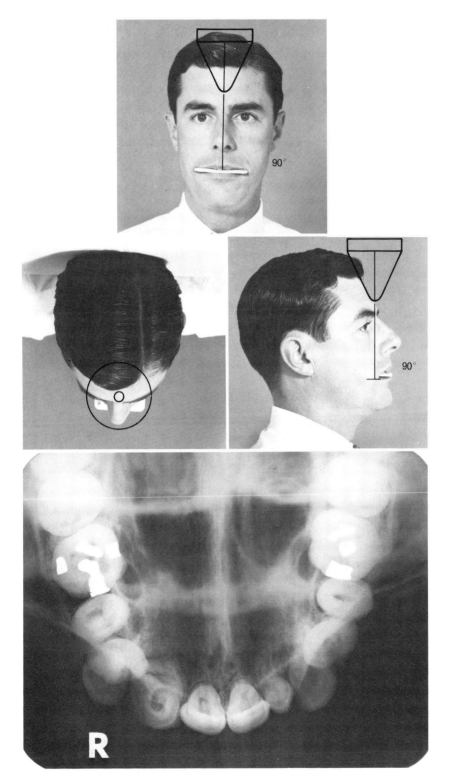

Fig. 13-15. Maxillary anterior projection and exposure. (From Silha, R. E. 1965. Dent. Radiogr. Photogr. **38:**37.)

niques have been described, as virtually any area may be visualized by varying the film position and the angulation of the tube. Description of some of the more popular views follows. Techniques and radiographic projections of these views, described by Silha (1965), are contained in Figs. 13-15 to 13-23.

Maxillary anterior projection. The maxillary anterior projection (Fig. 13-15) is termed "true occlusal" since the central ray strikes the film perpendicularly in two planes. The exposure time must be increased because the frontal portion of the skull is penetrated.

The occlusal plane and film plane should be parallel with the floor. The central ray is perpendicular to the film plane and is directed to the intersection of an imaginary line between the lingual surfaces of the first molars and the midsagittal plane.

Maxillary anterior modified projection. In the maxillary anterior modified projection (Fig. 13-16), the occlusal plane and film plane should be parallel with the floor. The central ray is directed along the midsagittal plane to the intersection of an imaginary line between the lingual surfaces of the first molars and the midsagittal plane. The vertical angulation is +75 degrees.

Maxillary posterior oblique projection. In the maxillary posterior oblique projection (Fig. 13-17), the occlusal plane and film plane should be parallel with the floor. The edge of the film should be parallel with the buccal surfaces of the maxillary teeth and project approximately ¼ inch. The central ray is directed through the apex of the lingual root of the first molar. The vertical angulation is +50 degrees.

Mandibular anterior projection. For a mandibular anterior projection (Fig. 13-18) the patient's head may be in any comfortable position that allows the central ray to be directed perpendicular to the film plane. The central ray is directed to a point where imaginary lines between the lingual surfaces of the first molars and the midsagittal plane intersect.

Mandibular anterior modified projection. The mandibular anterior modified

projection (Fig. 13-19) is facilitated by positioning the patient's head so that the occlusal and film planes are perpendicular to the floor. The angulation is −55 degrees. The central ray is directed between the apices of the central incisors.

Mandibular oblique projection. In the mandibular oblique projection (Fig. 13-20) the occlusal plane and the film plane should be parallel with the floor. The lateral edge of the film should be parallel to the buccal surfaces of the mandibular teeth, and the front end should project approximately ¼ inch out of the oral cavity. The central ray is directed at the apex of the mandibular second premolar. The vertical angulation is −50 degrees.

Lateral jaw, anterior body projection. For the anterior body projection of the lateral jaw (Fig. 13-21) the teeth should be in occlusion with the occlusal plane parallel to the floor. The middle of the film packet is positioned over the first premolar area. The central ray enters at a point ½ inch diagonally below the palpated angle of the mandible and emerges at the cervical line of the first premolar. The vertical angulation is −5 to −10 degrees.

Lateral jaw, posterior body projection. For the posterior body projection of the lateral jaw (Fig. 13-22) the teeth should be in occlusion with the occlusal plane parallel with the floor. The angle and posterior border of the ramus can be seen radiographically with a minimum overlapping of the adjacent structures if the patient's neck and the chin are extended forward. This action will bring the posterior border of the ramus anterior to the spinal column. When the patient is requested to assume this position, there is often a tendency to bring the chin up and forward. The maneuver will be of benefit only if the occlusal plane is maintained parallel to the floor. The middle of the film packet is over the third molar area and the lower edge of the film is parallel with the lower border of the mandible. The central ray enters at a point ½ inch diagonally below the palpated angle of the mandible and emerges at the crown of the third molar. The vertical angulation is approximately −10 degrees.

Text continued on p. 437.

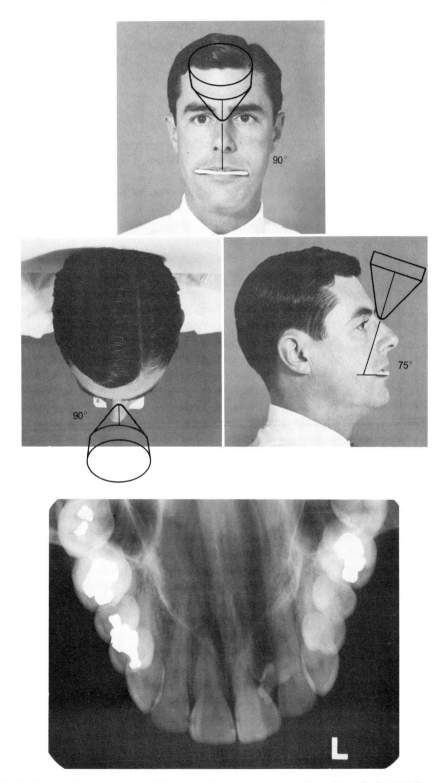

Fig. 13-16. Maxillary anterior modified projection and exposure. (From Silha, R. E. 1965. Dent. Radiogr. Photogr. **38**:38.)

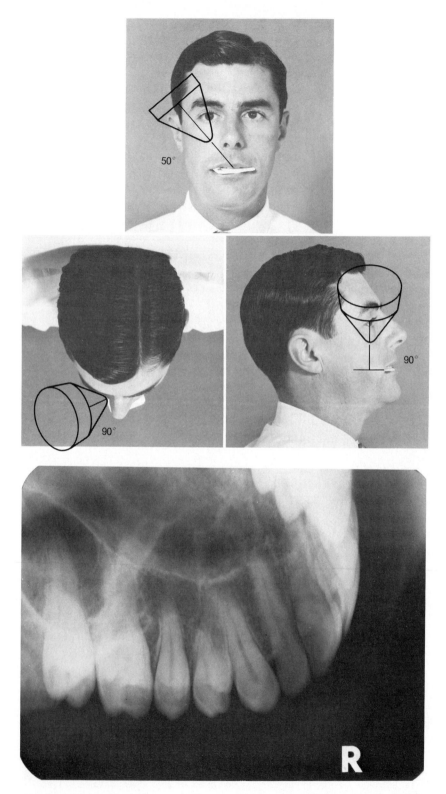

Fig. 13-17. Maxillary posterior oblique projection and exposure. (From Silha, R. E. 1965. Dent. Radiogr. Photogr. **38**:38.)

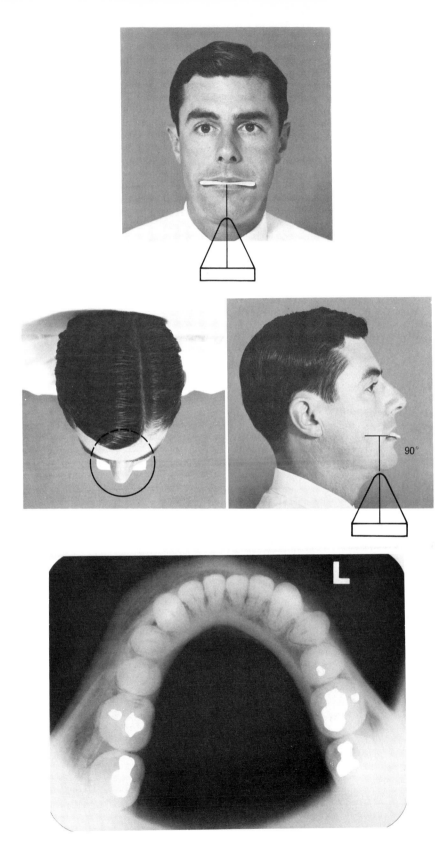

Fig. 13-18. Mandibular anterior projection and exposure. To present uniform illustrations, occlusal plane is shown parallel with floor and central ray is at an angle of −90 degrees. "Cone cutting" resulted here because patient had a short thick neck and cone had to be anterior to recommended position. (From Silha, R. E. 1965. Dent. Radiogr. Photogr. **38**:43.)

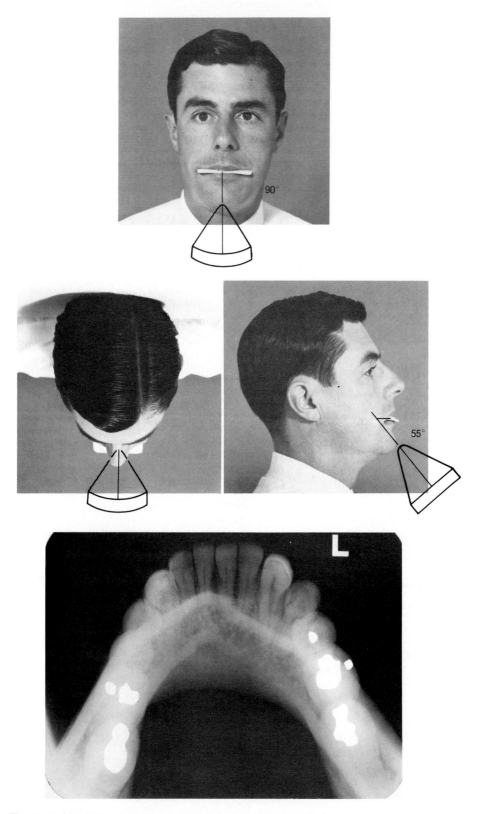

Fig. 13-19. Mandibular anterior modified projection and exposure. Shows occlusal and film planes parallel to floor and an angulation of −55 degrees. (From Silha, R. E. 1965. Dent. Radiogr. Photogr. **38**:43.)

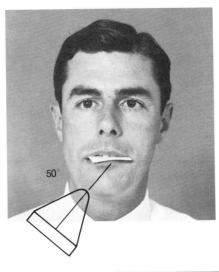

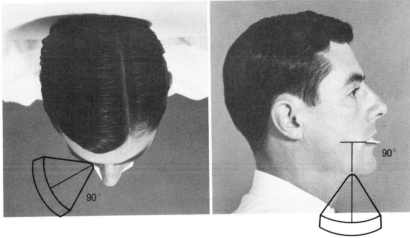

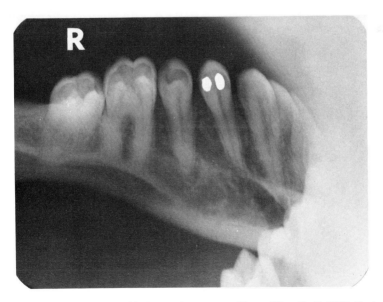

Fig. 13-20. Mandibular oblique projection and exposure. (From Silha, R. E. 1965. Dent. Radiogr. Photogr. **38**:44.)

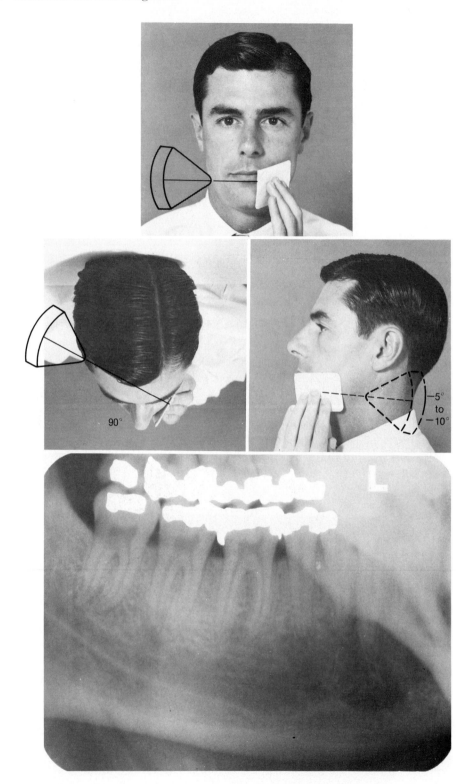

Fig. 13-21. Lateral jaw, anterior body projection and exposure. (From Silha, R. E. 1965. Dent. Radiogr. Photogr. **38:**44.)

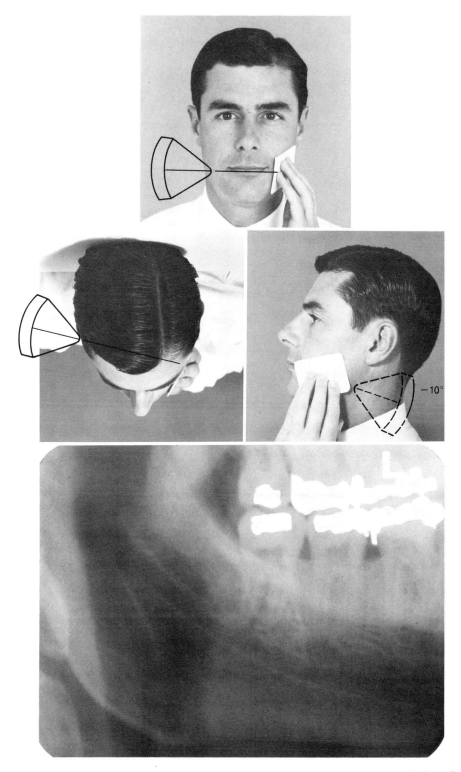

Fig. 13-22. Lateral jaw, posterior body projection and exposure. (From Silha, R. E. 1965. Dent. Radiogr. Photogr. **38**:51.)

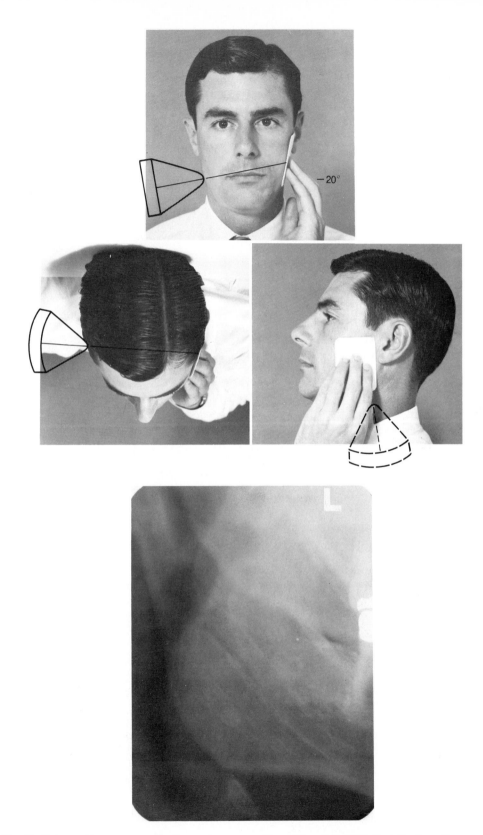

Fig. 13-23. Lateral jaw, ramus projection and exposure. (From Silha, R. E. 1965. Dent. Radiogr. Photogr. **38**:52.)

Lateral jaw, ramus projection. In the ramus projection of the lateral jaw (Fig. 13-23) the teeth should be in occlusion with the occlusal plane parallel with the floor. The neck and chin should be extended forward. The film is positioned with the long axis vertical and centered

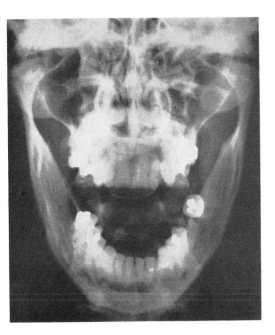

Fig. 13-24. Posteroanterior view taken with chin and nose on cassette and mouth wide open. Condyles and joint spaces are shown in sagittal plane.

over the ramus of the mandible. The central ray enters at a point ½ inch diagonally below the palpated angle of the ramus and emerges at the middle of the ramus on the opposite side. The vertical angulation is approximately −20 degrees.

Various other occlusal film techniques are described by Stafne (1974, p. 390-396), Williamson (1954), and Silha (1965).

Temporomandibular articulation

The temporomandibular joint (TMJ) and condyles may be shown by means of various projections. Some have already been discussed. Panoramic, posteroanterior, Townes, and base views all demonstrate the TMJ to varying degrees. Many specific techniques (Barton, 1955; Heusser, 1951) have also been designed to eliminate superimposition of anatomic structures that would normally obstruct adequate visualization of the joint. Examples of these follow.

Open posteroanterior projection. In the normal posteroanterior projection the condyle is only partly visualized when in the glenoid fossa; however, with the mouth open a more favorable view of the condyle and joint space may be obtained (Fig. 13-24).

Transorbital view. In the transorbital view (Figs. 13-25 and 13-26) the film is placed behind the patient's head extend-

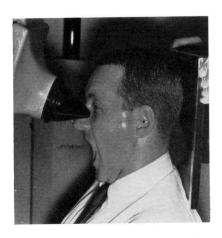

Fig. 13-25. Transorbital condylar projection.

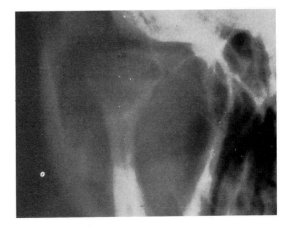

Fig. 13-26. Transorbital projection showing sagittal view of head and neck of condyloid process.

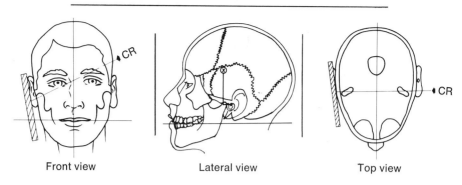

Front view   Lateral view   Top view

Fig. 13-27. Transcranial (Gillis) projection. (From Lewis, G. R. 1964. Dent. Radiogr. Photogr. **37:**8.)

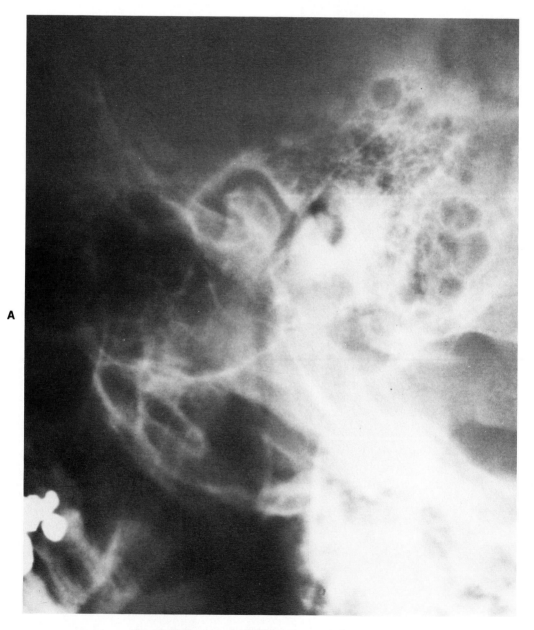

Fig. 13-28. Transcranial (Gillis) exposure. **A,** Closed position.

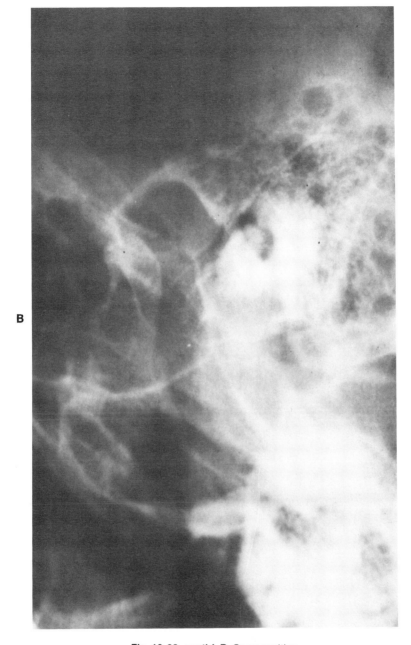

B

Fig. 13-28, cont'd. B, Open position.

ing laterally to the side to be examined. The film inclines to form an angle of approximately 20 degrees with the transverse or frontal plane of the head. The cone is placed gently at the inner canthus of the closed eye of the patient. The central ray is directed posteriorly, laterally, and downward through the median aspect of the orbit at approximately 30 degrees toward a point judged to be 1 inch below the condyle on the side to be examined. The resultant radiograph gives a relatively undistorted, somewhat enlarged, picture of the condyle in the sagittal plane. The zygomatic arch is also visible. Both sides should be taken in certain cases to afford an opportunity for comparison.

Transcranial or temporal views. (Gillis, 1935; Goncalves and Miller, 1974; Lewis, 1964.) Several techniques have been described for transcranial views, all of which vary somewhat at the point of entry of the central ray. The Gillis technique is representative of this group of lateral transcranial projections. The central ray enters ½ inch anterior and 2 inches superior to the ipsilateral external auditory meatus and is directed toward the contralateral TMJ (Figs. 13-27 and 13-28).

Tomography. Several tomographic techniques are currently in use; however, all utilize a similar principle of motion to obscure overlying structures. Both the film and tube move synchronously while the plane of interest remains stationary in the fulcrum point. The structures outside the fulcrum point are blurred by the movement of the tube, while the stationary plane of interest results in a relatively sharp image. By varying the type and amplitude of motion, varying degrees of detail as well as thickness of section may be achieved. Linear tomography is most commonly used; however, more complex movements such as a circular motion (zonography) and a polydirectional motion (hypocycloidal tomography) not only provide more detail, but sections as thin as 1 mm can be achieved for evaluation of the temporomandibular articulation (Coin, 1974; Markovic and Rosenberg, 1976).

Most radiographic techniques for the TMJ are designed to eliminate superimposed anatomic structures either by varying the angulation of the central ray or by utilizing the motion of the more refined technique of tomography. However, none gives any attention to the variations in morphology and angulation of the indi-

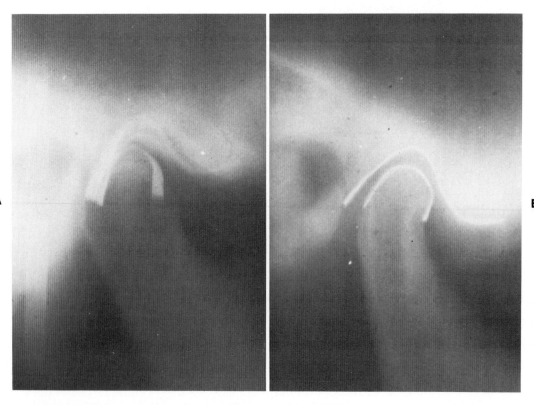

Fig. 13-29. A, Uncorrected and, **B,** corrected lateral tomogram of temporomandibular joint of dried skull. Lead foil marks center of condyle and fossa. Note distortion of uncorrected view. (Courtesy of Dr. D. M. Laskin.)

vidual condyles (Yale and Rosenberg, 1961). Yale (1969) and Yale and Rosenberg (1961) have emphasized the importance of this consideration so that the temporomandibular articulation may be viewed in an accurate, undistorted manner. To accomplish this, the technique of corrected TMJ laminagraphy or tomography was developed. Utilizing an inferosuperior (base) and posteroanterior view, measurements are made to determine the horizontal and vertical angulation of the condyles. Combining this information with the principles of tomography allows the plane of interest to be positioned so that the resultant radiograph provides both excellent detail and an undistorted view of the temporomandibular joint area (Figs. 13-29 to 13-31) (Goncalves and Miller, 1974).

Use of radiopaque media

Radiopaque substances are used for the investigation of a great variety of conditions, such as diseases of the bronchopulmonary apparatus, genitourinary tract, uterus and fallopian tubes, kidneys and ureter, and spinal canal.

In oral and maxillofacial surgery these media also have many uses, not only as aids in diagnosis but sometimes as local therapeutic agents, since they contain iodine, which is continuously set free in small quantities through decomposition of the substances by the inflamed tissue (Thoma, 1941).

In the diagnosis of oral disease the method is employed for the injection of fistulae and sinus tracts, making it possible to visualize their origin and cause. The injection of radiopaque media into cysts helps to differentiate them from tumors; in the maxilla, cysts may be visualized if invading the maxillary sinus (Fig. 13-32). The injection of salivary glands (Fig. 13-33) is important in the diagnosis of pathologic conditions (Mandel and Baurmash, 1965), and the injection of the intra-articular spaces of the temporomandibular joint (Fig. 13-34) can be used as an aid in the diagnosis of arthritic changes (Norgaard, 1947).

The following radiopaque substances can be used.

Lipiodol (Lafay, 1901) is an amber-colored liquid, faintly aromatic and tasteless. It is a chemical combination of elemental iodine and poppy-seed oil, containing 40% pure iodine by weight. At room temperature it is viscid, becoming much more fluid if heated to body temperature. It deteriorates when exposed to excess light, air, heat, or moisture. Discolored lipiodol should not be used, since

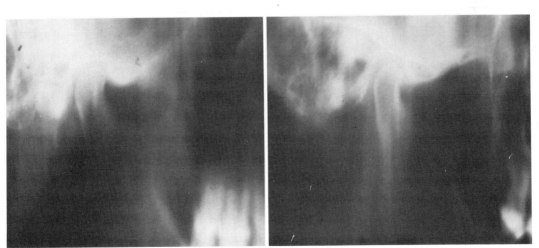

Fig. 13-30. A, Uncorrected and, **B,** corrected lateral tomogram of temporomandibular joint of normal patient. There is distortion of condyle and less definition of cortical surface in uncorrected view. (Courtesy of Dr. D. M. Laskin.)

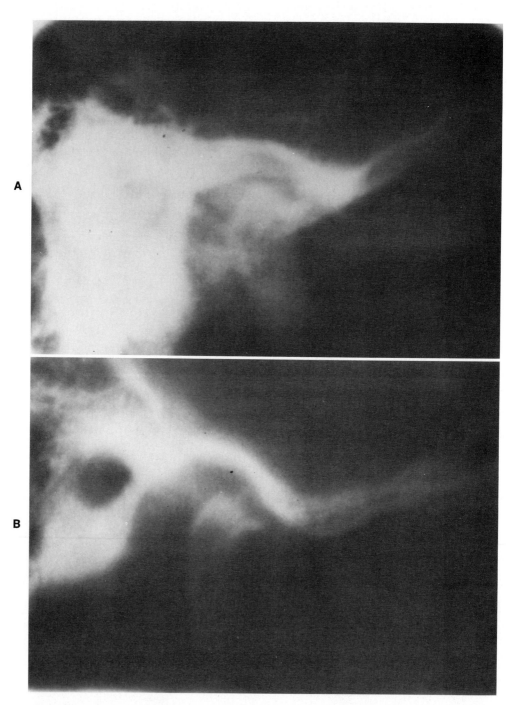

Fig. 13-31. A, Uncorrected and, **B,** corrected lateral tomogram of temporomandibular joint showing degenerative changes on condylar surface. Note greater clarity of corrected view.

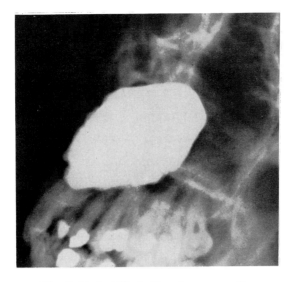

Fig. 13-32. Cyst filled with radiopaque media.

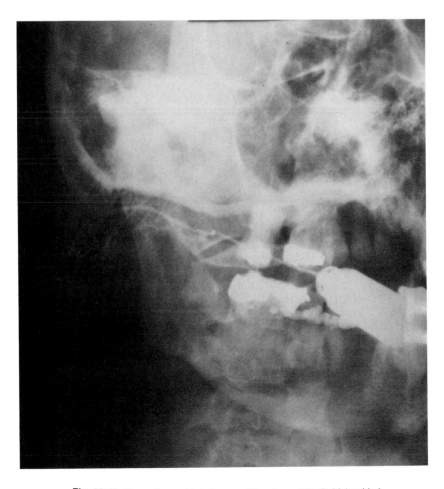

Fig. 13-33. Normal parotid sialogram. (Courtesy of Dr. D. M. Laskin.)

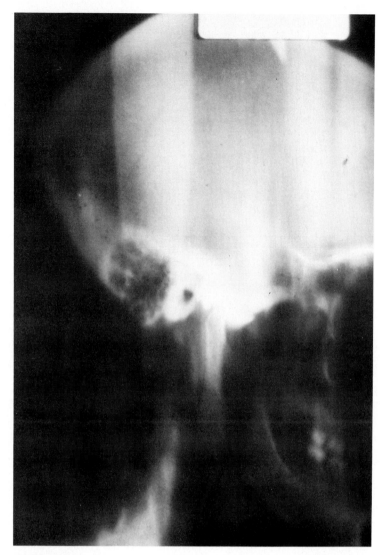

Fig. 13-34. Corrected lateral tomogram of temporomandibular joint with radiopaque media injected into upper compartment. (Courtesy of Dr. I. Pearlman.)

it is then irritating and may produce unpleasant symptoms. When fresh, however, it is nonirritating even to very delicate tissues and causes no pain or inflammation.

Because it has a high specific gravity, Lipiodol tends to gravitate to lower levels and fills the inferior part of a cavity first. Elimination from the tissues or closed cavities of the body is, as a rule, rather slow, ranging from several months to 2 years or more. Lipiodol may be diluted with two or three volumes of a refined

peanut or olive oil if a modification of its viscosity is desired; so diluted, it will still retain ample efficiency for use in radiographic diagnosis.

Ethiodol is the ether ester of iodized fatty acids of poppy-seed oil, containing 37% iodine. Because its viscosity is much less than that of Lipiodol, it is easier to inject and it will be absorbed and eliminated more quickly.

Renografin is another contrast medium, which has been recommended to produce arthrograms. It is preferable for the

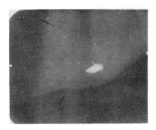

Fig. 13-35. Radiograph taken with dental film placed under upper lip to show foreign body located in soft tissue.

injection of joints since it is absorbed very rapidly in contrast to oil-based media.

The use of iodine-containing contrast media is contraindicated in patients with an idiosyncrasy to iodides. Cole and Nalls (1938) reported symptoms of iodism occurring in 10 patients of 600 in whom Lipiodol was injected, but the symptoms were not severe enough to cause alarm. The patient should be prevented from swallowing the expelled solution.

In case of suspected hemangiomas or when the extent or size of hemangiomas cannot be readily ascertained, the injection of Hypaque solution, a water-soluble radiographic contrast medium, allows visualization of the lesion and its tributary vessels. Harrigan, Fredrics, and Spiegel (1958) reported its use in such cases. The use of Hypaque for the study of the oral circulation by means of arteriography has been reported by Person, Dubowy, and Zeff (1959).

Localization techniques

Since an ordinary radiograph is a two-dimensional image of a three-dimensional object, it is often necessary to use more definitive techniques to localize teeth, pathologic processes, or foreign objects. When the pathologic entity is cystic, radiopaque media may be helpful (Fig. 13-32). Foreign bodies when large are not difficult to locate radiographically provided they are radiopaque. The lips, buccal mucosa, and often the floor of the mouth are accessible to this technique (Fig. 13-35).

Tangential or right angle exposures are often helpful. This technique employs two projections perpendicular to each other and directed at the object of interest. A good example is localizing an opacity seen on a lateral projection of the mandible. If this is combined with an occlusal projection, one may determine if the opacity is in the buccal mucosa or body of the mandible, or is perhaps a stone in the submandibular duct (Fig. 13-36).

Right angle procedures are not always feasible when locating teeth or foreign bodies within the jaws owing to inability to achieve proper angulation. If this is the case, the tube shift technique can be of great value (Wuehrmann and Manson-Hing, 1977). The principle of this technique involves moving or shifting the source of radiation (tube) while the x-ray film, object of interest, and a reference object of known position remain stationary. Two radiographs are taken with the tube in different positions. If the object of interest moves in the same direction as the tube, then it is closest to the film. If the object of interest moves in the opposite direction of the tube, then it is closest to the tube. For example, to determine the location of an impacted maxillary canine (object of interest) two projections are made, one of the canine-premolar area and the second of the canine–lateral incisor area. In this case the reference objects would be the premolar and lateral incisor. If on the radiograph the canine moved in the same direction that the tube moved, then the canine would be located toward the palate (closest to the film). If it moved in the opposite direction of the tube, the canine would be closest to the tube or in the labial aspect of the alveolus (Fig. 13-37). When an object of reference such as a tooth is not present, a needle or other radiopaque object of reference must be placed near the object of interest prior to the radiographic projection. This situation may occur when a foreign body or root tip is present in an edentulous area.

Xeroradiography

Xeroradiography is a relatively new method that can be used to visualize soft

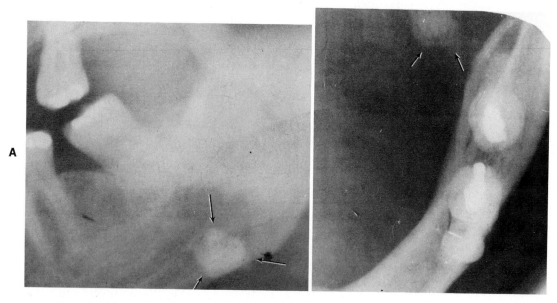

Fig. 13-36. A, Lateral projection of mandible showing opacity at mandibular angle. **B,** Occlusal projection discloses opacity present in retromylohyoid area.

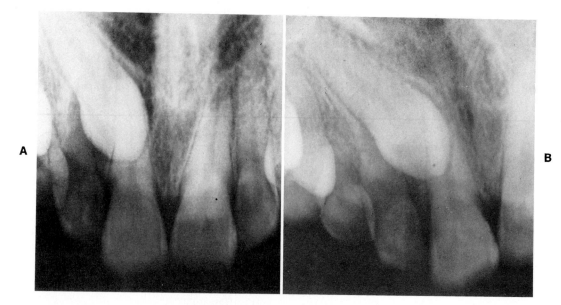

Fig. 13-37. Tube shift technique to locate position of impacted canine. **A,** Canine-lateral incisor view. **B,** Canine-premolar view. Note as tube shifts canine (object of interest) moves in same direction as tube. Therefore canine is closest to film (toward palate).

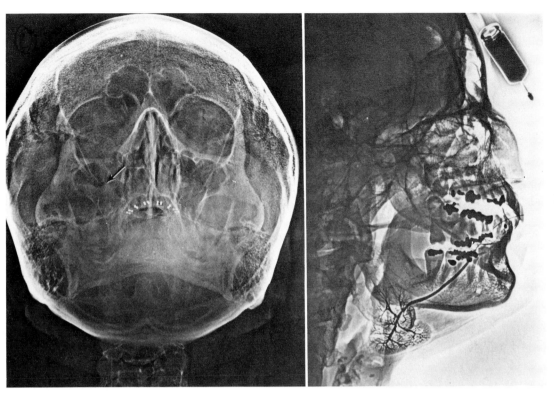

Fig. 13-38. Xeroradiographs. **A,** Waters projection showing classic trimolar fracture of right zygoma. Note air-fluid level in right antrum (arrow). **B,** Right lateral oblique projection showing submandibular gland xerosialogram. (From Olson, et al. 1976. J. Oral Surg. **34:**438.)

as well as hard tissues (Fig. 13-38). Its use has been suggested for localization of foreign bodies, determining the extent of oral lesions, sialography, examination of the temporomandibular joint, and cephalometry (Olson et al., 1976). The projection techniques are similar to those used for routine views, but the imaging process and developing procedure are different.

REFERENCES

Barton, E. J. 1955. Roentgenographic evidence of condylar neck fracture, Oral Surg. **8:**58.

Blackman, S. 1960. Rotational tomography of the face, Br. J. Radiol. **33:**408.

Blackman, S. 1961. Panagraphy, Oral Surg. **14:**1178.

Coin, C. G. 1974. Tomography of the temporomandibular joint, Dent. Radiogr. Photogr. **47:**23.

Cole, D. B., and Nalls, W. L. 1938. Twelve years' experience with iodized oil, Va. Med. Mon. **65:**336.

Gillis, R. R. 1935. Roentgen ray study of the temporomandibular articulation, J. Am. Dent. Assoc. **22:** 1321.

Goncalves, N., and Miller, A. M. 1974. Radiographic evaluation of defects created in mandibular condyles, Oral Surg. **38:**474.

Harrigan, W. F., Fredrics, H., and Spiegel, E. H. 1958. Case report of a cavernous hemangioma of the submaxillary triangle, Oral Surg. **11:**113.

Hudson, D. C., Kumpula, J. W., and Dickson, G. 1957. A panoramic dental x-ray machine, U.S. Armed Forces Med. J. **8:**46.

Ivy, R. H. 1917. Stereoscopic technique in dental and maxillary roentgenography, Dent. Cosmos **59:**723.

Lafay, L. 1901. Sur l'huile iodee biioduree et iodo-biioduree, Bul. Dermat. Sylph. Fourth Series, **2:**448.

Lewis, G. R. 1964. Temporomandibular joint radiographic technics — a comparison and evaluation of results, Dent. Radiogr. Photogr. **37:**8.

Lopez, J. 1976. Xeroradiography in dentistry, J. Am. Dent. Assoc. **92:**106.

Mandel, L., and Baurmash, H. 1965. Radiopaque contrast solution for sialography, J. Oral Ther. **2:**73.

Markovic, M. A., and Rosenberg, H. M. 1976. Tomographic evaluation of 100 patients with temporomandibular joint symptoms, Oral Surg. **42:**838.

Norgaard, F. 1947. Temporomandibular arthography, Copenhagen, Ejnar Munksgaard.

Olson, D. J., et al. 1976. The application of xeroradiography in oral surgery, J. Oral Surg. **34**:438.

Paatero, Y. V. 1961. Pantomography and orthopantomography, Oral Surg. **14**:947.

Person, P., Dubowy, J., and Zeff, S. 1959. Studies of the oral circulation, I. Preliminary report on external carotid arteriography, Oral Surg. **12**:371.

Potter, G. D. 1975. Radiographic analysis of the skull, Med. Radiogr. Photogr. **51**:2.

Silha, R. E. 1965. The versatile occlusal film, Dent. Radiogr. Photogr. **38**:36.

Silva, C. A. 1956. Stereoroentgenograms in dentistry, Oral Surg. **9**:757.

Smith, C. J. 1974. A comprehensive review of normal anatomic landmarks and artifacts as visualized on panorex radiographs, Oral Surg. **37**:291.

Stafne, E. C., and Gibilisco, J. A. 1975. Oral roentgenographic diagnosis, ed. 4, Philadelphia, W. B. Saunders Co.

Takeshi, O. 1975. Panoramic anatomy of maxillary sinus, Oral Surg. **39**:658.

Thoma, K. H. 1941. The use of radiopaque diagnostic media in roentgen diagnosis of oral surgical conditions, Am. J. Orthod. **27**:64.

Updegrave, W. J. 1963. Panoramic dental radiography, Dent. Radiogr. Photogr. **36**:75.

Updegrave, W. J. 1966. The role of panoramic radiography in diagnosis, Oral Surg. **22**:49.

Williamson, S. W. 1954. Occlusal radiography, Dent. Radiogr. Photogr. **27**:50.

Wuehrmann, A. H., and Manson-Hing, L. R. 1977. Dental Radiology, ed. 4, St. Louis, The C. V. Mosby Co.

Yale, S. H. 1969. Radiographic evaluation of the temporomandibular joint, J. Am. Dent. Assoc. **79**:102.

Yale, S. H., and Rosenberg, H. M. 1961. Laminagraphic cephalometry in the analysis of mandibular condyle morphology, Oral Surg. **14**:793.

Yale, S. H., and Rosenberg, H. M. 1975. The living skull, Dent. Radiogr. Photogr. **48**:3.

CHAPTER 14

Clinical laboratory diagnosis

Richard D. Zallen

The use of clinical laboratory tests constitutes an important part of the diagnostic evaluation of any patient, both from a general medical standpoint and in terms of specific conditions that may be related to the etiology of the pathologic process being considered by the oral and maxillofacial surgeon. It is essential, however, that these tests be used judiciously, not only because this will avoid unnecessary cost and discomfort, but also because it will avoid the confusion that can be created by positive or negative results of tests unrelated to the diagnosis being considered. Routine ordering of a large number of tests in the hope of finding sufficient positive data to establish a diagnosis generally is misleading and constitutes poor practice. A good rule to follow is that every laboratory procedure ordered should have a logical reason.

The following is a listing of the most commonly used laboratory tests with which the clinician should be familiar. A partial interpretation of these tests is given, but the reader should be aware that other disease states also may sometimes cause variations in the test results.

HEMATOLOGY

The routine blood examination consists of a hemoglobin and hematocrit determination and the complete blood count (CBC), which includes the red blood cell count, white blood cell count, differential white cell count, an estimation of platelet number, and a description of the blood smear. Other determinations are performed when specifically indicated.

Hemoglobin (Hb)

Hemoglobin is the oxygen-carrying material found in red blood cells. In females, it is normally in the range of 12 to 16 gm/100 ml of blood and in males 14 to 18 gm/100 ml of blood.

Hematocrit (HCT)

Hematocrit is a measurement of the packed red cell volume in a volume of blood. It is a simple laboratory test and is easily reproducible. The normal value is between 37% and 47% for females and between 40% and 52% for males. The hematocrit is valuable in evaluating polycythemia, anemia, and blood loss. A rule of thumb is that a four point loss or gain in hematocrit is roughly equal to the loss or gain of one unit or 500 ml of blood.

Red blood cell count (RBC)

The red blood cell count in adult males varies between 4.5 and 6.2 million cells/cu mm and in adult females between 4.5 and 5.5 million cells/cu mm. The red cell count provides a gross estimate of the body's oxygen-carrying capacity and is used in figuring the red cell indices, which are important in the diagnosis of various types of anemia.

Red cell morphology

A well-prepared smear of the peripheral blood, usually stained with a polychrome stain such as Wright's stain, can give a vast amount of information concerning the morphology of the red blood cells. Some terms used to describe alterations in size, shape, and staining characteristics follow.

normocytic normal size red blood cell
macrocytic large size red blood cell
microcytic small size red blood cell
normochromic normal hemoglobin content
hyperchromic greater than normal hemoglobin content
hypochromic smaller than normal hemoglobin content
anisocytosis refers to abnormal size of the red blood cells and includes both the microcytic and macrocytic cells
poikilocytosis refers to abnormal shapes of red blood cells and includes such descriptive terms as burr cells, sickle cells, target cells, spherocytes, and ovalocytes
target cells have a central area of hemoglobin with a pale zone around this and a normal staining periphery; found in sickle cell anemia and iron deficiency anemia
sickle cells found only in patients with either sickle cell trait or sickle cell anemia; red blood cell crescent shaped, owing to the presence of the abnormal hemoglobin S
burr cells cells with "spiny" crenated borders; usually result from technical problems in slide preparation but can be associated with advanced uremia
nucleated red blood cells normally found in the peripheral blood of the newborn; beyond this age, abnormal finding in the peripheral blood representing an abnormally large demand on the bone marrow to produce red blood cells; associated with infections and hypoxic conditions
polychromasia describes the staining quality of some young, mature red blood cells and is due to a mixture of hemoglobin and retained nuclear material

White blood cell count (WBC)

The white blood cell count is an extremely valuable laboratory study when dealing with infections or other diseases such as leukemia that affect the white cell series. The normal white count is between 5000 and 10,000 white cells/cu mm. Values above 10,000 are referred to as a leukocytosis, and values below 5000 are referred to as a leukopenia.

Differential white cell count

The differential white cell count is a cell type distribution of the total white blood cell count. On a well-prepared, Wright stained slide, 100 to 200 white cells are counted and the percent of each kind of cell is reported. The normal distribution of white cells is as follows: neutrophils (polymorphonuclear leukocytes), 50% to 70%; lymphocytes, 25% to 40%; monocytes, 3% to 8%; eosinophils, 1% to 4%; and basophils, 0% to 1%.

When referring to the differential count, the term "shift to the left" indicates an increase in the immature neutrophils, usually associated with an acute infection. A "shift to the right" means an increase in the number of mature neutrophils.

Platelet (thrombocyte) count

See p. 452.

Red cell indices

Red cell indices are very useful laboratory tools for measuring the size, shape, and hemoglobin content of the red cells. They utilize the hematocrit, hemoglobin, and red cell count determinations as a basis.

Mean corpuscular volume (MCV)

The mean corpuscular volume uses the hematocrit and red cell count to estimate the volume of the average red cell, as shown by the following equation.

$$MCV = \frac{HCT \times 10}{RBC}$$

The normal range is 82 to 98 cuμ; values below the normal indicate microcytic anemias and values above indicate macrocytic type anemias. Normocytic anemias fall in the normal range.

Mean corpuscular hemoglobin (MCH)

The mean corpuscular hemoglobin uses the hemoglobin content and red blood cell count to estimate the hemoglobin content of the individual red blood cell, as shown by the following equation.

$$MCH = \frac{Hb \times 10}{RBC}$$

The normal range is 27 to 32 micromicrograms ($\mu\mu$g), with values below this being suggestive of the microcytic anemias and values above being suggestive of the macrocytic type anemias.

Mean corpuscular hemoglobin concentration (MCHC)

The mean corpuscular hemoglobin concentration estimates the average amount of hemoglobin in 100 ml of packed red blood cells by using the hemoglobin and hematocrit determinations, as shown by the following equation.

$$\text{MCHC} = \frac{\text{Hb} \times 100}{\text{HCT}}$$

The normal range is 32 to 38 gm/100 ml. The MCHC is only elevated in hereditary spherocytosis and decreased in the microcytic type anemias.

Reticulocyte count

Reticulocytes are an immature form of red blood cell that represent a stage between the nucleated red blood cell and the mature red blood cell. Normally they account for 0.5% to 1.5% of red blood cells counted. Reticulocytes are found in large numbers when red cell formation is increased and are associated with the treatment of various anemias and blood loss.

Sedimentation rate (SR)

The normal values for sedimentation rate are 0 to 20 mm/hr for females and 0 to 10 mm/hr for males. It is a nonspecific test; above normal values usually mean that infections, infarctions, trauma, or tumors may be present.

COAGULATION TESTS

The coagulation mechanism originates from two pathways, the extrinsic and intrinsic, which then lead to the conversion of prothrombin to thrombin through the common pathway. Thrombin, in turn, activates fibrinogen to fibrin (Fig. 14-1).

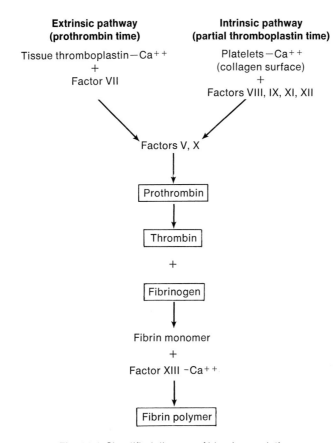

Fig. 14-1. Simplified diagram of blood coagulation.

The following is a list of coagulation factors:

   I. Fibrinogen
  II. Prothrombin
 III. Tissue thromboplastin
  IV. Calcium
   V. Accelerator globulin (AcG), Proaccelerin
 VII. Serum prothrombin conversion accelerator (SPCA)
VIII. Antihemophilic globulin (AHG)
  IX. Plasma thromboplastin component (PTC; Christmas factor)
   X. Stuart-Prower factor
  XI. Plasma thromboplastin antecedent (PTA)
 XII. Hageman factor
XIII. Fibrin stabilizing factor (FSF)

In order to evaluate the competency of these various pathways, a coagulation profile, including a prothrombin time, partial thromboplastin time, platelet count, bleeding time, and fibrinogen concentration, is ordered.

Prothrombin time (PT)

The prothrombin time measures the extrinsic and common pathways. The normal values are reported in either seconds or percentages. If the values are reported in seconds, the laboratory will give the patient's prothrombin time over the control time, with the normal range being between 11 and 15 seconds. If it is reported in percentages, the normal range is between 70% and 100%. The prothrombin time is prolonged in factor I, II, V, VII, and X deficiencies and occurs with anticoagulant therapy, cirrhosis, hepatitis, obstructive jaundice, colitis, celiac disease, sprue, and salicylate therapy.

Partial thromboplastin time (PTT)

The partial thromboplastin time measures the intrinsic and common pathways. The normal values are between 25 and 40 seconds. The partial thromboplastin time is prolonged in factor VIII, IX, XI, and XII deficiencies and in deficiencies of those factors necessary for the common pathway—I, II, V, and X. The partial thromboplastin time is also prolonged in patients undergoing heparin therapy.

Platelet count

The normal platelet count is between 150,000 and 400,000 cells/cu mm. Bleeding from thrombocytopenia rarely occurs until the count is below 60,000/cu mm.

Bleeding time (Duke)

The Duke bleeding time, although difficult to standardize and reproduce, nevertheless gives some information concerning vascular and platelet interaction. The normal bleeding time should not exceed 5 minutes and is usually prolonged in thrombocytopenia, von Willebrand's disease, and disorders of platelet function.

Fibrinogen

The normal level of fibrinogen is between 200 and 400 mg%; however, bleeding does not usually ensue until a level of 100 mg% is reached. Decreased levels of fibrinogen are found in hepatic disease and with circulating fibrinolysins.

• • •

The preceding five tests make up an initial coagulation profile that helps the clinician in determining the presence and cause of a bleeding diathesis. Other laboratory tests that may also be helpful include the following.

Tourniquet test (Rumpel-Leede)

The tourniquet test is a crude test used to study the capillary-platelet interphase. Classically the study consists of placing a blood pressure cuff on the upper arm and leaving it inflated for 5 minutes halfway between the patient's systolic and diastolic blood pressures. A positive test shows more than five petechiae in a 2.5 cm circle on the forearm in males and more than 10 petechiae in females. The test is not used routinely because of its poor correlation with the platelet count and the fact that petechiae are usually present in thrombocytopenia.

Clot retraction

Clot retraction represents a complex interaction between platelets, fibrin, and trapped red blood cells. The normal range for clot retraction is 48% to 64%. Clot retraction is deficient with thrombocytopenia and circulating fibrinolysins.

Clotting time

In theory, if the blood sample is drawn cleanly and there is no tissue thromboplastin contamination, the clotting time should measure the intrinsic and common pathways. In practice only severe factor deficiencies in these pathways cause a prolonged clotting time. The chief use for the clotting time is in the management of heparin therapy. The normal range for the Lee-White clotting time is 4 to 10 minutes.

Thromboplastin generation test (TGT)

The thromboplastin generation test is used to differentiate specific factor deficiencies in the intrinsic and common pathways, namely, factors VIII, IX, XI, XII, V, and X. The normal range is 12 seconds or less.

Prothrombin consumption test

The prothrombin consumption test measures the same factors as the thromboplastin generation test, but it is less sensitive and will not pick up mild factor deficiencies. The normal value is 20 seconds or longer.

BLOOD CHEMISTRY (AUTOMATED ANALYSIS, "SMA-12")

The SMA-12 (Sequential Multiple Analyzer-12) is a biochemical survey of 12 blood constituents that help in screening patients for a variety of diseases. The tests vary somewhat in different hospitals. Some substitute the electrolytes for uric acid, phosphorus, cholesterol, and glutamic pyruvic transaminase, and include a bilirubin determination. In screening for specific diseases or following their clinical course, individual tests should be ordered.

Total protein

The normal value for total protein is 6 to 8 gm/100 ml of serum. Increased total protein is usually associated with dehydration and dysgammaglobulinemic states. Decreased values are usually associated with hepatocellular disease, malabsorption disease, and starvation.

Albumin

The normal value for albumin is between 3.5 and 5 gm/100 ml. Increase in serum albumin is most often associated with dehydration. Decreases in serum albumin are associated with kidney diseases such as nephrosis and chronic glomerulonephritis, gastrointestinal diseases such as ulcerative colitis and protein losing enteropathy, and liver diseases such as Laennec's cirrhosis and hepatocellular damage secondary to hepatitis. Decreases are also found in some of the collagen diseases and in lymphatic and myelogenous leukemia.

Calcium

The normal value for serum calcium is between 8.5 and 10.5 mg/100 ml. Increased levels are associated most commonly with excessive osteolysis such as occurs in hyperparathyroidism and malignancy with bone metastasis. Decreased levels are associated with hypoparathyroidism, pseudohypoparathyroidism, tetany, hypoalbuminemia, acute pancreatitis, renal failure, and starvation. Since one third to one half of serum calcium is bound to protein, the total protein and serum albumin levels must be known before serum calcium levels can be interpreted.

Phosphorus (inorganic)

The normal value for serum phosphorus is between 2.5 and 4.5 mg/100 ml. Increased levels are associated with hypoparathyroidism, pseudohypoparathyroidism, secondary hyperparathyroidism caused by chronic renal failure, and metabolic acidosis. Decreased levels are associated with primary hyperparathyroidism, vitamin D deficiency, malabsorption diseases, and chronic antacid usage. A high phosphorous and low glucose level may be an artifact associated with an unrefrigerated sample.

Cholesterol

The normal cholesterol value is between 150 and 300 mg/100 ml. Increased levels of cholesterol are associated with idiopathic hypercholesterolemia and secondary hypercholesterolemia caused by nephrosis, chronic obstructive biliary disease, hypothyroidism, and diabetes. Decreased levels are associated with hyperthyroidism, malnutrition, and severe liver cell damage.

Glucose

The normal glucose value is between 65 and 110 mg/100 ml. Increased levels are associated with diabetes mellitus (see glucose tolerance test, p. 455), Cushing's disease, acromegaly, stress that increases the endogenous output of epinephrine and glucocorticoids, pheochromocytoma, acute and chronic pancreatitis, pancreatectomy, and hyperthyroidism. Decreased levels are associated with hypoglycemic medications, islet cell tumors of the pancreas, advanced cirrhosis or hepatitis, early diabetes mellitus, Addison's disease, functional hypoglycemia, and certain inborn errors of metabolism such as hereditary fructose intolerance, galactosemia, and maple syrup urine disease.

Uric acid

The normal uric acid value is between 2.5 and 8 mg/100 ml. Increased levels are associated with gout, renal failure, diets high in nucleoproteins, and diseases associated with increased breakdown of nucleoproteins such as leukemia, multiple myeloma, lymphoma, and hemolytic anemia. When hyperuricemia is associated with hypercholesterolemia, the incidence of myocardial infarction secondary to coronary artery disease is increased. Hyperuricemia is also associated with the use of diuretics and aspirin. Decreased levels are associated with the use of uricosuric drugs, Wilson's disease, and the use of adrenocorticotropic hormone (ACTH).

Creatinine

The normal creatinine value is between 0.7 and 1.4 mg/100 ml. Increases are associated with impaired kidney function and muscle diseases. Serum creatinine varies inversely with the glomerular filtration rate and is a more sensi-tive indicator of this rate than the blood urea nitrogen test (see p. 455). However, because some creatinine is secreted by the tubules, a normal serum creatinine does not mean renal filtration is not impaired. Another advantage of serum creatinine is that it is almost unaffected by diet.

Alkaline phosphatase

The normal adult alkaline phosphatase value is between 20 and 48 I mU/ml (1.5 to 4.5 Bodansky units; 4 to 13 King-Armstrong units). In the child the values are higher (5 to 14 Bodansky units; 15 to 30 King-Armstrong units). Increases in this enzyme are associated with hepatic obstruction, either intrahepatic or extrahepatic secondary to infection or tumor. The enzyme is also elevated as a result of osteoblastic activity associated with Paget's disease, hyperparathyroidism, osteoblastic tumors of bone, and osteogenesis imperfecta. The differentiation of hepatic and bone origin of alkaline phosphatase can be accomplished by analysis of the isoenzymes. Decreases are associated with hypophosphatasia, hypothyroidism, and malnutrition.

Lactic dehydrogenase (LDH)

The normal value of lactic dehydrogenase is between 90 and 200 mU/ml. Serum lactic dehydrogenase is a ubiquitous enzyme found in many tissues, including kidney, heart, skeletal muscle, liver, red and white blood cells, and skin. It is increased in various malignancies, inflammations, necrotic processes, and infections. Some of the most common diseases that are associated with increases in the enzyme are myocardial infarction, where the enzyme may remain elevated for 10 to 14 days, pulmonary embolus and pulmonary infarction, hepatitis, leukemia, lymphoma, and congestive heart failure. The enzyme has been divided into five isoenzymes that often can be used to identify the tissue of origin.

Glutamic oxaloacetic transaminase (SGOT)

The normal serum value of SGOT is between 10 and 50 mU/ml. Like LDH,

SGOT is found in many tissues, including heart, kidney, liver, skeletal muscle, and pancreas. The enzyme remains elevated in myocardial infarction from about 12 hours to 3 to 5 days. High elevations are also found in hepatitis, with moderate elevations occurring in cirrhosis and liver neoplasms. Slight elevations are seen with muscular trauma and after surgery.

Glutamic pyruvic transaminase (SGPT)

The normal serum value of SGPT is between 6 and 36 mU/ml. The values generally parallel those for SGOT but are more elevated in liver damage than myocardial damage.

OTHER BLOOD DETERMINATIONS

Blood urea nitrogen (BUN)

The normal value is between 10 and 20 mg/100 ml. Increases are associated with a decrease in the glomerular filtration rate (GFR); however, an approximately 30% to 40% decrease in GFR is needed before the BUN becomes elevated. Increases can also be associated with pre- and postrenal azotemia. Decreased levels are associated with advanced liver disease and low protein diets.

Bilirubin

Bilirubin is a breakdown product of hemoglobin. Its measurement is therefore important in evaluating for hemolytic anemias. Since it is removed from the blood by the liver through a process of conjugation to protein, it is also an important measure of hepatic function.

Bilirubin is measured in two forms: direct (conjugated) and total (conjugated and unconjugated). The difference between total and direct bilirubin represents the unconjugated form (indirect). Determining the type responsible for elevation of total bilirubin helps distinguish between hepatocellular and obstructive forms of liver disease.

The normal serum contains less than 0.8 mg of total bilirubin/100 ml. Of this, no more than 0.3 mg is unconjugated.

Acid phosphatase

The normal value of acid phosphatase is between 0.5 and 11 mU/ml (0.13 to 0.63 Sigma units). The prostate is rich in acid phosphatase and small amounts are also found in red blood cells, bone, kidney, liver, and spleen. An increase in acid phosphatase usually indicates that a carcinoma of the prostate has metastasized, especially to bone.

Amylase

The normal value of amylase is between 60 and 150 Somogyi units/100 ml. Increases are most often associated with diseases of the pancreas, such as acute pancreatitis, recurrent bouts of chronic pancreatitis, pancreatic duct obstruction secondary to a carcinoma, or spasm resulting from the use of opiates. Increases may also occur with salivary gland disease, bowel obstruction, and upper gastrointestinal surgery.

Glucose tolerance test (GTT)

When elevated glucose levels are found in the blood and/or urine, the glucose tolerance test (GTT) may be used to diagnose diabetes mellitus. This test is started with a patient who has been fasting overnight. After the patient ingests a glucose load, blood and urine specimens are taken at 30 minutes, 1 hour, 1½ hours, 2 hours, and 3 hours. Specimens are also taken prior to glucose ingestion.

The normal value for fasting blood sugar is between 65 and 110 mg/100 ml, with the fasting urine negative for glucose. From here the glucose level will climb to 160 mg/100 ml or less within 30 minutes to 1 hour, with a gradual decrease and return to fasting levels or slightly below at the 2 hour interval and a leveling off at the 3 hour interval. Urine samples are negative for glucose at the same time intervals.

The diabetic curve may show the fasting blood level at or near the upper limits of normal. Following the test dose, blood values do not come back to normal before the 2 hour interval. The 1 and 2 hour values are over 160 mg/100 ml, with the urine samples also positive for glucose at these intervals. Certain diseases will affect the GTT and must be considered before making a diagnosis of diabetes mellitus; these include hyperthyroidism,

Cushing's disease, poor absorption from the gastrointestinal tract, severe liver damage, and reaction to some medications.

Creatine phosphokinase (CPK)

The normal values range between 5 and 50 I mU/ml. Like other tissue enzymes, CPK is found in striated muscle, heart, and brain. Elevation of CPK with myocardial infarction generally parallels that of SGOT, rising quickly and peaking in 1 to 2 days. Increases are also associated with cerebral infarction and Duchenne type muscular dystrophy. An association between increased CPK levels and malignant hyperthermia has been described.

Serologic tests for syphilis

A number of screening tests for syphilis are available, which, if positive, must be further tested against more specific antigens. Examples of screening tests are the Venereal Disease Research Laboratory (VDRL), Kahn, and Hinton tests. These tests may give false positive results with lupus erythematosus, leprosy, malaria, infectious mononucleosis, hepatitis A, rheumatoid arthritis, and in narcotic addicts. More specific tests are the Reiter, *Treponema pallidum* immobilization (TPI), and fluorescent treponemal antibody absorption (FTA-ABS) tests. The last is the most sensitive test.

Australia antigen (hepatitis B surface antigen; HB_sAg)

Australia antigen can be identified in the laboratory and is a useful screening test to determine the presence or absence of the hepatitis B virus. It typically appears in the last few weeks of the incubation period and disappears with clinical recovery. In about 10% of cases, however, it may persist for months or years, indicating ongoing hepatic disease.

Transfused HB_sAg-positive blood causes severe hepatitis. Certain groups of patients have been identified as being high-risk carriers of HB_sAg; these include the mentally retarded and patients with Down's syndrome who are institutionalized, patients receiving renal dialysis, patients with immunologic defects, patients receiving numerous blood transfusions and blood derivatives, and chronic drug abusers who use the intravenous route. Serum antibody to HB_sAg indicates exposure at some time in the past. Failure to detect HB_sAg does not exclude type B hepatitis.

Iron

The normal vaues for iron range between 50 and 175 μg/100 ml, with males being slightly higher than females in this range. Serum iron is available for the formation of hemoglobin. Increases are associated with hemolytic anemias, hemochromatosis, and pernicious anemia. Decreased levels are found in iron deficiency anemias and anemias secondary to chronic infections.

Total iron binding capacity (TIBC)

The normal value is between 250 and 410 μg/100 ml. Increases are found in iron deficiency anemias and anemias secondary to blood loss. Decreased levels are associated with chronic infection and liver disease.

Serum osmolality

The normal values for serum osmolality range between 275 and 295 mOsm/L. Serum osmolality measures the total concentration of all particles in solution whether they are electrolytes or not. Increases are associated with excessive water loss, chronic renal disease with a rising BUN, increasing serum glucose levels secondary to diabetes mellitus, and diabetes insipidus. Decreases are associated with inappropriate antidiuretic hormone secretion (IADH) and Addison's disease.

Carbon dioxide (CO_2)

The normal value is between 24 and 32 mEq/L and reflects the amount of carbonic acid and bicarbonate in the blood. In acid-base balance, the CO_2 level must be evaluated in light of the other electrolytes and blood gases. In general, the bicarbonate level will be decreased in metabolic acidosis and respiratory alkalosis and increased in metabolic alkalosis and respiratory acidosis. This will be reflected by similar changes in CO_2 content of the blood.

SERUM ELECTROLYTES°
Sodium (Na)

The normal values of sodium range between 135 and 145 mEq/L. Hyponatremia is associated with cirrhosis, congestive heart failure, adrenal insufficiency, nephrosis, excessive use of diuretics, inappropriate antidiuretic hormone secretion, and water intoxication. Hypernatremia is usually caused by excessive loss of water in vomiting, diarrhea, severe sweating, and diabetes mellitus.

Potassium (K)

The normal value of potassium is between 3.2 and 5.5 mEq/L. Hypokalemia is usually associated with inadequate intake or losses from the gastrointestinal or the urinary tracts. The latter include vomiting, diarrhea, nasogastric suction, and use of diuretic medications. Hyperkalemia is associated with release of cellular potassium secondary to surgery, crush injuries, hemolysis of red blood cells, renal failure, and acidosis.

Chloride (Cl)

The normal value of chloride is between 95 and 105 mEq/L. Serum chloride levels usually follow those for serum sodium; however, chloride will be reduced in vomiting.

°See "Blood Chemistry," p. 453 for calcium and phosphorus; "Blood Gases," p. 458 for bicarbonate.

Magnesium (Mg)

The normal value of magnesium is between 1.5 and 2 mEq/L. Increases can be associated with renal failure and large doses of antacids that contain magnesium. Decreases are associated with alcoholism, diabetic acidosis, malabsorption, hypocalcemia, and hypokalemia.

LIPID PROFILE

Hyperlipoproteinemias can be subdivided into five types. In order to clinically distinguish these five types, a serum cholesterol, serum triglyceride level, and lipoprotein electrophoresis should be obtained (Table 14-1).

Cholesterol

See "Blood Chemistry," p. 453.

Triglycerides

The normal value of triglycerides ranges between 35 and 150 mg/100 ml of blood. Increased levels are associated with congenital hyperlipidemia, nephrotic syndrome, diabetes mellitus, and myocardial infarction.

Lipoprotein electrophoresis

The electrophoretic pattern consists of an alpha band, a prebeta band, and a beta band. Chylomicrons are not present on electrophoresis in normal patients but are present in type I and II hyperlipoproteinemias.

IMMUNOGLOBULINS
IgG

The normal value of IgG is between 800 and 1500 mg/100 ml of blood. IgG forms about 73% of the immunoglobulins

Table 14-1. Laboratory diagnosis of hyperlipoproteinemia

	Cholesterol	Triglycerides	Lipoprotein abnormality
Type I	Increased or normal	Markedly increased	Hyperchylomicronemia
Type II	Increased	Normal or slightly elevated	Hyperbetalipoproteinemia
Type III	Increased	Increased	Dysbetalipoproteinemia (broad beta band)
Type IV	Normal or increased	Increased	Hyperbetalipoproteinemia (dense beta band)
Type V	Normal or increased	Increased	Hyperchylomicronemia and hyperprebetalipoproteinemia

in normal serum. Increased levels are found in cirrhosis of the liver. Decreased levels are found in the nephrotic syndrome and in the antibody deficiency syndromes.

IgM

The normal value of IgM is between 50 and 120 mg/100 ml of blood. IgM forms about 7% of the total immunoglobulins in normal serum and is efficient in stimulating agglutination and phagocytosis.

IgA

The normal value of IgA is between 40 and 120 mg/100 ml of blood. IgA forms about 19% of the total immunoglobulins. IgA is found mainly in external secretions such as saliva, intestinal tract secretions, respiratory tract secretions, and lacrimal and nasal secretions. It appears that its main role is in the prevention of infections in various mucosal membranes.

BLOOD GASES

Blood gas determinations help in evaluation of acid-base balance and the degree of oxygenation. The studies are usually done on an arterial blood sample, but venous blood may be used. In addition to measurement of actual blood gases, determination of related factors such as pH and CO_2 combining power and calculation of blood bicarbonate and base excess permit identification of the clinical cause of acid-base disturbances and monitoring of subsequent treatment.

pH

The normal value for arterial pH is 7.40 with a range of 7.35 to 7.45. With venous blood the normal value is 7.36 with a range of 7.31 to 7.41. The acidity or alkalinity of the blood is measured by the pH. Values less than 7.35 indicate acidosis and those greater than 7.45 indicate alkalosis.

P_{CO_2}

The normal value for arterial blood ranges between 35 and 45 mm Hg and for venous blood between 41 and 51 mm Hg. P_{CO_2} refers to the pressure of dis-

solved CO_2 in the blood and is influenced by the lungs; increases secondary to hypoventilation represent respiratory acidosis and decreases secondary to hyperventilation represent respiratory alkalosis (see Chapter 9, p. 338).

Actual bicarbonate (HCO_3)

Bicarbonate can be calculated from the Henderson-Hasselbalch equation if the pH and P_{CO_2} are known. The normal values for both arterial and venous blood are 22 to 26 mEq/L. HCO_3 is not regulated by respiratory processes but is controlled by metabolic processes. Increases in the HCO_3 level are therefore associated with metabolic alkalosis and decreases are associated with metabolic acidosis (see Chapter 9).

Carbon dioxide combining power (CCP)

The carbon dioxide combining power of the blood is an indicator of the state of acid-base balance. Since all but about 5% of the CO_2 is derived from bicarbonate, it is actually a measure of alkaline reserve. The normal range is from 55 to 75 ml of CO_2/100 ml of plasma (24 to 29 mEq/L). Acidosis is shown by a decrease in CO_2 combining power and alkalosis by an increase.

Base excess

Base excess is another calculated value used to determine the state of acid-base balance. It represents the difference between theoretical and actual total CO_2 content of the blood. Normally it should be 0 with a range of ±2 mEq/L for either arterial or venous blood. A negative value below this signifies bicarbonate deficit and a positive value indicates bicarbonate excess. Therefore positive numbers represent metabolic alkalosis and negative values represent metabolic acidosis.

P_{O_2}

The normal value for arterial P_{O_2} is between 80 and 100 mm Hg and for venous blood between 35 and 40 mm Hg. Decreased levels of P_{O_2} are associated with various degrees of hypoxia and may be associated with respiratory acidosis secondary to impaired diffusion or shunting. Normal levels of PO_2 may be present in metabolic acidosis and alkalosis.

O_2 saturation

The normal value for arterial O_2 saturation is between 95% and 98% and for venous blood between 60% and 85%.

URINALYSIS

The urinalysis consists of a gross, chemical, and microscopic examination.

Gross examination

Color

The color of urine varies with its dilution and endogenous and exogenous pigment content. The normal color of urine is straw to amber; dilute urine is almost colorless, and concentrated urine is yellow to dark yellow. Examples of abnormal endogenous pigments are hemoglobin, which turns urine a red or reddish brown color; bilirubin, which turns it a greenish orange; urobilin, which turns it an orange-brown; and homogentisic acid, which turns it a brown to black color on standing. Red blood cells will give urine a smoky red to brown color. Examples of exogenous pigments that change the color of urine are beets, which turn urine red, and rhubarb, which turns it a yellow-brown.

Appearance

Normal urine is usually clear; however, amorphous phosphates and urates may form a whitish sediment. Bacteria can cause a cloudy urine and pus will usually give a white mucoid-like sediment.

Odor

Normal urine has a faint aromatic odor that is not unpleasant. If urine is allowed to stand without being refrigerated, the odor becomes heavy and unpleasant secondary to bacterial overgrowth. Odors from asparagus and fecal contamination are also characteristic.

Specific gravity

The specific gravity of urine depends on the state of hydration of the patient. In a dilute sample from a well-hydrated patient, the specific gravity will be under 1.010. In a concentrated sample (dehydrated patient), the specific gravity is usually above 1.020. Solutes such as protein and glucose will also elevate the specific gravity and should be suspected when there are high values.

Chemical examination

pH

Normal urine is usually acid, being in the range of 4.8 to 7.5. Acid urine results from the normal ability of the renal tubules to exchange hydrogen ions for sodium ions. Urine allowed to stand may become alkaline secondary to the liberation of ammonia by bacteria that split urea.

Protein

Normally the kidney tubules will reabsorb most of the protein in the glomerular filtrate. Approximately 30 to 100 mg of protein are lost in 24 hours. Increased transient losses of protein normally occur after strenuous exertion, in orthostatic proteinuria, and with fevers. Pathologic conditions that cause a constant proteinuria are hypertension, congestive heart failure, glomerulonephritis, pyelonephritis, and the nephrotic syndrome.

Glucose

The normal renal threshold is approximately 180 mg/100 ml of blood sugar. When this level is exceeded, glucose will appear in the urine. Glucosuria associated with hyperglycemia is usually secondary to diabetes mellitus but will also be seen with dextrose infusion, Cushing's disease, pheochromocytoma, ingestion of large amounts of glucose, stress, and increased intracranial pressure.

Ketone

Acetone, acetoacetic acid, and beta-hydroxybutyric acid are known as ketone bodies and are the breakdown products of fat metabolism. Increased ketone levels are found in diabetic ketoacidosis; starvation; fever; high fat, low carbohydrate diets; and dehydration.

Hemoglobin

Hemoglobinuria is the result of red cell hemolysis in the blood or in the urine specimen. Hemoglobinuria is found with hemolytic anemias and incompatible blood transfusions.

Bilirubin

Bilirubin in the urine is an indication of liver disease. Conjugated, direct acting bilirubin, when present in the urine, is usually associated with extrahepatic and intrahepatic obstruction and hepatocellular disease.

Urobilinogen

The normal value of urobilinogen is 1 Ehrlich unit or less in 2 hours or 0.5 to 4 units (0.05 to 2.5 mg) in 24 hours. Increased levels are associated with hepatocellular disease, whereas decreased levels are associated with obstructive jaundice.

Bence-Jones protein

Bence-Jones protein is an abnormal protein that is found 20% to 50% of the time in the urine of patients with multiple myeloma.

Microscopic examination

White blood cells

Occasionally white blood cells are found in the urinary sediment, with 1 to 5 white cells per high-power field being considered within normal limits. An increased urinary WBC count is usually suggestive of urinary tract infection.

Red blood cells

The normal range is from 0 to 1 cell per high power field. An increased red cell count, when not associated with menstrual flow, is usually associated with glomerulonephritis, renal infarction, nephrolithiasis, urethritis, prostatitis, blood dyscrasias, anticoagulant therapy, or excessive physical exertion.

Epithelial cells

Renal cells are indicative of kidney damage, whereas transitional cells indicate possible pathologic conditions in the renal pelvis, ureter, or bladder. Squamous cells originate from the superficial layers of the urethra and vagina and are of little diagnostic importance.

Casts

Casts are composed of protein material alone or a combination of protein material and cells. They are called casts because their shape is a replica of the internal diameter of the distal and collecting renal tubules where they are formed. There are three types: hyaline, blood, and epithelial. Hyaline casts occur with intrinsic renal disease, heart failure, shock, fever, and excessive exercise. The presence of red blood cell casts indicates glomerular damage or ruptured tubules. White blood cell casts are associated with renal infections. Epithelial cell casts usually indicate heavy metal poisoning, advanced glomerulonephritis, pyelonephritis, or malignant nephrosclerosis.

Crystals

The significance of crystals in the urine is not great. Depending on the urinary pH, various crystals may be precipitated. Their main importance is when one suspects nephrolithiasis or gout.

FECAL EXAMINATION

Occult blood

Blood in the stool is abnormal. The guaiac test is used to reveal blood that is not visible on gross examination. Usually bleeding from the upper gastrointestinal tract will produce black "tarry" colored stools, whereas bleeding from the lower gastrointestinal tract will usually show gross blood in the stool. The guaiac test is particularly useful in examining for asymptomatic lesions of the gastrointestinal tract.

Urobilinogen

The normal value of urobilinogen is between 40 and 300 mg/24-hour sample. Increased levels are due to hemolytic anemias, while decreased levels are associated with hepatic obstruction or hepatocellular disease and antibiotics that destroy the intestinal flora.

MICROBIOLOGIC EXAMINATIONS

Specimens from the oral cavity must be taken very carefully so as not to contaminate them with extraneous oral flora. For aerobic cultures, the swab must be placed directly in the lesion, wound, or fluid. Specimens from an abscess that are to be cultured anaerobically can be taken by cleaning the oral mucosa or skin, placing a needle into the abscess and withdrawing some material, then corking the needle and sending the needle and syringe to the laboratory. (See also Chapter 4.)

Smears

The material being submitted should be smeared on a glass slide and stained in an attempt to identify the type of organism (see Chapter 4). The routine stains include Gram stain, acid-fast stain, and stains for fungus.

Cultures

Routine cultures are done for aerobic, anaerobic, and acid-fast organisms as well as for fungi.

Antibiotic sensitivity test

The most widely used technique is the disc method, where the organism(s) cultured from the original specimen are grown in the presence of antibiotic-impregnated discs (see Chapter 4). The discs that develop a wide zone of bacterial inhibition around them indicate that the organism is sensitive to that antibiotic. This is an imprecise technique and the clinical situation should be considered along with the laboratory information.

LIVER FUNCTION TESTS

Because of the wide range of activities in the liver, hepatic function can be evaluated in a number of ways. These include measurement of alkaline phosphatase (p. 455), bilirubin (p. 454), and SGPT (p. 455). The bromsulphalein (BSP) test also is very useful in evaluating the status of the liver parenchymal cells. Normally there is less than 5% dye retention in the blood 1 hour after injection.

THYROID FUNCTION TESTS
Protein bound iodine (PBI)

The normal values for protein bound iodine range between 3.5 and 8 mg/100 ml. Increased PBI values are associated with hyperthyroidism, iodine-containing drugs, and pregnancy. Decreased values are associated with hypothyroidism, nephrotic syndrome, and severe liver disease.

Butanol extractable iodine (BEI)

The normal values for butanol extractable iodine are between 3.5 and 7.5 μg/100 ml. Increases and decreases of BEI parallel those of the PBI, with the one main advantage that inorganic iodine does not alter the BEI. Organic iodine, such as contrast media, will alter both the BEI and PBI.

Total thyroxine (T$_4$)

The normal value of total thyroxine is between 2.9 and 6.4 μg/100 ml. This test has the main advantage of not being affected by organic, nonthyroid iodine and mercurial diuretics.

T$_3$ uptake

The normal value for T$_3$ uptake is between 25% and 35%. T$_3$ uptake is increased in hyperthyroidism, conditions that produce decreased serum protein, and with certain drugs such as penicillin, salicylates, heparin, and dicumarol. Decreased values are associated with hypothyroidism, pregnancy, and estrogen therapy.

REFERENCES

Bauer, J. D., Ackermann, P. G., and Toro, G. 1974. Clinical laboratory methods, ed. 8, St. Louis, The C. V. Mosby Co.
Broughton, J. O. 1973. Understanding blood gases. In Hudak, C. M., et al. Critical care nursing, ed. 1, Philadelphia, J. B. Lippincott Co.
Brown, D. F. 1971. The diagnosis and treatment of hyperlipoproteinemia, The Heart Bulletin **20**:13.
Council on Dental Therapeutics. 1976. Type B (serum) hepatitis and dental practice, J. Am. Dent. Assoc. **92**:153.
Davidshon, I., and Henry, J. B. 1974. Todd-Sanford's clinical diagnosis by laboratory methods, ed. 15, Philadelphia, W. B. Saunders Co.
D'Eramo, E. M. 1973. The significance of serum studies (SMA-12), J. Oral Surg. **31**:795.
Harrison, T. R., et al. 1974. Principles of internal medicine, ed. 7, New York, McGraw-Hill Book Co.
LaRosa, J. C. 1972. Hyperlipoproteinemia, Postgrad. Med. **51**:62.
Levinson, S. A., and MacFate, R. P. 1969. Clinical

laboratory diagnosis, ed. 7, Philadelphia, Lea & Febiger.

Little, J. W. 1976. Detection and management of the potential bleeder in dental practice, J. Oral Med. **31**:11.

Mosley, J. W., and White, E. 1975. Viral hepatitis as an occupational hazard of dentists, J. Am. Dent. Assoc. **90**:492.

Page, L. B., and Culver, P. J. 1961. A syllabus of laboratory examinations in clinical diagnosis, Cambridge, Harvard University Press.

Raphael, S. S., et al. 1976. Lynch's medical laboratory technology, ed. 3, Philadelphia, W. B. Saunders Co.

Ravel, R. 1973. Clinical laboratory medicine, ed. 2, Chicago, Year Book Medical Publishers, Inc.

Schwartz, H. C., and Gracia, R. M. 1975. Malignant hyperthermia, J. Oral Surg. **33**:57.

Sparling, P. F. 1971. Diagnosis and treatment of syphilis, N. Engl. J. Med. **284**:642.

Tomasi, T. B. 1972. Secretory immunoglobulins, N. Engl. J. Med. **287**:500.

Wallach, J. 1974. Interpretation of diagnostic test, ed. 2, Boston, Little, Brown & Co.

Wells, B. B. 1967. Clinical pathology, ed. 4, Philadelphia, W. B. Saunders Co.

CHAPTER 15

Radionuclide diagnosis

Gary F. Gates

Nuclear medicine and diagnostic radiology both utilize ionizing radiation to obtain clinical information, but beyond that point the similarity of the two clinical specialties diminishes. Information resulting from a nuclear medicine examination is related to organ function, without which a specific radiopharmaceutical will not localize within a target organ. Diagnostic radiologic examinations, on the other hand, depend on the physical attenuating effects that anatomic structures have on a transmitted x-ray beam; the "shadows" cast upon photographic film by the transmitted beam do not necessarily indicate the functional status of the organ being studied. Thus nuclear medicine examinations reflect organ function, whereas diagnostic radiographic studies usually indicate anatomic relationships or abnormalities. Obviously some overlap exists such as intravenous urography (where kidney function is necessary for the concentration of an administered iodinated contrast agent and thus the desired radiographic image) or liver scanning (where the anatomic location and size of a liver tumor may be evident by radionuclide studies).

The information resulting from a nuclear medicine examination is unique and may not be obtained easily, if at all, by other means. The radiation exposure to the patient is usually very low and in certain instances is far less than the radiation received from a comparable radiographic examination (for example, radionuclide cystography versus x-ray cystography). Radiobiologic effects are apparent only with therapeutic doses of radionuclides.

The purpose of this chapter is to discuss those aspects of nuclear medicine that are pertinent to the main theme of this text: oral and maxillofacial surgery. A few basic remarks regarding the nature of radionuclides, radiopharmaceuticals, and instrumentation are necessary, but it is beyond the scope of this chapter to enter into a detailed discussion of these topics. Virtually all standard nuclear medicine textbooks devote large sections to these basic topics, and the reader is referred to such works if further information is desired (Blahd, 1971; Early, Razzack, and Sodee, 1979; Freeman and Blaufox, 1973a, 1973b, 1974, 1977; Freeman and Johnson, 1975; Gottschalk and Potchen, 1976; Rollo, 1977; Wagner, 1968, 1975).

BASIC PRINCIPLES
Radionuclides

All nonionized atoms consist of a nucleus surrounded by orbiting electrons (each of the latter having a -1 charge). The nucleus contains protons (with a $+1$ charge), neutrons (with a net zero charge), and various other subatomic particles and/or energy quanta not germane to this discussion. The nuclear particles are called nucleons while the entire nucleus containing all its nucleons is called a nuclide. The number of electrons in orbit around a nucleus equals the number of its protons in a nonionized atom, thereby maintaining electrical neutrality. The number and arrangement of orbiting electrons determine the chemical properties of an atom. The number of protons within a nucleus is represented by the atomic number, Z, which is written as a subscript preceding the chemical symbol of the element, while the atomic mass number, A, (that is, sum of the number of protons and neutrons) is indicated as a preceding superscript (for example, $^{131}_{53}I$).

Elements are defined on the basis of chemical properties, as determined by the orbiting electrons, but it is possible for an element to have varying numbers of neutrons within its nucleus. Nuclides having the same Z number but a different A number (because of variations in neutron content) are called isotopes. However, all isotopes of an element have identical chemical properties because the number and arrangement of orbital electrons is the same. Since all isotopic forms of a given element have the same Z number, indication of this numeric designation, in combination with the chemical symbol, is redundant and is usually deleted (for example ^{131}I).

A radionuclide is a radioactive form of an isotope that behaves chemically in a similar manner to its nonradioactive counterpart(s). However, the nuclear binding energy of a radioactive element is insufficient to hold the nucleus together, and consequently it disintegrates, releasing particles (for example, alpha or beta particles) of varying energy levels and/or electromagnetic radiation such as gamma rays. Detection of electromagnetic radiation emitting from a patient following administration of a radiopharmaceutical forms the basis for most diagnostic nuclear medicine imaging tests (for example, lung scans). Particulate radiations are utilized for internal therapy (for example, thyroid disease).

Radioactive decay is the process whereby the number of radioactive atoms of an element within a population is reduced through disintegration. The decay rate of a radioisotope population is constant and cannot be altered by physical or chemical means. The radioactive physical half-life ($T_{p\,1/2}$) is used to express this decay process and is defined as the time required for one half of the original num-

ber of atoms in a radioactive sample to decay. Most of the radionuclides used in nuclear medicine have a physical half-life ranging from seconds to a few days. In biologic systems, however, one must also consider the biologic half-life ($T_{b\,1/2}$), which is the time required for the body to eliminate one half of an administered radionuclide by a process of regular elimination. Obviously any radionuclide that is retained in the body for only a short period of time will have a relatively small radiobiologic effect regardless of the time parameter of its physical half-life. Consequently both physical and biologic half-lives must be taken into consideration when determining the radiobiologic effect of an administered radionuclide. The effective half-life ($T_{e\,1/2}$) is the result of such a dual half-life consideration and is defined as the time required for the radioactivity from an administered radionuclide to be reduced to 50% of its initial value as a result of the combined effects of the physical and biologic half-lives. The relationship of these three half-lives can be expressed as:

$$T_{e\,1/2} = \frac{(T_{p\,1/2})\,(T_{b\,1/2})}{(T_{p\,1/2}) + (T_{b\,1/2})}$$

Under no circumstances can the effective half-life exceed the physical half-life and in most circumstances it is less because of the biologic half-life. In dose estimate calculations the mean effective life ($\overline{T}_e$) is used in determining the absorbed radiation resulting from the total decay of a radionuclide:

$$\overline{T}_e = 1.44\ T_{e\,1/2}$$

As an example of the values derived when such determinations are made, the following results are presented using ^{131}I uptake within the thyroid of a presumably normal person (Early, 1979):

$$T_{p\,1/2} = 8\ \text{days}°$$
$$T_{b\,1/2} = 24\ \text{days}°$$
$$T_{e\,1/2} = 6\ \text{days}°$$
$$\overline{T}_e = 8.6\ \text{days}°$$

The decay rate of a radionuclide can

° Approximate values.

also be expressed as the number of nuclear disintegrations occurring per unit time. The curie, Ci, (named in honor of Marie Curie) is a standard unit of measurement of radioactive decay; one curie equals 3.7×10^{10} disintegrations per second (dps). The millicurie (mCi), which equals 3.7×10^7 dps, and the microcurie (μCi), which equals 3.7×10^4 dps, are the units most commonly used in nuclear medicine when calculating the activity of a radionuclide that will be administered to a patient. However, the curie is related to the number of nuclear disintegrations per second and not the energy or characteristics of the emitted radiation. The energy levels of particulate or electromagnetic radiation are expressed in thousands of electron volts (keV) or millions of electron volts (meV).

The radiation a patient receives from any procedure using ionizing radiation (that is, nuclear medicine, diagnostic radiology, or radiation therapy) is measured in terms of "rads." The rad (*radiation absorbed dose*) is the unit used to quantitate the energy deposited in tissues following radiation exposure. The rad is defined as the deposition of 100 ergs in 1 gm of matter. Calculations of absorbed dose can be quite complicated but the following are a few comparison values for various situations in order that one might have some perspective of absorbed doses.

1. Radiation therapy: up to 7000 rads in a few weeks to variably sized tissue volumes
2. Permissible dose for radiation workers: 5 rads of whole body radiation per year
3. ^{99m}Tc-labeled phosphate bone scan: 0.01 to 0.04 rads whole body radiation (O'Mara and Charkes, 1975; Webster, Alpert, and Brownell, 1974)
4. Lumbar spine radiographs (15-year-old): 0.15 rads whole body radiation (Webster, Alpert, and Brownell, 1974)

A decay scheme is a means of representing the important characteristics of a radionuclide's existence: its physical half-life, method of decay (indicating the energy levels released), and ultimate fate. For the sake of illustration, the simple decay scheme of ^{32}P will be shown:

$$^{32}_{15}\text{P} \; (\text{T}_{\text{p} \, 1/2} = 14.28\text{d})$$
$$\searrow \bar{\beta} \, 1.7 \, \text{meV} \, (100\%)$$
$$^{32}_{15}\text{S} \; (\text{stable})$$

This is a shorthand method of saying that ^{32}P has a physical half-life of 14.28 days and decays directly to stable (that is, nonradioactive) ^{32}S by releasing a 1.7 meV β- particle (electron). This is a simple example of beta decay. Other decay systems exist and many (including beta decay) are quite complex, yielding a variety of subatomic particles of multiple energy levels, plus electromagnetic radiation of varying energies, plus unstable (that is, radioactive) elements that in turn disintegrate.

Radiopharmaceuticals

Radiopharmaceuticals differ from other medically employed drugs since they generally elicit no pharmacologic response (owing to the minute quantities administered), and they contain a radionuclide. Some radionuclides may be administered in an elemental form (for example, ^{123}I for thyroid scanning), but in many cases the radionuclide is only part of a larger complex radiopharmaceutical. In many instances the radioactive element acts only as a "tag" to facilitate detection of the complex molecular structure to which it has been attached. Often the biologic and chemical behavior of the unlabeled material determines its use in a procedure, and the radionuclide "tag" may play no role in selective organ localization. Liver scanning is an example of this situation. Injected colloidal material (such as colloidal carbon, ^{198}Au colloid, ^{131}I or ^{99m}Tc-microaggregated albumin, ^{99m}Tc-sulfur colloid, and ^{113m}In-labeled colloids) are all phagocytized by the liver, producing a "liver scan"; the radionuclide "tag" merely allows external detection and does not have any special affinity for the liver. In other circumstances preferential uptake of an ionic form of a radionuclide will occur within specific organs, thereby forming the basis of a diagnostic procedure (for example, ^{123}I, ^{131}I, or ^{99m}Tc within the thyroid or ^{99m}Tc within the salivary glands or gastric mucosa). The following is a general outline of the methods of localization of certain radiopharmaceuticals commonly used in clinical organ imaging procedures (not all agents are included and some cannot be easily subcategorized) (Modified from Freeman and Blaufax, 1977).

A. Active transport
   1. Thyroid scans (^{131}I, ^{123}I, ^{99m}Tc pertechnetate)
   2. Renal scans (^{131}I-orthoiodohippurate)
   3. Hepatocellular liver scans (^{131}I-rose bengal)
   4. Pancreatic scans (^{75}Se-selenomethionine)
   5. Salivary gland scans (^{99m}Tc pertechnetate)
   6. Gastric mucosal scans (^{99m}Tc pertechnetate)
   7. Myocardial perfusion scans (^{201}Tl)
B. Colloid phagocytosis
   1. Reticuloendothelial liver, spleen, and bone marrow scans (^{99m}Tc or ^{111}In-labeled colloids)
C. Cell sequestration
   1. Spleen (heat-damaged ^{51}Cr or ^{99m}Tc-labeled red blood cells)

D. Capillary blockage
   1. Perfusion lung scans (^{99m}Tc or ^{111}In-labeled macroparticles)
E. Simple or exchange diffusion
   1. Bone scans (excluding phosphate-labeled agents)
   2. Brain scans (^{99m}Tc pertechnetate, ^{99m}Tc DTPA)
   3. Ventilation lung scans with radioactive gases ([81m]Kr, ^{133}Xe)
F. Physiochemical adsorption
   1. Bone scans (^{99m}Tc phosphates)
   2. Thrombus scans (^{131}I, ^{123}I-labeled fibrinogen)
   3. ? Gallium tumor/abscess scans (^{67}Ga citrate)
G. Compartmental localization
   1. Cardiovascular blood pool (^{131}I, ^{99m}Tc albumin, ^{99m}Tc-labeled RBC's, ^{111}In transferrin)

Technetium (Tc) 99m ("m" referring to "metastable," indicating that ^{99m}Tc decays by isomeric transition into ^{99}Tc) is the radionuclide currently used most frequently in clinical practice. This radionuclide emits a 140 keV gamma ray that is highly suitable for external detection by scintillation cameras and has no particulate emission (which in the case of an organ imaging test contributes no useful diagnostic information but may significantly increase the patient's absorbed

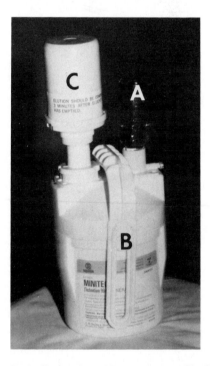

Fig. 15-1. Technetium 99m generator (Squibb). Sterile saline (supplied in bottle, *A*) is used to elute ^{99m}Tc from [99]Mo, which is enclosed in lead shielded case, *B*. The ^{99m}Tc is collected in glass vacuum bottle enclosed in lead case, *C*.

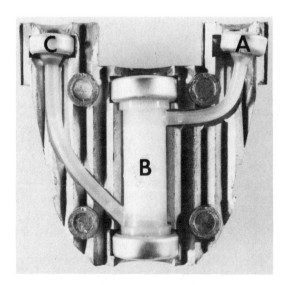

Fig. 15-2. Technetium 99m generator (Squibb). Alumina column, which contains [99]Mo, *B*, is shown with saline input, *A*, and vacuum output, *C*.

radiation dose). Technetium 99m has a 6-hour physical half-life and is obtained from a molybdenum (Mo) 99-technetium 99m "generator" (Figs. 15-1 and 15-2). This generator is a small lead-encased container that harbors a sterile alumina column onto which is fixed the parent radionuclide, ^{99}Mo. The daughter radionuclide, ^{99m}Tc, is separated from the parent by eluding the column with sterile saline. The exudate contains only ^{99m}Tc, since the ^{99}Mo is firmly attached to the powdered aluminum in the column. These generators are usually delivered on a weekly basis to a nuclear medicine department and can be eluded one or more times a day. Other similar generators are available such as the tin (Sn) 133–indium (In) 113m system.

^{99m}Tc can be administered intravenously as sodium pertechnetate (as for salivary gland, brain, thyroid, or gastric mucosal scanning) or following chemical combination with complex molecules (as with sulfur colloid for liver-spleen or bone marrow scanning, chelating agents for renal or brain scanning, albumin macroparticles for perfusion lung scanning, or phosphate complexes for bone scanning). Commercially available "kits" allow for easy preparation of these complex ^{99m}Tc-labeled radiopharmaceuticals within any nuclear medicine department. Other more specialized radionuclides or radiopharmaceuticals, such as thallium 201, xenon 133 (gas), ^{131}I-orthoiodohippurate, ^{131}I-rose bengal, gallium 67, ^{131}I, or ^{123}I, are usually ordered directly from a commercial manufacturer; these substances either require a reactor or cyclotron for production or need special compounding that is not practical for a hospital laboratory.

In general two types of images are produced in tests of organ visualization. The first and most desirable type occurs when an administered radiopharmaceutical selectively localizes in an abnormal region to a greater degree than it does in surrounding normal structures (that is, brain, bone, and gallium scanning). These tests produce a high "target-to-background" ratio, which contributes greatly to their accuracy. The second pattern of image presentation is the opposite of the first: the radionuclide accumulates in normal tissues to a greater degree than it does in abnormal areas (which may have decreased or absent uptake). Examples of this second type include liver, lung, and many thyroid scans. Small abnormal regions devoid of radionuclide may be "hidden" by surrounding adjacent normal areas, which have avidly accumulated radioactive material.

Instrumentation

Although a large variety of radiation detection instruments are available, this section will be limited to discussion of scintillation counters since they are the most widely used systems in clinical practice. In its simplest form the scintillation counter consists of a radiation detector containing a thallium-activated sodium iodide crystal that has been optically coupled to a photomultiplier tube. The hygroscopic crystal is enclosed in a lightproof, hermetically sealed, internal light-reflecting aluminum container (except where it is optically coupled to the photomultiplier tube). A lead-shielded case that is open at one end is placed over the detector assembly. Photons of electromagnetic radiation (usually gamma rays) penetrate the lightproof container in the region where the lead case has its opening and interact with the sodium iodide crystal producing blue-violet flashes of light (scintillations). Since the crystal is transparent to light, these scintillations reach the sensitive surface of the photomultiplier tube (photocathode) resulting in a release of a pulse of electrons (photoemission). This electron pulse is then amplified in a steplike fashion through a series of dynodes (usually 10) within the photomultiplier tube. Each dynode releases more electrons (secondary emission) than the number incident upon it so that at the end of this amplification sequence a single flash of light (scintillation) falling upon the photocathode may ultimately result in a burst of millions of electrons (voltage pulse). It is obvious why the photomultiplier tube has earned its name.

A system of proportionality exists

throughout the crystal-photomultiplier assembly:

1. The height of the final voltage pulse produced by the photomultiplier tube is ultimately proportional to the number of electrons released at the photocathode.

2. The number of electrons released by the photocathode is directly proportional to the intensity of incident light received from the crystal.

3. The intensity of scintillations within the crystal is directly proportional to the energy of the incident gamma ray.

4. Therefore the final voltage pulse height produced by the photomultiplier tube is directly proportional to the energy of the incident gamma ray.

The hole in the lead case surrounding the crystal (through which the gamma rays enter) usually contains or is covered by a lead collimator, which is an integral part of most detector systems. A collimator is a device for confining the dimensions of an incoming beam within a specified solid angle. These precision-matched lead appliances come in a variety of shapes and configurations depending on the function they are to serve. They are not lenses as in a photographic system but according to their size and shape can either restrict or enlarge fields of view (from which gamma radiation will interact with the crystal) and/or absorb and remove undesirable scattered radiation from the patient before it reaches the crystal. More will be said about collimators when discussing scintillation cameras.

The detector system so far discussed consists of a collimator, sodium iodine crystal, and photomultiplier tube. The last component is a "preamplifier," which matches the impedances between the photomultiplier tube and amplifier and provides a driving force so that the pulse characteristics will not be lost in the several feet of cable connecting the detector to the adjacent processing and display unit.

On entering the processing and display unit, the signal from the detector is directed to a linear amplifier. All the pulses are increased by a constant factor so that the final pulse remains proportional to the energy deposited in the crystal by the incident gamma ray. Thereafter the pulse is routed to a pulse height analyzer, which can be preset to select voltage pulses of a certain height and reject all others for further processing. This instrument, often in the form of a gamma spectrometer, can sort the spectrum of gamma energies and "count" or further process only those voltage peaks that correspond to the photon energy levels emitted by the administered radionuclide. The selected voltage pulses are then sent forward for display in a variety of ways such as:

1. Counts on a scaler (an electronic circuit that counts signal pulses from a radiation detector)

2. Needle deflection on a rate meter (which may be plotted on a strip chart recorder using either analogue or digital methods)

3. Organ image representation on either an oscilloscope or photographic film, or as dots on special types of paper

4. Computer processing for further extraction of information

Of the four general types of scintillation detection systems available, only two, the rectilinear scanner and scintillation camera, produce images of radionuclide distribution within an organ. The *stationary probe* (Fig. 15-3) is used mainly for tests of concentration of radionuclide within an organ (for example, thyroid uptake of radioiodine) or dynamic function studies (for example, older renograms). These probes yield numeric information as shown either on a scaler (as counts per present time or time required to obtain a predetermined number of counts) or as a tracing on a strip chart recorder. *Well counters* (Fig. 15-3) operate on the same basic principle but are designed for counting samples of body fluids or tissue specimens. They are now available as large automated instruments that can count hundreds of samples without interruption.

The *rectilinear scanner* (Fig. 15-4) was the first nuclear medicine organ imaging device. Although introduced over 20 years ago by Cassen, these instruments

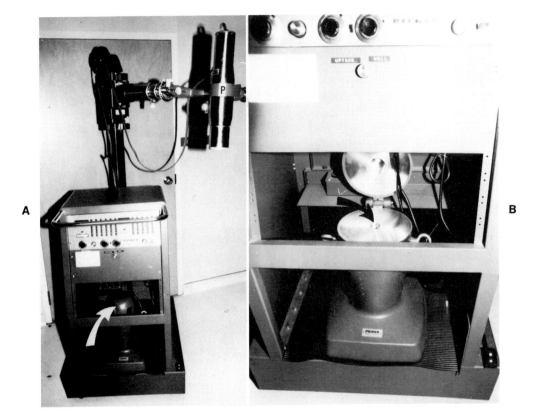

Fig. 15-3. Single probe scintillation counter (Picker). **A,** Scintillation probe, *P,* used for quantitating localized in vivo radionuclide activity such as during thyroid uptake determination. Arrow points to well counter used for in vitro assays. **B,** Top of lead encased well counter is open exposing central cavity ("well" shown by arrow into which glass tubes containing samples are placed). Both well and probe counters yield only numeric results relating to count rates, which are displayed in vertical rows on illuminated panel seen in **A.**

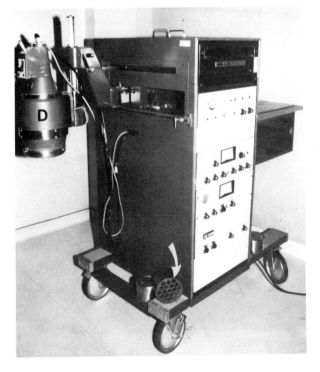

Fig. 15-4. Rectilinear scanner (Picker). Detector, *D,* moves back and forth over patient and detects emitted radiation, which is plotted on either x-ray film or paper. Arrow points to collimator, which is inserted into detector assembly; various collimators are used depending on energy of emitted gamma rays.

are still widely used in clinical practice. The rectilinear scanner produces a two-dimensional image of the distribution of radionuclide within an organ. This image is progressively built up by the systematic movement of the scintillation detection assembly back and forth across the region of interest, while it also moves in a cranial-to-caudad (or vice versa) direction. Since the detector "scans" the body by its simultaneous to-and-fro and top-to-bottom motions, the resultant image is called a "scan." However, the detector "sees" only a small region at any given moment, and the total picture is constructed slowly line by line until complete. The sodium iodine crystal is either 3 or 5 inches in diameter and 2 inches thick. Generally a focusing collimator is used, which permits only a restricted area to be optimally imaged at a given time. These lead collimators have holes arranged in a honeycomb fashion with the outer holes progressively angled inward (when viewed from the top) so that imaginary linear extensions of their individual central axes would converge at a predetermined point some distance from the face of the collimator. Newer rectilinear scanners have dual detection assemblies that face each other; this system allows for simultaneous scanning of both the front and back of a patient, thereby reducing the time necessary to complete a multiview study. Furthermore, when the total body is scanned (as with a bone scan) the image may be electronically minified so that the entire body is displayed on a single sheet of x-ray–like transparent film.

Rectilinear scanners have some limitations, two of which will be briefly discussed. First, they are generally slow in performing studies, which poses a practical problem for patients who are unable to lie still for extended periods of time (that is, children or critically ill patients). A second limitation is their inability to perform "dynamic" or "perfusion" studies; these examinations follow the course of a radionuclide during the initial few seconds following injection while it is in the blood vessels and before it has either localized in its target organ (for example, liver) or reached total-body

vascular equilibrium (for example, diolabeled albumin). These "dynam. studies are called nuclear angiogram (that is, nuclear angiocardiograms, nuclear cerebral angiograms, and so on) and are absolutely crucial in establishing some diagnoses. The rectilinear scanner, however, only records a "static" or equilibrium image and cannot follow the rapid vascular course of radionuclides during the first few seconds following their intravenous injection.

The *scintillation camera*, or *gamma camera*, (Fig. 15-5) was first introduced over 10 years ago by Anger and has undergone continual modification and de-

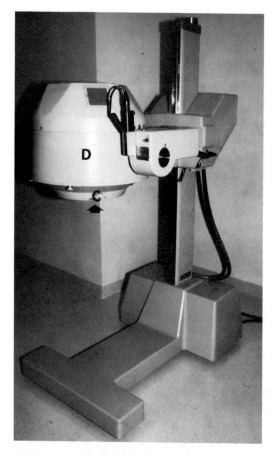

Fig. 15-5. Scintillation camera (Searle). Collimator, *C*, is bolted in front of detector, *D*. Unlike rectilinear scanners that contain only single photomultiplier tube, this camera has 37 photomultiplier tubes arranged in hexagonal array over crystal contained i detector assembly.

velopment since. Without a doubt it is the most versatile piece of organ imaging equipment in any nuclear medicine department. The camera is a stationary imaging device that produces a "picture" of an organ without movement of the detector (therefore the analogy to a photographic "camera" taking a "snapshot"). The camera has a much larger field of view than a rectilinear scanner and may image some organs in their entirety. Cameras can also process very high count rates (up to 100,000 counts per second in newer systems), thus producing rapid sequence images during the "dynamic phase" of an examination. The detector can be positioned in many angles to obtain special views (oblique and so forth) of an organ. Since the camera does not move or perform a scanning motion

(except in case of some specialized tomographic scanners that are beyond the scope of this discussion), the resultant image is not a "scan" but is called a "scintigram" or "scintiphoto."

The scintillation camera achieves its versatility by being constructed in a different manner than the rectilinear scanner. Its detector system is based on a large, thin (11 or 15 inches in diameter, ½ inch thick) thallium-activated sodium iodide crystal, which is optically coupled to multiple (19, 37, or even 61) photomultiplier tubes, which are arranged in a hexagonal configuration over the crystal. A scintillation occurring within the crystal is "viewed" by several photomultiplier tubes at the same time. The photomultiplier tubes are connected to the processing and display unit (Fig. 15-6),

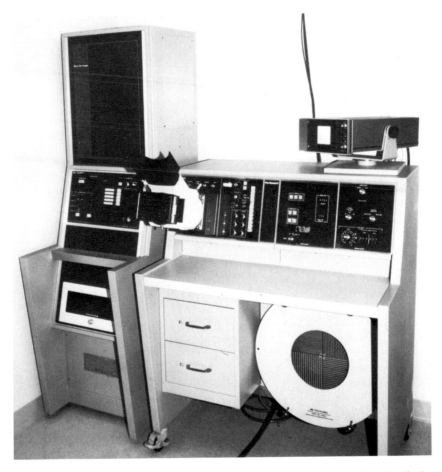

Fig. 15-6. Camera's control panel (short console) is placed next to multi-image – forming display unit (taller console), which produces multiple images on transparent, x-ray – like film.

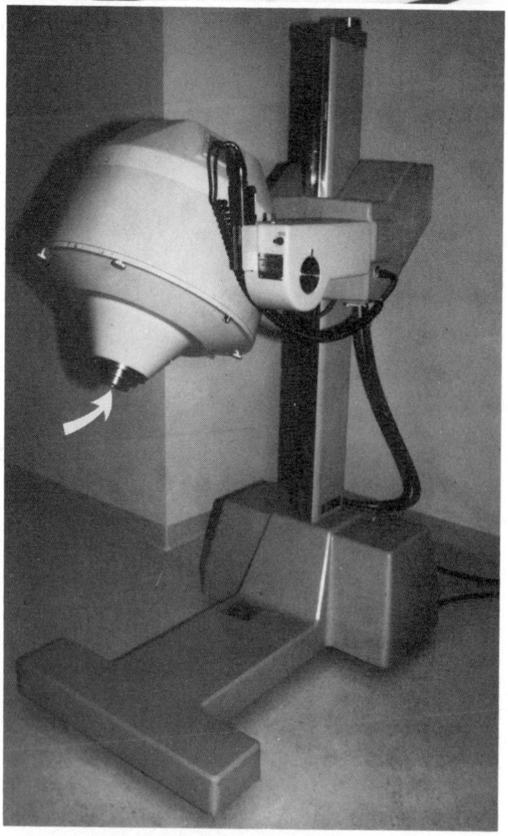

Fig. 15-7. Camera collimators. **A,** Multiple, thick-walled septa of medium energy, parallel-hole collimator viewed from top (arrow). **B,** Pinhole collimator in place. Apex of cone (arrow) is placed close to patient, resulting in magnification of part being examined.

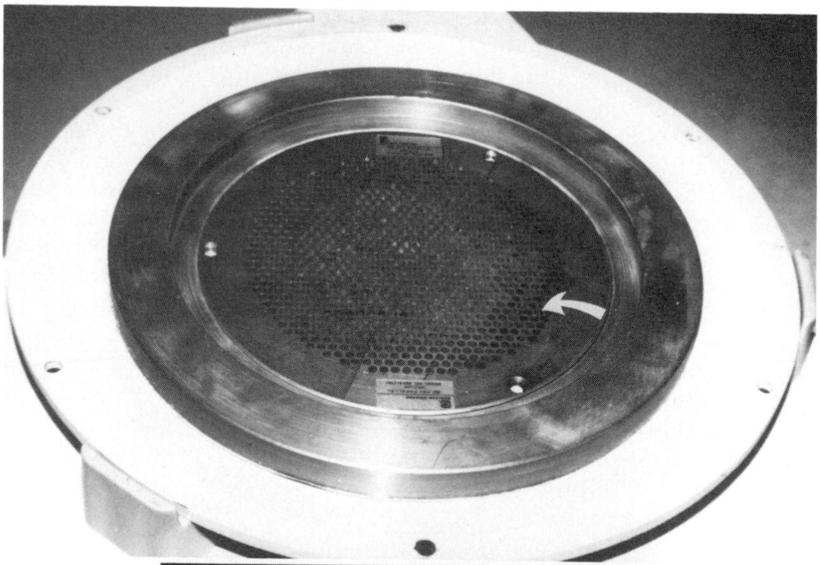

which identifies the position and brightness of each scintillation and then plots them on an oscilloscope in the same X-Y coordinates as they occurred in the crystal. The oscilloscope may be directly photographed, or the information may be sent to a digital computer for further image processing (and generation of time-activity curves in the case of dynamic studies).

Scintillation cameras have one limitation, however; their ½-inch thick crystal does not allow for optimal imaging using high-energy photons (such as the 511 keV emission from fluorine 18). High-energy gamma rays will penetrate the crystal without transferring all their energies into scintillations. In such circumstances the 2-inch thick crystal of the rectilinear scanner is needed to assure optimal imaging. The ½-inch thick camera crystal is very well suited, however, to lower and medium energy photons such as ^{99m}Tc, ^{123}I, ^{67}Ga, and so on.

A variety of special interchangeable collimators are available for cameras. With the exception of the pinhole collimator (a large cone, which has a single, small opening at the apex, fitted over the crystal surface), most collimators are heavy lead attachments containing multiple, precisely located holes (Fig. 15-7). Each collimator is designed for use with radionuclides of a specific energy range (as reflected in the thickness of the lead septa separating the various holes). When the collimator holes are all parallel with each other, the crystal will "see" an area equal to its diameter. If the holes diverge away from the center, a larger solid angle will be subtended and the crystal will "see" an area larger than its intrinsic diameter. Collimators in which the holes converge toward the central axis subtend a smaller solid angle; in this situation the entire crystal surface will "see" an area that in actuality has a smaller diameter than the crystal. Thus diverging collimators open up a larger area of view to the crystal but in doing so the object being imaged appears smaller than if a parallel-hole collimator were used. On the other hand, a converging collimator will result in a narrow field of view for the crystal but the object appears enlarged. A pinhole collimator produces a tremendous increase in size and resolution of objects that are much smaller than the crystal's diameter (for example, the thyroid gland).

The resolution of camera systems is generally better than that associated with rectilinear scanners. With new cameras it is possible to resolve line pairs ¹⁄₁₀ of an inch apart under experimental conditions, although the resolution in clinical situations is less because of surrounding radioactivity in the patient and a lesion's distance from the collimator surface (image resolution in a camera system decreases the further an object of interest is removed from the collimator). Generally speaking, an abnormality must be 1 to 2 cm in size before it can be imaged by standard nuclear medicine techniques.

Further engineering advances have produced a "moving table" (Fig. 15-8), which slowly but continually moves the entire patient before the camera to produce a single "total body" image (as during a bone scan). This image can be electronically minified to allow its presentation on a single sheet of transparent film. Advances in pulse height analyzers now allow simultaneous analysis of pulses derived from two different radionuclides administered at once or simultaneous analysis and utilization of multiple photo peaks from a single radionuclide (for example, ^{67}gallium).

CLINICAL PRACTICE

The clinical practice of nuclear medicine covers an enormous spectrum of examinations, all of which share one common feature—the use of a radionuclide. Nuclear medicine departments can perform various organ-imaging examinations (for example, bone scans), in vivo tracer studies (for example, thyroid uptake determinations), plus in vitro determinations (for example, radioimmunoassays). The purpose of this section is to describe those nuclear medicine studies that would be of most assistance to dental or medical practitioners who are treating patients with maxillofacial or oromandibular abnormalities. Most emphasis will

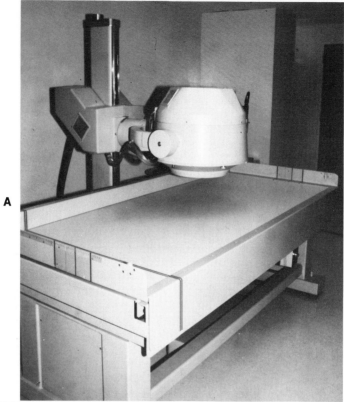

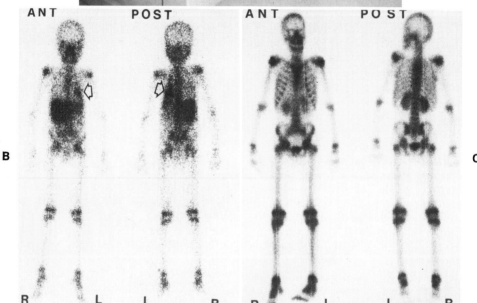

Fig. 15-8. Moving table. **A,** Large table beneath camera moves back and forth before detector. Electrical-mechanical synchronization results in "total-body image" as shown in **B** and **C. B,** Gallium 67 scan on child. Although some osseous uptake of gallium occurs, liver uptake is prominent and normal. Arrow points to site of radiation pneumonitis in which radionuclide accumulation occurred (normally gallium does not localize in lung tissue). **C,** Bone scan (^{99m}Tc pyrophosphate) on adolescent male. Convention dictates viewing any scan in same orientation as patient would be seen in life. Thus anterior scan has patient's right on viewer's left, while posterior scans are the reverse. Distribution of radionuclide in body is detected by image system and shown as "dots" on film (either black dots on transparent film or white dots on black background as with Polaroid film). Notice patient's skeleton with accentuated uptake at ends of long bones, which are sites of active growth. Kidneys and bladder are also seen on bone scans.

be placed on the detection of abnormalities in these anatomic regions, but for the sake of completeness, some attention must be devoted to those problems that may face any surgical patient. None of the following procedures needs any special equipment or radiopharmaceuticals other than those found in any modern community hospital. The greatest requirement is the close consultation between the nuclear medicine physician and his dental and medical colleagues.

Bone imaging

General background and radiopharmaceuticals

Of all the nuclear medicine tests available, bone imaging offers the greatest potential for evaluating the maxillofacial or oromandibular regions. Bone scanning developed because of the need to improve the accuracy of diagnostic radiographs in detecting skeletal abnormalities. The extent to which a destructive lesion must proceed before radiographic detection is possible was demonstrated by Borak (1942) and Wagner, Hunt, and Pendergrass (1945); these separate investigators drilled holes in isolated vertebrae and showed that cylindric defects up to 1 cm in diameter could exist in the spongiosa without apparent radiographic changes. Others confirmed that destructive vertebral lesions less than 1½ cm in diameter would probably not be identified by radiography (Ardran, 1951; Bachman and Sproul, 1955). According to the investigations of Borak and Ardran, 30% to 50% of vertebral depth must be lost before a corresponding radiolucency could be detected. These experimentally produced lesions, however, were cylindric; Edelstyn, Gillespie, and Grebbell (1967) showed that spheric lesions must destroy 50% to 75% of vertebral spongiosa to be visualized as radiolucencies. Overall it appears that up to 50% demineralization of bone must occur before consistent radiographic detection of density changes is possible on routine films.

Several radionuclides have been used as bone-seeking agents. These radiopharmaceuticals interact with hydroxy-apatite $(Ca_{10}[PO_4]_6[OH]_2)$ crystals in newly forming bone. Calcium 47 was first used by Bauer (1958) to study bone metabolism since it, like stable calcium, is incorporated in bone crystal. External detection disclosed increased amounts of ^{47}Ca in fracture sites and Paget's disease compared to normal bone. However, the high energy of its photon emission (1.31 meV) made bone scanning impractical. Strontium 85 was the first radionuclide to be widely used for clinical bone scanning. It appeared to be chemically similar to calcium and through cationic substitution (exchange) was incorporated into the hydroxyapatite crystal. Strontium 85 has some serious drawbacks, however: It has a long physical half-life[*] (64 days) resulting in a high-radiation exposure to the patient (whole body = 4.2 rads, bone = 36 rads). To minimize radiation exposure, low doses were injected (0.1 mCi in adults), which resulted in poor counting statistics and image degradation. Its 513 keV photon emission was too high for scintillation cameras. Lastly, the scanning procedure could not be started until 2 to 7 days following radionuclide administration and was commonly hampered by colonic and rectal accumulation, which often required repeated enemas.

Strontium 87m was substituted for ^{85}Sr, since it had a shorter physical half-life (2.8 hours), which resulted in a lower radiation exposure (whole body = 0.02 rads, bone = 0.08 rads) despite a higher administered dose (2 to 4 mCi in adults). Its 388 keV photon emission was still high for optimal utilization of a scintillation camera. A further drawback was the necessity for prompt imaging (owing to its short physical half-life) despite the slow blood clearance of the radionuclide; this resulted in a low target-to-background ratio. Strontium 87m was obtained from a relatively expensive ^{87}Y-^{87m}Sr generator.

The current interest in bone scanning is

---

[*]Data on various half-lives and absorbed doses from O'Mara, R. E., and Charkes, N. D. 1975. The osseous system. In Freeman, L. M., and Johnson, P. M., eds.: Clinical scintillation imaging, ed. 2, New York, Grune & Stratton, Inc., p. 537-599.

due in large part to the introduction of fluorine 18 (Blau, Bender, and Nagler, 1962). Unlike ^{85}Sr, ^{87m}Sr, or ^{47}Ca, fluorine 18 replaces the OH^- group in hydroxyapatite to form fluoroapatite crystals. This union is rapid and rather permanent. The ^{18}F is rapidly cleared from the blood by urinary excretion resulting in the highest target-to-background ratio of any bone-seeking radiopharmaceutical. Fluorine 18 has a very short physical half-life (1.87 hours) resulting in a low radiation dose (whole body = 0.04 rads, bone = 0.15 rads) despite a higher administered dose (1 to 10 mCi in adults). However, ^{18}F suffers two major drawbacks. The 110-minute physical half-life creates a logistic problem since a cyclotron is necessary for its production. Furthermore, the 511 keV photon emission does not allow for optimal gamma camera utilization.

Subramanian and McAfee in 1971 introduced ^{99m}Tc-tripolyphosphate for use in clinical bone scintigraphy. Since then many other complex phosphate molecules have been labeled with ^{99m}Tc and are widely available in kit form for clinical use. These agents probably react through the phosphorus groups by "sorption" onto the calcium of hydroxyapatite in bone, although they may also interact with certain large molecules such as fibrous or globular proteins (Jones, Francis, and Davis, 1976). Approximately 50% of the administered radiopharmaceutical is deposited in the osseous system within 3 hours of injection; the rest is rapidly excreted by the kidneys. The 140 keV photon emission of ^{99m}Tc is ideal for imaging by the scintillation camera. A physical half-life of 6 hours results in a low radiation exposure (whole body = 0.01 rads, bone = 0.045 rads) when using a 1 to 15 mCi dose in adults. Scanning is usually performed 2 to 4 hours following radionuclide administration. Thomas and coworkers (1978) have reported higher localized absorbed radiation doses to metaphyseal growth complexes in a series of children ranging in age from 4 to 16 years. The higher growth rates of those areas resulted in increased accumulation of ^{99m}Tc EHDP (Osteoscan); the dose to

the growth plate ranged from 0.8 to 4.7 rads when adjusted to an administered activity of 200 $\mu Ci/kg$. Adult radiation doses in comparable regions are lower since the growth activity is less than that of children (0.6 rads in adults according to Thomas, although variations may exist in dose estimates to the adult skeleton depending on the amount of radionuclide administered). Currently ^{99m}Tc-labeled phosphates are the preferred radiopharmaceuticals for bone scintigraphy. The adult radiation dose is small, although it is higher in localized growth centers in children. However, the benefits must be weighed against the risks (however small) for any diagnostic examination. Since virtually all bone scans are performed in patients with serious diseases, the small amount of absorbed radiation is clinically acceptable.

Bone is not a static organ system but is continually undergoing remolding and laying down of new hydroxyapatite crystals. Proliferating osteoblasts cause the hydroxyapatite crystals to be incorporated into a preformed osteoid matrix, which is the region where localization of bone-seeking radiopharmaceuticals occurs. Consequently, the entire skeleton will accumulate a bone-seeking radiopharmaceutical to various degrees. A bone scan, therefore, can depict regional versus generalized osteoblastic activity. A further influencing factor governing radionuclide accumulation is bone vascularity; poorly vascularized regions have less than expected radionuclide uptake despite the presence of osseous abnormalities that would otherwise result in increased accumulation (Siegel et al., 1976). Destructive bone lesions (for example, tumors, fractures, or infections) may appear to be osteolytic on radiograms, but in the vast majority of cases a reparative process consisting of new bone formation by osteoblasts is coexistent. This osteoblastic activity accounts for the increased accumulation of radionuclide in such areas. The neoplasm or infection in the bone does not accumulate the radioactive material. Occasionally some highly anaplastic, destructive tumors or indolent slow-growing lesions with minimal if any reactive bone formation may not have enough radionuclide accumulation to identify the region as being abnormal; this probably accounts for the 3% to 8% false-negative results obtained with bone scanning (O'Mara, 1974). Such highly destructive tumors include carcinomas of the breast, thyroid, and lung, reticulum cell sarcomas, and neuroblastomas (Charkes, Sklaroff, and Young, 1966; Gilday, Ash, and Reilly, 1977). It must be mentioned, however, that these tumors are more commonly associated with regional osteoblastic hyperactivity and focal areas of increased radionuclide accumulation. Bone scans of patients with widespread multiple myeloma may be falsely interpreted as normal since there is often diffuse osteoblastic hyperactivity throughout the skeleton without regional asymmetry.

Osteomyelitis may be identified by bone scanning as regions of increased radionuclide uptake, whereas radiographs may not become abnormal until several weeks following the clinical onset of symptoms (sometimes radiographs never become abnormal if the patient is started on antibiotic treatment). If a scintigram of the area in question is obtained immediately following radionuclide administration, a "blood pool" effect is present and localized hyperemia can be identified (Gilday, Paul, and Paterson, 1975). However, many tumors can also be associated with such hyperemia including Ewing's sarcoma and osteogenic sarcoma (Gilday, Paul, and Paterson, 1977). Similar hyperemia is not uncommonly seen with fractures. Handmaker and Leonards (1976) have reported that bone scans may become abnormal as early as the first 24 hours following the onset of symptoms. Recently, however, several investigators have reported cases of acute osteomyelitis in which there was diminished radionuclide uptake in the diseased bone (Handmaker and Leonards, 1976; Russin and Staab, 1976; Teates and Williamson, 1977). This is believed to result from localized bone ischemia secondary to the pressure of inflammatory debris compressing the nutrient arteries. In one case report a gallium scan was

abnormal 72 hours following a normal bone scan in a patient with osteomyelitis (Teates and Williamson, 1977), while in a similar patient repeat bone scans were abnormal at 1, 2, and 5 weeks following an initially normal study (Russin and Staab, 1976). The vast majority (over 90% to 95%) of patients with osteomyelitis will have an abnormal bone scan that is characterized by increased uptake of radionuclide in the abnormal region. Indications for performing bone scans in such patients, according to Handmaker and Leonards (1976), include:

1. Assessment of acute osteomyelitis and its response to therapy — scans should eventually return to normal
2. Osteomyelitis versus cellulitis — comparison of immediate postinjection scintigrams (vascular phase) with delayed ones (bone uptake phase) will show radionuclide uptake increasing with time in osteomyelitis and decreasing with cellulitis
3. Osteomyelitis versus synovitis or arthritis — more often than not, patients with early synovitis or pyogenic arthritis have normal bone scans during the early course of their diseases (although joint hyperemia may be evident on postinjection images)
4. Osteomyelitis versus infarction — acute bone infarctions will have reduced tracer uptake compared to the increased radionuclide concentration occurring in osteomyelitis. Eventually increased tracer uptake occurs with healing infarcts.
5. Osteomyelitis versus "periosseous disease" — chronic osteomyelitis, periostitis, "osteitis," sclerosing osteomyelitis of Garré, and sacroiliitis all produce abnormally increased radionuclide uptake

Abnormal bone scans should always be correlated with skeletal radiographs and the patient's history, since many benign bone disorders (for example, osteoid osteoma, melorheostosis, Paget's disease, arthritis, fractures, and osteomyelitis) may produce a "positive" bone scan (O'Mara, 1974). Furthermore, soft tissue accumulation of bone-seeking radiopharmaceuticals may occur in calcifying or necrotic lesions such as cerebral and myocardial infarctions, neuroblastomas, soft tissue tumoral calcifications of unknown origin, osteogenic sarcoma metastatic to the lung, diffuse pulmonary metastatic calcification caused by hypercalcemia or renal failure, calcified splenic infarctions associated with sickle cell anemia, myositis ossificans, and calcifying ovarian or hepatic tumors.

As shown by the experimental work cited at the beginning of this section, a great deal of bony destruction must have occurred before changes are detectable on routine radiographs. These destructive changes are measured in terms of grams of destroyed bone. However, a coexistent reparative process can be identified with incorporation of radionuclide in quantities as small as 10^{-13} gm (Fordham, 1976). The increased sensitivity of radionuclide bone imaging over skeletal radiography in detecting skeletal metastases is apparent in clinical practice where 10% to 40% of patients with skeletal metastases have normal skeletal radiographs at the time when a radionuclide bone scan is abnormal; conversely, less than 5% of bone scans are normal at a time when radiographs reveal localized skeletal abnormalities (DeNardo, Jacobson, and Raventos, 1972). The greater sensitivity of radionuclide bone imaging over skeletal radiography was confirmed by Pistenma, McDougall, and Kriss (1975); 28.5% of their 200 patients with biopsy-proven malignant diseases had false-negative skeletal radiographs, whereas only 1.5% of the bone scans were falsely negative. Despite their sensitivity, bone scans are nonspecific in their results. Many different types of abnormalities (for example, tumors, trauma, or infections) may result in an abnormal study. Therefore the patient's history, physical signs, and pertinent radiographs must be considered before rendering an interpretation of a bone scan. The following sections will illustrate the utility of skeletal scintigraphy in a variety of conditions affecting the maxillofacial area.

Maxillofacial scintigraphy

Basic principles. Bone scanning is a sensitive screening procedure for detecting metastatic neoplasia, especially when the primary tumor originated in the lungs, prostate, breast, head and neck, or lymphomatous tissues (DeNardo, Jacobson, and Raventos, 1972). It has also been advocated for detection of osteomyelitis and fractures, plus assessment of regional osteoblastic activity in a variety of benign conditions. Although much has been written about maxillofacial and skull radiography, there has been relatively limited experience in scintigraphic imaging of these areas. Bone scanning of the skull has been advocated for detection of metastases (Coleman et al., 1974; Jones et al., 1974), Paget's disease (Coleman et al., 1974; Miller et al., 1974; Preimesberger, Loken, and Shafer, 1974), primary hyperparathyroidism (Sy, 1974), and premature craniosynostosis (Gates and Dore, 1975). Several reports indicate the usefulness of maxillofacial bone scanning in the detection of many abnormalities, including adenocarcinoma of the lacrimal gland (Jones et al., 1974), meningiomas of the sphenoid ridge (McQuade and Higgins, 1974), osteomyelitis of the mandible (O'Mara and Charkes, 1975), ameloblastoma in the mandible (Olson and McCombs, 1977), dental disease (Arft, 1975; Garcia et al., 1977), craniofacial fibrous dysplasia (Fitzer, 1977), and invasion from adjacent neoplasms of the head, neck, and oropharynx (Mashberg et al., 1969; Vera et al., 1971). Alexander (1976) showed the utility of bone scanning in his series of benign and malignant mandibular abnormalities. Several investigators have reported that bone scanning of the maxillofacial region is a more sensitive means of detecting abnormalities than radiography (Alexander, 1976; Alexander, Alani, and Hansell, 1975; Gates and Goris, 1976).

Although abnormalities of the maxillofacial region are detectable by radionuclide bone imaging, anatomic localization may be imprecise or misleading unless multiple, properly positioned views are obtained. Radiographic positioning techniques can be modified or adapted to the scintigraphic examination, but resulting images may be initially difficult to interpret owing to the anatomic complexity of the facial structures that are being viewed in unfamiliar projections. Jones and Patton (1976) correlated the scintillation camera images of facial bones (using ^{99m}Tc-labeled phosphates) with radiographs of the same patient. Posteroanterior, lateral, Waters', and oblique views were used for both radiographic and scintigraphic studies. Brown and co-workers (1977) studied the anatomy of the facial bones of normal and abnormal patients using a single-photon emission tomographic system and ^{99m}Tc pyrophosphate. The tomographic effect was very useful in separating deep from superficial structures and in clearly defining regions of abnormality. Unfortunately, most institutions do not have such instruments.

Maxillofacial scintigraphic positioning techniques have been studied by obtaining transmission images using a dried skull placed in various projections and a ^{201}Tl (2 mCi) flood-field source (Gates and Goris, 1976). In this procedure ^{201}Tl is placed in a large, thin, disclike container and sealed to prevent the liquid radionuclide from leaking. This flat-field source is then placed beneath a scintillation camera and the dried skull interposed between the two. This results in an image-generating system analogous to diagnostic radiology. The gamma rays originate from a source behind the object being examined, penetrate the subject to varying degrees (depending on the attenuation encountered), and thereafter strike the crystal of the camera producing a "shadow" of the subject according to its attenuating characteristics. ^{201}Tl was chosen because its 69 to 80 keV emission was suitable for both photoelectric absorption by bone and detection by a scintillation camera. The skull was placed in various positions relative to the camera to simulate patient positions. Three anterior views (one straight view with the canthomeatal line perpendicular to the plane of the scintillation crystal, a second with the canthomeatal line shifted to form a 60 degree angle with the crystal surface, and a third similar to a Waters' projection with the canthomeatal line further shifted to 45 degrees), a 25-degree oblique orbital view

(similar to a Rhese projection) and a lateral scintigraphic view were obtained. ^{57}Co markers were placed at various anatomic landmarks on the skull so that precise interpretation of the transmission scintigrams was possible.

Fig. 15-9 shows the results of this positioning study; in addition to the dried skull with its transmission images, scintigrams of a patient in the same position are included for comparison on each panel. Fig. 15-10 shows how the patient was positioned for each of these views. The straight anterior view (Fig. 15-10, *A* corresponding to Fig. 15-9, *A*) was produced by placing the forehead and tip of the nose on the collimator. The angled anterior view (Fig. 15-10, *B* corresponding to Fig. 15-9, *B*) was achieved by placing the tip of the patient's nose and chin on the collimator. The Waters' view (Fig. 15-10, *C* corresponding to Fig. 15-9, *C*) was obtained by keeping the tip of the chin in contact with the collimator and tilting the head back so that the nose was a few centimeters off the collimator. The oblique orbital view (Fig. 15-10, *D* corresponding to Fig. 15-9, *D*) was obtained by positioning the plane of the orbital boundaries on the center of the collimator. The lateral view (Fig. 15-10, *E* corresponding to Fig. 15-9, *E*) was obtained in the usual manner. These views are easily reproduced, which allows for direct comparison of serial studies. Usually a high-resolution parallel-hole collimator is used, although a converging one may be substituted in small children. A pinhole collimator is occasionally used for "spot views" of localized regions.

Both transmission and clinical studies have shown the Waters'-like view shown in Figs. 15-9, *C* and 15-10, *C* to be the least valuable projection owing to facial foreshortening, which produces difficulties in separating small structures. The anterior view shown in Figs. 15-9, *B* and 15-10, *B* (canthomeatal line shifted to form a 60-degree angle with the crystal) was better than the straight anterior view (Figs. 15-9, *A* and 15-10, *A*) for evaluating the supraorbital and zygomatic areas. However, the straight anterior view was better for viewing the mandibular and

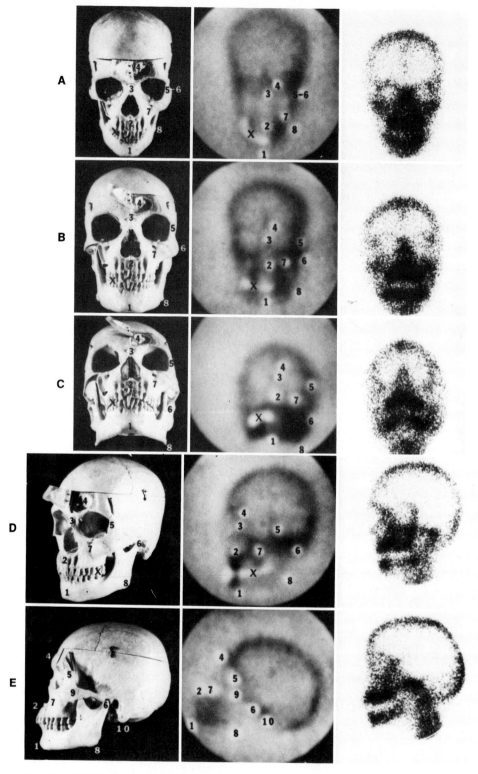

Fig. 15-9. 201 Thallium images of dried skull and similarly positioned patient studies using ⁹⁹ᵐTc polyphosphate. Anterior view with canthomeatal line perpendicular to camera, **A;** shifted to 60 degrees, **B;** and 45 degrees, **C;** 25 degree oblique orbital view, **D;** lateral view, **E.** ⁵⁷Co markers are placed on skull at mental protuberance, *1,* intermaxillary suture, *2,* internasal suture near nasion, *3,* frontal sinus, *4,* zygoma near zygomaticofrontal suture, *5,* mandibular condyle at temporomandibular joint, *6,* maxillary sinus, *7,* angle of mandible, *8,* zygomatic arch near zygotomaticotemporal suture, *9,* mastoid tip, *10,* and occlusal plane, *X.* (From Gates, G. F., and Goris, M. L. 1976. Radiology **121:**677.)

maxillary areas. The oblique orbital view (Figs. 15-9, *D* and 15-10, *D*) was more useful for mandibular and maxillary imaging than a lateral view (Figs. 15-9, *E* and 15-10, *E*), since superimposition of the two sides did not occur; it was also the best projection for orbital imaging. The lateral view proved useful in studying the body of the mandible, pterygopalatine fossa, and temporomandibular joint (TMJ) area while also displaying the maxilla and zygomaticofrontal regions.

Interpretation of any one view may be difficult if not misleading. Depending on patient positioning, anterior views may superimpose zygoma, mastoid, and TMJ areas; medial maxilla upon upper alveolar ridges; pterygopalatine fossa upon maxilla; and lesions in a single alveolar ridge upon each other. Oblique orbital and lateral views separate these areas but in turn superimpose other structures. A complete examination of the maxillofacial area often requires six views: both

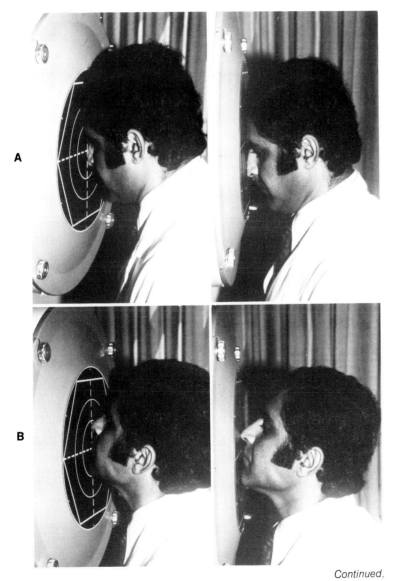

Continued.

Fig. 15-10. Patient-positioning techniques for maxillofacial scintigraphy. Patient views **A, B, C, D,** and **E** correspond to positioning used in obtaining Fig. 15-9 **A, B, C, D,** and **E,** respectively.

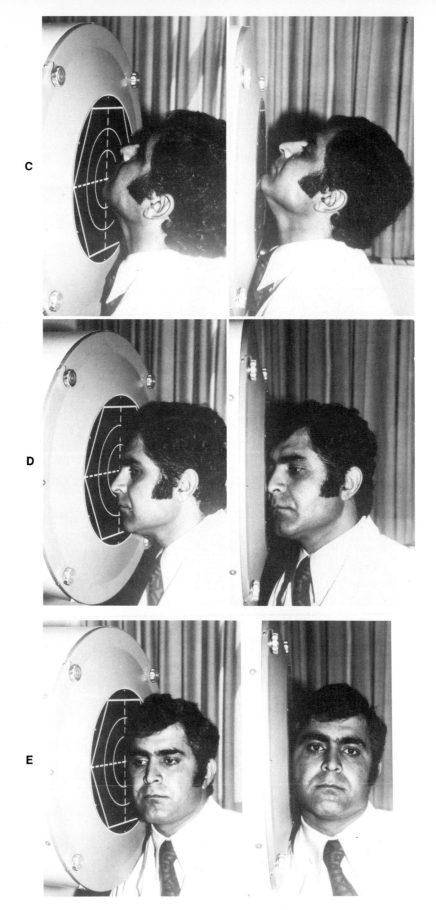

Fig. 15-10, cont'd. For legend see p. 481.

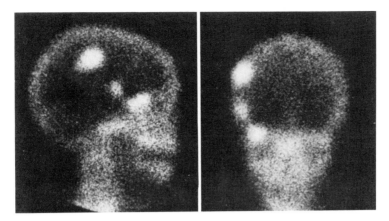

Fig. 15-11. Metastatic lesions of fibrous histiocytoma were imaged on ^{99m}Tc pyrophosphate scintigrams as regions of abnormal uptake in right calvarial and supraorbital areas (right lateral and anterior view shown).

oblique orbitals, both laterals, and two anterior images (preferably those shown in Figs. 15-9, *A;* 15-10, *A* and 15-9, *B;* 15-10, *B*). On occasion a Waters' view may be helpful. Some patients may not require all of these scintigraphic views for an abnormality to be confidently localized. However, multiple right angle and tangential views are often necessary to accurately localize a lesion because the close approximation of so many structures may produce an image that is too complex for interpretation based on single views alone. Furthermore, it is important to be aware of previous surgery or radiation therapy to the maxillofacial area since these treatment modalities may considerably alter the bone scintigraphic appearance. The 20 to 30 minutes necessary for obtaining multiple images will often yield valuable information and more than justify the additional effort. Careful patient positioning with multiple views allows for parallactic correlation of abnormalities and accurate anatomic localization, which is crucial if radiation therapy, biopsy, or corroborative radiographic studies are planned.

Tumor detection in general. Although the utility of bone scanning is not limited to the detection of malignancies, it would not be an exaggeration to say that at the present time most patients undergoing radionuclide imaging of the skeleton have, or are suspected of having, a neo-plastic disease. Accordingly it is fitting to introduce clinical bone scanning by illustrating its general use in tumor detection in the maxillofacial area. Specific anatomic regions will be discussed hereafter.

Most malignant neoplasms that spread to, or arise in, bone evoke an osteoblastic response, which accounts for the localization of bone-seeking radiopharmaceuticals in these areas. Fig. 15-11 illustrates the multiple sites of cranial spread of a fibrous histiocytoma; both calvarial and right supraorbital areas have focal regions of osteoblastic hyperactivity representing metastatic foci. Similar osteoblastic hyperactivity was seen in an adrenal carcinoma metastatic to the left maxilla and supraorbital area (Fig. 15-12) and an osteogenic sarcoma involving the central bony facial structures, especially the left maxilla (Fig. 15-13). Metastatic neuroblastomas may appear to be osteolytic on routine radiographs but usually have a significant osteoblastic component accounting for radionuclide localization; on occasion, however, a purely destructive lesion may not have an associated reparative component. The child in Fig. 15-14 had destructive bony lesions attributable to metastatic neuroblastoma involving the right maxilla and greater wing of the left sphenoid. These areas avidly accumulated radionuclide, but in the same patient metastases destroyed a portion of a vertebrae without producing an increase

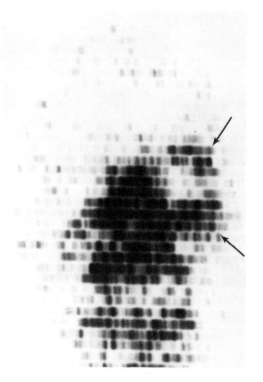

Fig. 15-12. Rectilinear scanner was used to perform bone scan on patient with metastatic adrenal carcinoma (arrows). Generally speaking, scanner images are not of same quality as gamma camera studies, although they are certainly diagnostic. Film recording system used here was opposite of Fig. 15-11, which explains black-white reversal.

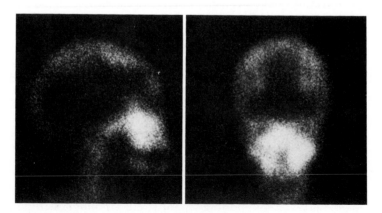

Fig. 15-13. Maxillary uptake in 23-year-old girl with metastatic osteogenic sarcoma. Central facial and possible skull accumulation is striking in its intensity.

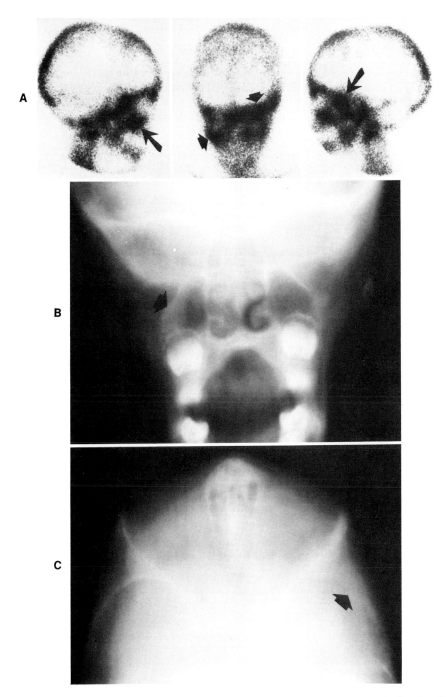

Fig. 15-14. Child with neuroblastoma metastatic to right maxilla and lesser wing of left sphenoid had both sites disclosed by bone scintigraphy. **A,** Arrows point to lesions. Anterior view shows both abnormalities. Lateral projections showed lesions to be of relatively greater intensity when affected side of skull was presented to scintillation camera, although abnormal radionuclide uptake in tumor region on opposite side could still be identified (that is, "shining through"). Facial tomograms showed thinning of lateral wall of right maxillary sinus with soft tissue density (tumor) within, **B,** frontal view, while basal view, **C,** showed erosion of lesser wing of left sphenoid.

in focal radionuclide accumulation. On the contrary, the involved bone had diminished radionuclide uptake, which indicated diminished reparative osteoblastic activity.

Skeletal scintigraphy is useful not only in detecting malignancy but also in planning therapy. The patient shown in Fig. 15-15 had carcinoma of the prostate metastatic to the facial area. If a straight anterior scan alone (top left) had been performed (as often might be the case in a "total body scan"), one would suspect that a single focus was present near the left zygoma. Multiple views disclosed two foci, however. The body of the zygomatic bone was involved in addition to the region of the zygomaticofrontal suture. As

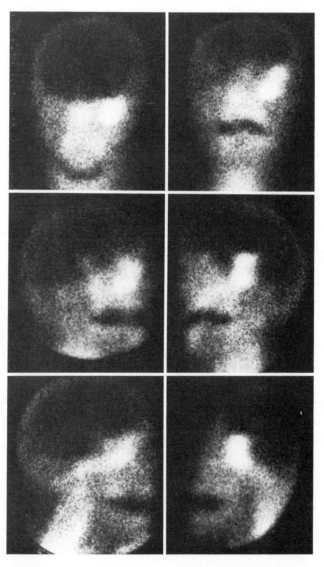

Fig. 15-15. Bone scintigrams of metastatic carcinoma of prostate shown in multiple views (straight and 60 degree angled views on top left and right, respectively; oblique orbital and lateral projections in middle and lower rows, respectively). Diagnosis of solitary metastasis would have probably been made if only straight anterior view had been obtained. Angled anterior and oblique orbital projections show two sites, however: one in body of left zygomatic bone and another in area of zygomaticofrontal suture. Radiation therapy portals were adjusted accordingly.

a result of this information, the radiation therapy portals were adjusted accordingly.

Often radionuclide studies will detect abnormal regions that cannot be seen on routine radiographs. Fig. 15-16 shows a 57-year-old woman with multiple metastases of breast carcinoma. The right supraorbital component of her juxtaorbital lesion had been irradiated and received a maximum dose. However, the zygomatic portion was untreated. Precise localization of the untreated area was crucial before additional radiation therapy to avoid reirradiating the maximally treated supraorbital area. This distinction could not be determined by radiography. Scintigraphy, however, showed increased radionuclide uptake in the untreated right zygoma while the treated supraorbital component had diminished uptake. On this basis radiation therapy portals could be determined.

Fig. 15-17 shows a 61-year-old female with diplopia and right facial pain in the distribution of the maxillary division of the trigeminal nerve. Bone scintigraphy showed an abnormal focus on the right side. If only a frontal or oblique view had been obtained, the abnormality could

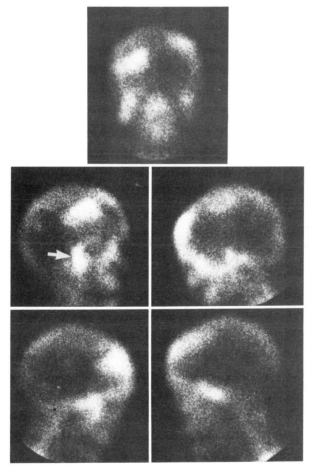

Fig. 15-16. Bone scintigrams of multiple metastases of breast carcinoma (straight anterior, oblique orbital, and lateral views from above downward). Only supraorbital component of right juxtaorbital lesion had been irradiated, leaving zygomatic portion untreated (arrow). Precise localization of untreated area was crucial to avoid reirradiating maximally treated supraorbital component. (From Gates, G. F., and Goris, M. L. 1976. Radiology **121:**677.)

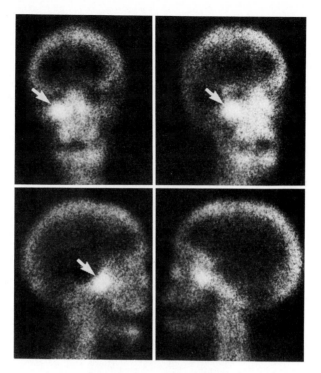

Fig. 15-17. Woman with diplopia and right facial pain in distribution of maxillary division of trigeminal nerve owing to breast carcinoma metastatic to greater wing of sphenoid forming posterior wall of pterygopalatine fossa. Sixty-degree angled anterior, right oblique orbital, and both lateral bone scintigraphic views shown. Abnormality (arrow) could have been mistakenly localized in maxillary sinus or zygoma if only frontal or oblique views were obtained. Lateral image showed it to be posterior to maxilla, however. Parallactic correlation of all three views correctly placed lesion. (From Gates, G. F., and Goris, M. L. 1976. Radiology **121**:677.)

have been mistakenly localized in the maxillary sinus or zygoma, respectively. The lateral image showed it to be posterior to the maxilla, but if only a lateral view had been obtained, the focus could have been mistakenly localized in the TMJ area (a possibility excluded by the frontal and oblique views). Parallactic correlation of all views placed the abnormality in the region of the pterygopalatine fossa (through which the maxillary division of the trigeminal nerve passes). Skull and sinus radiographs and cerebral angiography failed to disclose an abnormality. Surgical exploration of the area revealed a tumor implant from a previously undiagnosed carcinoma of the breast that had metastasized to the greater wing of the sphenoid, the latter forming the posterior wall of the pterygopalatine fossa.

Mandible. Tumors, fractures, and osteomyelitis may involve the mandible resulting in regional osteoblastic hyperactivity and focal accumulation of bone-seeking radiopharmaceuticals. Bone scanning is a very sensitive means of detecting regional mandibular abnormalities, which can be investigated further by radiography or biopsy.

A wide spectrum of tumors can involve the mandible. Fig. 15-18 shows a patient who had a squamous cell carcinoma arise in a dentigerous cyst, which was located in the right hemimandible. Prior to scintigraphy, the patient had a pathologic fracture through the region. Although the abnormality is well demonstrated on a conventional right lateral view, a pinhole collimator was used to obtain an even higher resolution image (lower right scintigram). The regions of reparative bone growth surrounded the carcinoma-containing cyst, which appeared as a centrally located area devoid of radionuclide.

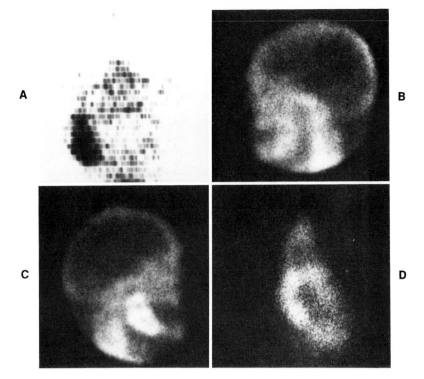

Fig. 15-18. Squamous cell carcinoma arising in mandibular dentigerous cyst. Rectilinear anterior scan, **A,** showed abnormal uptake of bone-seeking radiopharmaceutical in site of lesion (through which there was also pathologic fracture). Right lateral camera views with parallel-hole collimator, **C,** and pinhole collimator, **D,** gave excellent definition of reactive osteoblastic activity and its distribution. Lesion was not identified on left lateral view, **B.**

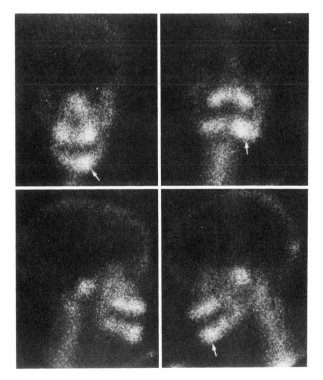

Fig. 15-19. Lymphoblastic lymphoma (arrows) arising in body of left hemimandible was identified on skeletal scintigram as region of increased radionuclide uptake (straight and angled anterior views, above, shown with both lateral views, below).

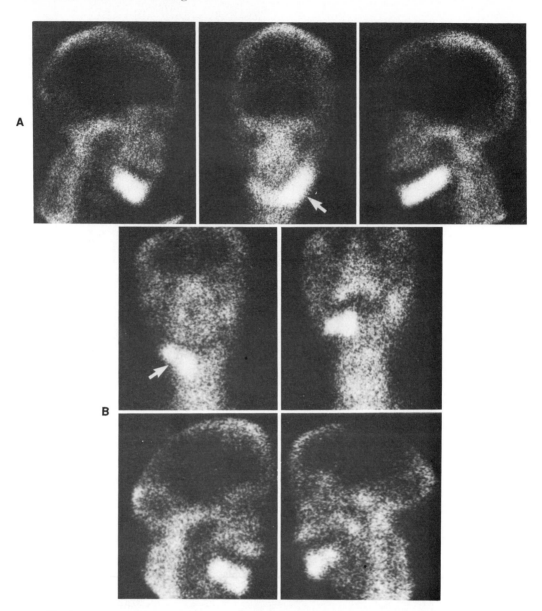

Fig. 15-20. A, Man with osteogenic sarcoma arising in body of left hemimandible had preoperative bone scintigram. Straight anterior view is between both lateral views. Correct localization of tumor (arrow) to involved half of mandible could not be accomplished by lateral views alone. **B,** Patient was restudied 1 month later following removal of left hemimandible. Straight and 60-degree angled anterior views shown over both lateral views. Without knowledge of patient's history, right hemimandible (arrow) could be called "hot" while absent left hemimandible might not be appreciated. (From Gates, G. F., and Goris, M. L. 1976. Radiology **121**:677.)

Other tumors involving the mandible can include lymphoblastic lymphomas (Fig. 15-19), ameloblastomas (Fig. 15-37), and osteogenic sarcomas (Fig. 15-20). Alexander (1976) has also shown abnormal mandibular scintigrams of patients having squamous cell carcinoma of the gingi-va, cementifying fibroma, fibrous dysplasia, and a radicular cyst (the latter presenting as a region devoid of radionuclide but surrounded by an area of increased uptake owing to reactive bone response to the expanding cyst).

Surgery or bone biopsy can drastically

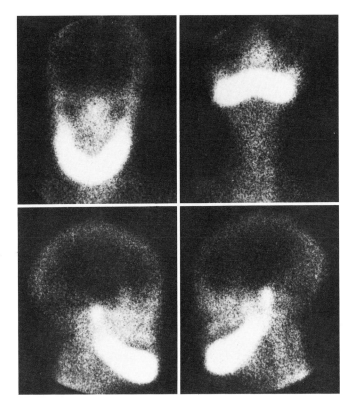

Fig. 15-21. Patient with adenocarcinoma of base of tongue and right tonsillar fossa had right hemiglossectomy and submandibular triangle dissection 2½ months prior to bone scintigraphy. Profuse radionuclide accumulation throughout mandible and both TMJ's was probably attributable to surgical manipulation (which also included hyoid resection and laryngeal suspension at mandible). Straight and 60-degree angled views shown over both lateral views. Notice how shifting canthomeatal line on anterior views drastically alters mandibular image. (From Gates, G. F., and Goris, M. L. 1976. Radiology **121:**677.)

alter the appearance of a bone scintigram. The patient shown in Fig. 15-20 had an osteogenic sarcoma arise in the left hemimandible. Correct identification of the abnormality could not be achieved by lateral views alone, since the intense radionuclide uptake in the left side would also be seen to some degree on the right lateral view (that is, the latter being a summated image of its own radionuclide content plus that "shining through" from the opposite side). An anterior view correctly localized the tumor, however (Fig. 15-20, A). The patient was restudied 1 month later; during the time interval between the two scintigraphic examinations, the left hemimandible had been surgically removed. Knowledge of the patient's history was crucial in this instance: the right hemimandible could

mistakenly be identified as the abnormal side (owing to the intensity of its radionuclide uptake), while the absent left hemimandible might not be appreciated, a feature that was radiographically obvious.

Surgery usually results in excessive radionuclide accumulation in the traumatized bony structures. However, extensive soft-tissue resection may also result in considerable radionuclide uptake in adjacent osseous structures, which is presumably due to periosteal reaction occurring secondary to surgical manipulation. The patient shown in Fig. 15-21 had an adenocarcinoma of the base of the tongue and right tonsillar fossa. She had a right hemiglossectomy and submandibular triangle dissection, which included hyoid resection and laryngeal suspension at the mandible. Two and a half months after surgery scintigraphy disclosed profuse radionuclide uptake throughout the mandible including the TMJ areas. Mandibular radiographs were normal and 17 months later she was without recurrence.

Radiation therapy has a profound affect on bone. During and immediately following therapeutic levels of radiation, radionuclide uptake in irradiated bone may be diffusely increased or decreased (Fordham and Ramachandran, 1974). The late effect is invariably one of greatly decreased radionuclide uptake (Bell, McAfee, and Constable, 1969; Fordham and Ramachandran, 1974; Gates and Goris, 1976; McNeil et al., 1973). The margins of such decreased uptake correspond exactly to the limits of the radiation field. If a radiation field incompletely covered a malignancy, adjacent untreated tumor will have increased radionuclide uptake compared to the treated area (Fig. 15-16). Response of a tumor to radiation therapy cannot be determined during or immediately after treatment since increased uptake could be due to any one or a combination of the following: acute radiation response, retrenchment of disease with healing of bone, or progressive disease (Fordham and Ramachandran, 1974). A 3-month interval following irradiation is usually adequate to allow assessment of response to therapy, but sometimes recurrent disease within the treatment area cannot be evaluated accurately by bone scanning.

Radiation therapy thus eventually results in decreased radionuclide uptake in irradiated bone, which in turn produces a scintigraphic image showing adjacent nonirradiated (and possibly normal) areas appearing with increased uptake by comparison. The patient shown in Fig. 15-22 had a carcinoma of the tongue treated with 7000 rads of megavoltage radiation several months prior to bone scintigraphy. The radionuclide uptake throughout the mandibular body was diminished, while the untreated mental protuberance continued to accumulate it in the normal manner. Without the knowledge of prior radiation therapy, the mental protuberance could be mistakenly diagnosed as abnormal because of its "increased" uptake of radionuclide (these changes in growth patterns were not radiographically evident). Depressed regional osteoblastic activity following radiation therapy may persist for years (up to 7 years in one of our patients).

Osteomyelitis provokes a reparative response that accounts for its detection via bone scanning. Fig. 15-23 shows a 16-year-old boy who had a 7-year history of chronic osteomyelitis of the left hemimandible. Regional hyperemia was shown on a scintigram that was obtained within a minute or two following radionuclide administration (Fig. 15-23, A). During this time the radiopharmaceutical was mainly within the vascular space. By the time delayed static views were obtained (2 to 4 hours following injection), the radionuclide had entered the hydration shell of the newly forming hydroxyapatite crystals and was indicating osteoblastic activity (Fig. 15-23, B). The extensiveness of the abnormality was more easily seen on the scintigrams than on corresponding radiographs (Fig. 15-23, C). The increased sensitivity of scintigraphy over radiography in detecting mandibular osteomyelitis was also reported by Alexander (1976).

Patients with fractures are not usually studied by bone scintigraphy unless a complication occurs such as nonunion of the fracture fragments, delayed union, avascular necrosis, or osteomyelitis. Repair within a fracture site starts within 24 to 48 hours following injury (Marty et al., 1976; Wendeberg, 1961). A fibrocallus forms across the fracture and joins the fragments. Cartilage is laid down within the callus and eventually undergoes transformation into bone. Following bony remodeling and repair the healed fracture may eventually be radiographically undetectable. Wendeberg (1961) studied the healing of tibial fractures using ^{85}Sr and observed three phases of bony repair as determined by external counting: (1) increased ^{85}Sr uptake within the fracture site occurred as soon as 24 to 48 hours following injury, (2) peak activity occurred at 6 to 8 months, and (3) increased activity could persist as long as 9

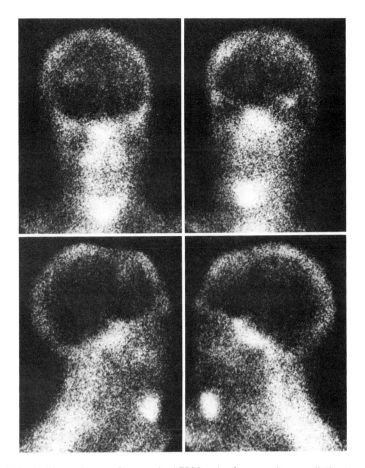

Fig. 15-22. Patient with carcinoma of tongue had 7000 rads of megavoltage radiation to area several months prior to this bone scintigraphic study. Straight and 60-degree angled anterior views over both lateral views. Radionuclide uptake throughout mandibular body is decreased while untreated mental protuberance, which normally accumulates radionuclide, looks "hot" by comparison. Mandibular radiographs were normal. (From Gates, G. F., and Goris, M. L. 1976. Radiology **121**:677.)

years. Nonosseous union of a fracture (using autografts or allografts as the experimental model) was characterized by decreased radionuclide uptake (Stevenson et al., 1974), whereas delayed union (Marty et al., 1976) or a viable bone graft (Alexander, 1976; Stevenson et al., 1974) may have increased uptake. Avascular necrosis has decreased radionuclide localization (Marty et al., 1976). The patient in Fig. 15-24 had systemic lupus erythematosus with diffuse vasculitis. She suffered an iatrogenic fracture of the left hemimandible at the time of dental extraction. This was subsequently complicated by osteomyelitis in the region and nonosseous union of the fracture frag-

ments. A bone scintigram was obtained to (1) determine the extent of osteomyelitis and (2) determine if any osseous reparative process (albeit on a cellular level) was ongoing in the fracture site. The scintigram showed heightened osteoblastic activity at the edges of the fracture but none between. Follow-up studies a month later were unchanged. Presumably a fibrous union bridged the gap between the fracture fragments, and the radiographically persistent gap in the mandible did not represent delayed union. The radionuclide accumulation at the edges of the fracture could be due to either a reparative response following trauma, osteomyelitis, or both.

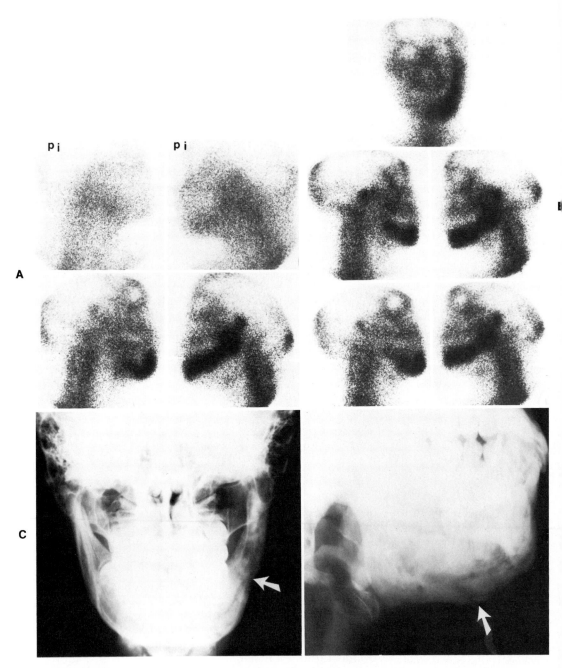

Fig. 15-23. Chronic osteomyelitis. **A,** Lateral scintigrams obtained within 2 minutes following injection of ^{99m}Tc pyrophosphate showed greater vascular component in left hemimandibular region compared to right (*pi* — postinjection images). Delayed images showed greatly increased uptake throughout left hemimandible indicating osteoblastic hyperactivity. **B,** Delayed static images in multiple projections showed extensiveness of abnormality (straight anterior, lateral, and angled lateral views from top to bottom). **C,** Radiographs showed destructive effects of osteomyelitis in left hemimandible (arrows).

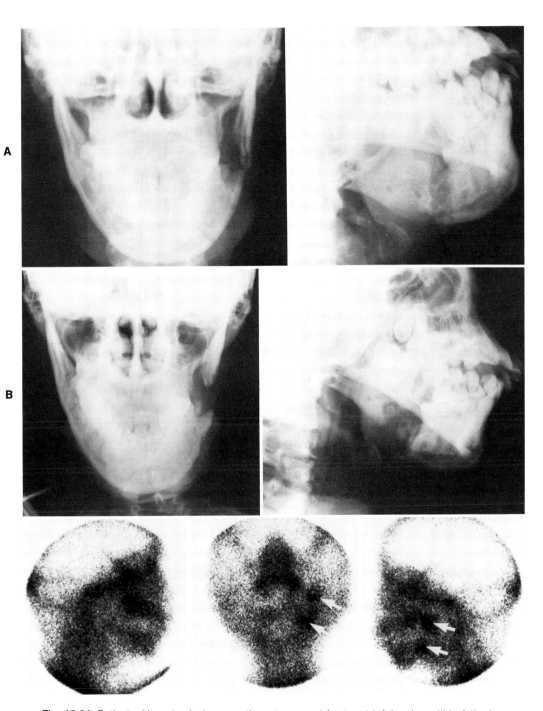

Fig. 15-24. Patient with systemic lupus erythematosus and fractured left hemimandible following dental extraction had complication of osteomyelitis in fracture site. **A,** Radiographs soon after injury. **B,** Six months later repeat radiographs showed continued bony resorption at fracture site. **C,** Bone scintigram was performed at that time to determine if there was any osteoblastic activity in gap between fragments. Radionuclide study revealed accentuated osteoblastic activity occurring on borders of fracture (arrows) but diminished uptake in between. This indicated nonosseous rather than delayed osseous union.

Metabolic diseases can also produce an abnormal mandibular uptake of a bone-seeking radiopharmaceutical. Sy (1974) reported a generalized increase in radionuclide uptake in the mandibles of patients with primary or secondary hyperparathyroidism. In addition Sy noted increased calvarial, sternal, and acromioclavicular uptake. Evens, Ashburn, and Bartter (1969) reported abnormal uptake of radionuclide in a patient with parathyroid carcinoma and a "brown tumor" (osteoclastoma) in the mandible.

Temporomandibular joint (TMJ) region. A painful TMJ can be studied by bone scanning. It may be difficult to differentiate between an abnormality in the head or neck of the condyloid process versus the articular tubercle or mandibular fossa of the temporal bone owing to the proximity of these structures. However, regional abnormalities may initially be detected by scanning before they are radiographically evident.

Referred pain in the TMJ region can be associated with dental disease as shown in Fig. 15-25. Dental abscesses may result in reactive bone formation and subsequent localization of a bone-seeking radiopharmaceutical. The patient in Fig. 15-25 had dental abscesses and also had previous dental extractions, both of which could account for localized radionuclide accumulation. Garcia and co-workers (1977) concluded that bone imaging was potentially useful for detecting incipient dental disease that was not readily identified on dental examinations and that scanning was a valuable adjunct to radiography in distinguishing active from inactive (arrested) disease.

The value of multiple views is brought out in Fig. 15-26, *A*, which shows TMJ uptake in a 17-year-old girl who had pain

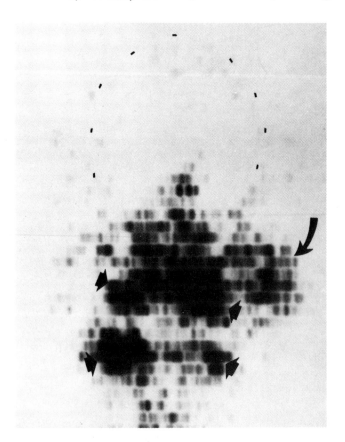

Fig. 15-25. Rectilinear bone scan of patient with painful TMJ (curved arrow) and multiple dental abscesses (short arrows).

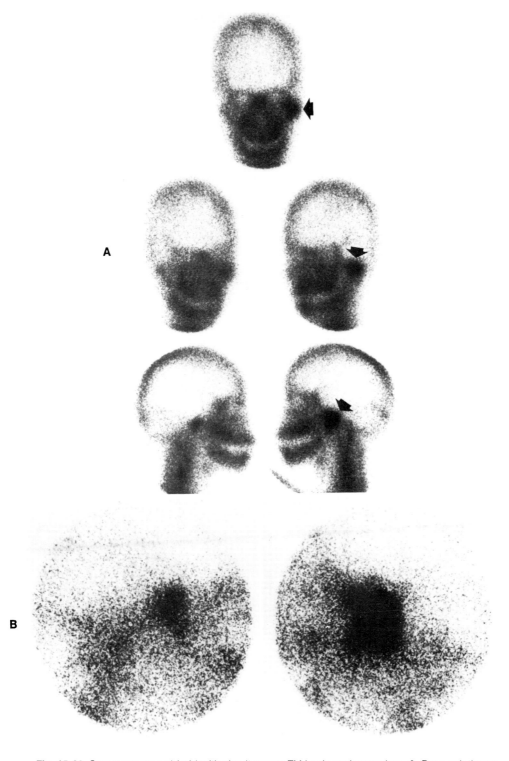

Fig. 15-26. Seventeen-year-old girl with simultaneous TMJ pain and gonorrhea. **A,** Bone scintigram (straight anterior, oblique orbital, and lateral views from top to bottom) showed increased radionuclide uptake in left TMJ (arrows). Compare with Fig. 15-15—pterygopalatine fossa uptake—to see how similar lateral views are; notice difference in oblique and anterior views, however, and how multiple projections are necessary for correct diagnosis. **B,** Lateral pinhole collimator views of TMJ further show increased radionuclide uptake in area.

Continued.

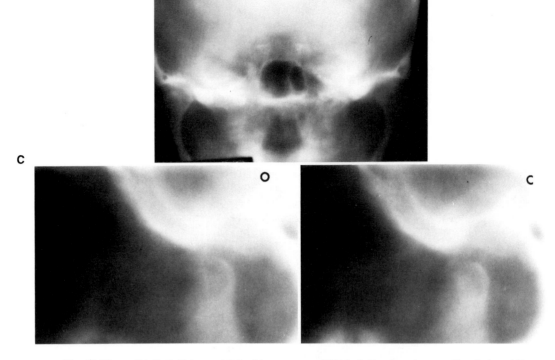

Fig. 15-26, cont'd. C, Anterior and lateral tomograms of TMJ's (latter done in open *O* and closed *C* mouth positions) showed anterolateral subluxation of mandibular head, which otherwise appeared normal.

in the area occurring at the same time she had a gonorrheal infection of the uterine cervix. The TMJ is superimposed over the sella turcica in the lateral views, but anterior and oblique views show it to be clearly separate from that midline structure (the asymmetric uptake on the lateral views is a further clue to its nonmidline origin). Pinhole collimator views (Fig. 15-26, *B*) showed diffuse uptake in the TMJ region. The radionuclide uptake in the TMJ region increased with time (as determined by comparing immediate postinjection views with delayed ones), indicating that osteoblastic hyperactivity was present in addition to regional hyperemia. Radiographic tomograms (Fig. 15-26, *C*) showed an anterolateral subluxation of the mandibular head on both open and closed mouth views, although the bony architecture appeared normal.

Tumors may also involve the TMJ region. Fig. 15-27 shows a patient with car-cinoma of the prostate metastatic to the head of the mandible. His mandibular radiographs were equivocal, but on the strength of the bone scan a regional biopsy was performed that disclosed the metastatic neoplasm.

As mentioned at the beginning of this subsection, the close proximity of the head of the mandible and adjacent portions of the temporal bone may produce difficulties when trying to differentiate between lesions in these contiguous areas. Fig. 15-28 shows a patient with carcinoma of the prostate metastatic to that portion of the petrous bone that is inferior to the internal auditory canal. Radionuclide uptake in this lesion was seen near the TMJ area on a lateral view, although anterior and posterior views showed the abnormality to be more medially located than expected for the usual TMJ localization. The patient also had additional metastases in the fourth and fifth cervical vertebral bodies as shown in Fig. 15-28.

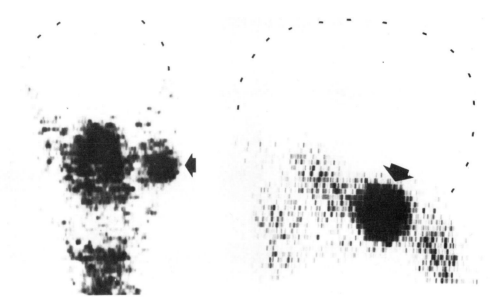

Fig. 15-27. Anterior and lateral rectilinear bone scans of patient with prostatic carcinoma metastatic to head of mandible. Radiographs were equivocal but biopsy was positive for tumor.

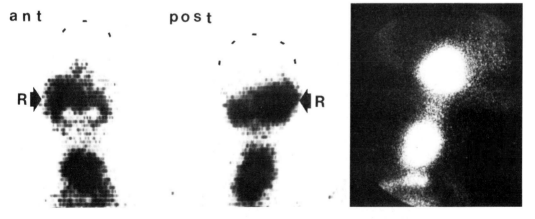

Fig. 15-28. Anterior and posterior rectilinear bone scans plus right lateral scintigraphic view of man with prostatic carcinoma metastatic to petrous bone inferior to auditory canal (as well as fourth and fifth cervical vertebrae). Arrows point to petrous lesion, which could be confused with TMJ tumor except for its inward extension.

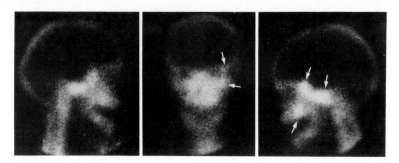

Fig. 15-29. Six-year-old child with rhabdomyosarcoma arising in left palate and extending into left maxillary sinus, left zygoma, and sella turcica. Bone scintigrams show multiple sites of abnormal radionuclide uptake corresponding to sites of bone destruction.

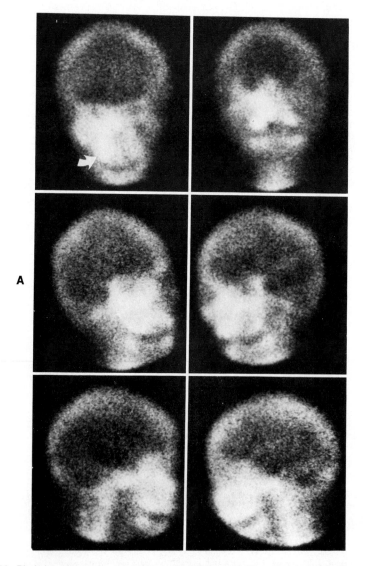

A

Fig. 15-30. Rhabdomyosarcoma in right maxillary sinus of 18-year-old girl. **A,** Bone scintigrams (straight and 60-degree angled, oblique orbital, and lateral views from top to bottom) show abnormal radionuclide uptake (arrow). **B,** Brain scan showed effects of tumor hypervascularity during late venous phase (second image on top, *V*), which persisted on immediate postinjection scintigram (PI image) but faded by the time delayed static image (DS image) was obtained 90 minutes later.

Paranasal sinuses. Tumors frequently occur in the paranasal sinuses and include carcinomas, fibrosarcomas (Fig. 15-38), and rhabdomyosarcomas (Fig. 15-29). Rhabdomyosarcomas not uncommonly arise in the head and neck region of children. Hornback and Shidnia (1976) reported that 27% of the rhabdomyosarcomas in their series of 45 children arose in the head and neck region (9% in the orbit, 18% elsewhere). Fig. 15-29 shows a rhabdomyosarcoma that originated in the left side of the palate in a 6-year-old child and extended to involve the left maxillary sinus, left zygoma, and sella turcica. Additionally, he had restricted motion of the left TMJ. Radiographs, including angiograms, showed bony destruction in the left maxilla and erosion on the left side of

the sella turcica. Regional hypervascularity in the right maxillary sinus harboring a rhabdomyosarcoma in another patient was well identified on a brain scan (Fig. 15-30). This vascularity persisted even on a scintigram obtained 3 hours following administration of ⁹⁹ᵐTc DTPA (diethylene-triaminepenta-acetic acid, a radiopharmaceutical that is neither a boneseeking or tumor-specific agent).

Sinusitis may also be seen on a brain scan as a hypervascular region. When the mucoperiosteum has been stimulated or actual osteomyelitis is present, a bone scan will also become positive. The patient in Fig. 15-31 had radiographs showing an air-fluid level in the left maxillary sinus and sclerosis in the left frontal sinus. Following trauma to the left frontal

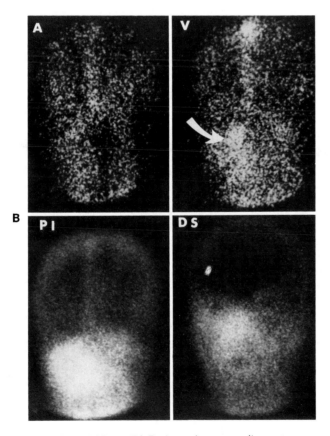

Fig. 15-30, cont'd. For legend see opposite page.

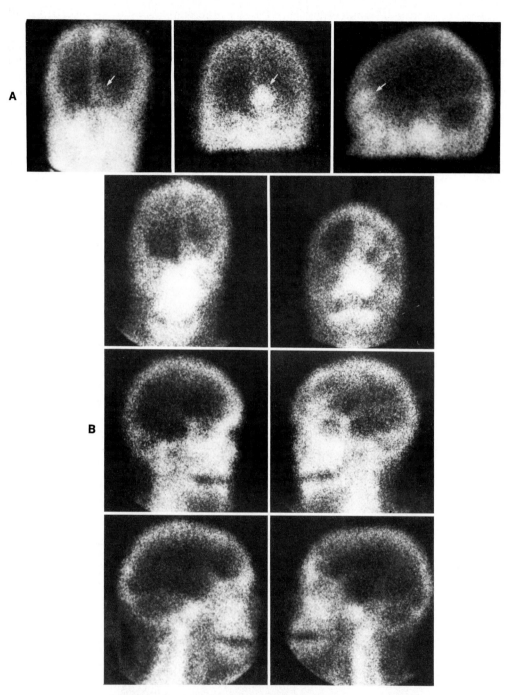

Fig. 15-31. Sinusitis and brain abscess. **A,** Brain scintigram showed slight uptake of ^{99m}Tc DTPA on immediate postinjection image (first picture on left), which greatly increased on delayed static views (middle and right images): uptake occurred in abscess located on superficial portion of left frontal lobe. Compare this sequence with Fig. 15-30, **B. B,** Bone scintigram (straight and 60-degree angled anterior, oblique orbital, and lateral views from top to bottom) showed radionuclide uptake in left maxillary and frontal sinus regions. Some uptake above frontal sinus could also have been caused by trauma.

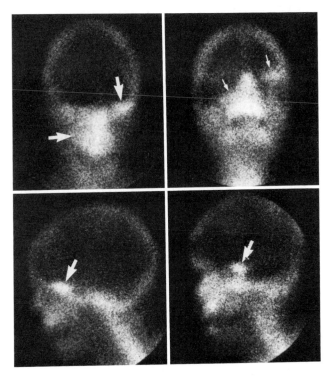

Fig. 15-32. Patient with right maxillary and left ethmoid sinusitis, parameningitis, and left orbital pseudotumor caused by lethal midline granuloma. Bone scintigrams (including straight and 60-degree angled views above; left lateral and oblique images below) showed left supraorbital and right maxillary radionuclide accumulation (arrows). Supraorbital component was lateral to frontal sinus. (From Gates, G. F., and Goris, M. L. 1976. Radiology **121**:677.)

sinus, the patient had pneumococcal meningitis and a brain abscess as shown on a brain scan (Fig. 15-31, *A*). Notice how the brain abscess increased in intensity with delayed imaging compared to simple hypervascularity (Fig. 15-30, *B*), which diminishes with time (see section on brain scanning). Bone scintigrams showed abnormal radionuclide uptake in the left maxillary and frontal sinuses; some of the uptake above the frontal sinus could also have been due to trauma.

Fig. 15-32 shows the bone scintigraphic study of a 66-year-old man with right maxillary and left ethmoid sinusitis and a left orbital pseudotumor attributable to a lethal midline granuloma. Skull and sinus radiographs (including tomography) showed a small fluid level in the right maxillary sinus, mucoperiosteal thickening in the left ethmoid sinus, and a soft-tissue density over the left orbit. The left supraorbital abnormality shown on the

bone scintigrams was not radiographically evident.

Fibrous dysplasia may also involve the facial region as shown in Fig. 15-33. The right maxillary radionuclide uptake corresponded to a region of fibrous dysplasia shown on radiographs. Correlation of radiographic and scintigraphic studies was important in this case since the bone scan was initially performed as a part of a metastatic screening survey in this 62-year-old man with lung carcinoma. This proves the point that regional abnormalities occurring on bone scans of tumor patients may not always be the result of neoplasia. Bone scans are sensitive indicators of osseous abnormalities but are also nonspecific and must be correlated with a patient's history, radiographs, and other studies.

Orbits. Orbital scintigraphy must be interpreted with the realization that the zygomaticofrontal suture commonly has

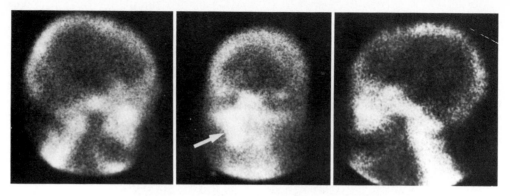

Fig. 15-33. Fibrous dysplasia in right maxillary region showing increased osteoblastic activity (arrow).

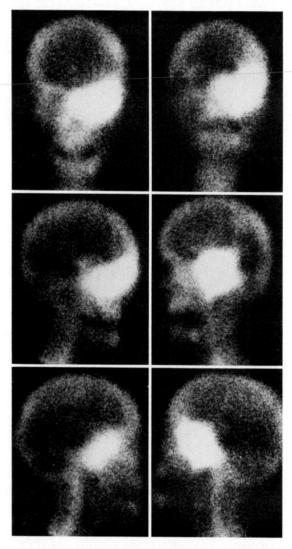

Fig. 15-34. Recurrent sphenoid ridge meningioma protruding through orbit of 57-year-old woman. Bone scintigraphic views include straight and 60-degree angled anterior, oblique, and lateral projections (top to bottom). Left oblique orbital view gives good definition of reactive osseous borders in relation to orbit, while anterior views show extent along sphenoid ridge. (From Gates, G. F., and Goris, M. L. 1976. Radiology **121:**677.)

increased radionuclide uptake in normal patients and must not be mistaken for an abnormal focus. Oblique orbital views are quite helpful in many circumstances as shown in Fig. 15-34. This 57-year-old woman had a recurrent sphenoid ridge meningioma that was protruding through the left orbit. The left oblique orbital view gave good definition of the reactive osseous borders in relation to the orbit. The anterior view showed the extent of the reactive change along the sphenoid ridge.

As shown in Fig. 15-35, enucleation

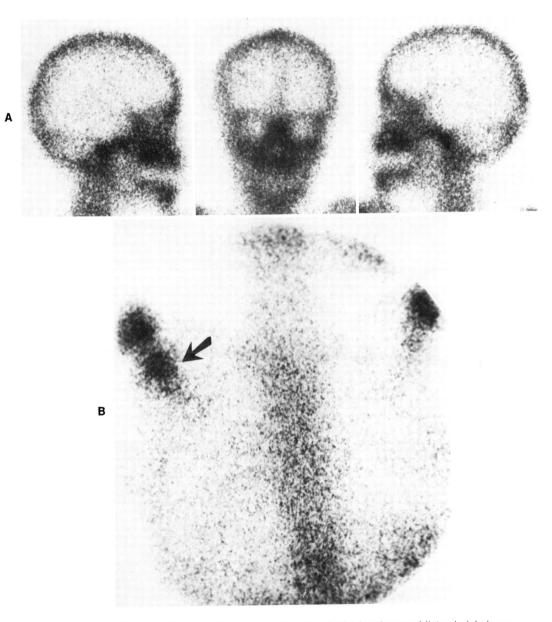

Fig. 15-35. A, Normal facial skeletal scintigrams in child who had undergone bilateral global enucleations for retinoblastoma. Tumor had metastasized to left glenoid fossa of scapula, however. **B,** Posterior view of upper torso with arrow pointing to metastatic site. Proximal humeral epiphyseal centers normally accumulate radionuclide and also appear "hot."

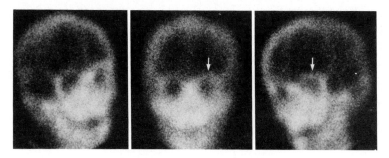

Fig. 15-36. Child who had retinoblastoma and left global enucleation. Following surgery left orbital abscess developed. Skeletal scintigraphy showed haziness over orbit associated with increased radionuclide uptake in left supraorbital ridge (arrow) owing to osteomyelitis.

may not result in abnormal bone uptake. This child had bilateral global enucleations for retinoblastomas. The tumor did not involve the orbit bones, and the surgery did not evoke an osteoblastic response. However, the tumor did metastasize to the glenoid fossa of the scapula.

Intraorbital infections following enucleation may result in osteomyelitis as shown in Fig. 15-36. This child had a left global enucleation for a localized retinoblastoma. Following surgery he developed an orbital abscess that was associated with supraorbital osteomyelitis as shown by bone scintigraphy. A repeat study was normal following antibiotic therapy.

Gallium

General background

Gallium (Ga) 67 citrate is the tumor-seeking radiopharmaceutical most commonly used in current clinical practice. Tumor localization of agents in this general class of radiopharmaceuticals (including ^{67}Ga citrate, ^{75}Se selenomethionine, ^{111}In transferrin, and ^{111}In bleomycin) results from the nonspecific physiologic changes occurring with a neoplasm's presence. These changes include localized increased blood volume, abnormal tumor circulation with increased microvascular permeability, increased affinity for radiotracer-labeled proteins in the metabolically active neoplastic site, and prolonged extravascular presence of radionuclide that may be secondary to impaired lymphatic drainage from the tumor region (Alderson, Krohn, and

Welch, 1976; Potchen et al., 1971). Three of the tumor-seeking radiopharmaceuticals are either plasma protein bound (that is, ^{67}Ga citrate or ^{111}In chloride, which attach to transferrin) or incorporated into the plasma protein fraction (that is, ^{75}Se selenomethionine) shortly after administration. The increased affinity of tumors for these plasma proteins is probably quite important in the tumor-localizing properties of these agents (Alderson, Krohn, and Welch, 1976). Although the exact mechanism of gallium uptake in neoplasms is unknown, radionuclide localized in tumor tissue has been identified in the intracellular lysosomes (Swartzendruber, Nelson, and Hayes, 1971). Indium 111 has been combined with the chemotherapeutic antibiotic bleomycin and used for tumor localization (Verma et al., 1973). However, the stability of this radiopharmaceutical has been questioned and the possibility raised that in vivo conversion of ^{111}In bleomycin to ^{111}In transferrin might occur.

Gallium 67 decays by electron capture (into stable ^{67}Zn) with a physical half-life of 78 hours. It emits four major gamma photons: 93 keV (45% abundance), 184 keV (24%), 296 keV (22%), and 388 keV (7%). The usual dose administered is 1 to 4 mCi. Imaging is started 48 to 72 hours later except when searching for infections, under which circumstances scanning may begin in 24 hours or less. It is a technical challenge to perform a scan when using a radionuclide that emits photons of multiple energy levels. The ideal method is to use equipment having three pulse height analyzers, which can be set to detect the 93, 184, and 296 keV photons but, if only dual peak capability is available, the two lower ones are generally used (Pinsky and Henkin, 1976). When using equipment that has only a single pulse height analyzer, two techniques may be used; either the 93 or 184 keV photons may be used with a scintillation camera (using a middle-energy collimator), or a large "window" (defined as the upper and lower energy ranges allowed to pass through a pulse height analyzer) may be used to encompass the 184 and 296 keV peaks when using a rectilinear scanner (Hoffer and Gottschalk, 1974; Pinsky and Henkins, 1976).

The biologic fate of ^{67}Ga is interesting and important. Following intravenous administration of the citrated form, ^{67}Ga^{++} is largely bound to plasma proteins including transferrin, lactoferrin, haptoglobins, and albumin (being loosely bound to the last). During the next week, 26% is excreted in the urine and 9% in the feces (McAfee and Subramanian, 1975); 18% of administered ^{67}Ga is localized in the skeleton and 5% in the active marrow. The highest tissue concentration occurs in the spleen (4%/kg), while the bone marrow averages 3.6%/kg compared to 2.6%/kg for bone (McAfee and Subramanian, 1975). Other organs that also accumulate ^{67}Ga include liver, kidneys, lacrimal glands, thymus, nasopharyngeal lymphoid tissue, postpartum breasts, male genitalia, and intestines, especially the colon. Hoffer (1977) reported that the affinity of ^{67}Ga for lactoferrin was greater than that for transferrin. Lactoferrin is normally found in high concentrations in human colostrum and milk, neutrophilic leukocytes, bone marrow, spleen, colon, tears, and genital, salivary, and nasopharyngeal secretions. Thus ^{67}Ga lactoferrin may account for normal radionuclide localization in these tissues or fluids (Hoffer, Huberty, and Khayan-Bashi, 1977). The biologic half-life of ^{67}Ga is 27 days. Total body radiation dose is about 0.7 rads and the bone marrow dose is 1.4 rads (McAfee and Subramanian and Esser, 1975).

Tumor uptake of gallium was first described by Dudley, Imire, and Istock (1950) but was initially believed to be restricted to bone tumors. Soft tissue tumor localization of radiogallium was first noted by Edwards and Hayes (1969, 1970) while evaluating this radionuclide for its possible use as a bone scanning agent. Tumor uptake of gallium varies according to different histologic types. The majority of patients with Hodgkin's disease will have increased gallium uptake in at least one of their tumor sites (Hoffer and Gottschalk, 1974). A national cooperative study of 141 patients with untreated Hodgkin's disease reported that in only 73% of the cases were all tumor sites detected by gallium scanning; however, 90% of the patients had at least one positive site and the false-positive rate was less than 5% (Johnson et al., 1974). Overall accuracy in detecting Hodgkin's tumor sites was highest in the neck and chest (83% to 85%) but less in the axilla (50% to 64%), abdomen (50% to 62%), and inguinofemoral areas (40% to 50%). Hodgkin's disease of the nodular sclerosing type was detected more often (74%) than other types. The same cooperative study group also evaluated gallium uptake in 167 untreated malignant lymphomas. Seventy-eight percent of the patients had at least one positive site of radionuclide uptake but only 51% of all histologically proven sites were identified by gallium scanning. However, the false-positive rate was about 1%. Accuracy in tumor detection varied according to body region: neck (53% to 55%), thorax (65% to 77%), abdomen (48% to 49%), and inguinofemoral region (38% to 55%). The best results were obtained with well-differentiated lymphocytic lymphomas (85% to 88%), while the worst were with poorly differentiated lymphocytic lymphomas (31% to 36%). Histocytic lymphomas were detected about as well as Hodgkin's disease (70% to 71%). In both Hodgkin's disease and lymphoma studies tumor sites were revealed by gallium scanning that were not initially detected or suspected by other means. Since the overall accuracy for detecting tumors in this general group is in the 70% to 75% range, it is obvious that gallium scanning cannot be the only staging technique used for patient evaluation. However, its very small (1% to 5%) false-positive rate is highly significant: an abnormal region seen on gallium scanning will have an overwhelming chance of representing neoplastic disease, some sites of which may have been unsuspected.

Gallium also accumulates in other tumors. Eighty-five percent of patients with untreated lung cancer had positive gallium scans for the primary lesion but only 80% for lymph node sites and 49% for proven metastasis in organs such as bone or brain (DeLand et al., 1974). The squamous cell carcinomas had a higher detection rate (81%) than adenocarcinomas (73%) and small cell carcinomas (70%). Thesingh and co-workers (1978) and Kinoshita and co-workers (1974) reported a greater uptake of ^{67}Ga by undifferentiated and squamous cell lung carcinomas than adenocarcinomas.

Over 90% of hepatomas are positive on gallium scans (Lomas, Dibos, and Wagner, 1972). Hepatoblastomas (Lomas, Dibos, and Wagner, 1972) also accumulate gallium as do certain benign hepatic tumors such as hepatocellular adenomas (Belanger, Beauchamp, and Neitzschman, 1975). Nonmalignant liver diseases such as cirrhosis do not usually show increased gallium accumulation. However, abscesses and inflammatory diseases may have increased uptake (to be discussed later).

Other tumors also accumulate gallium to varying degrees. Gallium accumulation in primary and secondary brain tumors was evaluated by Waxman and co-workers (1973) who reported that its uptake in these neoplasms was greater than that of ^{99m}Tc-pertechnetate, a conventional brain scanning agent; of 73 cases, gallium uptake exceeded technetium in 21, was less in 2, and equal in 50. Gallium scanning was also used in evaluating testicular tumors (95% accuracy) (Bailey et al., 1973), breast carcinomas (54% accuracy) (Richman et al., 1975), Ewing's sarcoma (positive in all primary sites) (Frankel et al., 1974), malignant mela-

noma (54% accuracy) (Milder et al., 1973), and head and neck tumors (to be discussed later). Gallium scanning is of little value in assessing genitourinary tumors, (except of testicular origin), neoplasms of the digestive tract, and thyroid carcinoma (Pinsky and Henkin, 1976). Although gallium scanning can detect skeletal metastases of breast carcinoma and bone tumors, it is inferior to bone scanning for such purposes.

Gallium scans can also be used to assess the effectiveness of radiation or chemotherapy on malignant disease as long as one remembers: (1) a negative gallium scan may not be absolute proof of the lack of disease since the tumor may not have accumulated gallium in the pretreatment state, and (2) therapeutic radiation doses as low as 200 to 400 rads may convert a "positive" gallium scan into a "negative" one. On the other hand, a positive gallium scan during or following therapy should be considered ominous as it may indicate residual or recurrent tumor.

For several years gallium has been known to accumulate in inflammatory foci such as abscesses. One hypothesis used to account for this phenomenon has been the belief that gallium is incorporated into polymorphonuclear leukocytes (PMN's), either by intracellular accumulation of ^{67}Ga lactoferrin (Hoffer, Huberty, and Khayan-Bashi, 1977) or by uptake within PMN lysosomes. Another possibility is that ^{67}Ga is carried by transferrin and/or other plasma constituents into the proximity of tissue proteins, which in turn bind the radionuclide more avidly and remove it from the carrier (Winchell, 1976). Neoplasms, areas of inflammation, and regions of ischemic infarction (in certain stages) have increased capillary permeability to macromolecules, which is a result of neovascularity with large intercapillary pores. Regional perfusion may be increased and lymphatic proliferation delayed (especially with tumors and inflammatory conditions), resulting in additional residence time of macromolecules in the interstitial fluid space. Increased regional macrophage activity may result in intracellular ingestion of the labeled macromolecules or their fixation on the cell surface with subsequent intracellular translocation of the radioactive tracer (Winchell, 1976). Winchell further believes that the binding macromolecule for ^{67}Ga is transferrin. He suggests that some cells have specific membrane receptor sites for transferrin-bound iron, which erroneously accept ^{67}Ga (or ^{111}In) from transferrin when attempting to engage in heme enzyme synthesis. Altered cell membrane permeability (as occurs in dead, dying, or traumatized cells) may also allow for intracellular penetration of a macromolecule that would otherwise be excluded (Winchell, 1976).

Tsan and co-workers (1978) reported that human PMN's had a greater affinity for ^{67}Ga than lymphocytes whereas red blood cells had no affinity. The PMN plasma membrane was shown to serve as a diffusion barrier. ^{67}Ga binds to the PMN surface membrane, but when its permeability was disrupted, intracellular gallium accumulation increased considerably. Tsan also studied ^{67}Ga distribution within experimental abscesses; only 20% of the radionuclide within an abscess was in intact PMN's, cellular debris, or bacteria while the rest was in a soluble, noncellular fraction. Tsan and co-workers (1978) propose that ^{67}Ga binds to the surface membrane of PMN's, which in turn move out of the circulation into inflammatory sites. ^{67}Ga may also diffuse into inflammatory sites where it is taken up by bacteria directly (owing to nonspecific binding and/or a carrier-mediated transport system) (Menon, Wagner, and Tsan, 1978).

Regardless of its method of localization ^{67}Ga uptake has been noted to occur in a variety of inflammatory conditions including abdominal abscesses, cholecystitis, pelvic inflammatory disease, granulomatous colitis, osteomyelitis, cellulitis, pneumonia caused by a variety of organisms including *Pneumocystis carinii*, pulmonary tuberculosis, lung abscesses, radiation pneumonitis, sarcoidosis, pneumoconiosis, bronchiectasis, and mycotic aneurysm (Kinoshita et al., 1974; Levenson et al., 1976; Michall and Coleman,

1977; Siemsen et al., 1976; Teates and Hunter, 1975; Waxman and Siemsen, 1975).

The results of gallium scanning can be correlated with other radionuclide imaging studies in an attempt to arrive at a more specific diagnosis of an abnormality. Such use of dual studies is exemplified by comparing conventional brain scans (using ^{99m}Tc in either ionic or compounded form) with gallium scans of the brain. Waxman and co-workers (1975) correlated ^{99m}Tc-pertechnetate and ^{67}Ga citrate brain scans performed in 93 patients with cerebral neoplasms and in 70 others with cerebral infarction or hemorrhage. There was a greater accuracy of tumor detection when using gallium as an imaging agent compared to technetium (96% versus 85%, respectively). All cerebral infarctions or hemorrhages were identified when using ^{99m}Tc. However, 67% of cerebral infarctions failed to concentrate ^{67}Ga while 27% had a much lower uptake compared to the ^{99m}Tc study. The two radionuclides were equivalent in 6% of infarction patients. Other investigators, however, have reported a 100% uptake of gallium in cerebral infarctions (Reba and Poulose, 1974). Waxman and Siemsen (1976) also compared ^{99m}Tc and ^{67}Ga brain scans for the detection of cerebral and cranial infections and reported that seven of 18 lesions were seen with gallium but not pertechnetate. However, three of the seven cases were skull lesions including osteomyelitis or mastoiditis.

Application to maxillofacial scanning

At the time gallium scans are usually performed (48 to 72 hours following its administration), radionuclide uptake is normally seen in the nasopharynx, liver, bone, spleen, lacrimal glands, salivary glands, and external genitalia (Fig. 15-8, *C*). The maxillofacial region can be successfully imaged using the same positioning techniques shown in Figs. 15-9 and 15-10. Ideally a scintillation camera having the capability of simultaneously utilizing the three lower photopeaks of ^{67}Ga offers the greatest versatility for clin-

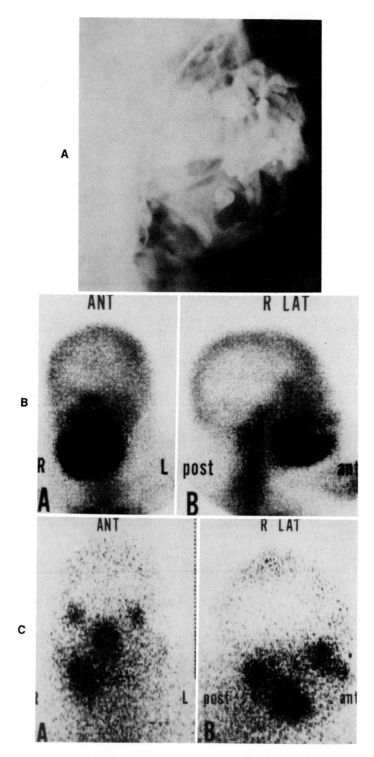

Fig. 15-37. A, Destructive features of an ameloblastoma in right hemimandible are shown radiographically. **B,** Bone scintigrams and, **C,** ^{67}gallium scans both show tumor well although bone study is probably superior in its detail. Bilateral gallium uptake near orbit has been attributed by some as representing lacrimal gland uptake. (From Olson, W. H. 1977. J. Nucl. Med. **18:**348.)

ical imaging. A medium energy collimator must be used.

Silberstein and co-workers (1974) studied 52 patients with squamous cell carcinoma of the head and neck region using ^{67}Ga and correctly predicted the presence or absence of disease with a 65% accuracy; however, nine of the 16 patients with falsely negative scans had preoperative irradiation. Twenty-three patients with lymphoreticular neoplasms were also studied with ^{67}Ga; scanning had an 87% accuracy in detecting these tumors. Silberstein concluded that ^{67}Ga had little value in the staging of squamous cell carcinoma of the head and neck but was useful in detecting lymphoma sites. Higashi and co-workers (1972), however, reported that all eight of their patients with maxillary sinus cancer had strongly positive ^{67}Ga scans. Higashi and co-workers (1972) also reported two cases of benign tumors of the submandibular gland, plus an ameloblastoma of the mandible, which did not accumulate ^{67}Ga; however, all four of their cases of sialadenitis had abnormal scans. Olson and McCombs (1977) described an ameloblastoma that was easily identified by both bone and gallium-67 scanning, but they concluded that bone imaging was the superior diagnostic radionuclide technique (Fig. 15-37).

In 1972 Higashi noted that ^{67}Ga uptake in malignant lung tumors diminished in proportion to the dose of megavoltage radiation delivered to the neoplasm. Higashi and co-workers later (1977a) used ^{67}Ga scanning to assess the effectiveness of radiation therapy (on occasion supplemented by chemotherapy) in 25 patients with malignant tumors of the maxillary sinuses, cervical lymph nodes, tonsils, tongue, pharynx, salivary gland, and thyroid. Pretreatment scans showed malignant lymphomas, anaplastic carcinomas, squamous cell carcinomas, and malignant melanomas accumulating more radionuclide than adenocarcinomas and adenoid cystic carcinomas. Posttherapy studies were performed 1 to 2 weeks following completion of treatment; in all instances (except in an unresponsive adenoid cystic carcinoma of the palate)

repeat studies showed reduced ^{67}Ga accumulation in the tumor site. Higashi and colleagues (1977a) observed that tumors that initially had strongly positive scans tended to have a more favorable response to therapy than those that had only equivocal or weakly positive scans. However, posttreatment scans were more important in determining prognosis; patients whose ^{67}Ga scans became negative after therapy remained free of tumor in the treated areas. If a lesion continued to accumulate ^{67}Ga following therapy (even if the scan looked improved compared to the pretreatment scan), the prognosis was worse and the likelihood of local recurrence was high. A singular exception was a radioresistant malignant melanoma of the maxillary sinus that continued to grow during therapy despite an "improving" posttherapy ^{67}Ga scan. Higashi's work (1977a) points out the importance of timing a patient's ^{67}Ga scan in relationship to radiation therapy, as does the work of Silberstein and co-workers (1974) with its "false-negative" postirradiation scans in instances of squamous cell carcinomas.

Higashi and co-workers (1977b) also reported on the utility of ^{67}Ga to separate patients with carcinoma of the maxillary sinus from those with chronic sinusitis. In either case radiographic differentiation may be difficult since sinus opacification and apparent bone destruction or erosion may be evident. All of Higashi's patients with squamous cell carcinomas of the maxillary sinus (a total of 14) plus those with epidermoid carcinomas, reticulum cell sarcomas, and malignant melanomas of the maxillary sinus (one in each tumor category) had strongly abnormal ^{67}Ga scans; one patient with an adenocarcinoma of the maxillary sinus had only a weakly positive study. On the other hand, five of seven patients with chronic maxillary sinusitis had negative ^{67}Ga scans, while a sixth had an equivocal study and the seventh a weakly positive scan. Sinus opacification and apparent bone destruction were radiographically evident in all seven (even by tomography). However, no actual bone destruction was found at the time of surgery on a patient with chronic sinusitis. The appar-

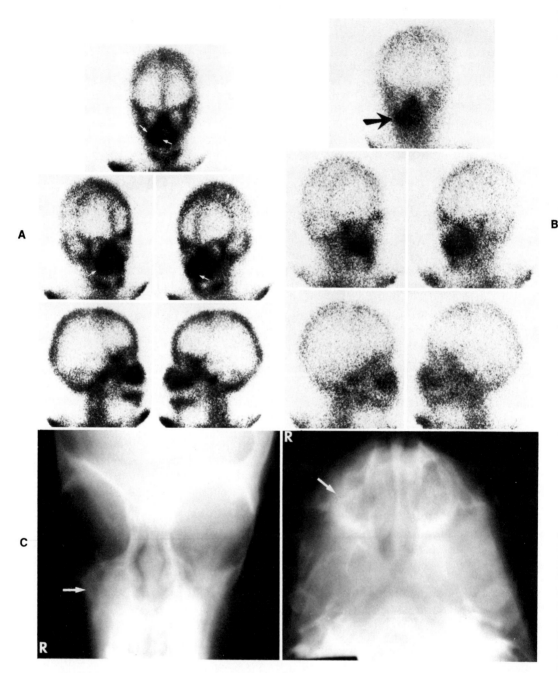

Fig. 15-38. Fibrosarcoma arising in right maxillary sinus of child was studied by both skeletal, **A,** and gallium scintigraphy, **B.** Same patient positioning was used for both studies (straight anterior, oblique orbital, and lateral views from top to bottom). Tumor could be localized by either method (arrows). Radionuclide uptake on bone study occurred as result of reparative osteoblastic response to destructive tumor in sinus, whereas gallium uptake occurred predominantly within neoplasm itself. **C,** Facial tomograms showed presence of tumor within sinus (frontal and basal views shown).

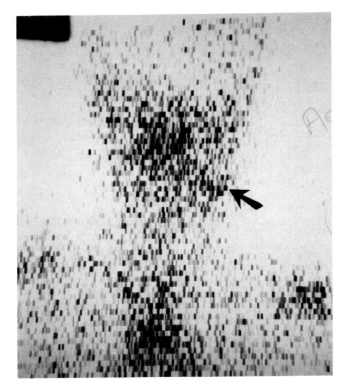

Fig. 15-39. Cervical lymph node enlargement caused by Hodgkin's disease detected by ^{67}gallium scanning. Upper chest with sternum is in lower field with shoulders laterally; arrow points to tumor in this anterior view.

ent bone destruction seen radiographically could be attributed to rarefying osteitis secondary to chronic inflammation (Towers and McAndrew, 1975) although its radiographic features were similar to the bone destruction associated with a malignant process. Higashi acknowledged the ability of ^{67}Ga to accumulate in both malignant and inflammatory sites and suggested that the discrepancy of radionuclide accumulation in this circumstance (that is, chronic sinusitis versus maxillary carcinoma) might be related to the higher metabolic activity of the tumor tissue. Higashi referred to Waxman and Siemsen (1975), who reported a greater accumulation of ^{67}Ga in patients with acute cholecystitis compared to those with chronic cholecystitis but acknowledged ^{67}Ga uptake in chronic sialadenitis (Higashi et al., 1972).

Gallium 67 is useful in tumor localization in general as shown in Fig. 15-38 where a fibrosarcoma of the maxillary sinus was seen by both bone and ^{67}Ga scintigraphy. Cervical lymph node involvement owing to lymphoma can be well demonstrated by ^{67}Ga (Fig. 15-39) while imaging of thyroid metastases is usually unsuccessful. Chest (Fig. 15-40) and abdominal malignancies (Fig. 15-41) as well as localized inflammations (Fig. 15-42) may be well demonstrated by ^{67}Ga scanning.

• • •

The development of specific tumor-seeking radiopharmaceuticals is one of the most promising areas of research in nuclear medicine. The potential for detecting small foci of tumor and perhaps indicating the response of a malignancy to therapy is the goal of many current investigations.

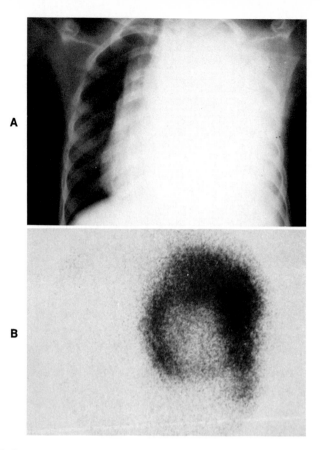

Fig. 15-40. Left chest mass in child owing to lymphocytic lymphoma. **A,** Cardiomediastinal structures are displaced to right by tumor. **B,** Anterior gallium 67 scintigraphy of chest showed uptake of radionuclide at tumor's periphery but none in center (compatible with avascularity and/or necrosis). Entire chest was included in field of view; right hemithorax contained no radiogallium (which is normal).

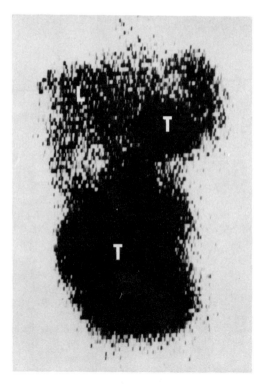

Fig. 15-41. Huge, dumbbell-shaped abdominal mass caused by Hodgkin's disease avidly accumulated ^{67}Ga (*T*, tumor). Normal liver, *L*, uptake is much less by comparison. Anterior scan shown extended from lowermost chest to lower pelvis.

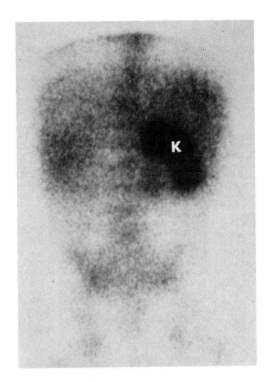

Fig. 15-42. Posterior scintigram showing right kidney, *K*, uptake of ^{67}Ga in patient with pyelonephritis.

Other nuclear medicine applications

A great number of radionuclide examinations besides bone and gallium scans can be performed. The purpose of this section is to briefly describe those studies that also could be useful to oral and maxillofacial surgeons. Topics that might be of less interest and less immediate application will be discussed only briefly, and the reader is referred to current textbooks or periodical reviews such as *Seminars in Nuclear Medicine* for further information.

Salivary glands

The salivary glands can be imaged following administration of ^{99m}Tc pertechnetate or radioactive iodine. [99m]Tc is the preferred agent owing to its low radiation dose and the desirability of its photon emission (which is highly suitable for scintillation camera imaging), despite the fact that it attains a saliva/plasma ratio only half that of radioiodine (Alexander

et al., 1966). Salivary gland scanning is made possible by the glandular ability to concentrate radionuclide before excreting it into the saliva; the human salivary/plasma ratio for radioiodine is 40:1 (Schiff et al., 1947). Radioiodine is secreted by the epithelium of the salivary gland's intralobar ducts (Burgen, Terroux, and Gouder, 1959; Cohen, Logothetopoulos, and Myant, 1955). Presumably pertechnetate secretion occurs in a similar manner. Salivary gland scanning, therefore, is both a functional and morphologic test. Tracer concentration depends on functional integrity of the intralobar ductal epithelium; following radionuclide concentration, imaging techniques directly display the secreting glandular parenchyma.

The technique of salivary gland scanning is quite simple. [99m]Tc pertechnetate is administered intravenously in doses ranging from 0.5 to 10 mCi. Routine studies probably require only 1 to 2 mCi (Schall and DiChiro, 1972), although some use up to 4 mCi (Gates, 1972). The total body radiation exposure resulting from 10 mCi of ^{99m}Tc is estimated to be 100 mR (McAfee et al., 1964). A vascular blush outlining the parotid glands is seen immediately following pertechnetate administration (Fig. 15-43) even if the glandular epithelium does not concentrate the tracer. The concentration phase begins within the first 10 minutes and represents the active accumulation of radionuclide by the ductal epithelium; this phase may be enhanced by administering pilocarpine nitrate, 20 mg subcutaneously (Tarkiainen, Stjernvall, and Tarkannen, 1970). The excretory phase begins 10 to 40 minutes following pertechnetate administration and represents the tracer being transported into the saliva and excreted into the oral cavity; this phase may be enhanced by lemon juice, tart candy, or oral administration of potassium perchlorate, 1 gm/70 kg (Mishkin and Freeman, 1975). Salivary excretion is blocked by the intramuscular administration of 0.8 to 1 mg of atropine 30 minutes prior to scanning (Gates, 1972). Scintigraphy is usually performed in the anterior projection although lateral views can be

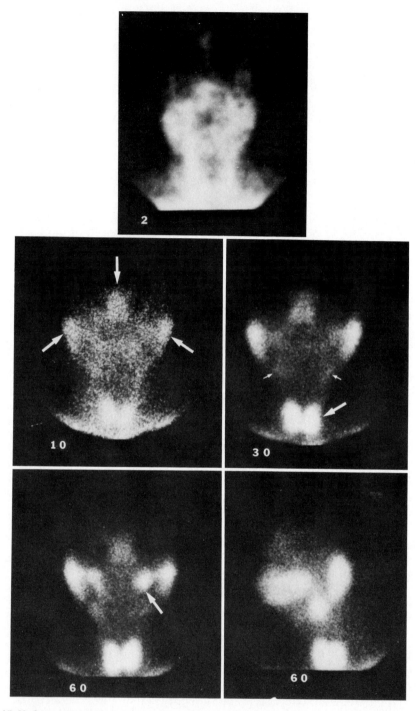

Fig. 15-43. Sequential anterior views during normal radionuclide salivary scintigraphy. Numbers indicate time in minutes following injection of ⁹⁹ᵐTc pertechnetate. Vascular phase occurred shortly after tracer injection as shown on 2-minute scintiphoto. Concentration phase occurred during first 10 minutes at which time nasal (midline arrow) and parotid gland (lateral arrows) uptake was evident. Thyroid was well seen by 30 minutes (large arrow) along with submandibular glands (small arrows). By 60 minutes excretion of ⁹⁹ᵐTc into saliva was occurring (arrows point to radionuclide in parotid ducts approaching oral cavity); anterior and left lateral views shown at 60 minutes. (Courtesy Dr. Ved Prakash, Palo Alto Verterans Hospital.)

obtained when indicated. It may be helpful to permanently identify landmarks such as the tragus, angle of the mandible, and lateral canthus on the scintigram for future reference.

Salivary scintigraphy is usually performed in patients suspected of having either tumors or inflammatory conditions involving the glands. Contrast sialography can differentiate, under the best conditions, benign from malignant tumors and both from inflammatory disease; it can also assess extrinsic from intrinsic glandular disease. These diagnoses, however, are made indirectly by observing secondary changes within the ductal system from which parenchymal abnormalities are inferred. Salivary scanning, on the other hand, is a means of directly imaging the secreting glandular parenchyma and assessing its functional status. This procedure should precede contrast sialography because of the latter's disruptive effects on glandular function (Schall and DiChiro, 1972).

The smallest salivary gland neoplasm detectable by scintigraphy is in the range of 1 to 2 cm in diameter. Primary glandular malignancies as well as metastases to the glands, abscesses, and cysts fail to accumulate pertechnetate and appear as regions devoid of radionuclide (that is, a "cold" nodule). The scintigraphy of a Warthin's tumor (cystadenoma lymphomatosum), however, is distinctly different from the primary malignancies, since this benign neoplasm actively accumulates radionuclide to a greater degree than surrounding normal glandular tissue (that is, is a "hot" nodule) as in Fig. 15-44. This feature is attributed to the ductal inclusions, from which the tumor is thought to arise, retaining their ability to concentrate pertechnetate (Schall and DiChiro, 1972). Warthin's tumors also have increased vascularity, which has been demonstrated by scintiangiography (Sagar, Piccone, and Meckelnburg, 1977). Oxyphilic adenomas (oncocytomas) have also been reported as actively concentrating pertechnetate so as to produce a "hot" nodule on scanning (Ausband, Kittrell, and Cowan, 1967); these neoplasms arise from glandular epithelium (Johns, Regizi, and Batsakis, 1977), which probably accounts for their tracer concentrating abilities. Gates (1972), however, reported an oxyphilic adenoma that was "cold" upon scanning. The mixed tumor (pleomorphic adenoma), which accounts for about two thirds of all salivary neoplasms, can appear either as a "cold" or "warm" (that is, uptake nearly equal to surrounding, normal gland) nodule as in Fig. 15-45.

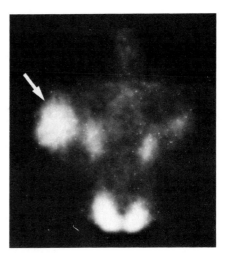

Fig. 15-44. Right-sided Warthin's tumor seen as area of increased radionuclide uptake (arrow) on ^{99m}Tc pertechnetate salivary scintigraphy. (Courtesy Dr. Ved Prakash, Palo Alto Veterans Hospital.)

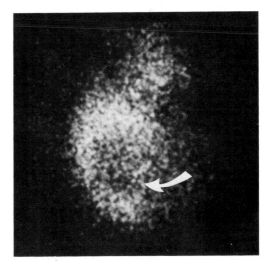

Fig. 15-45. Mixed tumor in right parotid (right lateral pinhole collimated scintigram) shown as region of diminished ^{99m}Tc pertechnetate uptake surrounded by normal gland. (Courtesy Dr. Ved Prakash, Palo Alto Veterans Hospital.)

Tumor location and size are also important in detection. A mixed tumor arising from a superficial portion of the parotid gland may be "hidden" owing to superimposed activity coming from deeper layers. A deep-seated tumor, on the other hand, may be recognized by the glandular distortion it causes. A small "cold" nodule completely surrounded by normal radionuclide-bearing tissue will probably not be identified. Scanning is useful not only in the detection of a salivary gland mass but in assessing residual or ectopic tissue following surgery or evaluating glandular function after radiation therapy or surgical denervation (Schall and DiChiro, 1972). Furthermore, neck and facial masses can be easily differentiated from salivary gland tissue.

Acute sialadenitis is associated with an increased concentration of pertechnetate, whereas decreased concentration occurs in chronic sialadenitis. The use of serial scintigraphy, however, discloses a variability in the scan appearance of various diseases with time. There is a great uptake of pertechnetate in parotid glands of patients with bacterial (staphylococcus) or viral (mumps) parotitis in the acute phase. This has been attributed to the hyperemia of infection and edema fluid compressing the intralobar ducts. A similar situation occurs in acute parotitis following sialolithiasis in which there is major ductal obstruction with retention of pertechnetate. Following antibiotic treatment, acute suppurative parotitis subsides and a subsequent scan appears normal. Scintigraphy of a patient in the convalescent stage of mumps, however, shows decreased or absent glandular tracer uptake occurring at a time when histopathologic studies reveal epithelial necrosis and lymphocytic infiltration (Schall and DiChiro, 1972). Chronic recurrent parotitis may have similar scintigraphic features owing to glandular fibrosis and cellular infiltration.

Sjögren's syndrome is a particular form of chronic sialadenitis in which the diagnosis requires two of the following three symptoms: xerostomia, keratoconjunctivitis sicca, and a connective tissue disease (usually rheumatoid arthritis). Serial studies in large patient groups have resulted in four classes of glandular function ranging from normal (class I) to complete loss of salivary function (class IV). Serial scintigraphic studies not only document progressive loss of function in untreated or unsuccessfully treated patients, but they can show return of function in those individuals successfully managed with cyclophosphamide (Schall and DiChiro, 1972). In Sjögren's syndrome the concentrating and excretory abilities of the parotid are gradually lost, as may be determined by comparing thyroid to parotid uptake ratios (Alarion-Segovia et al., 1971). Loss of glandular ability to discharge pertechnetate following perchlorate administration also characterizes Sjögren's disease (Mishkin and Freeman, 1975).

Tumor margination has also been a diagnostic aid in interpretation of salivary gland scintigrams (Gates, 1972). Smoothly marginated "cold" nodules are most likely to be benign neoplasms, cysts, or early preinvasive malignancies. Irregularly marginated "cold" nodules are likely to be primary or metastatic malignancies or occasionally Sjögren's syndrome or severe inflammation. Smoothly marginated "hot" nodules strongly suggest Warthin's tumor or less commonly an oxyphilic adenoma.

The overall accuracy of salivary gland scanning in 102 patients was assessed by Gates (1972); there were 22% false negatives but no false-positive scans. The sublingual, submandibular, and parotid glands can all be studied. The various scintigraphic results that are likely to be encountered are summarized in Table 15-1.

Gallium 67 citrate localizes in salivary glands. Several potential conditions resulting in such localization (infections, tumors, and so forth) have already been discussed in previous sections. However, some special conditions need to be mentioned. Patients who have undergone radiation therapy to the neck may have increased gallium uptake in the salivary glands included in the treatment field for the next year (Bekerman and Hoffer, 1975). This uptake is not associated with,

Table 15-1. Clinical uses of radionuclide salivary gland imaging

Abnormality	Scintigraphic appearance
Tumors	
Warthin's	Hot focus
Oxyphilic adenoma	Hot or cold focus
Mixed	Cold or warm focus
Malignant (primary or secondary)	Cold focus
Cysts	Cold focus
Abscesses	Cold focus
Sialadenitis	
Acute	Increased glandular uptake
Chronic	Decreased glandular uptake
Sjögren's syndrome	Glandular uptake initially normal, later decreased

and should not be confused with, recurrent neoplastic disease (Fig. 15-46). Bekerman also observed bilateral salivary gland uptake in two nonirradiated patients, one with chronic renal failure and the other with systemic lupus erythematosus. Gallium 67 uptake in parotid, anterior and posterior auricular, or high cervical lymph nodes might be mistaken for parotid gland uptake; similar gallium 67 accumulation in submandibular lymph nodes might be confused with salivary gland localization. Fig. 15-47 shows gallium 67 uptake in bilaterally enlarged lymph nodes in a child with the mucocutaneous lymph node syndrome. The similarity in location of these lymph nodes and the parotid glands is obvious.

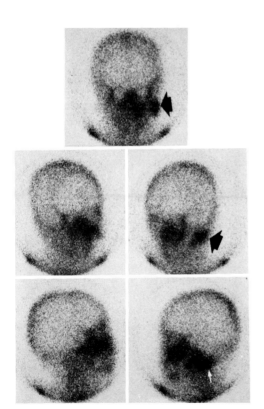

Fig. 15-46. Left parotid gland accumulation of ^{67}Ga in child who had radiation therapy to left maxillary sinus and contiguous facial areas for fibrosarcoma. Arrow points to parotid, which was irradiated; there was no neoplastic disease in area (straight anterior, oblique, and lateral views shown, top to bottom).

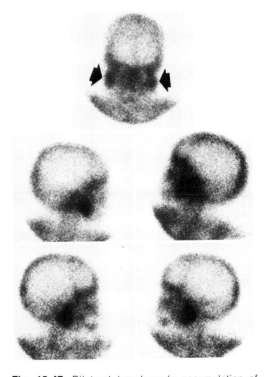

Fig. 15-47. Bilateral lymph node accumulation of ^{67}Ga in child with mucocutaneous lymph node syndrome. Arrows point to regions of abnormal gallium uptake, which must not be confused with parotid glands. This distinction might not be made on anterior views alone (See Fig. 15-46); oblique and lateral scintigrams aid in this differentiation (straight anterior, oblique, and lateral views shown, top to bottom).

Thyroid

The thyroid gland was the first organ in the body to be extensively studied with radionuclides. Consequently, a wealth of information regarding thyroid physiology and pathophysiology has been discovered in the past several decades. A great variety of in vivo (both imaging and non-imaging tests) and in vitro studies are available for thyroid assessment. This section will deal only with that aspect of thyroid disease that might be of practical significance to the oral and maxillofacial surgeon: the assessment of a neck mass.

Radioactive iodine (for example, ^{131}I or ^{123}I, both of which are used in clinical imaging) is taken into the thyroid by active transport and subsequently incorporated into thyroid hormone by the process of organification. [99m]Tc pertechnetate can also be used as an imaging agent since it is also trapped by the gland (but not organified). [123]I is administered orally to a fasting patient in either liquid or capsular form; ^{99m}Tc is injected intravenously. [123]I is the isotope of iodine currently preferred for clinical studies since it lacks the beta emission of ^{131}I, has a 13-hour half-life, and has a 159 keV gamma photon that is suitable for imaging with either a scintillation camera (using a pinhole collimator) or rectilinear scanner. The absorbed radiation dose to the thyroid from 100 μCi of ^{123}I is 0.5 to 2 rads, while the dose from 2.5 mCi of ^{99m}Tc is 0.5 to 1 rad (Atkins, 1975). These radiation figures are a vast improvement over those associated with ^{131}I, where a 50 μCi scan dose delivered 25 to 100 rads to the gland (Atkins, 1975).

The indications for thyroid imaging are varied and include evaluation of glandular size, position, and function; assessment of masses in the neck, base of the tongue, or mediastinum; functional assessment of thyroid nodules; and detection of functional metastases in patients known to have thyroid carcinoma. Many of these clinical problems will be discussed in the following paragraphs.

The growth and development of the thyroid must be understood before discussing some of the anomalies that may be present as neck masses. The thyroid is the first glandular structure to appear and develops as early as in the 2 mm embryo (six somite stage). The gland starts as a bulge in the ventral floor of the foregut. The thyroid diverticulum, an entodermal pocket, soon protrudes between the first pair of pharyngeal pouches and attaches to the pharynx by a narrow neck known as the thyroglossal duct. This latter primitive hollow structure connects the developing thyroid to the tongue, which is simultaneously organizing from the pharyngeal floor. The duct eventually becomes a solid stalk and breaks up by the sixth week, but its point of attachment to the tongue persists as the foramen cecum. The developing thyroid becomes a solid mass against the primitive aortic sac and soon assumes a bilobed shape. When set free from the atrophic stalk, the gland begins to be converted into an irregular mass of epithelial plates. By the seventh week the crescent-shaped thyroid is in a transverse position with a lobe on each side of the trachea. The follicles begin to form by the eighth week, acquire colloid during the third month, and soon afterward become functional. Anomalous development may result in persistent portions of the thyroglossal stalk giving rise to cysts, a median fistula opening in the neck, or accessory thyroid tissue. Improper failure to descend leaves the thyroid located near the base of the tongue (Arey, 1954).

Midline neck masses are clinical problems that are easily studied by thyroid scanning. The basic question to be answered is whether the mass contains functional thyroid tissue. Although a thyroglossal duct cyst is usually rounded and smooth to palpation, an accurate clinical distinction between it and aberrant thyroid tissue is not always possible. Both thyroglossal duct cysts and abnormally positioned thyroid tissue may be located in the sublingual or midneck region. Incomplete obliteration of the branchial clefts may also lead to cystic neck masses or even fistulae; cervical cysts are closed epithelial sacs derived from either ectodermal or entodermal tissue. The purpose of thyroid scanning is to identify the functional thyroid tissue present and be sure that a clinically suspected "thyroglossal duct cyst" is not a sublingual thyroid. Thus scanning should be performed preoperatively to avoid removal of a functioning sublingual thyroid, which would result in a permanent athyroid state. Fig. 15-48 shows an examination of a patient with a normal thyroid gland and a thyroglossal duct cyst; the cyst is not identified on the scintigram (since it contains no functional thyroid tissue capable of trapping iodine), but its location relative to the gland is indicated on a second scintiphoto by a cobalt 57 marker. Occasionally

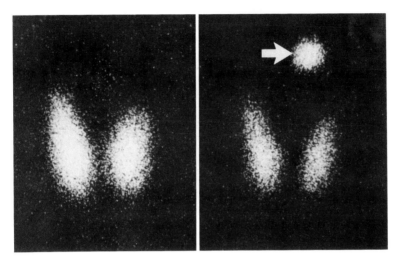

Fig. 15-48. [123]I scintigraphic study in child with nodule in neck (anterior, midline, and just above larynx). Thyroid was normally located and consisted of two lobes (left). Location of nodule relative to thyroid was determined by placement of [57]Co source over lesion during exposure of second scintiphoto (arrow on right). Nodule lacked functional thyroid tissue and thus did not accumulate [123]I. Thyroglossal duct cyst was removed at subsequent surgery. Scintillation camera with pinhole collimator was used in all thyroid studies shown.

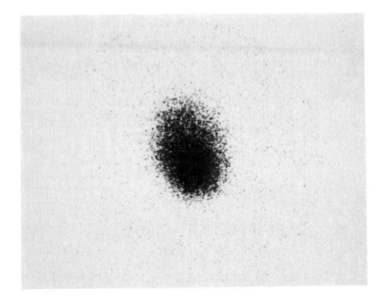

Fig. 15-49. Sublingual neck mass in child was evaluated by ^{123}I scintigraphy. Nodule avidly accumulated radioiodine and had 24-hour uptake of 12%. There was no other functional thyroid tissue present. Once it was determined that nodule was sublingual thyroid, surgery was not contemplated.

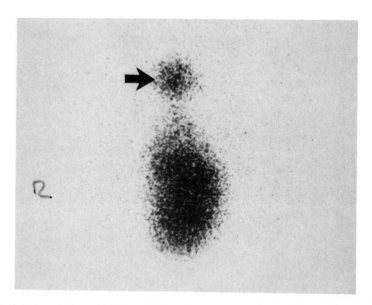

Fig. 15-50. Anterior midline nodule in neck (in same region as in patient shown in Fig. 15-48) was evaluated by ^{123}I scintigraphy. Nodule readily accumulated radioiodine as seen on scintigram. Second, smaller area was seen on scintiphoto to be located in sublingual region (arrow). Nodule could not be palpated in this second area. This situation represented incompletely descended thyroid with residual tissue in sublingual area (same region for latter as shown in Fig. 15-49). A 24-hour uptake value of 13% was determined. As in patient shown in Fig. 15-49, surgery was not contemplated.

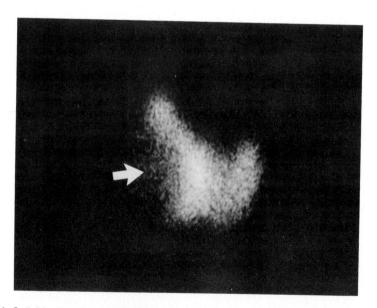

Fig. 15-51. Colloid adenoma was identified on ^{123}I scintigraphy as region devoid of radionuclide (since it lacked functional thyroid tissue necessary to trap radioiodine). This "cold" nodule produced distortion of middle and lower portion of right lobe of thyroid (arrow). Although nodule originated within thyroid, it is conceivable that extrinsic nodule adjacent to thyroid could produce similar defect.

a cyst can be directly anterior to a normal thyroid.

Aberrantly located, but otherwise normally functioning thyroid tissue will accumulate radionuclide, allowing scintigraphic detection. Such uptake differentiates an abnormally located thyroid from a cyst. The thyroid tissue may be rounded, compact, and solitary as shown in the sublingual thyroid in Fig. 15-49 or in several functional components as shown in Fig. 15-50. The thyroid function of the patients in Figs. 15-49 and 15-50 was normal.

Scintigraphy with radioiodine is commonly performed to evaluate a thyroid nodule. A nodule failing to accumulate radioiodine is classified as being "cold." Such solitary hypofunctioning or nonfunctioning nodules are usually cysts, adenomas (Fig. 15-51), degenerative areas, or focal thyroiditis. However, a carcinoma may also be seen as a "cold" nodule (Fig. 15-52). The overall incidence of

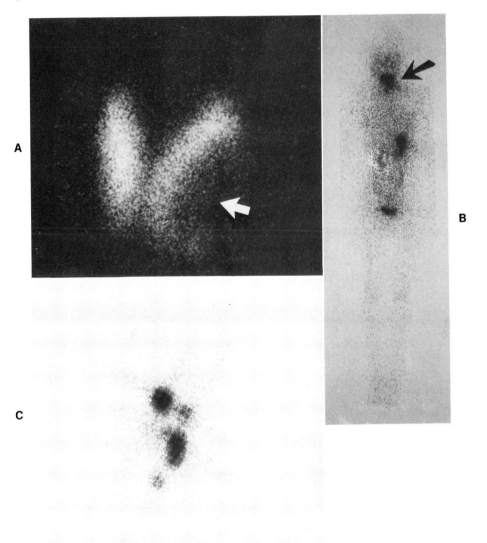

Fig. 15-52. A, Papillary-follicular carcinoma of thyroid may also be "cold" nodule as shown. Following thyroidectomy and removal of such malignancy, total body ^{131}I scintiscanning may be performed to search for metastases that take up radioiodine. **B,** Another patient had several metastatic regions in neck (arrow). Notice normal stomach, bowel, and bladder visualization. **C,** Anterior view of neck using parallel-hole collimator disclosed multiplicity of lesions.

malignancy in such "cold" nodules can be as high as 20% to 25%, but individual chances of malignancy vary according to age (higher chance of being cancer in younger individuals); sex (although overall incidence of thyroid cancer is higher in women, any given solitary "cold" nodule has a greater chance of being malignant in a male); rapid growth; laryngeal infiltration and/or cord paralysis and cervical adenopathy (features more commonly associated with malignancy); and response to suppression therapy (nodules disappearing following thyroid hormonal replacement are unlikely to be malignant) (Hoffer, Gottschalk, and Quinn, 1976). About 75% of thyroid malignancies are well-differentiated papillary, follicular, or mixed-cell types with good prognosis. Twenty percent are poorly differentiated, arise in older patients, and have a relatively poor prognosis. The remaining 5% are medullary carcinomas, which may arise from parafollicular cells of the thyroid and be hormonally active; these latter tumors have an increased familial incidence and may be associated with other endocrine tumors.

Following histologic diagnosis of thyroid cancer and surgery (usually a total thyroidectomy), follow-up scanning with ^{131}I may detect functioning metastases (Hoffer, Gottschalk, and Quinn, 1976) [131]I with its 8.1 day half-life is preferred in this instance since actual scanning is not started until 2 to 4 days following an oral administration of 3 to 5 mCi. This delay is necessary to allow normal excretion of ^{131}I to occur and thus lower the body background level to the point where metastases are identifiable. However, any remnant of normal functioning thyroid tissue will accumulate radionuclide to a greater degree than functional metastases. Thus it is important to ablate any residual thyroid tissue with a therapeutic dose of [131]I (usually a single 50 to 80 mCi dose of ^{131}I) and assure maximal thyroid-stimulating hormone (TSH) stimulation (achieved by temporarily withholding thyroid replacement from a thyroidectomized patient) prior to performing a total body ^{131}I scan. At least 70% of well-differentiated metastatic thyroid carcinomas will take up some radioiodine (Fig. 15-52), although less than 50% will have sufficient uptake to allow successful treatment with [131]I (Hoffer, Gottschalk, and Quinn, 1976).

Radionuclides other than radioiodine have been used to study thyroid cancer. Gallium 67 citrate does not accumulate in normal thyroid tissue; furthermore, it does not localize frequently enough in thyroid malignancies to warrant its routine clinical use (Kaplan et al., 1974; Heidendal et al., 1975). [99m]Tc pertechnetate has recently been used as a routine thyroid imaging radiopharmaceutical since in most cases ^{99m}Tc and ^{123}I give essentially similar information (^{99m}Tc is more readily available and cheaper than ^{123}I) (Arnold and Pinsky, 1976). However, some thyroid-image disparity is occasionally seen when comparing these two radionuclides. Arnold and Pinsky (1976) reported one case of a papillary-follicular carcinoma that appeared normal on an anterior ^{99m}Tc image but abnormal on a ^{123}I study; oblique views using either agent, however, showed the lesion. An additional 11 patients had focal areas of increased ^{99m}Tc uptake in regions that appeared normal on ^{123}I scintigraphy; the significance of this disparity was not known (Arnold and Pinsky, 1976). Other instances of increased ^{99m}Tc uptake have been reported to occur in various thyroid neoplasms including a poorly differentiated follicular carcinoma (O'Connor, Cullen, and Malone, 1977), papillary-follicular carcinoma (Turner and Spencer, 1976), follicular carcinoma (Massin, Planclon, and Perez, 1977), colloid adenoma (Massin, Planclon, and Perez, 1977), and Hürthle cell adenoma (Hirabayashi et al., 1975); radioiodine scans performed in these patients showed diminished areas of uptake. The cause of this disparity is not completely understood.

A major advantage of thyroid scanning with radioiodine is the determination of the iodine-trapping ability of a thyroid nodule. Cysts, many adenomas, degenerative areas, focal thyroiditis, and most carcinomas are identified as "cold" nodules on scanning. Some nodules may accumulate radioiodine and appear to be either "warm" (uptake similar to surrounding normal thyroid tissue) or "hot" (uptake exceeding normal thyroid). "Warm" nodules are generally TSH dependent whereas "hot" nodules are not; the probability of either being malignant is remote, especially with "hot" nodules.

It is important to determine if a "warm" or "hot" nodule is autonomous (that is, autonomous from TSH control) since an autonomously functioning nodule may develop into a toxic nodule, ultimately producing symptoms of hyperthyroidism. A nodule's autonomy can be determined by scanning following TSH suppression. Exogenous thyroid hormone (often given as triiodothyronine, T_3) is administered to suppress normal TSH output; repeat scanning will show diminished or absent radioiodine uptake in previously identified normal glandular tissue or nonautonomous nodules whereas autonomous nodules will still be imaged. The patient in Fig. 15-53 had a palpable nodule in the right lobe of the thyroid and was referred for ^{123}I scintigraphy with a diagnosis of "probable 'cold' nodule." The initial scintigram showed a

"hot" nodule present; its autonomy was demonstrated on a repeat study following TSH suppression. If only a "hot" nodule is initially imaged, the remaining, suppressed thyroid gland may be seen on a repeat study following TSH stimulation (given as an intramuscular injection of bovine TSH). A hyperfunctioning autonomous nodule may produce enough thyroid hormone to suppress endogenous TSH production to the point that the remaining, normal gland is nonfunctional. The TSH stimulation test causes this quiescent thyroid tissue to become metabolically active.

Thyroiditis (inflammatory lesions involving the thyroid) can be subdivided into three main groups: acute suppurative (for example, staphylococcal or streptococcal in origin), subacute (of uncertain etiology), or chronic. Hashimoto's or lymphocytic thyroiditis, which is probably an autoimmune disease, is the commonest form of chronic thyroiditis. Riedel's struma is another chronic form. The gland is temporarily incapable of trapping iodine and synthesizing hormone in patients with acute or subacute thyroiditis. Hashimoto's thyroiditis is usually seen as

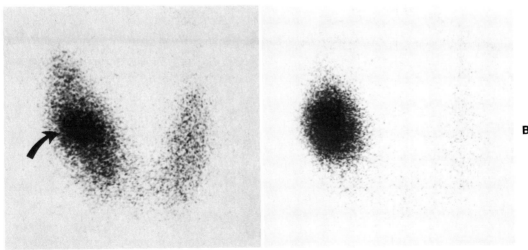

A **B**

Fig. 15-53. Patient with thyroid nodule was referred for ^{123}I scintigraphy with clinical diagnosis of "probable 'cold' nodule." **A,** Resultant scintigram showed focal "hot" region that corresponded to palpable nodule (arrow). Remaining thyroid areas had relatively poor uptake. **B,** Following short course of thyroid hormone, repeat scan was performed. "Hot" nodule was still evident (which indicated its autonomy from TSH control) but remaining thyroid tissue was not visualized (since it was suppressed). Probability of such an autonomous nodule being malignant is nil.

an enlarged nodular gland of several year's duration and should be considered when encountering a nontoxic nodular goiter. The scan pattern of Hashimoto's thyroiditis is variable; the gland may appear nearly normal or have regions of hypofunction or hyperfunction. The patient whose scan is shown in Fig. 15-54 was referred for thyroid scintigraphy because of a palpable nodule in the right lower pole. Scintigraphy with ^{123}I showed an enlarged right lobe with a hyperfunctioning nodule in the lower pole. Six- and 24-hour radioactive iodine (RAI) uptake determinations were 10% and 17%, respectively, as determined by a scintillation probe counter (Fig. 15-3, *A*). These values are measurements of the percentage of administered radioiodine, which is accumulated within the gland at specified times, and are an indication of the gland's trapping ability and general functional status. The RAI uptake determination is very dependent on the size of the plasma iodine pool. Ingested nonradioactive iodides (or injected, as with iodinated contrast agents used in radiography) expand the iodine pool and secondarily depress RAI uptake determina-

tions. Thus the normal values of 5% to 30% and 10% to 40% for 6- and 24-hour determinations, respectively, are based on a presumption of a normal iodine pool. These values have slowly been dropping over the years as the iodine pool in the general population has been slowly increasing (owing in part to the iodine content of commercially produced bread) and may vary somewhat from laboratory to laboratory. Determination of RAI uptake values are useful in Hashimoto's thyroiditis. In this disorder the gland is able to trap ^{123}I but cannot organify it; consequently, the free iodine content of the gland may be expanded (Hoffer, Gottschalk, and Quinn, 1976). Because of the suspicious appearance of the thyroid scintigram, the patient in Fig. 15-54 was brought back and given another dose of ^{123}I in order to perform a perchlorate discharge test. This test is based on the concept that perchlorate competitively inhibits iodine trapping and "flushes" free iodine from the gland (Hoffer, Gottschalk, and Quinn, 1976). Following radioiodine administration, an uptake determination is performed (2 to 6 hours later) to be followed by oral perchlorate

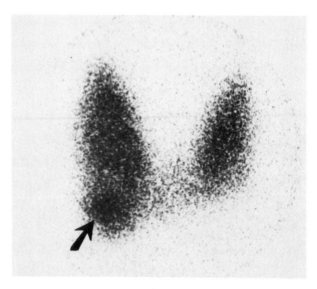

Fig. 15-54. Patient with Hashimoto's thyroiditis had ^{123}I scintigram because of palpable nodule in lower pole of right lobe of thyroid. Scintiphoto showed enlarged right lobe with accentuated uptake at tip of its lower pole plus small region of slightly reduced uptake between lower pole and midpoint. Nodule corresponded to region of accentuated uptake identified by arrow. Following oral administration of perchlorate, patient's ^{123}I uptake dropped over 50% in 1 hour.

administration and a second uptake determination 1 to 2 hours afterwards. Normally, iodine is rapidly organified once it enters the gland and is not exchangeable with the extrathyroid-free iodine pool; perchlorate administration will not alter the normal glandular iodine content (indirectly being studied in this instance by the RAI uptake test). In Hashimoto's thyroiditis or congenital enzymatic organification defects, however, the second determination will show a marked drop compared to the first as the intrathyroidal, nonorganified iodine passes out of the gland and cannot be replaced since the trapping mechanism is blocked by perchlorate. This patient's RAI uptake determination dropped over 50% in 1 hour following perchlorate administration.

Fig. 15-55 shows a ^{123}I scintigram of a euthyroid female who was first seen with a left-sided neck mass (the right lobe of the thyroid was not palpable). The scan showed the mass to correspond to an enlarged left lobe that had "warm" and "cold" nodules scattered throughout. The scan was unchanged from one obtained in the past and the mass was clinically stable. This represents agenesis of the right lobe of the thyroid with a nontoxic multinodular goiter on the left. The probability of a malignancy in this situation is much lower than if only a solitary nodule were present; the incidence of malignancy would increase if the patient were younger, however. Thyroid malignancies may coexist with other thyroid diseases including Hashimoto's thyroiditis, toxic adenomas, focal nodular hyperplasia, and metastases to the thyroid (Kim and Mattar, 1976; Livadas et al., 1977). Multiple "cold" nodules may also be seen in multifocal thyroiditis (perchlorate discharge test negative in this case).

Thyroid hemiagenesis is a rare condition; only 36 cases have been previously reported (Avramides et al., 1977). It occurs six times more commonly in females than males and involves the left lobe three times more commonly than the right. The etiology is not understood. Some suggest a double origin of the thyroid on the basis of its dual blood supply from the superior and inferior thyroid arteries (Das, 1962); a single, unpaired primordium originating from the endo-

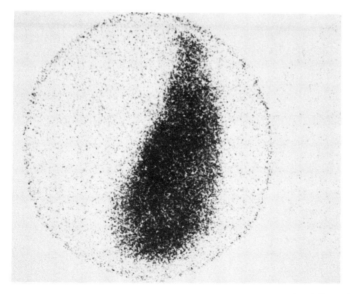

Fig. 15-55. Long-standing neck mass in woman proved to be nontoxic, multinodular goiter in solitary left lobe of thyroid (thyroid hemiagenesis).

derm as a pharyngeal diverticulum between the first and second branchial
arches, and two lateral anlagen forming
from the ventral portion of the fourth
branchial pouches, which ultimately
join with the medial section to form the
gland. The pharyngeal section supposedly contributes to the thyroglossal duct
while presumably the lower segments
form the lobes. Hemiagenesis occurs
even less frequently than total agenesis
(Avramides et al., 1977).

This section has dealt only with one
limited aspect of thyroid scanning—the
assessment of a neck mass. Conceivably,
an unknown neck mass might require the
combined use of salivary, gallium, and
thyroid scanning before full assessment
is completed. A substernal chest mass of
thyroid origin can also be detected by
scintigraphy, thus eliminating various
thoracic tumors or vascular abnormalities
from consideration. Symmetric enlargement of the gland as might occur with
Graves' disease or other thyroid abnormalities were not discussed, as a thyroid
etiology would usually be more obvious
and not pose a problem in the differential
diagnosis of a neck mass. Furthermore, a
variety of in vitro tests, including radioimmunoassays, have not been discussed as they are beyond the scope of
this section.

Brain

Radionuclide brain scintigraphy occurs
in two separate phases: dynamic and
static. Dynamic scintigraphy (scintiangiography) follows the cerebral course
of radionuclide during its early, vascular phase and is especially important
in detecting arteriovenous malformations (AVM's), early strokes, hypervascular brain tumors, and other abnormalities
that result in alterations of normal blood
flow through the brain. Static scintigraphy is mainly an assessment of the integrity of the blood-brain barrier, which may
be broken down by tumors, abscesses,
strokes, and so forth, although hypervascular lesions may be seen using blood
pool agents such as ^{131}I or ^{99m}Tc-labeled
albumin or red cells, or ^{113m}In transferrin.
A scintillation camera must be used for

dynamic studies, but either it or a rectilinear scanner is suitable for static examinations.

The sequence of brain scintigraphy is
relatively straightforward. Following the
positioning of a patient before a scintillation camera, a small volume of radionuclide is rapidly injected into an antecubital vein. The tracer's course through the
brain is recorded in rapid sequence on
photographic film or processed by a digital computer. ^{99m}Tc DTPA can be used as
a standard brain-imaging agent (up to 15
to 25 mCi in adults), which gives a 0.3 rad
total body dose (McAfee, Subramanian,
and Esser, 1975). ^{99m}Tc pertechnetate
may also be used, but premedication
with oral perchlorate to block the choroid
plexus is desirable since the latter will
show up on the subsequent pertechnetate brain scan and may prove to be a
diagnostic problem; such premedication
is unnecessary with ^{99m}Tc DTPA, however.

A further advantage of ^{99m}Tc DTPA
over pertechnetate is the shorter time
required from injection to onset of static
scanning. A 3 to 4 hour delay is necessary
when using ^{99m}Tc pertechnetate to assure
the highest accuracy in brain tumor detection (Gates, Dore, and Taplin, 1971),
whereas a 1 to 2 hour delay will be adequate for ^{99m}Tc DTPA. These delays are
necessary to achieve the high tumor-to-
normal brain count ratios that result in
greater tumor detectability. DTPA is
cleared from the body (mainly vascular
background) by the kidneys at a faster
rate than pertechnetate, thus allowing
earlier scanning without loss of accuracy.
Using an appropriate delay, radionuclide
brain scan accuracy in tumor detection is
as high as 93% (Gates, Dore, and Taplin,
1971). Brain tumor identification is based
on the localized disruption of the blood-
brain barrier by the neoplasm resulting
in an abnormal tracer accumulation in
the lesion (Fig. 15-56). Astrocytomas
(especially of higher grades), meningiomas, glioblastomas, acoustic neuromas,
and various metastatic carcinomas (including lung and breast), adenocarcinomas, and sarcomas are identifiable by
radionuclide brain scanning. New com-

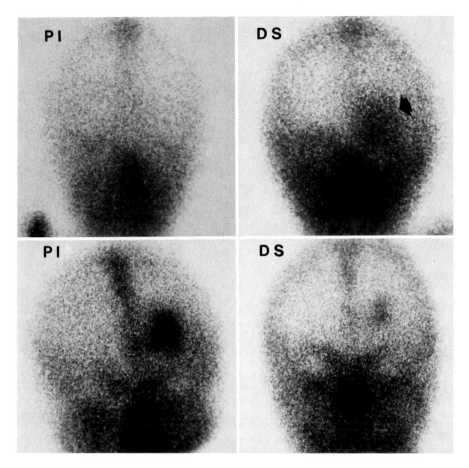

Fig. 15-56. Importance of proper time sequence for brain imaging is illustrated by comparing anterior scintigrams obtained immediately postinjection, *PI,* versus 1-hour delayed static, *DS,* image. Upper panel shows astrocytoma that was not evident on PI view but was well seen on DS images (arrow); this effect of improved tumor detection on delayed static views is also true for abscesses and strokes. Lower panel shows AVM that was well seen on PI view and then "faded" with time; this is typical for AVM.

puted tomographic (CT) brain scans have a somewhat higher accuracy in tumor detection (up to 96%).

Dynamic scintigraphy (an examination that cannot be performed by CT scanners) is crucial in evaluation of patients with AVM's or strokes of recent onset. Static radionuclide scans and CT brain scans may not always detect these abnormalities (Gates, Fishman, and Segall, 1977, 1978), which are grossly obvious on scintiangiograms (Fig. 15-57). Only 17% of static radionuclide brain scans are abnormal during the first week of an ischemic stroke, although 50% of hemor-rhagic infarctions may be positive during the same time. Most strokes produce abnormal static scans during the second or third week (Fig. 15-58) although up to 30% will remain negative on serial studies. The detection of a stroke on a static brain scan is improved following a 1 to 2 hour delay after ^{99m}Tc DTPA injection. The scintiangiogram may be abnormal throughout the entire scanning sequence, however, despite normal static studies; the radionuclide diagnosis thus may depend entirely on dynamic scintigraphy. A neoplasm should be suspected if a static brain scan is strongly positive

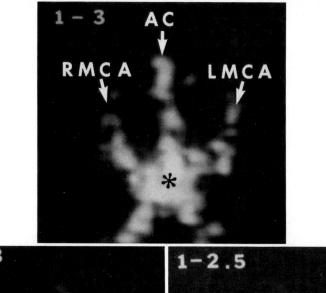

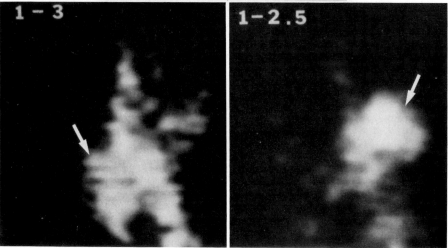

Fig. 15-57. Dynamic scintigraphy (scintiangiography) is effective means of visualizing intracerebral vessels. Top illustration is normal patient and shows anterior cerebral arteries, *AC,* left and right middle cerebral arteries, *LMCA* and *RMCA,* and circle of Willis area*; numbers indicate time interval in seconds following tracer arrival in brain shown on this computer processed picture. Lower left image shows lack of RMCA visualization in stroke patient (see Fig. 15-58) while lower right is AVM shown in Fig. 15-56. These images were obtained with same intravenously administered tracer used to perform static brain scintigrams.

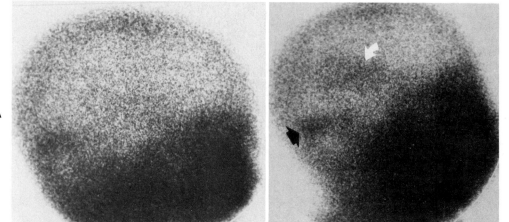

Fig. 15-58. One day following RMCA infarction patient had brain scintigram: dynamic phase was abnormal (Fig. 15-57, left lower image) but the delayed static view, **A,** was normal. **B,** Fourteen days later, repeat study was performed at which time delayed static image disclosed breakdown in blood-brain barrier that was in distribution of RMCA (white arrow): dynamic study was still abnormal (black arrow—normal venous sinuses).

during the first week of a presumed "stroke." In contradistinction to tumors and strokes, AVM's are best seen (if at all) on static brain scans obtained immediately following tracer injection since they rapidly "fade" with time owing to clearance of radionuclide from the vascular compartment (Fig. 15-56).

Hypervascular or hypovascular abnormalities in the great vessels of the neck are also detectable by scintiangiography. Traumatic occlusion of the carotid artery secondary to a transoral penetrating wound (Fig. 15-59), hypervascular neck metastases of thyroid carcinoma (Makler, Charkes, and Malmud, 1977), and chemodectomas of the jugular glomus (Alavi et al., 1976) have been identified by this procedure.

Subdural hematomas or hygromas are evident on radionuclide brain scans as crescent-shaped accumulations of tracer over the surface of the brain seen best on static anterior and posterior views (Fig. 15-60). As with cerebral infarctions, a subdural hematoma may not be evident on static scintigrams during the first week of its presence. Ninety percent of subdural hematomas may be identified if scanned 10 days or more following injury but only 50% if scanned sooner (Maynard, 1969), although scintiangiography may show a peripheral avascular area in the involved region. CT scanning has made a major contribution since it can differentiate blood (as in subdural hematomas) from cerebral spinal fluid (as in hygromas). Before attributing a crescentic uptake of radionuclide to a subdural hematoma, however, one must be sure that scalp hematomas and skull trauma are not present since they may produce similar scan features.

Inflammatory disease in the subdural

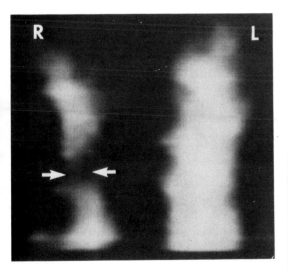

Fig. 15-59. Child fell while running and landed on pointed stick, which went into her mouth and through oropharynx. Stick pierced the right internal carotid artery resulting in thrombus formation and massive stroke. Several months later vascular surgeon wished to determine patency of carotid without having to initially perform arteriogram. Dynamic scintigraphy of neck (anterior view) showed narrowed, scarred right carotid (arrows point at site of old penetration); left side was normal. (From Gates, G. F. 1976. Proceedings Sixth Symposium on Sharing Computer Programs and Technology in Nuclear Medicine, 204-212.)

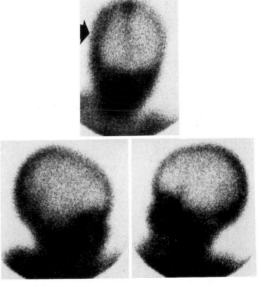

Fig. 15-60. Crescent-shaped area of peripheral radionuclide uptake, best seen on anterior or posterior views, is typical of subdural hematoma. Arrow points to abnormal region on this anterior view while right lateral view shows only slight haziness: frontal view accentuates difference between two sides. Membrane enclosing subdural hematoma is believed to accumulate radionuclide, causing scintigraphic abnormality.

space or over the surface of the brain can be detected by radionuclide scanning where the process is seen as a peripheral, superficial accumulation of tracer (Fig. 15-61). At the present time the role of CT scanning in such conditions is inconclusive; the CT scan performed in the patient shown in Fig. 15-61 did not correctly diagnose the subdural empyema that was present. Cerebral abscesses are also evident by brain scanning as shown in Fig. 15-31, *A*. Delayed scanning increases the probability of abscess, brain tumor, and cerebral infarction imaging. Hyperemia caused by scalp, skull, or sinus abnormalities may be identified as a regional area of nuclide uptake on a scintigram obtained immediately after tracer injection, but following a delay, the uptake will diminish in contradistinction to tumors, abscesses, and infarctions. A large AVM may also appear less obvious on delayed static images compared to an immediate postinjection scintigram. Dynamic scintigraphy of an AVM is diagnostic, however.

Cerebrospinal fluid (CSF) leakage into the nose or pharynx may be assessed following intrathecal administration of appropriate radionuclides such as ^{99m}Tc, ^{131}I albumin, or ^{111}In DTPA. Scintigraphy will show the site of leakage, which can be further localized by placing cotton pledgets in the drainage sites of different sinus cavities. The activity in the pledgets (determined after removal and placement in a well counter) can narrowly localize the drainage route of leaking CSF.

Lungs

The lungs were the last major organs to be visualized by radionuclide scanning owing to the lack of a suitable particulate

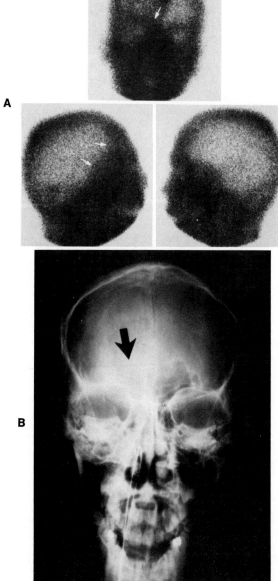

Fig. 15-61. A, Febrile comatose child had cerebral scintigram showing diffuse radionuclide uptake over anterior portion of right frontal lobe. Anterior view showed right-sided uptake to be accentuated in area of right frontal sinus (arrow). Right lateral view confirmed increased frontal uptake. Surgery was performed rapidly thereafter revealing subdural empyema in area shown to be abnormal on scintigram. Surface of brain was inflamed, which probably resulted in breakdown of blood-brain barrier (thus accounting for abnormal tracer accumulation); there was no membrane enclosing acute empyema. **B,** Child's skull radiograph shows right frontal (arrow) and ethmoid sinus opacification. Accentuated uptake in right frontal sinus seen on scintigraphy was probably result of hypervascularity. Computed tomographic scan done at same time failed to disclose empyema.

test material. In 1963 Taplin and associates introduced ^{131}I-labeled macroaggregated albumin (MAA) and described its use in performing perfusion lung scintigraphy. Since then, this test of regional lung perfusion has gained worldwide acceptance.

Perfusion lung scanning is based on the temporary occlusion of a tiny fraction of the pulmonary capillary bed by the intravenously injected radioaggregates. The particles used most commonly now are ^{99m}Tc-labeled MAA or microspheres (MSP). These particles vary in size from 10 to 90 μ for MAA to 10 to 45 μ for MSP. They exceed the diameter of the smallest capillary they encounter and thus temporarily impact in the pulmonary bed when injected in a systemic vein. The human lung has an average of 300 million pulmonary arterioles and 280 billion capillary units (Weibel, 1963). An injection of MAA may contain 400,000 particles less than 20 μ in size and 200,000 particles greater than 20 μ. Ninety-five percent are trapped in the lungs of individuals lacking right-to-left transcardiac or transpulmonary shunts (Gates and Goris, 1977), resulting in a temporary obstruction of only one in several hundred thousand capillaries by the small particles and one in 1500 arterioles by the larger particles. This small percentage of vascular blockage accounts for the huge safety margin of over 1000-fold for lung scanning in normal humans. The half-time removal rate of these biodegradable particles from the lungs is 3 to 5 hours (Gates and Goris, 1977). Once they undergo fragmentation, the tiny particles enter the systemic circulation and eventually undergo phagocytosis by the Küpffer cells of the liver.

In three circumstances caution should be used in performing perfusion scintigraphy. An allergy to human serum albumin (from which the particles are compounded) is an obvious contraindication. Scanning in cases of severe pulmonary arterial hypertension should be judiciously considered since the restricted caliber of the more proximal arterioles may trap a larger proportion of the injected radioaggregates, which in turn could further elevate pulmonary artery pressure. Large right-to-left shunts will allow a fraction of the radioaggregates to enter the systemic circulation, which then transiently impact in the capillary beds of the brain, kidneys, liver, and so forth. However, reduced amounts of these particles have been injected in cyanotic children for the purpose of quantitating cardiac shunting (Gates, 1974; Gates, Orme, and Dore, 1971, 1974, 1975). No adverse reaction has ever occurred following the administration of such low doses, the injected volume of which is as low as 0.1 ml.

The usual clinical indication for performing a perfusion lung scan is the suspicion of a pulmonary embolism. The embolism will produce a perfusion defect (which is usually segmental or subsegmental) on the scan since the vascular occlusion will block the peripheral passage of injected radioaggregates. It is important to perform the study soon after the onset of clinical symptoms and before radiographic changes may develop. It is essential that a chest radiograph be obtained at the same time as the perfusion lung scan to exclude obvious parenchymal pulmonary abnormalities such as pneumonia, atelectasis, infarction, or chronic obstructive airway disease. These conditions may also produce perfusion abnormalities (although not necessarily segmental or subsegmental in distribution). The probability of a pulmonary embolism producing a perfusion defect increases when the chest radiograph is normal. The most definite means of diagnosing a pulmonary embolism is by pulmonary angiography, which of course is an invasive procedure with an associated risk.

Repeat perfusion lung scans in patients with pulmonary emboli can vary from the initial studies because of continual showering of emboli or resolution following anticoagulant therapy (Fig. 15-62). James, Menn, and Moser (1978) reported rapid resolution of a documented massive pulmonary embolism within 51 hours of the start of the heparin therapy.

Ventilation lung scans are extremely useful when performed along with the perfusion studies. Many parenchymal

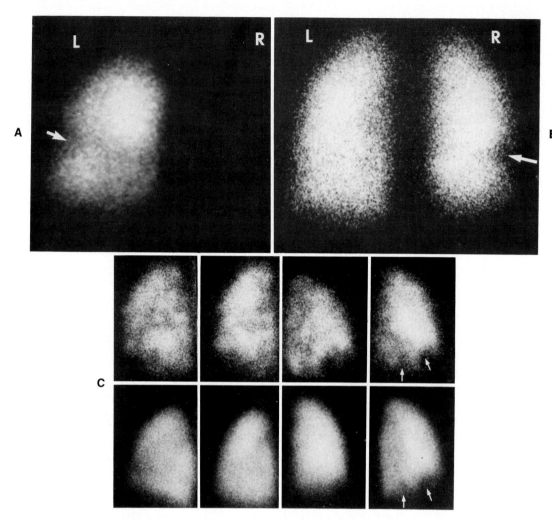

Fig. 15-62. A, Massive pulmonary embolization. This posterior perfusion lung scintigram was performed with ^{99m}Tc MAA a few hours after acute onset of dyspnea and chest pain. There was no pulmonary artery perfusion on right; left lung had several defects in lower lobe (one of which is indicated by arrow). **B,** Following anticoagulant therapy, repeat perfusion lung scintigram was performed 18 days later. Perfusion in left lung is normal. Right lung perfusion is nearly normal except for lower defect (arrow). **C,** Another patient with dyspnea and chest pain had perfusion lung scintigram shown on top row (left posterior oblique, left posterior, right posterior, and right posterior oblique views from left to right). She had multiple perfusion defects owing to showers of emboli. Three days later repeat study (lower row) showed nearly normal scan except for few persistent right basilar defects indicated by arrows on both studies.

lung diseases, such as obstructive airway disease, may result in perfusion defects. Taplin (1978) reports that in his experience obstructive airway disease is a far more frequent cause of radiographically unexplained perfusion abnormalities than is uncomplicated pulmonary embolization. Pulmonary ventilation can be assessed by use of radioaerosols or radioactive gases (that is, ^{133}Xe or ^{81m}Kr) as shown in Fig. 15-63. Under most circumstances, pulmonary embolization will initially produce a perfusion defect unaccompanied by any ventilatory disturbance (Fig. 15-64). Obstructive airway disease, however, produces matched ventilation and perfusion defects, many of which are neither segmental nor sub-

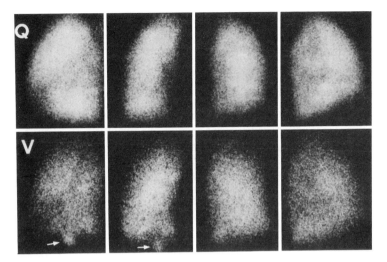

Fig. 15-63. Assessment of pulmonary ventilation, *V,* as well as perfusion, *Q,* can be crucial in diagnosis of pulmonary embolization. Upper row shows posterior perfusion images (left posterior oblique, left posterior, right posterior, and right posterior oblique views from left to right), while lower row shows ventilation obtained by using radiolabeled aerosol (^{99m}Tc-sulfur colloid), which patient inhales. Arrows point to tracer in stomach (owing to patient swallowing aerosol during procedure). This normal study had matched ventilation and perfusion (upper lobes appear to be not quite as well ventilated as perfused since patient was upright for ventilation portion but supine when MAA was injected).

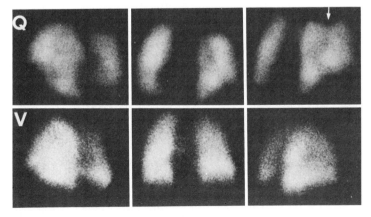

Fig. 15-64. Effects of acute pulmonary embolization are shown by perfusion defect in apex of right upper lobe in this woman (arrow in upper row) (left posterior oblique, left posterior, right posterior, and right posterior oblique views from left to right). Ventilation scan with radioaerosol was normal. Absent perfusion in ventilated lung region is typical of embolization.

segmental (Fig. 15-65). Matched ventilation-perfusion defects have rarely been reported in pulmonary embolization. Speculation has attributed these ventilatory defects to possible localized bronchospasm following embolization (Epstein et al., 1975); some investigators attribute this phenomenon to localized release of serotonin or histamine (Stein et al., 1973). Such ventilatory defects are rare and usually occur only transiently during the acute phase of the embolic episode. Alderson and co-workers (1978) reported an 8.7% incidence of such ventilatory defects occurring in their series of experimental embolization produced in dogs. These infrequent ventilatory abnormalities are not a common cause of ventilation-perfusion mismatching in clinical practice. Alderson's study showed perfusion images revealing the location of 83% of emboli that completely obstructed pulmonary vessels, but only 26% of those causing partial obstruction (presumably radioaggregates could "slip by" a partial obstruction and proceed to move out peripherally). Ninety-seven percent of emboli completely obstructing vessels over 2 mm in diameter were detected by scintigraphy but only 66% of those occluding smaller vessels. The combined use of perfusion and ventilation scintigraphy is the ideal way to study a patient suspected of having pulmonary embolization. Each individual embolus may not always be detected, but since multiple emboli occur in most patients, the probability is high that many of them will be identified by perfusion scintigraphy. The procedure is safe, accurate, and has a low radiation exposure (0.3 rads to the lung and 0.03 rads to the total body for 2 mCi ^{99m}Tc MAA; 0.05 to 0.5 rads to the lungs and 0 to 0.02 rads to the total body for ^{133}Xe) (McAfee and Subramanian and Esser, 1975).

Perfusion lung scintigraphy is also useful in detecting maldistribution of pulmonary flow owing to tumor impingement on major vessels, pulmonary arterial stenosis, or airway obstruction as might occur with an aspirated foreign body (Fig. 15-66). Regional alveolar hypoxia following endobronchial occlusion results in decreased arterial perfusion to the affected lung segment. The alveolar hypoventilation produces acute pulmonary arterial constriction with elevation of pulmonary artery pressure in the hypoxic lung (Apau, Saenz, and Siemsen, 1972). If a suspected endobronchial foreign body or its secondary gross ventilation changes are not radiographically evident, perfusion lung scanning is an easy screening

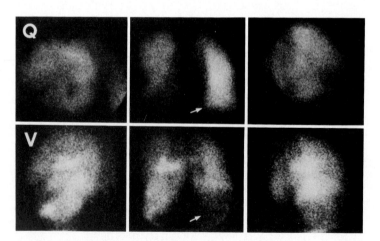

Fig. 15-65. Chronic obstructive pulmonary disease (COPD) may also produce multiple perfusion defects that are generally matched by ventilation abnormalities. Man in this illustration did not have pulmonary embolization but did have many areas of abnormal ventilation and perfusion caused by COPD; notice right lower lobe, which was perfused but not well ventilated (arrows).

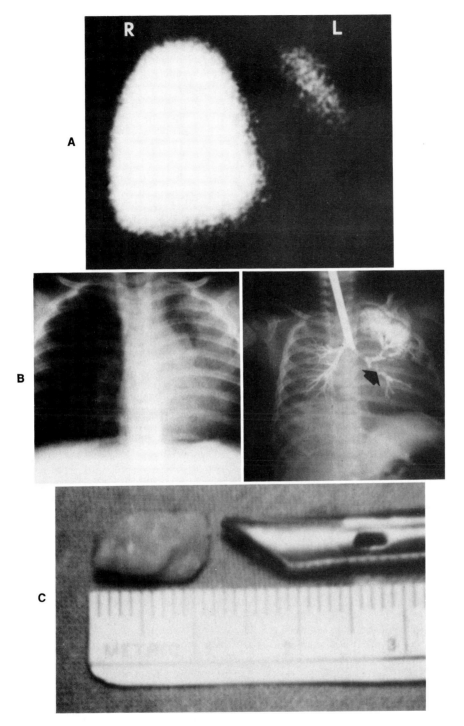

Fig. 15-66. A, Perfusion lung scan (anterior view) in child with chronic cough showed nearly complete absence of perfusion to left lung except for some to upper lobe. **B,** Chest radiograph showed overexpansion of right lung with volume loss on left side. Bronchogram showed normal patency of right side but endobronchial defect on left (arrow), which prevented contrast medium from entering lower lobe. **C,** Foreign body was removed and proved to be aspirated piece of carrot; perfusion defect was due to ventilatory abnormality in affected lung segment. (From Gates, G. F. 1974. Radionuclide scanning in cyanotic heart disease, Springfield, Ill., Charles C Thomas, Publisher.)

test to detect the regional circulatory abnormalities that might be associated with aspirated material.

Once a pulmonary perfusion defect compatible with a pulmonary embolism has been demonstrated, it is very helpful to know its origin. The deep veins of the legs are common sites of embolic origin and can be studied by either contrast venography (a diagnostic radiographic procedure using an iodinated contrast agent) or radionuclide venography. Ennis and Elmes (1977) reported a 95% agreement between radionuclide and contrast venography and a 100% accuracy of the radionuclide method in the diagnosis of popliteal, femoral, and iliac vein thrombosis. Ennis and Elmes' (1977) technique is particularly appealing since the dose of MAA, which would usually be administered in an antecubital vein, is simply divided and injected into a dorsal vein on each foot. Thus the patient receives the benefit of a venogram and perfusion lung scan without added radiation exposure. Recently ^{125}I fibrinogen (DeNardo et al., 1977) and ^{123}I fibrinogen (DeNardo and DeNardo, 1977) have been used in clinical practice. These agents are incorporated into the actual thrombus in the leg, the location of which can be determined by either external counting with a hand-held probe (^{125}I fibrinogen) or total body scintiscanning (^{123}I fibrinogen).

Liver

Following intravenous injection of a radionuclide-labeled colloidal particle (usually ^{99m}Tc-sulfur colloid), the material will undergo phagocytosis by the reticuloendothelial cells of the liver, spleen, and bone marrow. Eighty-five percent of the normal injected dose is thus accumulated by the Küpffer cells of the liver, 10% by the spleen, and 5% by the bone marrow. A 3 mCi dose of ^{99m}Tc-sulfur colloid delivers 0.9 rads to the liver and 0.06 rads to the total body (McAfee, Subramanian, and Esser, 1975).

If a neoplasm, abscess, hematoma, or cyst is located within the liver, the normal uniform hepatic deposition of radiocolloid will be disrupted. The region containing the mass will appear devoid of tracer since such abnormalities lack the Küpffer cells necessary for phagocytosis (Fig. 15-67). Liver scanning has about a 70% to 85% accuracy in the diagnosis of liver disease (Holder and Saenger, 1975; Lomonaco et al., 1975; Rasmussen et al., 1973), although some series report an over 90% accuracy (Rosenfield and Treves, 1974). Multiplicity of defects can represent metastatic malignancy, multiple cysts, or abscesses, while solitary defects can likewise represent primary or metastatic malignancies, a large abscess, or a solitary cyst. There is nothing characteristic about any particular defect that will reliably lead to a correct diagnosis regarding its etiology (with the possible exception of the rare hepatic adenoma that avidly accumulates radiocolloid and appears as a "hot" nodule).

Dynamic scintigraphy, however, can contribute greatly to a diagnosis. Hypervascular masses (for example, lesions receiving early increased hepatic artery perfusion) have been shown to be hepatoblastomas, hepatomas, hepatic adenomas, and cavernous hemangiomas or hemangioendotheliomas (Gates, Miller, and Stanley, 1978). Hypovascular masses are usually metastases, cysts, abscesses, or a huge primary hepatic tumor as listed above, which has undergone internal hemorrhage or necrosis (although a hypervascular rim may still persist). Hepatic ultrasonography can further define the nature of an hepatic mass and separate solid tumors from abscesses and cysts (Gates and Miller, 1977). Bryan and co-workers (1977) recommended radionuclide scanning as the screening test of choice for hepatic masses except in lymphoma patients where ultrasonography was suggested as the initial test. Ultrasonography was recommended as the next test to be used in studying scintigraphic abnormalities instead of CT body scanning.

A variety of other hepatic disorders can be evaluated by liver scanning, including cirrhosis, hepatitis, fatty infiltration, and diffuse granulomatous diseases. Furthermore, biliary patency can be evaluated by ^{131}I-rose bengal or the newer [99m]Tc-

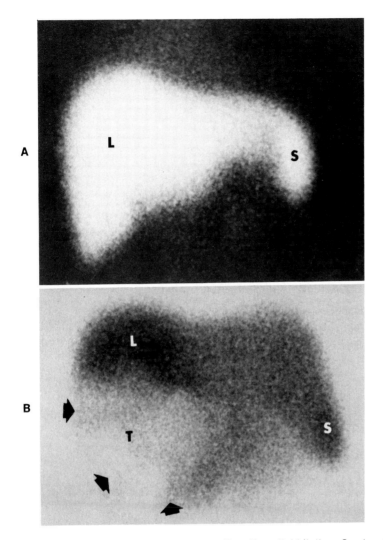

Fig. 15-67. A, Normal anterior liver scintigram using ⁹⁹ᵐTc-sulfur colloid (*L,* liver; *S,* spleen). **B,** Scintigram of patient with poorly differentiated sarcoma metastatic to right lobe. Tumor, *T,* is outlined with arrows; it does not accumulate sulfur colloid since it lacks normal Küpffer cells.

labeled biliary agents. The combined simultaneous use of liver-lung scanning (produced by two injections; one of radiocolloid and the other of radioaggregate) is useful in evaluating the right subdiaphragmatic space for a mass such as an abscess. The reader is referred to the literature for these applications.

Blood volume

The determination of a patient's blood volume is very helpful when planning fluid and/or blood replacement especially in extensively burned patients, those with cardiac or renal insufficiency, or postoperatively following extensive surgery. Currently the most common method used for making such a determination is based on the dilution of a 5 μCi dose of ¹²⁵I-human serum albumin (HSA). Ten minutes following intravenous administration of ¹²⁵I HSA, a venous blood sample is drawn and placed in a heparinized tube. A measured amount of blood is then counted in a well counter (Fig. 15-3, *B*) and compared to a sample of the injected dose (in the form of a standard). The dilution that occurs is directly proportional to total blood volume. Plasma volume can be similarly measured by counting a sample of plasma instead of blood. Normal values can be derived from nomograms based on body height and weight (Arnold, 1976) or based on weight alone (Maynard, 1969: total blood volume = 68 to 88 ml/kg, plasma volume = 39 to 44 ml/kg, RBC volume by interpolation = 30 to 38 ml/kg; Freeman and Blaufox, 1977: plasma volume for men = 36 to 66 ml/kg and women = 35 to 55 ml/kg). Unfortunately, there can be considerable normal individual deviation in plasma volume compared to population norms based on height and weight nomograms, thus resulting in a normal range varying as much as ±20% of the mean (Freeman and Blaufox, 1977). The test, however, is quite reproducible within any individual in a steady state (that is, repeat studies agree within 5%). Therefore it is best to perform serial studies in patients rather than relying on a single determination. Whenever possible, a preoperative determination should be done to serve as a baseline value for future comparison if significant postoperative fluid (including blood) replacement is anticipated.

Red cell mass can also be separately determined by drawing a sample of the patient's blood, labeling the RBC's with ^{51}Cr, and then reinjecting them. After waiting 10 minutes, a sample is withdrawn and RBC volume determined by the dilutional method. This is a more direct (and probably more accurate) means of determining RBC volume compared to subtracting ^{125}I-HSA determined plasma volume from similarly determined whole blood volume. It is a lengthy process, however, and many institutions use the ^{125}I HSA method alone.

The following is an example of the utility of performing serial blood volume determinations. The patient was a 14-year-old girl undergoing renal dialysis. Her nephrologists wished to know the changes in plasma volume that occurred immediately following dialysis. Thus whole blood and plasma volume determinations were performed immediately before and after renal dialysis using [125]I

HSA. A preinjection blood sample was taken before the second determination for the purpose of background subtraction (since both tests were performed within hours of each other on the same day). The red cell volume was estimated by subtracting plasma volume from whole blood volume.

	Predialysis	Postdialysis
Whole blood volume (ml)	3108	2079
Plasma volume (ml)	2706	1679
Red cell volume (ml)	402	400

The striking changes in plasma and whole blood volumes following dialysis are readily apparent. Equally important is the demonstration of an unchanged red cell volume, a feature that supports the accuracy of this test (red cell volume should not change following dialysis, only plasma volume: this radionuclide test showed that all changes in whole blood volume could be attributed to decreased plasma volume).

Heart

It is probably altogether fitting to conclude this chapter with a brief discussion of nuclear cardiology since this area is undergoing spectacular growth and opening new vistas in clinical medicine. Four basic types of procedures are available for clinical application: myocardial infarct imaging, myocardial perfusion studies, assessment of ventricular function, and cardiac shunt quantitation. Myocardial infarct imaging can be performed using standard bone scanning agents such as ^{99m}Tc pyrophosphate. There is an intramitochondrial accumulation of calcium in infarcted myocardial cells, which has been offered as an explanation for pyrophosphate accumulation in these regions. Scanning shows the infarcted region as a "hot spot," thus allowing for assessment of its extent.

Thallium 201 is currently used to assess ventricular perfusion. This agent may be given intravenously at rest or during exercise to detect regions of poor or absent myocardial perfusion, which appear as "cold" spots. Such abnormal areas may be due to ischemia or fibrosis.

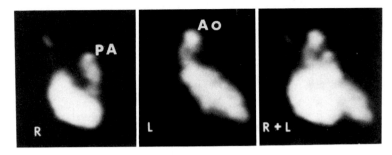

Fig. 15-68. Nuclear angiocardiogram showing right heart phase, *R*, with pulmonary artery, *PA*; left heart phase, *L*, with aorta, *Ao*; and composite of both images, *R + L*. Various parameters of cardiac function can be determined after such images have been generated. These computer processed images were obtained following intravenous injection of ^{99m}Tc pertechnetate.

This procedure is rapidly gaining acceptance as a screening procedure for coronary artery disease or chest pain prior to coronary arteriography.

Ventricular function is assessed following injection of either ^{99m}Tc pertechnetate or ^{99m}Tc-labeled albumin or red cells. The left ventricular ejection fraction is rapidly assessed; this value is useful in determining ventricular performance and can be used as a means of assessing response to therapy. Abnormalities in ventricular wall motion, such as aneurysms or regions of poor contractility, can also be detected during these studies.

Nuclear angiocardiography (Fig. 15-68) and detection of cardiac shunts are quite useful techniques in pediatric cardiology. A cardiac murmur may be assessed without resorting to cardiac catheterization. All of these studies mentioned previously may be performed, repeatedly if necessary, on an outpatient basis, allowing for continual follow-up on cardiac abnormalities (Alderman, 1976; Kan, Hopkins, and Carroll, 1977; McLaughlin, 1976; Spies, 1978; Wagner, 1976; Werner, 1977).

REFERENCES

Alarion-Segovia, D., et al. 1971. Radioisotopic evaluation of salivary gland dysfunction in Sjögrens syndrome, Am. J. Roentgenol. **112**:373.

Alavi, A., et al. 1976. Radionuclide angiography in evaluation of chemodectomas of the jugular glomus, Radiology **121**:673.

Alderman, E. L. 1976. Angiographic indicators of left ventricular function, J.A.M.A. **236**:1055.

Alderson, P. O., Krohn, K. A., and Welch, M. J. 1976. Radiopharmaceuticals. In Gottschalk, A., and Potchen, E. J., eds.: Diagnostic nuclear medicine, Baltimore, The Williams & Wilkins Co.

Alderson, P. O., et al. 1978. Ventilation-perfusion lung imaging and selective pulmonary angiography in dogs with experimental pulmonary embolism, J. Nucl. Med. **19**:164.

Alexander, J. M. 1976. Radionuclide bone scanning in the diagnosis of lesions of the maxillofacial region, J. Oral Surg. **34**:249.

Alexander, J. M., Alaui, A., and Hansell, J. R. 1975. Bone imaging in evaluation of jaw lesions, J. Nucl. Med. **16**:511. (Abstr.)

Alexander, W. D. et al. 1966. Comparison of the concentrating ability of the human salivary gland for bromine, iodine, and technetium, Arch. Oral Biol. **11**:1205.

Apau, R. L., Saenz, R., and Siemsen, J. K. 1972. Bloodless lung due to bronchial obstruction, J. Nucl. Med. **13**:561.

Ardran, G. M. 1951. Bone destruction not demonstrable by radiography, Br. J. Radiol. **24**:107.

Arey, L. B. 1954. Developmental anatomy, ed. 6, Philadelphia, W. B. Saunders Co., pp. 237-238.

Arft, S. C. 1975. Radioisotope bone scanning as a diagnostic aid relative to bone lesions of the jaws, Masters thesis, Horace H. Rackham School of Graduate Studies, The University of Michigan.

Arnold, J. E. 1976. Blood volume. In Gotteschalk, A., and Potchen, E. J., eds.: Diagnostic nuclear medicine, Baltimore, The Williams & Wilkins Co.

Arnold, J. E., and Pinsky, S. 1976. Comparison of ^{99m}Tc and ^{123}I for thyroid imaging, J. Nucl. Med. **17**:261.

Atkins, H. L. 1975. The thyroid. In Freeman, L. M., and Johnson, P. M., eds.: Clinical scintillation imaging, ed. 2, New York, Grune & Stratton, Inc.

Ausband, J. R., Kittrell, G. J., and Cowan, R. J. 1967. Radioisotope scanning for parotid oncocytoma, Arch. Otolaryngol. **93**:628.

Avramides, A., et al. 1977. Thyroid hemiagenesis, Clin. Nucl. Med. **2**:310.

Bachman, A. L., and Sproul, E. E. 1955. Correlation of radiographic and autopsy findings in suspected metastases of the spine, Bull. N.Y. Acad. Med. **31**:146.

Bailey, T. B., et al. 1973. A new adjuvant in testis tumor staging: gallium-67 citrate, J. Urol. **110**:387.

Bauer, G. C. H. 1958. Skeletal metabolism in humans studied with body surface counting of Sr-85 and Ca-47. In Exterman, R. L., ed.: UNESCO international conference on radioisotopes, Paris, 1957, vol. 4, New York, Pergamon Press, Inc.

Bekerman, C., and Hoffer, P. B. 1975. Salivary gland uptake of Ga-67 citrate following radiation therapy, J. Nucl. Med. **16**:514.

Belanger, M. A., Beauchamp, J. M., and Neitzschman, H. R. 1975. Gallium uptake in benign tumor of liver, J. Nucl. Med. **16**:470.

Bell, E. G., McAfee, J., and Constable, W. C. 1969. Local radiation damage to bone and marrow demonstrated by radioisotopic imaging, Radiology **92**:1083.

Blahd, W. H., ed. 1971. Nuclear medicine, ed. 2, New York, McGraw-Hill Book Co.

Blau, M., Bender, M. A., and Nagler, W. 1962. Fluorine-18: a new isotope for bone scanning, J. Nucl. Med. **3**:332.

Borak, J. 1942. Relationship between the clinical and roentgenological findings in bone metastases, Surg. Gynecol. Obstet. **75**:599.

Brown, M. L., et al. 1977. Facial bone scanning by emission tomography, J. Nucl. Med. **18**:1184.

Bryan, P. J., et al. 1977. Correlation of computed tomography, gray scale ultrasonography, and radionuclide imaging of the liver in detecting space-occupying processes, Radiology **124**:387.

Burgen, A. S. V., Terroux, K. G., and Gonder, E. 1959. Sites of transfer of sodium, potassium and iodine in the parotid duct system of the dog, Can. J. Biochem. Physiol. **37**:359.

Charkes, N. D., Sklaroff, D. M., and Young, I. 1966. A critical analysis of strontium bone scanning for detection of metastatic cancer, Am. J. Roentgenol. **96**:647.

Cohen, B., Logothetopoulos, J. H., and Myant, N. B. 1955. Autoradiographic localization of I-131 in the salivary glands of the hamster, Nature **176**:1268.

Coleman, R. E., et al. 1974. Efficacy of skull imaging in routine bone scanning, J. Nucl. Med. **15**:1185.

Das, P. 1962. Congenital absence of one thyroid lobe, J. Ind. Med. Assoc. **39**:302.

DeLand, F. H., et al. 1974. ^{67}Ga-citrate in untreated primary lung cancer: preliminary report of cooperative group, J. Nucl. Med. **15**:408.

DeNardo, G. L., Jacobson, S. J., and Raventos, A. 1972. ^{85}Sr bone scan in neoplastic disease, Semin. Nucl. Med. **2**:18.

DeNardo, G. L., et al. 1977. Assessment of conventional criteria for the early diagnosis of thrombophlebitis with the ^{125}I-fibrinogen uptake test, Radiology **125**:765.

DeNardo, S. J., and DeNardo, G. L. 1977. Iodine-123-fibrinogen scintigraphy, Semin. Nucl. Med. **7**:245.

Dudley, H. C., Imire, G. W., Jr. and Istock, J. 1950. Deposition of radiogallium (^{72}Ga) in proliferating tissues, Radiology **73**:571.

Early, J. P., Razzak, M. A., and Sodee, D. B. 1979. Textbook of nuclear medicine technology, ed. 3, St. Louis, The C. V. Mosby Co.

Edelstyn, G. A., Gillespie, P. J., and Grebbell, F. S. 1967. The radiological demonstration of osseous metastasis: experimental observations, Clin. Radiol. **18**:158.

Edwards, C. L., and Hayes, R. L. 1969. Tumor scanning with ^{67}gallium citrate, J. Nucl. Med. **10**:103.

Edwards, C. L., and Hayes, R. L. 1970. Scanning malignant neoplasms with ^{67}gallium, J.A.M.A. **212**:1182.

Ennis, J. T., and Elmes, R. J. 1977. Radionuclide venography in the diagnosis of deep vein thrombosis, Radiology **125**:441.

Epstein, J., et al. 1975. Acute pulmonary embolus associated with transient ventilatory defect, J. Nucl. Med. **16**:1017.

Evens, R. G., Ashburn, W., and Bartter, F. C. 1969. Strontium^{85} scanning of a "brown tumor" in a patient with parathyroid carcinoma, Br. J. Radiol. **42**:224.

Fitzer, P. M. 1977. Radionuclide angiography—brain and bone imaging in craniofacial fibrous dysplasia (CFD): case report, J. Nucl. Med. **18**:709.

Fordham, E. W. 1976. Bone scanning. In Gottschalk, A., and Potchen, E. J. eds.: Diagnostic nuclear medicine: Golden's diagnostic radiology, Baltimore, The Williams & Wilkins Co.

Fordham, E. W., and Ramachandran, P. C. 1974. Radionuclide imaging in osseous trauma, Semin. Nucl. Med. **4**:411.

Frankel, R. S., et al. 1974. Clinical correlations of ^{67}Ga and skeletal whole body radionuclide studies with radiography in Ewing's sarcoma, Radiology **110**:597.

Freeman, L. M. and Blaufox, M. D., eds. 1973a. Instrumentation in nuclear medicine. I, Semin. Nucl. Med. **3** (Jul).

Freeman, L. M., and Blaufox, M. D., eds. 1973b. Instrumentation in nuclear medicine. II, Semin. Nucl. Med. **3** (Oct).

Freeman, L. M., and Blaufox, M. D., eds. 1974. Radiopharmaceuticals, Semin. Nucl. Med. **4** (Jul).

Freeman, L. M., and Blaufox, M. D., eds. 1976. Physicians' desk reference for radiology and nuclear medicine 1977-78. Oradell, N.J., Medical Economics Co., p. 38.

Freeman, L. M., and Blaufox, M. D., eds. 1977. Advances in imaging instrumentation, Semin. Nucl. Med. **7** (Oct).

Freeman, L. M., and Blaufox, M. D. Physicians' desk reference for radiology and nuclear medicine, Oradell, N.J., Medical Economics Co. 1977-78, pp. 17-19.

Freeman, L. M., and Johnson, P. M., eds. 1975. Clinical scintillation imaging, ed. 2, New York, Grune & Stratton Inc.

Garcia, D. A., et al. 1977. Jaw imaging in clinical dental diagnoses, J. Nucl. Med. **18**:604. (Abstr.)

Gates, G. A. 1972. Radiosialographic aspects of salivary gland disorders, Laryngoscope **32**:115.

Gates, G. F. 1974. Radionuclide scanning in cyanotic heart disease, Springfield, Ill., Charles C Thomas, Publisher.

Gates, G. F., and Dore, E. K. 1975. Detection of

craniosynostosis by bone scanning, Radiology **115**:665.

Gates, G. F., Goris, M. L. 1976. Maxillary-facial abnormalities assessed by bone imaging, Radiology **121**:677.

Gates, G. F., and Goris, M. L. 1977. Suitability of radiopharmaceuticals for determining right-to-left shunting, J. Nucl. Med. **18**:255.

Gates, G. F., and Miller, J. H. 1977. Combined radionuclide and ultrasonic assessment of upper abdominal masses in children, Am. J. Roentgenol. **128**:773.

Gates, G. F., Dore, E. K., and Taplin, G. V. 1971. Internal brain scanning with sodium pertechnetate Tc-99m for tumor detectability, J.A.M.A. **215**:85.

Gates, G. F., Fishman, L. S., and Segall, H. D. 1977. Assessment of cerebral perfusion in childhood strokes, J. Nucl. Med. **18**:596.

Gates, G. F., Fishman, L. S., and Segall, H. D. 1978. Scintigraphic detection of congenital intracranial vascular malformations, J. Nucl. Med. **19**:235.

Gates, G. F., Miller, J. H., and Stanley, P. 1978. Scintiangiography of hepatic masses in childhood, J.A.M.A. **239**:2667.

Gates, G. F., Orme, H. W., and Dore, E. K. 1971. Measurement of cardiac shunting with technetium labeled albumin aggregates, J. Nucl. Med. **12**:746.

Gates, G. F., Orme, H. W., and Dore, E. K. 1974. Cardiac shunt assessment in children with macroaggregated albumin 99mTc, Radiology **112**:649.

Gates, G. F., Orme, H. W., and Dore, E. K. 1975. Surgery of congenital heart disease assessed by radionuclide scintigraphy, J. Thorac. Cardiovasc. Surg. **69**:767.

Gilday, D. L., Ash, J. M., and Reilly, B. J. 1977. Radionuclide skeletal survey for pediatric neoplasms, Radiology **123**:399.

Gilday, D. L., Paul, D. J., and Paterson, J. 1975. Diagnosis of osteomyelitis in children by combined blood pool and bone imaging, Radiology **117**:331.

Gottschalk, A., and Potchen, E. J., eds. 1976. Diagnostic nuclear medicine. In Robbins, L. L., ed.: Golden's diagnostic radiology, Baltimore, The Williams & Wilkins Co.

Handmaker, H., and Leonards, R. 1976. The bone scan in inflammatory osseous disease, Semin. Nucl. Med. **6**:95.

Heidendal, G. A. K., et al. 1975. Evaluation of cold areas on the thyroid scan with ⁶⁷Ga-citrate, J. Nucl. Med. **16**:793.

Higashi, T., et al. 1972. Clinical evaluation of ⁶⁷Ga-citrate scanning, J. Nucl. Med. **13**:196.

Higashi, T., et al. 1977a. Gallium-67 scanning in the evaluation of therapy of malignant tumors of the head and neck, J. Nucl. Med. **18**:243.

Higashi, T., et al. 1977b. Gallium-67 scanning in the differentiation of maxillary sinus carcinoma from chronic maxillary sinusitis, Radiology **123**:117.

Hirabayashi, S., et al. 1975. Inconsistent images of thyroid nodule scintigrams made with iodine and pertechnetate, J. Nucl. Med. **16**:918.

Hoffer, P. B., and Gottschalk, A. 1974. Tumor scanning agents, Semin. Nucl. Med. **4**:305.

Hoffer, P. B., Gottschalk, A., and Quinn, J. 1976. Thyroid in vivo studies. In Gottschalk, A., and Potchen, E. J., eds.: Diagnostic nuclear medicine, Baltimore, The Williams & Wilkins Co.

Hoffer, P. B., Huberty, J., and Khayan-Bashi, H. 1977. The association of Ga-67 and lactoferrin, J. Nucl. Med. **18**:713.

Holder, L. E., and Saenger, E. L. 1975. The use of nuclear medicine in evaluating liver disease, Semin. Roentgenol. **10**:215.

Hornback, N. B., and Shidnia, H. 1976. Rhabdomyosarcoma in the pediatric age group, Am. J. Roentgenol. **126**:542.

James, W. S., Menn, S. J., and Moser, K. M. 1978. Rapid resolution of a pulmonary embolus in man, West. J. Med. **128**:60.

Johns, M. E., Regezi, J. A., and Batsakis, J. G. 1977. Oncocytic neoplasms of salivary glands: an ultrastructural study, Laryngoscope **87**:862.

Johnson, G., et al. 1974. ⁶⁷Ga-citrate imaging in untreated Hodgkins disease: preliminary report of cooperative group, J. Nucl. Med. **15**:399.

Jones, A. E., et al. 1974. Brain scintigraphy with ⁹⁹ᵐTc pertechnetate, ⁹⁹ᵐTc polyphosphate, and ⁶⁷Ga citrate, Radiology **112**:123.

Jones, A. G., Francis, M. D., and Davis, M. A. 1976. Bone scanning: radionuclide reaction mechanisms, Semin. Nucl. Med. **6**:3.

Jones, B. E., and Patton, D. D. 1976. Bone scans of the facial bones: normal anatomy, Am. J. Surg. **132**:341.

Kan, M. K., Hopkins, B., and Carroll, C. F. X. 1977. Scintigraphic evaluation of suspected acute myocardial infarction, J.A.M.A. **238**:1637.

Kaplan, W. D., et al. 1974. ⁶⁷Ga-citrate and the nonfunctioning thyroid nodule, J. Nucl. Med. **15**:424.

Kim, E., and Mattar, A. G. 1976. Primary and secondary carcinoma with focal nodular hyperplasia in a multinodular thyroid, J. Nucl. Med. **17**:983.

Kinoshita, F., et al. 1974. Scintiscanning of pulmonary diseases with ⁶⁷Ga-citrate, J. Nucl. Med. **15**:227.

Levenson, S. M., et al. 1976. Abnormal pulmonary gallium accumulation in pneumocytis carinii pneumonia, Radiology **119**:395.

Livadas, D. P., et al. 1977. The coexistence of thyroid malignancy with autonomous hot nodules of the thyroid, Clin. Nucl. Med. **2**:350.

Lomas, F., Dibos, P. E., and Wagner, H. N., Jr. 1972. Increased specificity of liver scanning with the use of ⁶⁷Ga citrate, N. Engl. J. Med. **286**:1323.

Lomonaco, A., et al. 1975. Nuclear medicine and ultrasound correlation in diagnosis of disease of liver and biliary tree, Semin. Nucl. Med. **5**:307.

Makler, P. T., Charkes, N. D., and Malmud, L. S. 1977. Metastatic thyroid carcinoma presenting as a hypervascular neck lesion, Clin. Nucl. Med. **2**:192.

Marty, R., et al. 1976. Bone trauma and related benign diseases: assessment by bone scanning, Semin. Nucl. Med. **6**:107.

Mashberg, A., et al. 1969. Use of scintillation scanning for the early detection of bone involvement by squamous cell carcinoma of the oral mucosa: preliminary report, J. Am. Dent. Assoc. **79**:1151.

Massin, J. P., Planclon, C., and Perez, R. 1977. Comparison of 99mTc-pertechnetate and 131I in scanning of thyroid nodules, Clin. Nucl. Med. 2:324.

Maynard, C. D. 1969. Clinical nuclear medicine, Philadelphia, Lea & Febiger, pp. 66-69.

McAfee, J. G., and Subramanian, G. 1975. Radioactive agents for imaging. In Freeman, L. M., and Johnson, P. M., eds.: Clinical scintillation imaging, ed. 2, New York, Grune & Stratton, Inc.

McAfee, J. G., Subramanian, G., and Esser, P. D. 1975. Appendix: radionuclides used for imaging. In Freeman, L. M., and Johnson, P. M., eds.: Clinical scintillation imaging, ed. 2, New York, Grune & Stratton, Inc.

McAfee, J. G., et al. 1964. Technitium 99m pertechnetate for brain scanning, J. Nucl. Med. 5:811.

McLaughlin, P. 1976. Radionuclide imaging in cardiovascular disease: current indications, J.A.M.A. 236:2439.

McNeil, B. J., et al. 1973. Fluorine-18 bone scintigraphy in children with osteosarcoma or Ewing's sarcoma, Radiology 109:627.

McQuade, S., and Higgins, H. P. 1974. 99mTc-polyphosphate in diagnosing meningiomas of the sphenoid wing, J. Nucl. Med. 15:1205.

Menon, S., Wagner, H. N., Jr., and Tsan, M. F. 1978. Studies on gallium accumulation by inflammatory lesions. II. Uptake by *Staphylococcus aureus,* J. Nucl. Med. 19:44.

Michall, J. A., and Coleman, R. E. 1977. Localization of 67Ga citrate in a mycotic aneurysm, Am. J. Roentgenol. 129:1111.

Milder, M. S., et al. 1973. Gallium-67 scintigraphy in malignant melanoma, Cancer 32:1350.

Miller, S. W., et al. 1974. Technetium99m labeled diphosphonate bone scanning in Paget's disease, Am. J. Roentgenol. 121:177.

Mishkin, F. S., and Freeman, L. M. 1975. Progress in scintillation imaging. In Freeman, L. M., and Johnson, P. M., eds.: Clinical scintillation imaging, ed. 2, New York, Grune & Stratton, Inc.

O'Connor, M. K., Cullen, M. J., and Malone, J. F. 1976. A kinetic study of [131I] iodine and [99mTc] pertechnetate in thyroid carcinoma to explain a scan discrepancy, J. Nucl. Med. 18:796.

Olson, W. H., and McCombs, R. K. 1977. Positive 99mTc diphosphonate and 67Ga-citrate scans in ameloblastoma: case report, J. Nucl. Med. 18:348.

O'Mara, R. E. 1974. Bone scanning in osseous metastatic disease, J.A.M.A. 229:1915.

O'Mara, R. E., and Charkes, N. D. 1975. The osseous system. In Freeman, L. M., and Johnson, P. M., eds.: Clinical scintillation imaging, ed. 2, New York, Grune & Stratton, Inc.

Pinsky, S. M., and Henkin, R. E. 1976. Gallium-67 tumor scanning, Semin. Nucl. Med. 6:397.

Pistenma, D. A., McDougall, R., and Kriss, J. P. 1975. Screening for bone metastases: are only scans necessary? J.A.M.A. 231:46.

Potchen, E. J., et al. 1971. Pathophysiologic basis of soft tissue tumor scanning, J. Surg. Oncol. 3:593.

Preimesberger, K. F., Loken, M. K., and Shafer, R. B. 1974. Abnormal brain scan in Paget's disease of bone—confusion with subdural hematoma, J. Nucl. Med. 15:880.

Rasmussen, S. N., et al. 1973. Ultrasound in the diagnosis of liver disease, J. Clin. Ultrasound 1:220.

Reba, R. C., and Poulose, K. P. 1974. Nonspecificity of gallium accumulation: gallium-67 concentration in cerebral infarction, Radiology 112:639.

Richman, S. D., et al. 1975. Usefulness of gallium scintigraphy in primary and metastatic breast carcinoma, J. Nucl. Med. 46:996.

Rollo, F. D., ed. 1977. Nuclear medicine physics, instrumentation and agents, St. Louis, The C. V. Mosby Co.

Rosenfield, N., and Treves S. 1974. Liver-spleen scanning in pediatrics, Pediatrics 53:692.

Russin, L. D., and Staab, E. V. 1976. Unusual bone scan findings in acute osteomyelitis: case report, J. Nucl. Med. 17:617.

Sagar, V. V., Piccone, J. M., Meckelnburg, R. L. 1977. Dynamic flow study in Warthin's tumor of parotid gland, Clin. Nucl. Med. 2:404.

Schall, G. L., and DiChiro, G. 1972. Clinical usefulness of salivary gland scanning, Semin. Nucl. Med. 2:270.

Schiff, L., et al. 1947. Gastric and salivary excretion of radioiodine in man, J. Natl. Cancer Inst. 7:349.

Siegel, B. A., et al. 1976. Skeletal uptake of 99mTc-diphosphonate in relation to local bone blood flow, Radiology 120:121.

Siemsen, J. K., et al. 1976. Gallium-67 scintigraphy of pulmonary diseases as a complement to radiography, Radiology 118:371.

Silberstein, E. B., et al. 1974. Gallium-67 as diagnostic agent for detection of head and neck tumors and lymphoma, Radiology 110:605.

Spies, S. M. 1978. Radioisotope techniques in clinical cardiology, J.A.M.A. 239:1651.

Stein, N., et al. 1973. Airway responses to pulmonary embolism. In Moser, K. M., and Stein, M., eds.: Pulmonary thromboembolism, Chicago, Year Book Medical Publishers, Inc.

Stevenson, J. S., et al. 1974. Technetium99m-phosphate bone imaging: a method for assessing bone graft healing, Radiology 110:391.

Subramanian, G., and McAfee, J. G., 1971. A new complex of 99mTc for skeletal imaging, Radiology 99:192.

Swartzendruber, D. C., Nelson, B., and Hayes, R. L. 1971. 67Gallium localization in lysosomal-like granules of leukemic and nonleukemic murine tissues, J. Natl. Cancer Inst. 46:941.

Sy, W. M. 1974. Bone scan in primary hyperparathyroidism, J. Nucl. Med. 15:1089.

Taplin, G. V. 1978. Inhalation lung imaging with radioaerosols and gases (editorial), Appl. Radiol. (Nuclear Medicine) 7:119.

Taplin, G. V., et al. 1963. Scientific exhibit on radioalbumin aggregates for organ scanning, Tenth annual meeting of the Society of Nuclear Medicine, Montreal, June 26.

Tarkiainen, E., Stjernvall, L., and Tarkkanen, J. 1970. Pilocarpine as diagnostic aid in the scintilography of sialopathies, Acta Otolaryngol. 70:113.

Teates, C. D., and Hunter, J. G., Jr. 1975. Gallium scanning as a screening test for inflammatory lesions, Radiology 116:383.

Teates, C. D., and Williamson, B. R. J. 1977. "Hot and cold" bone lesion in acute osteomyelitis, Am. J. Roentgenol. **129**:517.

Thesingh, C. W., et al. 1978. Accumulation and localization of gallium-67 in various types of primary lung carcinoma, J. Nucl. Med. **19**:28.

Thomas, S. R., et al. 1978. Dose to the metaphyseal growth complexes in children undergoing ^{99m}Tc-EHDP bone scans, Radiology **126**:193.

Towers, J. F., and McAndrew, P. G. 1975. Maxillary sinusitis mimicking malignant disease, Oral Surg. **39**:718.

Tsan, M. F., et al. 1978. Studies on gallium accumulation in inflammatory lesions. I. Gallium uptake by human polymorphonuclear leukocytes, J. Nucl. Med. **19**:36.

Turner, J. W., and Spencer, R. P. 1976. Thyroid carcinoma presenting as a pertechnetate "hot" nodule, but without ^{131}I uptake, J. Nucl. Med. **17**:22.

Vera, R., et al. 1971. Determination of occult invasion of bone by adjacent tumor, Radiology **101**:125.

Verma, R., et al. 1973. ^{111}Indium-bleomycin: a new radiopharmaceutical for tumor scintigraphy, J. Nucl. Med. **14**:641.

Wagner, G. W., and Hunt, A. D., and Pendergrass, E. P. 1945. A study of the relative importance of the cortex and spongiosa in the production of the roentgenogram of the normal vertebral body, Am. J. Roentgenol. **53**:40.

Wagner, H. N., Jr., ed. 1968. Principles of nuclear medicine, Philadelphia, W. B. Saunders Co.

Wagner, H. N., Jr., ed. 1975. Nuclear medicine, Tucson, H. P. Books.

Wagner, H. N., Jr. 1976. Cardiovascular nuclear medicine: a progress report, Hosp. Pract. **11**:77.

Waxman, A. D., and Siemsen, J. K. 1975. Gallium gallbladder scanning in cholecystitis, J. Nucl. Med. **16**:148.

Waxman, A. D., and Siemsen, J. K. 1976. Gallium scanning in cerebral and cranial infections, Am. J. Roentgenol. **127**:309.

Waxman, A. D., et al. 1973. Differential diagnosis of brain lesions by gallium scanning, J. Nucl. Med. **14**:903.

Waxman, A. D., et al. 1975. Reliability of gallium brain scanning in detection and differentiation of central nervous system lesions, Radiology **116**:675.

Webster, E. W., Alpert, M. N., and Brownell, G. L. 1974. Radiation doses in pediatric nuclear medicine and diagnostic x-ray procedures. In James, A. E., Wagner, H. N., Jr., and Cooke, R. E., eds.: Pediatric nuclear medicine, Philadelphia, W. B. Saunders Co.

Weibel, E. R. 1963. Morphometry of the human lungs, New York, Academic Press, Inc., p. 81.

Wendeberg, B. 1961. Mineral metabolism of fractures of the tibia in man studied with external counting of Sr^{85}, Acta Orthop. Scand. Suppl. **52**:1-79.

Werner, J. A., et al. 1977. Acute myocardial infarction—clinical application of technetium 99m stannous pyrophosphate infarct scintigraphy (medical progress), West. J. Med. **127**:464.

Winchell, H. S. 1976. Mechanisms for localization of radiopharmaceuticals in neoplasms, Semin. Nucl. Med. **6**:371.

CHAPTER 16

Oral manifestations of systemic diseases

Daniel M. Laskin

There are a number of systemic diseases that can become important factors in oral and maxillofacial surgery by complicating the operation or retarding healing. Even a simple tooth extraction, usually performed in the office without great inconvenience or danger to the patient's life, becomes a formidable and serious undertaking if the patient has uncontrolled diabetes, cardiovascular disease, liver dysfunction, or a blood dyscrasia. It is therefore important to be aware of the oral manifestations of systemic diseases.

Besides the presence of unusual changes in the mouth, a careful history of previous illnesses and operations may yield important information. Complications that attended former operations or even the administration of anesthetics may be illuminating. Unless a patient is under the care of a physician from whom information may be obtained, a thorough physical examination is indicated whenever systemic conditions are suspected. In some cases, evaluation and treatment by a consultant internist may also be required. The oral and maxillofacial surgeon, however, should be familiar with the nature of such diseases, especially with the signs and symptoms they produce in the oral region and with the effect they may have on the course of surgical operations (see Chapter 17).

If there is any doubt regarding the patient's general health, he should be hospitalized. Of course the decision is also influenced by the seriousness of the operation, the incapacity that may result, and the supportive treatment that may be needed from trained attendants.

BLOOD DISEASES

Blood diseases very often produce signs in the oral cavity that can lead to their diagnosis. Serious complications may develop if the causes of these conditions are not recognized before an operation is performed. Primary or secondary uncontrollable hemorrhage may occur that can lead to exsanguination and result in death. Oral manifestations or even a suspicious history is an indication for laboratory tests (see Chapter 14) and possible examination by an internist or hematologist.

Hypochromic anemia

Many patients, especially middle-aged women, suffer from hypochromic anemia (see Chapter 17). This results in a diminished oxygen-carrying capacity of the blood. General anesthesia in adults is contraindicated if the hemoglobin is below 9 gm% (in children, 11 to 12 gm%). When general anesthesia is used, adequate oxygenation must be ensured.

Oral signs and symptoms. The oral tissues, especially the lips, are very pale. The tongue may be smooth on the sides and dorsum, or there may be only small areas affected by desquamation of the filiform papillae (Fig. 16-1). In addition,

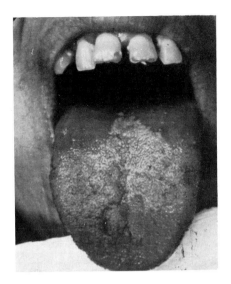

Fig. 16-1. Hypochromic anemia with localized atrophy of tongue.

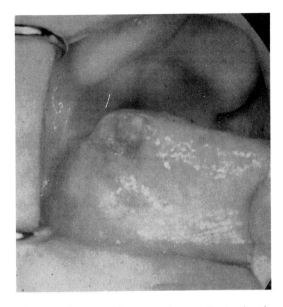

Fig. 16-2. Plummer-Vinson syndrome with atrophy of the lingual papillae and carcinoma.

muscular atrophy may cause a decrease in the size of the tongue. There is a predisposition to wound infection and ulceration. Septicemia has been reported to occur after extraction of infected teeth.

Treatment. Operative procedures should be preceded by corrective measures. Blood transfusions before the extraction of teeth or other surgery are recommended if treatment is urgent. Otherwise iron therapy is indicated (see Chapter 17).

Plummer-Vinson syndrome

Vinson described the Plummer-Vinson syndrome in 1922 and named it hysterical dysphagia. However, Plummer-Vinson syndrome is the name commonly used. It is also known as sideropenic dysphagia, a name suggested by Waldenström (1939) because the outstanding symptoms are iron deficiency, anemia, and dysphagia. Many patients also suffer from achlorhydria. The precancerous nature of the disease, however, must also be recognized (Watts, 1961).

Oral signs and symptoms. The lips are thin with a narrow vermilion border. The oral as well as the pharyngeal mucosa is pale and atrophied, and the tongue is smooth because of atrophy of the filiform papillae. Occasionally, leukoplakia

develops on the tongue, and angular cheilosis may be present.

Carcinoma may develop on the posterior part of the tongue or pharynx and esophagus in the late stages of the syndrome (Fig. 16-2). Ahlborn (1936) published an investigation of 150 patients with carcinoma of the upper alimentary tract and showed that 70% suffered from Plummer-Vinson syndrome. Cahn (1938) reported a case in which a large carcinoma had formed in the gingivolabial fold.

Treatment. Because Plummer-Vinson syndrome is often complicated by carcinoma, early diagnosis and treatment are of great importance. Ferrous sulfate or ferrous gluconate, 300 mg orally t.i.d., is the recommended therapeutic agent.

Pernicious anemia

This macrocytic, hyperchromic anemia usually occurs between the ages of 45 and 60 years. It is caused by a deficiency of an intrinsic factor secreted by the parietal cells of the fundus of the stomach. The mean corpuscular volume and mean corpuscular hemogloblin are increased, and the mean corpuscular hemoglobin concentration is normal. However, total hemoglobin is low. The blood is very fluid and yellowish in color. The red cell count often falls below 2,000,000. There is a leukopenia with relative lymphocytosis.

Oral signs and symptoms. At first the tongue is red in contrast to the yellowish color of the rest of the mucosa. Later, atrophy of the filiform papillae causes a characteristic smooth, waxy appearance. The tongue is never coated and therefore has a very clean appearance (Fig. 16-3).

The subjective oral symptoms are often distressing; the patient complains of an unbearable burning and sometimes of numbness. The condition is aggravated by extreme temperatures of food as well as salty and highly seasoned meals.

Treatment. The megaloblastic anemias are treated with preparations that stimulate erythrocyte maturation such as folic acid, vitamin B_{12}, and liver concentrates.

Aplastic anemia (pancytopenia)

This disease is characterized by a great diminution of all the blood elements caused by failure of the bone marrow to produce hematopoietic cells. Besides the idiopathic type there is a secondary form that is caused by toxic chemicals, irradiation, and radioactive substances. Among chemical substances, the injudicious use of chloramphenicol (Chloromycetin),

especially in children, should be mentioned. Aplastic anemia also occurs in osteosclerosis, marble bone disease (Albers-Schönberg disease), and with extensive bone metastases, all caused by reduction or elimination of bone marrow.

Oral signs and symptoms. The tongue is only rarely atrophic but is smooth and either burns or feels numb. Secondary mouth infections develop toward the end of the disease. Gingival bleeding may occur because of the associated thrombocytopenia (Lasser, Cametta, and Needleman, 1977).

Treatment. Transfusions of whole blood are essential if an operation must be performed without delay. They should be repeated postoperatively to bring the hemoglobin and red cell count back to normal.

Thrombocytopenic purpura

Both idiopathic and secondary purpura can occur. The main clinical manifestation is extravasation of blood beneath the skin. Petechial hemorrhages also are seen, especially in the moving parts such as the eyelids (Fig. 16-4). There may be bleed-

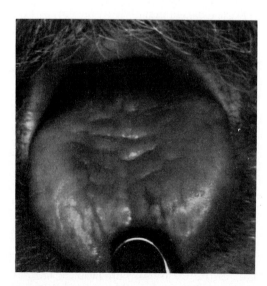

Fig. 16-3. Pernicious anemia causing glossitis and papillary atrophy.

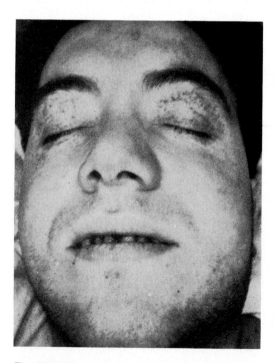

Fig. 16-4. Petechiae in idiopathic thrombocytopenic purpura.

ing from the gastrointestinal tract and epistaxis. Death can occur from intracranial hemorrhage.

Secondary thrombocytopenic purpura is generally caused by the prolonged use of certain drugs such as quinine (Levine, 1959), benzol, chloramphenicol, and others. Foshager (1964) reported a case in a 27-year old woman caused by prolonged use of quinidine sulfate. The patient complained of purplish lesions in the mouth and spontaneous bleeding. Laskin (1974) reported a case of a reaction from a single dose after being off quinidine for 10 months. Oral bleeding was also this patient's initial complaint. According to Sprague et al. (1952), secondary thrombocytopenic purpura results from an antigen-antibody reaction owing to a thrombocytopenic factor contained in the patient's plasma.

Diagnosis involves differentiation from other hemorrhagic diseases by hematologic examination. The bleeding time is prolonged if the platelet count is below 50,000, but the clotting time is normal. Because of the decrease in the number of platelets, clot retraction is poor.

Oral signs and symptoms. Slight trauma causes bleeding and petechial hemorrhages in the mouth (Fig. 16-5). Areas of ecchymosis on the palate (Fig. 16-6) or the buccal mucosa are common and often the first signs of the disease. Occasionally large hematomas may form on the palate

and buccal mucosa; on the ventral part of the tongue, as in a case reported by Beck (1962); and on the gingivae as shown in Fig. 16-7.

Treatment. Oral surgical procedures should be deferred until the platelet count is adequate. If an operation is necessary, transfusion of platelets is recommended before and during the procedure. Corticosteroid therapy and splenectomy are some of the therapeutic measures recommended for idiopathic purpura.

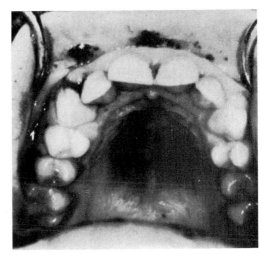

Fig. 16-6. Thrombocytopenic purpura with ecchymosis of palate.

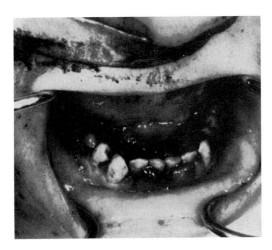

Fig. 16-5. Thrombocytopenic purpura with gingival hemorrhage.

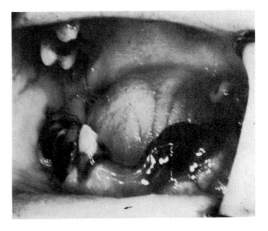

Fig. 16-7. Thrombocytopenic purpura with hematoma of mandibular gingiva.

Hemophilia

Hemophilia is the most difficult hemorrhagic disease to deal with (see also Chapter 17). True hemophilia is characterized by a prolonged clotting time, often as much as 2 to 3 hours. Interesting cases have been reported by Archer (1950, 1951), Steg and co-workers (1960), Israels, Lempert, and Gilbertson (1951), Mersky (1951), and Lucas and Geisler (1965) who discussed female bleeders.

Hemophilia at present can no longer be considered a single disease entity since there is evidence of the existence of at least two additional types with similar clinical and laboratory features. Frick (1954), investigating 55 patients whose disease had previously been diagnosed simply as hemophilia, found the clotting defect to be due to AHG deficiency in 45, PTC deficiency in six, and PTA deficiency in the remaining four.

Hemophilia A, *true hemophilia*, is a sex-linked, recessive, hereditary disease transmitted by females to male descendants. It is caused by a deficiency of antihemophilic globulin (AHG; factor VIII).

Aggeler and co-workers (1952) and White, Aggeler, and Glendenning (1953) described *plasma thromboplastin component (PTC) deficiency*, which is also a sex-linked recessive trait. All patients with factor IX deficiency are males. They have normal quantities of antihemophilic globulin. This variety is also known as hemophilia B or Christmas disease (Biggs and Douglas 1953).

Rosenthal, Dreskin, and Rosenthal (1953) described *plasma thromboplastin antecedent (PTA; factor XI) deficiency (hemophilia C)*. This type of hemophilia is not sex-linked; it is transmitted to both male and female descendants by female and probably male carriers. PTA-deficient plasma can be used to restore the AHG as well as PTC factors.

The characteristics of hemophilia are a prolonged clotting time, normal bleeding time, normal plasma prothrombin time, and abnormal partial thromboplastin time. The results of the various laboratory tests are further discussed in Chapters 14 and 17.

Combinations of the various deficiencies also occur. Soulier and Larrieu (1953) have described cases in which a combination of AHG and PTC deficiencies was present.

Oral signs and symptoms. The patient may complain of bleeding from slight causes such as use of the toothbrush (Fig. 16-8), and large clots may develop around the teeth (Fig. 16-9). In other instances the shedding and eruption of teeth may be associated with oozing of blood for days or weeks. Tooth extraction may give

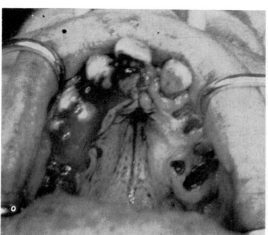

Fig. 16-8. Hemophilia. Hemorrhage from gingivae.

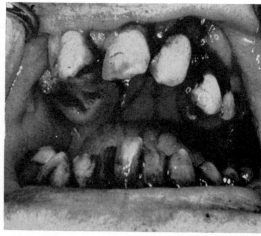

Fig. 16-9. Hemophilia. Spontaneous hemorrhage with clot formation.

the first indication of the disease; exsanguination is possible if proper treatment is not available (Fig. 16-10).

Treatment. Replacement of missing factors either by plasma or plasma fractions is the primary form of therapy. Factor VIII is found only in fresh plasma, but factor IX remains stable and active for long periods in stored plasma. Factor VIII can also be replaced by a cryoprecipitate (cryofactor VIII). Epsilon-aminocaproic acid (Amicar), a drug that blocks the action of fibrinolysin, has also been found to be helpful when given prior to and following dental extractions (Reed et al., 1964). Factor IX deficiency can be treated with fresh or stored plasma as well as by the use of prothrombin complex concentrates that contain factors VII, IX, and X. The high risk of hepatitis with the latter agent must be taken into consideration. Factor XI is replaced with fresh plasma. Current concepts in the management of oral surgical patients with hemophilia have been described by Mulkey (1976) and Sachs, Lipton, and Frank (1978).

The leukemias

Leukemia is a fatal disease that arises in the blood-forming organs and is characterized by an abnormal proliferation of the white blood cells and their precursors, with infiltration into the various tissues of the body. At some time during the course of the disease, abnormal white blood cells, sometimes in great numbers, appear in the circulating blood. This disease, therefore, is considered to be neoplastic in nature.

The oral and maxillofacial surgeon is frequently consulted by the patient before a physician is seen because of the local oral hemorrhage, ulcerations, and gingival hyperplasia, signs that have been termed "leukemic stomatitis." It is very important to recognize the oral manifestations of leukemia because of their early onset and the danger that results from surgical interference, which may be undertaken because the true condition has not been recognized. In acute leukemia, especially the monocytic type, swelling of the gingivae may be so severe that the teeth become covered (Fig. 16-11). When intraoral operations are performed, the wounds do not heal properly and there is extensive sloughing and gangrenous destruction of the soft tissue. Also, there is the danger of prolonged and massive bleeding. Submucosal hemorrhages may give rise to extensive ecchymosis and formation of hematomas. After tooth extraction, which should be undertaken only if absolutely unavoidable, oral ulcerations may increase, and surgical pro-

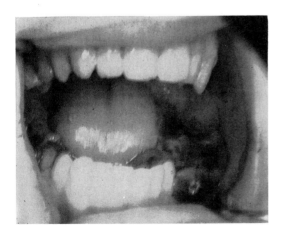

Fig. 16-10. Patient with hemophilia 6 days postoperatively showing oozing of blood and clot formation at site of tooth extraction.

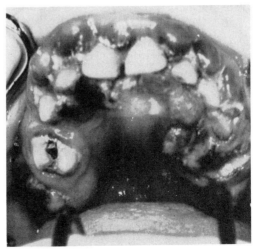

Fig. 16-11. Monocytic leukemia with ulceration, necrosis, and edema of gingiva.

cedures in general often precipitate a rapid downward course of the disease. Barnfield (1945), who studied 123 cases of various types of leukemia, found that the disease becomes more acute in about half of the patients undergoing dental operations.

Myelogenous leukemia

This form of leukemia is characterized by a widespread hyperplasia of the leukopoietic tissue. Both primitive myelocytes and adult neutrophilic, eosinophilic, and basophilic leukocytes may be increased in number, but the myelocyte is the main feature of the blood picture. Myeloblasts are more abundant than mature cells in acute leukemia, and in the terminal stage of the disease the white cell count may be as high as 400,000 to 500,000/cu mm of blood, with 95% to 99% of the cells of myeloid origin.

The disease may have an insidious onset. Later the spleen becomes enormously enlarged. Lassitude, progressive pallor, loss of weight, and gastrointestinal disturbances are common symptoms. Pain in the bones and anemia accompany the disease, which is fatal, although there may be remissions.

Oral signs and symptoms. The interdental papillae and later the gingivae become so greatly enlarged that they may cover the teeth almost completely. In the acute form there is a tendency for hemorrhage, and the mucosa shows a deep red or purplish discoloration. The teeth may be covered with blood clots (Fig. 16-12). Ulcerations are common. The loose gingival margin allows the establishment of periodontal infection and causes loosening of the teeth. There is severe fetor oris.

Lymphatic leukemia

In lymphatic leukemia the lymphoid cells proliferate in the bloodstream and accumulate in the tissues. The white cell count may be 100,000 or more, with 90% to 99% lymphoid cells.

The lymph nodes in various parts of the body enlarge, often to the size of a walnut, owing to the accumulation of lymphocytes. The spleen and liver may be palpable. Ecchymosis of the skin and hemorrhages are features. There is loss of weight and cachexia, with death frequently occurring in less than 5 years.

Oral signs and symptoms. In chronic lymphatic leukemia one may find extreme hypertrophy of the gingiva (Fig. 16-13), whereas in acute cases ulcerations may be the main feature. The patient is especially susceptible to Vincent's infection (Fig. 16-14).

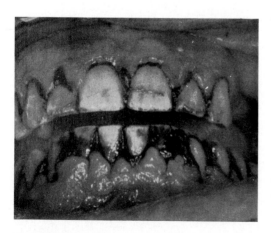

Fig. 16-12. Myelogenous leukemia with gingival hyperplasia and hemorrhage.

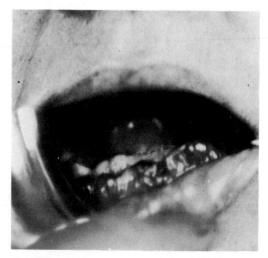

Fig. 16-13. Lymphatic leukemia with severe gingival hyperplasia.

Monocytic leukemia

This form of leukemia is comparatively rare. The leukocytes are only moderately increased (15,000 to 45,000); the primary feature is a marked increase in monocytes to about 70% to 90%.

Oral signs and symptoms. Monocytic leukemia also produces hyperplasia and ulceration in the mouth and hemorrhages from the gingiva (Fig. 16-11).

Treatment. Management of the leukemic patient is directed toward improving oral hygiene and reducing oral infection (Shepard, 1978). Any surgical procedures should be postponed until there is a period of remission.

Aleukemic leukemia

In this disease proliferation of the cells occurs in the hematopoietic tissues, but the cells fail to appear in the blood in increased numbers, although the finding of abnormal forms is characteristic. Any of the named white cells may be involved. It is considered a phase of the leukemic state and, when progressing, will later show the clinical and blood findings of one of the other forms of leukemia described (Fig. 16-15).

Agranulocytopenia

Agranulocytopenia, also called agranulocytosis or pernicious leukopenia, is characterized by fever and an almost complete absence of granular leukocytes; it is accompanied by a drop in the total white cell count. Drug therapy may be a causative factor, but there is also a recurrent type found in children. The mortality rate is 50% to 95%.

Oral signs and symptoms. A great variety of oral lesions occur. The only common characteristic is an absence of any local cause. Spontaneous hemorrhage is not uncommon (Fig. 16-16). Necrosis may be a feature and produces a nonspecific ulcerating stomatitis. Gangrenous lesions may involve the periodontium and bone. The lymph nodes may become enlarged. The patient may suffer considerable pain and have difficulty in swal-

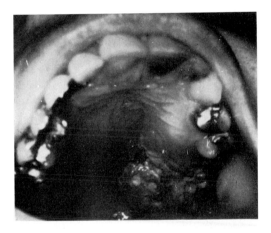

Fig. 16-15. Aleukemic leukemia with palatal swelling and ulceration.

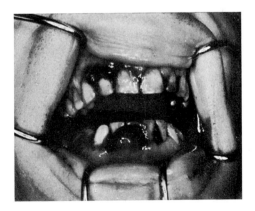

Fig. 16-16. Agranulocytopenia with spontaneous hemorrhages from gingival margins.

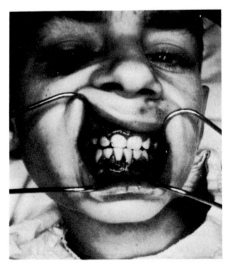

Fig. 16-14. Lymphatic leukemia with gingivitis owing to Vincent's infection. Note ecchymosis below eye.

lowing. Lesions in the throat give rise to agranulocytic angina.

Treatment. The drug suspected to cause the disease should be stopped. Good oral hygiene is important (see Chapter 17).

Hodgkin's disease

Hodgkin's disease was first described by Thomas Hodgkin in 1832. It is associated with loss of weight, weakness, pallor, and an enlarged spleen and liver. A continuous fever is common. Painless swellings appear in the neck or other sites where lymph nodes are present; these generally increase in size (Fig. 16-17). Although there is no characteristic blood picture, leukocytosis is usually present, often with slight anemia and eosinophilia.

Oral signs and symptoms. A patient with enlarged lymph nodes in the neck may be referred to the oral and maxillofacial surgeon. When there is a single node, a differential diagnosis from a branchial cleft cyst or submandibular gland enlargement must be made, generally by biopsy or excision. Multiple and bilateral

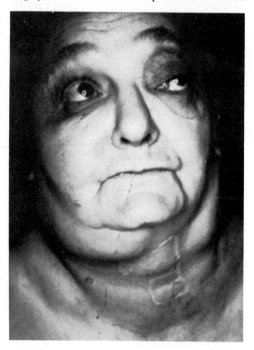

Fig. 16-17. Patient with swelling of neck from Hodgkin's disease.

enlargement (Fig. 16-17) is easier to recognize.

CARDIOVASCULAR DISEASES

Certain heart diseases can account for unexpected death during an operation (see Chapter 17). If nephritis is also present, an increase in the risk is noted. This risk may be greatly diminished by careful preoperative study and judicious selection and expert administration of anesthetic agents. The added risk caused by heart disease is generally proportional to the degree of decrease in the cardiac reserve. The degree of cardiac reserve may be determined by the amount of fatigue on moderate exertion or the experience of breathlessness or cardiac pain after exercise, the occurrence of dependent edema, and the complaint of nocturnal dyspnea.

Oral signs and symptoms. The color of the lips and oral mucosa may be changed significantly. Jacoby (1960) states that in early cases cyanosis may cause a bluish discoloration. Reduced blood circulation in cardiac insufficiency also produces a cyanotic, reddish violet color of the tongue as well as an increase in size. Dilation of the lingual veins may also be noted. Right-sided cardiac failure can cause distention of the cervical veins.

LIVER DISEASE

Patients with serious liver damage, such as occurs in advanced cirrhosis, often bleed spontaneously and excessively after operations (see Chapter 17). Such bleeding, in the presence of vomiting, may represent ruptured esophageal varices. Patients with liver damage should not be given drugs or anesthetic agents that are detoxified by the liver.

Oral signs and symptoms. In severe liver disease the tongue is dark red, smooth on the dorsal surface, and has no coating. The red color of the tongue contrasts with the yellow-colored (jaundiced) soft palate and gingiva. Rhagades of the lip are sometimes prominent. If prothrombin deficiency occurs, petechial hemorrhages and ecchymotic areas, as well as spontaneous gingival bleeding, may be noted.

KIDNEY DISEASE

Renal disease is often associated with a disturbance of the fluid and electrolytic balance, and impaired renal function limits or eliminates the ability to excrete waste products (see Chapter 17). When renal insufficiency occurs, urinary constituents are retained in the blood and the clinical picture of uremia develops. In the uremic state, the patient becomes drowsy, has intractable headaches and disturbances of vision, and may suffer from nausea and vomiting. Diarrhea, dyspnea, and edema are other symptoms. Coma may occur in the terminal stages.

Kidney disease requires a careful selection of anesthetic agents and drugs. Generally, those agents that are excreted through the kidneys should not be used, especially when the nonprotein nitrogen is high.

Oral signs and symptoms. In uremic stomatitis the oral mucosa is red and swollen and often covered by a pseudomembrane that can be detached, leaving a dry red surface. An offending fetor oris, the so-called ammonia breath, is a characteristic feature.

DIABETES MELLITUS

In diabetes mellitus the ability to utilize carbohydrates is diminished or lost because of faulty pancreatic activity (see Chapter 17). This produces hyperglycemia with glycosuria and polyuria, producing symptoms of thirst, hunger, emaciation, and weakness. There is also a lowered resistance to pyogenic infections.

Unexplainable complications may be due to unrecognized diabetes in patients who come to the office or outpatient clinic to have surgery performed. Schliack (1960) mentions an incidence of unrecognized diabetes among dental patients of 1.5%. O'Driscoll (1966) found that of 73 glycosurics, 11 were known diabetics and under treatment. Of the others, eight had blood sugar levels of over 120 mg/100 ml, whereas the rest had blood sugar levels below 120 mg/100 ml. Glucose tolerance tests revealed that, of these, six patients had moderately severe diabetes, whereas two were latent diabetics.

Oral signs and symptoms. The oral signs and symptoms of diabetes are not remarkable in the early stages. Severe gingival and periodontal disease is one of the most common findings. Gottsegen (1963) associated some cases of denture-sore mouths and denture intolerance with diabetes. Lowered resistance to infection is likely the cause of gingival abscesses. Healing of wounds is slow and often complicated. Ulcers and angular cheilosis may not heal until the diabetes is controlled. Belting, Hiniker, and Dummett (1964) stated that vascular occlusive disorders increase the severity of periodontal disease. Xerostomia is common and often the patient complains of burning of the tongue, but the red beefy tongue of diabetes is not often seen today. A sweet, fruity (acetone) breath is another characteristic occurring mostly in the advanced stages of the disease.

AMYLOIDOSIS

Amyloidosis is a degenerative disease affecting various tissues and organs of the body. In most cases the spleen, kidneys, liver, and adrenal glands are principally affected.

Primary amyloidosis, a rare disease, is characterized by massive deposition of amyloid in the mesodermal tissues. It forms nodules or discrete masses (amyloid tumors). Secondary amyloidosis is associated with chronic diseases such as multiple myeloma (Kraut et al., 1977), tuberculosis, bronchiectasis, osteomyelitis, and rheumatoid arthritis. Death generally occurs from cardiac or renal failure.

Oral signs and symptoms. Amyloidosis is a difficult disease to diagnose. Gingival biopsy is of considerable value in this regard (Schwartz and Olson, 1975). Selikoff and Robitzek (1947) found positive biopsies in 14 of 18 cases. Gorlin and Gottsegen (1949) recommended that the biopsy be taken from the mucobuccal reflection of the upper canine or premolar area, a strip 4 mm wide extending to the gingival margin and including the interdental papilla. It is excised down to the periosteum. Stained according to Lieb (1947) with crystal violet or methyl violet, the amyloid shows as a reddish

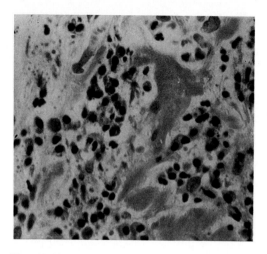

Fig. 16-18. Amyloidosis. Specimen from gingiva shows deposit in form of amorphous hyalinized material in papillary layer of corium. (Courtesy Dr. H. M. Goldman.)

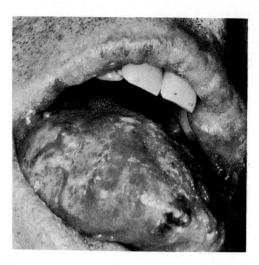

Fig. 16-19. Amyloidosis with ridged, hard tongue and nodular formations on dorsum. (From Cahn, L. R. 1957. Oral Surg. **10**:735.)

purple deposit in the perivascular areas (Fig. 16-18). Whereas many authors have reported satisfactory results from gingival biopsies, Symmers (1956), Cooke (1958), and Lovett, Cross, and Van Allen (1965) state that the procedure gives so few positive results that it is of little value.

Tillman (1957) describes various oral symptoms. The most common findings are related to the tongue, which may show firm ridges and nodules (Fig. 16-19). The buccal mucosa may also be involved.

SYSTEMIC REACTIONS TO HEAVY METALS

A number of the heavy metals can cause systemic reactions frequently associated with oral findings. In the mouth, the deposition of the metallic salts in the tissues can interfere with circulation, and the reduced resistance permits secondary invasion by bacteria. Secretion of some of the metals in saliva increases salivary flow and produces a metallic taste. The secreted metals may also be directly irritating to the tissues.

Lead poisoning

Lead poisoning is due to absorption of lead through the skin or respiratory or gastrointestinal tract. Painters are frequently affected as well as young chil-

dren who chew on painted objects. Anemia results, with stippling of erythrocytes. Clinical signs are pasty skin, lassitude, weakness, and constipation. The characteristic black-blue lead line along the gingival margin (halo saturninus) and the so-called lead breath (halitus saturninus) are common oral findings. The patients frequently complain of a sweet metallic taste and excessive salivation.

Bismuth poisoning

Bismuth may, if used over a long period of time, produce deposits in the gingival margins that cause a bluish black line, especially if gingivitis is present (Fig. 16-20). Similar deposits may occur on the cheeks and at the junction of the papillated dorsum of the tongue with the smooth ventral surface.

Argyria

Silver compounds are found in some nasal drops and sprays, and in former years were used to treat syphilis and gastric ulcer. Absorption of silver can cause permanent discoloration of the skin. The tissues have a gray color and the appearance can be confused with cyanosis. The sclera and conjunctiva may also be involved.

Orally, the mucous membranes will

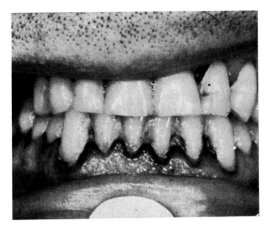

Fig. 16-20. Bismuth line.

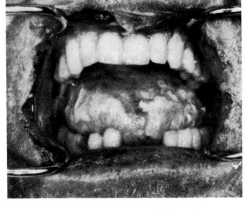

Fig. 16-21. Stomatitis medicamentosa.

also have a uniform gray color owing to the even distribution of the silver throughout the tissues. Despite the patient's appearance, there are few, if any, subjective symptoms.

Mercurialism (ptyalism)

Mercurialism can develop as a result of occupational contact or self-medication with mercury-containing drugs. The general symptoms include intestinal colic, diarrhea, headache, and insomnia. Renal symptoms may also develop.

The lips are dry, cracked, and swollen. Oral ulceration may develop and the tongue can become enlarged and painful. There is an excessive production of a viscid saliva and a metallic taste. The oral tissues may have a burning sensation. Enlargement of the salivary glands is not uncommon.

Aurism

Gold salts used in treating rheumatoid arthritis and some dermatologic diseases can cause systemic reactions in from 10% to 40% of patients. The usual findings are dermatitis and stomatitis. Auric stomatitis is characterized by vesiculation and ulceration of the mucous membranes. Purpura and neutropenia have also been reported.

ERYTHEMA MULTIFORME

Erythema multiforme is an inflammatory disease characterized by red mac-ules, papules, and occasionally vesicles or bullae, which are likely to recur. In the mouth, vesiculobullous lesions form with rapid onset, followed by necrosis of epithelium, ulceration, bleeding, and crust formation after a few hours.

The causes are viral conditions, systemic infections, malignant disease, and ingestion of drugs. The result of the last is known as stomatitis medicamentosa. The most common sites are the lips, cheeks, and tongue (Al-Ubaidy and Nally, 1976) (Fig. 16-21). Differential diagnosis should include benign mucous membrane pemphigoid and pemphigus (Kennett, 1968).

Generally, the oral lesions in stomatitis medicamentosa are not pathognomonic. A few drugs, however, produce symptoms that can be recognized. Among these are the granulomatous lesions resulting from iodides and the noninflammatory gingival hyperplasia seen in epileptic patients who have been given diphenytoin (Dilantin) sodium over a long period of time (Fig. 16-22).

Treatment. Prednisone, 10 mg t.i.d. for 2 to 3 days, with subsequent gradual dose reduction, has been recommended. Topical anesthetic mouthwashes and a bland, soft or liquid diet are also helpful in minimizing discomfort.

ALLERGY (See Chapter 6)

Susceptible people may become sensitized by foreign substances (allergens)

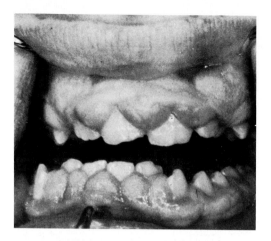

Fig. 16-22. Dilantin hyperplasia of gingivae.

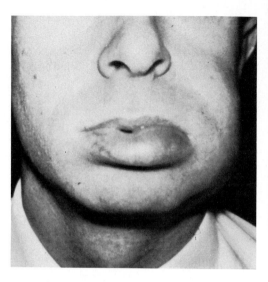

Fig. 16-23. Angioneurotic edema affecting cheek, simulating edema caused by dental abscess. (Courtesy Dr. H. M. Goldman.)

and develop specific antibodies against them; the antibodies combine with a body protein, which then produces a histamine-like reaction. In most instances the allergic reactions occur on the skin and mucosae of the body.

Some well-known allergies are to foods such as fish, lobsters, oysters, eggs, nuts, strawberries, and cheese. Food allergies, however, are sometimes actually drug allergies caused by contamination or additives. Milk, for example, may contain penicillin used to treat mastitis in cows. Honey may be contaminated with sulfa drugs the apiarist gives in sugar syrup to prevent or cure diseases of bees.

Drug allergies have become quite common. They are frequently produced by the antibiotics but also by other drugs. A careful history may reveal similar reactions to the drug when taken previously. A sudden appearance of the systemic symptoms after its use is characteristic. Withdrawal of the drug and replacement by another may confirm the diagnosis. In some cases the drug causing the allergic reaction may be a component of a combined medication. An example is a patient sensitive to procaine who was given procaine penicillin G by his dentist because of an infection and immediately went into anaphylactic shock.

Oral signs and symptoms. The oral mucosa may have a generalized redness or sometimes only reddish spots may

occur. Vesicles, blebs, and ulcerations may form, often in asymmetric distribution. There is no itching, as on the skin, but a burning sensation is frequently felt. The association with dermal urticaria and itching of the skin is significant. Angioneurotic edema is the most frequent oral symptom. Edematous, circumscribed, painless swellings may affect the lips or cheeks. The swelling is not symmetric and must be distinguished from that associated with submandibular or other dental abscesses (Fig. 16-23). The tongue, soft palate, and epiglottis may be involved. Spatz (1964) reported a case in which the reaction was so violent that it produced bulbous extravasation of blood. This resulted from dilation of small blood vessels and transudation of fluid into the submucosal and subcutaneous tissues. In serious cases with rapid onset the reaction may lead to death by asphyxiation before treatment can be given.

Treatment. In persons with urticaria and edema the administration of antihistamines often gives dramatic results. Corticosteroids, if given promptly, can effectively block the response and keep the patient relatively symptom free. In the more severe reactions, epinephrine given subcutaneously or intramuscularly is the agent of choice. It is better, of course, to avoid the specific drug causing the reaction and to make a correct diagnosis that will prevent another attack, which might be anaphylactic in nature.

PEUTZ-JEGHERS SYNDROME

Peutz (1921) and later Jeghers, Mc-Kusick, and Katz (1949) described a disease characterized by formation of polyps in the intestinal tract that may give rise to abdominal pain, bleeding, and peritonitis. The disease is hereditary and the polyps are described as being hamartomas, although malignant transformation has been reported.

Oral signs and symptoms. Melanotic pigmentations are found in the face and mouth. Fine spots develop around the lips, nostrils, and eyes. The mucosa of the cheeks is covered with characteristic round or oval, rarely confluent spots that are brown to black in color and measure 1 to 12 mm in diameter (Fig. 16-24). Sometimes they are seen on the mucosa of the lips but only rarely on the tongue, palate, and gingiva.

VITAMIN DEFICIENCIES

In vitamin deficiencies, retarded healing of both bone and soft tissues may result. In addition, the deficiencies can lower the resistance to infection so that secondary infections may occur, and often various mouth diseases develop that resist the accepted therapeutic measures.

Deficiencies rarely occur singly but manifest their presence in groups, such as the B-complex group and the fat-soluble vitamin group. They arise from inadequate intake, diminished absorption, increased need (as in pregnancy and infection with fever), increased destruction, and diminished utilization. Poor selection of food and destruction of the gastrointestinal flora by oral antibiotics are common causes of vitamin deficiency.

Ascorbic acid deficiency

In the severest form of ascorbic acid deficiency, scurvy results—a rather rare disease at present. In the past scurvy was caused by the lack of available fresh vegetables and fruit that contain vitamin C.

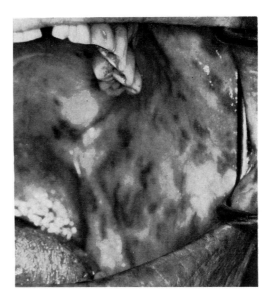

Fig. 16-24. Peutz-Jeghers syndrome with melanotic spots on buccal mucosa and hard palate. (Courtesy Dr. H. M. Goldman.)

Ascorbic acid deficiency produces hemorrhagic manifestations that are caused by failure of the intercellular material to bind the vascular endothelial cells. Clinically, the patient loses weight and develops secondary albuminuria and anemia. Hemorrhages into the skin and joints are common.

Oral signs and symptoms. Scorbutic stomatitis is characterized by gingival inflammation and classic enlargement of the gingival margins and interdental papillae. The gingivae have a purplish appearance and bleed easily. They become enlarged and cover the teeth almost completely (Fig. 16-25). Later, necrosis and infection may cause severe destruction involving the periosteum and periodontal tissues (Boyle, Bessey, and Wolbach 1937), and the teeth loosen because of the breakdown of the collagen fibers of the periodontal ligament. Occasionally large hematomas may form and gingival bleeding from slight trauma is common (Fig. 16-26). Vincent's infection often complicates the disease.

Treatment. The treatment for scurvy is ascorbic acid. The adult dose is 250 mg q.i.d. until signs disappear. A maintenance dose should then be given.

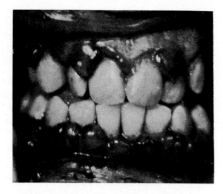

Fig. 16-25. Scurvy. Gingival hyperplasia of purplish color. (Courtesy Dr. I. Hirschfield.)

Vitamin B complex deficiency

An effort has been made to find specific symptoms for each component of the vitamin B complex, but even in well-established deficiencies there are almost always concomitant deficiencies in some of the other components present—even deficiencies of other types, such as iron.

Niacin deficiency

In its full-blown state niacin deficiency produces pellagra. Patients complain of sleeplessness, tiredness, absence of appetite, and loss of weight. Dermatologic manifestations and gastrointestinal disease may be prominent, as well as vertigo, headache, numbness, nervousness, palpitation, and mental depression.

Oral signs and symptoms. Gingivitis and stomatitis are seen in niacin deficiency; often ulcers form on the mucosa. The lips are reddened and cracked, and the mouth feels as if it were scalded. The ulcers may contain Vincent's organisms in enormous numbers. The tongue shows the most characteristic changes, resulting in the so-called Sandwith's bald tongue. This is caused by desquamation of the lingual papillae. In the beginning only the tip or sides of the tongue may be affected. Later, the entire tongue becomes fiery red and swollen and shows an eroded, beet-red surface; for this reason it is also spoken of as beefy tongue (Fig. 16-27). In the chronic stage the tongue shows fissuring and loss of substance caused by muscular atrophy.

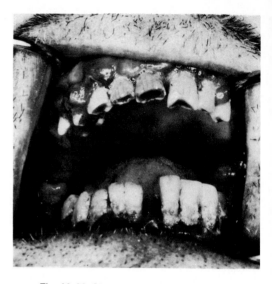

Fig. 16-26. Gingival hemorrhage in scurvy.

Treatment. During the active stage, 300 to 1000 mg/day of nicotinic acid in divided doses is recommended for niacin deficiency. If the patient suffers from serious intestinal disease, nicotinamide, 100 to 250 mg, is given subcutaneously two or three times a day.

Thiamine deficiency

Thiamine or vitamin B_1 deficiency results in beriberi with polyneuritis and bradycardia. The patient complains of loss of appetite and decrease of weight and strength, fatigue, muscular cramps, and diarrhea. Palpitation and shortness of breath are other symptoms. Burning, numbness, and tingling of the extremities are specific. Dry beriberi is differentiated from wet beriberi in which there is edema and serous effusions.

Oral signs and symptoms. The mouth lesions in thiamine deficiency are not distinctive. Gingivitis and edema of the oral mucosa may be accompanied by atypical types of facial neuralgia. The tongue and gingival tissues may have a satiny appearance and a rose color. Enlargement of the fungiform papillae and indentation markings along the periphery of the tongue are common. Vesicles may develop at the vermilion border and small cracks in the lips may also be pres-

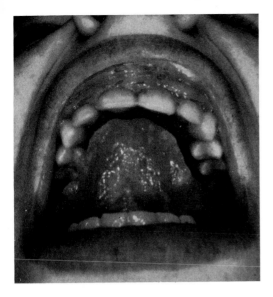

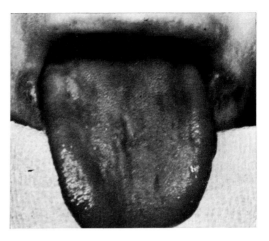

Fig. 16-28. Angular cheilosis with enlarged tongue.

Fig. 16-27. Pellagrous glossitis (niacin deficiency). Note eroded appearance of margin of tongue.

ent. A number of patients who complained of pain in the jaws, teeth, face, and tongue have been relieved by vitamin B_1 therapy. Goodman (1939) also found thiamine chloride to give relief in herpes zoster.

Treatment. For acute deficiency, injections of thiamine hydrochloride, 10 to 20 mg b.i.d., are recommended for adults. In some cases oral administration is as effective as intravenous or intramuscular administration, but usually parenteral use is preferred. It brings about more rapid improvement, and a deranged gastrointestinal tract can prevent the effective absorption of the drug. In chronic cases 5 to 10 mg is given twice a day.

Riboflavin deficiency

Riboflavin or vitamin B_2 deficiency is often a secondary manifestation occurring with other vitamin B deficiencies.

Oral signs and symptoms. In ariboflavinosis, cracks develop at the corners of the mouth. This is the typical picture of perlèche or angular cheilosis. Bacterial infection may occur and then these areas are likely to become larger. *Candida albicans* is a common secondary invader. The tongue may be enlarged and red, with slight enlargement of the fungiform papillae and loss of muscle tone (Fig. 16-

28). This may be accompanied by glossodynia.

Treatment. Whereas the effects of riboflavin deficiency yield promptly to riboflavin medication, it should be remembered that often other deficiencies may be present, such as iron or pyridoxine deficiency. In most cases riboflavin, 10 to 30 mg per day orally in divided doses, is given until a response is evident. Topical antibiotic or antifungal ointments, depending on the organism, are used for the cheilosis.

Pyridoxine deficiency

Pyridoxine or vitamin B_6 deficiency produces weakness, nervousness, and irritability. Seborrheic skin lesions about the eyes, nose, and mouth occur as well as erosions resembling the cheilosis seen in riboflavin deficiency. Glossitis and stomatitis similar to that occurring in niacin deficiency also develop in some patients.

Treatment. Oral administration of pyridoxine, 50 to 100 mg daily, is used to treat vitamin B_6 deficiency.

Vitamin B_{12} deficiency

The oral lesions of vitamin B_{12} deficiency are related to pernicious anemia (see p. 547).

Vitamin K deficiency

Antibiotics, especially if administered orally, may bring about a vitamin K deficiency through the elimination of the gastrointestinal bacteria that are involved in the formation of vitamin K. Secondary deficiency can also occur from malabsorption. Severe liver disease that inhibits prothrombin synthesis produces the same effect as vitamin K deficiency.

General symptoms are hemorrhages in any organ or tissue. Large areas of ecchymosis are frequently the first clinical manifestation. Scurvy, purpura, anemia, and leukemia must be ruled out in the differential diagnosis.

Oral signs and symptoms. Spontaneous gingival bleeding or ecchymosis can occur with vitamin K deficiency. Excessive bleeding during an operation, with ecchymosis and the development of hematomas, is also characteristic.

Treatment. Phytonadione (vitamin K) is the preparation of choice in vitamin K deficiency. In nonemergency situations, when absorption is not a problem, the medication can be given orally in a dose of 5 to 20 mg daily until symptoms of hypoprothrombinemia disappear. If absorption is a problem, the drug can be given intramuscularly in 10 mg doses. When there is an emergency bleeding situation, 10 to 50 mg is given intravenously at a rate of not more than 1 mg/minute.

SPECIFIC INFECTIONS

Specific diseases that can involve the jaws and oral tissues include tuberculosis, sarcoidosis, syphilis, granuloma inguinale, candidiasis, actinomycosis, aspergillosis, and leprosy, as well as some of the South American diseases that are now occasionally seen in other countries (see Chapter 4).

Tuberculosis
Tuberculosis of soft tissue

Tubercle bacilli that occur in the sputum of patients affected by pulmonary tuberculosis may invade a wound in the oral mucosa and produce a variety of lesions. Some are hypertrophic and are called tuberculomas; others appear as ulcers with ragged edges and undermined borders (Fig. 16-29). This is in contrast to the ulcer of squamous cell carcinoma, which usually has a firm rolled

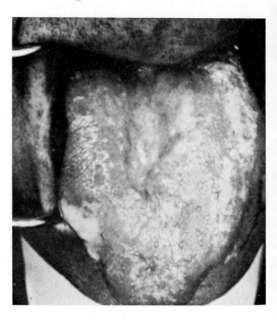

Fig. 16-29. Tuberculous ulcer of lateral border of tongue.

edge. The tongue is frequently affected because of injury by sharp, decayed teeth. The gingival tissues may also become infected.

Tuberculous bone infection

The jaw bone may be involved via a superficial ulcer or from the bacillus entering through a carious tooth or extraction wound. Sixty percent of all cases of tuberculosis of the jaws occur in children under 16 years of age, according to Pichler and Trauner (1948). Bone infections as the result of tuberculous infection, however, are rare (Sachs and Eisenbud, 1977). Tagliano (1947) pointed out that two locations in the mandible have great affinity for the tuberculous infection—the alveolar process and the angle of the jaw. Eleven cases reported by him affected the alveolar bone.

If the infection enters through a root canal, caseous foci develop that appear on the radiograph as radiolucent areas. These are often surrounded by a zone of sclerotic bone. A diagnosis can usually be established only by biopsy or microscopic examination of the tissue excised at operation. Although generally pulmonary tuberculosis precedes development of oral infection (Figs. 16-30 to 16-32), Tay-

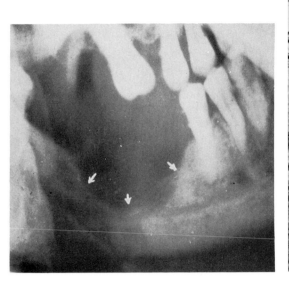

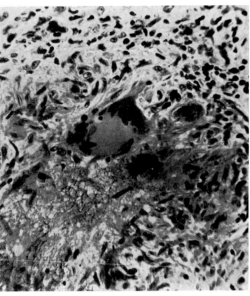

Fig. 16-30. Radiograph showing bone destruction from a tuberculous infection.

Fig. 16-31. Photomicrograph of biopsy from patient in Fig. 16-30 showing typical tuberculous lesion.

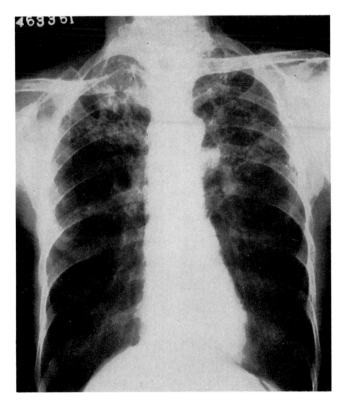

Fig. 16-32. Chest film of patient in Fig. 16-30 showing moderately advanced tuberculosis of both lungs.

lor and Booth (1964) reported a case of bilateral bone involvement without the lungs being affected.

Lymph node involvement

Cervical swellings caused by tuberculous infection are generally the result of invasion through the lymph channels, although hematogenous dissemination can occur. The lymph nodes at first are considerably enlarged, firm, and nontender but subsequently may undergo caseous necrosis and breakdown. Visible swellings can form in the submandibular or cervical regions (Figs. 16-33 to 16-35).

Treatment. General therapy consists of isonicotinic acid hydrazide (INH). This is the least toxic, most effective, and most easily administered drug. Usually it is combined with streptomycin or para-aminosalicylic acid (PAS). The oral lesions will usually heal as the general condition of the patient improves.

Treatment of tuberculous osteomyelitis should be conservative. Greatest reliance is placed on medical management. Loose teeth and sequestra should be removed and the wound packed to permit observation of the healing process.

Sarcoidosis

Sarcoidosis was first described by Hutchinson in 1898 and become known as Mortimer's malady, the name of his patient. Schaumann (1914) was the first to describe its generalized nature; he named the disease lupus pernio. It is also known as maladie Besnier-Boeck. Boeck (1899) himself suggested the name sarcoid or sarcoidosis.

The disease predominantly occurs in early adulthood. It is most common among northern Europeans and American Negroes. At one time sarcoidosis was considered to be of tuberculous or syphilitic origin. More recently it has been suspected of having a viral origin or to involve a disordered defense mechanism.

Lesions most commonly occur in the lungs, lymph nodes, liver, eyes, and skin. Involvement of the oral cavity is not as frequently observed. Bhaskar (1977) cited evidence of sarcoid in the parotid gland, soft palate, and cheek. Kerr (1965) reported a case with swelling of the submandibular and submental area and upper deep cervical lymph nodes, and Roche and Morris (1967) reported a case in the sublingual gland. Mandel and

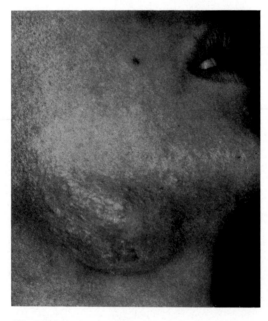

Fig. 16-33. Circumscribed submandibular tuberculous abscess.

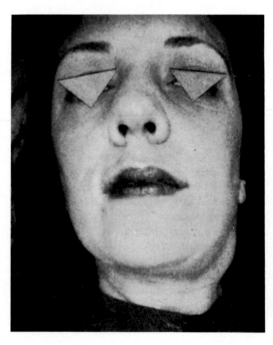

Fig. 16-34. Tuberculous lymphadenopathy.

Baurmash (1962) also reported sarcoid forming a gradually increasing, painless growth involving the submandibular region. Orlean and O'Brien (1966) reported a case involving the floor of the mouth and Tillman, Taylor, and Carchidig (1966) reported a case affecting the tongue, producing nodules and irregular lateral borders. A patient with sarcoidosis of the mandible has been reported by Betten and Koppang (1976).

The characteristic histopathologic findings are those of a granulomatous disease. Caseation is absent. Biopsy reveals nodules of epithelioid cells with inflammatory cells, especially lymphocytes, interspersed. There may be typical Langhans' giant cells present that are irregular in shape and occasionally contain so-called Schaumann's or asteroid bodies.

The *Kveim test*, an immunologic reaction, is positive in 50% to 85% of patients, but reactions occur in other diseases as well. The antigen is made from sarcoid lesions (spleen or lymph node) and is injected intradermally, where a sarcoid lesion will develop in about 4 weeks.

Treatment. Since this disease has a low mortality rate and is often self-limiting, many patients are not treated but are carefully watched. The use of antitubercular drugs is not indicated and is an unnecessary hazard in treating sarcoidosis.

Oral lesions have been treated surgically with good short-term results. Corticosteroid therapy has been used in some patients, but one should weigh carefully its possible benefits in treatment of a relatively benign disease against the complications known to accompany its administration.

Syphilis

This disease may be divided into congenital or acquired forms (primary, secondary, and tertiary stages). Except in the congenital form, the initial lesion is the so-called chancre. All other lesions follow chancre formation and involve many parts of the body. The disease is caused by infection with *Treponema pallidum*. Accidental infection is rare but may occur in the office, laboratory, or necropsy room.

Congenital syphilis

Congenital syphilis produces permanent defects. Linear scars, which are healed fissures, extend from the corners of the mouth, and are spoken of as rhagades. A saddle nose, prominent frontal bosses, and deafness are other evidences of the disease. The teeth show characteristic abnormalities: severe hypoplasia of the deciduous teeth, as well as the screwdriver permanent incisors and mulberry molars (Hutchinson's teeth), are pathognomonic.

Primary syphilis

Chancres in the oral region are found mostly on the lip (Fig. 16-36) and tongue. The lesions are almost always solitary

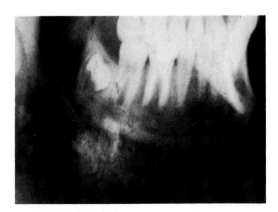

Fig. 16-35. Calcified tuberculous submandibular and cervical lymph nodes.

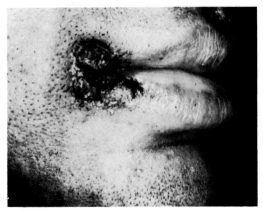

Fig. 16-36. Chancre of lip.

and have the appearance of an ulcer or tumefaction covered by thick, adherent, dark crusts. No pain is caused by the lesion, but the regional lymph nodes become enlarged. Dark-field examination shows the presence of *Treponema pallidum*. The chancre is highly infectious.

Secondary syphilis

The secondary lesions occur 6 to 12 weeks after the onset of the disease. Multiple, discrete, oval, grayish white, or reddish pink patches form on the buccal mucosa and tongue. They are surrounded by a slightly raised, reddish, inflammatory halo. These lesions are known as mucous patches. They are highly infective. Usually the patient develops generalized enlargement of the lymph nodes.

Diffuse glossitis is common in the early stages of the disease and causes atrophy of the lingual papillae. Hyperkeratosis may develop, which gives the tongue a glazed appearance and produces the so-called bald or glass tongue (Fig. 16-37).

Tertiary syphilis

Gummas usually develop within 3 to 10 years after the onset of the disease. They are deeply seated and often involve the underlying bone.

The solitary gumma produces a painless swelling most frequently found on the tongue, palatal mucosa, and uvula. Later central necrosis and ulceration develop. The deeply excavated lesion often is difficult to differentiate from carcinoma. The hard palate is one of the frequent sites of a solitary gumma (Figs. 16-38 and 16-39).

Diffuse involvement of the tongue often results in interstitial fibrosis and papillary atrophy. Leukoplakia frequently occurs in association with this type of glossitis. The incidence of carcinomatous change in these leukoplakic areas is relatively high.

In the mandible the gummatous process may resemble acute pyogenic osteomyelitis. The process may be so extensive that the teeth become loose. Large areas of the alveolar and basilar bone can become destroyed (Fig. 16-40). Meyer and Shklar (1967), in a study of 81 cases with oral manifestations of syphilis, described a tertiary syphilitic involvement of the mandible that produced such extensive bone destruction that spontaneous fracture occurred.

Treatment. Antisyphilitic treatment in all stages calls for large doses of penicillin. In tertiary syphilis involving the jaws removal of devitalized teeth and bone sequestra is indicated. Resulting defects should not be repaired until the disease is cured.

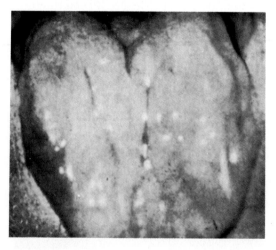

Fig. 16-37. Bald tongue in syphilis. (Courtesy Dr. Francis McCarthy.)

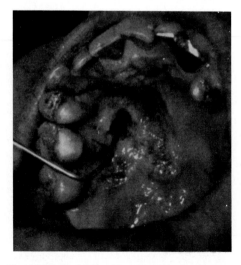

Fig. 16-38. Syphilitic ulcer with palatal perforation.

Candidiasis (moniliasis)

Candidiasis may be generalized, causing widespread infections not only of the skin but also of the respiratory passages and gastrointestinal tract. Localized lesions may also occur in various parts of the body, especially the axillary, submammary, and inguinal regions, and there is a vulvovaginal variety.

In the oral cavity the fungus produces candidal stomatitis, often spoken of as thrush (Figs. 16-41 and 16-42). The clinical features and histologic changes in 14 cases were described by Lehner (1964). It occurs most commonly in the mouth of young, poorly nourished infants. Woodruff and Hesseltine (1938) found that children born of mothers having fungi in the vagina have about 35 times greater chance of developing oral thrush than those born of noninfected mothers. Thrush, however, does not occur only in infants; it may be seen at all ages. The organism may remain latent and harmless and then suddenly become pathogenic. Candidiasis has been observed to occur in patients receiving antibiotic therapy. The antibiotics upset the bacteriologic balance of the mouth and allow fungi and yeasts to proliferate unhindered. It has also been suggested that riboflavin deficiency favors candidiasis, just as pellagra favors fusospirochetosis (Sebrell and Butler, 1938). This idea is prob-

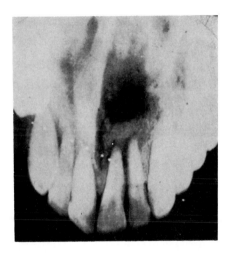

Fig. 16-39. Radiograph showing bone destruction by gumma.

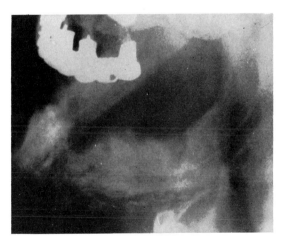

Fig. 16-40. Radiograph of syphilitic involvement of mandible.

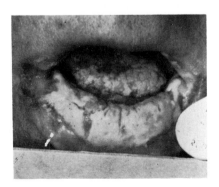

Fig. 16-41. Candidiasis of lip and tongue.

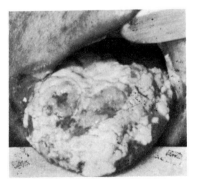

Fig. 16-42. Candidiasis of tongue.

ably related to the fact that the associated angular cheilosis (perlèche) is often secondarily infected by the fungus (see p. 561).

In young infants the infection is generally seen on the sides of the tongue and the cheeks. It produces soft, painless, pearly white, slightly elevated patches that resemble deposits of coagulated milk, but they adhere firmly so that the mucosa bleeds when they are removed. The condition resembles diphtheria except for its more extensive distribution.

Some forms of denture stomatitis may also be due to candidal infection. A diagnostic screening method has been described by Remmer and co-workers (1979).

Debilitated patients may also develop candidiasis. The lesions may spread into the respiratory and digestive tracts. Zimmerman, Frutschey, and Gibbes (1947) reported a case of candidal meningitis in which the disease extended either by way of the cribriform plate or a hematogenous route. A candida septicemia was reported by Dennis, Miller, and Paterson (1964).

Treatment. Nystatin and amphotericin B are the agents of choice for treating candidiasis (Campbell et al., 1960; Nairn, 1975). Because these agents are not well absorbed from the intestinal tract, oral lesions should be treated either topically or parenterally.

Actinomycosis

Actinomycosis is usually due to *Actinomyces israelii* (see Chapter 4), but in many cases an infection mixed with pyogenic bacteria is found. The fungus has a preference for growth in the fascia and the subcutaneous tissue. Actinomycosis should be suspected whenever subacute or chronic cellulitis, with or without sinus tract formation, does not improve after appropriate treatment, especially if the skin is raised by a swelling or a series of swellings. In a study by Dechaume and co-workers (1955), bacteriologic examination of 37 specimens from 32 patients with such disease disclosed in 10 the presence of *"Actinobacterium israelii"* and in 21 bacteria very close to actino-

myces (actinomyces-like organisms). Yellow granules were found in only five instances. The authors expressed their belief that failure to find *A. israelii* does not prove absence of actinomycosis. They may be few and difficult to discover, but later developments may confirm the clinical diagnosis. This was also pointed out by Glahn (1951). He distinguished two types; one was the classic type caused by *A. israelii* and the other a nontypical type for which he suggested the term "actinomycosis atypica."

Hertz (1960) employed the term "pseudoactinomycosis" for cases in which the smear shows only a few mycelia with other microorganisms. He (1955) also described a third form, a tender but painless tumorlike mass that contains grampositive rods of the actinomyces group and anaerboic streptococci.

When extending to the soft tissues of the face, the disease first produces a submandibular or a perimandibular abscess. Only later is the typical clinical picture of cervicofacial actinomycosis produced. This consists of a swelling caused by proliferation of the subcutaneous tissue containing an infiltrate in which multiple abscesses develop. The latter produce sinus tracts in the overlying, thinned-out skin, which has a bluish red color (Fig. 16-43). Pus discharged from these abscesses may contain sulfur

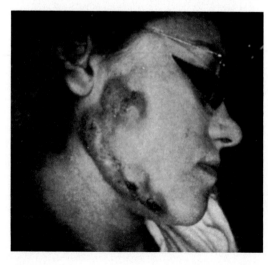

Fig. 16-43. Actinomycosis with multiple draining sinus tracts.

granules, which, when examined microscopically, disclose actinomyces colonies. The lymph nodes are generally not involved, although in mixed infections they may be enlarged and tender. However, cases have been reported in which the organism was found in the regional nodes. Dorph-Peterson and Pindborg (1954) reported a case of lingual actinomycosis. It formed an abscess that produced a nodule on the lateral aspect that was blue, smooth, and shiny (Fig. 16-44). After it was punctured, a considerable amount of yellow, thick pus escaped, which contained actinomyces-like gram-positive organisms. Zitka (1951) reported a case in which meningitis developed by extension, ending fatally, and cited cases reported in the German literature with metastatic involvement of the lungs, liver, kidney, and brain.

Actinomycosis of jaws

The anaerobic *Actinomyces* may invade the bone via the root canal of a carious tooth, a periodontal pocket, or via a tooth extraction wound, producing a radiolucent defect resembling osteitis in the radiograph (Fig. 16-45). The area may develop to considerable size and contain

granulation tissue, which, on microscopic examination, discloses the presence of colonies of actinomycetes. The lesions are generally of chronic character and symptomless, but in mixed infections exacerbations may occur. Sequestration is rare, but Breuer (1951) reported a case with sequestration at the inferior border of the mandible. In cases in which the bone is penetrated, the soft tissues surrounding the jaw may be extensively involved. A hard swelling develops, with trismus, and later multiple sinus tracts form and discharge pus in which sulfur granules that contain the organisms may be found. A case in which the alveolar process of the mandible was extensively involved was reported by Gold and Doyne (1952). A case of actinomycosis of the body of the mandible was described by Gruber (1953). In his case the infection started from an unerupted third molar and was associated with trismus, numbness of the lip, and swelling of the face.

In advanced cases the bone expands; this is the type that Pichler and Trauner (1948) spoke of as "actinomycoma." From the angle of the jaw the infection may spread to the condyle so that the joint may become involved. Breuer (1951) pointed out that in such cases fatal complications may occur by the disease breaking through the base of the skull to the brain.

Other organs of the body may be affected by actinomycosis. Otto (1954) described cases involving the gastrointestinal and urinary tracts, kidneys, testicles, eyes, and lungs, as well as the parotid gland.

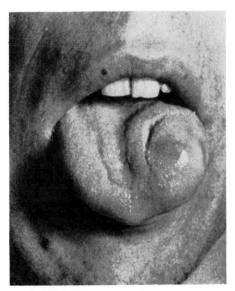

Fig. 16-44. Abscess caused by actinomycosis involving lateral part of tongue. (From Dorph-Peterson, L., and Pindborg, J. J. 1954. Oral Surg. **7:** 1178.)

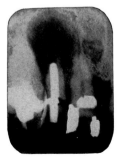

Fig. 16-45. Actinomycosis of maxilla.

Treatment. Antibiotic therapy gives excellent results. Penicillin was first used by Florey and Florey (1943) and Lyons (1943). In the early days the doses of the antibiotic were insufficient; large doses of the antibiotic are required. Penicillin G, 10 to 20 million units per day intravenously, should be given for at least 2 weeks. Oral penicillin V, 500 mg q.i.d., may then be substituted and continued for 3 to 6 months. Erythromycin, clindamycin, or tetracycline (Hinds and Degnan, 1955) can be used in patients allergic to penicillin. Adequate drainage should be established if abscesses occur. When the jaw is involved, removal of infected teeth, sequestra, and granulation tissue is indicated.

Blastomycosis

Blastomycosis is due to a specific infection that produces lesions in the skin and oral mucosa but may also affect all the large organs of the body. The South American form is caused by the fungus *Blastomyces brasiliensis* described in Chapter 4. It affects agricultural workers in coffee-growing regions, mainly in Brazil. Salman (1962) reported a case occurring in New York, and three other cases occurring in the United States were discussed by Joseph, Mare, and Irving (1966). All the patients had worked in South America, but the symptoms did not appear until years later, causing painful lesions in the mouth. However, the thought was expressed that these patients were not infected in Brazil, but that they had acquired the habit of chewing coffee beans or leaves and in this manner had contracted the disease later. Limongelli and co-workers (1978) recently reported a case of a patient who had lived in Venezuela, and reviewed the previous cases published in the United States.

North American blastomycosis is caused by *Blastomyces dermatitidis* (see Chapter 4). Cases have been reported by Mincer and Oglesby (1966) and Bell, Gamble, and Farrington (1969). Two cases occurring in Kentucky were recently reported by Page and co-workers (1979).

The oral lesions of both types of blasto-mycosis are similar. Small papular lesions are first seen that frequently occur on the cutaneous part of the lips. These become ulcerated and may resemble low-grade carcinoma (Fig. 16-46). Aubrey (1946) reported a case in which the gingiva of the mandible was involved. Marked gingival hyperplasia, which was painless and red, developed after extraction of a tooth. The regional lymph nodes were enlarged and hard. A small amount of pus was expressed, and biopsy examination lead to the diagnosis of blastomycosis. A week later lesions appeared on the legs.

Generally the regional lymph nodes are involved, simulating tuberculous adenitis and Hodgkin's disease. The lungs may become affected.

Treatment. Amphotericin B is the drug of choice in treating blastomycosis. Hydroxystilbamidine is used occasionally but must be administered with caution.

Histoplasmosis

Histoplasmosis, occurring especially in Panama, the Philippines, Argentina, Brazil, Honduras, Java, and more than 14 states of this country, is caused by the biphasic fungus *Histoplasma capsulatum* (see Chapter 4). Primary local lesions form that are nodular, ulcerative, or

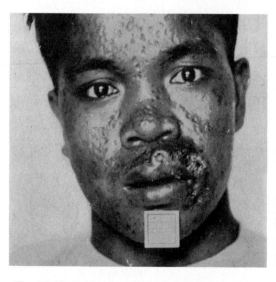

Fig. 16-46. Cutaneous blastomycosis causing papulopustular ulcers of the lips. (AFIP Acc. No. 68155.)

vegetative (Fig. 16-47). The tongue, lips, and cheeks are most frequently involved. There is also a disseminated type involving the lungs and other organs of the body (Boden, 1967).

Histologically, epithelioid cells and multinucleated giant cells, similar to Langhans' cells, are usually seen. The small organism, 1 μ to 5 μ, is oval or round and can be found in the cytoplasm of various phagocytic cells.

The disseminated form of histoplasmosis, when it occurs in children and elderly persons with debilitating disease, is often fatal. It affects the reticuloendothelial system producing involvement of lungs, bone marrow, spleen, and liver. Anemia and leukopenia are seen in the terminal stages. The white blood cell count may fall below 3000. In the healthy adult the disease may take a more chronic course. Silverman and co-workers (1955) recommend that the following steps be taken to make a diagnosis: skin test, complement fixation test, biopsy of oral lesions and lymph nodes, and cultures from blood, marrow, and organs showing involvement.

Treatment. Amphotericin B is the preferred treatment. Boden (1967) has outlined the therapeutic procedures.

Aspergillosis

This disease is caused by various species of *Aspergillus* (see Chapter 4). The lungs are the most common site of the infection. Hinson, Moon, and Plummer (1952) reviewed the literature and reported eight new cases.

Mehrotra (1965) reported a case occurring in the maxilla in a 50-year-old farmer who complained of a swelling of 3 years' duration. He had coughing associated with fever and hemoptysis. A spheric swelling, 4 cm in diameter, was found under the eye ("fungus ball"; aspergilloma). There was severe periodontal disease and heavy calculus deposits. Radiographs of the chest showed mottling in the right apex of the lung. In the face there was opacity of the maxillary sinus extending into the orbit. Tuberculosis was suspected and a biopsy was done. Epithelioid cells, giant cells, and elongated septate fungal hyphae were found.

Erlichman and Trieger (1978) have reported a case of aspergillosis in a patient receiving immunosuppressive drugs. With increased use of these agents, such cases may become more common.

Treatment. Aspergillosis is treated with amphotericin B.

Leprosy (Hansen's disease)

Leprosy is caused by *Mycobacterium leprae* (see Chapter 4), an acid-fast bacillus of high infectivity but low pathogenicity. It is not a common disease in the United States and most cases are found among immigrants from Africa, Southeast Asia, and South America.

The skin lesions usually present as numerous small macules, papules, or nodules. Invasion of peripheral nerves by the organisms frequently results in associated numbness. The face is commonly affected and the nasal, oral, and pharyngeal mucosa may be involved. Necrosis of the nasal cartilages can cause deformity and collapse. The oral lesions generally consist of nodular tumor masses that ulcerate as a result of trauma and secondary infection (Fitch and Alling,

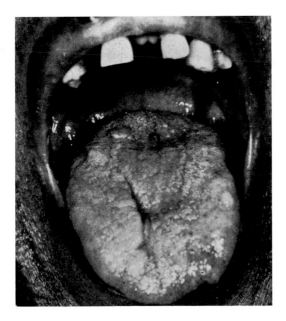

Fig. 16-47. Histoplasmosis of tongue causing swelling of dorsum and sides. (From Nutman, N. N. 1949. Oral Surg. **2:**1562.)

1962). The lips, tongue, and palate are the most commonly involved sites. Scarring of the lips may result in microstomia.

Sulfones are the drugs of choice for treatment of leprosy. Dapsone is the agent used most frequently. Long-term therapy is necessary, extending for as long as 2 years after the disease becomes inactive.

Granuloma inguinale

Granuloma inguinale is a chronic granulomatous disease that usually involves the genitalia. It is caused by the bacillus *Donovania granulomatis* (see Chapter 4). The oral lesions begin as painless nodules that subsequently break down to form ulcers with well-defined, elevated, granular margins (Ferro and Richeter, 1946). The lips, tongue, and gingiva may be involved. The gingival lesions may become confluent, resulting in a red, granular appearance. The diagnosis can be made by the demonstration of Donovan bodies in smears taken from the lesions. Treatment consists of tetracycline, 500 mg orally, four times a day for 10 to 14 days.

REFERENCES

Aggeler, P. M., et al. 1952. Plasma thromboplastin component (PTC) deficiency; new disease resembling hemophilia, Proc. Soc. Exp. Biol. Med. **79:**692.

Ahlborn, H. E. 1936. Simple achlorhydric anemia, Plummer-Vinson syndrome, and carcinoma of the mouth, pharynx and oesophagus in woman, Br. Med. J. **2:**331.

Al-Ubaidy, S. S., and Nally, F. F. 1976. Erythema multiforme, Oral Surg. **41:**601.

Archer, W. H. 1950. Hemophilias, the pre- and postoperative treatment, Oral Surg. **3:**1377.

Archer, W. H. 1951. Postextraction bleeding in a hemophiliac, Oral Surg. **4:**845.

Aubrey: Quoted from Burkett, L. W. 1946. Oral medicine, Philadelphia, J. B. Lippincott Co., p. 501.

Beck, L. 1962. Thrombocytopenic purpura, Oral Surg. **15:**148.

Bell, W., Gamble, J., and Garrington, G. 1969, North American blastomycosis with oral lesions, Oral Surg. **28:**914.

Belting, C. M., Hiniker, J. J., and Dummett, C. O. 1964. Influence of diabetes mellitus on the severity of periodontal disease, J. Periodont. **35:**476.

Betten, B., and Koppang, H. S. 1976. Sarcoidosis with mandibular involvement, Oral Surg. **42:**731.

Bhaskar, S. N. 1977. Synopsis of oral pathology, ed. 5, St. Louis, The C. V. Mosby Co.

Biggs, R., and Douglas, A. S. 1953. The thromboplastin generation test. J. Clin. Pathol. **6:**23.

Boden, R. A. 1967. Disseminated histoplasmosis with an oral lesion, Oral Surg. **23:**549.

Boeck, C. 1899. Multiple benign sarcoid of the skin, J. Cutan. Genito-Urin. Dis. **17:**543.

Boyle, P. E., Bessey, O. A., and Wolbach, S. B. 1937. Experimental production of diffuse alveolar bone atrophy type of periodontal disease by diets deficient in ascorbic acid, J. Am. Dent. Assoc. **24:**1768.

Breuer, J. 1951. Die Kieferknochen und Kiefergelenksaktinomykase und ihre Behondlung, Z. Stomat. **48:**26.

Cahn, L. R. 1938. The Plummer-Vinson syndrome facies: an oral pre-cancerous sign, Arch. Clin. Oral Pathol. **2:**308.

Campbell, J. B., et al. 1960. Activity of amphotericin B against *Candida albicans*, Oral Surg. **13:**1273.

Cooke, P. E. D. 1958. Biopsy procedures, Oral Surg. **11:**75.

Dechaume, M., et al. 1955. Cervicofacial actinomycosis, Rev. Stomatol. **56:**1.

Dennis, D., Miller, M. J., and Paterson, C. G. 1964. Candida septicemia, Surg. Gynecol. Obstet. **119:**50.

Dorph-Peterson, L., and Pindborg, J. J. 1954. Actinomycosis of the tongue, Oral Surg. **7:**1178.

Dozin, A. 1966. Amylase buccale, Actualités Odontostomatol. **75:**239.

Erichman, M. C., and Trieger, N. 1978. Aspergillus infection in a patient receiving immunosuppressive drugs, J. Oral Surg. **36:**978.

Ferro, E. R., and Richeter, J. W. 1946. Oral lesions of granuloma inguinale: report of three cases, J. Oral Surg. **4:**121.

Fitch, H. B., and Alling, C. C. 1962. Leprosy, oral manifestations, J. Periodontal. **33:**40.

Florey, M. E., and Florey, H. W. 1943. General and local administration of penicillin, Lancet **1:**387.

Foshager, V. D. 1964. Thrombocytopenic purpura following quinidine therapy, Oral Surg. **17:**401.

Frick, P. G. 1954. The relative incidence of antihemophilic globulin (AHG), plasma thromboplastin component (PTC) and plasma thromboplastin antecedent (PTA) deficiency, J. Lab. Clin. Med. **43:**860.

Giordano, N. D., et al. 1967. Dental extractions in hemophilic patients on aminocaproic acid prophylaxis, Oral Surg. **24:**171.

Glahn, M. 1951. The treatment of cervicofacial actinomycosis with special reference to penicillin therapy, Acta Chir. Scand. **102:**433.

Gold, L., and Doyne, E. E. 1952. Actinomycosis with osteomyelitis of alveolar process, Oral Surg. **5:**1056.

Goodman, M. J. 1939. Herpes zoster: treatment with thiamine chloride, Calif. Western Med. **51:**105.

Gorlin, R. J., and Gottsegen, R. 1949. The role of the gingival biopsy in secondary amyloid disease, Oral Surg. **2:**864.

Gottsegen, R. 1963. Dental considerations in diabetes mellitus, Dent. Abstr. **8:**278.

Gruber, M. D. 1953. Actinomycosis of the mandible, Oral Surg. **6:**292.

Hertz, J. 1955. Actinomycosis of the mandible, Acta Pathol. Microbiol. Scand. **36**:205.

Hertz, J. 1960. Actinomycosis: borderline cases, J. Int. Coll. Surg. **34**:148.

Hinds, E. C., and Degnan, E. J. 1955. Use of Achromycin and neomycin in the treatment of actinomycosis, Oral Surg. **8**:1034.

Hinson, K. F. W., Moon, A. J., and Plummer, N. S. 1952. Broncho-pulmonary aspergillosis, review and report of 8 new cases, Thorax **7**:317.

Hutchinson, N. 1898. Cases of Mortimer's malady, Arch. Surg. (London) **9**:307.

Israels, M. C. G., Lempert, H., and Gilbertson, E. 1951. Hemophilia in the female, Lancet. **1**:1375.

Jacoby, H. 1960. Veränderungen der Zunge in der Diagnostik des praktischen Arztes, Stuttgart, Schattaner.

Jeghers, H., McKusick, V. A., and Katz, K. H. 1949. Generalized intestinal polyposis and melanin spots of oral mucosa, lips, and digits, N. Engl. J. Med. **241**:993.

Joseph, E. A., Mare, A., and Irving, W. R. 1966. Oral South American blastomycosis in the United States of America, Oral Surg. **21**:732.

Kennett, S. 1968. Erythema multiforme affecting the oral cavity, Oral Surg. **25**:366.

Kerr, N. W. 1965. Sarcoidosis, Oral Surg. **20**:166.

Kraut, R. A., et al. 1977. Amyloidosis associated with multiple myeloma, Oral Surg. **43**:63.

Laskin, J. L. 1974. Oral hemorrhage after the use of quinidine: report of case, J. Am. Dent. Assoc. **88**:137.

Lasser, S. D., Cametta, B. M., and Needleman, H. L. 1977. Dental management of patients undergoing bone marrow transplantation for aplastic anemia, Oral Surg. **43**:181.

Lehner, T. 1964. Oral thrush or acute pseudomembranous candidiasis, Oral Surg. **18**:27.

Levine, S. 1959. Thrombocytopenic purpura due to quinine with oral symptoms, Oral Surg. **12**:692.

Lieb, E. 1947. Permanent stain for amyloid, Am. J. Clin. Pathol. **17**:413.

Ligmongelli, W. A., et al. 1978. Disseminated South American blastomycosis (paracoccidioidomycosis): report of case, J. Oral Surg. **36**:625.

Lovett, D. W., Cross, K. R., and Van Allen, M. 1965. The prevalence of amyloids in gingival tissue, Oral Surg. **20**:444.

Lucas, O. N., and Geisler, P. H. 1965. Dental extraction in an haemophilia A female, Br. J. Oral Surg. **2**:179.

Lyons, C. 1943. Penicillin treatment of surgical infections in the U.S. Army, J.A.M.A. **123**:1007.

Mandel, L., and Baurmash, H. 1962. Differentiation of submaxillary lymphadenopathy and submaxillary salivary gland pathology, Oral Surg. **15**:3.

Mehrotra, M. C. 1965. Aspergillosis of the maxilla, Oral Surg. **20**:33.

Mersky, C. 1951. The occurrence of hemophilia in the human female, Quart. J. Med. **20**:299.

Meyer, I., and Shklar, G. 1967. The oral manifestations of acquired syphilis, Oral Surg. **23**:45.

Mincer, H., and Oglesby, R. 1966. Intraoral North American blastomycosis, Oral Surg. **22**:36.

Mulkey, T. F. 1976. Outpatient treatment of hemophiliacs for dental extraction, J. Oral Surg. **34**:428.

Nairn, R. I. 1975. Nystatin and amphotericin B in the treatment of denture-related candidiasis, Oral Surg. **40**:68.

O'Driscoll, P. M. 1966. The incidence of and management of diabetics in oral surgery, Br. Dent. J. **4**:38.

Orlean, S. L., and O'Brien, J. J. 1966. Sarcoidosis manifesting a soft tissue lesion in the floor of the mouth, Oral Surg. **21**:819.

Otto, H. 1954. Ueber die vershiedenen Lokalisationen der Aktinomycesinfektion im menschlichen Körper, Z. Ges. Inn. Med. (Leipzig) **9**:578.

Page, L. R., et al. 1979. Blastomycosis with oral lesions, Oral Surg. **47**:157.

Peutz, J. L. 1921. A very remarkable case of familial polyposis, Nederl. Maandschr. Geneesk. **10**:134.

Pichler, H. and Trauner, R. 1948. Mund und Kieferchirurgie, part II vol. 1, Wien, Urban & Schwarzenberg, p. 137.

Reed, W. O., et al. 1964. The use of epsilon-aminocaproic acid in the management of dental extractions in the hemophiliac, Am. J. Med. Sci. **248**:184.

Remmer, R. P. et al. 1979. The role of *C. albicans* in denture stomatitis, Oral Surg. **47**:323.

Roche, W. C., and Morris, C. R. 1967. Sarcoidosis of sublingual gland, J. Oral Surg. **25**:77.

Rosenthal, R. L., Dreskin, O. H., and Rosenthal, N. 1953. New hemophilia-like disease caused by a deficiency of a third thromboplastin factor, Proc. Soc. Exp. Biol. Med. **82**:171.

Sachs, S. A., and Eisenbud, L. 1977. Tuberculous osteomyelitis of the mandible, Oral Surg. **44**:425.

Sachs, S. A., Lipton, R., and Frank, R. 1978. Management of ambulatory oral surgical patients with hemophilia, J. Oral Surg. **36**:25.

Salman, L. 1962. South American blastomycosis, Oral Surg. **15**:671.

Schaumann, J. 1914. Sur le lupus pernio, Soc. Francaise de Dermatologic et Syphilographic Zambaco.

Schliack, V. 1960. Serial examination of dental patients for determination of unrecognized diabetes mellitus, Dent. Abstr. **5**:437.

Schwartz, H. C., and Olson, D. J. 1975. Amyloidosis: a rational approach to diagnosis by intraoral biopsy, Oral Surg. **39**:837.

Sebrell, W. H., and Butler, R. E. 1938. Riboflavin deficiency in man, Public Health Rep. **53**:2282.

Selikoff, I. J., and Robitzek, E. H. 1947. Gingival biopsy for the diagnosis of generalized amyloidosis, Am. J. Pathol. **23**:1099.

Shepard, J. P. 1978. The management of oral complications of leukemia, Oral Surg. **45**:543.

Silverman, F. N. et al. 1955. Histoplasmosis, Am. J. Med. **19**:410.

Soulier, J. P., and Larrieu, M. J. 1953. Nouvelle méthode de diagnostic de l'hemophile, dosage des facteurs antihemophiliques A et B, Sang **24**:205.

Spatz, S. 1964. Angioneurotic edema of the maxillary region, Oral Surg. **18**:256.

Sprague, C. C., et al. 1952. Platelet transfusions and pathogenesis of idiopathic thrombocytopenic purpura, J. A. M. A. **150**:1193.

Steg, R. F., et al. 1960. Bleeding due to deficiency of

plasma thromboplastin antecedent (PTA) and plasma thromboplastin component (PTC), Oral Surg 13:671.

Symmers, W. St. C. 1956. Primary amyloidosis, J. Clin. Pathol. 9:187.

Tagliano, P. 1947. La Tuberculosi della Mandibula, Stomatologia 1:515.

Taylor, R. G., and Booth, D. F. 1964. Tuberculous osteomyelitis of the mandible, Oral Surg. 18:7.

Tillman, H. H. 1957. Oral manifestations of generalized systemic amyloid disease, Oral Surg. 10:743.

Tillman, H. H., Taylor, R. G., and Carchidig, E. 1966. Sarcoidosis of the tongue, Oral Surg. 21:190.

Vinson, P. P. 1922. Hysterical dysphagia, Minnesota Med. 5:107.

Waldenström, J., and Kjellberg, S. R. 1939. The roentgenological diagnosis of sideropenic dysphagia, Acta Radiol. 20:618.

Watts, J. M. 1961. The importance of the Plummer-Vinson syndrome in the aetiology of carcinoma of the upper gastrointestinal tract, Postgrad. Med. J. 37:523.

White, S. G., Aggeler, P. M., and Glendenning, M. B. 1953. Plasma thromboplastin component (PTC), a hitherto unrecognized blood coagulation factor, Blood 8:101.

Woodruff, P. W., and Hesseltine, H. C. 1938. Relationship of oral thrush to vaginal mycosis and incidence of each, Am. J. Obstet. Gynecol. 36:467.

Zimmerman, S. L., Frutschey, L., and Gibbes, I. H. 1947. Meningitis due to *Candida albicans* with recovery, J.A.M.A. 135:145.

Zitka, E. 1951. Klinische und therapeutische Erfahrungen bei cervicofacialer Aktinomykose, Oest. Z. Stomat. 48:11, 69.

CHAPTER 17

Implications of systemic diseases in the surgical patient

Victor J. Matukas

The astute oral and maxillofacial surgeon must be aware of systemic diseases that may have early or peculiar oral manifestations so that he may play a role in early diagnosis (see Chapter 16). He must also be aware of the reaction of the oral cavity to various systemic states and be prepared to manage oral surgical problems in this group of patients. He must further recognize various disease processes of a systemic nature that may influence the choice of therapy or those that represent a definite risk in surgical management. Additionally, it is expected that the modern oral and maxillofacial surgeon will have developed sufficient skills to recognize early systemic disease even if oral manifestations are not involved and thus expeditiously place the patient in the proper medical referral pattern. It is obvious that the attainment of these skills requires competent instruction and frequent reinforcement to be clinically useful.

RESPIRATORY DISEASES

From the standpoint of the oral and maxillofacial surgeon, it is useful to divide respiratory problems into three broad categories: (1) preexisting lung disease in patients having elective surgery, (2) respiratory problems accompanying trauma, and (3) postoperative respiratory complications.

Chronic lung disease

Conceptually, specific disease states of the respiratory system are not as important to the oral and maxillofacial surgeon as the degree of remaining respiratory function. This is true regardless of the pathophysiologic process by which function has deteriorated. In evaluating a patient with preexisting lung disease, several factors must be considered. These are: (1) What is the preoperative status of the patient? (2) What will the effects of the operation be on the patient? (3) Can the preoperative condition of the patient be reversed or improved prior to surgery? (4) What diagnostic and therapeutic measures should be used intra- and postoperatively to maintain adequate respiratory function.

In evaluating the respiratory system, the surgeon has certain modalities available to him. One must keep in mind, however, that the respiratory system works in conjunction with the cardiovascular and hematopoietic systems to supply oxygen to the tissues and rid them of carbon dioxide. Thus similar symptoms may be produced by disease states in any of these systems and they cannot be considered independently.

A history of long-standing emphysema, asthma, bronchitis, recurring pneumonia, viral respiratory infections, or recurring pneumothorax should be of considerable concern to the surgeon. However, the residual pulmonary reserve is more important than the type of disease, and, indeed, most patients with chronic lung disease probably have a combination of several of these pathologic states.

Certain specific factors are important in the evaluation of the respiratory system. Three important parameters are chronic cough, smoking, and exercise tolerance. Persistent coughing is not normal, and a history of early morning coughing may be very significant. One must diligently pursue questioning about this symptom as many patients feel that frequent coughing (smoker's cough) is unimportant. Generally, cough indicates upper airway irritation. It can be almost categorically stated that pulmonary dysfunction is present when a patient has smoked for 20 or more years. In some cases, dysfunction will be present with a much shorter smoking history.

Exercise tolerance is an important indicator of pulmonary as well as cardiac status. It is essential to remember when questioning about exercise tolerance that respiratory failure may be insidious and the patient may have voluntarily limited activity to a level where dyspnea does not occur. The answer to a question such as "Do you get short of breath?" will then be negative because the patient avoids exertion and thus never works hard enough to obtain that state. Eliciting an admission of a gradual limitation of physical activity may be a more significant finding. A useful classification of exercise tolerance is one advocated by McCarthy (1972) for evaluation of cardiac status since, as previously mentioned, the pulmonary and cardiac systems are interdependent.

Class I – Normal
Class II – Dyspnea with exertion
Class III – Dyspnea with normal activity (two flights of stairs or six blocks)
Class IV – Dyspnea at rest

Class III and IV patients are obviously high-risk individuals and require more extensive preparation prior to elective surgery.

There are certain very important physical parameters that should be considered in evaluating respiratory status. Heart and respiratory rate and the work of breathing should be assessed. A resting pulse of greater than 100 may be compensatory for hypoxemia caused by respiratory disease. It is obvious that other influencing factors such as infection, decreased cardiac output, or anxiety must be ruled out. Tachypnea with a rate of greater than 20 may also be compensatory for respiratory disease. In obstructive lung disorders the work of breathing is also increased and accessory muscles may be needed. Tidal volume may decrease and shallow rapid breathing may occur. The presence of asymmetric chest movements or splinting should be noted. The configuration of the chest should also be observed. A large barrel-shaped chest should make one suspicious of emphysema.

The character of the breath sounds is another important parameter in the evaluation of pulmonary status. However, many patients with extreme loss of respiratory reserve have relatively normal auscultatory examinations. Patients with emphysema exhange little air because of increased dead space and thus may have quiet chests to auscultation. Similarly, if obstruction is present and the patient is hypoventilating, enough air may not be moved to evoke a wheeze. The presence of abnormal sounds such as rales (collapsed or fluid-filled small airways), ronchi (fluid or mucus in large airways), and wheezing (obstruction) should be noted. Wheezing is particularly important because of the catastrophic nature of acute asthmatic attacks and the usual controllable nature of the disease prior to surgery.

There are two simple tests that also may be helpful in evaluating marginal cases of pulmonary disease. In the forced expiration test the time from maximum inspiration to maximum expiration is recorded. A figure of greater than 5 seconds is abnormal and probably merits use of pulmonary function tests. In the instance of a normal or high normal resting pulse, testing the response to mild exercise (one flight of stairs [15] at a brisk rate) may be revealing. A pulse of less than 120 with a return to normal in 1 minute indicates adequate cardiopulmonary reserve. Pulse rates between 120 and 140 are suspect, and a pulse rate greater than 140 represents a poor risk patient. The degree of dyspnea should also be noted.

Depending on the nature of the findings from the history and physical evaluation, the surgeon can order certain laboratory examinations that may be of value.

Chest radiograph

The chest radiograph may be relatively normal even in long-standing lung disease. However, most often effusions, infiltrates, nodules, and pleural accumulations will be detected. One should observe the pattern of pulmonary vasculature for signs of increasing pulmonary resistance. Also, patients with emphysema will typically have small, rather upright hearts and may show signs of right ventricular hypertrophy.

Hematocrit

Long-standing hypoxemia is a potent stimulus to increase red cell mass. Thus compensatory polycythemia may occur in long-standing respiratory disease and the hematocrit will be elevated.

CO_2 combining power

If the patient has alveolar hypoventilation and has retained CO_2 over a long period of time, a compensatory metabolic alkalosis will develop in response to respiratory acidosis. CO_2 is a potent stimulant for renal bicarbonate reabsorption and the CO_2 combining power may rise.

Arterial blood gases

The proper use of blood gas studies is mandatory in the evaluation of patients in any modern surgical practice. Hypoxemia may be due to alveolar hypoventilation, shunting (ventilation/perfusion abnormalities), or diffusion block. Hypoventilation is always accompanied by a corresponding increase in P_{CO_2} so that valid judgments can be made as to the nature of the respiratory problem. Decisions as to whether to institute medical therapy, relieve obstruction, increase oxygen, or mechanically assist ventilation can often be made from blood gas interpretation. It must be noted, however, that resting blood gases may be deceptively normal in patients with poor reserve and long-standing disease. A prudent course of action prior to surgery in patients with suggestive, but not conclusive, historical and physical findings is to measure resting baseline arterial blood gases and, if in doubt, also after exercise.

Pulmonary function tests

There are many complex examinations that are done by laboratories in major centers. The two most common and perhaps most useful to the surgeon are vital capacity and forced vital capacity. The former measures useful lung volume and generally indicates restrictive pulmonary disease. The latter measures the ability of the patient to move air irrespective of volume and thus is an indication of obstructive lung disease. Values of less than 70% of that predicted in either test represent poor risk patients for general anesthesia. It is very common to find impairment in both tests in patients with long-standing respiratory disease, and, in fact, pure obstructive or restrictive disease is rare.

Based on the data collected from the history, physical examination, and laboratory tests, the surgeon must make his diagnostic and therapeutic decisions (see also Chapter 9). Certainly measures to reverse or control respiratory disease prior to elective surgery can be instituted. General symptom-ameliorating medical measures prior to surgery, such as cessation of smoking, use of bronchodilators, antibiotics, and steroid therapy, should be considered. Also of great importance are preoperative physical measures such as postural drainage, vibropercussion, encouragement of deep coughing, and an increase in general ambulation and activity. Careful attention to such medical and physical details often makes the difference between a benign and stormy postoperative course.

Respiratory problems accompanying trauma

The major traumatic injuries that may be encountered that affect the respiratory system are lung contusions, rib fractures, hemopneumothorax, and flail chest.

Many of the diagnostic criteria already discussed for evaluating preexisting lung disease are also applicable in assessing chest trauma. However, with chest trauma the radiograph is one of the most useful adjuncts. Significant effusions secondary to contusions or rib fractures, hemopneumothorax, pneumonia secondary to splinting, and flail chest may all be apparent on the radiograph. Arterial blood gas measurements are very helpful in deciding whether to therapeutically intervene following trauma. Large effusions of fluid and blood generally should be drained by appropriately placed chest tubes. Small effusions coupled with satisfactory blood gas levels may be left to resorb. Although their primary injury may not be great, patients with rib fractures should be carefully observed because voluntary splinting owing to chest pain may lead to atelectasis and/or pneumonia.

The modern therapy for flail chest is positive pressure ventilation, usually with positive end-expiratory pressure and intermittent mandatory ventilation. The latter requires some form of airway control (endotracheal tube or tracheostomy) and a proper ventilator. Usually 7 to 14 days are required for stabilization of the chest and extubation. Most of the above conditions will require the utilization of appropriate consultation for proper management and decision about timing of therapy for associated maxillofacial injuries.

Postoperative pulmonary complications

The most common postsurgical respiratory complication is segmental atelectasis with ensuing infection. This particular problem is most often seen in patients with unrecognized preexisting lung disease, but it may also occur in otherwise healthy patients following general anesthesia. Typically the patient will suddenly develop low-grade fever and may or may not have auscultatory or radiographic findings of consolidation. Often these symptoms will be alleviated by physical measures such as the use of blow bottles, deep coughing, and ambulation. If frank pneumonia occurs, sputum smears, cultures, and antibiotic sensitivity tests should be obtained and the patient placed on appropriate antibiotics in addition to the physical measures just mentioned.

One of the most serious pulmonary complications that can follow severe trauma or major surgery has been referred to by a variety of names—shock lung, aspiration lung, wet lung syndrome, and so on. The current view is that the disease can be precipitated by a variety of pathologic processes, and the preferred name is acute respiratory distress syndrome. Among the possible etiologic factors is a direct toxic effect on the lung from inhalation of noxious agents, aspiration of foreign material, or fat embolism. More indirect etiologies have included shock, disseminated intravascular coagulation, and cerebral trauma. While the pathophysiology of this disease is not entirely clear, the initial lesion seems to be an increase in pulmonary capillary permeability. As the process continues, alveolar surfactant is destroyed and areas of atelectasis and fluid-filled alveoli develop. The net result is a severe diffusion defect, a ventilation/perfusion abnormality, and a physiologic shunting across the lung. Thus hypoxemia, which can only be partially corrected by increasing inspired oxygen concentration, develops. If the process continues, dyspnea occurs with tachypnea and tachycardia. The chest radiograph will show fluffy infiltrates usually beginning at the lung bases or peripheral areas. In the full-blown syndrome with profound hypoxemia, treatment consists of a closed oxygen system utilizing intubation, a volume-cycled ventilator, positive end-expiratory pressure, and FIO_2 (fraction of inspired oxygen) concentrations of 50% or greater. Steroids have also been suggested as being helpful. Treatment of the underlying cause of the disease is mandatory.

Obviously the treatment of these patients requires the help and guidance of physicians specially trained in the management of such matters. It is important for the surgeon to recognize the process in its early stages and take appropriate steps to reverse it. Not only is the disease acutely life threatening, but if it is not controlled early, the patient will develop chronic restrictive lung disease.

CARDIOVASCULAR DISEASES

It is obviously of great importance to evaluate the cardiovascular system prior to surgery. The diseases to be considered can be roughly classified as peripheral vascular or cardiac in origin. For the most part, the same considerations relative to evaluation of reserve mentioned for respiratory disease are also valid in considering cardiac disease. The same classification as outlined previously for respiratory reserve can be used. In the case of congestive heart failure, dyspnea is also the indicator of the reserve end point, and the patient is categorized as a Class I, II, III, or IV risk (see p. 576). With coronary artery disease, the presence of chest pain with varying degrees of exercise is a convenient end point and again a similar classification may be useful.

Peripheral vascular disease

The main entities to be considered with regard to peripheral vascular disease are advanced atherosclerosis and hypertension. A well-controlled hypertensive patient should offer no special problems for routine surgery but should probably be considered at least a Class II risk. Prolonged hypertension, however, causes multiple organ disease, and patients with a long history of high blood pressure should be evaluated very carefully. This group of patients may have left ventricular or biventricular failure caused by prolonged cardiac work against a high afterload. Some degree of renal failure may also be present owing to arteriosclerosis, or, conversely, renal failure may be the precipitating cause of the hypertension. Patients with hypertension may also be on a variety of drugs, the therapeutic potency of which depends on the degree of elevated pressure. Generally, the more potent drugs have more numerous side effects. The drugs used may range from mild diuretics to ganglionic-blocking agents.

Adequate control of hypertension should not be measured by normal standards, as this patient population may have become accustomed to high perfusion pressures and what would constitute proper blood pressure in a normotensive patient may be low for a patient with prolonged hypertension. On the other hand, elective surgery should certainly be postponed if the pressure is greatly elevated. This is especially true if the patient is symptomatic (that is, has dizzy spells, headaches, scotoma, and/or epistaxis).

Not only should the hypertension be controlled but, if possible, its etiology should be determined. Sometimes this will lead to the recognition of problems in other organ systems. A diagnosis of essential hypertension should be made with caution. For example, although not a common occurrence, one would not want to unknowingly perform an elective surgical procedure on a patient with a pheochromocytoma.

Certain clinical laboratory procedures are helpful in evaluating the cardiac patient. The electrocardiogram is perhaps the most useful. The chest radiograph is also a valuable diagnostic aid. Note should be made of heart size and signs of ventricular dilation or hypertrophy. The lung fields should be examined for prominent vasculature or signs of pulmonary edema.

The urinalysis and serum BUN and creatinine levels provide an indication of whether renal involvement may be present. Prolonged hypertension often leads to proteinuria and a decrease in the glomerular filtration rate. It is preferable to use the serum creatinine level as an estimate of the glomerular filtration rate rather than the BUN because the latter is influenced by numerous nonrenal factors. In evaluating kidney function it is important to remember that renal pathology can cause hypertension as well as be caused by it.

The initial workup may also include an intravenous pyelogram, measurement of urinary catecholamines and plasma renin levels, as well as other tests. These are primarily diagnostic tests to rule out correctable causes of hypertension and are not commonly employed in following the course of a diagnosed case of essential hypertension.

Patients with far advanced arteriosclerotic vascular disease may also be suffering from generalized organ failure caused by microangiopathy and general ischemic changes. Of paramount importance is the presence of coronary artery involvement (see p. 581) and the resultant angina, cerebral vascular changes, or both. The latter may produce changes ranging from generalized senility to transient ischemia to actual stroke. The transient ischemic attacks are characterized by brief motor or sensory deficits that may or may not leave permanent damage. A carotid bruit may be noted by auscultation. If such attacks are frequent or the bruit is significant, it may be wise to defer elective surgery until corrective endarterectomy is performed.

Cardiac diseases

Cardiac diseases can generally be categorized into three broad groups that are of significance to the surgeon: congestive heart failure, coronary artery disease, and diseases requiring antibiotic prophylaxis.

Congestive heart failure

Congestive heart failure may be right, left, or biventricular. Such states as prolonged hypertension, myocardial infarction, congenital heart disease, and long-standing pulmonary disease may ultimately either directly decrease the contractility of the heart or place undue work on a normal myocardium, thus leading to the syndrome of decreased cardiac output or failure. The underlying causative disease is of less importance than the fact that cardiac output may be low and myocardial reserve diminished. A sufficient degree of cardiac failure may secondarily cause cardiac arrythmias, which by themselves may be compatible with life but which add to the problem by causing insufficient ventricular filling and decreased reserve. The end result may be decreased cardiac output to a point that is incompatible with life.

Cardiac failure can be clinically assessed by estimating cardiac output at rest and the degree of reserve that is available to maintain adequate output with function. One of the best indicators of reserve is exercise tolerance (see p. 576). Other important historical factors are orthopnea, paroxysmal nocturnal dyspnea, dependent edema, cyanosis, chest pain, and cough.

The adequacy of performance of the cardiovascular system can be estimated from certain physical findings. Normal cardiac output at rest is 3.5 L/min/m^2. This most obviously increases when oxygen demand rises, as with trauma, fever, or exercise. Such factors as a strong pulse, warm and pink extremities, and adequate arterial blood pressure indicate the adequacy of output at the time of estimation. Other observations such as sufficient urinary output, circulation, and cardiac rhythm also are helpful in making this estimate. The other factor that must be considered is whether all available reserve is being used to maintain this output. If so, the patient may do well at rest but go into failure during stress. Basic reserve mechanisms that may be used to maintain cardiac function are increased rate and myocardial stroke volume to increase cardiac output, increased venous tone to increase cardiac preload, and selective increase in arteriolar resistance to effectively shunt perfusion from nonvital organs to the kidneys, brain, and heart. Thus the presence of tachycardia and cold and pale extremities, coupled with a history of dyspnea on exertion, should lead one to a diagnosis of compensated cardiac failure.

Certain generalizations can be made about arrythmias. For the most part, supraventricular arrythmias are not as hemodynamically embarrassing as those of the ventricle. In supraventricular arrythmias, the degree of decompensation is somewhat dependent on ventricular rate. If the ventricles are following atrial impulses at rates greater than 150, adequate diastolic filling is not present and cardiac output is decreased. Rates greater than 100 cannot be tolerated for long periods because of increased work and, therefore, increased oxygen demand on the heart.

The common atrial arrythmias are sinus tachycardia, fibrillation, and flutter. In sinus tachycardia the ventricles usually respond on a 1 to 1 basis, and vagal stimulation or sedation will usually slow the rate. Atrial fibrillation may be long-standing, and if the accompanying ventricular rate is less than 100, adequate cardiac output can usually be maintained. The pulse rate is irregularly irregular and an apical/radial pulse deficit may be noted. This event subsequently leads to inefficient, but generally adequate, perfusion. Quinidine or electrocardioversion may be employed to abolish the arrythmia. If conversion is unsuccessful, digitalis is employed to delay impulse conduction through the atrioventricular node and thus decrease the ventricular rate and increase diastolic filling.

Atrial flutter is a rarer condition, but more difficult to manage. The atria may be discharging at rates of 300/min or more and ventricular response will vary according to the degree of heart block. If a 2 to 1 block occurs with an atrial rate of 300, then the ventricular rate will be 150; if 3 to 1 it will be 100, and so on. Flutter should be converted early, if possible, as the ventricular rate in atrial flutter is difficult to control with digitalis. For example, adequate digitalization may convert a 2 to 1 block with a rate of 150 to 6 to 1 with a rate of 50. All the preceding represent hemodynamically compromised patients and elective surgery should be preceded by careful evaluation and precautions.

Ventricular arrythmias in contrast to those of atrial origin may be acutely life threatening. They range in order of severity from premature ventricular contractions to ventricular tachycardia to ventricular fibrillation to cardiac standstill. Hypoxemia, ischemia, acid/base disorders, electrolyte imbalance, and drugs are common causes of ventricular arrythmias and such conditions should be evaluated quickly and resolved when they develop.

Premature ventricular contractions may occur as occasional events and thus not be significant. They become significant if they exceed 6 to 8/min, show evidence of being multifocal, or come in sequential runs. All of these rhythms may lead to ventricular tachycardia or fibrillation. These rhythms may not be immedi-

ately fatal, but they must be controlled. Lidocaine given by intravenous bolus, followed by a constant drip, is the drug of choice. Adequate preparation must be made for cardiopulmonary resuscitation in such a situation.

Ventricular fibrillation is incompatible with life because of inadequate cardiac output and thus is equivalent to cardiac standstill. Cardiopulmonary resuscitation should be employed to maintain stable hemodynamics while defibrillation is accomplished (see Chapter 11).

Coronary artery disease

Coronary artery disease is another cardiac condition that must be evaluated prior to elective surgery. Angina pectoris is related to a discrepancy between myocardial oxygen demand and availability. Factors that increase oxygen demand are increased heart rate, myocardial contractility, and left ventricular wall tension. Thus oxygen demand will increase with hypertension, ventricular dilation and hypertrophy, and tachycardia. These states may be precipitated by drugs such as catecholamines, alpha-blockers, or digitalis. Under normal conditions, this increased oxygen demand is met by an increase in coronary artery circulation. Other factors such as hemoglobin concentration and alveolar/arterial oxygen differences are also important, but by far the major determinant of myocardial oxygenation is coronary artery blood flow. Since resistance is inversely related to flow, therapy of angina pectoris is usually designed to decrease coronary artery resistance in order to improve oxygenation of the myocardium.

Anginal attacks have classically been characterized as producing crushing substernal pain that radiates down the left arm. However, the pain associated with myocardial ischemia may vary from such a classic presentation to such variants as dyspnea and tightness in the chest to other more diffuse types of pain. Two factors are reasonably constant with each attack. The pain may become more severe as the disease progresses, but the pattern of pain tends to remain constant in any given person. The other relatively constant factor in true angina pectoris is a tendency toward pain after a fixed amount of exercise. Very often the patient will subconsciously not exceed this exercise limit and thus decrease the degree and number of episodes of pain. Because of this factor, careful questioning may be necessary to elicit a concrete history of true angina.

As the disease progresses, the amount of exercise necessary to produce pain decreases and the intensity of pain often increases. These increasing symptoms are a serious consequence and indicate progressive coronary artery disease. True angina at rest or nocturnal angina usually carries a grave prognosis and represents a patient who is a very poor risk for elective surgery.

The surgical management of a patient with either congestive heart failure or angina pectoris depends on the severity of the disease and the associated cardiac reserve. In the case of congestive heart failure the measured component is cardiac output, and in the case of angina it is coronary artery reserve. Class I and II patients can generally be managed for outpatient surgery without special precautions. Class IV patients in both categories represent a distinct risk and probably are not candidates for elective surgery. Class III patients, or patients with dyspnea on normal activity or angina under similar conditions, can be managed in the office but certain precautions should be taken. The judicious use of sedatives to decrease tissue oxygen demand may be helpful if oversedation to the point of respiratory depression is avoided. The use of concomitant oxygen therapy may be helpful to increase the arterial PO_2. It may be desirable to operate on the patient in a sitting position because of the problems of orthopnea in patients with congestive heart failure and decreased respiratory exchange in patients with diminished coronary artery blood flow. Prophylactic nitroglycerin may also be of value in patients with angina pectoris if given prior to anesthetic injection.

Patients who have a documented history of a myocardial infarction need special consideration in two areas. The first is the risk of precipitating a life-threatening event by elective surgery. During the first weeks following necrosis of cardiac muscle, rupture of a large infarct of the ventricular wall may occur. Later a ventricular aneurysm may be present because of a weakened ventricular wall. Pericarditis is an infrequent manifestation of transmural infarction. Depending on the vessel involved, various conduction problems may also occur such as atrial and ventricular arrythmias, bundle branch block, and various degrees of heart block. A common acute manifestation is congestive heart failure, which may range from mild to severe. If cardiac output falls below a critical level, evidence of clinical shock appears. The symptoms just mentioned may be transient or may persist to some degree. Because of the lability of the cardiac conduction system and the weakness of the ventricular wall immediately after infarction, it is probably a wise policy to avoid any elective surgery for a period of at least 6 months after a documented myocardial infarction. This allows sufficient time for scar formation to produce a stable ventricular wall and for electrical excitability of the conducting system to stabilize. After 6 months, the surgery patient can usually be managed on the basis of signs and symptoms that indicate the degree of residual damage. Common residual problems after infarction are ventricular failure, arrythmias, and persistent angina pectoris. A treatment plan should take into account the degree of persistent pathology.

Diseases requiring antibiotic prophylaxis

Cardiac diseases requiring antibiotic prophylaxis are of special interest to the oral and maxillofacial surgeon. This includes the group of patients who have rheumatic heart disease, congenital heart disease, or prosthetic cardiac or vascular appliances. All of these patients should be covered by appropriate antibiotic therapy prior to any oral surgery manipulation. Some controversy exists as to the need for antibiotic coverage in patients who have a known history of rheumatic fever as a child but have no residual clinical cardiovascular signs. In view of the serious consequences if subacute bacterial endocarditis should develop, it is perhaps a prudent policy to assume residual valvular vegetations are present and use prophylactic coverage.

Young patients and patients with high risk of recurrent streptococcal infections may also be on low doses of penicillin for prophylaxis against recurrences of rheumatic fever. The dosage employed is not sufficient to render protection against acute or subacute bacterial endocarditis in these patients and adequate supplementary antibiotics are recommended.

It has been estimated that 70% of all cases of subacute bacterial endocarditis and 90% of all cases of acute bacterial endocarditis are caused by alpha-hemolytic streptococci. If cases caused only by dental manipulation are considered, the incidence of this organism as a causative agent is probably higher. Since alpha-streptococci are sensitive to penicillin, this drug remains the agent of choice. The principles of prophylaxis are to have bactericidal blood levels of antibiotic at the time of surgery and for 2 days following (see Chapter 9, p. 330). There is no good evidence that maintaining antibiotic levels for a time prior to surgery is effective in decreasing the amount of bacteremia that occurs during the operation, and there is always the possibility that resistant strains will emerge. There remains some controversy as to whether antibiotics that include a gram-negative spectrum or that affect penicillin-resistant staphylococci should be used on patients who have been on long-term penicillin prophylaxis and who may have altered oral flora. In these cases cephalosporin, streptomycin, or penicillinase-resistant penicillin constitute a reasonable approach to the therapeutic problem.

Essentially the same antibiotic considerations hold true for patients with congenital heart disease and those with prosthetic valvular or vascular replacement. Some difference of opinion exists as to the adequate management of patients who have had coronary artery bypass procedures, an operation that is increasingly more common and thus likely to confront the oral and maxillofacial surgeon as a management problem. Insufficient data exist regarding this particular area, and therapy presently is dictated by local custom.

GASTROINTESTINAL DISEASES

There are several diseases of the gastrointestinal tract that are of direct importance to the oral and maxillofacial surgeon. Such diverse disorders as peptic ulcer, regional enteritis, pancreatitis, and ulcerative colitis may cause secondary problems if oral surgery is contemplated, particularly during acute exacerbations. Moreover, because of the relationship of stress to some of these conditions, anticipation of surgery or surgery itself may cause exacerbations.

Long-standing inflammatory disease of either the upper or lower bowel, with either chronic bleeding or multiple episodes of acute bleeding, may lead to an iron deficiency anemia. Additionally, patients of this type may be suffering from varying degrees of malnutrition ranging from protein depletion to both fat- and water-soluble vitamin deficiency. The effects of dietary changes resulting from oral surgery must also be considered in these patients. However, it would be relatively rare for the oral and maxillofacial surgeon to have to manage a surgical problem in a patient either rendered hypovolemic or in a state of electrolyte imbalance owing to long-standing bowel disease. Water and electrolyte imbalances are correctable and this should certainly be accomplished prior to any surgical intervention (see Chapter 9).

Malabsorption represents another disease state in which oral surgery care may need to be modified. Malabsorption represents a syndrome and may be caused by a wide variety of etiologic factors. Two basic types occur: either there is a basic defect in the lining of the intestinal mucosa with ensuing malabsorption, often of selected foods; or foodstuffs are not prepared properly in the intestine for absorption by a normal mucosa. An example of the first is celiac disease and of the second is pancreatic insufficiency.

Regardless of the cause, however, the clinical manifestations are similar. Diarrhea with foul bulky stools caused by unabsorbed fats is the most common symptom. These patients fail to thrive and weight loss is common. Of particular interest to the oral and maxillofacial surgeon is a tendency toward edema from decreased absorption of protein, osteoporosis owing to hypovitaminosis D, and bleeding owing to the malabsorption of fat-soluble vitamin K. The last leads to a decrease in synthesis of vitamin K–dependent factors by the liver. Various forms of anemia may also coexist owing to iron, B_{12}, and folate deficiency.

Prior to elective surgery, these patients should be evaluated for general health and nutrition as well as for anemia. A prothrombin time should be done routinely. Since the liver is intact, the patient will respond to parenteral vitamin K if an abnormal prothrombin time exists.

HEPATIC DISEASES

Hepatic disease is a relatively common ailment that may complicate oral and maxillofacial surgery. Two categories are of prime importance: one is the patient with hepatic failure caused either by obstruction or an altered metabolic process and the other is viral hepatitis.

Chronic failure

Chronic diffuse liver disease, that is, cirrhosis with a concomitant loss of hepatic function, is a common end point of many liver disorders. Since the liver is responsible for numerous metabolic processes, loss of functioning hepatocytes may lead to a variety of disease signs and symptoms. Important liver functions include regulation of carbohydrate, fat, and protein metabolism and thus hypoglycemia and wasting are signs of advanced liver disease.

Edema is common owing both to a decrease in albumin concentration and to salt retention because of a decrease in the deactivation of aldosterone by the liver. Factors I, II, V, VII, X, and XI are synthesized in the liver, and thus clotting abnormalities also may occur. The inability to absorb fat-soluble vitamins is also impaired because of the role of bile salts in their absorption. A decrease in vitamin K absorption may contribute to the bleeding tendencies seen in hepatic disease. If hepatic coma accompanied by an increase in serum ammonia occurs, platelet function may also be impaired and bleeding problems encountered.

Thus frequent symptoms of liver disease are jaundice, malnutrition, ascites and edema, portal hypertension, poor wound healing, decreased resistance to infection, and both bleeding and clotting abnormalities. Hepatomegaly may or may not be present. It must be emphasized, however, that the liver has large reserves, and a considerable amount of hepatic damage is necessary for clinically apparent, permanent metabolic changes to occur. If the etiologic agent is removed and sufficient stroma is not destroyed, hepatic regeneration usually occurs.

Common noninvasive tests that are used to evaluate residual hepatic function are as follows (see also Chapter 14).

Serum albumin

A decreased serum albumin concentration may indicate either volume expansion, starvation, or decreased synthesis by the liver. Decreased albumin levels based on decreased hepatic function usually occur late in the disease.

Prothrombin time

The prothrombin time test is one of the most practical determinations of residual hepatic function. Since the liver is responsible for the synthesis of many clotting factors necessary for a normal prothrombin time and since a large reserve exists with each factor, it is clear that a significant increase in prothrombin time indicates significant hepatic disease. Generally, in the absence of acute hepatobiliary disease, a normal prothrombin time probably indicates adequate hepatic reserve for most routine oral surgical procedures.

Serum bilirubin

In advanced hepatic disease, total serum bilirubin rises. Often the unconjugated fraction rises out of proportion to the conjugated fraction because of the inability of the liver to handle the products of hemoglobin catabolism. In the absence of hemolytic disease, increased bilirubin levels are indicative of either intrahepatic or obstructive liver disease.

Serum alkaline phosphatase

Both bone and liver disease will cause an increase in serum alkaline phosphatase. Since they are isoenzymes, biochemical techniques are available to distinguish the two. An elevation of liver alkaline phosphatase is associated primarily with obstructive rather than hepatocellular liver disease.

Serum transaminase levels

Increased serum levels of transaminase (serum glutamic-oxaloacetic transaminase, serum glutamic-pyruvate transaminase) indicate ongoing cellular necrosis and are common in acute liver disease. However, as extensive necrosis and replacement by fibrous tissue occurs, the serum levels may fall and the tests are generally of little value in long-standing chronic liver disease. They may also be elevated in any process involving cellular necrosis and are thus not specific for hepatic disease. Therefore interpretation based on these values depends on correlation with the clinical condition.

BSP retention

Bromsulphalein (BSP) is a dye that is taken up by hepatocytes and secreted with the bile. It is the most specific of the tests for remaining liver function, and normally after an injection of 5 mg/kg less than 5% is circulating after 60 minutes. However, the test is not without morbidity and requires careful clinical interpretation in the presence of jaundice, hypovolemia, and advanced age of the patient. It is a test probably best performed by a physician familiar with its complications and interpretations.

Infectious disease (viral hepatitis)

Of major concern to the practicing oral and maxillofacial surgeon is the management of the patient with viral hepatitis. Obviously patients with acute type A or type B hepatitis are poor surgical risks, highly infectious, and are not candidates for elective surgery. Viral hepatitis is presently thought to consist of at least two types—type A (infectious hepatitis) and type B (serum hepatitis). Symptoms of the two are similar, consisting of a prodromal period of 2 to 14 days of flulike symptoms generally followed by jaundice, nausea and vomiting, right upper quadrant tenderness, and fever.

There are several differences between the two types of the disease. Serum hepatitis has a longer incubation period and is considered to be a more serious illness with a mortality rate of up to 20% versus 0.01% in type A hepatitis. The presence of hepatitis B surface antigen (HB_sAg or Australia antigen) in the serum is the most common test used to differentiate between types A and B hepatitis. Type A is generally spread via the fecal/oral route while type B is primarily spread via contact with contaminated blood or secretion. The virus has been demonstrated in the blood in both types A and B during the incubation and acute stages but rarely during convalescence in type A and only occasionally in type B. Since certain segments of the world have up to a 20% incidence of HB_sAg-positive individuals who are without clinical symptoms of hepatitis, the relationship between the presence of antigen and infectivity is not clear. Certain cases of type B hepatitis will remain HB_sAg positive and may or may not have chronic active or relapsing hepatitis.

A major problem is the incidence of dentists who have contracted type B hepatitis presumably from so-called carriers, that is, asymptomatic patients who are HB_sAg positive. This is one reason why gloves should *always* be worn and instruments autoclaved. It behooves any oral and maxillofacial surgeon to obtain a clear history regarding hepatitis and to attempt to ascertain the type, duration, and whether the patient remains HB_sAg positive. Aside from the obvious morbidity and mortality to the dentist from contracting the disease, a certain number remain antigen positive and must, therefore, take special precautions during surgery because of the possibility that they may be carriers who can spread the disease to others.

GENITOURINARY SYSTEM
Renal failure

As with the cardiovascular system, it is more often the degree of renal function remaining that is of major importance to the surgeon rather than the specific cause of functional loss. A wide variety of disease states may lead to renal failure. Some are acute and may be encountered by the oral and maxillofacial surgeon during the management of acute trauma. Others are of a more chronic nature.

Acute renal failure

An example of a disease that can cause sudden renal failure is acute tubular necrosis. Other causes of acute renal failure, as manifested by depressed urine formation and inability to secrete a solute load, are hypovolemia and urinary tract obstruction. In prerenal disease the situation is reversed rapidly by rehydration and/or restoration of normal hemodynamics. However, if prolonged hypotension or hypovolemia occurs, prerenal dysfunction may lead to renal disease.

A wide variety of injuries may cause acute tubular necrosis. The common end point is tubular dysfunction and a depression in the glomerular filtration rate. In both prerenal and renal disease, oliguria is common and serum BUN and creatinine rise. The major metabolic defect, from the standpoint of elective surgery, is an inability to handle hydrogen ions and secrete potassium. Thus, if untreated, these patients are acidotic and hyperkalemic. The latter may lead to cardiac irritability and arrythmias if the patient is challenged by surgery. Since the tubules are not functioning well, sodium reabsorption is impaired and urine sodium concentrations tend to be elevated (>75 mEq/L). In prerenal azotemia, sodium is avidly reabsorbed in an attempt to compensate for the decreased vascular volume, and urinary sodium concentration tends to be low (<20 mEq/L). Thus, challenge by a volume load and urinary sodium determination is useful in distinguishing between the prerenal and renal disease in the face of acute oliguria.

If a diagnosis of acute tubular necrosis is made, treatment is directed toward restriction of fluids to prevent fluid overload. Generally this is accomplished by restricting fluids to insensible loss and instituting dietary restrictions of protein and potassium to decrease serum levels of urea and potassium. Sodium may or may not need restriction depending on the nature of the disease. If acidosis is severe (CO_2 combining power of less than 15), correction is necessary and is accomplished by giving bicarbonate either orally or intravenously. Hyperkalemia may need control by ion exchange resins—either by mouth or enema.

The oral and maxillofacial surgeon must recognize renal failure if it occurs, because prompt therapy is necessary to prevent morbidity or death. If the problem is transient, fluid and diet restrictions combined with control of potassium levels may lead to spontaneous recovery. However, if this therapy is inadequate, dialysis may be necessary to prevent the signs and symptoms of uremia. This can be accomplished by either peritoneal or hemodialysis. If the condition is prolonged or permanent, it may be necessary to place a shunt in the patient's arm for repeated hemodialysis.

Chronic renal failure

In patients with chronic renal failure, either secondary to acute failure or prolonged renal disease, both medical management and dialysis are often necessary. Dialysis usually is indicated when serum BUN cannot be maintained at less than 80 mg% or serum creatinine at levels of about 8 mg% by medical management. The latter represents a decrease in the glomerular filtration rate of about 85% and thus indicates considerable loss of renal function.

Patients who have received successful kidney transplants may have no signs of renal failure and have normal electrolyte, BUN, and creatinine levels. These patients are almost invariably on steroids and other immunosuppressive drugs and thus represent a management problem because of the effects of these drugs. Only if rejection of the transplant occurs do the signs of renal failure and symptoms of uremia appear. On the other hand, patients on hemodialysis tend to remain marginally uremic. The degree of symptom control depends on the degree of remaining renal function and the frequency of dialysis. If little renal function remains, the patient feels well after each dialysis but generally becomes marginally symptomatic by the time of the next treatment. Signs and symptoms such as nausea and vomiting, lethargy, weight loss, pallor, and effusions are common. In addition, anemia, hypertension, acidosis, and hyperkalemia are invariably found in these patients. They also exhibit abnormalities in platelet function that are manifested by prolonged bleeding times.

Anemia may be severe and hematocrits of 20 to 25 are not uncommon. If surgery is comtemplated, the patient can be transfused to obtain a hematocrit of 30 or above but invariably this is transient and the value falls after surgery. Hypertension is usually controlled by drug therapy, and the degree of control should be evaluated and taken into consideration prior to elective surgery. Acidosis may be controlled by oral bicarbonate but is immediately corrected by dialysis. The same is true of serum potassium concentrations, which, while clinically controlled by ion exchange resins, can immediately be corrected by dialysis by controlling the potassium concentration in the dialysis bath. In total renal failure, if ion exchange resins are not used, it is not unusual for serum potassium to rise from 3.5 mEq/L immediately after dialysis to levels of 5 or 6 mEq/L 2 days later.

Thus in the management of patients with chronic renal failure, bleeding, hypertension, decreased resistance to infection, anemia, fluid overload, acid/base disturbances, and electrolyte imbalances are problems that require consideration prior to surgery. It is usually wise to schedule needed surgery on the same day as dialysis, since this represents the time of the patient's optimum metabolic status. Prophylactic antibiotics may be indicated, taking into account the inability to secrete or filter these drugs. Anemia may be temporarily corrected for surgery but is not permanently correctable, and infusion of fresh platelets may help if bleeding is encountered during surgery. The latter effect is usually transitory, however, as the defect is thought to result from acquired platelet dysfunction caused by an accumulated by-product in the serum. One further consideration is the fact that heparin is used during the dialysis procedure and it must be ascertained that the effects of the drug are reversed prior to surgery.

HEMATOPOIETIC SYSTEM
Anemia

The first consideration for the surgeon is establishment of the fact that anemia exists and its degree of severity. Since anemia is a symptom rather than a disease, a search for an underlying cause of the process is necessary. By definition anemia can be considered a decrease in the total circulating hemoglobin, which, if severe enough, cannot adequately meet the needs of the tissues for oxygen. The serum hemoglobin concentration or packed cell volume may or may not be decreased depending on the circulating blood volume of the patient. Symptoms may be present only when the oxygen demands of the body exceed the ability of circulating hemoglobin to meet these needs.

The signs and symptoms of anemia can be considered in three broad categories: (1) physiologic adaptation to the process, (2) symptoms common to all anemias owing to hypoxemia, and (3) certain symptom constellations that are not common to all anemias.

The primary physiologic compensation that takes place in all anemias is related to the cardiovascular system. In an attempt to compensate for the anemia, cardiac output may increase and the patient may develop a tachycardia with concomitant increased blood flow. Flow murmurs may be detected if the cardiac output increases sufficiently. Shunting of blood from the nonessential organs may also occur and skin coolness and pallor may be present. An increase in the respiratory rate in an attempt to increase the arterial oxygen concentration may also occur.

Symptoms of all anemias include fatigue, weight loss, lethargy, and pallor of mucous membranes. Other specific causes of anemia produce a variety of symptoms specific for each disease. Examples would be the abdominal or extremity pain in sickle cell disease and the peripheral neuritis often found in B_{12} deficiency. It must also be remembered that symptoms are dependent to some extent on the rapidity of development of the disease. Thus a very low hemoglobin level may produce few symptoms if it is the result of a chronic process, and conversely acute symptoms may be manifest if the disease develops quickly. This observation has surgical significance as patients with chronic anemia tend to tolerate surgical and anesthetic procedures more satisfactorily than those with acute anemia.

For purposes of discussion, it is useful for the surgeon to consider the etiology of anemia in three broad categories—iron deficiency anemia, hemolytic anemia, and marrow suppression or replacement anemia. History and symptoms are important in the differential diagnosis of these processes, but certain laboratory tests are mandatory for specific delineation of etiology (see also Chapter 14).

Red cell count, hemoglobin concentration, hematocrit. The red cell count, hemoglobin concentration, hematocrit establish the diagnosis of anemia but not the etiology of the disease.

Red cell indices. The two most useful indices are the mean corpuscular volume and mean corpuscular hemoglobin. The use of these parameters classifies the type of anemia as microcytic, normocytic, or macrocytic and hypochromic or normochromic. These indices provide valuable information since certain inferences as to etiology can be made on this basis alone.

Blood smear. A well done and correctly read smear is essential to the diagnosis of anemia. Judgment as to variation in shape, size, and hemoglobin concentration is made, and the presence of abnormal cells is noted.

Serum iron. Low levels of serum iron usually reflect iron deficiency anemia—generally secondary to chronic blood loss. However, patients with the anemia of chronic disease often will also have low serum iron concentrations but still show normal total iron binding capacity owing to a concomitant decrease in serum transferrin. In contrast, true iron deficiency anemia causes a decrease in serum iron and an increase in the total iron binding capacity.

Total iron binding capacity. Total iron binding capacity is an indirect test of serum iron. It depends on normal levels of transferrin for accuracy. If iron stores are low and transferrin levels normal, extra binding sites for transferrin are available and the binding of exogenously administered iron will be high. The results must be correlated closely with serum iron concentrations to establish a diagnosis.

Reticulocyte count. A truly elevated reticulocyte count is usually indicative of hemolytic disease with vigorous bone marrow response. However, the results must be correlated with the red cell count to assure the true value. For example, a reticulocyte count of 3% with a red cell count of 2.5 million will fall to 1.5% if the red cell count rises to 5 million.

Bilirubin. In cases of hemolytic anemia, increases in unconjugated bilirubin occur early, with a rise in both fractions later in the disease as the liver conjugates the additional amount of bilirubin presented to it. The ratio of unconjugated to conjugated bilirubin then generally remains high throughout the subsequent course of the disease. However, isolated bilirubin levels must be interpreted with reference to clinical symptoms and other laboratory values.

Iron deficiency anemia

Iron deficiency is almost always a result of chronic blood loss. In young females a common cause is excessive menstrual flow and inadequate iron replacement. Unexplained iron deficiency in men should always lead to a high degree of suspicion of occult malignancy of the gastrointestinal tract. Any elective surgery should be curtailed prior to a diagnosis of the anemia and correction of the condition if the hemoglobin concentration is low.

Hemolytic anemia

Hemolytic anemias may be either intrinsic, whereby the defect lies in the red cell itself and its life span is shortened, or extrinsic, whereby the red cell is normal but excessive hemolysis occurs owing to circulating red cell antibodies. The signs and symptoms of the disease will depend on the rate of red cell production by the bone marrow and the ability of the liver to handle the excess bilirubin. It is, therefore, possible to have a hemolytic process but no clinical anemia or jaundice. In most hemolytic anemias decreased oxygen-carrying capacity is the major symptom, but in such conditions as sickle cell disease, acute episodes of abdominal and limb pain are also present because of sludging and microinfarction. In contrast to patients with iron deficiency anemias, those with many forms of hemolytic anemia are subject to acute crises that may be precipitated by the stress of an elective surgical procedure, drugs, or hypoxia.

Marrow suppression anemia

The third form of anemia is due to lack of red cell production by the bone marrow. This may result from a general deficient factor necessary for red cell synthesis such as B_{12} or folic acid. Replacement of marrow by another substance such as fat or tumor may also occur, or a nonspecific suppression of bone marrow may be present such as develops in drug-induced aplastic anemia. Marrow suppression may be selective for one group of cells such as granulocytes, or it may be total with a decrease in all products of marrow formation. Symptoms of the process will, therefore, vary from only those of anemia to defects in white cell production with loss of ability to mount an inflammatory response, to bleeding problems because of lack of platelet production. Thus management of a patient for elective surgery must take into account which elements

are reduced, and appropriate therapy must be instituted prior to surgery. The diagnosis of marrow suppression owing to B_{12} or folate deficiency can sometimes be suspected in cases of megaloblastic anemia. A bone marrow biopsy is often necessary for definitive diagnosis.

Regardless of the etiology any decrease in hemoglobin, and thus reduction in oxygen-carrying capacity, must be evaluated prior to surgery. A hematocrit of 30 or a hemoglobin of 10 generally is considered adequate to proceed with semi-emergency surgery. Ideally for purely elective cases, hematocrit values of 35% to 45% and hemoglobin values of 12 to 15 gm are desirable. In some cases prolonged correction of the condition is impossible. In total marrow failure or renal failure, patients may clinically maintain hematocrits of 15% to 25% without undue symptoms. Transfusions of packed red cells will transiently raise the level to normal, but it quickly falls after surgery. It is good policy to transfuse these patients to a level of 30% for an elective procedure, realizing that this is a temporary event to tide them over the acute effects of the operation.

White cell disorders

Disorders of white cells that are of significance to the surgeon fall roughly into two classes. The first is the management of patients with leukemia, be it granulocytic, lymphocytic, or monocytic. The second is the management of patients who have marrow suppression with a decrease in circulating white cells. In many cases the difference between the two from the viewpoint of the oral and maxillofacial surgeon is not great, for the net effect is a decrease in the ability to mount an inflammatory response. In many leukemias the total white count may be elevated but the neoplastic cells are abnormal and incapable of functioning in their normal role in combating infection. The cell type involved in the leukemic process is not as significant as whether the disease is acute, chronic, or in remission. The effects of chemotherapy may also require major modifications in management.

Leukemia

Acute leukemia is a progressively fatal illness with a projected life span of months to 3 years after the diagnosis. However, with modern multiple drug therapy for this disease, it is common for remissions to occur, whereby the patient has relatively normal marrow and blood values for a long period. Early signs are fever, lethargy, bleeding, and lymphadenopathy. Gingival lesions characterized by bleeding and swelling are an early sign of leukemia. This is especially true in the monocytic type. All needed surgical work should be done during periods of remission and can usually be accomplished without complication if appropriate precautions are taken. Ideally, surgery and dentistry should take place when the diagnosis is first made, prior to drug therapy. However, in acute leukemia the onset is usually so sudden that the patient already has platelet deficiency, white cell dysfunction, and anemia by the time the diagnosis is made. The first remission usually offers the best opportunity to remove oral sepsis.

Chronic leukemia, especially lymphocytic, has a generally better prognosis and may often be managed for a number of years without chemotherapy. In all forms of chronic leukemia, the patient develops symptoms similar to those seen in acute leukemia but the disease usually evolves gradually.

The principles of surgical therapy for patients with chronic leukemia are identical to those for acute leukemia but opportunity to perform necessary oral and maxillofacial surgery or dentistry can be found more frequently either prior to drug therapy or during remission. Again, with an adequate platelet count and normal white and red cell count, surgical procedures can usually be accomplished without undue hazard. If faced with an emergency procedure in a patient in the acute phase of leukemia, or a patient with severely suppressed marrow from drug therapy, platelet transfusions may be needed and intravenous broad-spectrum antibiotic coverage is indicated. It may be necessary to perform surgery on patients with platelet counts in the range of 25,000 because of the difficulty in achieving normal platelet levels owing to circulating platelet antibodies.

Marrow suppression

The considerations for management of patients with marrow suppression are similar to those already outlined for leukemia. Surgical therapy depends on whether the marrow suppression is total (pancytopenia) or selective (agranulocytosis). In any event, the missing blood components must be brought to acceptable levels prior to any elective surgery. A rule of thumb would be a hematocrit of 30%, white cell count of 4000/cu mm, with a normal differential count and greater than 50,000/cu mm normal platelets. These objectives may be difficult to obtain and certain compromises may be necessary if the condition warrants the risk.

Bleeding and clotting abnormalities

Abnormalities of hemostasis may be divided into two broad areas of dysfunction: bleeding and clotting problems. The former is present when abnormalities of the vessel wall or qualitative or quantitative platelet problems occur. The latter results from a deficiency in one of the factors necessary for the formation of a viable clot. The missing factor may be part of the extrinsic, intrinsic, or common pathway of clotting (see p. 451, Chapter 14). In certain states, that is, von Willebrand's disease, patients may show abnormalities in both of these parameters.

As a general rule, bleeding problems tend to be less severe than clotting defects. The severity of the latter depends largely on the quantity of missing factor. In the case of most factor-deficient states, severe spontaneous hemorrhage does not occur until only 3% to 5% of the normal level is present. Spontaneous hemorrhage might be absent, but patients may bleed after surgical or traumatic insult with factor levels of 5% to 20%. For the most part, levels of any clotting factor above 20% are acceptable for most surgical procedures.

There are basically three steps required for hemostasis following tissue injury. The first is a vascular response with reflex contraction of the smooth muscle of the vascular wall. The second is platelet aggregation at the point of injury. These two phases create a mechanical block against further blood loss. Following this, fibrin formation occurs, mediated by both the intrinsic and extrinsic pathways.

Vessel wall and platelet abnormalities usually manifest themselves in a history of prolonged bleeding following cuts or minor surgery and as mucous membrane bleeding and petechiae. It is rare to find such serious signs as spontaneous hemarthrosis in patients with isolated bleeding abnormalities. The presence of such a finding should lead to a high index of suspicion of a clotting abnormality with a factor deficiency of 95% or greater. However, patients with undiagnosed clotting problems may present for surgical care with deficiencies of 85% to 95%. These patients may have a history of prolonged bleeding after surgery and easy bruisability but not have the full-blown symptoms often noted with classic hemophilia. Nevertheless, following dental extractions, serious prolonged hemorrhage may occur. Typically this is not manifested by acute hemorrhage but rather by immediate homeostasis after surgery followed by poor clot formation, clinical breakdown of the clot, and oozing. Over a period of days these patients may require numerous blood transfusions to replace the missing factor.

Certain laboratory tests are valuable to the surgeon in determining the suitability of a patient for surgery. More sophisticated analysis is often required for a specific diagnosis of the particular disorder. Some common and useful screening tests follow (see also Chapter 14).

Bleeding time

The Duke or Ivy technique may be used to ascertain bleeding time. Each hospital has a standardized technique and the normal values for any given hospital or laboratory must be known prior to interpretation of the results. As mentioned earlier, prolongation of the bleeding time may occur in vessel wall disorders or with platelet dysfunction.

Platelet count

An estimate of the number of circulating platelets can be made by examining the stained blood smear. There should be about five to six platelets per high-power field. If this is not the case, a quantitative count is necessary. Greater than 75,000/cu mm will give relatively normal hemostasis and greater than 50,000/cu mm is adequate for surgery if careful attention is given to surgical technique. A platelet count will not reveal a qualitative platelet abnormality, and the presence of an abnormal bleeding time with a normal platelet count may require qualitative platelet function studies.

Prothrombin time

Abnormalities in the prothrombin time are an indication of a deficiency in factors I, II, V, VII, and X. Thus this test measures the extrinsic and common pathway of clotting. Results may be reported as related in time to the control or with reference to a standardized curve relating to percent of normal activity. Since the relationship of percent activity to time is not linear, it is more accurate to relate to the latter prior to surgery. Therapeutic anticoagulation is usually 20% to 25% of normal. This value represents a reasonable compromise between coagulation and spontaneous hemorrhage. Levels below 15% are dangerous in that spontaneous bleeding may occur.

Partial thromboplastin time

The partial thromboplastin test depends on all the intrinsic pathway factors—VIII, IX, XI, and XII as well as factors I, II, V, and X. It is, therefore, prolonged in the most common hemophilic states—factor VIII, IX, and XI deficiencies. A normal control value is between 25 and 40 seconds.

Fibrinogen

The normal value for fibrinogen is from 200 to 400 mg%. Active hemorrhage may occur as levels fall to 100 mg% or less. Mild deficiency may occur in liver disease, but very low levels are seen primarily in disseminated intravascular coagulation.

It is most important to establish an exact diagnosis in a patient with a bleeding or clotting disorder. The condition may be congenital or acquired. An example of the former is hemophilia and of the latter is a patient taking anticoagulants. After the diagnosis has been made, the next considerations are the risks and potential morbidity of surgery versus the benefits of the procedure. There are obvious emergency cases when correction of the state and surgery must be done, but elective surgery on severe hemophiliacs is unwarranted.

If surgery is necessary after the diagnosis is made, the patient should be brought to an acceptable state of hemostasis prior to intervention. In the case of vessel disease based on malnutrition or vitamin C deficiency, this may be accomplished by proper diet. Platelet dysfunction or deficiency must be recognized and, if grossly inadequate, platelet transfusions are given. Surgery is generally safe at a level of about 50,000/cu mm, but such a level may be essentially unobtainable if the patient has previously had multiple platelet transfusions and, therefore, high levels of circulating antibody. In such cases, levels of 25,000/cu mm may be practical. Since the half-life of infused platelets ranges from hours to 3 days, more than one transfusion may be necessary to maintain hemostasis after surgery.

Factor deficiencies may be replaced in some cases by fresh frozen plasma, but if the number of units required is large, excessive fluid volume may be a problem. Factor concentrates are available and are now the preferred method of administration. Safe levels vary with the factor employed but generally satisfactory results are obtained at 20% of normal. The amount of time the patient must be kept at acceptable levels is somewhat controversial, but it is generally agreed that the day of surgery and about 6 days after surgery represent critical times for hemorrhage. In the former, primary hemostasis is the consideration, while in

the latter it is bleeding from vascular granulation tissue.

After proper diagnosis, the number of replacement units must be calculated. Since with most factors one unit represents the amount of factor in 1 ml of normal plasma, this calculation is made by using 5% of the body weight in grams as an estimate of the plasma volume; that is, the desired increase in percent $\times$ 0.05 $\times$ the body weight in grams. For example, assuming 0 factor to begin with and a prescribed level of 30% for a 70 kg person, the calculation becomes 0.3 $\times$ 0.05 $\times$ 70,000 for a value of 1050 units. Depending on the half-life of the factor, transfusions are given at 12 to 24 hour intervals. Recently work has been reported using ϵ-aminocaproic acid, which blocks the conversion of plasminogen to plasmin, as a therapeutic adjunct.

A particularly dangerous state exists in patients who have circulating inhibitor rather than an absolute factor deficiency. Since the inhibitor is an antibody, steroids may reduce its effect, but usually large concentrations of factor replacement at more frequent intervals are required to override its effect. A common and easy guide to effectiveness is following the patient's partial thromboplastin time.

For patients receiving sodium warfarin (Coumadin), a prothrombin level of 30% or greater (or 1.5 times the control level) is considered safe. This can usually be obtained by simply stopping or reducing the dose for a few days prior to surgery if the patient has normal liver function and was properly anticoagulated. One hundred percent activity is not necessary and may be dangerous because of hypercoagulability owing to rebound. Parenteral vitamin K is usually not necessary, and it may be difficult to judge the proper dose and effects of vitamin K. Four to twelve hours are usually required for an effect after parenteral administration of vitamin K. If the prothrombin time is prolonged because of liver disease, the effects are not reversible by vitamin K and fresh frozen plasma may be required to replace all missing factors that are liver dependent.

NEUROLOGIC SYSTEM

Diseases of the neurologic system are of importance both in the management of surgical patients and in diagnosis of facial pain. The former type of condition may represent a crisis such as an acute stroke or seizure or a management problem such as seen in patients with Parkinson's disease or cerebral palsy. In the latter situation, such factors as vascular conditions and central tumors must be ruled out in the diagnosis of facial pain.

Cerebrovascular diseases

Patients with advanced cerebrovascular disease are at risk from a stroke caused by embolism or hemorrhage. These patients may have a history of numerous transient ischemic attacks, have carotid atheromatous plaques, and usually have evidence of advanced atherosclerotic disease elsewhere as well. Stroke can also occur in the presence of otherwise normal vessels if aneurysms occur in the cerebral vasculature. Symptoms of permanent or transitory motor or sensory loss, dysphasia, scotoma, and generalized dementia may indicate an underlying problem with the cerebral vasculature. The avoidance of hypertension owing to anxiety is important. It is also critical that patients with cerebrovascular problems not be made hypoxic or hypercapnic because the latter conditions cause an increase in intracranial pressure.

Seizure disorders

Seizure disorders may be focal neocortical, temporal lobe, or subcortical in origin. Neocortical seizures may range from severe motor to purely sensory. Temporal lobe seizures are sensory without a motor component and subcortical seizures may be sensory or motor. Since seizures are caused by uncontrolled firing of neurons with recruitment of surrounding groups of neurons, the area involved will determine the type of seizure. Causes range from congenital disorders or birth trauma to vascular and metabolic disturbances. Patients on regulatory medications should be maintained on these medications prior to and during surgery. In the case of general anesthesia, when oral intake is prohibited, the patient may have to be switched to a parenteral drug. If on phenytoin (Dilantin), an alternative is to give the next day's total dose at midnight prior to surgery and supplement with parenteral barbiturates or diazepam. Should seizures occur, they are usually self-limiting except for status epilepticus. The latter condition may be life threatening if not brought under control.

ENDOCRINE DISEASES

Pituitary

Disorders of the pituitary gland may involve either the anterior or posterior lobe or the entire gland. In addition, the disorder may be limited to a specific group of cells within one lobe. Since the anterior pituitary gland is responsible for the production of trophic hormones governing the function of other endocrine glands, symptoms of over- and underproduction are complex and depend on the type of cell and the other glands involved. The anterior pituitary gland contains alpha cells that produce prolactin and growth hormone, beta cells that produce thyroid-stimulating hormone, and gonadotropin and chromophobic cells. ACTH is thought to be produced by beta and/or chromophobic cells. Needless to say, patients who have loss of pituitary function either from trauma, tumor, or hemorrhage must be on replacement therapy to survive. Thus these patients are metabolically labile and require careful control and attention prior to any surgical intervention. If pituitary loss is total, the patient will be on either estrogen or androgen, thyroxine, and cortisone to supply the end organ's product rather than the trophic hormone itself. Special provisions must be made prior to surgery for steroid and thyroid replacement during surgery. These patients are sensitive to general anesthetics and narcotics, and most surgical procedures should be accomplished in the hospital under careful monitoring and control. When selective destruction of cells has occurred, management will depend on which target organ is decreased in function.

Hypopituitary coma may occur following surgery or anesthesia. Because of the lack of appropriate hormones, water intoxication with hyponatremia and hypoglycemia are immediate and urgent problems. Symptoms are hypotension, hypothermia, bradycardia, and sweating if hypoglycemia is present. Therapy is directed at cortisol replacement, water restriction, and relief of cerebral edema, as well as general attention to mechanical life support measures.

Disorders of the posterior pituitary involve symptoms relating to water and salt imbalance. Hypofunction (diabetes insipidus) is characterized by excessive water loss and the production of dilute urine. This eventually leads to hypernatremia. If the patient is conscious and the thirst center intact, adequate water intake is usually maintained by the oral route. In comatose patients proper fluids must be given parenterally, guided by vital signs and serum and urine osmolarities. These patients will respond to exogenous sources of antidiuretic hormone (vasopressin, ADH) if the disease is not nephrogenic in origin.

The other common syndrome with which the surgeon must be familiar is inappropriate ADH secretion. In this syndrome the tubules reabsorb large amounts of water and thus cause severe hyponatremia and urine with increased osmolarity. The treatment is water restriction. If symptoms of hyponatremia (serum levels less than 115 mEq/L) occur, hypertonic saline solution may be given. The syndrome may occur after trauma and may or may not be permanent.

Thyroid

Most diseases of the thyroid gland that lead to a hyper- or hypoactive state are well controlled by the time of elective surgery. When the patient is euthyroid, there is little risk involved in surgery. The diagnosis of hypo- and hyperfunction of the gland is made on historical, physical, and laboratory findings.

While the cellular actions of thyroid hormone (T_3 and T_4) are not entirely clear, certain generalizations can be made. These hormones cause an increased release of free fatty acids from adipose tissue and an increased rate of amino acid incorporation into protein. At greatly increased levels, a catabolic state is produced and the actions are similar to those of epinephrine. Increased thyroid hormone levels are usually caused by hyperplasia or tumors of the gland. The symptoms include a hypermetabolic state with sensitivity to catecholamines, catabolic effects on protein, tachycardia, diarrhea, and heat intolerance.

Decreased thyroid hormone levels may be caused by destruction of the gland or inability of the pituitary to produce its trophic hormone. Symptoms of hypofunction are water and mucopolysaccharide retention; slowing of metabolic processes leading to bradycardia, constipation, and lethargy; and hypothermia. Untreated hypothyroid patients respond poorly to stress and myxedema coma may occur. If this does occur, immediate parenteral administration of thyroid hormone may be necessary. Generalized life support measures are also indicated. Hyperthyroid patients may be pushed into thyroid storm by similar events. Again, the event is life threatening and control of the hyperpyrexia and tachycardia with high-output cardiac failure is necessary.

Pancreas
Diabetes mellitus (hyperglycemia)

Diabetes mellitus (hyperglycemia), caused by a relative or absolute insulin lack, is of great importance to the oral and maxillofacial surgeon. For purposes of assessing surgical risks, diabetes can be classified into three broad groups. The first is the adult onset diabetic who is controlled by diet or oral hypoglycemic agents. The second is the diabetic who is well controlled by insulin and does not have the sequelae of long-standing disease. The third is the "brittle," usually juvenile onset, diabetic whose metabolic needs are labile.

Most elective surgery can be accomplished without problems or special precautions in the first type. Stable insulin-dependent diabetics require some thought, and numerous regimens have been suggested to manage these patients for surgery (see also Chapter 9). For outpatient minor surgery, nothing more is usually required than the patient's usual insulin dose and ascertaining that this is covered with adequate calories. For general anesthesia, the patient's nutritional status, hydration, and electrolyte status should be optimal prior to surgery. The principles of management are to provide at least 200 gm of carbohydrate with adequate insulin to cover this need on the day of surgery. It is considered prudent to allow a relative hyperglycemia to occur rather than risk the acute effects of hypoglycemia. One half of the patient's normal insulin dose may be given the morning of surgery and intravenous glucose begun. Blood and urine sugars are monitored and additional insulin added after surgery, if needed. Every attempt should be made to return the patient to his preoperative oral intake as soon as feasible. Consideration of antibiotic coverage should be given because of the susceptibility of diabetics to staphylococcal and mixed gram-negative infections.

Very brittle diabetics, and those who have sequelae of long-standing disease such as renal failure, retinopathy, and generalized vascular disease, require very careful monitoring for any surgical procedure. The principles of management are identical to those indicated for the stable diabetic but much more rigid control is indicated. A sliding scale using crystalline insulin based on serial blood sugar determinations may be necessary. It is probably unwise to perform purely elective surgery on patients of this type.

Hypoglycemia

Hypoglycemia is manifested by agitation and apprehension secondary to compensatory epinephrine release. The patient is nervous, sweaty, and has tachycardia. As the blood glucose declines, the patient may lapse into a coma. Blood sugar levels required to produce symptoms vary and are dependent on the rapidity of the drop in concentration. It is this state that must be avoided during surgical management, and it is prudent to allow blood sugars of 175 to 225 mg%, with 1+ or 2+ urines, to develop if ketosis is not present.

On the other hand, severe stress, trauma, and infection may increase the insulin requirements of a diabetic, and ketoacidosis becomes a problem in a previously controlled patient. Clinical features are vomiting, tachypnea, Kussmaul breathing, dehydration, and circulatory collapse. It must be remembered that high blood glucose levels are not the major clinical consideration but rather ketoacidosis with its ensuing effects on the acid/base and electrolyte status of the patient. Also, in a long-standing diabetic, the renal threshold may be increased owing to a decrease in the glomerular filtration rate and thus higher levels of serum glucose may be required for urine glucose to become positive. Immediate laboratory tests for urine and serum glucose and acetone, serum electrolytes (potassium and bicarbonate), blood urea nitrogen, hematocrit, and arterial blood gases are indicated. A baseline electrocardiogram is helpful. Special attention is directed to base reserve (HCO_3) and problems of hypokalemia during correction of hypoglycemia. The therapeutic goals are restoration of normal carbohydrate, fat, and protein metabolism by insulin; replacement of fluids and electrolytes lost in the process; and the restoration of normal hemodynamics and acid/base and electrolyte status.

Parathyroid

Symptoms of parathyroid gland disease relate to either overproduction or underproduction of parathormone. Parathormone controls the normal blood level of calcium and phosphorus. Serum calcium levels are raised secondary to bone resorption and serum phosphorus levels are depressed by increased phosphorus secretion by the kidney. Thus the hallmark of hyperfunction is elevated serum calcium (greater than 11.5 mg%) and normal or depressed serum phosphorus. This latter finding often is useful in delineating hyperparathyroidism from other causes of hypercalcemia.

Hyperparathyroidism

Hyperparathyroidism is usually the result of a parathyroid adenoma or parathyroid hyperplasia. Occasional metastatic tumors produce a parathyroid-like substance. Symptoms depend both on the absolute serum calcium level and the rapidity of the disease. Hypercalcemia produces lethargy, muscle weakness, gastrointestinal disturbances, and polyuria. Renal stones, bone pain and resorption, and peptic ulcer are common. The diagnosis may be difficult in a mild case. The importance to the oral and maxillofacial surgeon is the recognition of potential giant cell lesions and bone changes of the jaw as part of the metabolic process and the avoidance of surgery in the hypercalcemic patient. If surgery is necessary, serum calcium should be controlled prior to operation by intravenous saline solution and diuretics, phosphates, or mithramycin.

Hypoparathyroidism

Hypoparathyroidism may be idiopathic or the result of a tumor or surgical ablation. The most common cause is inadvertent removal during thyroidectomy. Symptoms are related to a decrease in ionized serum calcium and increased phosphorous levels. Tetany and convulsions may be present. Neurologic symptoms such as confusion and memory loss may also occur. Therapy consists of oral vitamin D_2 (calciferol) rather than calcium. Controlled patients offer no therapeutic risk. If convulsions or frank tetany appear, it may be necessary to raise the calcium level acutely by the administration of parenteral calcium gluconate.

Adrenal

Disorders of the adrenal gland may be due to medullary or cortical dysfunction. The medulla is responsible for the production of epinephrine, while the cortex produces glucocorticoids, mineralocorticoids, and androgens.

Disorders of the adrenal medulla

The most important medullary disease to the oral and maxillofacial surgeon is the pheochromocytoma. This tumor may also be extramedullary and may produce both epinephrine and norepinephrine. Symptoms are commonly related to episodic attacks of hypertension and other signs of epinephrine release. Occasionally the symptoms are persistent but this is relatively uncommon. Thus the symptoms may resemble those of hypoglycemia. Diagnosis is made by measurements of urinary free catecholamines and the by-products of catecholamine metabolism. Provocative tests with histamine or tyramine are dangerous and should not be used. Symptoms can be controlled by alpha blockers such as phentolamine. A patient with an undiagnosed or uncontrolled pheochromocytoma is obviously very labile and a poor risk for any surgical procedure. If surgery is necessary, the risks must be weighed and preparation made for control with phentolamine.

Diseases of the adrenal cortex

Diseases of the adrenal cortex may be related to overproduction (Cushing's syndrome) or underproduction (Addison's disease). Generally the problem is related to glucocorticoid (cortisol) production, but hyperaldosteronism and adrenogenital syndromes do occur. It is the first that is of greatest concern to the surgeon.

Increased levels of glucocorticoids may be due to a pituitary adenoma, adrenal tumor, or iatrogenic, owing to therapeutic exogenous sources. The symptoms are diabetes, sodium and water retention with potassium excretion, and hypertension. Fatty redistribution occurs as well. A tendency to osteoporosis, poor wound healing, purpura, and mood changes are also common regardless of the cause. The diagnosis of spontaneous Cushing's syndrome is based on laboratory tests and may be made from various stimulation and suppression tests. These patients are poor surgical risks, and if surgery is necessary, careful attention must be given to carbohydrate metabolism, hypertension, and sodium and potassium levels. Problems of bleeding and poor wound healing must also be considered.

Adrenal suppression, either caused by exogenous steroids or destruction of the pituitary gland or adrenal cortex, leads to symptoms of muscle wasting, salt and water loss, potassium retention, and hypoglycemia. If the disease is of adrenal origin (Addison's disease), there is a reflex increase in ACTH secretion by the pituitary gland and hyperpigmentation may occur. This is due to the similarity between ACTH and melanocyte-stimulating hormone. Surgery should not be attempted on patients who show symptoms of Addison's disease as they are very labile and shock can readily occur. Most patients will have been diagnosed prior to surgery, however, and will be receiving replacement therapy.

The principles of management of patients with hypoadrenalism are similar regardless of cause. However, a daily maintenance dose of 20 to 30 mg of cortisol equivalent may be insufficient for the patient to withstand the rigors of stress imposed by trauma or surgery. Since the maximum normal adrenal output is 200 to 300 mg of cortisol daily, comparable exogenous doses may be necessary for preventing addisonian shock. Generally, patients who have had therapeutic steroids for longer than 2 weeks within the year prior to surgery can be considered to have some degree of adrenal suppression, and the use of exogenous steroids should be considered prior to surgery. All fluid and electrolyte deficits should be corrected and cortisol equivalent given on the day of surgery (see Chapter 9, p. 332 and Chapter 11, p. 389). The dose is then gradually reduced, depending on the degree of stress and condition of the patient. For minor procedures 200 mg in divided doses on the day of surgery followed by maintenance doses is often sufficient.

IMMUNOLOGIC DISEASES
Immune deficiency states

A deficiency in immunity may be congenital or acquired. In addition, the defect may be partial or complete, and there may be specificity whereby only certain types of immunoglobulins are involved. Generally, however, primary disorders in immunoglobulin synthesis involve antibody synthesis, lymphocyte function, or both (see also Chapter 6). In the former, humoral antibodies are deficient, and patients are very prone to acute bacterial infections. In the latter, a basic deficit in delayed hypersensitivity occurs and fungus disease and tuberculosis are serious side effects. Patients with problems such as DiGeorge's syndrome or Swiss-type immunologic deficiency are born with the disease and often do not survive. Others develop immunologic deficiencies later in life and if only one class of immunoglobulins is involved, or the deficiency is not complete, may be relatively asymptomatic. Acquired forms of deficiency may be secondary to certain disease states such as lymphomas, Hodgkin's disease, multiple myeloma, and the like. Other types of acquired deficiency are based on the use of chemotherapeutic drugs that nonselectively depress humoral antibody production and lymphocyte function.

The management of these patients for surgical procedures is primarily a matter of control of infection. It makes little difference whether the condition is congenital or acquired unless there is hope of reversing the process prior to surgery. In the case of humoral antibody suppression, gamma globulin from pooled human plasma will enhance resistance to infection to some degree and should be considered in a patient who requires surgical intervention. Very little can be done for patients who have a deficiency in lymphocyte function. Generally, long-term prophylactic antibiotics are not indicated but are of value prior to surgery, especially if the wound is nonsterile. Since the normal body defenses are not operative, the antibiotic of choice should be bactericidal.

Allergy

The problem of allergy and hypersensitivity is also of importance. Patients with a long history of atopic disease such as asthma, hay fever, and dermatitis are often allergic to numerous substances. These patients also often have hyperreactive smooth muscle and tend to develop bronchospasm after minor pulmonary irritation. Repeated bouts of asthma or respiratory infection may also leave residual pulmonary dysfunction. A history of true allergic reaction to any medication must be heeded as repeated exposure to the antigen may precipitate true anaphylaxis characterized by intense bronchospasm and shock. In surgical practice, penicillin and the para-aminobenzoic acid – derived local anesthetics have been the prime offenders in the past. One would be wise to ascertain that previous contact resulted in true allergy, as many reported episodes of allergic reactions to drugs represent simple syncope or nausea. A history of such symptoms as rash or rales and wheezing is important in making this determination. One must also bear in mind that drugs such as penicillin, sulfonamides, aminoglycosides, and salicylates may cause serum sickness type reactions on the first exposure. Usually a period of 7 to 10 days occurs prior to symptoms (hives, joint pain, fever), and subsequent administration of the drug provokes an accelerated reaction.

Collagen diseases

There are a wide variety of relatively common disease states of unknown etiology that have in common multiple immunologic abnormalities. Systemic lupus erythematosus, rheumatoid arthritis, scleroderma, and Sjögren's syndrome all fall into this pattern. Many cases cannot be neatly classified and the symptom complex is termed by some as collagen vascular disease. Symptoms involve numerous organ systems but generally are primarily joint or vascular in nature. Many of the organ system symptoms may be attributed to a secondary vasculitis. No unifying theory of causation is presently proven, but the complex is thought by most clinicians to be on an autoimmune basis. Therapy for the entire group is primarily supportive and depends on the degree and site of involvement. Many of these patients are on steroids and some may be on other immunosuppressive drugs as well. Proposed surgery on these patients should take into account the therapeutic drugs and their side effects and the degree of organ failure encountered. Pulmonary, cardiovascular, and renal diseases are commonly found in these patients.

REFERENCES

American College of Surgeons, Committee on Trauma. 1972. Early care of the injured patient, Philadelphia, W. B. Saunders Co.

American College of Surgeons, Committee on Pre- and Postoperative Care. 1971. Manual of preoperative and postoperative care, Philadelphia, W. B. Saunders Co.

Boedeker, E. C., and Dauber, J. H. 1974. Manual of medical therapeutics, Boston, Little, Brown & Co.

Brainerd, H. et al. 1970. Current diagnosis and therapy, Los Altos, Lange Medical Publications, Inc.

Condon, R. E., and Nyhus, L. M. 1975. Manual of surgical therapeutics, Boston, Little, Brown & Co.

Harvey, A McG., et al. 1972. The principles and practice of medicine, New York, Appleton-Century-Crofts Educational Division/Meredith Corp.

McCarthy, F. M. 1972. Emergencies in dental practice prevention and treatment, ed. 2, Philadelphia, W. B. Saunders Co.

Schwartz, S. I. 1969. Principles of surgery, New York, McGraw-Hill Book Co.

Shires, G. T. 1966. Care of the trauma patient, New York, McGraw-Hill Book Co.

PART FOUR

CONTROL OF PAIN AND ANXIETY

CHAPTER 18

Psychologic aspects of pain and anxiety control

Matisyohu Weisenberg

In our society one of the automatic ways of arousing a negative reaction is to mention a trip to the dentist. Especially singled out is the oral and maxillofacial surgeon. It does not take more than a brief visit to the patient waiting area to sense this fear and anxiety. A consequence of this reaction, especially as it relates to pain, is avoidance of dental care to the extent possible and a potential behavior problem patient when care no longer can be avoided. Estimates from a variety of sources indicate that 12 to 20 million people in the United States do not seek dental care because of fear of pain (Crockett, 1963; Freidson and Feldman, 1958; Rayner, 1976). Cole (1961) in his study of dentists in military service found that 29% of dentists themselves said they usually fear pain before receiving dental care, and 58% answered "yes" to the question, "Is going to the dentist an unpleasant experience for you?" In a study of patients seeking outpatient emergency care where most treatment was provided by oral surgeons, Weisenberg and co-workers (1975) reported that 72.6% of patients expected at least some degree of pain during treatment, with 19.2% reporting an expectation of severe pain.

In turn, when patients evaluate performance, Kriesberg and Treiman (1963) in their study of 1862 adults found that the dentist's skill in minimizing pain and his concern about causing pain were the most important criteria used. McKeithen (1966), similarly, found the rated attribute of the best dentist to be his ability to reduce fear and pain.

Although it is no longer fashionable in American dentistry to deliver care without use of at least local anesthesia, often this is not adequate. Local anesthesia itself usually deals with only one aspect of the problem of pain control—the sensory component. The fear and anxiety that are part of the motivational component of pain are usually left unsolved. The injection itself often adds to the anxiety associated with dentistry. In fact, in a study of the heart action of children undergoing operative procedures and extractions, Myers, Kramer, and Sullivan (1972) actually found a significant number of arrhythmias, the greatest effects occurring just prior to anesthetic injection. Srp and Kominek (1963) found an increased pulse and respiration rate when patients were shown the syringe or when they received an injection. In addition, telling the assistant, "The forceps, please," also produced a significant increase. Messer (1977) reports similar findings with the most extreme stress reactions occurring just before local anesthetic injection.

Concern with psychologic status can have a major positive influence on the patient regardless of the pharmacologic ingredients used. Thompson (1974) from the dentist's perspective has said, "Occasionally the dentist will learn that he can make some patients more comfortable by the things he says and does than by the medication he uses" (p. 59). Pollack (1966), for example, conducted a study with 500 dental patients on the effects of a topical anesthetic applied prior to injection of a local anesthetic. Half of the group received a topical anesthetic, while the other half received a placebo. Each half was further subdivided so that one group received a strong suggestion that the topical would be effective while the other group was not told anything. More calm ratings were given to the suggestion group. The study indicated that the suggestion of the operator was the most important factor in obtaining or failing to obtain anesthesia.

Even when pharmacologic means are used to control pain, the psychologic status of the patient will often determine their chemical effectiveness. Beecher (1959, 1972) has cited many examples supporting this assertion. The greater the stress, the more effective are placebos. There are certain drugs such as morphine that work for pain of pathologic origin (which is usually accompanied by anxiety) but that fail to work for experimentally produced pain (which has little anxiety). "Thus, we can state *a new principle of drug action:* some agents are effective only in the presence of a required mental state" (Beecher, 1972, p. 178).

In addition to the problems of acute pain, dentists have increasingly become involved in chronic situations, that is, pain of the face and neck region that is often unrelated to the teeth. Recent statements have indicated the psychophysiologic nature of many of these complaints (Laskin, 1969). For example, in an analysis of symptoms and clinical findings obtained from 170 consecutive patients seen at their TMJ-Facial Pain Clinic, Marbach and Lipton (1977) found that 80% of all patients complained of pain in the face; yet 60% of all the patients had negative radiographic findings. Even when positive radiographic findings were obtained, Greene and Markovic (1976) found that psychotherapeutic treatments were associated with favorable outcome.

It thus seems that behavioral psychologic aspects of pain and anxiety control can be extremely important in oral and maxillofacial surgery. One must deal with the entire patient and not just the patient's teeth and surrounding tissues. It is no longer a question of whether the patient has "real" pain, that is, based on a demonstrable, physiologic-organic lesion, or if it is "imaginary," that is, of a psychologic origin, since there is no demonstrable lesion. There is currently a recognition that all pain perception involves important psychologic processes whether or not there is a demonstrable lesion. It would be desirable, therefore, to understand how to conceptualize behavioral aspects of pain and anxiety control and how to apply techniques to deal with these in oral and maxillofaical surgery. It is to this conceptualization that we now turn.

Definition of pain and anxiety

Defining pain is not just an intellectual exercise, as definitions have led to specific methods of control often to the disadvantage of the patient and to the frustration of the health provider. Pain is a complex phenomenon. It is often defined as a reaction related to actual or impending tissue damage on the basis of the stimuli that arouse it and on the basis of the responses measured to indicate evidence of its presence. Sternbach (1968), for example, defines pain as an abstract concept that refers to "(1) a personal, private sensation of hurt; (2) a harmful stimulus which signals current or impending tissue damage; (3) a pattern of responses which operates to protect the organism from harm" (p. 12). Examination of pain phenomena, however, indicates that this or any other definition is inadequate.

Sensory approaches to pain, mainly through laboratory study, have made a major contribution to its scientific analysis. This has led to the development of finely controlled methods for exploration of the pain phenomena. However, studies that emphasize mainly sensory components of pain also have great limitations as demonstrated by clinical experience and as a result of the exclusion from study of the so-called motivational-emotional components of pain. For example, the definition of pain as reaction to actual or impending tissue damage implies that the greater the tissue damage, the greater the reaction. Aside from the problem of spatial summation, the classic study of Beecher (1956) has demonstrated how the setting can affect the reaction more than the actual tissue destruction. Of 215 men seriously wounded in battle, only 25% wanted a narcotic for pain relief. In comparison, in civilian life with a similar surgical wound made under anesthesia, over 80% of the group wanted pain relief. Beecher attributes the difference in reaction to the significance assigned to the wound rather than to the extent of physical tissue damage. In battle the wound meant a ticket to safety, while in civilian life the surgery meant disaster.

Another example of this paradoxical aspect of pain is causalgia (a burning pain associated with deformation of nerves by bullets and other high velocity missiles) that persists months after the tissue damage has healed.

Simplistic, stimulus-response views of pain as merely a sensation imply a simplistic clinical view in treatment, often with unfavorable outcomes. Pain looked at as any other sensation suggests that there are straightforward pain pathways. To stop pain all that is needed, therefore, is to interrupt this pathway. Surgical results, however, indicate a rather disappointing record of success (see Weisenberg, 1975, section 7). There are also examples of pain for which no apparent stimulus can be demonstrated. In instances of central pain there is an absence of observed pathology of the nerves, spinal cord, or brain sufficient to account for the pain and there is an unfavorable treatment result with peripheral surgical procedures in most cases (Loeser, in press).

Emotional and psychologic factors can cause pain. Psychiatric illness, especially depression, has been associated with complaints of pain (Spear, 1967; Sternbach, 1974). Thirty-eight percent of patients with pain and 40% of patients

without pain at a medical clinic were found to be there because of psychologic illness (Devine and Merskey, 1965).

To deal with problems of a simplistic stimulus-response definition of pain Merskey (1968) suggests that pain be viewed as an unpleasant experience primarily associated with tissue damage, and that it be described in such terms even when damage is not apparent. Psychogenic pain is caused mainly or wholly by psychologic factors, while organic pain is caused mainly or wholly by physical causes. Psychogenic pain occurs under three main circumstances: (1) in hallucinations, for example, schizophrenia; (2) pain owing to muscle tension caused by psychologic factors, for example, myofascial pain-dysfunction syndrome, tension headache; (3) conversion hysteria. From the patient's view, the subjective experience of psychogenic or organic pain may not be different.

Importantly, pain reactions often convey a great deal more than a signal that tissue damage is occurring. As Szasz (1957), Zborowski (1969), and others have pointed out in discussing human reactions to pain, communication aspects are frequently overlooked. Pain reactions can mean "Don't hurt me," "Help me," "It's legitimate for me to get out of my daily responsibilities," "Look, I'm being punished," "Hey, look, I am a real man," "I'm still alive." Woodforde and Fielding (1970) have argued that cancer has a great deal less pain associated with it than is commonly assumed. Much of the prescribing of potent analgesics and narcotics is based on a feeling of hopelessness, helplessness, and a desire to have a reason to maintain doctor-patient contact.

Pain and anxiety are usually associated with each other. The general conclusion is that the greater the anxiety, the greater the pain (Sternbach, 1968). Therefore control and reduction of anxiety not only permit a more pleasant dental visit, but help reduce pain as well. Although pain and anxiety are strongly related in many instances, their relationship is still not fully understood. Thus prescribing only diazepam or teaching muscular relaxation will not automatically result in the absence of pain.

Anxiety, too, is a complex concept. It has been used to refer to a state based on the particular environment in which the person finds himself at the moment (state anxiety). It has also been used to refer to a trait (trait anxiety), that is, to a personality attribute reflecting the status of the person generally (Spielberger, Gorsuch, and Lushene, 1970). Paul and Bernstein (1973) refer to anxiety as a complex response involving subjective feelings of apprehension and tension associated with sympathetic physiologic arousal. Arousal can be due to an external stimulus source or to the memory of a past experience. In common with pain, anxiety is perceived as uncomfortable and it leads to behaviors that will reduce it. When avoidance of the source of arousal is used as the means to reduce anxiety, the anxiety reaction is usually strengthened (Mowrer, 1950; Bandura, 1969). If a patient has successfully avoided dental care because of anxiety, his avoidance response becomes strengthened and his anxiety reaction is likely to be greater when dental care can no longer be avoided.

Pain and anxiety control have a great deal in common. Local anesthetic injections alone as used in dentistry are not enough. Over the past 10 years there has been an increase in clinical demonstration and experimental studies that have viewed pain as a complex psychologic phenomenon related to anxiety. Behavioral approaches have become a significant part of pain and anxiety control. Techniques include greater use of stress- and anxiety-reducing procedures such as relaxation, desensitization, hypnosis, biofeedback, modeling, and a variety of cognitive strategies. In other instances patients are taught that they can control and contain the influence of pain on their lives even when the sensation of pain itself cannot be eliminated completely. The amount of general anesthesia, surgical intervention, and the number of pills prescribed and consumed for pain and anxiety control have consequently gone down with the use of such behavioral approaches.

THEORETIC APPROACHES TO PAIN

Theories of pain ideally should account for the range of pain phenomena. However, as with definitions, no single pain theory is currently adequate to account for all pain phenomena. Each approach still leaves a great many unknowns. Many theories have focused on the neurophysiologic structures related to pain. Two main approaches that are still current are the specificity and pattern theories of pain.

Specificity theory refers to a pain system based on a specific set of peripheral nerve fibers that are nociceptive in function (see Mountcastle, 1974). At the periphery are sets of free nerve endings, A-delta and C fibers, associated with two qualities of pain, short-latency pricking pain and long-latency burning pain, respectively. Although temporal and spatial patterns may contribute to what is perceived, afferent impulses in these A-delta or C fibers are both necessary and sufficient peripheral input to evoke painful sensations in the human being. Pricking pain impulses enter the dorsal spinal cord where they synapse and ascend via the anterolateral system to thalamic centers and from there to somatic sensory areas of the cerebral cortex. Burning pain impulses follow a similar course into the anterolateral system but project to different thalamic, hypothalamic, and cortical areas. These latter projections seem to account for the affective, autonomic reaction to pain impulses. The nature, location, and interactions of higher pain centers are still not clearly spelled out (Mountcastle, 1974).

The pattern theory opposes the notion that pain has its own set of specialized receptors. It proposes that pain perception is based on stimulus intensity and central summation (Goldscheider, 1894). Crue and Carregal (1975), recent advocates of this approach, argue that there is no need to speak of pain as a primary sensory modality. Therefore there are no pain endings, pain fibers, or pain neurons in the peripheral nervous system. There is no such thing as a pain stimulus, only stimuli that are painful. Pain is a result of the summation of a spatial and temporal pattern of input.

Melzack and Wall (1965, 1970) and Melzack (1973) after critically examining specificity and pattern theories reject both notions. Specificity is viewed as making unwarranted physiologic assumptions and not adequately accounting for pain phenomena, while pattern theory is described as running counter to physiologic facts. They reject specificity but accept specialization. Specialization can be found at receptor sites such as A-delta and C fibers that respond to particular types and ranges of physical energy. However, specialization is not specificity. Specificity implies responding to one and only one kind of stimulus. Calling specific receptors pain fibers implies a direct connection from the receptor to a brain center where pain would always be perceived. This is an unwarranted physiologic assumption. There are a small number of fibers that respond only to intense stimulation; however, this does not mean they are pain fibers that always produce pain when stimulated. At various levels of energy stimulation there are many things happening. Aside from the activation of specific fibers, changes occur in the total number of neurons responding as well as in their temporal and spatial relationships. However, a pattern theory of pain by itself appears to contradict physiologic evidence.

The gate-control theory of pain contains elements of both specificity and pattern theories. It attempts to account for psychologic influences on pain perception as well as such clinical findings as spread of pain and persistence of pain after tissue healing. Conceptually, gate-control theory proposes a dorsal spinal gating mechanism in the substantia gelatinosa that modulates sensory input by the balance of activity of small diameter (A-delta and C) and large diameter (A-beta) fibers. Activity of large fibers closes the gate and prevents synaptic transmission to centrally projecting T (transmission) cells, while small diameter fibers open the gate and facilitate T-cell activity once a critical level is reached. Small fiber activity is believed responsible for prolongation of pain and spread to other parts of the body. A central control trigger can also influence the gate. Thus cognitive processes can either open or close the gate.

The exact mechanism involved in gate-control is still not clear. Mendell and Wall (1964) and Hillman and Wall (1969) speak of pre- and postsynaptic effects. A single electrical stimulus delivered to small fibers produces a burst of nerve impulses followed by repetitive discharges in the spinal cord. Successive electrical stimuli produce a burst followed by discharges of increasing duration after each stimulation. Successive electrical stimulation of large fibers produces a burst of impulses followed by a period of silence after each pulse. These studies form much of the mechanical basis of the gate-control theory.

More than with any other theory, Melzack and Wall (1970) have emphasized the different aspects of pain perception. Pain has a sensory component similar to other sensory processes. It is discriminable in time, space, and intensity. However, pain also has an essential aversive-cognitive-motivational and emotional component that leads to behavior designed to escape or avoid the stimulus. Different neurophysiologic mechanisms have been described for each system. The fibers that project to the ventrobasal thalamus and somatosensory cortex are partly involved in the sensory-discriminative aspects of pain. Fibers that project to the reticular formation, medial intralaminar thalamus, and limbic system are related to the aversive-cognitive-motivational and emotional component of pain that leads to escape behavior. Higher cortical areas are involved in both discriminative and motivational systems, influencing reactions on the basis of cognitive evaluation and past experience. More than any other theoretical approach, gate-control emphasizes the tremendous role of psychologic variables and how they affect the reaction to pain. Especially with chronic pain, successful pain control often involves changing the motivational component while the sensory component remains intact. Hypnosis, anxiety reduction, desensitization, attention, distraction, as well as other behavioral approaches can be effective alternatives and supplements to pharmacology and surgery in the control of pain.

However, the gate-control theory has come under harsh criticism. "I think, therefore, that one ought at this stage to strongly support Schmidt in his attempt to prevent the gate hypothesis from taking root in the field of neurology" (Iggo, 1972, p. 127). A key element in the gating mechanism is the differential response of large and small fibers. Investigators have failed to confirm the Mendell and Wall (1964) study, whereby C fibers produce hyperpolarization of presynaptic terminals with resulting presynaptic facilitation. Instead, both A and C fibers have been found to produce depolarization, which is the accepted mechanism of presynaptic inhibition (Franz and Iggo, 1968; Vyklický et al., 1969; Zimmerman, 1968). "With a natural painful stimulus, we have found no evidence for the existence of a presynaptic gating mechanism activated by painful stimuli such as that proposed by Melzack and Wall" (Vyklický et al., 1969, p. 186).

Dyck, Lambert, and O'Brien (1976) have presented clinical evidence that fiber size does not control, facilitate, or inhibit pain as proposed by gate-control theory. Friedreich's ataxia involves a greatly decreased number of large diameter fibers without the production of neuropathic pain. Patients with inherited amyloidosis and sensory neuropathy have a selective decrease or absence of A-delta and C fiber potentials with pain as a common feature. Pain seems to be related more to the rate of fiber degeneration than to the selective loss of large or small fibers as hypothesized by Melzack and Wall (1970).

Melzack (1975a) has argued that a greater role must be assigned to higher level mechanisms. It is possible in disease, with selective loss of large or small fibers, that higher centers become more important in determining pain perception. It is also possible that even in the healthy person the gating mechanism itself is mostly determined by these central processes rather than by peripheral mechanisms. Wall (1976), in an attempt to counter criticism of the gate-control theory, has argued that the 1965 presentation contained much speculation and was never intended to be a complete and final theory. Recent evidence does lend support to the theory. Although Burgess (1974) and Iggo (1974) discovered fibers in the A-delta group and in the C group that responded only to tissue damaging high-intensity pressure, this does not resolve the problem of how an individual perceives pain. Other fiber categories also respond to injury-producing stimuli. Even the specific nociceptive A-delta and C fibers respond to stimuli that are not usually nociceptive in character. Light pressure stimulation produces a nociceptive reaction once fibers have been sensitized by damage, heat, or a particular chemical environment. Therefore understanding specificity in simple terms is still not possible. In terms of the balance of large and small fibers, recent evidence, Wall argues, does not show that a preferential loss of large diameter fibers leads to pain. However, it does seem that pain is not felt if small fibers are missing. Functional predictions, Wall claims, should not be made only on the basis of morphologic observations. Small fibers really could be regenerated large fibers. Secondly, although fibers may appear intact morphologically, there can be disturbance at the receptors, in transmission, or at central endings. For example, no agreement yet exists regarding morphologic changes that occur in peripheral fibers with trigeminal neuralgia. Yet, it is known that a specific low-threshold afferent stimulus evokes pain.

Regardless of the accuracy of the specific wiring diagrams involved, the gate-control theory of pain has been the most influential and important current theory of pain perception. It ties together many of the puzzling aspects of pain perception and control. It has had profound influence on pain research and the clinical control of pain. It has generated new interest in pain perception, stimulating a multidisciplinary view of pain for research and treatment. It has been able to demonstrate the tremendous importance of psychologic variables. Still, there is little doubt that research will produce changes in the original gate-control conceptions.

Psychologically oriented theories

Following Sternbach (1968), no specific view is taken regarding monistic-dualistic views of the body. Linguistic parallelism is used instead. Sometimes it is easier to talk of pain in neurologic-physiologic terms, while at other times it is easier to talk of pain in psychologic terms. Psychologically oriented theories have been written mainly to account for reactions in chronic pain that have been refractory to routine medical/dental treatment.

Engel (1959) has spoken of "psychogenic" pain and the pain-prone patient based to a large extent on his experience with atypical facial pain patients. In Engel's view, although pain can be viewed in neurophysiologic terms, it is a psychologic phenomenon. Pain perception may require an external stimulus at an early stage of development. However, with the development of a psychic organization for pain perception the experience of pain no longer requires external stimulation just as visual or auditory sensation can occur without sensory input. Such pain without external stimulation can be felt in some part of the body and from the patient's view is no different from pain based on external stimulation. Pain has special interpersonal meaning related to concepts of good and bad and success and failure. Pain becomes an important way of dealing with guilt.

According to Engel, pain-prone patients may show some or all of the following: (1) conscious or unconscious guilt with pain providing atonement, (2) a background predisposing to use of pain as punishment, (3) a history of suffering, defeat, and intolerance of success, large numbers of painful injuries, operations, and treatments, (4) pain as a replacement for loss or threat of loss of a relationship, (5) a tendency toward a sadomasochistic type of sexual development with pain occurring over sexual conflict, (6) pain location related to unconscious identification with a love object in which the pain either is the one suffered by the love object or is aroused by conflict with the love object, (7) psychiatric diagnoses that include conversion hysteria, depression, hypochondriasis, or occasionally paranoid schizophrenia.

Szasz (1955, 1957) talks of pain as arising as a consequence of threatened loss of or damage to the body. The communication aspects of the pain are extremely important in understanding reactions to pain. At the first level are the straightforward facts that the clinician requires to evaluate the physical symptom. The second level involves use of the pain complaint as a cry for help. It is tied to the first level. At the third level of communication pain can be viewed as a symbol of rejection, where the request for help has been frustrated. Pain complaints can become a form of aggression and a means of atoning for guilt.

In a later publication, Szasz (1968) refers to l'homme douloureux who has made a career out of his pain. Such individuals give up their former careers as attorneys, businessmen, models, and so forth when they fail or are no longer sustained by them to take on a career of suffering. It is the caretakers' responsibility to recognize such people and refrain from treating them, for the doctor can also help in the creation of the sick man. The career, chronic pain patient does not wish to give up his suffering.

Merskey and Spear (1967) reviewed and evaluated these as well as other psychiatric theories of pain pointing to the difficulties involved in obtaining evidence to support them. They conclude that each approach has some value but none of them is adequate to explain pain phenomena.

Based on his own research, Merskey (1968) describes the modal psychiatric patient with pain as a lower-class married woman that possibly once was but no longer is pretty; was never keen on sexual intercourse; has a history of repeated negative physical findings, many with conversion symptoms in addition to pain; and relates a sad tale of a hard life and depression that does not respond to antidepressant drugs.

Anxiety, hysteria, hypochondriasis, depression

Spear (1967) reported on the results of a study of pain in psychiatric patients. Pain is found in some 45% to 50% of such individuals. Pain as a symptom appeared with the highest incidence in patients with anxiety states. Pain is also associated with a history of surgical operations, other somatic symptoms, and overt anxiety. No association was found between pain and overt depression, overt agitation, and, in females there was no association between pain and dysmenorrhea. Patients were grouped into those suffering from depressive illness and those suffering from anxiety/hysteria. Those with pain associated with depression showed a positive prognosis, while those with pain associated with anxiety/hysteria showed a poor prognosis, at least on a short-term basis.

In Merskey's (1965a, b) studies of psychiatric patients, pain was associated most frequently with neurosis, especially hysteria; it was relatively rare in schizophrenia or endogenous depression. Nearly all the pain patients were married, came from large families, had problems of frigidity and unsatisfactory sex lives, and showed a great deal of resentment toward others. They had an excess of bodily symptoms and a special concern with their bodies.

Pilling, Brannick, and Swenson (1967) suggest that pain seems to function in place of anxiety and depression. Patients with pain were seen less often with depression and anxiety. These patients may use pain or other organic symptoms in place of depression and anxiety.

Pilowsky, Chapman, and Bonica (1977) found that pain clinic patients yielded a low degree of depressive affect, with few patients showing a depressive syndrome. Perhaps the pain does function in place of depression. Pilowsky, Chapman, and Bonica (1977), however, prefer to emphasize the importance of a greater conviction of disease and somatic preoccupation, a reluctance to consider health problems in psychologic terms, and a denial of life's problems. The Pilowsky, Chapman, and Bonica pattern is referred to as abnormal illness behavior (see later section).

These findings raise questions concerning the widespread use of antidepressant medication in pain control (see Sternbach, 1974). It is possible, as Taub (1975) has argued, that although the medication is called antidepressant, its effectiveness in pain control has little to do with classically defined depression.

Sternbach (1974) deals with both psychogenic pain patients as well as with patients with organic lesions for whom surgery is not appropriate or from whom expressions of pain are greater than would be expected. Sternbach disagrees with Szasz regarding l'homme douloureux. Contrary to Szasz, Sternbach feels that the career pain patients do suffer terribly and would like to give up their suffering. Four classes of patients have been defined on the basis of their Minnesota Multiphasic Personality Inventory Profiles (MMPI): (1) The *hypochondriasis* pattern (highest on the hypochondriasis scale) displays extreme somatic preoccupation. It is more common among somatogenic than psychogenic patients. It is possible that Szasz's l'homme douloureux would fit into this group. It should also be noted that hypochondriacal patients were classed as treatment failures in the pain clinic program. (2) *Reactive depression* profiles consist of patients with high depression scores who are willing to admit that the pain has "gotten them down." These patients respond well to antidepressant medication. (3) *Somatization* reaction profiles are associated with patients who present the psychosomatic V. They are high on the hypochondriasis and hysteria scales and relatively low on the depression scale. These patients focus on bodily symptoms to avoid latent depression. This pattern occurs in both psychogenic and somatogenic pain patients. Such patients have adjusted to their pain and derive satisfaction from the sick role. Moderate treatment success has been obtained in this group. (4) *Manipulative reaction* profile patients have clear physical findings. They show an elevated psychopathic deviate scale. The patient uses his symptoms deliberately to manipulate others. This pattern was observed in a group of patients who had litigation pending.

Anxiety as a trait has been studied in the laboratory as well as in the clinic. Sternbach (1968) has reviewed some of these studies and concluded, as have others, that the greater the anxiety, the greater will be the reaction to painful stimulation. In addition, for certain individuals, anxiety can produce chronic, heightened muscle tension that may result in pain in the related muscles. However, as mentioned earlier, anxiety is an ambiguous concept. It undoubtedly relates to the reaction to pain. How it relates to pain perception and reaction is still not clear.

Rugh and Solberg (1976) in their review of psychologic factors in temporomandibular (TMJ) pain and dysfunction report several studies that indicate greater anxiety among TMJ patients, although this increased anxiety is not as high as in pathologically anxious or neurotic individuals. Similar data have been presented by Schwartz, Greene, and Laskin (1979). For a particular type of TMJ dysfunction, myofascial pain-dysfunction (MPD) syndrome, Laskin (1969) postulates a psychophysiologic theory to explain its etiology. The higher level anxiety for these patients leads to greater and more sustained muscle activity, which leads to spasm and pain. Once this has occurred, a spasm-pain-spasm cycle perpetuates chronic pain in the muscles of mastication.

Not all studies demonstrate higher anxiety in patients with TMJ dysfunction. Marbach and co-workers (1978) studied patients with idiopathic facial pain (IFP) and did not find higher levels of either state or trait anxiety when compared to other types of facial pain patients undergoing treatment. It is possible to explain the Marbach and co-workers (1978) results in a variety of ways. One possibility is that facial pain patients may not have heightened anxiety all the time. They merely use their facial musculature as a reaction to stress when they are placed in situations that do make them anxious. This is the concept of response stereo-

typy referred to by Lacey, Bateman, and Van Lehn (1953) and Shipman, Heath, and Oken (1970). Mercuri, Olson, and Laskin (1979) found that MPD patients exposed to experimental stress had a significantly greater increase in muscle activity in the masseter than control subjects, which lends support to the concept of response specificity. Under stress some people react with one bodily system while others react with another system. Facial pain patients use their facial apparatus, while ulcer patients use their gut. Only under stress is it possible to see this difference. Indeed, there is evidence showing night bruxing following stress experience during the day (see Rugh and Solberg, 1975).

Lack of replication has occurred when discussing other psychiatric approaches based on personality traits as related to chronic pain. Rugh and Solberg (1976) report a variety of personality traits associated with TMJ patients. These include the Engel view discussed earlier. Other researchers report that TMJ patients have conflicts related to dependency. They maintain a rigid self-concept of normalcy, are perfectionist in nature, and are reluctant to admit the smallest fault. The many studies reviewed, however, do not provide for a consistent personality type associated with TMJ pain. A variety of personality types seem to be susceptible to the problem. These results suggest that although these psychiatric approaches can be helpful, they must be used with caution as applied to any one individual patient.

Abnormal illness behavior

To deal with the various and at times ambiguous psychiatric terms used to describe the chronic pain patient, Pilowsky and Spence (1975, 1976a, b) introduced the concept of abnormal illness behavior. Illness behavior refers to the way an individual perceives and reacts to symptoms of all kinds. Psychiatric syndromes such as hypochondriasis, conversion reaction, neurasthenia, and malingering are all included under the concept of abnormal illness behavior. There is an inappropriate reaction by the patient to his symptoms and to the careful explanation of his doctor. A factor analytic study of an Illness Behavior Questionnaire (IBQ) has yielded seven main factors. The first factor relates to a phobic concern about one's state of health. There is also an element of interpersonal alienation blaming others for difficulties. The second factor relates to a conviction of disease to the point of rejecting the doctor's opinion. Other factors relate to a somatic versus a psychologic perception of illness, difficulty in expressing feelings, acknowledgment of anxiety and depression, admission of life problems, and irritability. Chronic pain patients can be classified according to their responses on this 62 item yes—no scale. Patients with pain that did not respond to conventional treatment were found to be more convinced as to the presence of disease, more somatically preoccupied, and less likely to accept reassurance from the doctor. There was no relationship found between abnormal illness behavior and degree of organic pathology (Pilowsky and Spence, 1976a).

Although none of these theoretic statements concerning pain is complete in and of itself, they all point to factors to be considered in evaluating a patient who comes for treatment. As Chapman (1977) has pointed out, complaints of pain reflect not only tissue damage but a variety of dimensions of human suffering. With chronic pain, life problems and secondary gain for the invalid role become very important. Treatment is not usually accomplished by simple, technical intervention alone. Other considerations include medication, habits, physical and social activity, and disturbed circadian or other biologic rhythms.

Cultural and racial reactions to pain

Differences in the reaction to pain among cultural and social groups have received a substantial amount of study. They are important for many reasons. They indicate, first of all, that there is no "correct" way in which an individual should react to pain. Being aware of this is important since it can affect clinical diagnosis and choice of treatment, as well

as add to our understanding of pain processes. Zola (1966) and Marbach and Lipton (1978), for example, have shown that different cultural social groups present similar problems in a different manner. Differences in cultural attitudes also can affect psychophysical and autonomic functioning as demonstrated by Tursky and Sternbach (1967) and Sternbach and Tursky (1965) in their studies of reactions to the pain of electric shock.

The study of cultural reactions to pain can result in *stereotypes* based on lack of sufficient research or poor methodology. For instance, Chapman and Jones (1944) conducted a study of a "group of Northern European stock; the remainder included 25 Southern Negroes, 15 Ukrainians and 30 of Jewish and other Mediterranean races" (p. 81). All subjects were tested for pain perception and pain reaction threshold using radiant heat. Eighteen of the 25 Negroes and a corresponding number of "northern Europeans" were compared. Negroes perceived pain at a lower level and had tolerance levels closer to pain perception level than the Northern Europeans. The "Mediterranean races" were closer to the Negroes, although they were more apt to protest being subjected to so intense a stimulus.

These findings, or "myths" as Zborowski (1969) calls them, seem to have persisted for many years despite the obvious overgeneralizations made on the basis of "18 Southern Negroes" and an unspecified but small number of "Mediterranean types." More recent studies show different results. Merskey and Spear (1964) found no difference in pain reactions of 28 white and 11 Afro-Asian male medical students using the pressure algometer. Winsburg and Greenlick (1968) found no difference in rated pain reaction between black and white obstetric patients.

The interaction process between experimenter and subject or clinician and patient are important elements usually neglected in pain research. For example, would Chapman and Jones (1944) have obtained the same results if they had used a black experimenter? In a recent clinical study of whites, blacks, and orientals using a deep pain tolerance test (Woodrow et al., 1972), it was found that whites tolerated the greatest amount of pain, orientals the least, with blacks in between. This seems most surprising considering the well-known stereotype of the stoic oriental. This again raises the issue of how the conditions of testing and the tester influenced the outcome. This same issue is raised regarding acupuncture when researchers speculate on the extent to which its effectiveness depends on the Chinese geographic and cultural surroundings.

Many groups have been studied. These include Italians, Irish, Jews, and Yankees (Sternbach and Tursky, 1965; Zborowski, 1969; Zola, 1966), blacks (Chapman and Jones, 1944; Merskey and Spear, 1964; Weisenberg et al., 1975; Woodrow et al., 1972), Eskimos and Indians (Meehan, Stoll and Hardy, 1954), Puerto Ricans (Weisenberg et al., 1975) and an assortment of anthropologic studies of groups around the world (see Wolff and Langley, 1968). Major differences among these groups seem to be related to the reaction or tolerance component of pain rather than to the threshold discrimination of the pain sensation as demonstrated in the Sternbach and Tursky (1965) study. Using magnitude estimation procedures, they found that ethnic group differences disappear (see section on measurement). Underlying attitudes and anxiety reactions appear to be a major source of these differences in pain tolerance. In a study of black, white, and Puerto Rican dental patients (Weisenberg et al., 1975), for example, use of four variables in a multiple discriminant analysis, two anxiety and two attitudinal, were adequate to permit correct groupings in 18 of the 24 Puerto Ricans, 12 of the 25 blacks, and 16 of the 24 whites. Significant differences among these groups were obtained on trait anxiety (Spielberger, Gorsuch, and Lushene, 1970) and dental anxiety (Corah, 1969). Attitude differences were also obtained reflecting relative willingness either to deny or avoid dealing with the pain or to get rid of the pain. This is shown by response to such items as "The best way to handle pain is to ignore it," or "It is a sign of weakness to give in to pain," or "When I am sick I want the doctor to get rid of the pain even before he finds out what the trouble is." Puerto Rican patients showed the strongest endorsement of these items, the whites the weakest; blacks were in between.

In treating pain, even with medication, concern for anxiety and attitudinal reactions can influence outcomes by making the patient more comfortable and by enhancing the effectiveness of an anesthetic. In the Weisenberg and co-workers (1975) study, Puerto Rican females displayed the highest level of anxiety. It would be likely, therefore, that they would benefit most in pain relief from reassurance, placebos, or other means that would reduce anxiety. For black patients who are concerned with self-esteem, the attitude and mannerisms of the dentist could facilitate pain relief. The dentist might make the patient aware of how well he is tolerating the pain and of the appropriateness of reacting to the pain without being thought of as less of a person.

Weisenberg (in press) reviewed these studies and placed them into a theoretic framework. Differences in sociocultural reactions to pain can be viewed from a theory of social comparisons (Festinger, 1950, 1954). Basically, the theory states that there exists a drive to test the validity of a person's judgment and opinions of the outside world. When outside sensory means for evaluation are reduced, the individual turns toward his social environment for validation of his judgments. Since pain is a private ambiguous situation, comparison with others helps to determine what reactions are appropriate. Is it permissible to cry? Does one have to "grin and bear it?" When is it permissible to ask for help? When is it appropriate to mask the pain with analgesics? People learn to express their reactions by observing the reactions of others. The models chosen are those who are similar to oneself, while those too divergent are rejected (Bandura and Whalen, 1966). Craig and Weiss (1971, 1972) and Craig and Neidermayer (1974) have demonstrated how pain tolerance is subject to the social influence of models in a laboratory situation (see later section).

The first important source of comparison is the family that transmits the cultural norms to its children. As Shoben and Borland (1954) have shown in their study of dental fears, the experiences and attitudes of one's family toward dental care are the most important factors determining whether the person will react with anxiety to dental treatment, avoid it for a long time, and be uncooperative in the chair. Johnson and Baldwin (1968) also found that children whose mothers had high anxiety scores showed more negative behavior during an extraction than children of mothers with low anxiety scores.

As mentioned earlier, pain reactions often convey a great deal more than a signal that tissue damage is occurring. Szasz (1955, 1957) and others have pointed out in discussing human reactions to pain that communication aspects are frequently overlooked. Within cultural and racial groupings there is a greater similarity in the manner in which individuals communicate with each other.

Different meanings can be fostered through social and cultural environmental factors. The social influence process can have a great effect on reactions to pain. Pain reactions can become reinforced independently of the original physiologic sensation and tissue damge connotation. Members of cultural groups learn some sensations are to be tolerated; others are not. Some are labelled as painful; others are not. Knowledge of the different meanings of pain can serve as the basis for effective control and therapy.

MEASURING PAIN

Pain measurement is a most difficult yet important task. It enables us to understand the basic concepts of pain, to produce a proper clinical diagnosis, and to determine the effectiveness of medication or other means of intervention. Beecher (1959, 1972) has been one of the strongest advocates of systematic quantitative double-blind research to understand the effects of clinical intervention

strategies on pain perception. He has distinguished between the original pain sensation and the psychic processing of the sensation known as the *reaction component*. Three major classes of reaction identified by Beecher are: (1) skeletal muscle reactions, (2) autonomic nervous system reactions, and (3) processing of the original stimulus by the central nervous system, which determines the absence or presence of suffering. Most clinically effective pain drugs such as narcotics, according to Beecher, affect the reaction component, that is, the psychic processing, of the original pain sensation.

Two points in the process of measurement have been singled out: (1) threshold and (2) tolerance. *Threshold* refers to the point where an individual first perceives the stimulation as painful. *Tolerance* refers to the point where the individual is not willing to accept stimulation of a higher magnitude or to continue to endure stimulation at a given level of intensity. Threshold has been associated mainly with physiologic factors, whereas tolerance has been associated with psychologic variables such as attitudes and motivation (Gelfand, Gelfand, and Rardin, 1965). The difference between threshold and tolerance has been called *pain duration* or *pain sensitivity range*. Most studies have found that threshold and tolerance measures are correlated but that threshold and pain sensitivity range are not (Merskey and Spear, 1964; Tursky, in press; Wolff and Jarvik, 1963). Such correlations suggest that lower levels of pain stimulation might to some extent be used to predict to higher levels without the necessity of inflicting subjects with higher levels of pain stimulation. Melzack (1976), however, has argued that higher levels of stimulation produce behaviors that are qualitatively different from those obtained at lower levels of stimulation.

Much of the data and many of the techniques used to elicit pain reactions have come from laboratory study. These have clinical limitations. For example, laboratory type tests of pain threshold and pain tolerance preoperatively do not necessarily relate to postoperative need for analgesics (Parbrook, Steel, and Dalrymple, 1973). Beecher (1959, 1963, 1972) has argued that it is not possible to equate laboratory pain with clinic pain produced by pathologic processes. Whereas, in the clinic morphine can be extremely effective in reducing pain reactions, in the laboratory morphine cannot be distinguished from saline. Whereas, in the clinic placebos are effective with approximately 35% of the cases, in the laboratory this percentage is reduced to 3.2. The missing ingredient in the laboratory is the anxiety associated with the disease process and the threat of disfigurement or death. Reducing pain reactions in the clinic often involves reducing anxiety. The laboratory presents a different context in which the complexity of the pain response is partially ignored. It may not, thus, be possible to generalize results from the laboratory to the clinic.

Reliance on verbal reports of pain raises questions regarding the terms used to assess and evaluate pain. This question is especially important in clinical pain where health providers rely on patient reports without resort to other forms of measurement or comparison. Pain can be described as burning, aching, stabbing, splitting, pounding, nagging, cramping, and so forth. Pain can also be intolerable, unbearable, awful, distressing, excruciating, severe, and so on. What are the relationships between these different expressions of pain? Melzack and Torgerson (1971) and Melzack (1975b) developed a pain scale, the McGill Pain Questionnaire. They categorized 102 pain terms into three classes: (1) sensory quality descriptors in terms of temporal, spatial, pressure, thermal, and other properties, for example, pounding, spreading, crushing, burning, and aching; (2) affective quality descriptors in terms of tension, fear, and autonomic properties, for example, exhausting, awful, and nauseating; (3) evaluative terms that describe the intensity of the total experience, for example agonizing, excruciating, and miserable. Each term was judged by groups of 20 judges to determine the degree of agreement of classification. Intensity relationship within classes were then

judged by 140 students, 20 physicians, and 20 patients. Substantial agreement was obtained in classifying the many different terms used to describe pain.

Development of descriptor scales can make possible meaningful clinical questionnaires using terms that are spaced appropriately. It becomes possible to say a *strong* pain is almost twice as great as a *moderate* pain while an excruciating pain is more than four times as great (Tursky, 1976). Melzack and Torgerson (1971) and Melzack (1975b) suggest that when used with spatial and temporal variables, it should be possible to reliably categorize distinct pain syndromes as found in the various disease classifications so that more appropriate diagnosis and treatment could be performed. Dubuisson and Melzack (1976) using the McGill Pain Questionnaire were able to demonstrate differences among constellations of words for eight clinical syndromes. Eight diagnostic categories were developed on the basis of which 77% of the patients were correctly classed. When information such as sex, age, spatial location of pain, and analgesic drugs was added to the verbal descriptions, 100% of patients were correctly classed. Verbal descriptions characteristic of toothache include the following qualities: (1) sensory—throbbing (50%), boring (50%), sharp (50%); (2) affective—sickening (40%); (3) evaluative—annoying (50%); and (4) temporal—constant (60%), rhythmic (40%).

Regardless of the measurement method to be used, it is important to standardize carefully the procedures on an adequate sample under controlled conditions. In the clinic it is easy to fall into the acceptance of a particular approach because it seemed to predict well for one or two patients. After completing a rigorous test of the predictive power of a procedure based on one or two patients, it can be quite shocking to the clinician to see how little validity it has. Rogers (1971) described a simple blink test as a method for the physician to distinguish those patients who have severe pain from those who are overreacting. Three cases are presented to show the test's effectiveness. Weisenberg (unpublished data) included this test as part of a study of cultural and racial reactions to pain. The blink test did not correlate with anxiety measures or differentiate racial and ethnic groups. Furthermore, it yielded a standard deviation that was larger than the mean showing that it held little discriminative power.

Related clinical measures

As previously mentioned, factors other than the description of the pain itself enter into the evaluation of the patient. Merskey (1974) recommends inclusion of an assessment of patient personality as well as an assessment of severity of pain and responses of the patient to stimuli. For chronic pain patients a widely used personality measure is the MMPI mentioned previously (Sternbach, 1974). Test administration is easy although it requires time on the part of the patient. Computer scoring and interpretation are also readily available. Even hand scoring requires no more than 20 minutes. The Pilowsky and Spence (1976a) measure of illness behavior (see earlier section) is another easily administered scale that can be extremely useful in guiding the choice of clinical treatment.

When dealing with the chronic pain patient, Sternbach (1974) recommends careful observation of the manner in which the patient responds as well as attention to what is said. Does the patient demand, whine, flatter, and so forth? What emotional response does the patient elicit from the interviewer — bravery, sympathy, irritation? Major areas of information that are useful in understanding the role of the pain in the patient's life and secondary gain related to the pain include: (1) evaluation of the patient's work environment, (2) a careful assessment of the patient's medication history, and (3) involvement of litigation and an evaluation of how the patient would live if he did not have the pain.

Chapman (1977), in addition, asks the patient to maintain a diary of what he does at home, hour by hour, for several days. Important aspects of the diary are the amount of active versus passive (resting, reclining) time, changes in sleep patterns, sexual activity, and social activity.

For patients who are frightened of dental care Corah (1969) has developed a simple four-item Dental Anxiety Scale. Items are: How would you feel if you would have to go to the dentist tomorrow? How do you feel when you are waiting your turn in the dentist's office? How do you feel in the dentist's chair when he is getting ready to drill? How do you feel when you are in the dentist's chair and the dentist is preparing the instruments to scrape your teeth around the gums? Three out of four items have response choices of (a) relaxed, (b) a little uneasy, (c) tense, (d) anxious, (e) so anxious that I sometimes break out in a sweat or almost feel physically sick. It would be a simple matter to add questions to these response choices regarding any kind of treatment of interest to the dentist. This scale is readily subject to a response bias in the direction of social desirability to appear in a favorable light. However, most patients (with the exception of adolescents) will readily admit fear of the dentist.

Weisenberg (unpublished data) has used a Fear Inventory to permit assessment of the fears patients have regarding dental treatment (see boxed material on opposite page). The items listed in the inventory contain dental situations that Gale (1972) found as sources of fear. The inventory can be used to pinpoint specifics of patient fears, to develop a hierarchy of fears, and to assess success of intervention strategies at reducing patient fear.

When dealing with young children, an assessment of the mother's own anxiety regarding dental care has been found to relate strongly to the child's reaction (Bailey, Talbot and Taylor, 1973; Johnson and Baldwin, 1968). In assessing the likelihood of having a behavioral problem as a result of dental treatment, age is an important factor. Hawley and co-workers (1974) found that over one third of all children exhibited negative behavior. Half of all the behavior problems occurred in children under 3, while few occurred past the age of 7. Negative behavior was found to be related to the

FEAR INVENTORY

The items in this questionnaire refer to things and experiences that may cause fear or other unpleasant feelings in the dental office. Please answer each item with your first impression as it is most likely to be accurate. Remember there are no right or wrong answers.

Name _____ Date of birth _____ Date _____

1. In the past 2 years, how often did you visit a dentist? Check the statement that applies to you.
   - ☐ a. Not at all
   - ☐ b. One time
   - ☐ c. Two times
   - ☐ d. Three times
   - ☐ e. Four times
   - ☐ f. More than four times

2. In general, which statement best describes how you feel when you go to the dentist's office? Check only *one*.
   - ☐ a. I look forward to it as a pleasant experience.
   - ☐ b. I feel a little uncomfortable.
   - ☐ c. I feel somewhat tense.
   - ☐ d. I feel moderately anxious.
   - ☐ e. I feel quite anxious.
   - ☐ f. I feel very anxious.
   - ☐ g. I feel absolutely terrified.

3. Check each item in the column that describes how much you are disturbed by it nowadays.

	Not at all	A little	A fair amount	Much	Very much
Dentist tells you he is through	☐	☐	☐	☐	☐
Dentist asks you to rinse your mouth	☐	☐	☐	☐	☐
Dentist is cleaning your teeth	☐	☐	☐	☐	☐
Making another appointment with the nurse	☐	☐	☐	☐	☐
Dentist squirts water in your mouth	☐	☐	☐	☐	☐
Dental assistant places a bib on you	☐	☐	☐	☐	☐
Calling a dentist to make an appointment	☐	☐	☐	☐	☐
Dentist places cotton in your mouth	☐	☐	☐	☐	☐
Dentist looks at your chart	☐	☐	☐	☐	☐
Getting in your car to go to the dentist	☐	☐	☐	☐	☐
Dentist cleans your teeth with steel probe	☐	☐	☐	☐	☐
Thinking about going to the dentist	☐	☐	☐	☐	☐
Dentist is putting in the filling	☐	☐	☐	☐	☐
Getting in the dentist's chair	☐	☐	☐	☐	☐
Nurse tells you it is your turn	☐	☐	☐	☐	☐
Dentist is laying out his instruments	☐	☐	☐	☐	☐
Sitting in the dentist's waiting room	☐	☐	☐	☐	☐
Dentist squirts air into a cavity	☐	☐	☐	☐	☐
Dentist laughs as he looks in your mouth	☐	☐	☐	☐	☐
Having a probe placed in a cavity	☐	☐	☐	☐	☐
Dentist is giving you a shot	☐	☐	☐	☐	☐
Dentist holds a syringe and needle in front of you	☐	☐	☐	☐	☐
Dentist tells you that you have bad teeth	☐	☐	☐	☐	☐
Dentist is drilling your tooth	☐	☐	☐	☐	☐
Dentist is pulling your tooth	☐	☐	☐	☐	☐
Other (specify)	☐	☐	☐	☐	☐

mother's prediction of uncooperative behavior, high maternal anxiety, the child's belief that he had a dental problem, the child's ignorance of what the dentist really does, and the child's contact with others who have had an unpleasant dental experience.

REDUCING PAIN AND ANXIETY

Cognitive strategies

Suggestion and placebo phenomena

Suggestion, as most health practitioners know, can be very important in achieving pain and anxiety control. In the Pollack (1966) study mentioned earlier the dentist's suggestion was more important than the chemical agent used.

Placebo responsiveness has been well documented throughout the literature. Beecher (1972) has shown that 35% of patients with pathologic pain will obtain relief with placebos. The greater the anxiety, the greater is the relief from placebo medication. Placebo relief seems to be based partially on the unwritten contract between doctor and patient that states the doctor is going to do all he can to relieve the patient's suffering. If he (the doctor) believes the treatment will work and the patient leaves with the expectation that it will work, then anxiety is relieved and the patient seems to heal himself.

That expectations of relief influence outcome was demonstrated in a controlled study of audioanalgesia. Gardner and Licklider (1959) and Gardner, Licklider, and Weisz (1960) had used music and white noise effectively in suppressing pain in 5000 dental operations. They had proposed that the music promotes relaxation while the noise directly suppresses pain. Many dentists quickly jumped on the bandwagon and purchased expensive noise and stereo equipment. As Melzack (1973) describes it, with some dentists and on some patients the results were dramatic. However, with other patients it did not work at all. Many dentists became quickly disillusioned. In a controlled laboratory study Melzack, Weisz, and Sprague (1963) were able to demonstrate that auditory stimulation did not abolish cold pressor pain. They compared three groups of subjects. Group 1 received strong auditory stimulation but no suggestion about the purpose of the music and noise. Group 2 received strong auditory stimulation together with strong suggestions of effectiveness. Group 3 received strong suggestion but only a low-frequency hum rather than strong auditory stimulation. Each group served as its own control having received cold pressor stimulation without any sound prior to group assignment. Group 2 produced a substantial increase in pain tolerance, while neither group 1 nor group 3 did in comparison to their control stimulation periods. What the audio stimulation did was divert attention away from cold pressor pain when accompanied by strong suggestion. Therefore, used by a dentist who could relate well to his patients, it was effective. For dentists who could not build up expectations of effectiveness, it did not work.

Melzack and Perry (1975) built on these results in a clinical study of alpha training, hypnosis, and suggested benefits. Three groups of chronic pain patients were compared. Group 1 was provided with alpha training with explicit suggestions that it would help control pain. Patients were also given hynotic training that included progressive relaxation and ego strengthening instructions. Group 2 was provided with the hypnotic training only, while group 3 was given the alpha training only. Results indicated that the combination hypnosis-alpha training significantly relieved pain from the baseline measures. Fifty-eight percent of the patients reported a decrease in pain of 33% or greater. Hypnosis alone achieved substantial but statistically insignificant change from baseline, while alpha alone was ineffective. The authors interpret the combined procedure as consisting of alpha training as a distractor of attention combined with relaxation, suggestion, and a sense of control over pain. The increase in percentage alpha production alone, a measure often used to indicate relaxation, was not adequate.

The placebo effect can be extremely powerful. In a signal-detection analysis of placebos, Feather, Chapman, and

Fisher (1972) showed that the major effects were not on sensory perception but on the willingness to label the sensation as pain. With the administration of the placebo drug subjects were told that there might be some side effects such as sleepiness or sluggishness. A significant number of side effects were indeed reported. In a classic example of the strength of placebo suggestion, patients suffering from nausea and vomiting were able to obtain relief with ipecac, a known emetic (Wolf, 1950).

Stroebel and Glueck (1973) have proposed a Placebo-Active Therapy Index (PATI) model to predict treatment success as a function of the combination of the placebo effects and the active components of a therapeutic intervention. The PATI score as applied by Stroebel and Glueck to biofeedback consists of the patient's active score based on his ability to achieve voluntary control and the patient's expectancy score based on his enthusiasm and confidence in the procedure. Current effectiveness of treatment and long-term success are predicted by the ratio of the active score to his expectancy score. Unbalanced conditions, when one component is high and the other component is low, predict current effectiveness but are unstable for a long-term prognosis. Biofeedback training for pain control will most likely be successful on a long-term basis when a relative balance is obtained between a patient's active control and his placebo expectancy scores.

Evans (1974a) has analyzed placebo treatment data collected by McGlashan, Evans, and Orne (1969) as a function of chronic or state anxiety. Placebo reaction that resulted in increased pain tolerance was associated with state anxiety reduction. This result was especially notable for subjects with chronic anxiety. Increased anxiety following the ingestion of the placebo drug resulted in decreased pain tolerance. In an earlier paper Evans (1967) did not find placebo reaction to be associated with personality measures of suggestibility.

Evans (1974b) reports the relative efficiency of placebos to drugs such as mor-phine, propoxyphene (Darvon), or aspirin as 0.54 to 0.56. That is, a placebo is 56% as effective as morphine. The effectiveness of a placebo is directly proportional to the active analgesic agent to which it is being compared. A placebo is usually more effective in relieving severe pain. The properties of the placebo mimic the drug to which it is being compared. Effects of the placebo and the comparison drug usually interact and are additive. Higher placebo dosages are more effective than lower doses. Injections are more effective than orally administered placebos. Placebos are also more effective when described to patients as a powerful drug than when described as an experimental drug. They are more effective when given by a health provider who is more likely to use drugs.

Laskin and Greene (1972) demonstrated the effectiveness of a placebo capsule dispensed by prescription and enhanced by a suggestive name. Twenty-six of 50 patients (52%) with MPD syndrome reported improvement in their condition with symptoms of pain and tenderness affected most. Long-term (6 months to 8 years) evaluation of patients indicated no difference between those who positively responded to placebo therapy or other forms of therapy. Only 6 out of 100 patients followed-up for a variety of different therapies reported that their MPD problem was not under control (Greene and Laskin, 1974).

The doctor-patient relationship is an important element in the effectiveness of placebo therapy. As was mentioned with biofeedback, however, placebo's effects are not only related to drugs. Goodman, Greene, and Laskin (1976) demonstrated that two mock equilibrations for MPD syndrome were effective in producing total or near total remission of symptoms in 16 (64%) of 25 patients. Thirteen of the patients for whom follow-up was possible remained symptom-free 6 to 29 months later. Successfully treated patients actually did have a variety of occlusal disharmonies that remained untreated. Goodman, Greene, and Laskin argue that it is the strong positive suggestion that is likely to be responsible for the success of those who provide routine occlusal therapy for MPD syndrome.

Thompson (1974) has provided numerous practical examples of suggestion that the clinician can use in a dental practice to deal with pain and anxiety. Careful use of language can describe accurately what the patient is to experience without arousing unnecessary anxiety and at the same time produce an important doctor-patient bond based on trust and credibility. Both verbal and nonverbal communications (grunts, frowns, and so forth) can influence the patient. Not just what is said but the tone in which it is said becomes important, for example, kindness, friendship, sincerity. Instead of saying "Tell me *when* it hurts," suggesting that it will, Thompson recommends, "If you think any of this procedure might bother you, raise your hand and I'll stop."

For the patient who is about to have a tooth extracted Thompson (1974) recommends careful explanation and assurance. One approach not recommended would be to start with lengthy explanations, such as "This tooth is really locked into the bone and I'm going to have a hard time removing it. This is a real tough one. I won't be surprised if you have trouble after this extraction. You're going to have a mighty sore jaw and I don't know how much swelling and discoloration you can expect. Get this prescription filled on your way home . . . it's for the pain. I'm concerned about development of a dry socket or infection. If your jaw starts to ache, be sure to call me and get in here at once." (p. 67).

Contrast the former with the approach recommended by Thompson. Explanation should include the notion that the tooth is encased in a socket that has a cartilaginous character somewhat like the end of the nose. This substance can be compressed to allow an instrument to be slipped in next to the tooth to pop it out. With a more difficult extraction the patient can be told that the tooth can be removed in one piece or to make it easier pieces can be removed separately. When removing pieces of tooth separately, the patient can be advised that it may take longer but it is simpler and allows heal-

ing to occur faster. Complimenting and reassuring the patient are important. "Since you stayed so comfortable and relaxed, bleeding and disruption of the tissues were minimal. This permits the circulation to be very active in that area and new cells will quickly replace the ones that were disturbed during the extraction. Healing should be rapid and uneventful, with a good solid clot in the socket to protect it and encourage proper healing. Rest and proper nutrition stimulate the healing process, so be sure that you get both. You must be pleased to be rid of that painful, offensive tooth, so that your body can be totally healthy once more. In a few days you will probably have forgotten all about this experience, except when your tongue accidentally goes looking at its new space" (p. 66).

These latter instructions are similar to those a dentist might give with the patient in a hypnotic trance. However, even without a formal hypnotic induction they can be effective.

Hypnosis

How do suggestion and placebo phenomena relate to hypnosis? To answer this question a clarification of the meaning and effects of hypnosis is required. There is little doubt that regardless of the theoretic arguments concerning the reality of hypnosis, it is an effective technique to be used in dentistry. Jacoby (1960) reports on 308 dental patients with whom he has successfully used hypnosis. Procedures included exodontic, operative, prosthetic, periodontal surgical, endodontic, and techniques to increase the acceptance of dentistry. Tape-recorded instructions for trance induction were used for more than half the cases. After the fourth visit it was not even necessary to give the patient a directed suggestion to relax. Patients seemed to do so on their own initiative.

Erickson (1966) has emphasized that hypnosis is used mainly as a means of fixing patients' attention and creating a responsive mental state to enable them to benefit from their own unrealized potential. Erickson presents unusual case examples in which he has achieved relief from the pain of cancer. Sarcedote (1970) has used such techniques as time distortion, hypnoplasty (changing the aching area into something else), and partial and total amnesia for the hypnotic relief from chronic pain. Orne (1974) has also reported success using hypnosis for the relief of cancer pain. He attributes success to anxiety reduction, the hope of relief provided by the physician, and the fact that something is being done. He also reports success using hypnosis for relief of organic pain but not for psychogenic pain.

What is hypnosis and how does it work? Chaves and Barber (1974) have argued that hypnosis does not place a person in a different state from being awake. Essentially, Barber has removed much of the glamour and magical notions associated with hypnosis by the use of carefully controlled laboratory research in which he has been able to demonstrate many of the same results claimed for hypnosis with awake simulators or with highly motivated subjects (see Barber, 1965).

What Chaves and Barber have stressed is that many of the claims of hypnosis are based on a readiness on the part of the individual to accept suggestions and not on some magical trance powers that certain individuals possess to influence others. Many experimental studies of hypnosis do not assess the contributions of the separate variables they use in obtaining the effect. There are suggestions that certain physiologic effects will occur. Instructions are given to maximize motivation to accept suggestion. Suggestions are given for relaxation. Subjects are asked to close their eyes and so forth. Each of these variables contributes to produce a person who is highly motivated to accept suggestion without postulating that a separate state has been attained. Much of what is done under hypnosis could also be done with the awake individual.

Barber and Hahn (1962), for example, asked subjects to immerse their hands in 2° C water for 3 minutes. One group received hypnotic induction and suggestions of hand anesthesia. A second group

was asked to imagine a pleasant situation. A third group was simply exposed to the painful stimulation, while a fourth group was asked to immerse in water at room temperature. The hypnotic or pleasant imagery groups did not yield differences either on subjective reports of pain or on four physiologic measures. Both were equally effective in reducing subjective pain reports, respiratory irregularities, and forehead muscle tension compared to the noninstructed control group. However, compared to the room temperature group the hypnotic analgesia and pleasant imagery groups reported higher levels of pain and showed elevated levels of skin conductance and faster heart rates.

Chaves and Barber (1974) argue that the spectacular results claimed for surgery under hypnosis are due to heightened motivation and an increased readiness to accept suggestions from the physician with the accompanying reduction in fear and anxiety. Hypnotic effectiveness in pain control thus depends mainly on a positive doctor-patient relationship. Aside from the increased motivation to increase tolerance, it must be realized that most surgical pain is due to the pain of incision. Deeper tissues and organs are not as sensitive to pain. Local anesthetic, a frequent concomitant of hypnosis, is used to deaden the pain of the incision. With little anxiety the surgery proceeds painlessly.

Although Barber and Chaves have accomplished a great deal in changing hypnosis from the status of magic to science, many investigators disagree with their conclusions and regard hypnosis as something real.

Hilgard (1973) has approached hypnosis on the basis of different levels of consciousness. There seem to be different systems of cognitive functioning so that even though the pain stimulus is able to reach one level of consciousness it is blocked from the more immediate level of awareness. That is, the person does perceive the pain stimulus at some lower level when the "hidden observer" is asked if it is painful. However, he is capable of keeping it from coming to the level of awareness that makes it distressing.

From a Melzack and Wall (1970) point of view both Barber and Hilgard stress the effects of hypnosis on the motivational-affective system of pain control. Both view hypnosis as producing an increased readiness to respond to suggestion. Chaves and Barber feel that there is no such thing as a trance state. Little is to be gained over the "waking" state by use of hypnotic induction techniques. Hilgard, however, does feel that there is a state called hypnosis and that there are response differences in the individual when he is hypnotized or awake. Orne (1974), too, feels that hypnosis is a real phenomenon that cannot be explained away by saying that subjects are trying to please the experimenter. Clinically, inducements would be hard to find to convince unhypnotizable subjects to undergo major surgery merely to please the surgeon.

Hypnosis seems to be most effective when there is the presence of anxiety. Shor (1962) found that without anxiety he could not distinguish between hypnotic and faking subjects in reaction to electric shock on six physiologic variables. Both placebo and hypnotic treatments seem to involve suggestion, expectation of successful outcome, and anxiety relief. It would seem, therefore, that they might be the same. However, McGlashan, Evans, and Orne (1969) have demonstrated that hypnotic reactions contain placebo reactions plus something more. A group of highly hypnotically susceptible subjects and a group of nonhypnotizable subjects were each exposed to three separate treatments while undergoing ischemic muscle pain. The first session involved baseline reactions. The second session involved hypnotic analgesia, while the third session involved a placebo drug given under double-blind conditions. Placebo and hypnotic reactions were uncorrelated for the highly susceptible subjects, while for the nonhypnotizable subjects they were highly correlated. Hypnosis has a placebo component. However, it also produces a greater effect in response to the suggestion that subjects will not experience pain.

Relaxation, biofeedback, desensitization

Both relaxation and desensitization procedures have become widely accepted as a means of reducing anxiety and eliminating fear. Desensitization, or systematic desensitization as referred to by Wolpe (1969), involves the pairing of anxiety-arousing stimuli with relaxation or other anxiety-countering procedures. These countering procedures serve to reduce the anxiety arousal. The attempt is to substitute relaxation for arousal, one response for another, and is referred to as counterconditioning. To the extent to which anxiety and pain are related, reducing anxiety also reduces the reaction to pain. Wolpe (1969) has suggested further that relaxation is antagonistic to the elicitation of anxiety. A person cannot be relaxed and anxious at the same time. It would follow, therefore, that relaxation should increase pain tolerance.

Folkins and co-workers (1968) studied the effects of four conditions on stress reaction: (1) an analogue desensitization process, (2) relaxation, (3) cognitive rehearsal of the upcoming event, and (4) control group. Stress reaction was measured by heart rate, skin conductance, and self-report. Cognitive rehearsal and relaxation were both effective in reducing reactions to a stressor film, but cognitive rehearsal was slightly superior.

Paul (1969) compared the effects of relaxation training, hypnosis, and self-relaxation groups on a paper and pencil measure of anxiety and on four physiologic measures of arousal. Both relaxation training and hypnosis produced greater changes in reduced anxiety than controls. Greater decreases were obtained for relaxation for heart rate and tonic muscle tension, systems not usually under voluntary control.

Bobey and Davidson (1970) compared the effects on female subjects of four group conditions: (1) relaxation, (2) increased anxiety produced by a tape of screams of women in labor, (3) cognitive rehearsal of the upcoming stimulation, and (4) control group. Subjects were given radiant heat and pressure algometer stimulation. Results indicated that the relaxation group yielded the highest tolerance scores, the anxiety and cognitive rehearsal groups were second, while the control groups yielded the lowest tolerance scores. With pressure stimulation, only the relaxation condition was significantly different from controls. There were some interesting experimenter effects. With the male experimenter all of the treatment groups differed from controls, while for the female experimenter only relaxation differed from controls. With female subjects, it seems that the male experimenter was more effective in producing reduced pain reaction.

McAmmond, Davidson, and Kovitz (1971) compared the effectiveness of relaxation, hypnosis, or controls in reducing the reaction to pressure algometer stimulation and the injection of anesthetics in dental phobics. For subjects with high baseline skin conductance levels, relaxation was most effective in reducing stress reactions. Hypnosis did not differ from controls. For subjects with a medium or low skin conductance baseline, relaxation was not effective. The hypnosis group rated their treatment as most effective, while the control group rated their treatment as least effective. Five month follow-up indicated that all subjects in the hypnosis group returned for dental treatment, while five of ten in the control group and only one of the relaxation group returned for care.

Lehrer (1972) assessed the effectiveness of relaxation, increased tension, or no instruction in terms of tonic physiologic activity and habituation of skin potential responses to electric shock. Both the relaxation and no instruction group subjects relaxed more and habituated to shock more quickly than the increased tension subjects. The relaxation group subjects did not substantially differ from the no instruction group. The author hypothesized that perhaps the anxiety was not sufficiently high to produce differences between groups.

Gessel and Alderman (1971) have taught relaxation to patients with myofascial pain-dysfunction (MPD) syndrome. MPD patients who have facial pain because of overactivity of the masticatory muscles appear to have higher chronic levels of muscle tension. Jacobsonian relaxation was taught in from 1 to 27 sessions. Six of eleven patients, those with an absence of depression, showed good results. Patients with depression were not helped.

Relaxation can be an effective procedure for increasing pain tolerance. However, experimental results indicate that it is not always the most effective procedure. The conditions under which it should optimally affect pain reaction must still be clarified. A better understood definition of how anxiety affects pain will probably also clarify the role of relaxation.

Detailed relaxation instructions are available from a variety of sources including Jacobson (1938), Wolpe (1969), Bernstein and Borkovec (1974), and Rimm and Masters (1974). A variety of commercially made audio cassette tapes also are readily available.

The basic concept associated with teaching relaxation is to be able to provide the patient with a means of learning something negative, what not to do. This is done by taking one muscle group at a time, showing the patient where the tension is and what it feels like. Patients are asked to tense the muscles of that group followed by a request to cease the tensing activity in order to produce relaxation. The patient is asked to pay particular attention to the difference in sensation between tension and relaxation. An example of a set of relaxation instructions can be seen in the boxed material on p. 622.

Relaxation training as described in many of the above-mentioned studies was mostly of brief duration. As used by Jacobson (1938) and even Wolpe (1969) relaxation training can require as much as several months for some patients to achieve muscle control. Biofeedback procedures represent a technologic advance that allows for shortening the amount of time necessary to learn relaxation as well as control of other body functions. For example, in a laboratory experiment, Green and co-workers (1969) found that 7 of 21 subjects were able to achieve a very

---

SAMPLE OF RELAXATION INSTRUCTIONS*

Have patient sit in the dental chair, back straight, head on a line with his back, and his arms and hands on the arms of the chair.

Instruct patient

- Wrinkle your forehead, then relax it. Pay attention to the difference in how your muscles feel when they are tight or when they are relaxed. (Repeat last sentence periodically.)
- Squeeze your eyes tight, then relax them.
- Wrinkle your nose up, then relax it.
- Put a forced smile on your face, then relax it.
- Put your tongue hard against the roof of your mouth. Tight . . . now relax.
- Tighten your jaws and/or clench your teeth. Hard . . . now relax.
- Pucker your lips. Now relax.
- Tense your neck, so that you can feel it tense in the front and in the back. You can do this by putting your chin down on your chest and then lifting it against resistance as if someone were pushing it down.
- Tense your right arm and hand, putting it in front of you. Also, clench your fist. Relax.
- Do the same with your left arm and hand. Relax.
- Extend your right foot out and tense your thigh, leg, and point your toe outward. Relax.
- Do the same with your left leg. Relax.
- Sit forward in the chair a little. Bend your elbows and put them behind your back and try to get them to touch each other. Feel the tension. Relax.
- Tighten your chest, your abdomen. Relax.
- Below the waist, tighten your thighs, your buttocks. Relax.
- Now, close your eyes and take a deep breath. As you exhale, slowly try to relax your body starting with your forehead, going down to your toes. Also, while you exhale, say the word "relax."
- Now, begin to concentrate on slow breathing, in . . . out . . . in . . . out . . . very slowly. While you continue slow breathing, go through your entire body relaxing all the muscles in it. (Mention all the body parts as listed earlier, pausing between each to allow patient to relax. Often patients may find it easier to relax with eyes closed.)

---

*Modification of instructions prepared by J. R. Cautela, Ph.D.

---

high level of muscle relaxation in less than 20 minutes of a single session when they were provided with EMG feedback. Budzynski and Stoyva (1969) also found that even in a single session mean EMG levels for a control group ran 70% above those of their experimental group.

Interestingly, Fowler and Kraft (1974) have demonstrated that patients and normal individuals are not able to estimate levels of muscle tension accurately. Yet chronic muscle tension is associated with clinical pain. Biofeedback can be extremely helpful for such tension-related pain. With MPD syndrome patients or with dental phobics who are reluctant to

admit having tension, biofeedback becomes an immediate, relatively objective means for showing both patient and doctor that the patient is indeed tensing his facial muscles. It is then possible to proceed with appropriate therapy.

Gessel (1975) reported the successful treatment of 15 of 23 MPD syndrome patients using EMG biofeedback. Surface electrodes were attached over the temporalis and masseter areas on the affected side. Sessions lasted 30 minutes. Those who failed to achieve relief of symptoms via biofeedback were successfully treated with tricyclic antidepressant medication. Although this latter group of patients had been able to continue with their principal day-to-day activities, they did show some degree of clinical depression.

For some patients, using relaxation procedures can be adequate to permit an experience of dentistry without excess anxiety. For others, however, a form of desensitization would be in order. One approach, as used by Weisenberg and Stilwell (1974), starts with pinpointing the specific aspects of the dental situation that elicit fear. The Weisenberg Dental Fear Inventory (p. 615) can be used for this purpose. These situations are then placed into a fear hierarchy with 1 being the most feared and 10 being the least feared as shown below.

Sample dental fear hierarchy

10 – Dentist cleans your teeth with steel probe
9 – Dentist uses rubber dam
8 – Dentist squirts air into a cavity
7 – Dentist is pulling your tooth
6 – Having a probe placed in a cavity
5 – Dentist tells you that you have bad teeth
4 – Dentist might consider you a baby
3 – Dentist is giving you a shot
2 – Dentist is drilling your tooth
1 – The anticipation of pain while being treated

Patients are next taught relaxation procedures while sitting in the dental chair. Once patients can achieve a deep state of relaxation, the actual stimuli of the fear hierarchy are presented briefly (approximately 45 seconds), starting with the least feared item on the hierarchy. When the use of actual dental stimuli are not possible, the patient is asked to use imagination and visualize the scene. A given stimulus is presented until it no longer produces an anxiety reaction. The next item on the hierarchy is then presented. This process is continued until the entire hierarchy is exhausted. It is then desirable to follow up with dental care as soon as possible.

The anxiety reaction can be seen directly by means of muscle tension when biofeedback procedures are used. Without biofeedback it is possible to train a patient to respond in SUDs (Subjective Units of Disturbance), units going from 0 (no anxiety) to 100 (anxiety as high as possible), after each stimulus presentation.

Bandura (1977) is of the opinion that desensitization via imagery reduces autonomic reactions to imagined threats but less so to real threats. It is only when imagination is followed by actual performance desensitization that the fear is eliminated. Thus dental treatment following an imagined desensitization procedure would be of the utmost importance in eliminating a dental fear to achieve what Bandura refers to as a sense of self-efficacy, that is, the belief that the patient has the ability to remain calm during the dental procedure.

There is another important aspect of desensitization that can be used by any practitioner without resorting to the formal procedures just described. That is, it is desirable to introduce the easiest, least traumatic procedures first and save the more difficult treatment for later. This permits the development of a doctor-patient relationship of trust and confidence and, as a consequence, a degree of lowered anxiety.

With children, Ayer (1973) has described a procedure using emotive imagery to counter the fear of injection. Children were first taught to imagine a yapping dog. Injections were given while the children were imagining the dog yapping.

Weisenberg and Epstein (1973) described how a variety of fear-reducing techniques were used to permit the dentist to successfully treat a 26-month-old girl. Techniques included brief desensitization, forced exposure (child physically placed in the chair), reward for staying in the chair, modeling (observing her older sister), and rehearsal (playing dentist at home). Use of these procedures in three brief (15 minute) appointments avoided treatment via general anesthesia, which is always an added risk.

Cognitive dissonance and attribution theory

Zimbardo and co-workers (1966, 1969) tested derivations from the theory of cognitive dissonance to show how commitment choice and justification can affect pain reactions. The theory states that when an individual experiences one or more behaviors or cognitions that are dissonant with each other, a tension state is established that motivates the person to reduce dissonance (Festinger, 1957). When a person knows that electric shock is painful and yet of his own free choice commits himself to endure more electric shock, he has acted to create dissonance. Dissonance can be reduced by increasing the justification for the commitment or by reducing the perception of the shock as not being so painful. Subjects were tested in a two-part experiment. All subjects were asked to learn lists of words by serial anticipation. Part I consisted of the learning task with painful electric shock given randomly to all subjects except those in one control group. Part II involved commitment to continue the study for either high justification (low dissonance) or low justification (high dissonance). Control subjects either were given shock at the same painful level in Part II or were given shock at a lower level. A third control group received a low level of shock in both Parts I and II. Dependent measures consisted of verbal ratings of shock, skin conductance, and number of learning trials to criterion. On all three measures high-dissonance subjects performed comparably to the control group that was given shock at a lowered level, while low-dissonance subjects performed like the control group that had high shock levels maintained in Part II. Cognitive controls thus acted in the same way as physically changing the stimulation.

Nisbett and Schachter (1966) manipulated attributions concerning the source of body arousal to increase pain tolerance to electric shock. Attribution theory states that people seek causes or explanations for the observed events that take place around them. The state of bodily arousal of subjects was attributed either to a "drug" (really a placebo) ingested prior to stimulation or to the shock under either high or low fear conditions. For the low fear group only, subjects who attributed their increased arousal to the drug tolerated over four times the level of

shock as subjects who attributed their arousal to the shock (1450 vs 350 microamperes, respectively).

Davison and Valins (1969) showed how pain tolerance can be increased when subjects are taught to attribute pain tolerance changes to their own efforts as opposed to the effects of a pill. Subjects were first tested for shock pain tolerance after which they were given a "drug" and retested with the shock physically reduced. Half the subjects were told that they had been given a placebo. All subjects were then retested. Those subjects who were told they had received a placebo, and hence were able to attribute their behavior change to their own efforts, tolerated more shock on the last trial than those who thought they had received a drug and thus attributed their improved ability to tolerate pain to the medication.

Attribution of control as caused by internal rather than external factors has been used as a key factor in the treatment of low back pain patients (Gottlieb et al., 1975). Patients with low back pain exhibit a learned helplessness as a result of their disability, which tends to become reinforced by masses of medication and dependency on others. Patients are taught self-regulation rather than drug regulation for dealing with their problems as part of a comprehensive treatment program.

Fordyce, Fowler and De Lateur (1968) utilized techniques derived from learning principles to deal with pain reactions based on learned helplessness in their treatment of a woman who had suffered from back pain for 18 years. She had undergone four major surgical operations without relief. She was taking four or five habit-forming drugs each day and could not remain active continuously for more than 20 minutes without reclining. Treatment essentially involved breaking the contingency between cry of pain and relief while at the same time increased physical activity was reinforced. At the end of 30 days she was able to maintain continuous out-of-bed activity for at least 2 hours. After hospital discharge, with continuous outpatient visits, she was able to maintain her increased activity level and her pain complaints ultimately ceased. Undoubtedly, pain relief did not eliminate the sensation of pain. Instead, the patient was taught to cope and function despite her pain. On a 22-month follow-up of 31 patients similarly treated, Fordyce and co-workers (1973) found that measures of reduction in perceived pain, interference of pain with normal activities, and the reduction in reclining time remained significantly changed from preadmission but not significantly changed from time of discharge.

Control and choice

A variety of studies have shown how control over the pain situation can reduce subject stress and pain reactions. Bowers (1968) has argued that lack of control increases anxiety and hence results in larger pain and stress reactions. Subjects informed prior to shock tolerance measurement that they would be able to avoid electric shock tolerated it at a level more than twice as high as those who thought shock was random. Postexperimental ratings of shock painfulness did not differ for each group.

Staub, Tursky, and Schwartz (1971) related control to predictability. Uncertainty increases anxiety and results in less pain tolerance, while reduction of uncertainty increases tolerance. Subjects given control over the intensity and timing of shocks tolerated higher levels before rating them as uncomfortable compared to no-control subjects. Loss of control after it had been given to subjects resulted in lower intensities of shock being rated as uncomfortable. No-control subjects produced large heart rate responses at all levels of intensity, while control subjects made more differentiated responses, reacting mainly to the most intense shocks.

The issue of control and predictability, as with other areas of pain perception, is not entirely clear. Corah (1973) tried to replicate a study showing that a control device introduced into the dental operatory would produce more cooperative behavior. Twenty-four children, ages 6 to 11, were provided with a two-button green-red light device to use during treatment. The control-device group showed less response to high arousal procedures as measured by GSR and slightly more response during low arousal procedures compared to a no-control group. Behavioral ratings of each group did not differ. These results are not entirely clear regarding the effectiveness of control.

In an analysis of control as a variable, Averill (1973) showed that it has been used to refer to behavioral control, cognitive control, or decisional control. He states that it is difficult to conclude that there is a direct relationship between stress and control. Other factors that must be considered include the presence or absence of feedback that tells the subject how well he is controlling, the subject's ability to tolerate the information necessary for control, and what appears as larger short-term stress reactions but long-term adaptation. It seems that control is an important variable in pain reduction. However, who should be given control, for example, patient or health provider, may vary depending on the goals or circumstances. Long-term gain may require greater immediate arousal as seen in the literature on preparation for surgery.

These questions also relate to the role of anxiety and coping style in pain perception. Coping style refers to the characteristic way an individual uses defenses in dealing with stress. DeLong (1970) has shown that avoiders (those who mainly use denial-type defenses), copers (those who use defenses to deal actively with the stress), and nonspecific defenders (those in between) differ in response to the information provided regarding upcoming surgery. For the avoider, for example, having a minimal amount of prior information and trusting that the dentist is in charge and will control the details can be preferable to knowing how to control things himself (DeLong, 1970). The coper, on the other hand, may want to feel more in charge himself. Placebo responses may reduce anxiety (Evans, 1974a) by producing a feeling that something is being done to control even if it is not the patient that is exerting control. It thus becomes important for the dentist to exert clinical judgment in deciding what to tell his patient and how much control to give him. It is likely that anxiety is thus reduced once the patient is provided reassurance that control is being exerted by someone, either the patient himself (if he can) or the dentist (if the patient finds it too difficult to accept this responsibility). Further support may be gathered for this view by an examination of the literature on advanced preparation in reducing pain reactions.

Advanced preparation for pain

Preparation for surgery has been credited with reducing severity of postoperative outcomes. Egbert and co-workers (1964) prepared one group of patients by a preoperative visit. They were told about the preparation for anesthesia, the time and approximate duration of the operation, and warned that they would wake-up in the recovery room. They were also told they would feel pain, how severe it might be, and how long it would last. The patients were reassured that feeling pain was normal after abdominal surgery and that there were ways by which they would be able to cope with the pain through relaxation procedures, by use of a trapeze, and by instructions on how to turn their bodies. They were also told they could ask for medication if it was needed. Compared to a control group, the specially instructed patients requested significantly less narcotic following surgery and were sent home an average of 2.7 days earlier.

Baldwin and Barnes (1966) studied 8- to 14-year-old patients who had to undergo dental extraction. They used the "Draw a Person" test and measured the size of the figure drawn at various points in the extraction process. When compared to a baseline nonstress period, they obtained a shrinking in the size of the drawing following the announcement to the patient of the impending procedure with a further reduction prior to surgery. Postsurgery, the drawings returned to the original baseline size. Control group subjects maintained a consistent drawing size.

One group of subjects was given from 4 to 7 days between the time of the announcement of the extraction and the extraction itself, while a second group was not notified until the day of the event itself. Children in the waiting period group were actually given the choice of prior warning or no prior warning. Every one of the children preferred advanced warning, while only half of the parents of the children preferred advanced warning. The reasons given by the children were such things as the need "to think about it," "to get ready for it," or "to ask my friends about it." Parents who wanted their children warned gave similar reasons.

Those parents who did not want their children warned mentioned reasons such as "he'll just get scared," or "why make him worry." Many of these parents, however, were expressing their own fears in such additional statements as "dentists scare me to death" or "I'm glad I'm not him." They wanted to avoid advance warning because of their inability to handle their own anxieties.

The comparison of human figure drawing size for the two groups (waiting period—no waiting period) showed significant differences in the postsurgical drawings. While both groups showed a constriction prior to surgery, the waiting-period group showed an increase in size postsurgery, while the no-waiting period group remained constricted and began to show an increase in figure size only in the follow-up period 1 month later.

What are the crucial ingredients that go into patient preparation? Janis (1958) has emphasized anxiety. There is an optimal relationship between the amount of suffering expected and the amount obtained that seems conducive to a feeling of mastery of a difficult situation and to speed of recovery. The optimal degree of worry or anxiety prior to the stressful event is best reached when the patient receives realistic information and is able to listen and accept what is being told to him. This occurs when the patient experiences a moderate level of anxiety. The credibility of the practitioner is enhanced and the patient is helped to prepare for the event.

The moderate fear group in the Janis study had been better informed prior to surgery and felt worried before surgery. Fewer in this group became angry, resentful, or emotionally upset following surgery. They had time to build up psychologic defenses prior to surgery. Without the "work of worrying," Janis describes a different sequence of events. There is little anticipatory fear. Thus there is no mental rehearsal of the impending danger. Lack of rehearsal results in feelings of helplessness when the danger manifests itself. In turn, this results in feelings of disappointment in protective authorities, intense fear, anger, and "victimization"—the sense of deprivation, loss, and suffering from a stressful experience.

Unfortunately, subsequent studies have not supported Janis' emphasis on fear and anxiety. Cohen and Lazarus (1973) have emphasized the importance of coping strategies in dealing with the stress of surgery. Unlike Janis, they feel that denial would be a beneficial strategy to use when the outcome is expected to be positive.

What the critical ingredients are still requires greater clarification. A period of advanced notice with prior information and coping techniques, however, does seem to help (Johnson, Dabbs, and Leventhal, 1970). The amount of detail, the temporal spacing of advanced information, and the personality disposition of the subject will also affect the outcome (Andrew, 1970; DeLong, 1970). Copers (those who attempt to deal with stress) and those called nonspecific defenders (those who use both coping and avoiding strategies) seem to be able to accept more detailed information than avoiders (those who try to deny or avoid dealing with stress) (DeLong, 1970).

Information regarding the sensations to be experienced seems to be more effective in reducing distress than information regarding the procedures to be used (Johnson, 1973; Johnson and Leventhal, 1974). For example, Johnson, Kirchoff, and Endres (1975), in a study of cast removal, found that children exposed to a brief tape recording that included the sound of the saw and a description of the sensations of heat, flying chalk, and so forth showed less distress and resistance to the procedure compared to a group only told of the procedure or not told at all.

From these studies it is apparent that careful preparation for oral and maxillofacial surgery is an important element that can hasten recovery and increase confidence and trust between doctor and patient. This preparation is prevented (1) if the event is too sudden, (2) if the patient suppresses information or otherwise denies his own vulnerability, (3) if no prior warning is given, or (4) if false assurances are given. The patient has to be given realistic information at the level that he is capable of absorbing. He need not be shown every last gory detail; only such information as relates to his expected experiences during and after surgery. If his level of anxiety is already too high, he can be helped by use of such techniques as relaxation, hypnosis, or other means of desensitization. To ignore the inevitable outcomes of an impending event is to invite hostility, loss of credibility, and retardation of the recovery process.

There are situations facing the surgeon, however, when there is no time for advanced preparation. These situations require a greater effort on his part to pay attention to factors in the doctor-patient relationship that can affect the outcome. As mentioned earlier, careful use of language, consideration of the patient as a person, relaxation and especially distraction, and careful definition of the sensations to be experienced can be extremely helpful in reducing anxiety and pain reactions.

Modeling

Modeling refers to the notion that a person can anticipate the consequences of a behavior without having to personally experience it. Bandura (1971) is of the opinion that most learning occurs via modeling rather than on a trial and error basis. Neufeld and Davidson (1971) demonstrated that the vicarious rehearsal of watching another person experience an aversive stimulus did not differ from the cognitive rehearsal of listening to the procedure described in detail. Both were equally effective in reducing pain reactions to radiant heat stimulation.

In a series of studies Craig and his co-workers showed how modeling can be used to change the ratings subjects give to electric shock stimulation. Craig and Weiss (1971) had subjects rate the intensity of incremental shocks when observing the rating of a confederate model. In one condition, the model tolerated a great deal of shock before labeling it as painful, while in a second condition he tolerated a great deal less before terming it painful. The high-tolerance group of subjects rated as painful shock of a mean intensity of 8.65 milliamperes. The control subjects yielded a mean of 6.35 milliamps. The low-tolerance group rated a mean of 2.50 milliamps as painful, some 70% less intense than the high-tolerance group. Furthermore, Craig and Neidermayer (1974) were not able to demonstrate any heart rate or skin conductance differences between high- and low-tolerance groups. The authors claim that this shows that the subjects were not merely masking subjective discomfort. However, it is possible that the physiologic indicators were not adequately discriminative to show differences.

Another study (Craig and Weiss, 1972) complemented the first by using a constant nonaversive shock. Each one of a group of subjects was paired with a model who rated the nonaversive shocks as increasingly painful. Compared to a control group, the model-paired subjects began to report ratings of painful to shock levels usually judged as nonaversive.

It is likely that dentists can readily relate to similar experiences. There are patients who react as if in pain when given nonpainful stimulation such as being touched with a probe. This occurs especially when anxiety is high; there is an expectation of painful treatment and the patient has little information as to what is about to happen.

Modeling is one way of providing advanced information as to what will occur during treatment. It also permits the patient to see how someone who is similar to himself can cope with the treatment without excess anxiety and stress reaction. Models should have some degree of similarity to the patient and should give a fairly realistic reaction, not suppress all response.

Vernon (1974) exposed hospitalized patients ages 4 to 9 to one of two films. One group saw children receiving injections without experiencing pain or expressing emotion. A second group saw a more realistic film in which children moderately reacted to the injections. A third group did not see any film. Reactions to actual injection were rated in a hospital setting. Those who saw the unrealistic film appeared to experience most pain while those who saw the realistic film exhibited least pain.

In dentistry several studies have shown how modeling can be effective. Machen and Johnson (1974) demonstrated how preschool children (36 to 65 months of age), who were introduced to dentistry through a modeling procedure, compared to a control group, showed greater cooperative behavior over a series of three appointments that included restorative work. Ghose and co-workers (1969) showed that older children can serve as models for younger siblings age 4 and above.

CONCLUDING COMMENT

Recent years have seen an increased concern for the control of pain and anxiety. New techniques as well as a variety of older available approaches have received prominence. Current views perceive pain as a complex phenomenon that includes a sensory and a motivational component. The motivational component has the stronger association with suffering. It includes memories of past experiences and involves a strong element of interpersonal communication. It is not adequately controlled by simple local injections of anesthesia.

Pain and anxiety control have been strongly linked so that the presence of anxiety usually leads to a stronger pain reaction. Behavioral strategies mainly influence the motivational component of pain. They can effectively be used to deal with both pain and anxiety. Behavioral techniques include suggestion, relaxation, placebos, biofeedback, desensitization, hypnosis, distraction, advanced preparation, modeling as well as a variety of cognitive strategies. Their effectiveness as techniques is lessened by automatic machine-like application and is greatly potentiated by interpersonal factors. It behooves the surgeon to become familiar with their use so that the association of surgery, pain, and discomfort need not remain fixed in the mind of patients.

REFERENCES

Andrew, J. M. 1970. Recovery from surgery with and without preparatory instruction for three coping styles, J. Pers. Soc. Psychol. **15:**223.

Averill, J. R. 1973. Personal control over aversive stimuli and its relationship to stress, Psychol. Bull. **80:**286.

Ayer, W. A. 1973. Use of visual imagery in needle phobic children, J. Dent. Child. **40:**125.

Bailey, P. M., Talbot, A., and Taylor, P. P. 1973. A comparison of maternal anxiety levels with anxiety levels manifested in the child dental patient, J. Dent. Child. **40:**277.

Baldwin, D. C., Jr., and Barnes, M. L., 1966. The psychological value of a presurgical waiting period in the preparation of children for dental extraction, Europ. Orthodont. Soc. Rep. Congr. **42:**297.

Bandura, A. 1969. Principles of behavior modification, New York, Holt, Rinehart & Winston.

Bandura, A. 1971. Analysis of modeling processes. In Bandura, A., ed.: Psychological modeling, Chicago, Aldine-Atherton.

Bandura, A. 1977. Self-efficacy: toward a unifying theory of behavioral change, Psychol. Rev. **84:**191.

Bandura, A., and Whalen, C. K. 1966. The influence of antecedent reinforcement and divergent modeling cues on patterns of self-reward, J. Pers. Soc. Psychol. **3:**373.

Barber, T. X. 1965. Physiological effects of "hypnotic suggestions": a critical review of recent research (1960-64), Psychol. Bull. **63:**201.

Barber, T. X., and Hahn, K. W., Jr. 1962. Physiological and subjective responses to pain producing stimulation under hypnotically-suggested and waking-imaged "analgesia," J. Abnorm Soc. Psychol. **65:**411.

Beecher, H. K. 1956. Relationship of significance of wound to the pain experienced, J.A.M.A. **161:**1609.

Beecher, H. K. 1959. Measurement of subjective responses: quantitative effects of drugs, New York, Oxford University Press, Inc.

Beecher, H. K. 1963. Quantification of the subjective pain experience, Proc. Am. Psychopath. Assoc. **53:**111.

Beecher, H. K. 1972. The placebo effects as a non-specific force surrounding disease and the treatment of disease. In Janzen, R., et al., eds.: Pain: basic principles, pharmacology, therapy, Stuttgart, Georg Thieme Verlag.

Bernstein, D. A., and Borkovec, T. D. 1974. Progressive relaxation training, Champaign, Ill., Research Press.

Bobey, M. J., and Davidson, P. O. 1970. Psychological factors affecting pain tolerance, J. Psychosom. Res. **14:**371.

Bowers, K. S. 1968. Pain, anxiety and perceived control, J. Consult. Clin. Psychol. **32:**596.

Budzynski, T. H., and Stoyva, J. M. 1969. An instrument for producing deep muscle relaxation by means of analog information feedback, J. Appl. Behav. Anal. **2:**231.

Burgess, P. R. 1974. Patterns of discharge evoked in cutaneous nerves and their significance for sensation. In Bonica, J. J., ed.: Advances in neurology: international symposium on pain, New York, Raven Press.

Chapman, C. R. 1977. Psychological aspects of pain patient treatment, Arch. Surg. **112:**767.

Chapman, W. P., and Jones, C. M. 1944. Variations in cutaneous and visceral pain sensitivity in normal subjects, J. Clin. Invest. **23:**81.

Chaves, J. F., and Barber, T. X. 1974. Hypnotism and surgical pain. In Barber, T. X., Spanos, N. P., and Chaves, J. F., eds.: Hypnosis, imagination and human potentialities, Elmsford, N. Y., Pergamon Press, Inc.

Cohen, F., and Lazarus, R. S. 1973. Active coping processes, coping dispositions, and recovery from surgery, Psychosom. Med **35:**375.

Cole, L. A. 1961. Attitudes towards dental treatment: a motivational analysis, J. Philippine Dent. Assoc. **14:**20.

Corah, N. L. 1969. Development of a dental anxiety scale, J. Dent. Res. **48:**596.

Corah, N. L. 1973. Effect of perceived control on stress reduction in pedodontic patients, J. Dent. Res. **52:**1261.

Craig, K. D., and Neidermayer, H. 1974. Autonomic correlates of pain thresholds influenced by social modeling, J. Pers. Soc. Psychol. **29:**246.

Craig, K. D., and Weiss, S. M. 1971. Vicarious influences on pain-threshold determinations, J. Pers. Soc. Pschol. **19:**53.

Craig, K. D., and Weiss, S. M. 1972. Verbal reports of pain without noxious stimulation, Percept. Mot. Skills **34:**943.

Crockett, B. 1963. Dental survey: Southeastern State College, J. Okla. Dent. Assoc. **51:**25.

Crue, B. L., Jr., and Carregal, E. J. A. 1975. Pain begins in the dorsal horn—with a proposed classification of the primary senses. In Crue, B. L., Jr., ed.: Pain: research and treatment, New York, Academic Press, Inc.

Davison, G. C., and Valins, S. 1969. Maintenance of self-attributed and drug-attributed behavior change, J. Pers. Soc. Psychol. **11:**25.

DeLong, R. D. 1970. Individual differences in patterns of anxiety arousal, stress-relevant information and recovery from surgery, Unpublished doctoral dissertation, University of California, Los Angeles.

Devine, R., and Merskey, H. 1965. The description of pain in psychiatric and general medical patients, J. Psychosom. Res. **9:**311.

Dubuisson, D., and Melzack, R. 1976. Classification of clinical pain descriptions by multiple group discriminant analysis, Exp. Neurol. **51:**480.

Dyck, P. J., Lambert, E. H., and O'Brien, P. 1976. Pain in peripheral neuropathy related to size and rate of fiber degeneration. In Weisenberg, M., and Tursky, B., eds.: Pain: therapeutic approaches and research frontiers, New York, Plenum Publishing Corp.

Egbert, L. D., et al. 1964. Reduction of postoperative pain by encouragement and instruction of patients, N. Eng. J. Med. **270:**825.

Engel, G. L. 1959. "Psychogenic" pain and the pain-prone patient, Am. J. Med. **26:**899.

Erickson, M.H. 1966. The interspersal hypnotic technique for symptom correction and pain control, Am. J. Clin. Hypn. **8:**198.

Evans, F. J. 1967. Suggestibility in the normal waking state, Psychol. Bull. **67:**114.

Evans, F. J. 1974a. Placebo analgesia: suggestion, anxiety and the doctor-patient relationship, Paper presented at annual meeting of the American Psychosomatic Society, Philadelphia.

Evans, F. J. 1974b. The placebo response in pain reduction. In Bonica, J. J., ed.: Advances in neurology: international symposium on pain, New York, Raven Press.

Feather, B. W., Chapman, C. R., and Fisher, S. B. 1972. The effect of a placebo on the perception of painful radiant heat stimuli, Psychosom. Med. **34:**290.

Festinger, L. 1950. Informal social communication, Psychol. Rev. **57:**271.

Festinger, L. 1954. A theory of social comparison processes, Hum. Relat. **7:**117.

Festinger, L. 1957. A theory of cognitive dissonance, Evanston, Ill., Row, Peterson & Co.

Folkins, C. H., et al. 1968. Desensitization and the experimental reduction of threat, J. Abnorm. Psychol. **73:**100.

Fordyce, W. E., Fowler, R. S., and De Lateur, B. 1968. An application of behavior modification technique to a problem of chronic pain, Behav. Res. Ther. **6:**105.

Fordyce, W. E., et al. 1973. Operant conditioning in the treatment of chronic pain, Arch. Phys. Med. Rehabil. **54:**399.

Fowler, R. S., and Kraft, G. H. 1974. Tension perception in patients having pain associated with chronic muscle tension, Arch. Phys. Med. Rehabil. **55:**28-30.

Franz, D. N., and Iggo, A. 1968. Dorsal root potentials and ventral root reflexes evoked by nonmyelinated fibers, Science **162:**1140.

Freidson, E., and Feldman, J. J. 1958. The public looks at dental care, J. Am. Dent. Assoc. **57:**325.

Gale, E. N. 1972. Fears of the dental situation, J. Dent. Res. **51:**964.

Gardner, W. J., and Licklider, J. C. R. 1959. Auditory analgesia in dental operations, J. Am. Dent. Assoc. **59:**1144.

Gardner, W. J., Licklider, J. C. R., and Weisz, A. Z. 1960. Suppression of pain by sound, Science **132:**32.

Gelfand, D. M., Gelfand, S., and Rardin, M. W. 1965. Some personality factors associated with placebo responsivity, Psychol. Rep. **17:**555-562.

Gessell, A. H. 1975. Electromyographic biofeedback and tricyclic antidepressants in myofascial pain-dysfunction syndrome: psychological predictors of outcome, J. Am. Dent. Assoc. **91:**1048.

Gessell, A. H., and Alderman, M. M. 1971. Management of myofascial pain dysfunction syndrome of the temporomandibular joint by tension control training, Psychosomatics **12:**302.

Ghose, L. J.: 1969. Evaluation of sibling support, J. Dent. Child. **36:**35.

Goldscheider, A. 1894. Ueber den Schmerz in physiologischer und klinischer hinsicht, Berlin, Hirschwald.

Goodman, P., Greene, C. S., and Laskin, D. M. 1976. Response of patients with myofascial pain dysfunction syndrome to mock equilibration, J. Am. Dent. Assoc. **92:**755.

Gottlieb, H. J., et al. 1975. A successful treatment program for chronic back pain patients, Symposium presented at the meeting of the American Psychological Association, Chicago.

Green, E. E., et al.: 1969. Feedback technique for deep relaxation, Psychophysiology **6:**371.

Greene, C. S., and Laskin, D. M. 1974. Long-term evaluation of conservative treatment for myofascial pain-dysfunction syndrome, J. Am. Dent. Assoc. **89:**1365.

Greene, C. S., and Markovic, M. A. 1976. Response to non-surgical treatment of patients with positive radiographic findings in the temporomandibular joint, J. Oral Surg. **34:**692.

Hawley, B. P., et al. 1974. The first dental visit for children from low socioeconomic families, J. Dent. Child. **41:**376.

Hilgard, E. R. 1973. A neodissociation interpretation of pain reduction in hypnosis, Psychol. Rev. **80:**396.

Hillman, P., and Wall, P. D. 1969. Inhibitory and excitatory factors influencing the receptive fields of lamina 5 spinal cord cells. Exp. Brain Res. **9:**284.

Iggo, A. 1972. Critical remarks on the gate control theory. In Janzen, R., et al., eds.: Pain: basic principles, pharmacology, therapy, Stuttgart, Georg Thieme Verlag.

Iggo, A. 1974. Activation of cutaneous nociceptors and their actions on dorsal horn neurons. In Bonica, J. J., ed.: Advances in neurology: international symposium on pain, New York, Raven Press.

Jacobson, E. 1938. Progressive relaxation, Chicago, University of Chicago Press.

Jacoby, J. D. 1960. Statistical report on general practice hypnodontics; tape-recorder conditioning, J. Clin. Exp. Hypn. **8:**115.

Janis, L. L. 1958. Psychological stress, New York, John Wiley & Sons, Inc.

Johnson, J. E. 1973. Effects of accurate expectations about sensations on the sensory and distress components of pain, J. Pers. Soc. Psychol. **27:**261.

Johnson, J. E., and Leventhal, H. 1974. Effects of accurate expectations and behavioral instructions on reactions during a noxious medical examination, J. Pers. Soc. Psychol. **29:**710.

Johnson, J. E., Dabbs, J. M., and Leventhal, H. 1970. Psychosocial factors in the welfare of surgical patients, Nurs. Res. **19**:18.

Johnson, J. E., Kirchoff, K. T., and Endres, M. P. 1975. Deferring children's distress behavior during orthopedic cast removal, Nurs. Res. **75**:404.

Johnson, R., and Baldwin, D. C., Jr. 1968. Relationship of maternal anxiety to the behavior of young children undergoing dental extraction, J. Dent. Res. **47**:801.

Kriesberg, L., and Treiman, B. R. 1963. Dentists and the practice of dentistry as viewed by the public, J. Am. Dent. Assoc. **64**:806.

Lacey, J. I., Bateman, D. E., and Van Lehn, R. 1953. Atonomic response specificity, Psychosom. Med. **15**:8.

Laskin, D. M. 1969. Etiology of the pain-dysfunction syndrome, J. Am. Dent. Assoc. **79**:147.

Laskin, D. M., and Greene, C. S. 1972. Influence of the doctor-patient relationship on placebo therapy for patients with myofascial pain-dysfunction (MPD) syndrome, J. Am. Dent. Assoc. **85**:892.

Lehrer, P. M. 1972. Physiological effects of relaxation in a double-blind analog of desensitization, Behav. Ther. **3**:193.

Loeser, J. D. In press. Mechanisms of central pain. In Weisenberg, M., ed.: The control of pain, New York, Psychological Dimensions, Inc.

Machen, J. B., and Johnson, R. 1974. Desensitization, model learning and the dental behavior of children, J. Dent. Res. **53**:83.

Marbach, J. J., and Lipton, J. A. 1977. The relation of diagnosis to treatment in the facial pain patient, N.Y. State Dent. J. **43**:282.

Marbach, J. J., and Lipton, J. A. 1978. Aspects of illness behavior in patients with facial pain, J. Am. Dent. Assoc. **96**:630.

Marbach, J. J., et al. 1978. Facial pains and anxiety levels: considerations for treatment, J. Prosthet. Dent. **40**:434.

McAmmond, D. M., Davidson, P. O., and Kovitz, D. M. 1971. A comparison of the effects of hypnosis and relaxation training on stress reactions in a dental situation, Am. J. Clin. Hypn. **13**:233.

McGlashan, T. H., Evans, F. J., and Orne, M. T. 1969. The nature of hypnotic analgesia and placebo response to experimental pain, Psychosom. Med. **31**:227.

McKeithen, E. J. 1966. The patient's image of the dentist, J. Am. Coll. Dent. **33**:87.

Meehan, J. P., Stoll, A. M., and Hardy, J. D. 1954. Cutaneous pain threshold in native Alaskan Indian and Eskimo, J. Appl. Physiol. **6**:397.

Melzack, R. 1973. The puzzle of pain, New York, Basic Books, Inc., Publishers.

Melzack, R. 1975a. An update of the gate control theory, Paper presented at the American Association for the Advancement of Science Symposium on pain control, New York.

Melzack, R. 1975b. The McGill Pain Questionnaire: major properties and scoring methods, Pain **1**:277.

Melzack, R. 1976. Pain: past, present and future. In Weisenberg, M., and Tursky, B., eds.: Pain: therapeutic approaches and research frontiers, New York, Plenum Publishing Corp.

Melzack, R., and Perry, C. 1975. Self-regulation of pain: the use of alpha-feedback and hypnotic training for the control of chronic pain, Exp. Neurol. **46**:452.

Melzack, R., and Torgerson, W. S. 1971. On the language of pain, Anesthesiology **34**:50.

Melzack, R., and Wall, P. D. 1965. Pain mechanisms: a new theory, Science **150**:971.

Melzack, R., and Wall, P. D. 1970. Psychophysiology of pain, Int. Anesthesiol. Clin. **8**:3.

Melzack, R., Weisz, A. Z., and Sprague, L. T. 1963. Strategies for controlling pain: contributions of auditory stimulation and suggestion, Exp. Neurol. **8**:239.

Mendell, L. M., and Wall, P. D. 1964. Presynaptic hyperpolarization: a role for fine afferent fibres, J. Physiol. **172**:274.

Mercuri, L. G., Olson, R. E., and Laskin, D. M. 1979. The specificity of response to experimental stress in patients with myofascial pain-dysfunction syndrome, J. Dent. Res. **58**:1866, 1979.

Merskey, H. 1965a. The characteristics of persistent pain in psychological illness, J. Psychosom. Res. **9**:291.

Merskey, H. 1965b. Psychiatric patients with persistent pain, J. Psychosom. Res. **9**:299.

Merskey, H. 1968. Psychological aspects of pain, Postgrad. Med. J. **44**:297.

Merskey, H. 1974. Assessment of pain, Physiotherapy **60**:96.

Merskey, H., and Spear, F. G. 1964. The reliability of the pressure algometer, Br. J. Clin. Psychol. **3**:130.

Merskey, H., and Spear, F. G. 1967. Pain: psychological and psychiatric aspects, London, Baillière Tindall.

Messer, J. G. 1977. Stress in dental patients undergoing routine procedures, J. Dent. Res. **56**:362.

Mountcastle, V. B. 1974. Pain and temperature sensibilities. In Mountcastle, V. B., ed.: Medical physiology, ed. 13, St. Louis, The C. V. Mosby Co.

Mowrer, O. H. 1950. Learning theory and personality dynamics, New York, The Ronald Press Co.

Myers, D. R., Kramer, W. S., and Sullivan, R. E. 1972. A study of the heart action of the child dental patient, J. Dent. Child. **39**:99.

Neufeld, R. W. J., and Davidson, P. O. 1971. The effects of vicarious rehearsal on pain tolerance, J. Psychosom. Res. **15**:329.

Nisbett, R. E., and Schachter, S. 1966. Cognitive manipulation of pain, J. Exp. Soc. Psychol. **2**:227.

Orne, M. T. 1974. Pain suppression by hypnosis and related phenomena. In Bonica, J. J., ed.: Advances in neurology: international symposium on pain, New York, Raven Press.

Parbrook, G. D., Steel, D. F., and Dalrymple, D. G. 1973. Factors predisposing to postoperative pain and pulmonary complications, Br. J. Anaesth. **45**:21.

Paul, G. L. 1969. Physiological effects of relaxation training and hypnotic suggestion, J. Abnorm. Psychol. **74**:425.

Paul, G. L., and Bernstein, D. A. 1973. Anxiety and

clinical problems: systematic desensitization and related techniques, Morristown, N.J., General Learning Press.

Pilling, L. F., Brannick, T. L., and Swenson, W. M. 1967. Psychologic characteristics of psychiatric patients having pain as a presenting symptom, Can. Med. Assoc. J. **97**:387.

Pilowsky, I., and Spence, N. D. 1975. Patterns of illness behavior in patients with intractable pain, J. Psychosom. Res. **19**:279.

Pilowsky, I., and Spence, N. D. 1976a. Pain and illness behavior: a comparative study, J. Psychosom. Res. **20**:131.

Pilowsky, I., and Spence, N. D. 1976b. Is illness behavior related to chronicity in patients with intractable pain? Pain **2**:167.

Pilowsky, I., Chapman, C. R., and Bonica, J. J. 1977. Pain, depression and illness behavior in a pain clinic population, Pain **4**:183.

Pollack, S. 1966. Pain control by suggestion, J. Oral Med. **21**:89.

Rayner, J. F. 1976. Pain control as a factor in preventive health care. In Weisenberg, M., ed.: Pain: new perspectives in therapy and research, New York, Plenum Publishing Corp.

Rimm, D. C., and Masters, J. C. 1974. Behavior therapy: techniques and empirical findings, New York, Academic Press, Inc.

Rogers, J. G. 1971. Blink test to establish threshold for reaction to pain, Postgrad. Med. **49**:108.

Rugh, J. D., and Solberg, W. K. 1975. Electromyographic studies of bruxist behavior before and during treatment, J. Dent. Res. **54**:L563, (Abstr.).

Rugh, J. D., and Solberg, W. K. 1976. Psychological implications in temporomandibular pain and dysfunction, Oral Sci. Rev. **7**:3.

Sarcedote, P. 1970. Theory and practice of pain control in malignancy and other protracted or recurring painful illnesses, Int. J. Clin. Exp. Hypn. **18**:160.

Schwartz, R. A., Greene, C. S., and Laskin, D. M. 1979. Personality characteristics of patients with myofascial pain-dysfunction (MPD) syndrome unresponsive to conventional therapy. J. Dent. Res. **58**:1435.

Shipman, W. G., Heath, H. A., and Oken, D. 1970. Response specificity among muscular and autonomic variables, Arch. Gen. Psychiatr. **23**:369.

Shoben, E. J., and Borland, L. 1954. An empirical study of the etiology of dental fears, J. Clin. Psychol. **10**:171.

Shor, R. C. 1962. Physiological effects of painful stimulation during hypnotic analgesia under conditions designed to minimize anxiety, Int. J. Clin. Exp. Hypn. **10**:183.

Spear, F. G. 1967. Pain in psychiatric patients, J. Psychosom. Res. **11**:187.

Spielberger, C. D., Gorsuch, R. L., and Lushene, R. E. 1970. Manual for the State-Trait Anxiety Inventory, Palo Alto, Calif., Consulting Psychologists Press.

Srp, L., and Kominek, J. 1963. The reaction of children to dental treatment, Odontol. Revy **14**:178.

Staub, E., Tursky, B., and Schwartz, G. E. 1971. Self-control and predictability: their effects on reactions to aversive stimulation, J. Pers. Soc. Psychol. **18**:157.

Sternbach, R. A. 1968. Pain: a psychophysiological analysis, New York, Academic Press, Inc.

Sternbach, R. A. 1974. Pain patients: traits and treatment, New York, Academic Press, Inc.

Sternbach, R. A., and Tursky, B. 1965. Ethnic differences among housewives in psychophysical and skin potential responses to electric shock, Psychophysiology **1**:241.

Stroebel, C. F., and Glueck, B. C. 1973. Biofeedback treatment in medicine and psychiatry: an ultimate placebo? Semin. Psychiatr. **5**:378.

Szasz, T. S. 1955. The nature of pain, Arch. Neurol. Psychiatr. **74**:174.

Szasz, T. S. 1957. Pain and pleasure, New York, Basic Books, Inc., Publishers.

Szasz, T. S. 1968. The psychology of persistent pain: a portrait of l'homme douloureux. In Soulairac, A., Cahn, J., and Charpentier, J., eds.: Pain: proceedings of the international symposium on pain, New York, Academic Press, Inc.

Taub, A. 1975. Factors in the diagnosis and treatment of chronic pain, J. Autism Child. Schizo. **5**:1.

Thompson, K. 1974. The role of suggestion in dental practice. In Bennet, C. R., Conscious sedation in dental practice, ed. 2, St. Louis, The C. V. Mosby Co.

Tursky, B. 1976. The pain perception profile: a psychophysical approach. In Weisenberg, M., and Tursky, B., eds.: Pain: therapeutic approaches and research frontiers, New York, Plenum Publishing Corp.

Tursky, B. In press. The measurement of pain reactions: laboratory studies. In Weisenberg, M., ed.: The control of pain, New York, Psychological Dimensions, Inc.

Tursky, B., and Sternbach, R. A. 1967. Further physiological correlates of ethnic differences in responses to shock, Psychophysiology **4**:67.

Vernon, D. T. A. 1974. Modeling and birth order in responses to painful stimuli, J. Pers. Soc. Psychol. **29**:794.

Vyklický, L., et al. 1969. Primary afferent depolarization evoked by a painful stimulus, Science **165**:184.

Wall, P. D. 1976. Modulation of pain by nonpainful events. In Bonica, J. J., and Albe-Fessard, D., eds.: Advances in pain research and therapy, New York, Raven Press.

Weisenberg, M., ed. 1975. Pain: clinical and experimental perspectives, St. Louis, The C. V. Mosby Co.

Weisenberg, M. In press. Cultural and racial reactions to pain. In Weisenberg, M., ed.: The control of pain, New York, Psychological Dimensions, Inc.

Weisenberg, M., and Epstein, D. 1973. Patient training as an alternative to general anesthesia, N.Y. State Dent. J. **39**:610.

Weisenberg, M., and Stilwell, N. 1974. The use of biofeedback in the treatment of dental phobia, Paper presented at the annual meeting of the Eastern Psychological Association. Philadelphia.

Weisenberg, M., et al. 1975. Pain: anxiety and attitudes in black, white and Puerto Rican patients, Psychosom. Med. **37**:123.

Winsburg, B., and Greenlick, M. 1968. Pain responses in Negro and white obstetrical patients, J. Health Soc. Behav. **8:**222.

Wolf, S. 1950. Effects of suggestion and conditioning on the action of chemical agents in human subjects, J. Clin. Invest. **29:**100.

Wolff, B. B., and Jarvik, M. E. 1963. Variations in cutaneous and deep somatic pain sensitivity, Can. J. Psychol. **17:**37.

Wolff, B. B. and Langley, S. 1968. Cultural factors and the response to pain: a review, Am. Anthropol. **70:**494.

Wolpe, J. 1969. The practice of behavior therapy, Elmsford, N.Y., Pergamon Press, Inc.

Woodforde, J. M., and Fielding, J. R. 1970. Pain and cancer, J. Psychosom. Res. **14:**365.

Woodrow, K. M., et al. 1972. Pain differences according to age, sex and race, Psychosom. Med. **34:**548.

Zborowski, M. 1969. People in pain, San Francisco, Jossey-Bass, Inc. Publishers.

Zimbardo, P. G., et al. 1966. Control of pain motivation by cognitive dissonance, Science, **151:**217.

Zimbardo, P. G., et al. 1969. The control of experimental pain. In Zimbardo, P. G., ed.: The cognitive control of motivation, Glenview, Ill., Scott, Foresman & Co.

Zimmerman, M. 1968. Dorsal root potentials after C-fiber stimulation, Science **160:**896.

Zola, I. K. 1966. Culture and symptoms: an analysis of patients' presenting complaints, Am. Sociol. Rev. **31:**615.

CHAPTER 19

Local anesthesia

Louis G. Mercuri

Local or regional anesthesia, as a therapeutic modality, may be defined as a transient, regional loss of sensation to a painful or potentially painful stimulus, resulting from a reversible interruption of peripheral conduction along a specific neural pathway to its central integration and perception in the brain.

There are many ways to interrupt peripheral nerve conduction leading to local anesthesia. Some of these methods may result in nerve tissue damage leading to a permanent anesthesia or paresthesia; thus these methods would not be useful therapeutically. Such methods include direct mechanical trauma to a nerve, prolonged hypothermia, local anoxia of nerve tissue, and chemical irritation such as by alcohol or phenol, all of which destroy nerve tissue. To be useful clinically, an agent must provide a transient, reversible blockade of peripheral stimuli. The local anesthetics have this capability and, therefore, are to date the most widely used drugs.

The local anesthetic drugs have been used as a mode of pain control in dentistry and medicine for over 85 years. With the current increased use of sedation techniques as forms of pain and anxiety control, the need for local anesthesia has not decreased. It must be remembered that the sedated patient is still conscious and will react to painful stimuli unless these stimuli are properly blocked by a local anesthetic. If the sedated patient experiences pain, the doctor should not interpret this as inadequate sedation; rather it is a reaction to pain resulting from incomplete local anesthesia. The patient should not be given an increased dose of the sedative agent because this brings him closer to the realm of light general anesthesia. This not only defeats the purpose of conscious sedation but also can lead to possible complications. That is why good local anesthetic technique is stressed as the cornerstone for effective pain and anxiety control. This chapter is designed to acquaint the practitioner with the techniques of local anesthesia, its pharmacology, physiology, and a rationale for its safe and effective use.

CLASSIFICATION OF LOCAL ANESTHETIC AGENTS

Many compounds that have local anesthetic properties are too toxic to tissues to be useful clinically. The clinically useful local anesthetic agents are classified into three groups—esters, amides, and hydroxyl-type compounds.

The molecular structure of compounds with local anesthetic properties is basically the same. There is an aromatic, lipophilic group joined to an intermediate chain that is either an ester or amide. The intermediate chain is then attached to a hydrophilic secondary or tertiary amino group (Fig. 19-1). The hydroxyl class lacks the hydrophilic amino group and is therefore insoluble in water. These agents are useful only as topical anesthetics. The metabolism of local anesthetics is also based on the type of linkage between the aromatic and intermediate chain moieties (see Chapter 5).

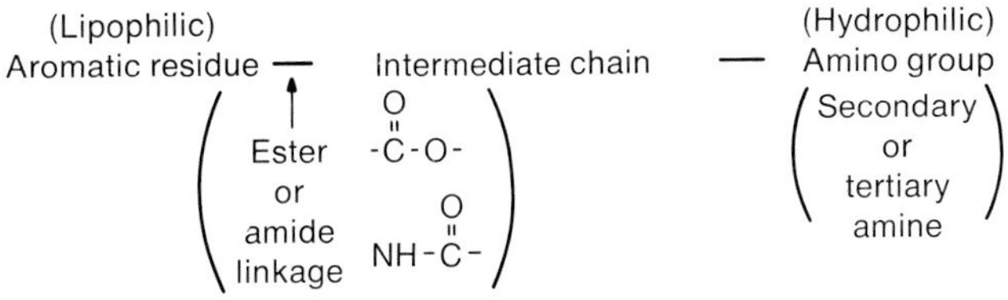

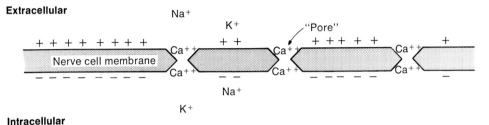

(Lipophilic)
Aromatic residue —   Intermediate chain   —   (Hydrophilic)
Amino group

$$
\begin{pmatrix}
\text{Ester} & \overset{\text{O}}{\underset{\|}{\text{-C-O-}}} \\
\text{or} & \\
\text{amide} & \overset{\text{O}}{\underset{\|}{\text{NH-C-}}} \\
\text{linkage} &
\end{pmatrix}
$$

$$
\begin{pmatrix}
\text{Secondary} \\
\text{or} \\
\text{tertiary} \\
\text{amine}
\end{pmatrix}
$$

Fig. 19-1. Basic molecular structure of local anesthetic agents.

Extracellular

Na+

K+   "Pore"

Nerve cell membrane

Na+

K+

Intracellular

Fig. 19-2. Nerve cell membrane at rest.

$$RMP = \frac{\left[K^+\right]_{In}}{\left[K^+\right]_{Out}} = -70\ mv$$

Fig. 19-3. Resting membrane potential (RMP) is determined by ratio of concentration of potassium ions inside nerve cell ([K+]in) to concentration of potassium ions outside nerve cell ([K+]out).

The potency as well as the toxicity of a local anesthetic agent depends on its chemical structure. For example, an increase in molecular weight within a homologous series increases the potency. Changes in the aromatic or amino portion of the molecule, which alter the lipophilic and hydrophilic properties, respectively, alter the partition coefficient and protein binding properties and change duration of action. As the partition coefficient increases or the percentage of protein-bound molecules rises, the duration of action increases. Therefore it is possible, by altering the basic molecular structure, to synthesize chemically new, more potent, longer acting, but sometimes more toxic local anesthetic agents.

BASIC PHYSIOLOGY OF NERVE CONDUCTION

To understand the mechanism of action of local anesthetics a short review of the basic physiology of nerve conduction is in order. Hodgkin and Huxley (1952) have proposed an electrophysiologic theory to explain this process. According to their concept, the nerve cell lies in a milieu of body water and the major extracellular cation in this milieu is sodium. The major intracellular cation is potassium (Fig. 19-2). At rest, the ratio of potassium ions inside the nerve cell to those outside the nerve cell is approximately 30:1. Based on this ratio, the potential across the nerve cell membrane is −50 to −70 millivolts. This is called the resting membrane potential (Fig. 19-3). As a result of this distribution of ions, the outside of the nerve cell membrane has a positive charge in relation to the negative charge of the inside of the nerve cell membrane.

There have been many hypotheses relating to the composition of membranes in the body. It is not the purpose of this discussion to study the merits of each. The reader is offered the following references should he desire to pursue this subject (Benson, 1966; Danielli and Davson, 1936; Gorter and Grendel, 1925; Green and Perdue, 1966; Lucy, 1964; Robertson, 1959; Singer and Nicolson, 1972; Sjostrand, 1964; Stein and Danielli, 1956). For simplicity, the nerve cell membrane will be considered as a porous structure with calcium ion acting as a "gate" within its pores. At resting membrane potential this "gate" is closed and therefore impermeable to sodium and potassium ions (Fig. 19-2).

When excitation of a nerve occurs and a threshold potential is reached, calcium ions are "displaced" from these pores, the "gate" opens, and sodium ions rush into the nerve cell altering the transmembrane potential. The inside of the nerve cell membrane becomes positive relative to the outside of the membrane (reversal of polarity). This reversal of polarity is called depolarization, and an action spike potential is formed that is propagated along the nerve cell membrane. In myelinated nerves this action potential is propagated along the nerve fibers from node of Ranvier to node of Ranvier by the process of saltatory conduction. When maximum depolarization has occurred (milliseconds), the permeability to sodium ion decreases, calcium ion "returns" to the pores in the nerve cell membrane, the "gate" closes, and the process of repolarization occurs. Repolarization brings the transmembrane potential as well as the resting membrane po-

tential back to their original levels. Repolarization involves a decrease in movement of sodium ions into the nerve cell and an increase in permeability to potassium ions with a resultant diffusion of potassium to the outside. These ionic events restore the transmembrane potential to the resting level of -70 millivolts. Finally, sodium is actively transported out of the nerve cell, and potassium is actively transported into the cell to return these ions to their original concentrations (Fig. 19-4).

HYPOTHESIZED MECHANISM OF ACTION OF LOCAL ANESTHETICS

Clinically useful local anesthetic agents are commercially available as the solutions of acid salts of weak bases. The local anesthetic weak base (BNHOH) must be combined with a strong acid (HCl) in order to make the acid salt (BNHCl) that is soluble for use in solution (Fig. 19-5, *a*). For this solution (BNHCl) to act as a local anesthetic, however, it must dissociate into the free base. A basic environment, found in normal tissue, is necessary (Fig. 19-5, *b*). As stated previously, the amino, hydrophilic portion of the local anesthetic molecule may exist as a secondary or tertiary amine. This charged amino group (BNH+) further dissociates outside the nerve sheath (Fig. 19-5, *c*). This results in a nonionized lipophilic molecule (BN). At normal tissue pH, the dynamics of this

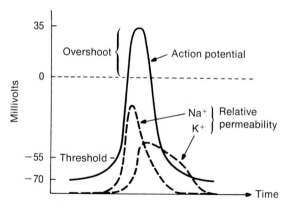

Fig. 19-4. Sequence of electrochemical events after excitation of nerve cell membrane. (From Schwartz, H. C. 1974. J. Am. Dent. Assoc. **89**:159).

equilibrium reaction take it to the right, yielding more nonionized molecule (BN) from the local anesthetic.

The nonionized lipophilic local anesthetic molecule (BN) diffuses readily through the lipid composed nerve sheath. After this molecule passes into the interstitial fluid between the nerve sheath and the nerve cell membrane, it enters into another equilibrium reaction with free hydrogen ion found here. This free hydrogen ion is liberated from buffer system reactions occurring in the area (Fig. 19-5, *d*). This reaction results in the formation of an ionized hydrophilic form of the local anesthetic molecule (BNH +). This molecule then passes through the "pores" in the nerve cell membrane, displaces the calcium "gate," and provides a more impermeable "gate" to the influx of sodium ion (Fig. 19-5, *e*). Therefore, when an impulse reaches this point, sodium ion influx is stopped, depolarization is halted, and nerve conduction beyond this point stops.

This hypothesis has been studied and tested by many investigators (Aceves and Machne, 1963; Blaustein and Goldman, 1966; Condouris, 1961; Hille, 1966; Kuperman et al., 1968; Narahashi et al., 1969; Papahadjopoulos, 1972; Ritchie et al., 1965; Shanes et al., 1959) and to date appears to be the most logical answer to the mechanism of action of the local anesthetic agents. It also helps to explain the failure of local anesthetic agents to completely block nerve conduction from an infected area (see also Chapter 5). An area of infection produces a high concentration of hydrogen ions, since it is an acidic environment. As previously stated, a basic environment is essential for the proper dissociation of local anesthetic agents after injection into tissue. After injection of a local anesthetic into an area of infection (Fig. 19-6), reaction (*b*) takes place but at a much slower rate. In normal tissue this dissociation reaction rapidly tended to go to the right (Fig. 19-5, *b*), whereas in the infected tissue an equilibrium is established with the reaction not going to completion. Further, since there is such an abundance of hydrogen ions in the infected tissue, the equilibrium of reaction (Fig. 19-6, *c*) by the law of mass action also shifts to the left. Therefore formation of the nonionized lipophilic molecule (BN), which is necessary for diffusion across the nerve sheath, is at a minimum. If there is little or no nonionized lipophilic molecule (BN) to diffuse through the sheath, there will be little or no ionized

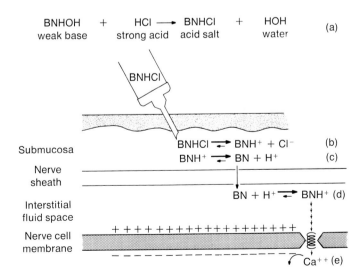

Fig. 19-5. Hypothesized mechanism of action of local anesthetic agents at normal tissue pH.

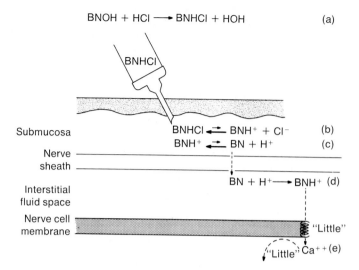

Fig. 19-6. Hypothesized mechanism of decreased activity of local anesthetic agents in environment with high hydrogen ion concentration (low tissue pH, that is, infection).

hydrophilic molecule (BNH +) formed to act at the nerve cell membrane to block conduction (Fig. 19-6, *d, e*).

PHARMACOKINETICS OF LOCAL ANESTHETICS

In the discussion of any drug the four basic elements of pharmacokinetics must be considered. These are absorption, distribution, metabolism, and excretion (see also Chapter 5).

Absorption

Since all local anesthetic agents except cocaine are vasodilatory, they are rapidly absorbed into the bloodstream after injection. There are certain factors, however, that may influence this absorption.

Presence or absence of vasoconstrictors in the solution

Vasoconstrictors are added to the solution of local anesthetic agents to counter their vasodilatory effect. This allows the local anesthetic agent to remain in the area of the nerve for a longer period, increasing not only the profoundness of the anesthesia but also the duration of action.

Tissue pH

The influence of tissue pH has been discussed previously. In extreme tissue alkalosis, the nonionized lipophilic local anesthetic molecule (BN) forms very rapidly and can diffuse directly into the bloodstream before it can reach the nerve.

Site of administration

If the solution of local anesthetic is injected into a highly vascular area, it will be absorbed more rapidly. Direct intraarterial or intravenous injection obviously also results in rapid drug removal.

Total dose administered

The more of the local anesthetic agent injected, the longer some will remain in the area. However, this effect is counterbalanced by the possibility of approaching toxic doses.

Distribution

Since the local anesthetic agents are absorbed into the bloodstream, they are ultimately distributed throughout the body. These agents are demonstrable in highest levels in vascular-rich organs—the brain, heart, liver, kidneys, and skeletal muscle.

Transplacental distribution to the fetus occurs by passive diffusion but is limited by the degree of protein binding of the particular agent in the mother's serum.

The more tightly bound to the protein in the maternal serum, the less the fetus receives.

Metabolism

The metabolism of the local anesthetic agents is directly related to their chemical structure, especially to the amide or ester linkage between the aromatic ring and the intermediate chain of the molecule (Fig. 19-1). Those agents with the ester-type linkage (that is, procaine and tetracaine) are metabolized by a pseudocholinesterase formed in the liver and found in the plasma. Those compounds with the amide-type linkage are metabolized in the liver by a hydrolytic process. Therefore patients with impaired liver function may not be able to rapidly metabolize the local anesthetic leading to a prolonged increase in blood level and possible toxic reactions.

Excretion

The kidney is the main excretory organ for most of the local anesthetic agents. Ninety percent of the drug is excreted as metabolites, whereas 10% is excreted unchanged in the urine.

ARMAMENTARIUM
Syringe

The breech or side-loading, metal, sterilizable syringe is the one most commonly used in oral surgery practice. The harpoon attached to the plunger allows penetration into the rubber stopper of the cartridge of local anesthetic solution. This maneuver makes the unit of syringe and cartridge an aspirating instrument. The use of nonaspirating syringes is not recommended. Disposable, single-use, plastic aspirating syringes may also be used.

Needles

In modern dental and medical practice, there is no place for reusable needles for the injection of local anesthetic agents. The small expense and the safety of single-use disposable needles make them unquestionably superior to reusable needles. A 25-gauge, 1⅝ inch, unibevel presterilized disposable needle is ideal for most standard intraoral local anesthesia techniques. The 25-gauge bore allows for good aspiration and the 1⅝ inch length discourages penetration with the needle to the hub, which could result in breakage of the needle in the mucosa should the patient move unexpectedly.

Cartridges

The standard 2 ml size dental cartridge of local anesthetic provides 1.8 ml of solution (0.2 ml of space is taken up by the rubber stopper). These cartridges contain a sterile solution but are not sterile outside. If immersed for long periods in an alcohol solution in an attempt to sterilize the outside of the cartridge, there is a possibility of the alcohol diffusing through the rubber diaphragm at the metal cap end, contaminating the anesthetic and possibly leading to chemical neurolysis of an injected nerve.

Since immersion or heat and gas sterilization are not feasible, it is suggested that contamination of the cartridges be minimized by storage in a sterile container and by wiping them with an alcohol-soaked sponge prior to use. Particular attention should be paid to the metal capped diaphragm end of the cartridge during this maneuver. If an absolutely sterile technique is necessary, the anesthetic can be obtained in ampules or multiple dose vials and used with a standard hypodermic syringe.

TECHNIQUES OF ADMINISTRATION
Infiltration anesthesia

In this method, the anesthetic solution is injected into the mucous membrane or beneath the skin. Anesthesia is induced by the action of the anesthetic agent on terminal nerve fibers. The method, therefore, is also called terminal or peripheral anesthesia. Its action is limited to a small area, and a considerable amount of solution must be injected when a large field is to be anesthetized.

In the maxilla and anterior mandible, with their thin cortical plates, the local anesthetic solution will penetrate the bone by traveling through the haversian canals. These canals are numerous and the apices of the teeth are near the surface. Therefore infiltration anesthesia will anesthetize the teeth, the solution affecting the dental nerves before they enter the apical foramen and periodontal tissues. This is not the case in the posterior mandible with its thick cortical plate in the buccal segments.

Infiltration anesthesia is often used in conjunction with general anesthesia not only to reduce pain impulses but especially to decrease bone bleeding when a vasoconstrictor has been added to the anesthetic solution.

Subcutaneous or submucosal injection technique

For anesthesia of the soft oral tissues or the skin overlying the jaws, the subcutaneous or submucosal method gives good results. The site where the needle is to be inserted is dried and prepared with an antiseptic solution. The needle is passed deep into the tissue, which is generally very loose; therefore little pressure is required to inject the solution. The needle is advanced slowly, aspirating and injecting until it is inserted to a point short of the hub. It can then be partially withdrawn and advanced in another direction or withdrawn completely and reinserted at a different place. Quite a large area can be covered by one puncture if the needle is long enough. Anesthesia develops in 3 to 5 minutes.

Supraperiosteal injection technique

The solution is injected supraperiosteally as close to the bone as possible so that it will penetrate through the haversian canals. This method is usually more successful in children and young adults, with their thin bone, than in older persons with denser and thicker bone. This is the anesthesia technique of choice in the maxilla because of the character of the bone and, as previously mentioned, it can also be used in the mandibular incisor area. In children, it can also be used in the posterior mandible to anesthetize the deciduous molars.

Conduction or block anesthesia

Conduction or block anesthesia is best suited for mandibular procedures, extensive maxillary procedures, or extensive maxillofacial soft and hard tissue procedures. This technique provides a much larger anesthetic field than the infiltration techniques. Conduction anesthesia may be produced by both intraoral and extraoral methods.

Inferior alveolar nerve block

The inferior alveolar nerve block injection is made intraorally into the pterygomandibular space (Fig. 19-7). This space is filled with connective tissue that has the potential to expand when a volume of solution is injected into it. The inferior alveolar nerve and blood vessels pass through this space prior to their entrance into the mandibular foramen. Block of the inferior alveolar nerve produces anesthesia of the hemimandible, the mandibular teeth, and half of the lower lip and chin. In combination with a lingual nerve block and long buccal nerve block, the lingual mucosa and gingiva, anterior part of the tongue, and floor of the mouth are also anesthetized.

Technique. The depth of the coronoid notch of the anterior border of the ramus of the mandible is palpated with the thumb or forefinger. The pterygomandibular raphe is then located. These landmarks form the legs of an inverted triangle with the apex at the retromolar pad. The syringe is brought into the mouth diagonally over the opposite premolar area so that the tip of the needle enters the mucosa overlying the pterygomandibular space at the center of this triangle. It is most important that the needle be lateral to the pterygomandibular raphe so as not to penetrate the medial pterygoid muscle. The needle is inserted until bone is contacted. Should this lead to a shallow insertion (anterior to the lingula) because of the angle of the ramus to the body of the mandible, the needle should be directed more posteriorly to a point behind the lingula where the opening of the mandibular foramen lies. This is done by moving the syringe to the canine or incisor area and inserting it deeper. When the needle is properly positioned, the piston of the syringe is pulled back to aspirate and three fourths of the solution

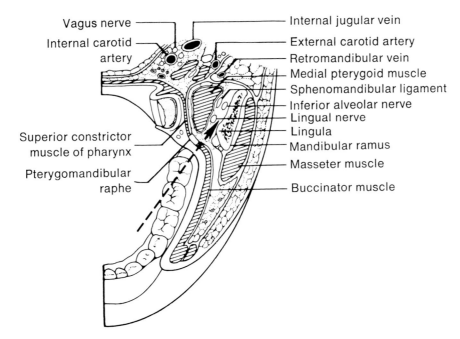

Fig. 19-7. Oblique section through head with mouth open. Arrow indicates path of needle insertion for inferior alveolar nerve block injection.

in the cartridge is deposited. The needle is withdrawn half way, aspirated, and the remainder of the solution is injected to anesthetize the lingual nerve. The needle is then completely withdrawn from the tissue. The long buccal nerve may be blocked by injecting a small amount of solution into the sulcus opposite the mandibular third molar.

For those patients requiring inferior alveolar nerve block who are unable to open their mouths, an extraoral approach can be used. In this technique the height and width of the ramus are first approximated; the mandibular foramen lies about in the center of the ramus inferosuperiorly and anteroposteriorly. The needle is inserted just below the middle of the lower border of the ramus and advanced on the medial aspect in contact with the bone parallel to the posterior border until it is about 3 to 4 mm above the midpoint of the ramus. This places the needle just lateral to the entrance of the inferior alveolar nerve into the mandibular foramen. The mandibular nerve can also be anesthetized extraorally as part of a total trigeminal third division block (see p. 643).

Mental nerve block

The mental and incisive nerves are the terminal branches of the inferior alveolar nerve. The mental nerve exits the mandible via the mental foramen, which lies approximately at the apex of the mandibular second premolar tooth halfway between the alveolar border and lower border in the dentulous patient. By depositing local anesthetic solution into the mental foramen, sensory conduction is blocked from the mental nerve that supplies half of the lower lip, chin, and gingiva and the incisive nerve that supplies the canine, lateral incisor, and central incisor ipsilaterally.

Technique. The mental foramen is located radiographically and by palpation in the region of the apex of the mandibular second premolar. Since this foramen opens posterosuperiorly, entrance into it by the needle tip must be from a downward, inward, and forward direction. With the jaws closed and the lips relaxed to facilitate access, the needle penetrates the mucosa in the area of the mesial aspect of the first molar and a small amount of anesthetic solution is deposited. The tip of the needle is then used as a probe to locate the entrance of the foramen. Once in the foramen, aspiration is done and the solution is injected slowly.

Lingual nerve block

The lingual nerve can be easily blocked during the procedure for anesthetizing the inferior alveolar nerve (see preceding discussion). It also can be blocked by injecting just superior to the mylohyoid ridge in the third molar region. The lingual nerve block produces anesthesia of the anterior two thirds of the tongue, the floor of the mouth, and the mucosa on the lingual aspect of the mandible.

Maxillary nerve block

The maxillary nerve, or second division of the trigeminal nerve, may be blocked intraorally as it courses through the pterygomaxillary space on its way from the foramen rotundum into the inferior orbital fissure. Access to this space intraorally is obtained via the greater palatine foramen and canal. Block of this nerve anesthetizes the maxillary teeth and supporting soft tissue and bone, the maxillary sinus, and lateral wall of the nasal cavity. The soft tissue of the face supplied by the inferior palpebral, lateral nasal, and superior labial nerves is also anesthetized, since these are the terminal branches of the maxillary nerve.

Technique. The greater palatine foramen is located at the junction of the horizontal and vertical processes of the hard palate in the area of the distal of the second molar. A standard 25-gauge, 1⅝ inch dental needle attached to an aspirating syringe is used.

The index finger is used to palpate the area described. Generally, a slight depression can be felt. The needle is inserted into the palatal mucosa in a posterolateral direction at the level of the distal half of the first molar and after aspiration a small quantity of local anesthetic is injected. This will anesthetize the anterior palatine nerve almost immediately, allowing for relatively painless probing for the greater palatine foramen. Once the foramen has been found, the needle is carefully inserted up the greater palatine canal to within 2 mm of the hub. Care should be taken to advance the needle slowly, aspirating as the needle is advanced and making sure the needle stays within the confines of the canal. After complete insertion to the level described, slow injection after aspiration is performed until the whole cartridge is emptied. The needle is withdrawn slowly and the patient allowed to remain undisturbed for 10 minutes. An infrequent occurrence is spasm of the internal maxillary artery resulting in a blanching of the face over the distribution of the lateral nasal, inferior palpebral, and superior labial arteries. This will cause no discomfort to the patient and the condition will pass within a short time without sequelae (Mercuri, 1979).

Posterior superior alveolar nerve block

The posterior superior alveolar nerve can be anesthetized as it divides into its two branches to enter the bone at the posterolateral aspect of the maxillary tuberosity. The internal branch is sensory to the maxillary molar teeth except for the mesiobuccal root of the maxillary first molar. The external branch is sensory to the gingiva of the buccal surface of the maxillary molar teeth.

Technique. A standard 1⅝ inch, 25-gauge dental needle on an aspirating syringe is used. The tip of the needle penetrates the mucobuccal fold opposite the third molar area and is advanced in a superomedial direction hugging the bone. The needle is inserted for a distance approximately half the height of the maxilla. After proper aspiration, the solution is deposited slowly in the area.

Infraorbital nerve block

With this procedure, anesthesia of the terminal branches of the infraorbital nerve, the inferior palpebral, lateral nasal, and superior labial nerves, is obtained. If the solution reaches the infraorbital canal, the anterior superior alveolar nerve supplying the canine, lateral, and central incisor teeth is also anesthetized.

Intraoral technique. The infraorbital foramen may be palpated below the infraorbital rim. It lies in a line with the superior orbital notch, pupil of the eye in direct anterior gaze, maxillary second premolar tooth, and mental foramen. The opening faces downward, forward, and inward. The needle is inserted intraorally slightly buccal to the depth of the vestibule opposite the apex of the root of the maxillary second premolar and directed superiorly. It will slide along the anterior surface of the maxilla and contact the superior aspect of the infraorbital foramen. The forefinger of the opposite hand is used to palpate the foramen as the needle is introduced and directed into place. A cartridge of local anesthetic solution is deposited after aspiration. Symptoms of anesthesia are numbness in the upper lip, lower eyelid, and side of the nose. This, however, is only a sign that the terminal branches have been anesthetized and is not an indication of anesthesia of the incisor and canine teeth. The mucosa of the palate is not affected, and a supplementary injection at the nasopalatine foramen is necessary (see "nasopalatine nerve block").

There is also an alternative technique for injection of the infraorbital nerve intraorally. This technique involves penetration of the mucosa in the area of the apex of the ipsilateral canine and passing the needle toward the roof of the infraorbital foramen in a direction bisecting the mesioincisive angle of the ipsilateral central incisor. The advantages of this technique are that it lessens the possibility of inadvertently entering the orbit and permits deeper penetration into the canal since the direction is more parallel with it.

Extraoral technique. The extraoral technique allows the needle to be introduced directly into the infraorbital canal. Entrance into the foramen is especially important if alcohol injections are used for neurolysis in treatment of trigeminal neuralgia. The extraoral method is more precise, since the anesthesia does not depend on diffusion of the solution into the canal. The direction of the infraorbital canal varies considerably. Its course is quite frequently curved, and it proceeds slightly upward and outward. Sometimes there are accessory foramina.

The skin is cleansed and the foramen located using the landmarks described previously. The needle is inserted at about a 45 degree angle through the skin medially and inferiorly to the foramen to compensate for the thickness of overlying tissue, and a small amount of anesthetic solution is injected. The tip of the needle is used to palpate for the opening of the foramen. Once found, keeping in mind the foramen and canal are oriented in a medial to lateral direction, the needle is advanced slowly into the canal. Aspiration and injection follow. The area anesthetized is the same as that affected by the intraoral method. The canine and incisor teeth may be more predictably anesthetized, since the solution is deposited directly into the canal in an area close to the anterior superior alveolar nerve.

Nasopalatine nerve block

The nasopalatine nerve is sensory to the palatal mucosa from canine to canine. The nerve emerges from the incisive foramen beneath the incisive papilla in the midline just behind the maxillary central incisors.

Technique. It is not recommended that the needle penetrate the incisive papilla directly as this is extremely painful. Rather the tip of the needle should be placed in the depression surrounding the incisive papilla, and a small amount of solution is injected until the papilla blanches. This makes entrance into the incisive foramen less uncomfortable. Unless surgery is to be performed in the anterior palate, injection further into the canal is not necessary.

Extraoral blocks of the second and third division of the trigeminal nerve

Extraoral nerve blocks are useful for the oral and maxillofacial surgeon when faced with trismus, maxillofacial trauma, or infection. Anesthesia over the sensory distribution of the second and third divisions of trigeminal nerve may be obtained easily with proper technique.

Technique. In performing an extraoral block of the second and third division of the trigeminal nerve, the anatomic landmarks used are the zygomatic arch, the temporomandibular joint, the sigmoid notch, and coronoid process of the mandible. A surgical preparation of the skin is done in the area of these landmarks and a sterile marking pencil or methylene blue dye is then used to outline them.

A small skin wheal is raised with local anesthetic at the center of the sigmoid notch (Fig. 19-8). A 25-gauge spinal needle marked to 4.5 cm is inserted at this point perpendicular to the skin, which in this area of the face is not necessarily perpendicular to the midsagittal plane of the head. Having the patient open the mouth, if possible, facilitates passage of the needle through the sigmoid notch. The needle is directed medially until contact is made with the lateral pterygoid plate (Fig. 19-9, *a*). For the second division block, the needle is then withdrawn slightly and directed superiorly and anteriorly toward the pterygomaxillary fissure (Fig. 19-9, *b*). The needle should never be inserted beyond the 4.5 cm mark. Local anesthetic solution, 3 to 5 ml, is deposited after aspiration.

In the case of the third division block, the same technique is followed except that the spinal needle is marked to only 4 cm, and after touching the lateral pterygoid plate the needle is redirected superiorly and posteriorly to the depth of the 4 cm mark to the foramen ovale (Fig 19-10). Again 3 to 5 ml of local anesthetic is deposited after aspiration. The patient is allowed to remain undisturbed for 8 to 10 minutes to obtain the maximum anesthetic effect.

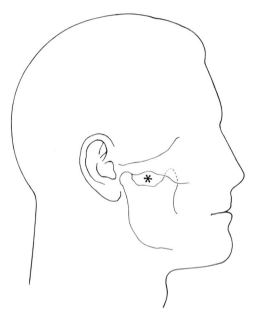

Fig. 19-8. Landmarks for extraoral penetration for injection of second and third divisions of trigeminal nerve.

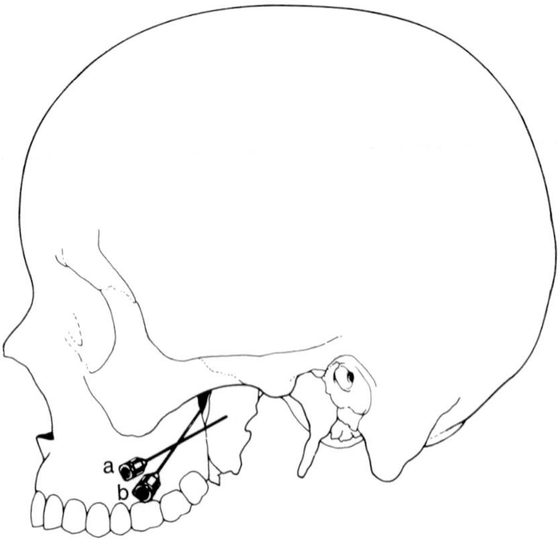

Fig. 19-9. Two positions of needle for extraoral injection of maxillary division of trigeminal nerve in pterygomaxillary fissure. (Redrawn from Sicher, H., and DuBrul, E. L. 1975. Oral Anatomy, ed. 6, St. Louis, The C. V. Mosby Co.)

COMPLICATIONS

Local complications

Complications at the site of injection of a local anesthetic agent are not common. Most complications are avoidable when one has a thorough knowledge of the anatomy of the site to be injected and when proper aspiration and injection techniques are used.

Hematoma

Although a hematoma may develop during any injection, and particularly when an injection is made into a foramen that contains blood vessels, the injection technique most commonly associated with hematoma formation is the posterior superior alveolar nerve block or "high tuberosity" injection. The needle passes behind the maxillary tuberosity and is directed toward the pterygomaxillary fissure. It was believed for a long time that the hematoma was due to laceration of the pterygoid venous plexus; however, since the venous system is a low pressure system, laceration of a vein would not result in the rapid hematoma formation that is seen. Therefore Sicher (Sicher and Du-Brul, 1975) has suggested that it is the posterior superior alveolar artery that is the source of the hematoma. The tip of the needle shears this vessel as it enters the bone resulting in rapid hematoma formation. This is manifested as a sudden swelling of the buccal area of the face.

The treatment is immediate application of pressure and ice packs to the face in the area of swelling. The patient should be advised of the situation and not alarmed. If the patient is not medically debilitated by any disease process or drugs that decrease the body's resistance to infection, these hematomas pose no problem and will resolve in 7 to 10 days. In a patient with a decreased tolerance to infection, antibiotic therapy is advisable to prevent infection. A hematoma when organizing has no circulation and acts as a perfect culture medium for any organism introduced into it from the oral cavity by the needle.

Needle breakage

Needle breakage should never be a problem provided certain basic principles are not violated. First, only disposable needles should be used and never

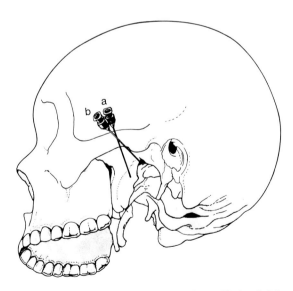

Fig. 19-10. Two positions of needle for extraoral injection of mandibular division of trigeminal nerve at foramen ovale. *a,* Initial contact with lateral pterygoid plate. *b,* Redirection of needle postero-superiorly. (Redrawn from Sicher, H., and DuBrul, E. L. 1975. Oral Anatomy, ed. 6, St. Louis, The C. V. Mosby Co.)

reused. Second, needles should never be bent prior to or during injection. Third, a needle should never be inserted in tissue up to the hub.

Should a needle break, and the third principle has not been violated, the broken end may be grasped with a hemostat and removed easily. If the needle has broken and is completely buried in tissue, the patient should be advised not to move or talk. Anteroposterior and lateral radiographs should be taken to localize the broken fragment. A second needle may be introduced to facilitate localization. When the relationship of the localizing needle and broken fragment has been established radiographically, dissection to retrieve the broken needle is carried out. This may prove to be extremely difficult.

An instrument that can be used in such situations is the image intensifier fluoroscopy unit found in the operating rooms of most hospitals that have an active orthopedic surgery service. The area of the broken needle is fluoroscoped and probed with a localizing needle until the broken fragment is contacted. Dissection is carried out along the localizing needle to the broken fragment. This direct vision technique makes what is often a difficult procedure much easier.

Transient or permanent paresthesia or anesthesia

Complete or incomplete interruption of conduction along the course of a nerve resulting in anesthesia or paresthesia is a rather uncommon complication of local anesthesia techniques. When it does occur, it is usually due either to direct trauma to the nerve by the needle tip or to the injection of the local anesthetic solution directly into the nerve causing pressure or ischemic necrosis. There is no way to avoid this other than by careful injection technique. As mentioned previously, prolonged storage of local anesthetic cartridges in alcohol solution may result in diffusion of alcohol into the cartridges through the metal cap rubber diaphragm. When this contaminated solution is injected, it can result in neurolysis causing a permanent paresthesia or anesthesia.

Infection

Infection should not be a problem with the use of disposable needles and careful aseptic handling of cartridges and syringes. Should infection occur, it is treated with antibiotics, heat, and incision and drainage if indicated. An attempt should be made to trace the cause and this situation should be corrected.

Tissue necrosis

Tissue necrosis at the site of injection of a local anesthetic solution may be seen most commonly in areas of tightly attached mucosa, such as in the region of the anterior palatine nerve. This is most likely related to the volume of solution injected and possibly the vasoconstrictor resulting in tissue ischemia and necrosis (Guinta, 1975). The ulceration is generally painful and systemic analgesics, topical anesthetics, and bland diet are helpful. Oral "bandage" preparations are of some benefit in relief of pain but do not seem to alter healing time. The lesion usually resolves in 7 to 14 days.

Postinjection pain

The most common causes for prolonged postinjection pain are either subperiosteal injection of the solution or tearing of the periosteum by the tip of the needle. Both of these can be avoided by good technique. Infiltration anesthesia should be given supraperiosteally, not subperiosteally. Checking the needle tip for barbs before each injection is also important in the prevention of periosteal damage and resultant postinjection pain.

Excessive concentrations of vasoconstrictor can also cause ischemic necrosis and pain. Concentrations of epinephrine of 1:100,000 (or equivalent concentrations of other vasoconstrictors) are sufficient for most purposes.

Postinjection trismus

Postinjection trismus is related to the tearing of a masticatory muscle by penetration of the needle during injection or the injection of the anesthetic solution directly into the muscle. In the latter situation, both the anesthetic solution (Benoit, 1978a,b and the vasoconstrictor can have adverse effects. The most commonly involved muscle is the medial pterygoid during inferior alveolar nerve block. This problem can be avoided by good injection technique. Staying lateral to the pterygomandibular raphe during penetration of the mucosa will avoid the medial pterygoid muscle, since this muscle lies medial to the raphe (Fig. 19-7).

Should this complication occur, no further injections into the area should be attempted until the trismus has resolved. Muscle relaxants and the use of moist heat are of some benefit in relieving muscle spasm. Soft diet is recommended; exercise of the jaw should be avoided. Infection must be considered in the differential diagnosis of postinjection trismus and can be ruled out by the signs and symptoms. Occasionally, the trismus may last up to 2 months in severe cases (Brooke, 1979).

Postinjection herpetic lesions

A postinjection herpetic phenomenon is occasionally seen over the terminal distribution of a previously anesthetized nerve. The most common site is the terminal distribution of the inferior alveolar or superior labial branch of the trigeminal nerve. It is usually seen in patients with a history of recurrent herpes labialis; therefore it may be related to arousal of dormant herpes virus particles by the trauma of injection. The treatment is symptomatic and no scarring occurs.

Skin blanching

Blanching of the skin over the terminal distribution of the anesthetized nerve in association with sharp pain during injection is related to spasm of the artery that accompanies the nerve at the point of injection. This spasm is in response to trauma to the vessel by the needle or more commonly to intra-arterial injection. It is usually a transient phenomenon and the patient should be advised not to be alarmed. No treatment is necessary.

Systemic complications
Toxicity

Generally, the more potent a local anesthetic agent is, the greater its toxicity.

The toxic dose for most agents used in oral and maxillofacial surgery is between 300 and 500 mg (about 5 mg/kg). In a standard 1.8 ml dental cartridge of a 2% solution of local anesthetic, there is 36 mg of the drug (20 mg/ml × 1.8 ml = 36 mg). Therefore, the injection of 10 cartridges of a 2% solution would be in the range of toxicity. Obviously, the precise toxic level varies with the age, weight, and condition of the patient as well as site and rapidity of injection and concentration of the vasoconstrictor, all of which affect absorption.

Two body systems are mainly affected by toxic levels of circulating local anesthetic drugs—the cardiovascular system and the central nervous system (Covino, 1972a, b). While the sequence of physiologic events described in the following section is dynamic in its occurrence, the events are presented in a stepwise manner for clarity.

Cardiovascular effects. At nontoxic levels there is no appreciable systemic cardiovascular effect from the injection of a local anesthetic. As toxic levels are approached, however, blood pressure is affected. Since most of the local anesthetics are vasodilators, blood pressure is decreased owing to a decrease in peripheral resistance (Blood pressure = total peripheral resistance × cardiac output). This is followed at increasing levels by a decrease in myocardial contractility, since local anesthetics also affect nerve conduction in the heart. This results in a decreased heart rate that will result in a decreased cardiac output (Cardiac output = heart rate × stroke volume). This further decreases the blood pressure.

The heart contains its own intricate neuronal conduction system that also can be inhibited or completely blocked by local anesthetic agents (that is, lidocaine therapy for arrhythmia). At toxic levels, depression of intracardiac nerve conduction can result in atrioventricular dissociation, ventricular rhythm, ventricular fibrillation, and ultimately cardiac standstill.

Central nervous system effects. Simply stated, the central nervous system contains facilatory neurons (nerves that mediate function) and inhibitory neurons (nerves that modify function, allowing for smoothness of action).

At nontoxic therapeutic levels, the local anesthetic agents have no effect on the central nervous system. However, the conduction of inhibitory neurons is usually blocked by local anesthetic agents as they reach toxic levels, resulting in unmodified action of the facilatory neurons (that is, convulsive-like movements). As the dose increases further, the facilatory neurons are also blocked resulting in cessation of function. Certain amide-type agents (that is, lidocaine) affect primarily facilatory neurons; hence, depression is seen rather than excitation (de Jong, Robles, and Corbin, 1969).

The respiratory system is affected by central nervous system depression, which can result in respiratory arrest. Therefore at toxic levels of local anesthetic agents, both respiratory and cardiac arrest may be seen. For this reason all persons using these agents must have resuscitative equipment available and be trained in cardiopulmonary resuscitation.

Toxic reactions are generally preventable by avoiding intravascular injections through the use of aspiration and by limiting dosage to reasonable quantities.

Hypersensitivity (allergy)

Hypersensitivity to local anesthetics can present a problem to the oral and maxillofacial surgeon. Allergy is manifested by skin rash, urticaria, edema, and in its full-blown state by anaphylaxis. On careful questioning concerning the manifestations of this allergy, many patients who claim allergy to the local anesthetics will say they "passed out" or "fainted" or that their heart beat "faster." Very few will state they developed a skin rash, itched, swelled, or went on to anaphylaxis as a result of an injection of local anesthetic. Therefore this type of patient may be eliminated as allergic to local anesthetics and classified under idiosyncratic reactors on the basis of the history.

In the patient whose history reveals the signs and symptoms of true allergy after injection of a local anesthetic, there are a number of approaches that can be used. If it can be determined that the reaction was in response to procaine or another ester-type anesthetic, an amide-type can be substituted. If the reaction supposedly was to an amide-type agent, several alternatives are available:

1. Have the patient skin-tested for reaction to the specific local anesthetic to be used. Since these anesthetics use methylparaben, a para-aminobenzoic acid (PABA) derivative, as a preservative, it rather than the anesthetic may be the allergen. Because ester-type local anesthetic agents are also PABA derivatives, one of these drugs may have been the original sensitizing agent.

2. If the allergy is due to the methylparaben, cardiac lidocaine, which does not contain methylparaben, can be used.

3. If the allergy is to the anesthetic, a 10% solution of diphenhydramine hydrochloride (Benadryl), which has local anesthetic properties as well as being an antihistamine (Bass, 1970), can be used.

Anyone using the local anesthetic agents must be aware of the possible complication of anaphylaxis and be prepared to handle it. Anaphylactic shock is a life-threatening reaction. The signs and symptoms are rapidly occurring and progressive. The patient may experience urticaria, abdominal cramping, vomiting, diarrhea, and incontinence. This is accompanied by respiratory distress, cyanosis, hypotension, cardiovascular collapse, and unconsciousness. Treatment must be rapid and succint (see Chapter 11). The patient is placed in a supine position and the airway is controlled. Oxygen is administered and it may be necessary to ventilate the patient manually. Epinephrine (0.3 to 0.5 mg) is given immediately either subcutaneously or intravenously. An antihistamine and a steroid may also need to be administered. Cardiopulmonary resuscitation is started if necessary. Generally, the patient should be transported to the hospital in an ambulance as soon as possible.

Idiosyncratic reactions

Idiosyncrasy is an abnormal reaction to a normal dose of a drug. These reactions are extremely variable and unpredictable. They may resemble toxic or allergic reactions but differ in terms of etiology. Some of the unusual or bizarre symptoms occasionally noted may also fit into this category but many have an emotional rather than a pharmacologic basis.

Treatment of idiosyncratic reactions will vary with the symptoms and is often the same as the therapy used for similar conditions classified as toxic or allergic in origin. Of prime importance in all instances is maintenance of the airway and support of respiration and circulation.

Syncope has frequently been considered an idiosyncratic reaction. Although theoretically the intravascular injection of a local anesthetic containing a vasoconstrictor could result in fainting, more often syncope is pyschogenic in origin, resulting from fright or anxiety.

Syncope

Syncope is the most common adverse reaction to injection of a local anesthetic. Patients may faint at the thought, sight, or penetration of the needle. This reaction can often be prevented by having the patient in a semireclining position with the legs elevated 10 degrees and the back elevated 30 degrees at the time of injection. Most of the new reclining dental chairs provide this position. The semireclining position keeps blood that would normally be pooled in the splanchnic region and legs when the patient is seated upright available to the general circulation and avoids cerebral hypoxia.

Prevention of anxiety-induced syncope may also be accomplished by explaining what is to be done, by the use of a topical anesthetic, and by good injection technique. Certainly holding the syringe in front of the patient's face while palpating for landmarks is an excellent anxiety inducer and may lead to syncope. Use of sedation may be considered should syncope at injection be a persistent problem.

Should syncope occur the patient should be placed in the Trendelenburg position (head down, feet elevated), oxygen should be administered, and the pulse and blood pressure should be monitored. This will usually result in a rapid recovery. Inhalation of aromatic spirits of ammonia can be helpful in stimulating the patient and elevating blood pressure. Should hypotension persist, use of a vasopressor such as phenylephrine may be necessary (see Chapter 11).

VASOCONSTRICTORS

The addition of a vasoconstrictor to a local anesthetic agent offers the following advantages:

1. The vasoconstrictor increases the duration of action and profoundness of the anesthetic by decreasing absorption into the bloodstream. As stated previously, all local anesthetics, with the exception of cocaine, are vasodilators; hence, their absorption is enhanced without the addition of vasoconstrictor agents.
2. The vasoconstrictor decreases the toxicity of local anesthetic drugs by extending the time of absorption of the injected bolus over a longer period.
3. The vasoconstrictor acts as a vascular tourniquet, decreasing blood loss in the area of surgery and providing a drier field.

The vasoconstrictors used in local anesthetic solutions are all sympathomimetic agents and produce their effect by stimulating local alpha-adrenergic receptors in the walls of arterioles in the area of injection. The agents commonly used in the order of decreasing potency are as follows: epinephrine, norepinephrine, nordefrin (Cobefrin), levonordefrin (Neo-Cobefrin) and phenylephrine (Neo-Synephrine). Other than differences in potency, the local and systemic effects of these agents are essentially the same. Toxic reactions are manifested by palpitations, tremors, headache, restlessness, hypertension with tachycardia, or in some cases bradycardia.

In order to produce systemic effects when injected into the tissues, a dose of 0.3 to 0.5 mg of epinephrine is necessary. In a standard 1.8 ml dental cartridge of local anesthetic containing 1:100,000 epinephrine, there is 0.018 mg (1 gm/ 100,000 ml × 1000 mg/1 gm × 1.8 ml = 0.018 mg). Therefore more than 10 cartridges would have to be injected before the systemic effects of the vasoconstrictor would occur. The exact amount depends on the age, weight, and condition of the patient.

There has been considerable controversy about the use of a vasoconstrictor in local anesthetics administered to patients with a history of cardiovascular disease. Based on the report of the joint meeting between the American Dental Association and the American Heart Association (Report, 1964), it has been recommended that not more than 0.2 mg of vasoconstrictor be used in patients with heart disease undergoing local anesthesia for dental procedures. The small amount of exogenous vasoconstrictor in a properly administered local anesthetic generally benefits these patients by producing a profoundness of anesthesia and a longer duration of action than can be obtained with vasoconstrictor-free solutions. The amount of catecholamine endogenously secreted by these patients as a result of pain and anxiety when the profoundness and length of the anesthetic are decreased by the omission of the vasoconstrictor is obviously greater than the small amount injected. Certainly, this has a more devastating effect on the cardiovascular system.

There are instances, however, when local anesthetic solutions containing vasoconstrictor agents should be used with caution. These include patients with a recent history of myocardial infarction or cerebrovascular accident, those taking medication to control hypertension, or those on maintenance doses of cardiac glycosides, phenothiazines, or MAO inhibitors. Caution means using a minimum dose of vasoconstrictor, administered after proper aspiration to ensure against intravascular injection. The combination of a local anesthetic agent without vasoconstrictor and one with vasoconstrictor in a 3:1 ratio of cartridges is suggested.

The absolute contraindication to the use of a local anesthetic solution containing a vasoconstrictor is in a patient with untreated hyperthyroidism. These patients are exquisitely sensitive to sympathomimetic agents and a thyroid storm may be produced.

REFERENCES

Aceves, J., and Machne, X. 1963. The action of calcium and of local anesthetics on nerve cells, and their interaction during excitation, J. Pharmacol. Exp. Ther. **140**:138.

Bass, K. D. 1970. Tissue response to diphendydramine hydrochloride, J. Oral Surg. **28**:335.

Benoit, P. W. 1978a. Reversible skeletal muscle damage after administration of local anesthetic with and without epinephrine, J. Oral Surg. **36**:198.

Benoit, P. W. 1978b. Microscarring in skeletal muscle after repeated exposures to lidocaine with epinephrine, J. Oral Surg. **36**:530.

Benson, A. A. 1966. On the orientation of lipids in chloroplast and cell membranes, J. Am. Oil Chem. Soc. **43**:265.

Blaustein, M. P., and Goldman, D. E. 1966. Competitive action of calcium and procaine on lobster axon: a study of the mechanism of action of certain local anesthetics, J. Gen. Physiol. **49**:1043.

Brooke, R. I. 1979. Postinjection trismus due to formation of fibrous band, Oral Surg. **47**:424.

Condouris, G. A. 1961. A study on the mechanism of action of cocaine on amphibian peripheral merve, J. Pharmacol. Exp. Ther. **131**:243.

Covino, B. G. 1972a. Local anesthesia. I, N. Engl. J. Med. **286**:975.

Covino, B. G. 1972b. Local anesthesia. II, N. Engl. J. Med. **286**:1035.

Danielli, J. F., and Davson, H. A. 1936. A contribution to the theory of permeability of thin films, J. Cell. Physiol. **9**:89.

de Jong, R. H., Robles, R., and Corbin, R. W. 1969. Central actions of lidocaine-synaptic transmission, Anesthesiology **30**:19.

Gorter, E., and Grendel, R. 1925. On biomolecular layers of lipid on the chromocytes of the blood, J. Exp. Med. **41**:439.

Green, D. E., and Perdue, J. F. 1966. Membranes as expressions of repeating units, Proc. Natl. Acad. Sci. U.S.A. **55**:1295.

Guinta, J., et al. 1975. Postanesthetic necrotic defect, Oral Surg. **40**:590.

Hille, B. 1966. Common mode of action of three agents that decrease the transient change in sodium permeability in nerves, Nature **210**:1220.

Hodgkin, A. L., and Huxley, A. F. 1952. A quantitative description of membrane current and its application to conduction and excitation in nerve, J. Physiol. **117**:500.

Kuperman, A. S., et al. 1968. Action of procaine on calcium influx from frog nerve and muscle, Nature **217**:673.

Lucy, J. A. 1964. Globular lipid mycells and cell membrane, J. Theor. Biol. **7**:360.

Mercuri, L. G. 1979. Intraoral second division nerve block, Oral Surg. **47**:109.

Narahashi, T., et al. 1969. Cationic forms of local anesthetics block action potentials from inside the nerve membrane, Nature **223**:748.

Papahadjopoulos, D. 1972. Studies on the mechanism of action of local anesthetics with phospholipid model membranes, Biochem. Biophys. Acta **265**:169.

Report of a working conference jointly sponsored by the American Dental Association and the

American Heart Association. 1964. Management of dental problems in patients with cardiovascular disease, J. Am. Dent. Assoc. **68:**333.

Ritchie, J. M., et al. 1965. The effects of the nerve sheath on the action of local anesthetics, J. Pharmacol. Exp. Ther. **150:**160.

Robertson, J. D. 1959. The ultrastructure of cell membranes and their derivatives, Biochem. Soc. Symp. **16:**3.

Schwartz, H. C. 1974. Local anesthesia, J. Am. Dent. Assoc. **89:**157.

Shanes, A. M., et al. 1959. Anesthetic and calcium action on the voltage clamped squid giant axon, J. Gen. Physiol. **42:**793.

Sicher, H., and DuBrul, E. L. 1975. Oral anatomy, ed. 6, St. Louis, The C. V. Mosby Co., p. 435.

Singer, S. J., and Nicolson, G. L. 1972. The fluid mosaic model of the structure of cell membranes, Science **175:**720.

Sjostrand, F. S. 1964. A new ultrastructure element of the membranes in mitochondria and some cytoplasmic membranes, J. Ultrastruct. Res. **9:**340.

Stein, W. D., and Danielli, J. F. 1956. Structure and function in red cell permeability, Discuss. Faraday Soc. **21:**238.

CHAPTER 20

Conscious sedation

Norman Trieger

In many oral and maxillofacial surgical offices there is a discernible movement away from the frequent use of full general anesthesia toward some form of conscious sedation. The choice between either local anesthesia or general anesthesia has gradually given way to the concept of rendering patients *comfortable, cooperative,* and *conscious* with appropriate sedatives and tranquilizers, while relying on regional anesthesia to effectively block painful stimuli. This serves to allay apprehension and anxiety, which are closely interrelated with the experience of surgical pain (see Chapter 18).

Although there are a number of methods to effect conscious sedation, most surgeons rely on the intravenous route to produce rapid and titratable results. Other methods include inhalation sedation with nitrous oxide and oxygen and the less controllable forms of oral and intramuscular premedication. In addition to the variability of individual response to orally administered sedatives, the time required for onset of effect is inconstant and duration often extends well beyond the surgical appointment. Although preoperative intramuscular medication is routinely given in the hospital before a general anesthetic, the situation in the office, which involves an ambulatory patient, is obviously different and requires different criteria and approaches.

Each patient needs to be evaluated individually to determine the best anesthetic method to facilitate the proposed surgical procedure. Practitioners should become familiar with a variety of management techniques so as to avoid stereotyping every patient into a single anesthetic treatment. Medical and psychologic evaluation will indicate which anesthetic regimen is best suited to that individual patient.

INDICATIONS AND LIMITATIONS OF CONSCIOUS SEDATION

First and foremost in the selection of an anesthetic technique is the consideration of patient cooperation. Patients who are too young to comprehend or are compromised mentally or emotionally are not good candidates, since it is necessary that local infiltration or nerve block anesthesia be used in conjunction with conscious sedation. Although the level of tolerance to pain may be raised with systemic premedication or intraoperative sedation and narcotic administration, this is still inadequate for the degree of pain relief required for surgery. Ordinarily, the combination of conscious sedation plus local anesthesia is adequate for successful, pain-free surgery. True allergy to local anesthetics may justify their avoidance, and preference should then be given to a general anesthetic. True allergy, however, is very rare especially when one uses the amide-type anesthetics.

Often when general anesthesia is used for a surgical procedure, it is because several goals are sought: analgesia, to render the patient pain free; amnesia, to minimize recall of a stressful event; and sedation or tranquilization to control fear and apprehension. Deep muscular relaxation is usually not required. These goals

652

can be readily achieved without loss of consciousness by the use of sedation combined with local anesthesia.

There are a number of advantages that may accrue from the use of conscious sedation rather than general anesthesia. When properly used, conscious sedation does not cause the patient to lose his protective reflexes, which invariably attend the unconsciousness of general anesthesia. With the patient lightly sedated the need for additional personnel immediately attending the patient is reduced. The standard anesthesia–oral surgery team of a minimum of three may be reduced to only the surgeon and an assistant after the patient has been sedated. Assessing the patient's level of responsiveness as well as other physiologic functions is easier in the conscious patient who is capable of rational response to question and command. Nevertheless, it is important to monitor even the conscious patient carefully to ascertain that vital functions and protective reflexes are not significantly obtunded by overdosage or adverse drug effects. It has been shown that laryngeal reflexes may be easily obtunded even in the conscious patient receiving diazepam, and aspiration of foreign material does occur (Healey and Vickers, 1971).

If the intravenous sedative technique is based on sound pharmacologic principles of titration, where the least amount of drug needed to achieve the desired effect is used, then complications secondary to individual variability and overdosage can be minimized. When intravenous sedation is used, the concept of individual titration is important and we should dismiss the erroneous idea of "average dose." While the concept of "average dose" readily applies to large groups, it is inappropriate when directed to an individual patient, especially when the method of intravenous administration permits careful titration for that individual.

TECHNIQUES OF CONSCIOUS SEDATION

Oral and intramuscular routes of administration are of necessity based on "average dose" concepts, with special consideration given to altering that dose based on the size, age, or weight of the patient. Chloral hydrate, 25 to 50 mg/kg, is commonly used for oral premedication in children. Barbiturates such as secobarbital (Seconal) and sodium pentobarbital (Nembutal) have long been used for preoperative medication in both children and adults. The recommended dose is 100 to 200 mg for adults and 3 to 5 mg/kg for children. Hydroxyzine hydrochloride (Atarax) or hydroxyzine pamoate (Vistaril) provides sedation and relief of anxiety as well as antiemetic and antihistamine effects. The recommended dose for adults varies from 25 to 100 mg. For children 1 mg/kg is used. Diazepam (Valium) also produces tranquilization and some muscular relaxation. For adults approximately 5 to 10 mg is recommended preoperatively.

Although oral premedication is easiest to take, its effect is subject to some delay in onset and will vary based on absorption, metabolic rate, and so on. It will, of course, outlast the duration of the surgical appointment and may be of further concern during the postoperative period. In addition to its pharmacologic effect, oral premedication serves a very useful function as a placebo. The message to the patient is clear—"I acknowledge your apprehension and will provide you with some help." This often serves the important function of enhancing rapport and improving cooperation.

Intravenous sedation

While methohexital is used to induce most outpatient general anesthetics, it is not the best agent to use for conscious intravenous sedation—the margin between being awake and relaxed versus being unconsciousness is very narrow. It has also been well documented that when methohexital is used for general anesthesia there is a 40% to 75% increase in heart rate (Allen, 1973; Campbell, Gregg, and Levin, 1976), as well as other physiologic changes such as a decrease in total peripheral resistance and stroke volume (Allen, 1973). Other untoward effects include occasional laryngospasm, postinduction apnea, and hiccoughing.

These troublesome changes are not seen when the patient receives conscious sedation.

The use of multiple drugs to effect conscious sedation has been advocated by many (Bennett 1976, 1978; Drummond-Jackson, 1970; Greenfield, 1976; Jorgensen and Hayden, 1967; Shane, 1975). Recently, it has been shown that the use of intravenous narcotics such as fentanyl or meperidine, even in low dosage, can cause respiratory depression, which is dose-related. The pH decreases, the P_{CO_2} increases, and P_{O_2} decreases (Campbell, Gregg, and Levine, 1976; Greenfield and Granada, 1974). The changes are small but significant, although not readily recognized clinically in the healthy patient. Fortunately, these cardiorespiratory depressive changes are reversed with the narcotic antagonist naloxone (Greenfield and Granada, 1974).

There are other disadvantages to using intravenous narcotics; their effect on the baroreceptors may enhance the hypotensive response and lead to postoperative postural collapse, nausea, and vomiting. In susceptible people, the narcotics also cause a histamine release, which may produce local effects at the venipuncture site or systemic effects such as bronchospasm (Hayden and Scott, 1974).

Although narcotics have long been used to supplement other sedative agents in conscious sedation techniques (for example, Jorgensen technique, 1967), the rationale for their use, considering the drawbacks, should be questioned. Since local anesthesia is a necessary part of any conscious sedation regimen, narcotics to block painful stimuli are not required. As a sedative, they have limitations and far better sedative and tranquilizing agents with fewer side-effects are available.

Intravenous diazepam sedation

The most widely used agent for conscious sedation is diazepam (Valium). It has pronounced tranquilizing and amnesic effects (Driscoll et al., 1972; Flinn, Wineland, and Peterson, 1975; Gregg, Ryan, and Levin, 1974) and a wide margin of safety. The safest way to give diazepam is slowly into a large vein. Although the manufacturer advises against mixing diazepam with any other solution, it can be effectively and safely given through a saline infusion, which also serves to minimize the "burning" the patient may experience at the venipuncture site. The burning pain is produced by the propylene glycol vehicle containing the diazepam, which is irritating to the vessel wall, especially if infused rapidly. By clinical experience as well as in vitro studies (Grower, Ayer, and Getter, 1976; Trieger, 1974), it has been shown that the whitish precipitate that occurs when diazepam is infused into a running saline line rapidly redissolves in the bloodstream and is again pharmacologically active. Increments of 2 to 2.5 mg of diazepam are added per minute until patients show evidence of relaxation by postural changes reflecting decreased tension and by verbal acknowledgment that they now feel more relaxed. Some of these changes are subtle, unlike the hypnotic effects seen with intravenous barbiturates. Although the "Verrill sign" (ptosis of the upper lid to cover the pupil approximately halfway) has been widely used as an end point for titration of diazepam (Drummond-Jackson, 1970), its discoverer never intended it to be used this way. Verrill's sign reflects deep sedation with some attendant central nervous system and respiratory depression.

If careful titration of the drug into a running saline infusion is practiced, safety is increased. Older patients are very susceptible to diazepam and smaller doses are required. With this technique it is important to bear in mind that more drug can always be given if required. There is no need to withdraw the needle or to permit the system to become blocked with a clot; a slow saline drip through a 21-gauge butterfly needle is maintained, providing ready access for additional drug or any emergency medication.

The development of thrombophlebitis in 1% to 3% of cases receiving diazepam is a small but significant complication. The incidence of thrombophlebitis with diazepam may be considerably higher

(15% to 18%) when a specific search is undertaken in postoperative patients (Gelfman and Driscoll, 1977). It is rarely a serious complication and is usually treated symptomatically with local heat and mild analgesics. The vessel will usually become rechannelized in 4 to 6 weeks. Unlike thromboses in lower limb veins, those in upper limbs are very rarely associated with pulmonary embolism (Hoare, 1974).

Diazepam serves to decrease circulating catecholamines and thereby diminish cardiac irritability and arrhythmias (Driscoll, et al., 1972; Saunders and Jenkins, 1973; Van Loon, 1968). It has only minimal effects on the cardiovascular system, usually resulting in minor changes in blood pressure, heart rate, and respiration. In large doses, diazepam causes a mild increase in heart rate as a compensatory change for the decreased peripheral resistance (Dalen et al., 1969; Dixon et al., 1973). Large doses of diazepam produce slight respiratory depression primarily by a decrease in tidal volume (Dalen et al., 1969; Dundee and Wyant, 1974; Dunsworth et al., 1975).

Recovery is rapid, with return of normal psychomotor function within the hour (Driscoll et al., 1972; Trieger, 1974). However, a delayed effect is experienced, with the serum level showing an increase approximately 6 hours later as the drug comes back out of the muscle and fat stores and is slowly metabolized (Baird and Hailey, 1972; Dundee and Wyant, 1974; Gelfman et al., 1979; Kortilla and Linnoila, 1975). The patient must be cautioned to avoid alcohol and other depressant drugs and refrain from driving or operating dangerous machinery.

There are two specific contraindications to the use of diazepam; hypersensitivity, which is rare, and acute narrowangle glaucoma. The latter is a very uncommon form of glaucoma that usually causes intense pain and constitutes an ophthalmologic emergency.

Jorgensen technique

The Jorgensen intravenous technique has been widely used to produce conscious sedation since 1945. It involves the intravenous administration of pentobarbital (Nembutal), 50 mg/ml, given until slight drowsiness is reported by the patient. An additional 10% of the dose already given is then infused. A second syringe containing meperidine (Demerol), 25 mg, and scopolamine, 0.32 mg, then replaces the first syringe. The contents of the second syringe are infused slowly based on a formula that is related to the amount of pentobarbital originally required to achieve drowsiness—the first cortical sign of depression. If it took 100 mg of pentobarbital, then 25 mg of meperidine is infused. If only 50 mg of pentobarbital was used, then 12.5 mg of meperidine is added. The toal dose of meperidine never exceeds 25 mg. Long-term clinical experience has been satisfactory and physiologic studies of cardiorespiratory changes support the effectiveness and safety of this technique of conscious sedation. (Everett and Allen, 1971a, b; Jorgensen and Hayden, 1967).

Shane technique

The Shane technique (Shane, Carrel, and Vandenberge 1974; Shane, 1975) is an example of multidrug-induced deep sedation, with the patient phasing in and out of unconsciousness. It employs five drugs and considerable verbal conditioning. The patient receives alphaprodine hydrochloride (Nisentil), hydroxyzine hydrochloride (Vistaril, Atarax), atropine, and methohexital (Brevital) in addition to local anesthetic blockade. Recently, the technique has been modified so that the hydroxyzine is given intramuscularly 20 minutes preoperatively.

This technique has been recommended for extensive dental reconstruction in an attempt to provide total dentistry in one sitting. It does not lend itself to short procedures, which are the most common need in oral surgical practice. Shane's approach to short procedures is to use intravenous diazepam plus methohexital, atropine, and local anesthetics. This modification has also been popularized by Foreman (1972) and Drummond-Jackson (1970). Berns (1963) had advocated the use of secobarbital sodium (Seconal), meperidine hydrochloride, and increments of methohexital plus local anesthesia.

Other techniques

Other techniques of multiple-drug sedation are also available (Greenfield, 1976). Greenfield uses scopolamine, diazepam, meperidine or fentanyl, plus nitrous oxide/oxygen, methohexital (0.2% drip) as needed, and local anesthesia. With such techniques, patients fade in and out of unconsciousness. It is therefore imperative that those using these techniques be knowledgeable and equipped to manage the unconscious patient. It is also advisable to administer supplementary oxygen by nasal mask whenever multidrug sedation including narcotics is used.

Dissociative analgesia

Greenfield (1976) has described the use of ketamine hydrochloride, a drug that alters the patient's awareness of his surroundings but does not produce the typical state of unconsciousness. The patient is "dissociated" from his environment into a state of catalepsy and experiences analgesia and amnesia. A revised weight-dosage relationship has been established by Greenfield and is based on intramuscular administration (see Chapter 21). At these dosage levels, consciousness is generally maintained together with protective reflexes and stable vital signs. The duration of effect varies from 20 to 40 minutes. Recovery is generally smooth and uneventful, with a very low incidence of nausea and vomiting and a high degree of retrograde amnesia. Premedication includes scopolamine to inhibit the secretions produced by ketamine. At higher dosage, ketamine is known to produce psychotomimetic effects, including hallucinations, through the recovery period and occasionally there are delayed bizarre disturbances (Allen, Boas, and Everett, 1974).

Neuroleptanalgesia

The introduction of a fixed drug combination, Innovar, containing an extremely potent, short-acting narcotic analgesic fentanyl (Sublimaze) and a long-acting, potent tranquilizer, droperidol (Inapsine),

has found limited usefulness in ambulatory oral surgical practice. These drugs are available separately, and fentanyl has been incorporated into regimens of conscious sedation. It has great analgesic potency, rapid onset, and a duration of 30 to 60 minutes. Used alone it produces a significant incidence of nausea and respiratory depression. If minute quantities of droperidol are added (10 to 15 μg/kg of body weight), it may be used for ambulatory patients without unduly prolonging recovery (Greenfield, 1976) (see also Chapter 21).

Other agents

Pentazocine (Talwin) is a non-narcotic analgesic that has been used for conscious sedation by oral and maxillofacial surgeons. It is a morphinelike drug with agonistic and antagonistic properties. It is more efficacious when given intravenously or intramuscularly and less depressant than morphine on both the cardiovascular and respiratory systems. It is reversible by naloxone (Narcan) (Greenfield and Granada, 1974). One of its major drawbacks is the high incidence of hallucinations, and it should be used with diazepam or some other sedative drug (Dundee and Wyant, 1974).

Two newer drugs related to diazepam may be of interest to the oral and maxillofacial surgeon. Flunitrazepam has 10 times the potency of diazepam and lasts slightly longer. There is somewhat less burning reported on administration; however the incidence of phlebitis is slightly higher than that reported for diazepam (Dundee and Wyant, 1974). Lorazepam (Atavar) is a long-acting drug that may be useful for preoperative sedation the night before. At bedtime 4 mg by mouth leads to a comfortable night's sleep. Intravenously 4 mg yields 6 hours of amnesia compared to 10 to 20 minutes for diazepam (Dundee and Wyant, 1974). Neither flunitrazepam nor lorazepam are yet available for use in the United States.

Inhalation sedation—nitrous oxide-oxygen

The principal advantage of the use of N_2O in conscious sedation is the rapidity of onset *and* the rapidity of recovery.

Signs and symptoms of psychosedation begin within 40 to 60 seconds, and the level of sedation can be very readily altered. Recovery to the presedation state occurs within 2 to 3 minutes after turning off the nitrous oxide (Trieger et al., 1971). No other sedative agent nor any other route of administration offers such flexibility. Inhalation sedation serves as a valuable adjunct to control anxiety in the conscious patient. This is accomplished by the effects created by N_2O in the central nervous system and by its potent effect as a placebo. It diminishes sensitivity to noxious stimuli in the conscious and responsive patient even in the absence of true analgesia (Langa, 1968). It does not, however, substitute for local analgesia when the procedure is a painful one nor does it fill the need for a full general anesthetic even when the patient is unconscious.

Unlike prior use of nitrous oxide, where unconsciousness was sought, the aim of inhalation sedation is to alter mood and perception without rendering the patient unconscious. Generally, this can be achieved with levels of nitrous oxide below 50%. Hypoxia is obviated and the likelihood of excitation, nausea, and vomiting is also reduced significantly. The technique calls for a gradual titration of nitrous oxide after 100% oxygen has been started and the patient's tidal volume observed. Patient variability in response to nitrous oxide is very great, requiring individual titration rather than arbitrary or predetermined dosage levels.

Initially there is a significant decrease in cardiac output, which then returns to normal levels as the total peripheral resistance progressively increases. Eisele and Smith (1972), Eisele and co-workers (1976), and others (Everett and Allen, 1971) have shown that inhalation of 40% nitrous oxide by patients with coronary artery disease causes significant depression of myocardial performance. In an in vitro study, Price (1976) showed that myocardial contractility is significantly reduced by 50% nitrous oxide.

There are few contraindications to the use of nitrous oxide-oxygen sedation. Nasal obstruction, upper respiratory infections, and allergic rhinitis all preclude the use of this technique. One of the most significant contraindications to this modality of psychosedation is emotional instability. Because this method causes some perceptual distortions, it is unwise to involve schizoid patients. It is far better when dealing with patients who are emotionally disturbed to maintain their tenuous contact with the reality of the treatment situation.

Recently, another important contraindication to N_2O has been publicized (Millard and Corbett, 1974). Nitrous oxide has been found to be teratogenic and its use is to be avoided in pregnant women. Indeed, concern has been expressed about the effect of even trace amounts of nitrous oxide present as air contaminants in the operatory, and various means of minimizing or disposing of these contaminants have been proposed (Allen, Adams, and Scaramella, 1976; Witcher et al., 1975).

Rectal sedation

Rectal sedation techniques are used mainly in young children (see also Chapter 21). Because of the unpredictability of absorption rate, it is difficult to accurately determine the dosage that will provide sedation, and the child frequently is either inadequately calmed or enters into an anesthetic plane. Moreover, recovery periods tend to be prolonged. Techniques combining inhalation and intravenous agents have been found to be more predictable and effective for the young combative child or retarded individual (Carrel, 1968).

Procedures for rectal sedation have been described by Behrman et al. (1955), Budd et al. (1965), and Chayen and Sarnat (1973).

REFERENCES

Allen, G. D. 1973. Minor anesthesia (Chalmers J. Lyons Memorial Lecture), J. Oral Surg. **31:**330.

Allen, G. D., Adams, D., and Scaramella, J. 1976. An inhalation analgesia circuit to minimize nitrous oxide pollution, Anesth. Prog. **23:**7.

Allen, G. D., Boas, R. A., and Everett, G. D. 1974. Modification of cardiovascular effects of ketamine by diazepam, Anesth. Prog. **21:**8.

Baird, E. S., and Hailey, D. M. 1972. Delayed recovery from a sedative: correlation of the plasma levels of diazepam with clinical effects after oral and intravenous administration, Br. J. Anaesth. **44:**803.

Behrman, S. J., et al. 1955. Rectal thiopental sodium anesthesia for the ambulatory child patient, J. Oral Surg. **13**:125.

Bennett, C. R. 1976. Conscious sedation as an alternative to general anesthesia, N.Y. State Dent. J. **42**:351.

Bennett, C. R. 1978. Conscious sedation in dental practice, ed. 2, St. Louis, The C. V. Mosby Co.

Berns, J., 1963. Twilight sedation—a substitute for lengthy office intravenous anesthesia, J. Conn. State Dent. Assoc. **37**:1.

Budd, D. C., et al. 1965. Methohexital for rectal basal narcosis, Anesth. Analg. **44**:222.

Campbell, R. L., Gregg, J. M., Levin, K. J. 1976. Cardiorespiratory effects of a balanced anesthetic technique in out-patient general anesthesia, J. Oral Surg. **34**:399.

Carrel, R. 1968. A supplement to an intravenous amnesia technique in pedodontic cases, Anesth. Prog. **15**:39.

Chayen, M. S., and Sarnat, H. 1973. Rectal premedication for small children, Anesth. Analg. **52**:837.

Dalen, J. C., et al. 1969. The hemodynamic and respiratory effects of diazepam (Valium), Anesthesiology **30**:259.

Dixon, R. A. et al. 1973. Intravenous diazepam in dentistry: monitoring results from a controlled clinical trial, Br. J. Anaesth. **45**:202.

Driscoll, E. J., et al. 1972. Sedation with intravenous diazepam, J. Oral Surg. **30**:332.

Drummond-Jackson, S. L. 1970. Intravenous anaesthesia, ed. 4, London, SAAD.

Dundee, J., and Wyant, G. M. 1974. Intravenous anaesthesia, Edinburgh, Churchill Livingstone.

Dunsworth, A. R., et al. 1975. Evaluation of cardiovascular and pulmonary changes during meperidine-diazepam anesthesia, J. Oral Surg. **33**:18.

Eisele, J. H., and Smith, N. 1972. Cardiovascular effects of 40% nitrous oxide in man, Anesth. Analg. **51**:956.

Eisele, J. H., et al. 1976. Myocardial performance and N_2O analgesia in coronary-artery disease, Anesthesiology **44**:16.

Everett, G. B., and Allen G. D. 1971a. Simultaneous evaluation of cardiorespiratory and analgesic effects of nitrous oxide-oxygen inhalation analgesia, J. Am. Dent. Assoc. **83**:129.

Everett, G. B. and Allen, G. D. 1971b. Simultaneous evaluation of cardiorespiratory and analgesic effects of intravenous analgesia using pentobarbital, meperidine and scopolamine with local anesthesia, J. Am. Dent. Assoc. **83**:115.

Flinn, F. J., Wineland, P., Peterson, L. J. 1975. Duration of amnesia during sedation with diazepam and pentazocine: preliminary report, J. Oral Surg. **33**:23.

Foreman, P. A. 1972. Psychosedation: intravenous route. In McCarthy, F. M., ed.: Emergencies in dental practice, Philadelphia, W. B. Saunders Co.

Gelfman, S. S., and Driscoll, E. J. 1977. Thrombophlebitis following intravenous anesthesia and sedation; an annotated review, Anesth. Prog. **24**:194.

Gelfman, S. S., et al. 1979. Comparison of recovery tests after intravenous sedation with diazepam-methohexital and diazepam-methohexital and fentanyl, J. Oral Surg. **37**:391.

Greenfield, W. 1976. Anesthesiology in dentistry—past, present and future, Anesth. Prog. **23**:4.

Greenfield, W., and Granada, M. G. 1974. The use of a narcotic antagonist in the anesthetic management of the ambulatory oral surgery patient, J. Oral Surg. **32**:760.

Gregg, J. M., Ryan, D. E., and Levin, K. H. 1974. The amnesic actions of diazepam, J. Oral Surg. **32**:651.

Grower, M. F., Ayer, W. A., and Getter, L. 1976. Solubility of injectable Valium in plasma and saline, Anesth. Prog. **23**:45.

Hayden, J., Jr., and Scott, E. 1974. A significant histamine response to fentanyl: report of a case, Anesth. Prog. **21**:84.

Healey, T. E. J., and Vickers, M. D. 1971. Laryngeal competence under diazepam sedation, Proc. Soc. Med. **64**:85.

Hoare, A. M. 1974. Pulmonary embolus after diazepam sedation, J.A.M.A. **230**:210.

Jorgensen, N. B., and Hayden, J. 1967. Premedication local and general anesthesia in dentistry, Philadelphia, Lea & Febiger.

Kortilla, K., and Linnoila, M. 1975. Psychomotor skills related to driving after intramuscular administration of diazepam and meperidine, Anesthesiology **42**:685.

Langa, H. 1968. Relative analgesia in dental practice: inhalation analgesia with nitrous oxide, Philadelphia, W. B. Saunders Co.

Millard, R. L., and Corbett, T. H. 1974. Nitrous oxide concentrations in the dental operatory, J. Oral Surg. **32**:593.

Price, H. L. 1976. Myocardial depression by nitrous oxide and its reversal by calcium, Anesthesiology **44**:211.

Saunders, B. A., and Jenkins, L. C. 1973. Cardiac arrhythmias of central nervous system origin: possible mechanism and suppression, Can. Anaesth. Soc. J. **20**:617.

Shane, S. M. E., 1975. Principles of sedation, local and general anesthesia in dentistry, Springfield, Ill., Charles C Thomas, Publisher.

Shane, S. M., Carrel, R., and Vandenberge, J. 1974. Intravenous amnesia—an appraisal after seven years and 10,500 administrations, Anesth. Prog. **21**(2):36.

Trieger, N. 1974. Pain control, Chicago, Quintessence Publishing Co.

Trieger, N., et al. 1971. Nitrous oxide—a study of physiological and psychomotor effects, J. Am. Dent. Assoc. **82**:142.

Van Loon, G. R. 1968. Ventricular arrhythmias treated by diazepam, Can. Med. Assoc. J. **98**:785.

Witcher, C., et al. 1975. Development and evaluation of methods for the elimination of waste anesthetic gases and vapors in hospitals, Cincinnati, U.S. Department of Health, Education and Welfare, National Institute of Occupational Safety and Health, Division of Field Studies and Clinical Investigations.

CHAPTER 21

General anesthesia

William Greenfield

Experience in anesthesiology constitutes a significant part of the training of the oral and maxillofacial surgeon. Through the use of techniques that can be applied to ambulatory patients, surgical procedures are performed in the office that otherwise would require hospitalization for reasons other than complexity of the surgery or medical status of the individual. The methods used are generally technically and pharmacologically less complex than those used in the hospitalized patient. The relative safety and efficiency of these methods have been well documented in the literature (ASOS Anesthesia Morbidity and Mortality Survey, 1974; Lytle, 1974).

EARLY HISTORY AND DEVELOPMENT OF GENERAL ANESTHESIA

Dentistry's involvement in the history of anesthesia is, of course, well known. Following the controversy between Drs. Wells, Morton, Jackson, and Long for the title of "discoverer of anesthesia," it remained for the American Dental Association (in 1864), followed by the American Medical Association (in 1872), to officially grant the title to Wells by formal resolutions to that effect. Although Morton cannot be called the discoverer of anesthesia, he most certainly introduced anesthesia as a practical procedure, and to the everlasting credit of the dental profession it was these two dentists who gave to mankind one of its greatest discoveries, the use of surgical anesthesia. Additionally, it should be noted that Dr.

Morton was also the first specialist in the administration of anesthesia, the first manufacturer of anesthetic equipment, and the first teacher of anesthesiology. It was a physician, Dr. Carl Koller, who first discovered the use of local anesthesia by anesthetizing the eye with a solution of cocaine, but interestingly enough, the first application of local anesthesia by injection again involved dentistry. Dr. William Halstead, a prominent New York surgeon, employed a syringe to inject cocaine for a dental procedure, blocking the inferior alveolar nerve. The technique of block anesthesia was first taught in this country by Dr. Guido Fischer, a German dentist, who was brought here in 1914 specifically for that purpose.

As new anesthetic drugs and agents appeared, they were clinically evaluated for inclusion in dental practice. Ethyl chloride was introduced toward the end of the nineteenth century as an anesthetic, was widely used in dentistry for about 50 years, and then was virtually discarded because of the advent of safer agents. Ethylene enjoyed a brief period of use in the early part of the twentieth century; cyclopropane, being explosive like ether, was never incorporated into dental practice. Divinyl ether (Vinethene) was first used in dentistry in 1933 and was widely used until relatively recently. Trichloroethylene (Trilene), introduced at about the same time, was also used extensively.

Through the first half of the twentieth century, techniques of pain control in dentistry consisted of either local anesthesia or inhalation general anesthesia, using nitrous oxide and the various volatile agents available. The introduction of intravenous barbiturate anesthesia opened an entirely new chapter in anesthesia in dentistry as well as in medicine. Several early pioneers in dentistry can be singled out for specific contributions in this area. Intravenous barbiturate anesthesia with hexobarbital (Evipal), was first used in dentistry in 1932 by S. L. Drummond-Jackson of London, some time before the introduction of thiopental (Pentothal) in the United States by Dr. John S. Lundy. Drummond-Jackson was also the first dentist to use intravenous barbiturates for restorative dentistry as well as oral surgery. Dr. Adrian Hubbell, who had studied with Lundy, and Dr. Harold Krogh, were early pioneers in the introduction and teaching of intravenous barbiturate anesthesia in office oral surgery practice. A major innovation in intravenous pain control techniques was achieved in 1945, when Dr. Niels Jorgenson introduced a method to obtain light sedation using a combination of barbiturate, narcotic, and belladonna in conjunction with local anesthetic block. This, plus a resurgence of interest in subanesthetic (analgesic or sedative) mixtures of nitrous oxide and oxygen, laid the groundwork for an expanded spectrum of techniques for pain control in dentistry, ranging from local anesthesia to inhalation and intravenous sedation, to neurolept and dissociative techniques, to general anesthesia, with many variations and combinations.

Definitions

The word "anesthesia," coined by Oliver Wendell Holmes in 1847, implies the absence of all sensations, as opposed to "analgesia," which is a diminution (or more properly absence) of the sensation of pain. One can then distinguish between local and general analgesia as well as between local and general anesthesia, with general anesthesia implying the loss of consciousness as well. By definition (*Guidelines for Teaching the Comprehensive Control of Pain and Anxiety in Dentistry,* American Dental Association, 1971), the conscious patient is one who has intact protective reflexes, including the ability to maintain an airway and is capable of rational response to question or command.

APPLIED RESPIRATORY AND CARDIOVASCULAR PHYSIOLOGY

While application of all of the basic sciences is involved in anesthesiology, clinical use of general anesthesia deals primarily with a combination of applied physiology and applied pharmacology, with a good working knowledge of respiratory and cardiovascular physiology being of paramount importance.

In simple terms, respiration provides an exchange of gases between the blood and the body cells whereby carbon dioxide is continually eliminated and oxygen is supplied to the tissues. Additionally, respiration is an important factor in the regulation of body temperature and acid-base balance. Most of the respiratory tract, including the nose, mouth, pharynx, larynx, trachea, bronchi, and bronchioles, acts simply as a conduit for the passage of air from the atmosphere to the deeper recesses of the lung, with the actual gas exchange taking place in the alveolar ducts, alveolar sacs, and alveoli. As a result, all of the air in the conducting passages is dead-space air that does not undergo gaseous exchange with the blood. The alveolar air in the lower respiratory passages makes up a volume of about 3 L.

Lung volumes and gas exchange

In an average adult, the volume of air exchanged during each inspiration or expiration while at rest is approximately 500 to 700 ml and is termed "tidal volume." About one third of this volume fills the dead space in the conducting passages and the rest mixes with the alveolar air. A maximal inspiration can provide an additional 2.5 to 3 L (inspiratory reserve volume), while a maximal expiration can expel an additional 1.5 to 2 L. The vital capacity is the sum of these three volumes, constituting a maximal inspiration followed by a maximal expiration, and is about 5 to 6 L in the average adult (Fig. 21-1).

In the ventilating portion of the lung,

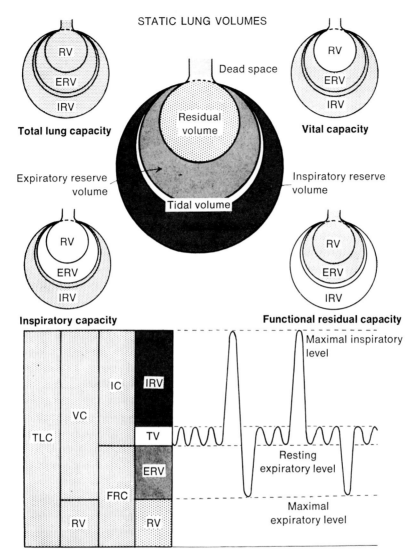

STATIC LUNG VOLUMES

Fig. 21-1. Lung volumes. (Reproduced with permission from Comroe, J. H., Jr., et al. The lung: clinical physiology and pulmonary function tests, ed. 2. Copyright © 1962 by Year Book Medical Publishers, Inc., Chicago.)

the alveolar gases are separated from the capillary blood by two thin endothelial membranes, and gases diffuse through this dual membrane based on differences in individual pressure gradients. Gas molecules move from an area of higher tension to one of lower tension, and in a mixture of gases, such as in air, each gas acts independently of the others. Dalton's law of partial pressures states that the total pressure is equal to the sum of the partial pressures. Following a normal inspiration, there is a mixing of gases in the conducting passages and in the alveoli, and the inspired, alveolar, and expired gases will have a different percentage composition and partial pressure. The pressure of water vapor is an additional factor that must be considered.

The diffusion of gases between alveolar air and the capillary blood constitutes the ventilating portion of external respiration, with each gas having its individual coefficient of solubility in the blood plasma. Owing to the difference in pressures, there is a diffusion of gases and venous blood is converted to arterial blood, which carries gases to the tissue cells. At the cellular level, after oxidative processes have occurred, there is a decrease in oxygen tension and an increase in carbon dioxide tension, resulting in another diffusion of gases referred to as internal respiration.

Blood combines with oxygen in two ways: (1) in physical solution in the plasma as dissolved oxygen and (2) in chemical combination with hemoglobin as HbO_2. The total amount of oxygen in arterial blood is about 20 ml/100 ml of blood, of which only about 0.3 ml is carried in physical solution in the plasma. In both cases, the amount of oxygen taken up depends on the Po_2 to which the plasma or blood is exposed. A graph of percent saturation of hemoglobin with oxygen plotted against Po_2 is not a straight line, but an S-shaped curve (Fig. 21-2), indicating that arterial oxygen tension does

not fall much below normal values even when there is pulmonary disease severe enough to cause a definite difference between the Po_2 of alveolar gas and of arterial blood.

Factors controlling respiration

The mechanics of respiration are divided into an active inspiratory effort originated by nervous impulses, in which the diaphragm descends and the intercostal muscles contract causing an enlargement of the thoracic cage; an expiratory effort that is primarily a passive process in which the muscles relax to their original positions; and a pause before the next active inspiration.

The respiratory center in the brain consists of three specific bilateral regions. The inspiratory and expiratory centers are located in the caudal third of the medulla, and the pneumotaxic center (respiratory inhibiting center) is located

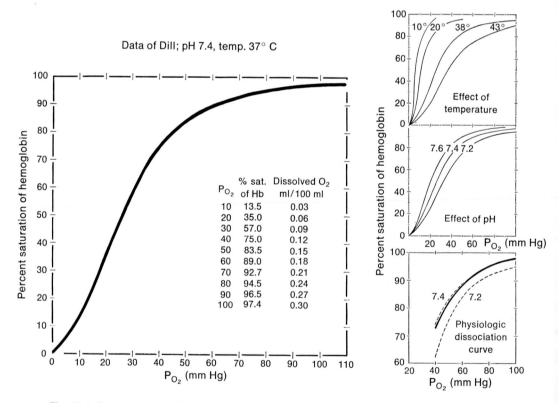

Data of Dill; pH 7.4, temp. 37° C

Po_2	% sat. of Hb	Dissolved O_2 ml/100 ml
10	13.5	0.03
20	35.0	0.06
30	57.0	0.09
40	75.0	0.12
50	83.5	0.15
60	89.0	0.18
70	92.7	0.21
80	94.5	0.24
90	96.5	0.27
100	97.4	0.30

Fig. 21-2. Oxygen-hemoglobin dissociation curve. (Reproduced with permission from Comroe, J. H., Jr., et al. The lung: clinical physiology and pulmonary function tests, ed. 2. Copyright © 1962 by Year Book Medical Publishers, Inc., Chicago.)

in the pons. The inspiratory center cells discharge automatically and rhythmically, initiating each inhalation by causing contraction of the inspiratory muscles as well as by sending impulses to the pneumotaxic center. The pontine neurons carry impulses to the expiratory center, which then sends inhibiting impulses back to the inspiratory center. The pneumotaxic center is thought to help bring about a more rhythmic respiratory pattern.

There are various chemical, physical, and nervous factors that affect the respiratory center. The normal respiratory center is exquisitely sensitive to a rise in arterial PCO_2. Any condition producing a slight increase in the partial pressure of carbon dioxide in the blood will directly stimulate the respiratory center, which responds promptly with an increase in tidal volume and alveolar ventilation. A 2 to 3 mm increase in PCO_2 increases ventilatory volume fourfold, while a 4 to 5 mm increase in PCO_2 produces a tenfold increase in ventilatory volume. Higher quantities of carbon dioxide (above 10%) are intolerable to the patient, since a 12 mm increase in PCO_2 will produce anesthesia, and a 16 mm increase will cause marked depression of the respiratory center. Conversely, any condition that causes a decrease in the partial pressure of carbon dioxide in the blood will decrease respiratory activity. Voluntary hyperventilation for a 3 to 5 minute period will be followed by a period of apnea, which is usually self-limiting.

A decrease in the partial pressure of oxygen in the blood (hypoxemia, anoxemia) will cause an increase in tidal volume and some increase in respiratory rate. This effect is not mediated by the respiratory center, which is depressed by a decrease in PO_2, but is due to peripheral reflexes initiated in the chemoreceptors of the carotid and aortic bodies. These bodies are attached directly to the ascending aorta and the external carotid artery and respond to slight changes in the composition of the arterial blood as it flows rapidly past them. The chemoreceptors are primarily affected by a decrease in PO_2 but also respond to carbon dioxide excess and H-ion increase through involuntary reflex control.

Physical factors influencing the respiratory center are temperature, blood pressure, and air pressure within the lungs. An increase in temperature will increase respiratory rate, and a decrease in temperature will decrease the rate. An increase in blood pressure will stimulate pressure receptors (pressoreceptors) in the carotid sinus and aortic arch sending impulses to the expiratory center, which in turn sends inhibiting impulses to the inspiratory center. A decrease in blood pressure will increase the respiratory rate. Inflation of the lungs stimulates stretch receptors in the lung tissue, also sending impulses to the expiratory center inhibiting inspiration. This important reflex is called the Hering-Breuer reflex.

Anoxia, or total lack of oxygen, is not a condition one encounters in clinical practice, since there is always some oxygen remaining in the lungs. However, hypoxia (an inadequate supply of oxygen) is frequently an insidious cause of many problems. Five basic types of hypoxia can be distinguished:

1. Hypoxic hypoxia is due to a diminution of oxygen in inspired air.
2. Stagnant hypoxia is due to a slowing of the circulation, as in shock or cardiac insufficiency.
3. Anemic hypoxia is due to a decrease in the oxygen-carrying capacity of the blood, as in a reduction in red cells or in amount of available hemoglobin.
4. Histotoxic hypoxia is due to an infection that limits the utilization of oxygen in the tissues.
5. Demand hypoxia is due to an increased BMR that requires a greater than normal supply of oxygen, as in a high fever.

Many mechanical and chemical effects that take place during general anesthesia can cause hypoxia. Almost all anesthetic agents are respiratory depressants, and it is always advisable to assist respiration periodically. Additionally, partial obstruction of the airway may result in a diminution of tidal volume and in hypoxia. Chronic hypoxia will eventually have a deleterious effect on cardiovascular dynamics, reducing cardiac output.

AUTONOMIC NERVOUS SYSTEM AS RELATED TO ANESTHESIOLOGY

Although the entire nervous system is of vital interest to the anesthesiologist, since all anesthetic drugs affect the nervous system to varying degrees, the autonomic nervous system is of special significance in general anesthesia where the patient is rendered unconscious.

The autonomic nervous system is anatomically a portion of the peripheral nervous system, but physiologically and pharmacologically it acts as a separate functional unit. This system is concerned with the automatic bodily functions and regulates visceral organs, circulation, respiration, digestion, excretion, and reproduction. It is divided into two portions. The sympathetic system, derived from the eighth cervical to the twelfth thoracic nerves and the first three lumbar nerves, is termed the "thoracolumbar division." The parasympathetic system, derived from the third, seventh, ninth, and tenth cranial nerves and the second, third, and fourth sacral nerves, is termed the "craniosacral division."

The sympathetic division prepares the body for stressful situations and increases its activities during times of stress. The parasympathetic division is concerned with the conservation and restoration of energy and does this by such functions as slowing the heart rate, lowering blood pressure, and aiding in alimentation.

General anesthesia is a controlled, reversible, progressive paralysis of the central nervous system, during which the medulla is bypassed temporarily as the depressing effect of the anesthetic is exerted on the brain and spinal cord from above downward. The suitability of a drug as an anesthetic agent depends on its ability to depress the higher centers with minimal change in the autonomic nervous system. Since some anesthetic agents mimic the effects of impulses from the sympathetic nervous system and some mimic those from the parasympathetic nervous system, we may classify them as sympathomimetic or parasympathomi-metic. The autonomic drugs may be further classified as sympatholytic or parasympatholytic, based on whether the principal effect is one of stimulation or depression.

THEORIES OF GENERAL ANESTHESIA

Numerous theories seeking to explain the action of anesthetics have been advanced. Even as some of the older ones have been discarded, modern investigative methods have given us new insights into drug action. When many theories exist concerning the causation of one complex process, there is a possibility not only that all are wrong but also that all are right. Much of the recent work in this area tends to support a multiple causation theory. Observation of the great differences in capabilities among the several substances used today in clinical anesthesia lends credence to such a view. Ether is a superb analgesic, halothane is a poor one; cyclopropane produces muscular relaxation, nitrous oxide produces none; trichloroethylene can cause excellent analgesia without affecting rationality; the patient receiving thiopental, although completely unconscious, may have no analgesia. All of these agents are called general anesthetics yet their individual abilities vary widely. It is doubtful that their mode of action is the same.

The older Meyer-Overton theory, noting that all anesthetics are soluble in fat, relates the degree of fat solubility to anesthetic potency and then observes that nervous system cells are rich in lipid (fatty) compounds. This explains why safe anesthetic drugs affect the nervous system more than other systems or organs. However, it does not help to explain how the effects are produced within the nerve cell.

Pauling (1961) has suggested that by promoting the persistence of so-called clathrates (orderly arrangements of water molecules in geometric relationships to one another), anesthetic molecules may allow the buildup of microcrystals of water, not dissimilar to ice, on cellular membranes. The presence of such crystals would interfere with electrical potential transfers along nerve cell membranes, "shorting" the action currents and stopping nervous system function. Involvement of enzyme receptor sites with these microcrystals might explain the observed derangement of function in organs other than those of the nervous system.

Featherstone and co-workers (1961) have presented evidence that because anesthetics are also highly soluble in proteins, the smaller molecules may, if present within the partially enclosed spaces existing within the coils of helically or conglomerately arranged long protein molecules, deform the overall shape of these structures just sufficiently to prevent their normal function in metabolic processes. It should be remembered that enzymes, on which most bodily functions depend, are protein in nature.

Miller (1961) has published results of experiments verifying that when anesthetic molecules dissolve in the fats of cell membranes, water molecules are simultaneously incorporated in the membrane structure, altering its density and the spatial arrangement of the lipid molecules composing its substance. Such alterations presumably could change membrane permeability by blocking the ingress of nutrients and the egress of harmful metabolites and by slowing cellular function.

The many avenues being explored are examples of the modern approach to understanding anesthetic action at the cellular level. Since the experiments or calculations seeking to verify these three new theories were each done with different drug models, they support the possibility of different modes of action for different types of anesthetics.

BASIC CONCEPTS OF GENERAL ANESTHESIA FOR THE AMBULATORY PATIENT

While techniques of conscious sedation are widely employed in office practice (see Chapter 20), general anesthesia is still required for certain categories of patients. Most general anesthetics in dentistry are given by oral and maxillofacial surgeons, but there is an ever-increasing group utilizing general anesthesia for general dentistry. Today the great majority of dental procedures, under either general or local anesthesia, are performed on ambulatory patients in the office. Statistics indicate that there are more anesthetics administered in dental offices than in all of the hospitals combined (Wylie and Churchill-Davidson, 1972).

Patients usually are admitted to hospitals for one or more of the following reasons: (1) the procedure is of an extensive surgical nature that is beyond the scope of office management; (2) the patient requires special preoperative or postoperative management or nursing care owing to some preexisting condition; (3) the patient requires special general anesthetic management. The last category usually involves the question of time. Many oral and maxillofacial surgeons, for example, will manage a short procedure under general anesthesia in their offices, but they will admit patients requiring procedures that they feel will take longer than a fixed arbitrary time to a hospital.

It is important to simulate as closely as possible in the office the conditions that prevail in a hospital for the management of surgical procedures under general anesthesia. It has been said that no matter how minor the surgical procedure may be, there is no "minor" general anesthesia—use of a general anesthetic is always a "major" procedure.

The three basic cornerstones of sound anesthetic management in the office are (1) adequate background and training, (2) adequate personnel, and (3) adequate equipment and facilities.

Background and training of the operating team are of primary importance. It has been long advocated, and the American Dental Association has adopted as part of a standard *Guidelines for Teaching the Comprehensive Control of Pain and Anxiety in Dentistry,* that a dentist should have a minimum of 1 year's training in anesthesiology, beyond the predoctoral level, prior to using general anesthesia in practice. Oral and maxillofacial surgery training programs incorporate such training. Additionally, there are hospitals throughout the country where dentists who are not oral surgeons may obtain residency training in anesthesiology. The interest in, and availability of, such programs is constantly increasing.

The operating team should consist of at least three people: the surgeon and two trained assistants. There must be adequate equipment and facilities to cope with any problem that may arise. Such things, for example, as well-functioning anesthetic equipment and suction are of course taken for granted, as is adequate lighting. A well-organized emergency tray should be readily available, and all personnel should be completely familiar with its contents. Recovery rooms should also be equipped with adequate suction, a source of oxygen, and ready access to all emergency equipment. The anesthetic management of the office patient can simulate hospital management in every respect, and there need be no compromise with ideal conditions. A well-trained team, operating in a well-equipped office, can provide the highest level of care in general anesthesia for the ambulatory patient.

The control of pain for office procedures has traditionally been achieved with either local anesthesia or general anesthesia. Within relatively recent years, however, the scope of anesthesia has been greatly expanded by the addition of many other modalities, with the result that the delineation of analgesia (diminution of pain without the loss of consciousness) from anesthesia (loss of all sensations including consciousness) is no longer as clear as it once was. Often when "general anesthesia" is requested for a particular procedure, careful analysis will reveal that what is actually required are the following: analgesia, so that the patient may be free of pain; amnesia, especially retrograde amnesia, so that the patient will not recall what occurred during the procedure; tranquility, or mental calmness, with absence of fear and apprehension; and some degree of cortical depression, ranging from mild sedation to sleep. All of these objectives can often be achieved without the loss of consciousness (see Chapter 20).

PREANESTHETIC ASPECTS
Evaluation and selection of patients

In selection of patients for office anesthesia, a careful history and physical evaluation are mandatory. They should be both subjective and objective, including evaluation of vital signs. An example of a form often used to record this information is seen in Fig. 21-3. The subjective portion consists of a series of questions, aimed primarily at determining the status of the patient's cardiovascular and respiratory systems but also including a review of past medical and surgical history, the patient's allergic status, and whether the patient is taking any medications or is under medical care for some preexisting systemic disease. A careful selection of patients is important, since it is generally recognized that only physical status class I patients and certain class II patients are suitable candidates for general anesthesia in the office. By definition, these would be patients free from organic disease or patients in whom ordinary physical activity does not cause undue fatigue or dyspnea. This category may include, for example, well-controlled diabetics, patients with well-compensated valvular heart disease provided it is not associated with hypertension, or patients with hypertension not complicated with other cardiovascular disease. Excluded from this category would be any of the following:

1. The extremes of age—very small children or patients past an arbitrary age of 60, in whom arteriosclerotic changes are inevitable

2. Very obese patients (It is well known that obesity predisposes to cardiovascular disease, impaired liver function, and postoperative thromboembolic phenomena, in addition to airway and respiratory problems during general anesthesia.)

3. Patients with congenital defects (These are often multiple and may include congenital cardiac defects of which the patient is unaware.)

4. Patients with more than one preexisting systemic disease, since this can compound potential problems (for example, a diabetic patient with hypertension)

Name _____ M F___ Age_____ Weight_____ Date_____

Review of past and present medical history:

Check one

	yes	no

1. Are you presently under a physician's care? _____
2. When did you last eat or drink? _____
3. Have you ever been a patient in a hospital? _____
4. Do you have a cough or cold? _____
5. Do you smoke, and how much? _____
6. Do you or did you ever have high blood pressure? _____
7. Have you ever been told that you have low blood pressure? _____
8. Are you able to carry on your daily activities without difficulty? _____
9. Do you experience any shortness of breath or chest pains? _____
10. Do you ever feel dizzy or have fainting spells? _____
11. Do your ankles swell? _____
12. Have you ever been told that you are anemic? _____
13. Do you have any history of prolonged bleeding? _____
14. Have you ever been told that you have kidney trouble? _____
15. Have you ever been treated for liver trouble, hepatitis or jaundice (yellow skin or eyes)? _____
16. Do you drink alcoholic beverages, and if so, how much? _____
17. Do you have or have you had hay fever? _____
    asthma? _____
    tuberculosis? _____
    rheumatic fever? _____
    diabetes? _____
18. Have you ever been told that you are allergic to any drugs (e.g. Penicillin, Novacaine, Aspirin)? _____
19. Are you now or have you recently been taking any drugs such as Cortisone, Rauwolfias, Anticoagulants, Thyroid, etc.? _____
20. Have you ever had any serious illnesses or operations? _____
21. Are you pregnant at this time? _____
22. Have you ever been treated for narcotic addiction? _____
23. Have you ever had a general anesthetic? _____
24. Is there anything else significant in your medical history or anything unusual about your physical condition that should be called to the doctor's attention? _____

Physical evaluation:

1. Blood pressure: _____
2. Pulse: Rate _____ Quality: _____ Rhythm _____
3. Respiration: Rate _____ Depth: _____ Rhythm _____
4. Temperature: (where pertinent) _____
5. Laboratory values: Blood: Hb. _____ Hct. _____
                       Other: _____

                       Urinalysis: Sp. gr. _____
                                    Sugar _____
                                    Albumin _____
                                    Other _____
6. Phys. status classification _____
7. Premedication (drugs, dosages, route of admin.) _____

8. Pertinent notes regarding patient management: _____
_____
_____
_____
_____
_____

                       Signature: _____

Fig. 21-3. Preanesthetic patient history and physical evaluation record.

5. Patients with upper respiratory infection (The primary problem is that many reflexes become hyperactive and are not obtunded until the patient is brought to a much deeper level of surgical anesthesia than is usually required. For example, pharyngeal reflexes are often not obtunded until the third plane of stage III, and patients may cough, gag, and "buck" until brought to this level.)

None of the office procedures performed by the oral and maxillofacial surgeon is a true emergency in the medical sense, so it is not absolutely essential to give a general anesthetic to any patient that does not fit the categories outlined.

Preparation of the patient

Ambulatory patients scheduled to be treated under general anesthesia should receive specific instructions regarding necessary preparation for anesthesia and surgery. The patient should not have had food or water for 6 to 8 hours before the comtemplated procedure and should be accompanied by a responsible adult who will also escort him home. If the procedure is scheduled for the morning, the patient is to have nothing by mouth after midnight, and if scheduled for the afternoon, he may have a clear liquid breakfast early in the morning. Patients should be instructed to void just prior to the procedure.

Premedication

After obtaining a careful history and doing a physical evaluation of the patient, it may be decided that the patient should be medicated preoperatively. Obviously, premedication is not necessarily indicated for every patient. As a matter of fact, there are those, such as Goldman (in Hunter, 1971), who feel that dental outpatients should not be premedicated. If a patient is to be premedicated, it should be for some specific effect that the surgeon would like to obtain.

In determining dosage of premedicating drugs, several factors must be taken into consideration: age of the patient, weight, physical status, and type of anesthetic to be used. Another important consideration is the timing of the premedica-

tion, with regard to the initial onset and peak effect, as well as the duration of action. For example, if a child is premedicated at home and it takes an hour to reach the office, after which the patient is kept waiting for another hour before being seen, the timing of the premedication is obviously poorly planned.

Effects to be obtained from premedication

Diminution of fear and apprehension. Several classes of drugs are available that produce diminution of fear and apprehension. It must be understood, however, that the true sedatives are not analgesic in any sense—they do not raise the pain threshold and should not be used to reduce pain. They can, however, aid the psychic portion of the pain experience if given in conjunction with an analgesic.

The most widely used group of sedatives is the barbiturates. Depending on the dose and the route of administration, the effect obtained can range from sedation (a mild state of cortical depression), to hypnosis (sleep), to basal narcosis (a degree of central nervous system depression just short of a surgical level of general anesthesia), to severe cortical depression and death. We are interested primarily in sedation. The long-acting barbiturates (such as phenobarbital) and intermediate-acting barbiturates (such as butabarbital) are not used very much in outpatients because of their long duration of effect. Short-acting barbiturates are usually preferable for sedation because of their rapid onset and short duration. Of this group, pentobarbital (Nembutal) and secobarbital (Seconal) are the two most commonly used. If the medication is given orally, one may expect some initial action in 15 to 30 minutes, a peak effect in 45 minutes, and a duration of effect of about 2 to 4 hours. Pentobarbital and secobarbital are detoxified by the liver and eliminated by the kidneys. The two drugs are very similar, and the usual adult hypnotic dose is 100 to 200 mg, with the sedative dose being half of this amount.

There is a tendency to believe that the only useful drugs are those that are new, expensive, and much advertised. One of the oldest sedatives is chloral hydrate, which was first introduced over 100 years ago and now has had a resurgence of use. It is inexpensive, well tolerated, and has a wide margin of safety. For effective sedation, the usual adult dose is 1 to 2 gm. It is marketed as Noctec, in both elixir and capsule form.

Of the ultrashort-acting barbiturates, virtually all of the drugs in this category, with the exception of thiopental (Pentothal), are administered exclusively by the intravenous route. Thiopental may also be administered rectally.

Another group of drugs commonly used to allay apprehension is the tranquilizers, or antianxiety drugs. These drugs are prescribed more frequently today than any other class. The group may be divided into three main categories: rauwolfia derivatives, phenothiazine derivatives, and "minor" tranquilizers.

While the classic sedatives, such as the barbiturates, act by depressing the central nervous system starting at the cortical level, the tranquilizers relieve anxiety primarily by a specific depression of subcortical levels, such as the reticular activating system, which are involved in regulating states of wakefulness. Since they do not act on the cortex, they do not make people sleepy; the usual effect produced can best be described as "tranquilization" rather than sedation.

The rauwolfia derivatives, such as Serpasil and Raudixin, are used primarily in the treatment of hypertension, and as a side-effect they produce sedation and tranquility. Accordingly, they have very little place in a discussion on premedication.

The phenothiazines, such as promethazine (Phenergan), propiomazine (Largon), chlorpromazine (Thorazine), promazine (Sparine), perphenazine (Trilafon), trifluoperazine (Stelazine), and a host of others, are powerful tranquilizers with many other pharmacologic effects. They have antihistamine action, are potent antiemetics, and potentiate other drugs such as narcotics and hypnotics in addition to their ability to tranquilize. The list of potential side effects of the phenothiazines is very long and includes parkinsonian-like seizures, agranulocytosis, dizziness, headache, emotional changes, and postural hypotension, among others.

The "minor" tranquilizers are those that produce a mild calmness and relieve apprehension, without any major side effects. Drugs falling into this classification include the benzodiazepine compounds such as diazepam (Valium) and chlordiazepoxide (Librium), hydroxyzine (Vistaril and Atarax), meprobamate (Miltown and Equanil), chlormeganone (Trancopal), phenaglycodol (Ultran), and many others. For use in ambulatory patients, these drugs are best given over a period of several days prior to treatment in order to build up an adequate blood level. The benzodiazepines, like meprobamate, were originally developed as centrally-acting skeletal muscle relaxants.

Control of preexisting pain. Of the available analgesics, the narcotics are most commonly used for premedication. These drugs relieve pain by depressing the cortex and raising the pain threshold. The narcotics possess other advantages in that they remove the psychic response to pain and produce euphoria, as well as sedate the patient (see p. 682).

Diminution of salivary secretions. The drugs most commonly used as antisialagogues are the belladonna alkaloids, specifically atropine and scopolamine. Both drugs share certain effects but also have certain differences (see p. 682).

Obtunding of nausea. Where a specific indication exists, antiemetics can be used as premedicants. Among the drugs used for this purpose are antihistamines such as dimenhydrinate (Dramamine) or diphenhydramine (Benadryl); phenothiazines such as prochlorperazine dimaleate (Compazine), promethazine (Phenergan), or chlorpromazine (Thorazine); and drugs with specific antiemetic activity such as trimethobenzamide (Tigan).

• • •

In addition to the preceding four effects of premedication that are often desired for ambulatory patients, whether their management will be under local or general anesthesia, there are two other aspects of significance that should be considered if general anesthsia is to be used. These additional effects are lowering of the basal metabolic activity (BMR) and obtunding of parasympathetic (vagal) effects.

Lowering of the basal metabolic activity. By lowering the basal metabolic rate, oxygen consumption is decreased, thereby diminishing the likelihood of hypoxia. The sedatives and hypnotics are useful in this regard.

Obtunding of parasympathetic (vagal) effects. Certain vagal reflexes are undesirable in patients undergoing general anesthesia. Preoperative administration of atropine can be useful in obviating this situation. The argument is often advanced, however, that the amount of atropine administered generally is too low to achieve all the desired effects. While it is true that the dose of atropine that would be necessary to completely obtund the vagus is six or seven times the usual physiologic dose (3 to 4 mg of atropine is required to obtund all vagal effects), this is not an all-or-none response, and a very definite EKG effect can be seen following use of 0.4 mg of atropine.

• • •

Any of the routes of administration (oral, rectal, intramuscular, or intravenous) may be used for preoperative medication of the patient, bearing in mind that the oral route is the least dependable and the parenteral route is the most dependable. Any of the drugs mentioned in this discussion can be used alone or in combination with other drugs, provided that one is thoroughly familiar with their actions, interactions, and side effects (Dukes, 1978). The subject of drug interactions, in particular, is a very important one and a number of texts have been published on the subject (*Evaluation of Drug Interaction*, 1973; Martin, 1971). Moreover, premedicated patients should be escorted to and from the office by a responsible adult, and they should not be permitted to drive themselves.

Technique of venipuncture

Venipuncture is a relatively simple maneuver when proper attention is given to technique and armamentarium. All of the necessary materials should be at hand before starting the venipuncture — tourniquet, syringe, needle, and alcohol sponges, as well as several strips of tape if the needle is to be maintained in place. The venipuncture site is first selected. The left arm is generally used, since the surgeon usually stands to the right of the patient. Although the antecubital fossa is the anatomic region most commonly selected, the needle is much more easily maintained in position if inserted anywhere in the forearm between the wrist and elbow, since movements of the arm then would not dislodge the needle as easily or cause perforation of the vein if the arm were bent. Other sites often used are the back of the hand and the medial surface of the wrist. A thorough knowledge of the topical anatomy of the arm is helpful in this regard.

After selection of the injection site, the tourniquet is applied approximately 2 to 3 inches proximal to that point. The tourniquet should be tight enough to obstruct venous return but not cut off the arterial blood supply, so that the radial pulse can still be palpated. If rubber tubing is used as a tourniquet, it is held in place by looping one of the ends underneath in such a way that it can be released with one hand. The free ends should not project toward the venipuncture site, but away from it so as not to obstruct vision. Also, the tourniquet should be stretched before applying it to the arm so that the skin is not stretched with the tourniquet. The vein is made to stand out as much as possible in several ways. The arm is lowered so that venous return is diminished; the patient is told to open and close the fist several times so that muscular action pumps more blood into the vein; recognizing that veins have valves, the vein is "milked" centrally.

The needle and syringe are then picked up and tested for patency. Generally a 20-gauge, 1½-inch needle is used. The venipuncture site is cleansed with an alcohol sponge. The vein is then held taut with the thumb of the free hand (Fig. 21-4, A), and the needle is inserted through the skin alongside the vein, bev-

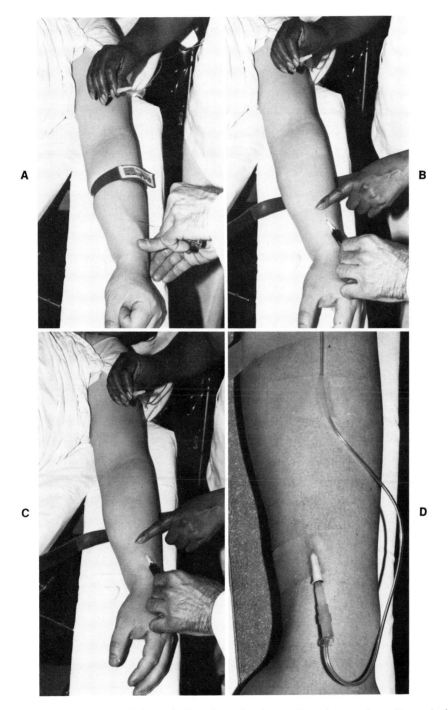

Fig. 21-4. Venipuncture technique. **A,** Tourniquet in place with syringe and needle ready for venipuncture. Note fixation of vein and assistant holding end of plastic tubing. **B,** Venipuncture accomplished and tourniquet released. Note assistant applying pressure with index finger over tip of needle. **C,** Tape placed over hub of needle. **D,** Syringe replaced with plastic tubing and fixation tapes applied.

el side up, at a 45-degree angle to the skin, for half the length of the needle. The vein is then pierced and the needle threaded into the vein for a quarter of the needle's length. This places the fulcrum of the needle in the skin and not in the vein, in the event of any slight movements of the needle. The thumb that had been fixing the vein is then placed on the hub of the needle, aspiration is performed to be certain the needle is in the vein, and the tourniquet is released (Fig. 21-4, *B*)). If the needle is not in the vein, the tourniquet must be released prior to withdrawing the needle from the arm, otherwise there is a strong likelihood of producing a hematoma. If the needle is to be maintained in position, a strip of tape is placed over the hub of the needle, an assistant holds a finger over the skin at the tip of the needle to prevent backflow of blood (Fig. 21-4, *C*), and the syringe is disengaged from the needle and replaced with the tip of the tubing from the intravenous set. The tubing is looped and another strip of tape is placed 6 to 8 inches further up to fasten the tubing to the skin (Fig. 21-4, *D*).

AGENTS FOR GENERAL ANESTHESIA
(see also Chapter 5)
Inhalation agents

Many gaseous and liquid anesthetics are in frequent use today, and current clinical investigation of additional compounds shows promise of adding others to the total. Agents in more common use will be discussed briefly, and for more extensive information the reader is advised to consult a standard text on anesthetics such as Dripps and co-workers (1977), Atkinson and Rushman (1977), or Cullen and Larsen (1974).

Nitrous oxide

The first compound employed in modern general anesthesia, nitrous oxide, exceeds all other anesthetics in the number of times that it is used annually. It has one outstanding property to recommend it—an excellent ability to produce analgesia. Only light anesthesia can be produced without severe oxygen restriction, and muscle relaxation must be obtained

by other means. Supplementation with other agents is required to achieve deeper planes of anesthesia. The unmatched ability to produce analgesia even in very low concentrations, however, makes nitrous oxide an extremely useful agent.

Nitrous oxide is nonirritating, sweet-smelling, and colorless and is the only inorganic gas used to produce anesthesia in man. It is not flammable or explosive but will support combustion of other agents. It is rapidly absorbed from the alveoli, and since it does not combine with hemoglobin, it is carried in simple solution in the blood. It does not undergo any chemical combination within the body and is eliminated unchanged through the lungs as rapidly as it is absorbed. Nitrous oxide is a weak anesthetic, and while some patients can be brought to an unconscious level by mixtures of nitrous oxide and oxygen containing at least 20% oxygen, it is generally preferable to precede its use by induction of anesthesia with an intravenous agent or by supplementation with a more potent inhalation agent to ensure a satisfactory level of oxygenation in the inspired mixture. As long as minimum physiologic concentrations of oxygen (20% or greater) are used, there is no contraindication to the use of nitrous oxide.

Ethyl chloride

Being an extremely potent and simple anesthetic to administer, ethyl chloride has been used extensively in dentistry since the early 1900's, particularly in children, as a fine spray on an open mask. It is a clear fluid that is not irritating to the respiratory mucosa, and concentrations of 3% to 5% in inspired air produce surgical anesthesia. Its major disadvantages are that it is explosive and depresses both cardiac output and peripheral vascular tone. Overdosage can result relatively easily because of the manner of application, particularly following a deep inspiration of a highly concentrated vapor after breath-holding. With the advent of more precise and easily controlled agents, the use of ethyl chloride for the production of anesthesia has largely been abandoned.

Fluroxene (Fluoromar)

Fluroxene is fluorinated ether, with many of the characteristics of diethyl ether. It is a flammable liquid with a mild ether-like odor that produces a high incidence of postoperative nausea and vomiting as well as stimulation of salivary secretions. There is rapid induction and recovery, but precision vaporizers must be used. A concentration of 4% to 8% is required for induction and 2% to 4% for maintenance. It is regarded by many anesthesiologists as possessing no distinct advantages over diethyl ether, and it has not been used extensively for outpatient procedures.

Diethyl ether

Ether is a colorless liquid with major advantages as an anesthetic because of its ability to maintain respiration and circulation while producing excellent muscular relaxation. It has a wide margin of safety but has not been used for dentistry or oral surgery to any extent because of its flammability, disagreeable odor, and tendency to produce protracted nausea and vomiting. Ether has played a very important historic role in anesthesia but is rarely used today.

Halothane (Fluothane)

Halothane is a colorless and very volatile liquid that is nonflammable and non-explosive. It is stored in amber-colored bottles with thymol added as a stabilizer. The agent was introduced for clinical use in England in 1956 and in the United States in 1958. It is a very potent anesthetic and must be administered with vaporizers that are accurately calibrated and temperature compensated. Induction of anesthesia is smooth and rapid, as is recovery. For induction, 2% to 3% concentration is required, and 0.5% to 1% is used for maintenance, generally in a mixture of nitrous oxide and oxygen. Postoperative nausea and vomiting are minimal, and a fair degree of muscular relaxation is produced. Halothane depresses respiration and blood pressure as well as cardiac

output, but this is dose-related. As with other halogenated agents, arrythmias are often produced, particularly during induction and recovery and in deep anesthesia. With use of epinephrine and norepinephrine, ventricular arrythmias can occur that may sometimes turn into ventricular fibrillation; it is therefore advisable to avoid the use of these drugs concurrently with halothane. Some anesthesiologists, however, such as Snow (1972) feel that epinephrine may be employed with halothane but that caution should be exercised. If a vasopressor drug is needed, phenylephrine (Neo-Synephrine), methoxamine (Vasoxyl), or methamphetamine (Methedrine) may be used safely.

Much has been written regarding the relationship of halothane to liver damage. Halogenated hydrocarbons have always been suspect as hepatotoxins because of the well-known association between chloroform and the development of acute yellow atrophy. Many retrospective studies of liver complications with halothane have been conducted, the most extensive of which was the National Halothane Study of the National Institutes of Health (1969). Data were collected from 34 institutions for the period 1958 to 1962, involving 856,500 administrations of all commonly used anesthetics. Halothane compared favorably with other anesthetics in overall death rate and in death rates adjusted for variations in age, sex, preoperative physical status, and operation. Fatal postoperative massive hepatic necrosis was rare and generally associated with other factors. There is overwhelming evidence that halothane is not poisonous to the liver, but it is becoming clear that in a few patients hepatic necrosis sometimes occurs when halothane is administered for a second time within a short interval. Some laboratory results suggest that the causative mechanism might be an immune reaction. Accordingly, many authorities (Cullen and Larsen, 1974; Mushin et al., 1971) suggest avoiding repeated administration of halothane in the same patient over short intervals (within 3 to 6 months) and recommend omitting halothane in patients with known liver or biliary tract disease.

The results of extensive experience with halothane indicate that the agent has a definite place in outpatient anesthesia.

Methoxyflurane (Penthrane)

First introduced into clinical practice in 1959, methoxyflurane is a fluorinated ethyl methyl ether that is the most potent and least volatile inhalation agent available. It is a clear, colorless liquid with a characteristic fruity odor, not flammable or explosive, and it produces a high degree of analgesia. As with other halogenated inhalation agents, methoxyflurane is parasympathomimetic, so that blood pressure, pulse rate, cardiac output, and respiration are depressed. It minimally sensitizes the heart to catecholamines. Reports have indicated the possibility of postanesthetic hepatic and renal involvement, which appear to be related to the dose and duration of exposure and production of a metabolite. Induction and recovery with methoxyflurane is quite slow, and some patients exhibit skin pallor postoperatively. For ambulatory patients, methoxyflurane is best used for maintenance following induction with some other agents, keeping the concentration very low and thus making use of the analgesic and relaxant properties of the drug. Methoxyflurane and all other halogen-containing agents should be avoided in patients with a history of cirrhosis or other liver disease (Snow, 1972).

Enflurane (Ethrane)

Following the introduction of halothane and methoxyflurane, much work has been devoted to the development of a halogenated compound approaching the features of an ideal anesthetic agent. Enflurane is more closely related to halothane than methoxyflurane and is a halogenated methyl ethyl ether. It is a nonflammable clear liquid that produces a rapid induction by inhalation. Only a small amount (2%) undergoes biotransformation, which hopefully should avoid renal dysfunction, and thus far liver toxicity has not been reported. At higher concentrations, enflurane tends to produce electroencephalographic changes that are characteristic of seizure activity, but a study by Trieger and co-workers (1975) on ambulatory patients did not demonstrate any unusual muscular activity such as twitching or jerking. Trieger's study also indicated that recovery time following enflurane anesthesia in outpatients was more rapid than with intravenous anesthesia when the modified Bender motor gestalt test was used, and the study concluded that it was an effective, readily controllable, and safe anesthetic for outpatient use.

Isoflurane (Forane)

Isoflurane, an isomer of enflurane, is the newest of the halogenated anesthetic agents, first synthesized in 1965, and has been found to have useful clinical properties. Cardiac contractility and performance are not altered with isoflurane anesthesia, and cardiac output is unchanged. Animal studies suggest that isoflurane undergoes minimal or no metabolism, and a recent study by Holaday and co-workers (1975) supports the view that it is subject to little or no biotransformation in man. This may be of significance since delayed toxic reactions following general anesthesia have generally been ascribed to three mechanisms, all dependent on biotransformation of the anesthetic. One is that a toxic metabolite may be formed in sufficient quantity to injure susceptible tissues, as appears to be the case in interference with renal function by methoxyflurane. A second mechanism depends on irreversible oxidation of fixed cellular elements by intermediate products of biotransformation. The third mechanism involves the formation of an antigen by the condensation of a fragment of the parent drug with a cellular protein, to which the body responds by formation of cell-mediated antibodies. The occasional occurrence of hepatic necrosis following exposure to halothane has been ascribed to this mechanism. Isoflurane is currently undergoing extensive clinical evaluation that seems most encouraging, but it must be noted that very recent data submitted by Corbett (1976) and others suggest that it may have carcinogenic properties in mice.

Intravenous agents

Thiobarbiturates (Pentothal, Surital)

Thiopental (Pentothal) and thiamylal (Surital) are very similar in their actions and almost impossible to tell apart; one being the sulfur analogue of pentobarbital and the other the sulfur analogue of secobarbital. With the introduction into clinical practice of the ultrashort-acting barbiturates in the mid-1930's, patient preference for the intravenous technique of anesthesia grew rapidly, with the result that virtually all general anesthetics in adults are started intravenously regardless of the anesthetic subsequently used for maintenance. Generally a 2% to 2.5% aqueous solution of thiopental is used for intermittent injections, and a 0.4% to 0.5% solution is administered for continuous infusion by drip. The barbiturates produce unconsciousness primarily by blocking the central brain stem core (reticular activating system), but they can produce any degree of central nervous system depression ranging from mild sedation to coma. Since the barbiturates are very poor analgesics, they are generally supplemented with inhalation anesthetic agents such as nitrous oxide to induce and maintain surgical anesthesia. Induction with intravenous barbiturates is rapid and pleasant, and dissipation of effects depends more on redistribution from brain to other tissues than on biotransformation. The barbiturates depress the respiratory center and the myocardium reducing cardiac output. The metabolic biotransformation rate is only 10% to 15% per hour, so that patients awaken within 5 to 10 minutes following one single dose of intravenous barbiturate owing to the redistribution from brain and other fatty tissues to lean tissues. If additional increments are added, more drug is then stored in the body and lean as well as fatty tissues begin to get saturated.

In patients with severe bronchial asthma, intravenous barbiturates should be used with caution since they are parasympathomimetic, and they are absolutely contraindicated in patients with porphyria. Although it is difficult to define overdosage, if more than 1 gm of thiopen-tal is required, it probably would be best to substitute another technique.

Methohexital (Brevital)

Methohexital, an oxybarbiturate, was first used clinically in 1955. It is highly alkaline, as are the thiobarbiturates, with a pH of about 11. Since it is approximately two to two and a half times as potent as thiopental or thiamylal it is used in a 1% solution and a 0.2% drip infusion. It is quite similar in actions to the thiobarbiturates, but patients appear to be more mentally alert following the use of methohexital, so it is used extensively in outpatient procedures. Hiccups occasionally occur, but they usually do not last long and are of no clinical significance. In general, bearing in mind the greater potency of methohexital, it can be used in exactly the same manner as the thiobarbiturates.

Other intravenous agents

Hexobarbital (Evipan) is an oxybarbiturate similar to methohexital. It was the first intravenous agent in wide use as a general anesthetic since it was introduced in Europe prior to the introduction of thiopental. It is not in wide use today because it produces adverse side effects and a relatively long recovery period.

Hydroxydione (Viadril) is one of a large group of steroids that have been found to produce general anesthesia, and it is probably the most satisfactory of the group for this purpose. It was the first steroid used to any extent to produce anesthesia in man that had no hormonal effects. It has achieved only modest success owing in large part to the high incidence of local irritation with intravenous injection.

Rectal agents

When an anesthetic drug is to be administered rectally, the patient should first be given a soapsuds enema to empty the rectum and provide more even absorption of the drug. Rectal anesthetic agents are generally administered to children, and, depending on the dosage, they can produce depression ranging from sedation or hypnosis to basal narcosis to unconsciousness. Since absorption can be rapid and unpredictable, patients should not be left unattended after the drug has been administered. Tribromoethanol (Avertin) was one of the early rectal agents, but rectal thiopental is the drug now most commonly used to produce basal narcosis.

For preanesthetic sedation or narcosis, a dose of 10 to 15 mg of rectal thiopental per pound of body weight is generally used; this will generally produce a light sleep within 10 minutes. For basal narcosis, about 20 mg per pound of body weight is required. It must be stressed that the patient should be watched carefully, since the protective reflexes may be lost, the patient may become obstructed, and respiration may be depressed. This technique is used only as a premedicant; it is then followed with inhalation and/or intravenous anesthesia.

TECHNIQUES OF GENERAL ANESTHESIA FOR THE AMBULATORY PATIENT
Pediatric anesthesia

The vast majority of general anesthetics for oral surgical procedures in children on an outpatient basis are conducted with inhalation anesthesia, generally utilizing halothane, nitrous oxide, and oxygen. A full face-mask is used for induction and, if the procedure is short, maintenance is accomplished with the same agents using a nosepiece. On occasion, where there is difficulty in maintaining an airway with a nosepiece alone (in children or adults), a nasopharyngeal tube may be inserted and the nosepiece placed over it (Fig. 21-5). If the procedure is lengthy, an intravenous infusion may be started and the patient may be maintained on intravenous barbiturates in addition to inhalation agents.

Adults

In adults, induction is generally accomplished with an intravenous barbiturate (generally methohexital, 1%). Unless specifically contraindicated, the venipuncture is started with atropine as a vagolytic agent. The patient is maintained with methohexital supplemented with inhalation agents. The use of a di-

lute infusion of barbiturate (0.2% methohexital) in addition to concentrated barbiturate (1% methohexital) is an excellent technique that permits patients to be maintained at a smooth and even level of anesthesia. Armamentarium found to be convenient and useful for this technique is shown in Figs. 21-6 and 21-7.

A thorough discussion of general anesthesia in dentistry may be found in Monheim's text on the subject, as revised by Bennett (1974).

Endotracheal intubation

Oral surgery patients are rarely intubated on an elective basis in the office, as opposed to hospital management where intubation is routine. There are several reasons for this, one being that patients that are intubated must be carried at deeper levels of anesthesia than is commonly done in office practice. Intubation is not a method of anesthesia, it is merely a technique for maintaining an airway. Intubation should be performed where there is difficulty in maintaining an airway with other techniques, or where there will be many loose particles, fragments of teeth, debris, or excessive bleeding so as to cause a threat of aspiration. The endotracheal catheter is introduced, preferably through the nose, and once intubation is completed, the airway remains patent and aspiration is prevented by packing the pharynx around the tube. The technique of nasal endotracheal intubation is illustrated in Fig. 21-8.

Monitoring

All patients should be carefully monitored. Monitoring allows continuous determination of (1) the patient's physiologic status, especially the status of his cardiovascular and respiratory systems, which is determined by an evaluation of vital signs; and (2) the level or depth of anesthesia, which is determined by evaluating the presence or absence of various reflexes in addition to observation of vital signs.

In an early discussion of ambulatory patient monitoring, Greenfield (1966) noted that only the exceptional office using gen-

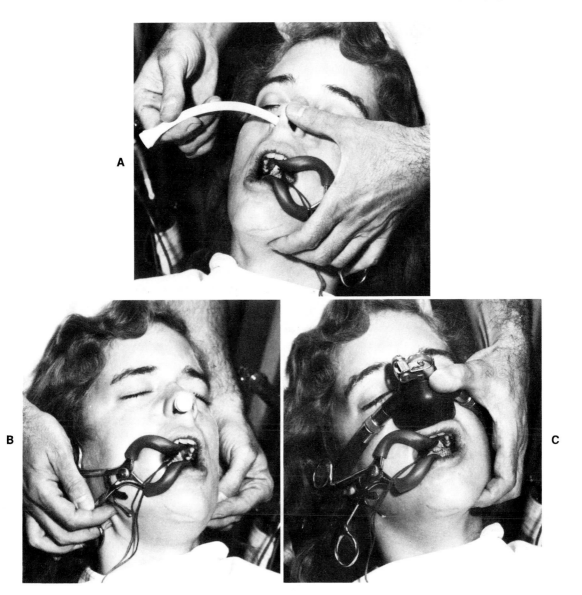

Fig. 21-5. Use of nasopharyngeal tube. **A,** Insertion of tube into nostril. **B,** Tube in place. **C,** Nosepiece positioned over nasopharyngeal tube.

eral anesthesia employed a cardiac monitor. This is no longer true, and today the use of cardiac and other electronic monitoring devices is widespread, as reported by Trieger (1976). However, then, as now, electronic or mechanical aids are not meant to replace the clinical acumen of the anesthesiologist but to serve primarily as a means of providing additional information about the status of the patient

so that any necessary changes can be effected in the anesthetic management. Monitoring mechanisms range from a finger on the pulse, to a precordial stethoscope, to an electronic stethoscope with audible amplification, to a finger plethysmograph for pulse rate and rhythm, to sophisticated electrocardiographic monitoring. Many anesthesiologists feel that the best indication of the integrity of the

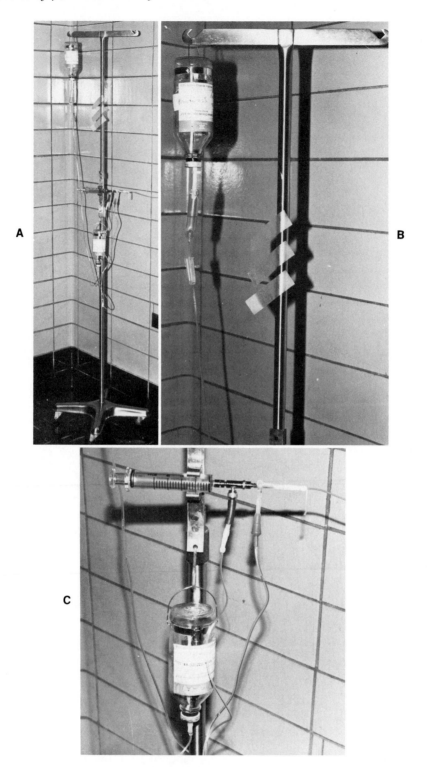

Fig. 21-6. Use of IV pole with syringe holder assembly attached. **A,** Overall view of pole and complete assembly, with syringe, valves, and solutions. **B,** Close-up of upper portion of pole with bottle of dilute barbiturate solution suspended. **C,** Close-up of lower portion of pole with syringe holder assembly, valves, and bottle of concentrated barbiturate solution.

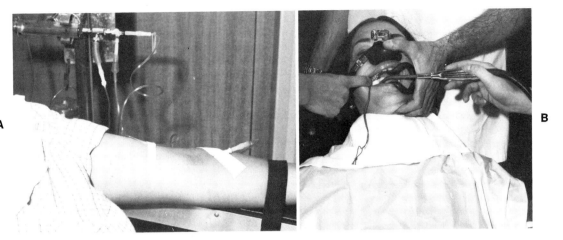

Fig. 21-7. Office team approach to general anesthesia for ambulatory patient. **A,** Intravenous line inserted and arm fastened to armboard. **B,** Team approach to ambulatory patient management: surgeon, anesthetist, and assistant.

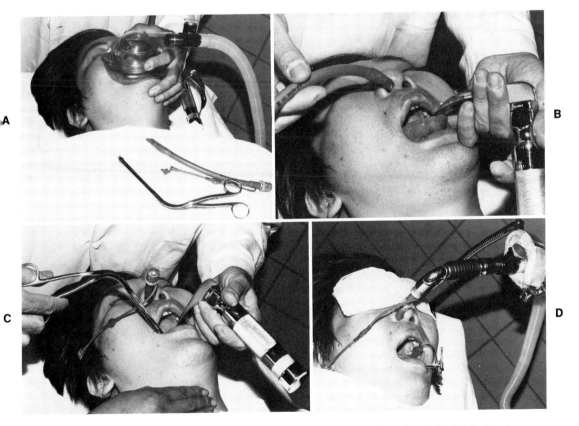

Fig. 21-8. Nasal endotracheal intubation technique. **A,** Patient induced and ready for intubation. **B,** Introduction of nasotracheal tube with laryngoscope in position. **C,** Passage of tube past vocal cords facilitated with Magill forceps; assistant is stabilizing larynx. **D,** Tube taped in position and connected to valve assembly.

cardiovascular system is the adequacy of local tissue perfusion, which can be tested quickly by finger pressure on any accessible skin area and then noting capillary refill time. Regardless of the system used, continuous monitoring gives added insight into the vital functions of the patient, and we are rapidly approaching the time when electrocardiographic monitoring will be standard practice in office as well as hospital anesthesia.

Office light anesthesia techniques

While general anesthesia is still widely used as a standard technique for certain categories of patients (those who cannot or will not cooperate to any degree whatsoever, true allergies to local anesthetics, severe gagging problems, small children, and so on), there seems to be no doubt that the movement in the United States is toward those techniques of pain control that keep the patient at a conscious level but fulfill the objectives of producing analgesia, amnesia, and sedation. A thorough discussion of techniques of intravenous sedation is presented in Chapter 20. Basically, all of these techniques make use of various combinations of drugs (barbiturates, narcotics, tranquilizers, belladonnas) via various routes of administration to bring the patient to a relaxed and sedated state just short of unconsciousness. It should be noted, however, that with most of these techniques, particularly those using combinations of drugs, patients generally drift in and out of consciousness. Accordingly, anyone using this type of technique should be knowledgeable in general anesthesia.

Neurolept and dissociative anesthesia

With the light anesthesia techniques, which some authors have referred to as techniques of "psychosedation," the patient usually has some awareness of his or her surroundings, and the analgesia obtained is generally inadequate to perform a surgical procedure without the addition of local anesthesia.

More recently, several drugs have been introduced that produce, in addition to the effects previously outlined, a state of psychic detachment of the individual from his environment—a total indifference to the surgical procedure being performed, often without the loss of consciousness. This state has been termed "neuroleptanalgesia," and may be defined as a state of central nervous system depression with tranquilization and intense analgesia, produced without the use of barbiturates or volatile agents. A related term that has come into use is "dissociative analgesia," produced by drugs that "dissociate" the patient from his environment into a state of catalepsy, in addition to producing analgesia and amnesia. If unconsciousness is also induced, the terms "neuroleptanesthesia" or "dissociative anesthesia" could more properly be applied. Definitions for the state of consciousness vary, but since levels of depression of the central nervous system are generally determined by the presence or absence of various reflexes, one can accept the fact that from a neurologic point of view an individual is conscious if the protective reflexes (pharyngeal, laryngeal, and so on) are active and the individual is in harmony with his or her surroundings. As opposed to conventional anesthetic agents, these drugs act on subcortical levels of the brain, producing these effects while leaving cortical and vital protective functions relatively intact. The prime example of a dissociative agent is ketamine HCl, which can be administered intramuscularly or intravenously and produces analgesia so profound that no supplementary agents are required. Studies (Greenfield and Granada, 1974) have indicated that the most effective manner of utilization of ketamine for ambulatory patients is at a greatly reduced dosage range, far below that recommended by the manufacturer. A revised weight-dosage relationship based on intramuscular administration has been established as follows:

Weight	Revised weight-dosage relationship for ketamine (intramuscular dosage)
Up to 50 lb	0.5 to 1.0 mg/lb
50 to 100 lb	1.0 to 1.5 mg/lb
Above 100 lb	1.5 mg/lb plus N_2O-O_2 (50:50)

At these dosage levels, dissociative analgesia is produced, consciousness is generally maintained together with protective reflexes, and vital signs are stable. The duration of effect varies from 20 to 40 minutes and can be prolonged by the addition of N_2O-O_2 in a 50:50 mixture. Recovery is generally smooth and uneventful, with a very low incidence of nausea and vomiting and a high degree of retrograde amnesia. The only premedication suggested is scopolamine to inhibit the copious secretions produced by ketamine, which probably accounts for the nausea and vomiting often produced in unpremedicated patients receiving higher doses of ketamine. It must be emphasized that ketamine is not a conventional drug and that conventional guidelines for anesthetic management cannot be directly applied. When using conventional anesthetic agents, one expects specific actions to be followed by specific results. When a barbiturate is injected, for example, one expects the patient to go almost immediately into a relaxed or nonresponding state. If such a response does not occur, the inference is that not enough agent has been administered, and a higher dosage is needed. In using dissociative drugs, this typical response does not take place and there are few physical changes discernible in the patient except for the characteristic cataleptic state produced. This does not mean, however, that analgesia is not present and that additional drugs should be administered. At the reduced dosage levels suggested, there are virtually none of the undesirable postoperative psychotomimetic effects often encountered with higher dosage levels. However, since this is an unconventional drug, the same effect cannot always be predictably duplicated from patient to patient. After prolonged study, it is apparent that the most reliable effect is produced in children, with the least satisfactory result in adults or adolescents weighing more than 100 pounds. Most of these patients can, however, be successfully managed by the addition of nitrous oxide and oxygen in sedative mixtures.

Apart from its use in oral and maxillofacial surgery, there are many other potential applications of ketamine to ambulatory patients. In many emergency room procedures, such as suturing lacerations, manipulation and closed reduction of fractures, and various painful diagnostic procedures, ketamine can be of great value, particularly in children. It can also be used, when properly applied, in restorative dentistry for unmanageable patients.

After an initial widespread surge of interest in ketamine for anesthesia in hospitalized patients, the unpredictability of effect coupled with the high incidence of stormy recovery periods caused the drug to fall into relative disuse. However, at reduced dosage levels, ketamine has a definite usefulness in ambulatory patients, often where no other drug is suitable, and it will no doubt find its own place in the overall scheme of patient management.

Neuroleptanalgesia is generally produced by using Innovar, a combination of fentanyl (Sublimaze), an extremely potent synthetic narcotic derived from meperidine (Demerol), and droperidol (Inapsine), a potent tranquilizer and antiemetic, in a fixed mixture of 50:1 of droperidol to fentanyl (2.5 mg/ml of droperidol: 0.05 mg/ml of fentanyl). Innovar can be used for premedication or for induction of anesthesia, but studies have indicated that its use is probably best confined to hospitalized patients because of prolonged and unpredictable recovery time and depressant effects on respiration. The components of Innovar are, however, available separately and, by varying the doses of fentanyl and droperidol, a new range of usefulness for the ambulatory patient can be achieved.

Fentanyl has an analgesic potency that is 50 to 100 times that of morphine and 1000 times that of meperidine, and since it has a short duration of action (30 to 60 minutes intravenously) as well as a rapid onset, it is particularly suitable for ambulatory patients. As with all potent narcotics, the possibility of respiratory depression exists, and fentanyl when used alone produces a significant incidence of nausea. When droperidol is added to fentanyl in a mixture such as Innovar, there is no nausea, but it must be kept in mind that the addition of droperidol to fentanyl prolongs recovery time and potentiates respiratory depression in addition to producing a detached and lethargic state. Accordingly, if droperidol is to be used in ambulatory patients, it is best administered in minute quantities, by diluting one ml (2.5 mg) of droperidol in 250 ml of saline solution to produce a concentration of 0.01 mg (10 μg/ml). At this concentration, droperidol can be used, following appropriate doses of fentanyl, at a dosage range of 10 to 15 μg/kg of body weight, in conjunction with local anesthetic blocks and N_2O-O_2 to produce analgesia, sedation, and a high degree of retrograde amnesia.

Other drugs used in general anesthesia

Belladonnas

The belladonnas, atropine and scopolamine, have been included in the previous discussion of premedication. While some authors, such as Allen (1970), question the routine use of atropine for premedication, it should be kept in mind that certain vagal reflexes are undesirable in the anesthetized patient. Since atropine is a more potent vagolytic agent than scopolamine, it would be advisable to start the intravenous infusion with atropine whenever a patient is to be given a general anesthetic with which he is to be brought to and maintained at a surgical level. On the other hand, if a patient is to receive a form of intravenous sedation, as previously described, it would be more desirable to give such a patient scopolamine, since scopolamine produces a high degree of psychic sedation and amnesia and inhibits much of the nausea associated with narcotics. Additionally, scopolamine potentiates the barbiturates and the narcotics and is a more potent antisialogogue than atropine. The adult dosage for both atropine and scopolamine is the same, 0.4 to 0.6 mg intravenously. Belladonnas, particularly scopolamine, should not be used in patients with glaucoma.

Narcotics

The use of narcotics in the anesthetic management of the ambulatory oral and maxillofacial surgery patient is a fairly common and long-standing practice. Narcotics have been used in various ways, alone or in conjunction with other drugs, for medication before general anesthesia or for intravenous sedation techniques. Morphine is generally not used in ambulatory patients owing to the high degree of depression produced. When a long-acting narcotic is required, meperidine (Demerol) is used most commonly. Meperidine is about one tenth as potent as morphine and produces fewer side effects and less respiratory depression. When meperidine or any other narcotic is administered intramuscularly, the analgesic effect is apparent in about 15 minutes and the maximum effect in 45 minutes. When given intravenously, the analgesic effect becomes apparent immediately and the full effect is reached in 15 minutes. If a narcotic such as meperidine is administered intravenously, it should be given in small increments to determine the patient's requirements, and there is rarely any indication for a dose higher than 50 mg. The effects may persist for up to 2 hours. Short-acting narcotics in common use include fentanyl (Sublimaze) and alphaprodine (Nisentil). Pentazocine (Talwin) can also be used. Fentanyl is an extremely potent analgesic with approximately 50 to 100 times the activity of morphine. It has a rapid onset and short duration of action (30 to 60 minutes when given intravenously). Alphaprodine is also a potent narcotic with a similarly short duration of action when administered intravenously. Pentazocine is a potent analgesic as well as a weak narcotic antagonist with a relatively short duration of action when administered intravenously. A dose of 50 mg of meperidine is approximately equivalent to 0.1 mg of fentanyl, 25 mg of alphaprodine, or 25 mg of pentazocine.

Narcotic antagonists

When narcotics are used as part of an anesthetic regimen in hospitalized patients, it is common practice to use a narcotic antagonist postoperatively to partially reverse the depressant effects of the drugs and to hasten the recovery period.

Until quite recently, the use of narcotic antagonists has never had a significant role in the management of ambulatory patients, owing partly to a common belief that no significant respiratory depression is produced by narcotics in ambulatory patient techniques and partly to the fact that most narcotic antagonists exhibit agonistic properties of their own. While nalorphine HCl and levallorphan tartrate have respiratory and circulatory depressant effects similar to those of narcotics, a more recently introduced narcotic antagonist, naloxone HCl (Narcan), differs from other antagonists in that it does not have agonistic properties of its own, does not induce tolerance or possess abuse potential, and, when administered to a patient who has not had a narcotic, acts as a placebo. Clinical studies by Greenfield and Granada (1974) have shown that narcotics such as fentanyl and meperidine, as commonly used in ambulatory patient management, can produce significant respiratory depression that is generally not clinically evident. Since narcotics are widely used in techniques of intravenous sedation as well as general anesthesia, and since naloxone will reverse any respiratory depression produced without any significant adverse effects, the use of naloxone postoperatively should be considered whenever a narcotic is used in ambulatory patient management. Cardiorespiratory effects of outpatient anesthetic techniques are discussed further by Campbell (1976).

Muscle relaxants

There are two basic groups of muscle relaxants: depolarizing agents, of which succinylcholine chloride is the most widely used, and nondepolarizing agents, which include curare and its analogues. The receptor area of the muscle cell membrane at the myoneural junction during the resting state is polarized, indicating a difference in electrical potential between the two sides of its surface membranes. When an impulse is propelled along the nerve axon, acetylcholine is released, the surface membrane is depolarized, and the muscle contracts. Ordinarily, the acetylcholine is then rapidly metabolized and the membrane again becomes repolarized. The muscle relaxants produce a neuromuscular blockage in one of two different ways.

The depolarizing drugs produce an initial action resembling that of acetylcholine so that depolarization and muscle contraction are produced, and continued presence of the drug keeps the membrane in a depolarized state producing muscular relaxation. As a result, muscle fasciculation is a characteristic of the depolarization block. Succinylcholine is a short-acting drug with a rapid onset and is metabolized within approximately 3 minutes. The nondepolarizing drugs act by preventing acetylcholine from reaching the receptor area of the muscle cell membrane, so that there are no fasciculations. Tubocurarine, gallamine, and decamethonium are nondepolarizing agents that act in this manner and are much longer acting than succinylcholine. In ambulatory patients, succinylcholine is used in the treatment of laryngospasm and in endotracheal intubation where required. Since it paralyzes all striated muscles, including the muscles of respiration, it produces apnea and should only be used by those skilled in artificially ventilating patients.

Factors influencing choice of anesthesia

Apart from preference of the patient, which is a significant factor and should be given consideration, the other factors to be considered in the selection of anesthesia include: (1) the physiologic status of the patient, (2) the nature and length of the contemplated procedure, (3) the pharmacologic effects of the drugs used, and (4) the anesthetist's familiarity and skill with the drugs and technique to be used.

Until relatively recently, pain control techniques consisted of either local anesthesia or general anesthesia. As already indicated, we now have available a broad spectrum of techniques and drugs for controlling pain and apprehension. The patient's history and physical evaluation determine to a large extent the drugs and techniques to be used. For example, one should avoid administering parasympathomimetic drugs to a patient with bronchial asthma. Similarly, in a patient with liver or kidney disease, one would exclude drugs with hepatotoxic or nephrotoxic properties or drugs that are metabolized in the liver or excreted by the kidneys. Elderly and debilitated patients require minimal drug concentrations and generally should be treated with conscious sedation techniques rather than general anesthesia on an ambulatory outpatient basis. Children and others who cannot or will not cooperate at all, and whose physical status does not present any contraindication, will probably require a general anesthetic. As a rule, one attempts to use the simplest form of pain control compatible with the safety and comfort of the patient.

The subject of drug interactions is assuming greater and greater significance. With increasing numbers of patients under routine multiple drug therapy, the possibility for interaction among drugs is considerable, and this of course includes anesthetics. A thorough review of the current status of the more common drug interactions is of prime importance to anyone who administers anesthetic drugs (Dukes, 1978; Martin, 1971).

SIGNS AND STAGES IN GENERAL ANESTHESIA

Guedel's classification

In administering an anesthetic, we must have signposts as guides in the determination of depth of anesthesia. Although others have suggested signs to divide depth of anesthesia into stages and planes, the classification of Guedel (1951) (Fig. 21-9) has been accepted the world over. Guedel's criteria were based on respiration, eyeball movement, and the presence or absence of various reflexes. In 1943, Gillespie added other criteria for determination of depth such as secretion of tears, response to skin incision, and evaluation of pharyngeal and laryngeal reflexes. While the stages were first described for ether anesthesia in unpre-

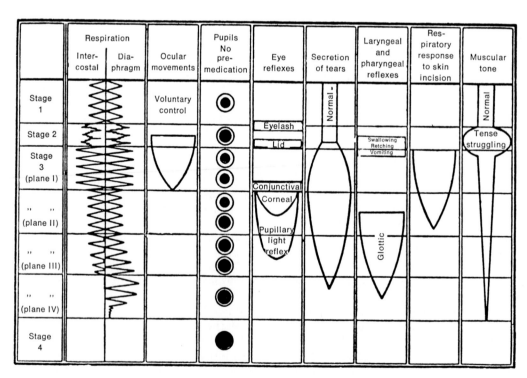

Fig. 21-9. Levels of disappearance of reflexes based on Guedel's classification. (From Lee, J. A. 1973. Synopsis of anesthesia, ed. 7, Baltimore, The Williams & Wilkins Co.)

medicated patients, they can be used with modification for all agents and can be recognized during both induction of and recovery from anesthesia.

Stage I – analgesia

Analgesia lasts from the beginning of induction until loss of consciousness. Respiration is quiet but often irregular. Reflexes are still present. Amnesia for the events occurring in part of this stage is common, even though consciousness and rationality may have appeared to be present. Loss of the eyelash reflex (blinking in response to stroking of the eyelashes) is a useful guide to the patient's entering stage II.

Stage II – excitement or delirium

Excitement or delirium lasts from the loss of consciousness to the onset of surgical anesthesia. The patient is unconscious and uncooperative. He or she may talk incoherently and move the limbs gently or violently. Respiration is irregular. Breath-holding often occurs; the irregular respiration may result in irregular intake of inhalation anesthetics. Reflexes are active. Retching frequently occurs and, if the stomach is not empty, vomiting may result. Aspiration of vomitus in this stage is a common complication. Quick and smooth progress through this stage will make these reactions less exaggerated and decrease the incidence of complications resulting from them. The eyelid reflex (immediate closure of the upper eyelid when it is gently raised) disappears when the patient goes from stage II to stage III, plane 1.

Stage III – surgical anesthesia

Surgical anesthesia extends from the onset of regular (automatic) respiration until respiratory failure occurs from an excessive concentration of anesthetic agent in the central nervous system. This stage is commonly divided into four planes.

Plane 1. In plane 1 movements of the extremities cease and respiration becomes regular; the eyelid reflex is lost. Vigorous, incoordinate eyeball movements are seen. The pharyngeal reflex disappears late in this plane, but the laryngeal reflex is still present. The conjunctival reflex (constriction of the eyelid if the conjunctiva is touched) is lost at the bottom of plane 1.

Plane 2. In plane 2 the eyes become fixed centrally, and pupillary size decreases. Muscle tone is decreased, but all muscles of respiration are still functioning. The laryngeal reflex is abolished. The corneal reflex (constriction of the eyelid if the cornea is touched) is lost during plane 2.

Plane 3. In plane 3 the pupillary light reflex is lost. There is the onset of intercostal muscle paralysis. Respiration is largely diaphragmatic. Muscle relaxation is present.

Plane 4. In plane 4 respiration gradually becomes more depressed with increasing diaphragmatic paralysis. A tracheal tug may be present.

Stage IV – medullary paralysis with respiratory arrest and vasomotor collapse

In medullary paralysis, the pupils are widely dilated and the skin is cold and ashen. The blood pressure is very low and the pulse feeble. Respiration is gasping and finally ceases.

These stages are usually well defined with ether or chloroform, but they are less clearly marked when cyclopropane or halothane are used. If anesthesia is induced with an intravenous barbiturate, the stages become telescoped, and the patient passes rapidly into stage III, plane 2 or deeper, depending on the dose given. The intermediate stages are not recognized.

When general anesthesia is administered in the office, it is advisable to be certain that the patient is brought to an adequate depth of anesthesia (surgical stage) at the start of the procedure, to avoid the difficulties often associated with lighter anesthesia. When the patient is too lightly anesthetized, all of the undesirable reflexes (pharyngeal, laryngeal, and so on) are most active. Also, the highest level of endogenous epinephrine is being liberated at these light levels and so is most likely to produce arrythmias in reacting with halogenated anesthetic agents such as halothane. As the operation progresses and the cumulative depressant effects of the anesthetics exert their influence, less anesthetic agent will be required and the level can be lightened.

Woodbridge's classification

Woodbridge (1958) reassessed the various levels of anesthesia in terms of depression of the central nervous system and delineated four components of the anesthetic state: unconsciousness, loss of sensation, loss of motor power, and elimination of reflex activity. Depending on what is required for the particular procedure and for the well-being of the patient, any desired effect or combination of these effects can be produced by varying the anesthetic agents and drugs used.

A few additional comments are in order with regard to signs of anesthesia. As Schwartz, Ngai, and Papper (1957) have pointed out, no one sign should be depended on, but the situation as a whole should be considered. Where two signs do not indicate the same depth of anesthesia, the more vital signs (blood pressure, pulse, respiration) should be relied on. For example, if the eyeballs indicate first plane of the third stage but respiration indicates third plane, it should be assumed that the latter sign is correct and one should react accordingly. Also, when administering an anesthetic, a certain stage of anesthesia does not necessarily have to be reached, but rather one should produce the best operating conditions for the particular procedure consistent with the patient's safety, and as little drug as necessary should be used to attain these conditions.

POSTANESTHETIC MANAGEMENT

Following a general anesthetic the central nervous system is depressed, and even if a patient is conscious the protective reflexes are somewhat obtunded. The patient must be observed carefully during the immediate postoperative period to ensure that respiration is adequate, the airway remains patent, and vital signs remain stable. In addition, bleeding should be under control so that blood or secretions will not go back into the pharynx. The patient should not be left unattended. When the patient has recovered sufficiently so that his motor coordination and compensatory mechanisms have been restored, he can be moved with careful assistance from the operating room to the recovery room, but never unescorted. Office patients should never be brought to the recovery room until the protective reflexes have returned.

In the recovery room, the patient should be under continuous observation until ready to be discharged. In general, a patient should be left in the recovery room for a period of time at least as long as the procedure and discharged only in the custody of a responsible adult after postoperative instructions have been given. Since there is interference with motor coordination as well as alertness, patients should not be permitted to drive until the following day. If at all possible, food and drink should be delayed for a few hours postoperatively, with the diet then consisting of mostly liquids for 12 hours.

PREVENTION, RECOGNITION, AND MANAGEMENT OF COMPLICATIONS AND EMERGENCIES
Respiratory complications
Airway obstruction

Obstruction of the airway may be partial or complete and is the most frequent complication of general anesthesia. It may be due to a foreign body, excessive mucus, the tongue falling back into the pharynx, or vomiting. In a patient with an obstructed airway, there will be increased respiratory effort with very little or no respiratory exchange. Obstruction must be corrected immediately before proceeding further with the case.

Respiratory depression

Depression of respiration must be differentiated from obstruction. In contrast to obstruction, there is very little or no respiratory effort in a patient with depressed respiration, in addition to very little or no respiratory exchange. It may be due to overdosage of a drug or anesthetic agent, too rapid administration of an anesthetic agent, or chronic hypoxia. If apnea occurs, or respiratory depression is suspected, vital signs should be checked and the level of anesthesia lightened.

Laryngospasm

Laryngospasm is usually partial rather than total, producing a high-pitched crowing noise. It is most commonly caused by irritation of the pharynx by blood, mucus, foreign body, or irritating anesthetic gases during light levels of anesthesia. In treating a laryngospasm, oxygen should very gently be insufflated past the vocal cords, and at the same time the level of anesthesia should be deepened, preferably with intravenous barbiturates. If this is unsuccessful, a muscle relaxant (succinylcholine) is administered intravenously, bearing in mind that respiration will have to be controlled until the effect of the drug is worn off since the patient will be paralyzed.

Bronchospasm

Most bronchospasms are total spasms, similar to an acute asthmatic attack, in which there is a complete closure of the bronchi. Treatment consists of administration of a bronchodilator, such as aminophylline (7.5 gr) slowly intravenously, or epinephrine if the bronchospasm is allergic in origin. A bronchospasm is a frightening and difficult problem to manage, and one should treat an active asthmatic having general anesthesia with great caution.

Vomiting

General anesthesia should not be administered on an ambulatory basis if a patient has recently eaten, since a minimum of 4 to 6 hours is needed for food to pass through the stomach and the emotional status can prolong the time greatly. If vomiting does occur, the patient should be placed in Trendelenburg position, the head should be turned to the side, and the vomitus aspirated. Following removal of the vomitus, 100% oxygen should be administered prior to continuing with the case.

Circulatory complications

The circulatory problems encountered most frequently in ambulatory patients are changes in pulse rate (tachycardia, bradycardia), changes in cardiac rhythm, and changes in blood pressure (hypertension, hypotension). The most common cause of most of these problems is chronic hypoxia, which can cause tachycardia and hypertension as well as arrhythmias. Vagal stimulation will often cause bradycardia in a patient that has not received atropine, while hypotension is often produced by deeper levels of anesthesia.

The most serious complication, cardiac arrest, may be due to either asystole or ventricular fibrillation and is reviewed thoroughly in Chapter 11.

Neurologic complications

The most common neurologic complications are convulsions and emergence delirium, both of which are probably due to hypoxia and hypercapnea. Emergence delirium is a stage of excitement during recovery from anesthesia, and it may require sedation with a tranquilizer or a narcotic given intravenously.

Hyperpyrexia

As techniques become more sophisticated, we must also learn to cope with more sophisticated problems. Malignant hyperthermia was first reported by Denborough in 1962; he described a fulminant crisis triggered by potent inhalation anesthetics, with the outstanding features being high fever, tachypnea, tachycardia, cyanosis, and rigidity of the skeletal muscles. It occurs most frequently in apparently healthy young adults and children and has a mortality rate over 65%. Much has been learned about this disease in only a few years and a distinct familial trait in many cases implies dominant inheritance. In some families the serum creatinine phosphokinase (CPK) is clearly higher than normal. Britt (1974) feels that the key to success in the management of acute crises is early recognition and cessation of all potent inhalation agents, hyperventilation with oxygen, and immediate and vigorous cooling. Schwartz and Garcia (1975), as well as others, have reported on this frightening syndrome in the oral surgery and dental literature.

Composition and use of emergency drug tray

A well-organized emergency drug tray should be maintained in the office, together with all other necessary armamentaria, such as sterile syringes and needles, tourniquet, and so on. Before elaborating on the contents of the drug tray, several general considerations should be mentioned. The number of drugs should be kept to a basic minimum and one should, of course, be familiar with the pharmacology of each drug. All office personnel should be familiar with the location of the drug tray — periodic practice drills help in this regard. The drugs should be checked frequently and should not be outdated. Also, since an emergency will require rapid action, it is possible that one may inadvertently pick up and administer the wrong drug. Wherever possible, therefore, every drug on the tray should be one that will not kill the patient if inadvertently given at the wrong time. One should also have available a suction apparatus and a source of oxygen.

Table 21-1 is a list of drugs, in different categories, that may be used for the complications indicated. Only one drug in each category is necessary on the drug tray.

In an emergency most drugs should be administered intravenously. If a venipuncture cannot be made, several alternatives are possible. If two or three times the intravenous dose is administered intramuscularly, together with 1 or 2 ml of hyaluronidase, an intravenous effect can be achieved. The injection may also be made sublingually to get rapid absorption.

Potential hazards related to trace anesthetic gas contaminants

In recent years, there have been references in the literature indicating that the presence of trace amounts of residual inhalation anesthetics in hospital operating rooms may have a deleterious effect on the health of operating room personnel. Large scale epidemiological studies (Cohen et al., 1974; Cohen, 1976) have shown that female operating room personnel demonstrate an increased incidence of spontaneous abortion and certain types of carcinoma. Birth defects in their offspring, as well as in the offspring of the nonoccupationally exposed wives of male anesthetists, are also increased. Preliminary studies in dentistry reported by the same group (1975) appear

Table 21-1. Drugs for an anesthesia emergency drug tray

Category	Drug	Dosage	Indication
Antihistamines	Benadryl	10-50 mg	Mild allergic reactions
	Chlortrimeton	10 mg	
Barbiturates	Nembutal	50-100 mg	Toxic overdose (local
	Seconal	50-100 mg	anesthetic)
Steroids	Solu-Cortef	100 mg	Severe allergic reactions
	Decadron	4-8 mg	(adrenal insufficiency)
Vasopressors	Methedrine	10-20 mg	Hypotension
	Vasoxyl	10-20 mg	
Bronchodilators	Isuprel	Nebulizer (0.2 mg)	Allergic or asthmatic conditions
	Aminophylline	0.25-0.5 gm	
	Epinephrine	0.2-0.5 ml (1:1000)	Anaphylactic shock or very severe allergic reaction *only*
	Nitroglycerin	1/150-1/200 gr sublingually	Angina pectoris
	Atropine sulfate	0.4-0.6 mg	Bradycardia
	Succinylcholine	40-60 mg	Laryngospasm

to indicate significant variations in the health of exposed individuals. While a direct cause-effect relationship has not yet been definitely established, sufficient data have been presented to indicate that a health hazard may exist and that all inhalation anesthetics are suspect. While no "safe" concentration can yet be clearly defined, it is desirable to maintain an office environment containing the lowest concentrations reasonably attainable. These have been cited by Whitcher and others (1975, 1977) as no more than 50 ppm N_2O, 0.5 ppm halothane, and other potent agents in proportion to the concentrations administered. Devices for sampling and analyzing gas concentrations for use in air monitoring programs are available, as well as equipment for scavenging and reducing occupational exposure of personnel to inhalation anesthetic agents. A thorough review of this subject can be found in a special section of the October 1977 issue of the *Journal of the American Dental Association* entitled, "Trace Inhalation Anesthetics in the Dental Office."

Medicolegal aspects

The legal right for a dentist to administer general anesthesia emanates from the dental practice acts of the individual states, with some states specifically granting this right and others implying it by not prohibiting its use. Anesthesiology is part of the practice of dentistry as it is part of the practice of medicine, and the laws of licensure bestow on the dentist the privilege of using general anesthetics as an integral part of dental practice. Additionally, the law holds a practitioner to account for competence and responsibility in the degree of performance.

We are witnessing major changes in the involvement of both state and federal regulatory agencies in the dental profession with particular reference to anesthesiology. Several of the state dental boards have adopted regulations requiring special certification for the administration of general anesthesia and sometimes other forms of pain control, in which the requisite background and training is clearly delineated. It has long been clear that responsible professional control over the use of outpatient general anesthesia will become mandatory. Self-government to protect the interests of the public is a professional obligation that practitioners must assume, together with a well-organized and non-self-serving evaluation and peer review mechanism such as that embodied in the *American Association of Oral and Maxillofacial Surgeons Office Anesthesia Emergency Self-Evaluation Manual*. A clear example of this type of responsibility is to be found in Ohio, where dentistry and oral and maxillofacial surgery organizations, together with the state dental board, jointly developed a set of regulations governing the use of general anesthesia in dentistry in 1974. The Ohio law can serve as a prototype for those states currently involved in or considering the planning of special legislation on the regulation of general anesthesia in dentistry.

Hospital management of ambulatory patients — ambulatory care facility

While the major focus of anesthesia in oral and maxillofacial surgery is on office procedures, our efforts to constantly upgrade the level of patient care in terms of safety and efficiency in providing anesthesia and pain control for ambulatory patients is shared by medicine, where outpatient general anesthesia is currently undergoing extensive evaluation as one of the concepts of the future. In 1966, Cohen and Dillon pointed out that hospital outpatient general anesthesia can provide a means of increasing efficiency of patient care while at the same time decreasing costs. In children particularly, the advantages of outpatient management have been recognized, and pediatric surgery without admission to the hospital has been advocated for many years. Steward (1975) has described a complete protocol for the management of pediatric anesthesia on an outpatient basis, and the American Society of Anesthesiologists (1973) has published *Guidelines for Ambulatory Surgical Facilities*. Variously termed "surgicenters," "day care sur-

gery," and "ambulatory admissions," facilities for performing anesthesia and surgery on an outpatient basis have prolifer-
ated. The procedures include general
surgery, urology, ophthalmology, otolo-
gy, and plastic surgery, and the basic
principles and techniques are comparable to those used for outpatient oral and
maxillofacial surgery.

REFERENCES

Allen, G. D. 1970. The indiscriminate use of atropine, Anesth. Prog. **17:**1.

ASOS anesthesia morbidity and mortality survey.
1974. J. Oral Surg. **32:**733.

Atkinson, R. S., and Rushman, G. B. 1977. A synopsis of anesthesia, ed. 8, London, John Wright &
Son, Ltd.

Bennett, C. R. 1974. Monheim's general anesthesia
in dental practice, ed. 4, St. Louis, The C. V.
Mosby Co.

Britt, B. A. 1974. Malignant hyperthermia: a phar-
macogenetic disease of skeletal and cardiac muscle, N. Engl. J. Med. **290:**20.

Campbell, R. L., et al. 1976. Cardiorespiratory effects of a balanced anesthetic technique in outpatient general anesthesia, J. Oral Surg. **34:**399.

Cohen, D., and Dillon, J. B. 1966. Anesthesia for
outpatient surgery, J.A.M.A. **196:**1114.

Cohen, E. N. 1976. Anesthetics and cancer, Anesthesiology **44:**6.

Cohen, E. N., et al. 1974. Occupational exposure
among operating room personnel: a national
study. Report of an ad hoc committee on the
effects of trace anesthetic agents on the health
of operating room personnel, Anesthesiology
41:321.

Cohen, E. N., et al. 1975. A survery of anesthetic
health hazards among dentists: report of an ad hoc
committee on the effects of trace anesthetic
agents on the health of operating room personnel,
J. Am. Dent. Assoc. **90:**1291.

Comroe, J. H., et al. 1962. The lung, ed. 2, Chicago
Year Book Medical Publishers, Inc.

Corbett, T. H. 1976. Cancer and congenital anomalies associated with anesthetics, Ann. N.Y. Acad.
Sci. **271:**58.

Cullen, S. C., and Larsen, P., Jr. 1974. Essentials of
anesthetic practice, Chicago, Year Book Medical
Publishers, Inc.

Denborough, M. A., et al. 1962. Anesthetic deaths
in a family, Br. J. Anaesth. **34:**395.

Dripps, R. D. et al. 1977. Introduction to anesthesia—the principles of safe practice, ed. 5, Philadelphia, W. B. Saunders Co.

Dukes, M. N. G. 1978. Side effects of drugs—annual
2, Amsterdam, Excerpta Medica.

Evaluations of drug interactions, ed. 1. 1973. Washington, D.C., American Pharmaceutical Association.

Featherstone, R. M., et al. 1961. Interactions of inert
anesthetic gases with proteins, Anesthesiology
22:977.

Gillespie, N. A. 1943. The signs of anesthesia,
Anesth. Analg. **22:**275.

Greenfield, W. 1966. Monitoring of the ambulatory
patient under general anesthesia, Anesth. Prog.
13:1.

Greenfield, W. 1973. Neuroleptanalgesia and
dissociative drugs, Dent. Clin. North Am.
17:263.

Greenfield, W., and Granada, M. G. 1974. The use
of a narcotic antagonist in the anesthetic management of the ambulatory oral surgery patient, J.
Oral Surg. **32:**760.

Guedel, A. E. 1951. Inhalation anesthesia, ed. 2,
New York, The Macmillan Co.

Guidelines for ambulatory surgical facilities. 1973.
Park Ridge, Ill., American Society of Anesthesiologists.

Guidelines for teaching the comprehensive control
of pain and anxiety in dentistry. 1971. Chicago,
American Dental Association, Council on Dental
Education.

Holaday, D. A., et al. 1975. Resistance of isoflurane
to biotransformation in man, Anesthesiology **43:**3.

Hunter, A. R., and Bush, G. H. 1971. General anesthesia for dental surgery, Springfield, Ill., Charles
C Thomas, Publisher.

Jones, T. W., and Greenfield, W. 1977. Position
paper of the ADA Ad Hoc Committee on Trace
Anesthetics as a Potential Health Hazard in Dentistry, J. Am. Dent. Assoc. **95:**751.

Lytle, J. J. 1974. Anesthesia morbidity and mortality
survey of the Southern California Society of Oral
Surgeons, J. Oral Surg. **32:**739.

Martin, E. W. 1971. Hazards of medication, Philadelphia, J. P. Lippincott Co.

Miller, S. L. 1961. A theory of gaseous anesthetics,
Proc. Natl. Acad. Sci. USA **47:**1515.

Mushin, W. W., et al. 1971. Post-halothane jaundice
in relation to previous administration of halothane, Br. Med. J. **2:**18.

National halothane study: a study of the possible association between halothane anesthesia and postoperative hepatic necrosis. 1969. Bethesda, Md.
National Institutes of Health.

Office anesthesia emergency self-evaluation manual. 1978. Chicago, American Association of Oral
and Maxillofacial Surgeons.

Pauling, L. 1961. A molecular theory of general
anesthesia, Science **134:**15.

Schwartz, H., Ngai, S. H., and Papper, E. M. 1957.
Manual of anesthesiology, Springfield, Ill.,
Charles C Thomas, Publisher.

Schwartz, H. C., and Gracia, R. M. 1975. Malignant
hyperthermia, J. Oral Surg. **33:**57.

Snow, J. C. 1972. Anesthesia in otolaryngology and
ophthalmology, Springfield, Ill., Charles C
Thomas, Publisher.

Steward, D. J. 1975. Outpatient pediatric anesthesia, Anesthesiology **43**(2):268.

Trace inhalation anesthetics in the dental office.
1977. J. Am. Dent. Assoc. **95:**749.

Trieger, N., et al. 1976. Anesthesia monitoring of
the ambulatory patient, Anesth. Prog. **23:**3.

Whitcher, C., et al. 1975. Development and evaluation of methods for the elimination of waste anesthetic gases and vapors in hospitals, GPO Stock

No. 1733-0071 2.15, Washington, D.C., U.S. Government Printing Office.

Whitcher, C., et al. 1977. Control of occupational exposure to nitrous oxide in the dental operatory, J.A.D.A. **95:**763.

Woodbridge, P. D. 1958. Changing concepts concerning depth of anesthesia, Anesthesiology **18:**536.

Wylie, W. D., and Churchill-Davidson, H. C. 1972. A practice of anesthesia, ed. 3, London, Lloyd-Luke Ltd.

Index